Coronary Heart Disease

Zeev Vlodaver · Robert F. Wilson · Daniel J. Garry
Editors

Coronary Heart Disease

Clinical, Pathological, Imaging, and Molecular Profiles

Springer

Editors
Zeev Vlodaver
Division of Cardiovascular Medicine
University of Minnesota
Minneapolis, MN, USA
zeev.vlodaver@gmail.com

Daniel J. Garry
Division of Cardiovascular Medicine
University of Minnesota
Minneapolis, MN, USA
garry@umn.edu

Robert F. Wilson
Division of Cardiovascular Medicine
University of Minnesota
Minneapolis, MN, USA
wilso008@umn.edu

ISBN 978-1-4614-1474-2 e-ISBN 978-1-4614-1475-9
DOI 10.1007/978-1-4614-1475-9
Springer New York Dordrecht Heidelberg London

Library of Congress Control Number: 2011943085

Printed on acid-free paper

Springer is part of Springer Science+Business Media (www.springer.com)

This book is dedicated to our wives

Dalia P. Vlodaver
Betsy Wilson
Mary G. Garry
For their encouragement, devotion and support.

Preface

Coronary Heart Disease

Clinical, Pathological, Imaging, and Molecular Profiles

This book will present a comprehensive picture of ischemic heart disease to those who, either as practitioners, students or investigators, deal with the varied facets of this complex subject. It has meaning to the fields of clinical cardiology, thoracic surgery, pathology, and cardiovascular molecular research.

After introductory chapters on the anatomy of the coronary blood vessels and cardiac development, several chapters will consider stress echo and nuclear diagnostics tests, noninvasive imaging and coronary angiography in ischemic heart disease, with techniques, indications, and examples of normal and abnormal patterns. In most instances, angiograms are paired with labeled line drawings, which help the initiated in the reading of films. Specific chapters will deal with congenital anomalies of the coronary arteries, which may engender states of ischemic heart disease.

The principal thrust of the work concerns the main arena of ischemic heart disease, namely, coronary atherosclerosis. The pathology of coronary atherosclerosis will be presented in conjunction with the results of anatomic, noninvasive imaging and angiographic studies. Related chapters on atherogenesis will present new insights into the pathophysiology of the vulnerable plaque, role of progenitor cells in vascular injury, inflammation and atherogenesis, and genomics of vascular remodeling.

Major chapters will discuss the subject of angina pectoris, acute coronary syndromes, healed myocardial infarction and congestive heart failure, catheter-based and surgical revascularization, and surgical treatment of myocardial infarction and its sequelae. Final chapters will present therapies for refractory angina; metabolic syndromes and coronary heart disease; coronary heart disease in women; and prevention and regression of atherosclerosis.

What is unique in this book is that many of the chapters will be case material from which profiles of the various manifestations are obtained through correlation of clinical, imaging, and pathological studies. The quality of the authors' contribution to this book will provide an immense depth to the book as they have hands on experience and are national leaders in their field of cardiac pathology, clinical cardiology, and cardiovascular molecular research. This book will present a comprehensive and real picture of the complexities of ischemic heart disease, both to the practitioners, who deal with it in day-to-day practice with its problems, and to the students, residents, and investigators who try to develop firm concepts regarding the varied states observed in this common condition and preparing them to the future advances in coronary heart disease.

Minneapolis, MN, USA

Zeev Vlodaver, M.D.
Robert F. Wilson, M.D.
Daniel J. Garry, M.D., Ph.D.

Acknowledgments

We wish to recognize four pillars of medical science whose important contributions to cardiovascular medicine are reflected in our book.

To Jesse E. Edwards, MD, a world-renowned, pioneering, and leading cardiac pathologist who had an extraordinary passion for teaching. He was professor of pathology at the Mayo Clinic in Rochester, Minn., and at the University of Minnesota, Minneapolis. He taught many medical students, pathologists, cardiologists, cardiac surgeons, and visiting medical experts from around the world. Dr. Edwards housed an enormous collection of autopsied hearts at United Hospital, St. Paul, Minn., known as the Dr. Edwards' Cardiovascular Registry that became a principal resource for his illustrated reference books: "An Atlas of Acquired Diseases of the Heart and Great Vessels" (1961), and "Congenital Heart Disease" (1965). He also co-authored nearly 800 journal articles and 14 books. Dr. Vlodaver pays special acknowledgment to Dr. Edwards who was his teacher, mentor and "inspirational force in his medical life." He died in 2008 at the age of 96.

C. Walton Lillehei, MD, world-renowned as the "Father of Open-Heart Surgery," was professor of surgery at the University of Minnesota. In 1952, he participated in the world's first successful open-heart operation using hypothermia, performed at the University of Minnesota, and in 1954, he performed the world's first open-heart surgery using cross-circulation. In 1958, Dr. Lillehei was responsible for the world's first use of a small, portable, battery-powered pacemaker; he also developed and implanted the world's first prosthetic valve in 1966. Thousands of cardiac surgeons over the world are indebted to Dr. Lillehei for his monumental contributions. Dr. Lillehei died in 1999 at the age of 80.

Kurt Amplatz, MD, professor of radiology for more than 40 years at the University of Minnesota, retired in 1999. A pioneer in cardiovascular interventional radiology, he is well known for his many inventions which bridged medical disciplines and included devices such as high-resolution x-ray equipment, heparin-coated wires, specially shaped cardiac catheters, and vascular occlusive devices. Although retired, he continues to improve patients' lives through the development of new technologies.

Howard B. Burchell, MD, cardiologist, professor of medicine at the Mayo Clinic in Rochester and chief of cardiology at the University of Minnesota. He was editor-in-chief of the journal Circulation from 1965-1970, a tenure marked by rapid advances in cardiac pacing and electrophysiology. Teaching and writing with a central theme of sound scientific evidence were hallmarks of Dr. Burchell's career. He passed away in 2009 at the age of 101.

We also extend our gratitude to the many specialists who have contributed generously to this book with considerable experience in their specialty areas.

We acknowledge and thank Jane Hutchins-Peterson, Stephanie Esperson and Andrea Silverman for their outstanding help and for handling the flow of material from the writers to the publisher.

We recognize with deep appreciation Barb Umberger for her dedication in the editing of the manuscript in the minutest detail to ensure the high quality of this project.

Our sincere thanks to Howard Gillbert for his invaluable illustrations and other artwork.

Our gratitude to Michael Griffin, developmental editor, Springer Publishing, for his tireless and utmost attention to all details needed for the production of the book.

We wish to acknowledge the support of and encouragement by Andrew Moyer, Senior Editor of Clinical Medicine, at Springer, and his predecessors Melissa Ramondetta and Frances Louie, for their enthusiasm for this project in bringing it to reality.

Minneapolis, MN, USA

Zeev Vlodaver, M.D.
Robert F. Wilson, M.D.
Daniel J. Garry, M.D., Ph.D.

Contents

Contributors

Richard W. Asinger, MD Department of Medicine, Hennepin County Medical Center, Minneapolis, MN, USA

Fouad A. Bachour, MD, FSCA1 Department of Medicine, Hennepin County Medical Center, Minneapolis, MN, USA

Michael Bolooki, MD University of Minnesota, Minneapolis, MN, USA

Marcelo F. Di Carli, MD,FACC Chief, Division of Nuclear Medicine and Molecular Imaging, Department of Radiology and Medicine, Brigham and Women's Hospital, Boston, MA, USA

Gladwin S. Das, MD Cardiovascular Division, University of Minnesota, Minneapolis, MN, USA

Sharmila Dorbala, MD, MPH Division of Nuclear Medicine and Molecular Imaging, Department of Radiology, Brigham and Women's Hospital, Boston, MA, USA

Emily R. Duncanson, MD Department of Jesse E. Edwards Registry of Cardiovascular Disease, United Hospital, St. Paul, MN, USA

Daniel Duprez, MD, PhD Cardiovascular Division, University of Minnesota, Minneapolis, MN, USA

James R. Dutton, BSc, PhD Stem Cell Institute, University of Minnesota, Minneapolis, MN, USA

Gary S. Francis, MD Division of Cardiovascular Medicine, University of Minnesota, Minneapolis, MN, USA

Santiago Garcia, MD Department of Cardiology, University of Minnesota, Minneapolis VA Medical Center, Minneapolis, MN, USA

Daniel J. Garry, MD, PhD Division of Cardiovascular Medicine, University of Minnesota, Minneapolis, MN, USA

Mary G. Garry, PhD Lillehei Heart Institute, University of Minnesota, Minneapolis, MN, USA

Daniel J. Hellrung, DO, PhD Mercy Hospital, Department of Internal Medicine, Coon Rapids, MN, USA

Timothy D. Henry, MD Minneapolis Heart Institute Foundation, Minneapolis, MN, USA

Jamie L. Lohr, MD Division of Pediatric Cardiology, University of Minnesota Amplatz Children's Hospital, Minneapolis, MN, USA

Joseph M. Metzger, PhD Department of Integrative Biology and Physiology, University of Minnesota, Minneapolis, MN, USA

Xiaozhong Shi, PhD Lillehei Heart Institute, University of Minnesota, Minneapolis, MN, USA

Jennifer L. Hall, PhD Department of Medicine, Lillehei Heart Institute, University of Minnesota, Minneapolis, MN, USA

Ranjit John, MD Division of Cardiothoracic Surgery, University of Minnesota Medical Center–Fairview, Minneapolis, MN, USA

Thomas Knickelbine, MD, FACC, FSCAI Minneapolis Heart Institute, Minneapolis, MN, USA

Frank D. Kolodgie, PhD CVPath Institute, Gaithersburg, MD, USA

Christopher B. Komanapalli, MD Surgery, Division of Cardiovascular and Thoracic Surgery, University of Minnesota Medical Center–Fairview, Minneapolis, MN, USA

Balaji Krishnan, MD, MS Department of Medicine, Division of Cardiovascular Medicine, University of Minnesota Medical Center–Fairview, Minneapolis, MN, USA

Elena R. Ladich, MD CVPath Institute, Gaithersburg, MD, USA

John R. Lesser, MD Department of Cardiology, Minneapolis Heart Institute, Abbott Northwestern Hospital, Minneapolis, MN, USA

Department of Cardiology, Minneapolis, MN, USA

Kenneth Liao, MD, PhD University of Minnesota, Minneapolis, MN, USA

Shannon M. Mackey-Bojack, MD Department of Jesse E. Edwards Registry of Cardiovascular Disease, United Hospital, St. Paul, MN, USA

Cindy M. Martin, MD Division of Cardiovascular Medicine, University of Minnesota, Minneapolis, MN, USA

Edward O. McFalls, MD, PhD Department of Cardiology, University of Minnesota, Minneapolis, VA Medical Center, Professor of Medicine, Minneapolis, MN, USA

Graham T. McMahon, MD, MMSc Division of Endocrinology, Harvard Medical School, Diabetes and Hypertension, Brigham and Women's Hospital, Boston, MA, USA

Michael Sean McMurtry, BASc, MD, PhD Department of Medicine, University of Alberta Hospital, Edmonton, AB, Canada

Eric M. Meslin, PhD Indiana University School of Medicine, Indianapolis, IN, USA

Evangelos D. Michelakis, MD, PhD Department of Medicine, University of Alberta, Edmonton, AB, Canada

Masataka Nakano, MD CVPath Institute, Gaithersburg, MD, USA

Marc C. Newell, MD Minneapolis Heart Institute, Abbott Northwestern Hospital, MHI Cardiology, Minneapolis, MN, USA

Fumiyuki Otsuka, MD CVPath Institute, Gaithersburg, MD, USA

Ryan J. Palacio, BA Department of Anesthesiology, University of Minnesota Medical School, Minneapolis, MN, USA

Rita C.R. Perlingeiro, PhD, MSc, BSc Lillehei Heart Institute, Department of Medicine, University of Minnesota, Minneapolis, MN, USA

Ganesh Raveendran, MD Cardiovascular Division, University of Minnesota, Minneapolis, MN, USA

Susan J. Roe, MD Department of Jesse E. Edwards Registry of Cardiovascular Disease, United Hospital, St. Paul, MN, USA

Mohammad Sarraf, MD Cardiovascular Division, University of Minnesota Hospital, Minneapolis, MN, USA

Jason C. Schultz, MD University of Minnesota Medical Center-Fairview and Minnesota Cardiovascular Division, Minneapolis, MN, USA

Robert S. Schwartz, MD Minneapolis Heart Institute, Minneapolis, MN, USA

Gautam R. Shroff, MBBS Department of Medicine, Hennepin County Medical Center, Minneapolis, MN, USA

Jonathan M.W. Slack, MA, PhD Stem Cell Institute, University of Minnesota, Minneapolis, MN, USA

Margo Tolins-Mejia, MD, FACC Department of Cardiology, Mercy/Unity Medical Centers, Minneapolis, MN, USA

Jay H. Traverse, MD Department of Cardiology, University of Minnesota Medical School, Minneapolis Heart Institute at Abbott Northwestern Hospital, Minneapolis, MN, USA

Uma S. Valeti, MD, FACC Cardiovascular Division, Department of Medicine, University of Minnesota, Minneapolis, MN, USA

Renu Virmani, MD CVPath Institute, Gaithersburg, MD, USA

Zeev Vlodaver, MD Division of Cardiovascular Medicine, University of Minnesota, Minneapolis, MN, USA

Robert F. Wilson, MD Division of Cardiovascular Medicine, University of Minnesota, Minneapolis, MN, USA

Saami K. Yazdani, PhD CVPath Institute, Gaithersburg, MD, USA

Chapter 1
Anatomy of Coronary Vessels

Zeev Vlodaver and John R. Lesser

Anatomy of the Coronary Vessels

In the normal heart, oxygenated blood is supplied by two coronary arteries that form the first branches of the aorta. The origin of the left and right coronary arteries from the aorta is through their ostia positioned in the left and right aortic sinuses of Valsalva, located just distal to the right and left aortic cusps, respectively, of the aortic valve.

In about half of the population, a third artery, the conus artery (CA), also originates from the aorta. Diagrams of the main coronary arteries and their important branches are shown in Fig. 1.1.

In addition, there are two types of cardiac veins: (1) the large veins, which run in the epicardium and terminate in the coronary sinus (CS), and (2) the thebesian veins, small "tributary veins" which terminate directly in either the left atrium (LA) or right atrium (RA).

Left Coronary Arterial System

Left Main Coronary Artery

The left main coronary artery (LM) branches from the upper part of the aortic sinus and runs toward the left, under the LA appendage. After a short course, the LM branches into two vessels: the left anterior descending coronary artery (LAD) and the left circumflex artery (CX) (Figs. 1.2 and 1.3).

The LM is most often 0.5–1.5 cm long; when it is less than 0.5 mm long, it is considered to be short. Angiographic measurements of coronary length are probably less accurate than postmortem pathologic studies, due to underestimation of the effects of rotation, angulation, and foreshortening.

In some hearts, the LM exhibits a trifurcation at its origin instead of the usual bifurcation. This third artery, termed ramus intermedius (RI) or ramus diagonalis, acts functionally as a circumflex artery, supplying a portion of the obtuse margin of the heart (Figs. 1.4 and 1.5).

Anterior Descending Coronary Artery

The LAD runs in the anterior interventricular sulcus, usually as a direct continuation of the LM, and extends toward the apex, terminating in the apical part of the crux (Figs. 1.6 and 1.7).

Z. Vlodaver, MD (✉)
Division of Cardiovascular Medicine, University of Minnesota, Minneapolis, MN, USA
e-mail: zeev.vlodaver@gmail.com

J.R. Lesser
Department of Cardiology, Minneapolis Heart Institute, Abbott Northwestern Hospital, Minneapolis, MN, USA

Z. Vlodaver et al. (eds.), *Coronary Heart Disease: Clinical, Pathological, Imaging, and Molecular Profiles*,
DOI 10.1007/978-1-4614-1475-9_1, © Springer Science+Business Media, LLC 2012

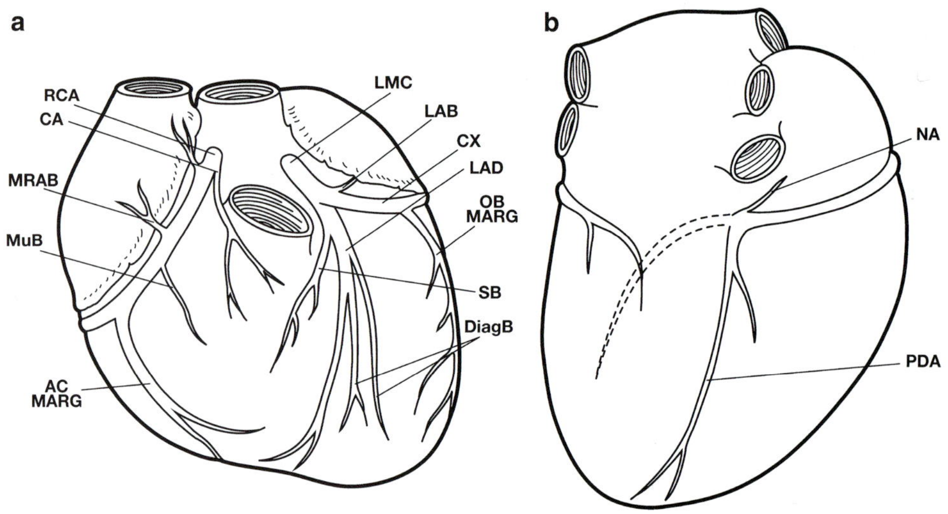

Fig. 1.1 Diagrams of the main coronary arteries and their branches as seen from the anterior (**a**) and posterior (**b**) aspects of the heart. This illustration shows the common phenomenon in which the right posterior descending artery (RPDA) arises from the terminal branch of the right coronary artery (RCA)

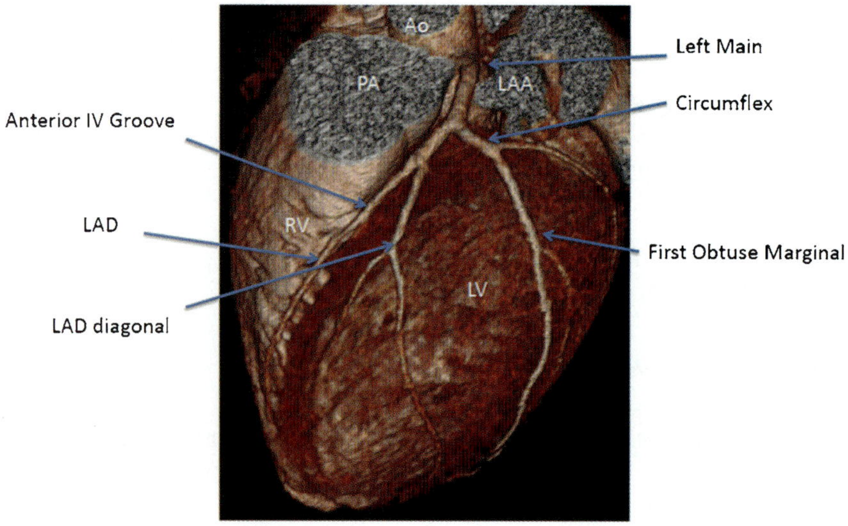

Fig. 1.2 Volume-rendered image shows the left main coronary artery (LM) arising from the aorta and bifurcating into the left anterior descending (LAD) and circumflex (CX) arteries and their branches

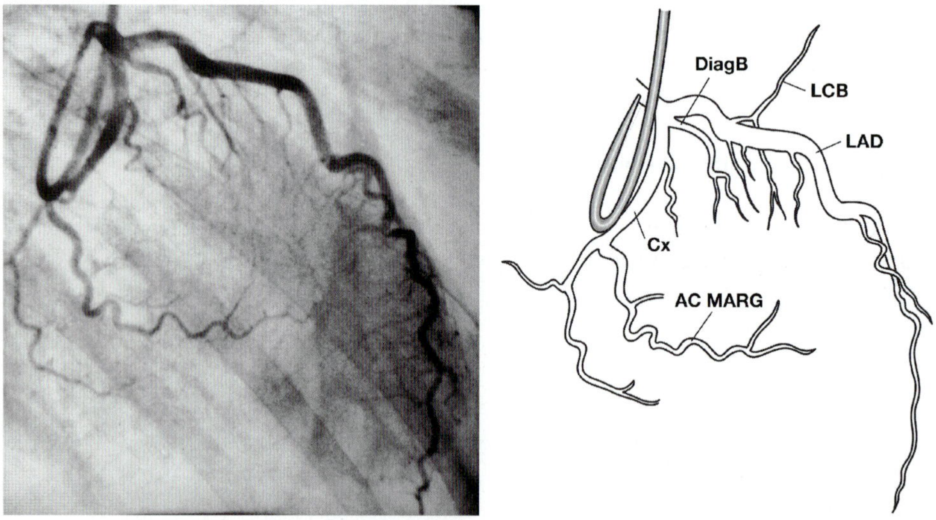

Fig. 1.3 LC arteriogram in the right anterior oblique (RAO) view showing the classic distribution of the left coronary arterial system

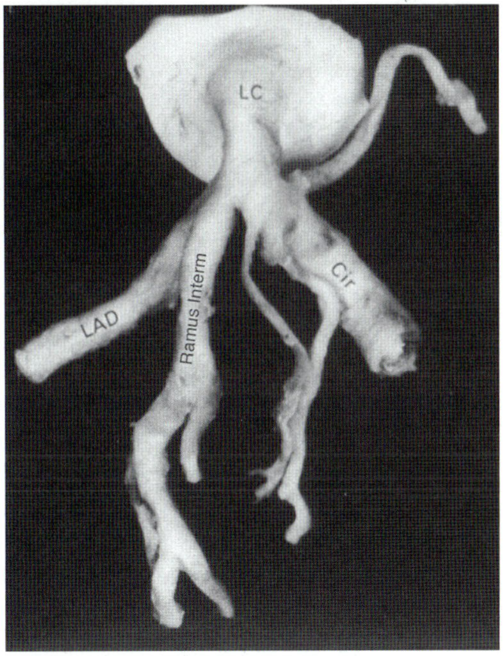

Fig. 1.4 Gross specimen of a portion of the aortic wall, the left main coronary artery (LM) proceeding from it, and branches of the LM. The LM measured 1.6 cm, which is normal. The branching is unusual because there is trifurcation of the LM into the left anterior descending artery (LAD), circumflex artery (CX), and a large branch ramus intermedius. The branch from the upper aspect of the CX is an atrial branch. The lower two branches of the CX are obtuse marginal branches (OMs)

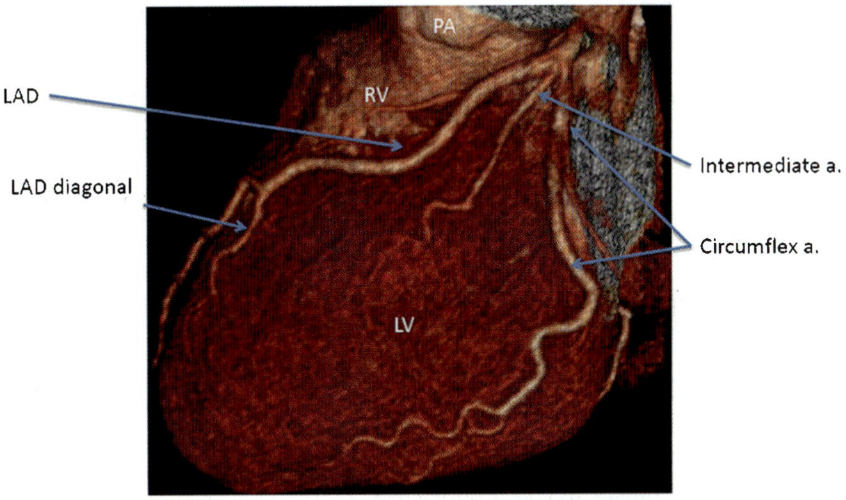

Fig. 1.5 Volume-rendered image shows the ramus intermediate branch arising between the left anterior descending artery (LAD) and circumflex artery (CX), resulting in trifurcation of the LM

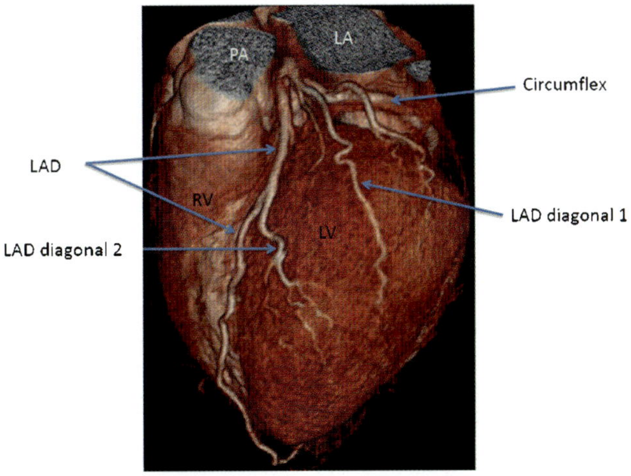

Fig. 1.6 Volume-rendered image illustrating the left anterior descending artery (LAD) and two diagonal branches arising from the left aspect of the artery and coursing over the left anterior aspect of the left ventricle

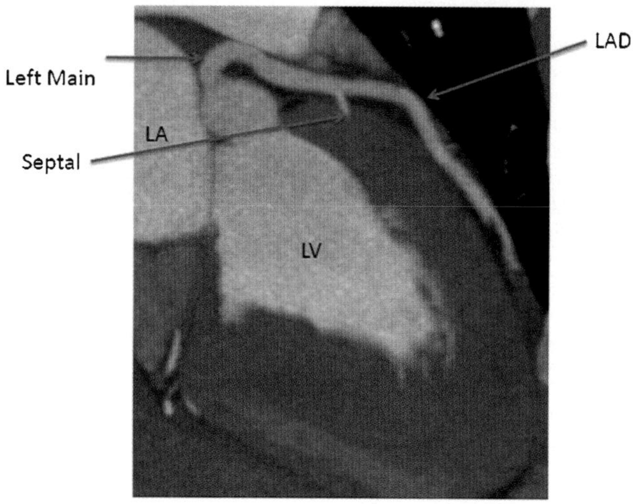

Fig. 1.7 Multidetector computed tomography angiography, long axis view, illustrating a septal branch of the left anterior descending artery (LAD) which penetrates the basal aspect of the ventricular septum anteriorly

The common branches of the LAD, proximally to distally, are (1) the septal branch (SB), which penetrates the basal aspect of the ventricular septum anteriorly (Fig. 1.7), and (2) one or more diagonal branches (Diag Bs), one proximal to the other, which arise from the left aspect of the LAD and course over the left anterior aspect of the LV. If two Diag Bs are present, the larger is usually first. In some cases, the width of the first Diag B may be equal to or exceed that of the LAD.

Left Circumflex Coronary Artery

The CX is one of the LM's two terminal branches. It arises at a sharp angle from the left side of the LM and courses forward under the LA appendage to enter the left atrioventricular (AV) sulcus, a position corresponding to the base of the mitral valve (Fig. 1.2).

Considerable variations occur in the course of the CX. In some instances, the artery terminates at the obtuse marginal branch (OM), which runs from the AV sulcus toward the apex along the lateral wall of the left ventricle (LV).

In other instances, the CX, after giving off the OM, continues in the left atrioventricular sulcus and terminates near the base of the crux, given off atrial branches and, occasionally, the sino-atrial branch.

Unusually Long Left Main Coronary Artery

According to Lewis et al., the length of the LM in 25 patients selected at random from a series of 354 arteriograms ranged from 7.5 to 20.5 mm ($M = 12.8$ mm) [1]. These findings are similar to those reported from the pathological studies of Baroldi and Scomazzoni [2].

Figure 1.8 depicts the features of an unusually long LM.

Short Left Main Coronary Artery

The practical significance of a short LM is that it may complicate perfusion of the left coronary arterial system during operative procedures, as in aortic valve replacement. Especially with a short LM and despite apparent optimal placement, the cannula may perfuse either the LAD or the CX, but not both, causing myocardial ischemia with resulting ventricular arrhythmias, myocardial infarct, or both.

Furlong et al. [3] observed that the angle of bifurcation of the LM is increased when LVH is present, as a result of upward displacement of the CX. This process may accentuate the problem of cannulating the left system when the main artery is short [3]. Figure 1.9 illustrates coronary angiographic features of a short LM.

A coronary artery is considered "short" when its intrinsic structure is uniformly narrow and it has a shorter course than usual. When a short artery is present, the region of the heart usually supplied by this artery is perfused through branches from the other coronary arteries. As a rule, only one of the coronary arteries is short – either the right or a branch of the left.

In the absence of other disease, a short artery is functionally insignificant.

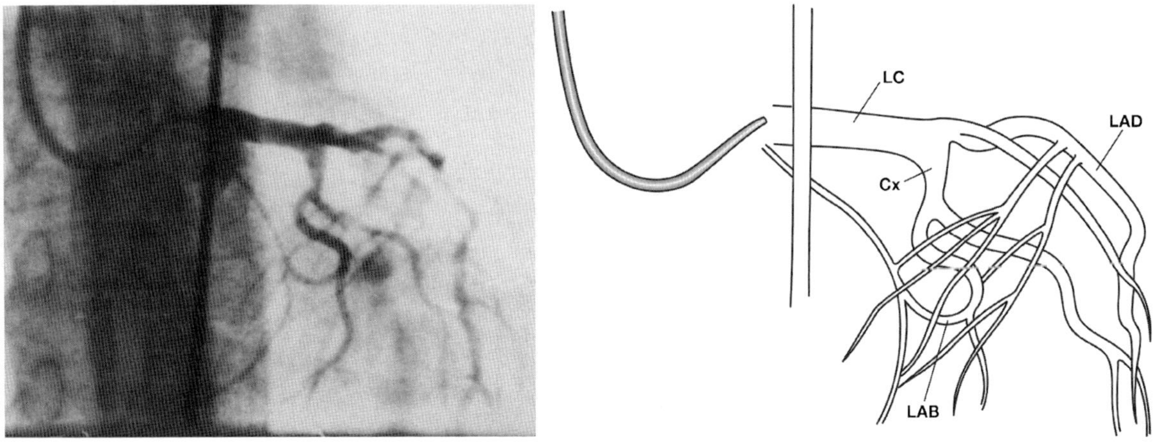

Fig. 1.8 LC arteriogram in the anterior posterior (AP) view showing a long LM, measuring approximately 30 mm

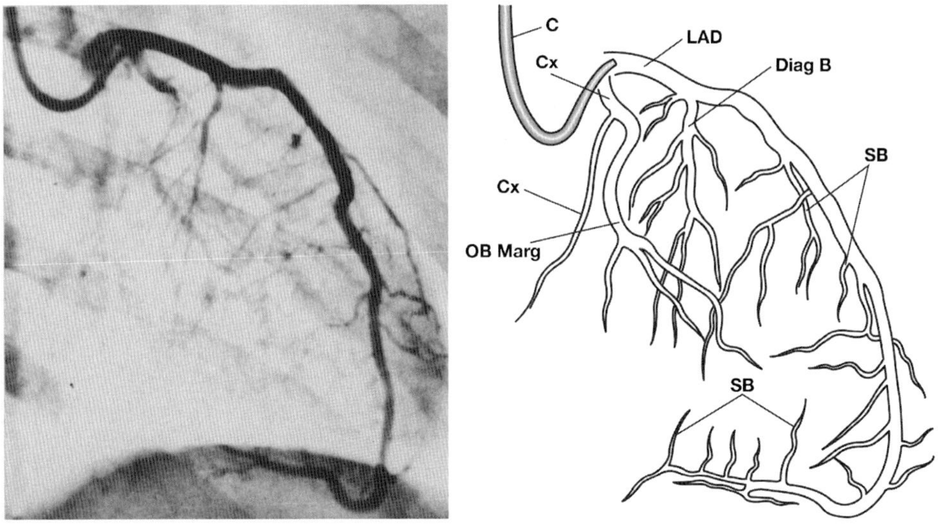

Fig. 1.9 LC arteriogram in RAO view showing a short LM

It should be recognized, however, that during both arteriography and surgery, it has been difficult to determine whether a narrow artery harbors disease or is congenital.

Short Left Anterior Descending Artery

Figure 1.10 shows a coronary arteriogram for a 44-year-old man with hypercholesterolemia. The arteriogram showed a large CX, while the LAD was short and terminated in small branches.

Short Circumflex Artery

Figures 1.11 and 1.12 pertain to a 10-year-old asymptomatic girl with familial hyperlipidemia. The ECG was normal. Coronary arteriography showed no lesions, and only two indistinct short vessels were noted in the anticipated location of the CX.

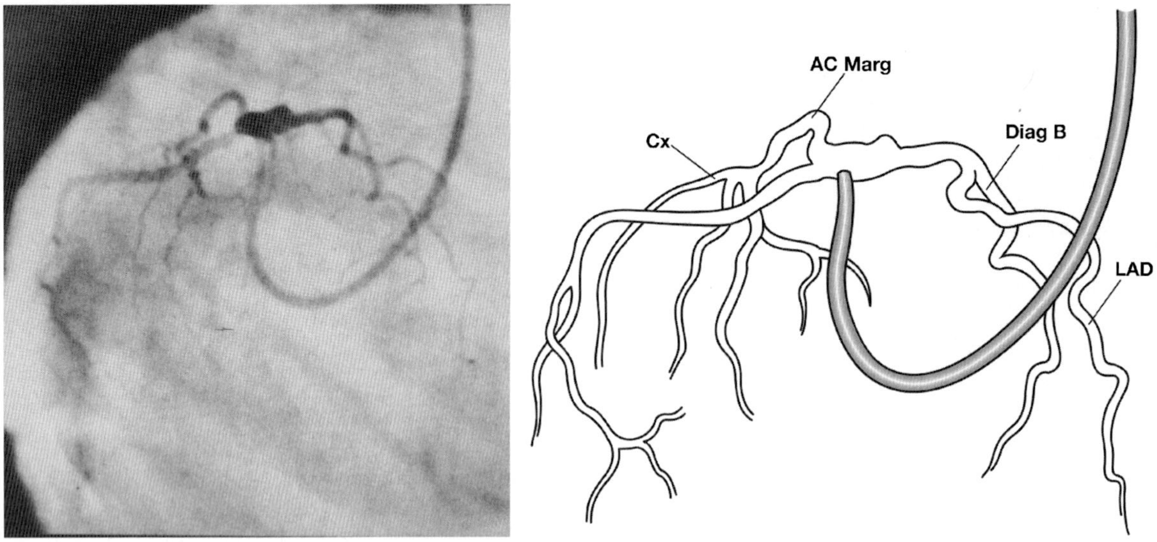

Fig. 1.10 Arteriogram in a lateral view showing a left coronary artery with a short left anterior descending artery (LAD)

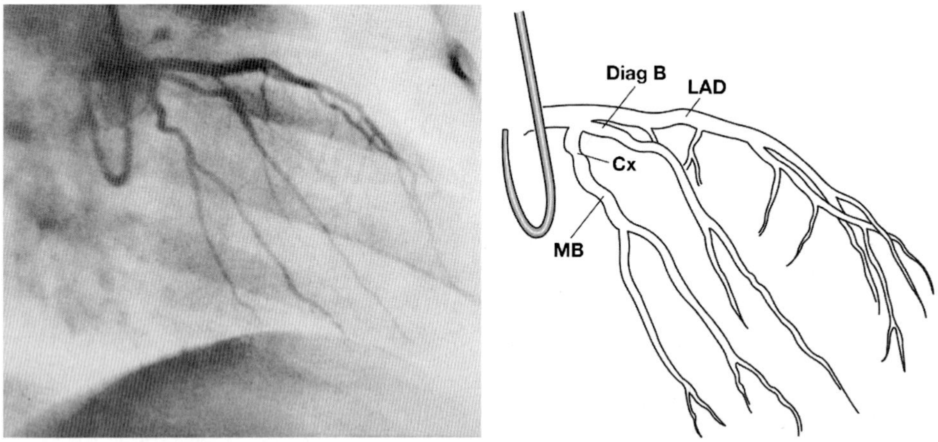

Fig. 1.11 RAO view of LC arteriogram shows a short circumflex artery (CX) leaving the left AV groove shortly after its origin and dividing into two obtuse marginal branches (OMs)

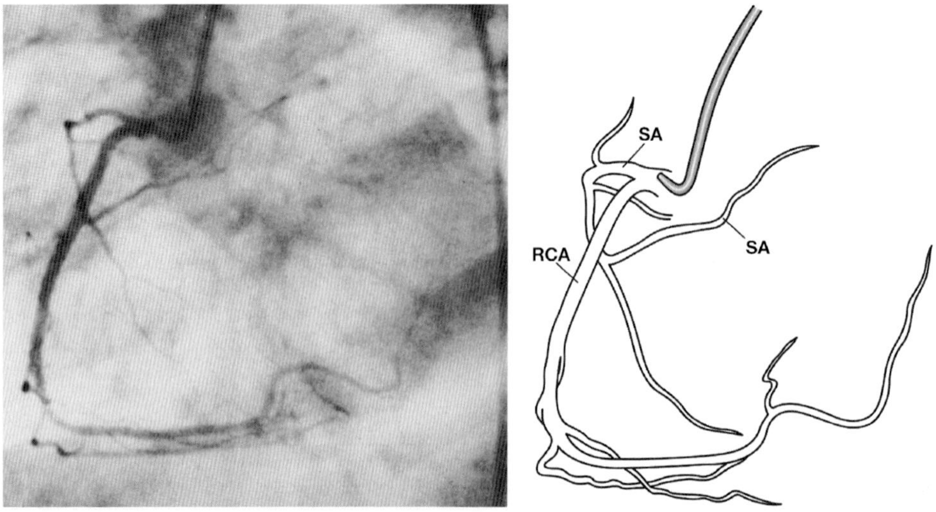

Fig. 1.12 Left anterior oblique (LAO) view of RC arteriogram shows unusual preponderance of the RCA. This artery continues in the atrioventricular (AV) groove toward the left ventricle (LV)

Right Coronary Arterial System

The right coronary artery (RCA) arises from the upper part of the right aortic sinus; as it leaves the aorta, it points somewhat anteriorly and proceeds toward the right, between the pulmonary artery to its left and the right atrium to its right, to enter the right AV sulcus. It then passes along the right AV sulcus past the acute margin of the heart to the base of the posterior (post) interventricular sulcus (the "crux").

The RV terminates at the crux about 10% of the time [4], but it is far more common for the artery to form a sharp U-shaped turn, and continue in the crux toward the cardiac apex as the right posterior descending artery (RPDA).

Several branches of the RCA have been given names. The conus artery (CA), when it does not begin from the aorta, appears as the first branch of the RCA and supplies the right ventricular infundibulum. Usually (about 55% of the time), the next major branch arising from the RCA is the sinus node artery (SA), which runs posterior to the RA appendage and proceeds upward toward the junction of the superior vena cava (SVC) and the RA [5]. In its course, the sinus node artery supplies branches to the RA. Past the origin of the SA, another right atria branch usually arises, often called the mid-right atrial branch (MRAB).

The RCA also gives off two or more branches to the free wall of the right ventricle (RV), the muscular branches (MuBs). The largest branch of the RCA runs along the acute margin of the RV. Called the acute marginal branch (AC Marg), it supplies the anterior and diaphragmatic wall of the RV.

In many hearts, the RCA terminates as the RPDA. However, it is also common for the RCA to terminate by dividing into two branches: the RPDA and a right posterior atrioventricular branch (RPAV). The latter courses in the left AV sulcus for varying distances and then proceeds over the lateral wall of the LV, where it terminates. In some cases, an accessory posterior descending artery (LPDA) originates from the RPAV and courses over the diaphragmatic surface of the LV from its base toward the apex.

The artery of the AV node, the so-called nodal artery (NA), usually arises from the RCA just proximal to the origin of the PDA. It proceeds upward to penetrate the atrial septum for supplying the AV node.

All of the classic branches of the RCA are illustrated in Figs. 1.13–1.15.

Short Nondominant Right Coronary Artery

The term "short nondominant RCA" characterizes an unusually short course of this artery: one that's only a few millimeters in length and does not reach the region of the crux. Figure 1.16 shows a diagram of a short nondominant RCA. Figure 1.17a, b pertains to a woman who died of obstructive biliary tract disease. The RCA was small and did not reach the right cardiac margin. Figure 1.18 shows a short nondominant RCA as seen in volume-rendering techniques with cardiac computed tomography angiography (VRT–CCTA). Images in Figs. 1.19 and 1.20 are from a 58-year-old woman with atypical chest pain. Coronary arteriography showed a short and narrow RCA, but no obstructive lesions.

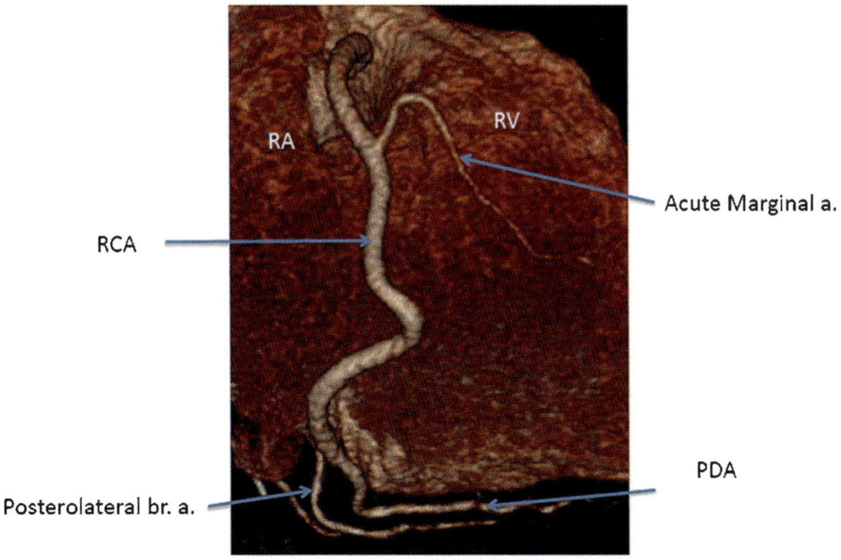

Fig. 1.13 Volume-rendered image in RAO orientation portrays all classical branches of the right coronary artery (RCA)

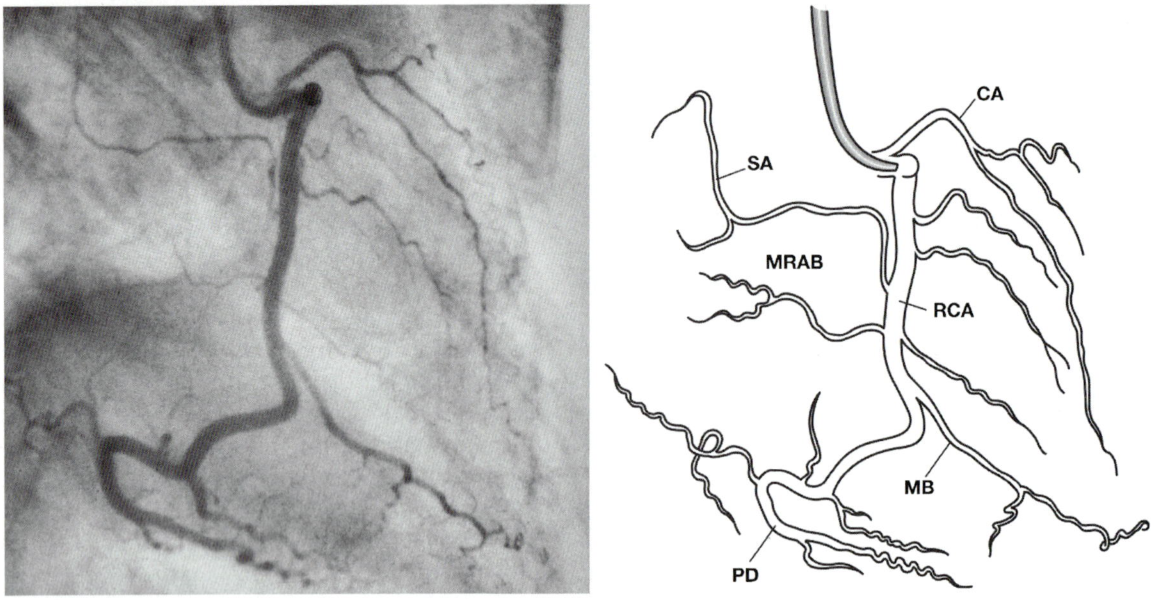

Fig. 1.14 RC arteriogram in RAO, which branches as indicated. Beyond the origin of the posterior descending artery (PDA) is a prominent right posterolateral (RPL) branch extending to the lateral wall. In this example, the conus artery (CA) arises from the right coronary artery (RCA)

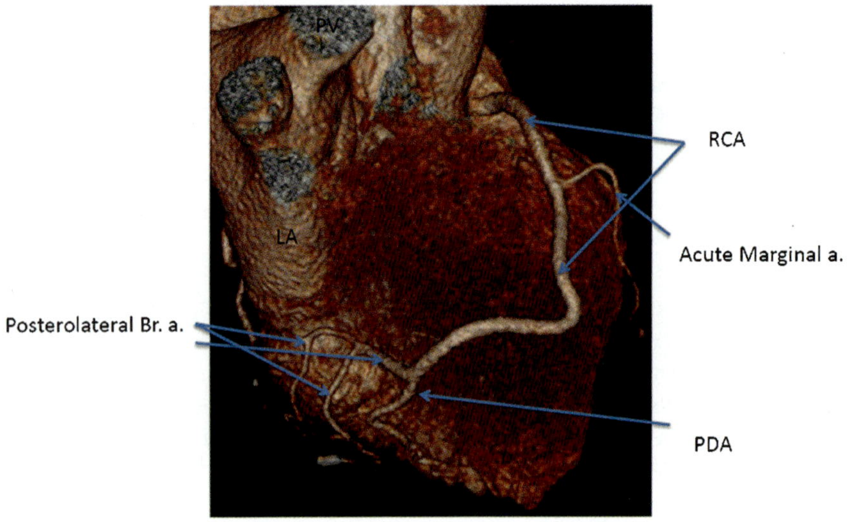

Fig. 1.15 Volume-rendered image, lateral wall of the RV, showing the RCA and its branches

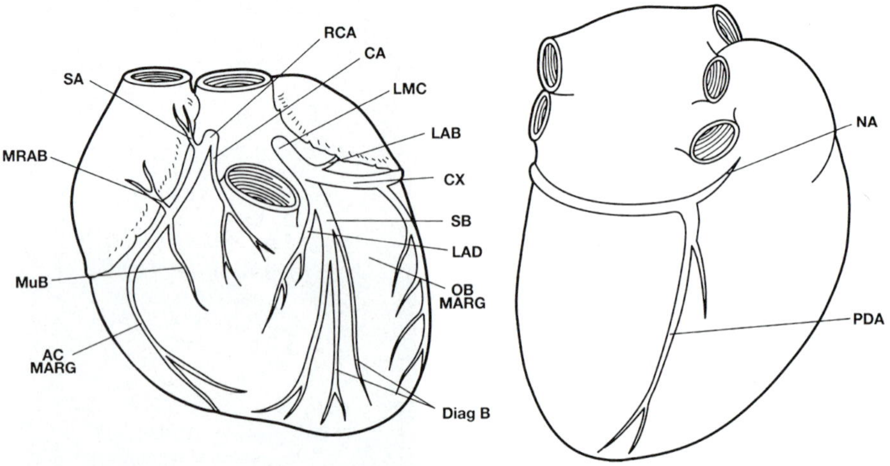

Fig. 1.16 Diagram of a short nondominant right coronary artery (RCA)

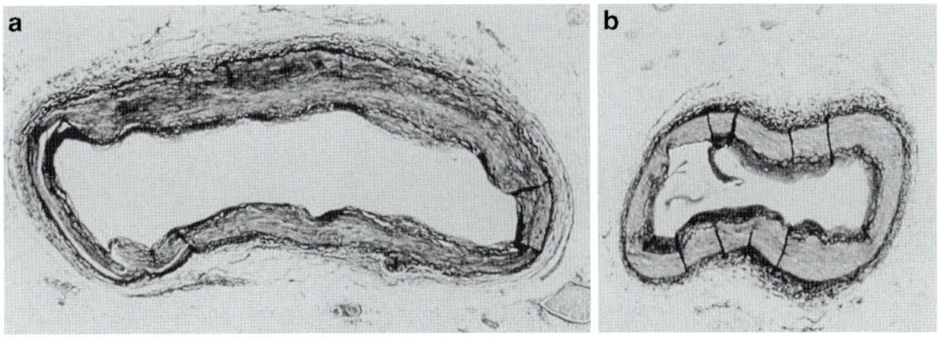

Fig. 1.17 Photomicrography of coronary arteries, each 1 cm from origin, in a case with short RCA. Elastic tissue stain ×18. (**a**) Left anterior descending artery (LAD) shows minimal intimal thickening. (**b**) RCA. The vessel shows a smaller caliber than the left anterior descending artery (LAD). Its structure is normal

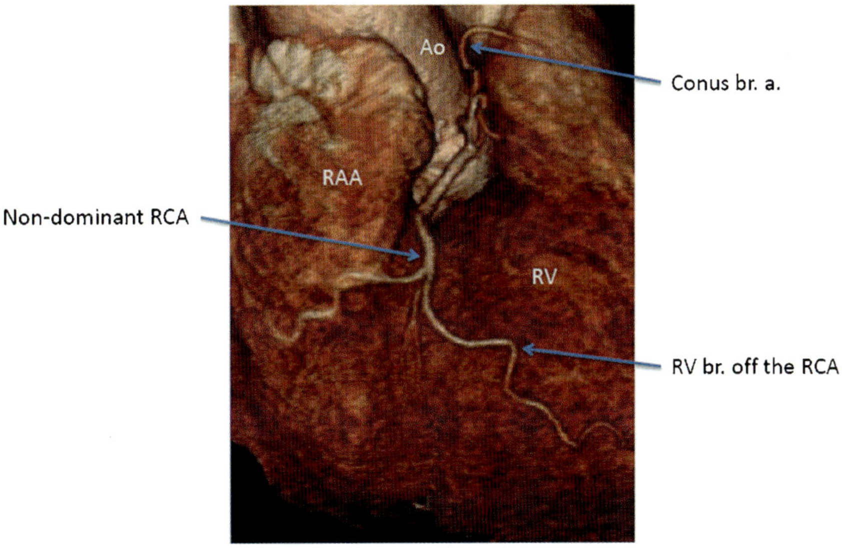

Fig. 1.18 Volume-rendered image illustrating a short, nondominant right coronary artery (RCA)

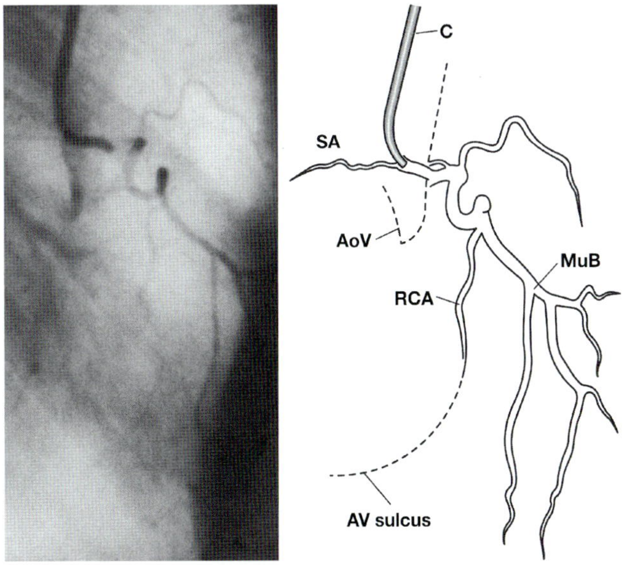

Fig. 1.19 RC arteriogram in lateral view. Only a small, short nondominant RCA vessel is seen in the atrioventricular (AV) sulcus

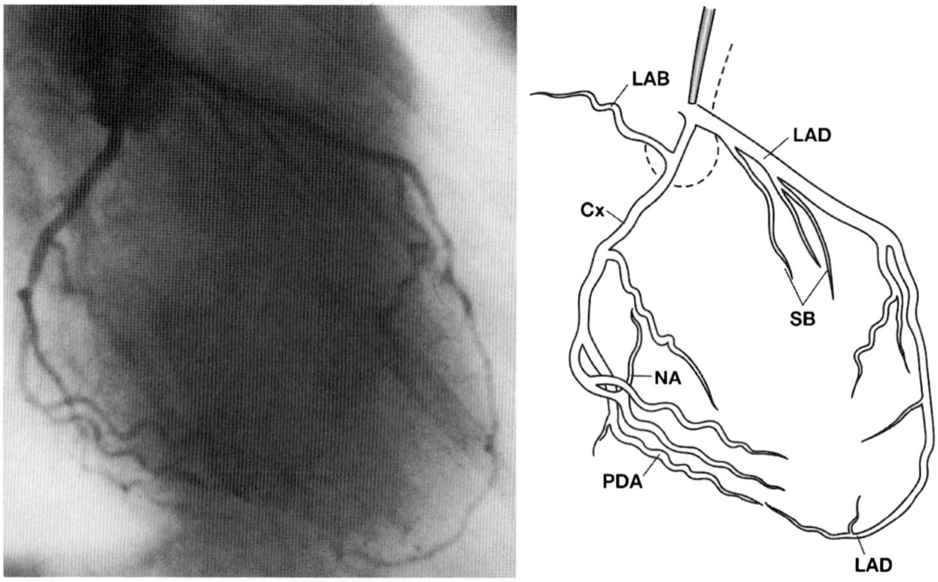

Fig. 1.20 LC arteriogram in RAO view, from patient illustrated in Fig. 1.20, demonstrating left predominance on which the entire basilar portion of the heart is supplied from the posterior descending artery (PDA), which arises from the circumflex artery (left dominant). The left anterior descending artery (LAD) curves around the apex to participate in supply of the inferior wall

Atrial Coronary Arterial Supply

In about half of the population, the sinus node artery is a branch of the proximal part of the CX. The artery courses along the anterior wall of the LA, beneath the LA appendage, to reach the anterior aspect of the RA and then the sinus node.

Another important atrial branch arising from the proximal portion of the CX is the LA artery. This artery supplies the lower portion and most of the posterior wall of the LA. The SA is sometimes enlarged in cases of mitral valvular disease, in which the LA is enlarged.

The branches that supply the atria may be of particular importance in supplying collateral flow when there is obstructive disease of the coronary arteries. The arterial supply to the atria may be demonstrated by CCTA or selective coronary arteriography.

Kugel's artery is prominent in instances of coronary arterial obstruction, and may be viewed as an abnormal secondary enlargement of a vessel. It runs posteriorly through the atrial septum and anastomoses with the nodal branch of the RCA. Its usual source is the proximal portion of the CX [6] (Fig. 1.21).

Atrial Supply from the Left Coronary System

The left arterial branch (LAB) of the CX is commonly visualized using CCTA or coronary arteriograms (Fig. 1.22). This branch may be clearly seen in rare instances where the LA is enlarged. In the case shown in Fig. 1.23, the patient, a 58-year-old woman, showed LA enlargement secondary to mitral stenosis. Origin of the sinus node artery from the LC system is demonstrated in Figs. 1.24 and 1.25.

Atrial Arterial Supply from the Right Coronary System

In most circumstances, demonstration of Kugel's artery indicates the presence of obstructive coronary arterial disease. The unusual instance shown in Fig. 1.26 is from a patient with normal coronary arteries as seen in the coronary arteriogram. CCTA illustrating the SA nodal artery from RCA is shown in Fig. 1.27.

Fig. 1.21 Sinus node artery (SA) arising from the LM

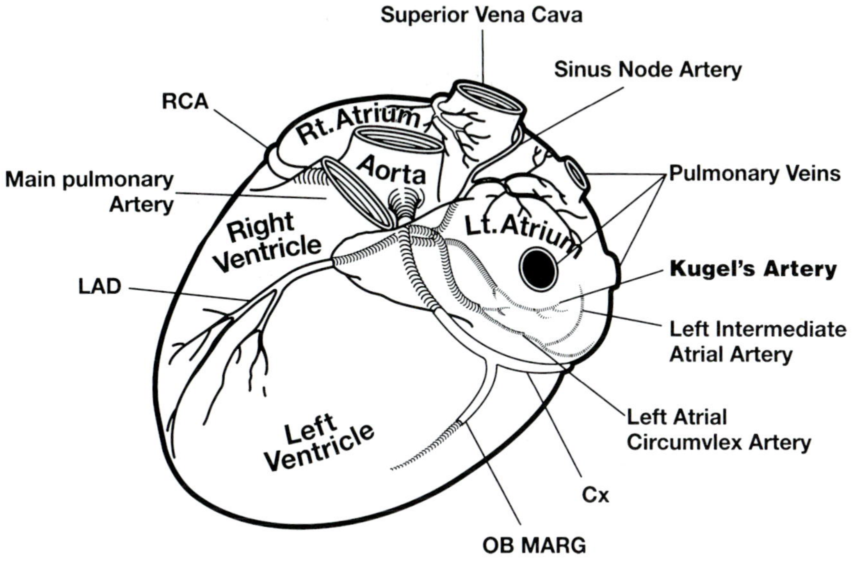

Fig. 1.22 Volume-rendered image illustrates left atrial branch from the circumflex artery (CX)

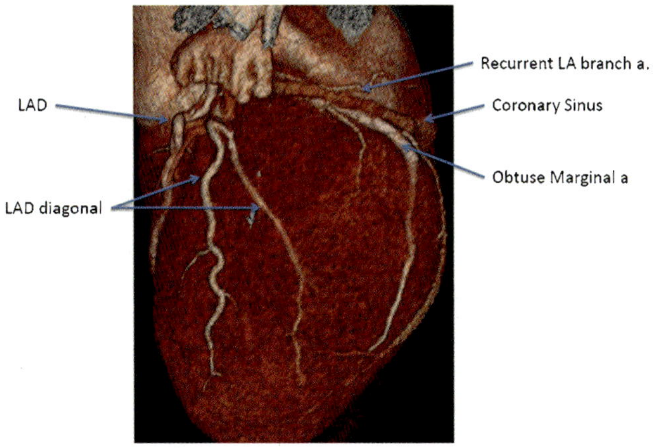

Fig. 1.23 LC arteriogram in lateral view shows a prominent left arterial branch (LAB) from the circumflex artery (CX)

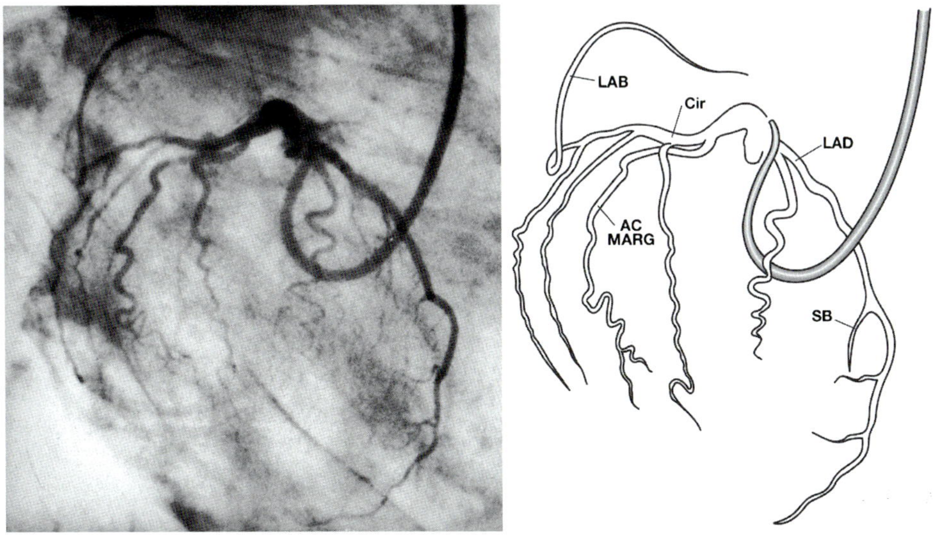

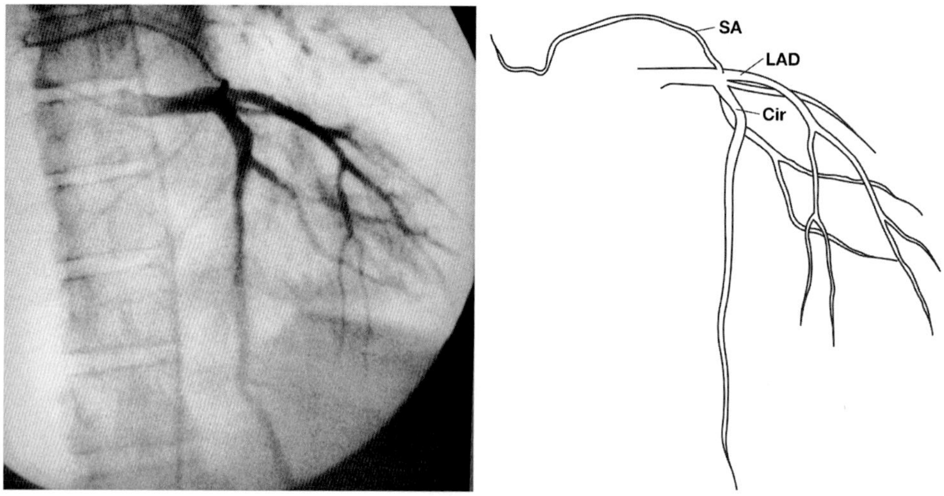

Fig. 1.24 Origin of the sinus node artery (SA) from the circumflex artery (CX) is portrayed in this LC arteriogram (frontal view)

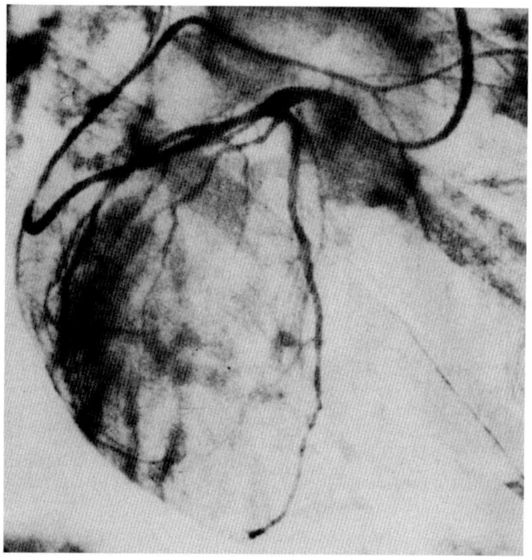

Fig. 1.25 Left anterior oblique (LAO) view of normal LC arteriogram. Unusually large left arterial branch (LAB) of the circumflex artery (CX) gives rise to the sinus node artery (SA)

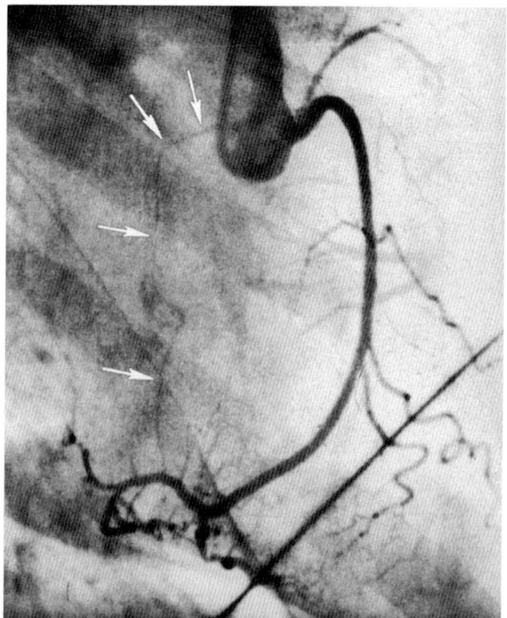

Fig. 1.26 RAO view of normal RC arteriogram in which a Kugel's artery arising from the proximal RCA (*arrows*) is demonstrable. The artery is in the center of the illustration

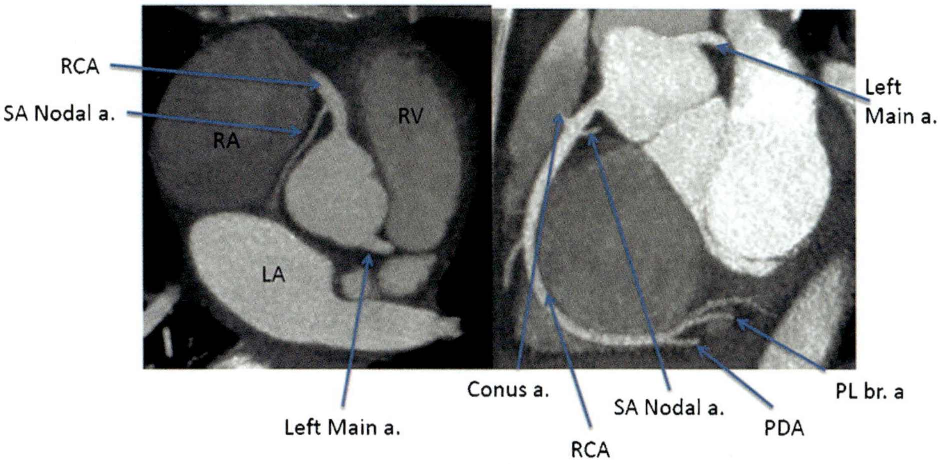

Fig. 1.27 (**a**) Axial CCTA image showing sinus node artery (SA) originating from the right coronary artery (RCA). (**b**) LAO orientation

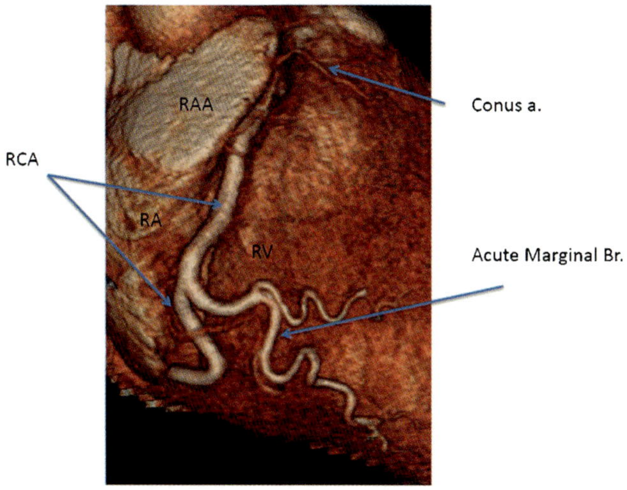

Fig. 1.28 Volume-rendered image in RAO orientation, illustrating the conus artery originating from the right coronary artery (RCA)

The Conus Artery

The conus artery supplies the outflow tract of the right ventricle. This vessel varies in size and arises from either the RCA or aorta. Figures 1.15, 1.18, and 1.28 show the conus artery arising from the RCA. When it arises from the aorta, the CA is sometimes called the "third coronary artery," [7] and its origin is in the right aortic sinus just anterior to the origin of the RCA (Figs. 1.29 and 1.30). It is a small artery with a lumen of less than 1 mm in diameter, and it courses the epicardium over the RV infundibulum.

The conus artery may play a significant role in the presence of obstructive coronary atherosclerosis. It may become an important collateral channel as it joins branches from the proximal portion of the LAD to form the Vieussens' circle.

Occasionally, in instances of the tetralogy of Fallot, the CA is particularly important in supplying blood to the RV and, sometimes, to the LV. During surgical repair, it could be accidentally injured, resulting in myocardial ischemic complications. Infrequently, the CA may communicate with an accessory branch of the pulmonary trunk (PT). In this way, it underlies a left-to-right shunt.

Coronary Dominance

The term "coronary dominance" was introduced by Schlesinger in 1940 [8]. The "dominant" coronary artery is the one that gives rise to the posterior descending artery, traversing the posterior interventricular sulcus, and supplying the posterior part of the ventricular septum and, often, the posterolateral wall of the left ventricular wall.

The RCA is dominant in approximately 70% of humans [9]. If the circumflex artery terminates in the posterior descending artery, left dominance is present (Figs. 1.31–1.33). This is seen in 15% of cases. In the remaining 15%, the posterior

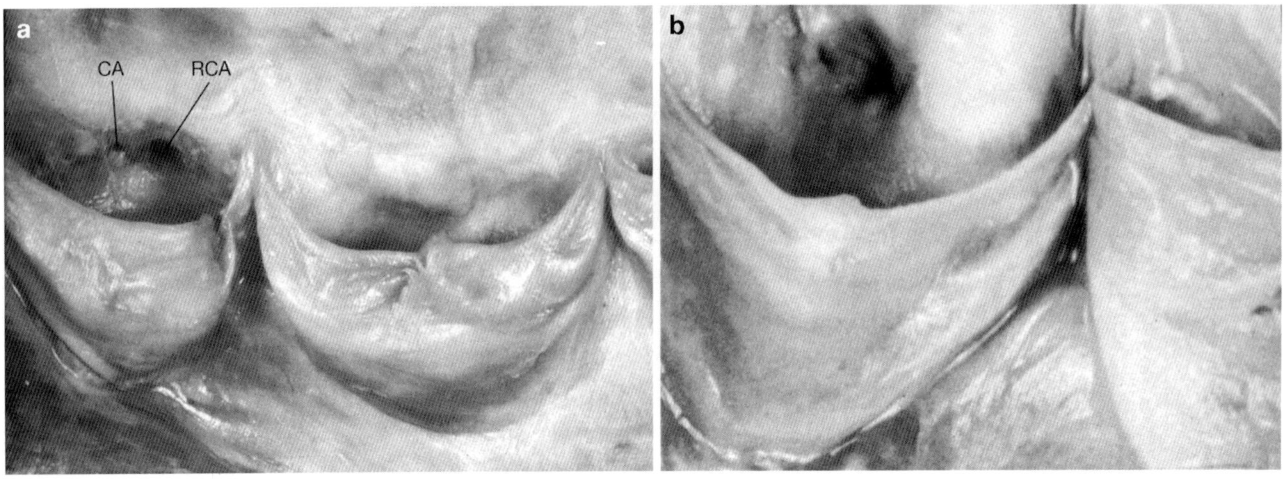

Fig. 1.29 Portions of the aortic valve in two cases. (**a**) A single conus artery (CA) arises from the ostium of the right coronary artery (RCA). (**b**) Two conus arteries (CAs) arise independently from the aorta anterior to the RCA

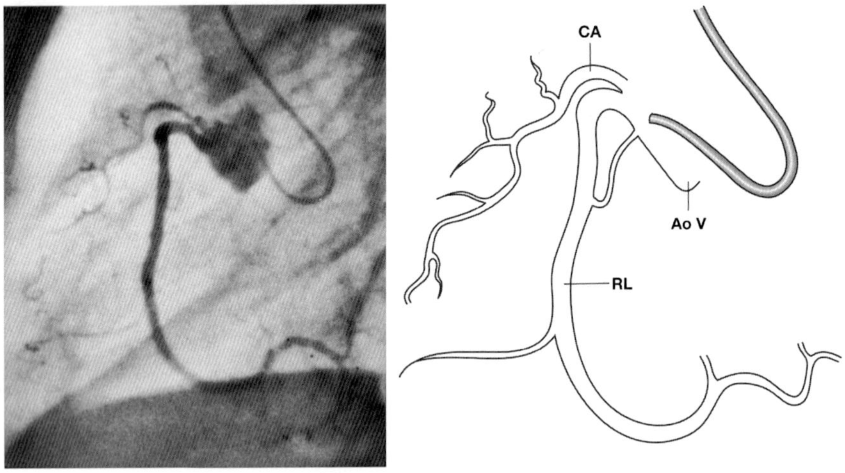

Fig. 1.30 RC arteriogram in lateral view shows independent origin of the conus artery (CA) from the right aortic sinus. The latter demonstration depends on reflux of contrast material into the right aortic sinus and subsequent opacification of the CA

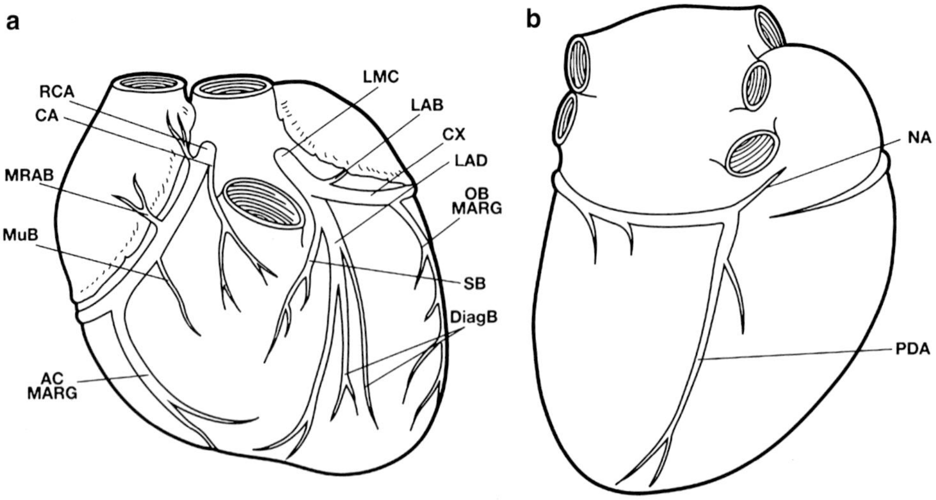

Fig. 1.31 A variation in distribution of the coronary arteries, occurring in about 15% of the population, in which the left posterior descending artery (LPDA) is represented as the terminal branch of the circumflex artery (CX) (left dominant circulation). (**a**) Anterior and (**b**) posterior aspects

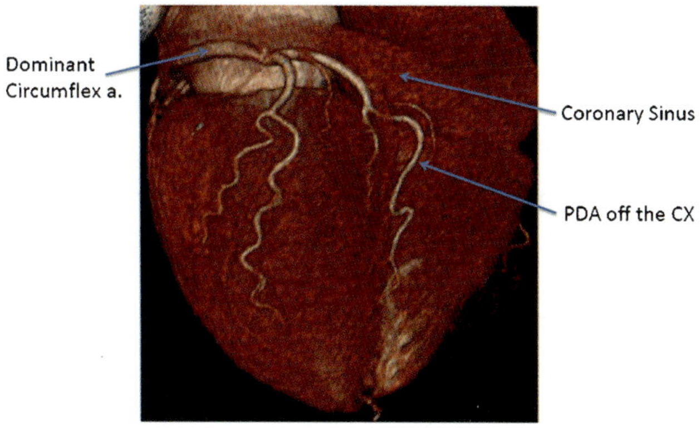

Fig. 1.32 Volume-rendered imaging in posterior orientation shows the inferior surface of the heart. A left-dominant system is depicted. The posterior descending artery (PDA) arises from the circumflex (CX) artery

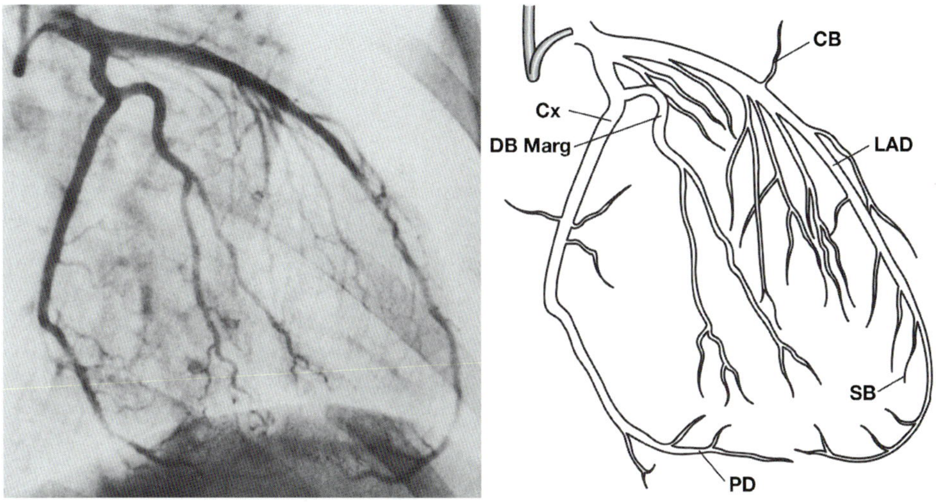

Fig. 1.33 LC arteriogram shows the circumflex artery terminating in the LPDA (left dominant)

septum is supplied by branches arising from both the right coronary and left circumflex arteries. In the latter situation, the circulation is said to be "balanced" and the posterior descending artery is either dual or absent [10], being supplied by a network of small branches.

It should be noted that anatomic dominance does not imply physiologic dominance. Although the RCA is usually dominant, the left coronary artery almost always supplies a greater myocardial mass [11].

The Coronary Veins

The veins of the heart fall into two major groups. One includes veins that tend to accompany the arteries; these are epicardial veins, which drain into the coronary sinus (Fig. 1.34). The other group is known collectively as the thebesian system, a variable number of small veins that open directly into the atria.

The coronary sinus courses parallel to the CX in the left atrioventricular sulcus and enters the posterior aspect of the right atrium (Fig. 1.35). Its orifice is partly covered by the thebesian valve, and this may render catheterization of the coronary sinus difficult. The major tributaries of the CS are the anterior interventricular vein, the posterior interventricular vein, and the left marginal vein.

The anterior interventricular vein, or great cardiac vein, begins at the apex of the heart and courses parallel to the LAD in the anterior interventricular sulcus (Fig. 1.36).

The posterior interventricular vein, or middle cardiac vein, begins at the apex posteriorly, courses parallel to the posterior descending artery in the crux, and ends in the terminal portion of the coronary sinus (Fig. 1.37). The left marginal vein, or posterior vein, begins at the posterior surface of the LV and follows the CX to terminate in the coronary sinus.

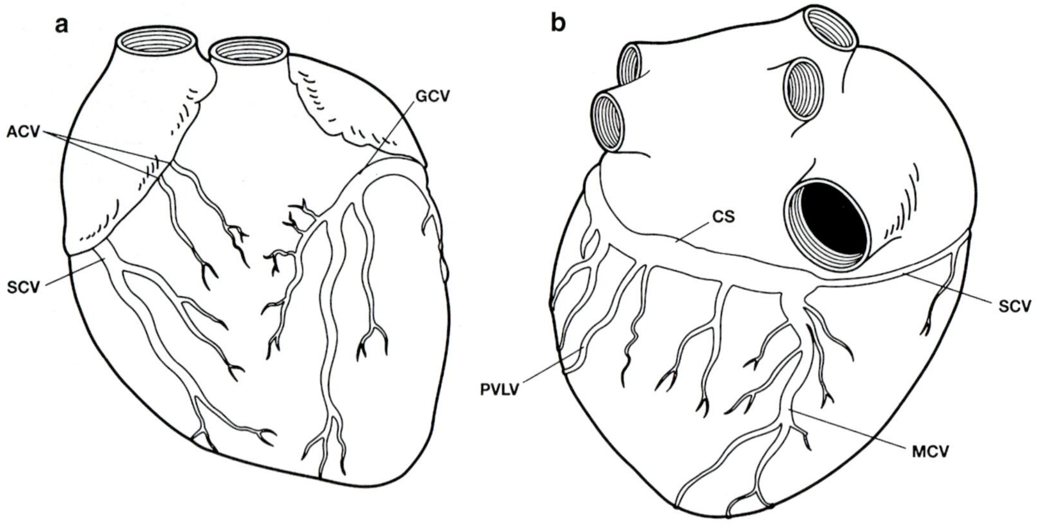

Fig. 1.34 Anterior (**a**) and posterior (**b**) veins of the heart show the positions of the major cardiac veins

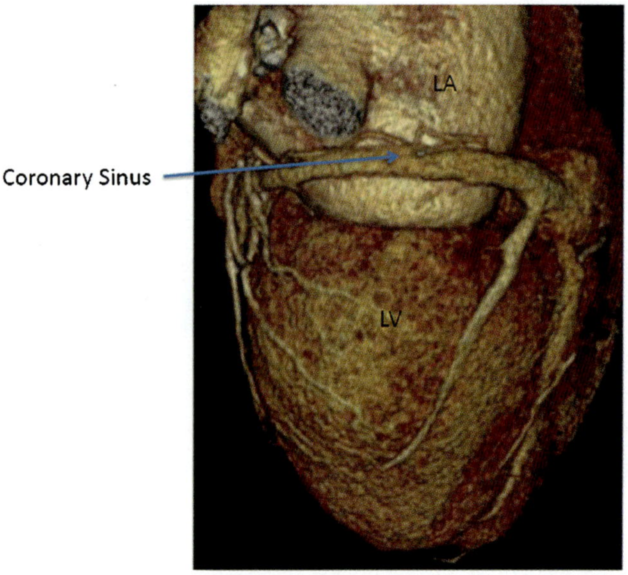

Fig. 1.35 Volume-rendered image with posterior orientation shows the coronary sinus running parallel to the circumflex artery

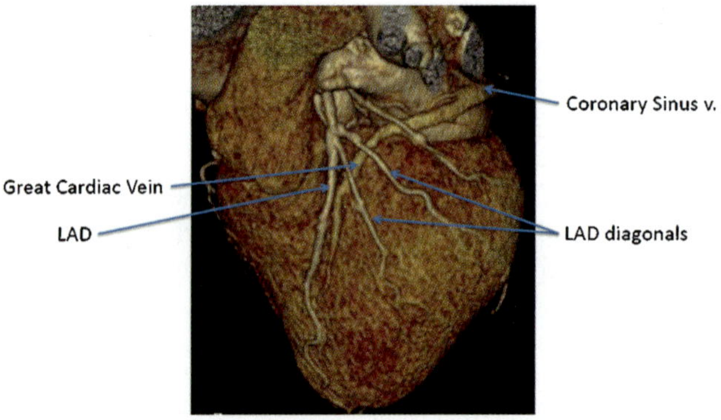

Fig. 1.36 Volume-rendered image in LAO cranial orientation showing the great cardiac vein that begins in the apex of the heart and courses parallel to the left anterior descending artery (LAD) in the IV sulcus and terminates in the coronary sinus

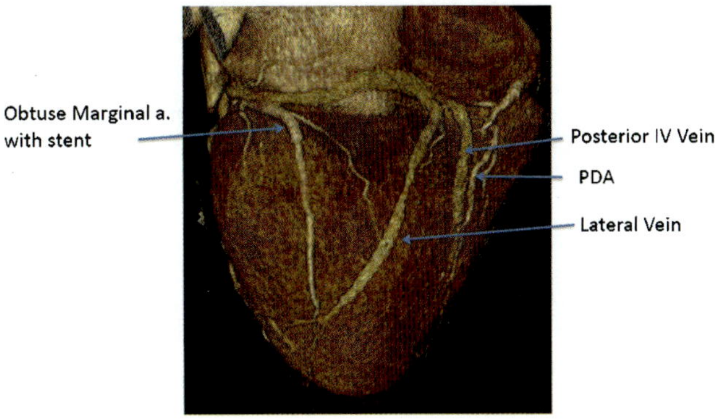

Fig. 1.37 Volume-rendered image with posterior orientation illustrates the posterior interventricular septum vein, which courses parallel to the PDA in the crux and ends in the terminal portion of the coronary sinus

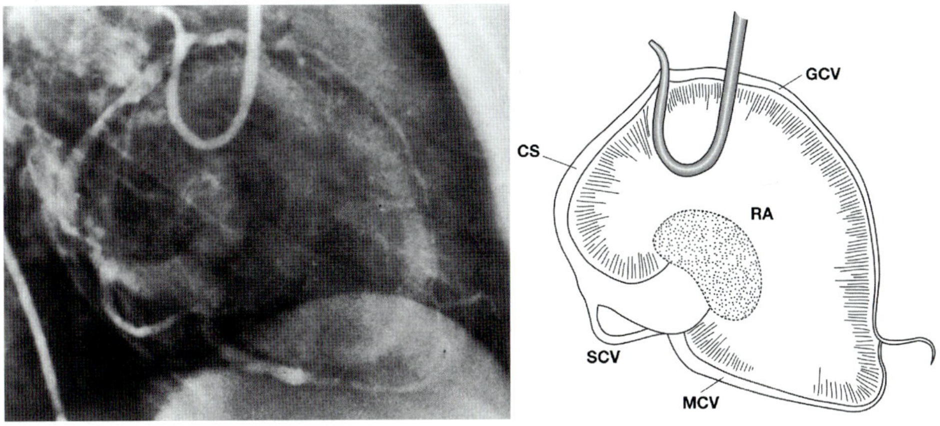

Fig. 1.38 Lateral view outlining the coronary sinus and the major epicardial veins

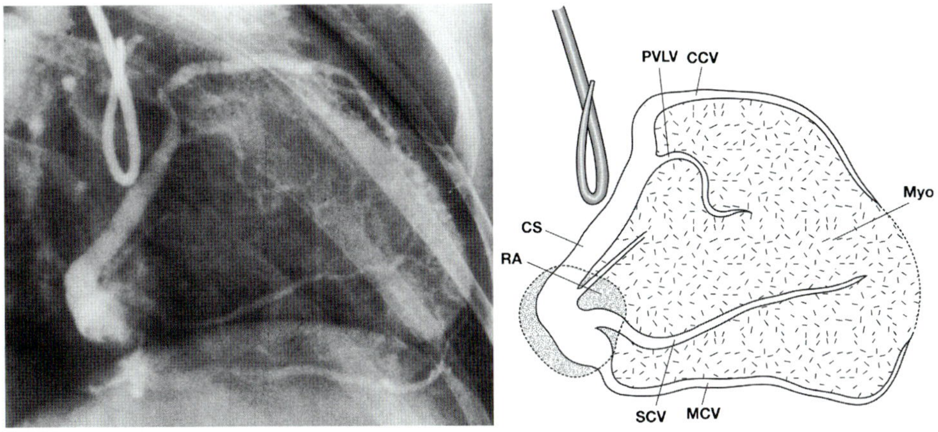

Fig. 1.39 RAO view showing highlights of the epicardial system of cardiac veins

The small cardiac vein (SCV) begins over the lateral wall of the RV and enters the right AV sulcus. The anterior cardiac vein runs from the wall of the infundibulum and empties into either the RA or SCV.

Among the smaller veins is Marshall oblique vein, which lies over the posterior wall of the LA and represents a vestige of the left SCV.

A fairly common variation is the left SCV remaining patent and terminating in the lateral aspect of the coronary sinus. In this circumstance, the CS is greatly enlarged.

Opacification of the epicardial cardiac veins may be observed in late phases of coronary arteriograms. The coronary arteriograms in Figs. 1.38 and 1.39 illustrate the main cardiac veins during this late stage.

Glossary of Acronyms

For quick reference, following is a list of acronyms used in this chapter and throughout the book. It is based on terminology used in Scanlon et al. [12]

Left coronary artery	
CX	Left circumflex artery (also: Prox CX, Mid CX)
Diag	Diagonal branch (also: 1st Diag, 2nd Diag)
LAB	Left atrial branch
LAD	Left anterior descending coronary artery
LAV	Left atrioventricular branch
LM	Left main coronary artery
LPDA	Left posterior descending artery
LPL	Left posterolateral branch
RI	Ramus intermedius branch
OM	Obtuse marginal branches of left circumflex
Septal branch	Septal branch (also: 1st septal branch)
Right coronary artery	
AC MARG	Acute marginal
Inf Septal	Inferoseptal artery
MuB	Muscular branch
MRAB	Mid-right atrial branch
NA	Artery of AV node (nodal artery)
RCA	Right coronary artery (also: Prox RCA, Mid RCAQ, Dist RCA)
RPAV	Right posterior atrioventricular artery
RPDA	Right posterior descending artery
RPL	Right posterolateral
SA	Sinus node artery

References

1. Lewis CM, Dagenais GR, Friesinger GC, et al. Coronary arteriographic appearances in patients with left bundle-branch block. Circulation. 1970;41:299.
2. Baroldi G, Scomazzoni G. Coronary circulation in the normal and pathologic heart. Washington DC: Office of the Surgeon General, Department of the Army; 1967. p. 9, 35.
3. Furlong MB, Gardner TJ, Gott VL, et al. Myocardial infarction complicating coronary perfusion during open-heart surgery. J Thorac Cardiovasc Surg. 1972;63(2):185.
4. James TN. Anatomy of the coronary arteries. Hoeber: New York; 1961. p. 51.
5. James TN. Anatomy of the coronary arteries and veins. In: Hurst JW, editor. The heart. 3rd ed. New York, NY: McGraw-Hill; 1974. p. 35–52.
6. Wilson WJ, Lee GB, Amplatz K. Biplane selective coronary arteriography via percutaneous transfemoral approach. Am J Roentgenol Radium Ther Nucl Med. 1967;100:332–8.
7. Schlesinger MJ, Zoll PM, Wessler S. The conus artery: a third coronary artery. Am Heart J. 1949;38:823.
8. Schlesinger MJ. Relation of anastomotic pattern in pathologic conditions of the coronary arteries. Arch Pathol. 1940;30:403–15.
9. Alwork SP. The applied anatomy of the arterial blood supply to the heart in man. J Anat. 1987;153:1–16.
10. Allwork SP. Angiographic anatomy. In: Anderson RH, Becker AE, editors. Cardiac anatomy. London: Churchill Livingstone; 1980.
11. Feiring AJ, Johnson MR, Kioschos JM, et al. The importance of the determination of the myocardial area at risk in the evaluation of the outcome of acute myocardial infarction in patients. Circulation. 1987;75:984–7.
12. Scanlon PJ, Faxon DP, Audet AM, et al. ACC/AHA guidelines for coronary angiography: a report of the American College of Cardiology/American Heart Association Task Force on Practice Guidelines (Committee on Coronary Angiography): developed in collaboration with the Society for Cardiac Angiography and Interventions. J Am Coll Cardiol. 1999;33:1756–824.

Chapter 2
Cardiac Development and Congenital Heart Disease

Jamie L. Lohr, Cindy M. Martin, and Daniel J. Garry

Technology has revolutionized the clinical diagnosis, medical management, surgical repair, and palliation of both congenital and acquired heart disease over the last 60 years. Despite this progress, congenital heart disease (CHD) remains the most common cause of death in infancy due to a birth defect. In addition to CHD, acquired heart disease can progress to heart failure, and the number of hospitalizations for heart failure in the adult population continues to increase. Advances in treatment for congenital and acquired heart disease will require the development of molecular and regenerative therapies; these treatment modalities require an enhanced understanding of the genetic and molecular control of normal cardiac development.

Cardiac Development

The heart is the first organ to form in the developing vertebrate embryo [1]. Establishing a functional circulatory system is required for survival during development. Defects in the heart and vasculature, along with chromosomal abnormalities, are commonly associated with early pregnancy loss [2]. Although the human heart is fully formed and functional before the end of the first trimester of pregnancy, cardiac maturation continues through fetal and neonatal life.

Cardiac Embryology

Specification of the Cardiac Mesoderm and Heart Tube Formation

Precardiac cells are specified in the third week of human gestation during the process of gastrulation, when molecular signals from the endoderm, along with other factors, direct the anterior mesoderm to form a cardiac fate. This anterior and lateral mesoderm forms bilateral heart tubes that coalesce and fuse in the midline of the folding embryo. This single linear heart tube begins to beat in a peristaltic wave at 22–23 days gestation in the human embryo, and blood flow can be observed by Doppler imaging at 4–5 weeks gestation [3]. The straight heart tube is formed by early cardiac mesoderm and consists of a primitive myocardium lined with a thin layer of endothelial cells. A layer of extracellular matrix or "cardiac jelly" is secreted by the myocardium and separates the myocardium and endocardium [4, 5].

The epicardial cells of the heart arise during the fourth and fifth weeks of gestation from the proepicardium, a mass of cells in the dorsal mesoderm near the inflow region of the heart tube. These cells migrate over the heart tube to contribute to the connective tissue of the myocardium and epicardium and give rise to the coronary arteries [6, 7].

J.L. Lohr, MD (✉)
Division of Pediatric Cardiology, University of Minnesota Amplatz Children's Hospital, Minneapolis, MN, USA
e-mail: lohrx003@umn.edu

C.M. Martin, MD • D.J. Garry, MD, PhD
Division of Cardiovascular Medicine, University of Minnesota, Minneapolis, MN, USA

Z. Vlodaver et al. (eds.), *Coronary Heart Disease: Clinical, Pathological, Imaging, and Molecular Profiles*,
DOI 10.1007/978-1-4614-1475-9_2,

These cells are the precursors to all cell layers of the coronary arteries and are the focus of studies pertaining to the genesis of the vasculature and the susceptibility to coronary vascular disease. In addition, recent studies suggest that they may be global progenitor cells, capable of differentiating into epicardial and myocardial interstitial cells, smooth muscle cells, and cardiomyocytes [7, 8].

Formation of the Vascular System

The primitive vascular system develops simultaneously with the heart tube. The arterial and venous systems are bilaterally symmetric, with paired aortic arches and paired anterior and posterior cardinal veins. Early during embryonic development, the paired dorsal aortas fuse to form a single thoracoabdominal aorta. The dual aortic arches and paired venous return persist until 6–8 weeks of human development; thereafter, asymmetric regression ultimately results in establishment of the adult vascular pattern [3].

Cardiac Looping

Between 22 and 28 days of human gestation, the beating heart tube elongates by the addition of cells from the second heart field [4, 5]. The second heart field is a region of mesoderm lining the pharynx and foregut in the embryo [4]. Second heart field cells from the pharyngeal region are added to the cranial outflow portion of the heart, and cells from the foregut are added to the inflow region or sinus venosus [4, 5]. This elongation and narrowing of the heart tube is accompanied by rightward looping, which brings the inflow region of the heart to a cranial position just behind the developing outflow tract. This highly conserved process of rightward looping establishes the anatomical relationships required for normal cardiac chamber formation and septation. The process of looping is dependent on normal secondary heart field and left–right axis determination in the embryo. Defects in the looping process are associated with severe forms of CHD, including inflow and outflow tract defects [4, 9].

Chamber Formation and Septation

Cardiac septation begins during the looping phase at approximately week 4 of human gestation [3]. The elongated, looping heart tube contains visible narrowings demarcating the cardiac regions from cranial to caudal: the conotruncus (distal and proximal outflow tracts), the ventricular chambers, the atrioventricular sulcus, the primitive atrial chamber, and the sinus venosus. The fifth week of human gestation is associated with induction of the endocardium at the atrioventricular sulcus by the myocardium to form endocardial cushions. The endocardial cushions of the atrioventricular canal enlarge and divide the canal into a right and left component. The presumptive right and left ventricles begin to enlarge asymmetrically and form trabeculations in the myocardial walls. The right component of the atrioventricular canal expands along with the right ventricle to allow blood from the sinus venosus to enter the right ventricle directly [3, 4].

The atrial and ventricular septae form and fuse with the endocardial cushions to complete septation of the cardiac chambers. Atrial septation occurs during the fifth week of human development through formation of the septum primum, a thin septum that divides the atrium and fuses with the endocardial cushions. This septum develops an opening termed the foramen secundum, which enables shunting of oxygenated blood from the placenta to the fetal myocardium and brain. The septum secundum is a thicker, muscular septum that forms during the fifth and sixth weeks of gestation, and overlaps the septum primum, also fusing with the endocardial cushions. The septum secundum develops an oval opening or foramen; regression of the septum primum allows it to form the flap-like valve of the foramen ovale [3].

Ventricular septation occurs during the same time period and is completed by the eighth week of gestation. The four portions of the ventricular septum close by varied mechanisms. The muscular ventricular septum gains prominence through the dilation and trabeculation of the enlarging ventricles and grows by cellular proliferation [3]. The inlet, membranous, and outflow septums are closed by the merging of the bulbar ridges on the inner curvature of the heart with the endocardial cushions and extension of this tissue to the muscular septum to close the membranous portion of the septum. Similar extension of tissue to the outflow tract cushions forms the outlet or aortopulmonary septum [3]. Failure of complete ventricular septation is the most common form of CHD [10].

Cardiac Outflow Tract Formation and Innervation

In addition to the primary and secondary heart fields, and the proepicardium, a fourth set of cells, the cardiac neural crest cells (CNCs), contribute to outflow tract septation and parasympathetic innervation of the developing heart [5]. This population of cells is formed in the dorsal neural tube between the otic placode and third somite. These CNCS have a unique identity and molecular signature [4, 11]. Neural crest cells migrate from the neural tube, through the branchial arches and second heart field, and into the cardiac outflow tract, where they help form the spiral septum that separates the aorta and pulmonary artery. CNCs also migrate to the venous pole of the heart, where they help in the formation of the anterior parasympathetic plexis, which provides cardiac innervation [12].

Formation of the Valves and Conduction System

Formation of the semilunar and atrioventricular valves occurs following septation and is complete by week 10 of gestation [13]. The cardiac valves originate from the endocardial cushions at the atrioventricular canal and outflow tract. The valve leaflets are connective tissue covered with endocardium that elongates and becomes thin and fibrous during cardiac development and maturation [14]. Cardiac valves have increased cellular proliferation during development but become relatively quiescent in adulthood [14]. Initial cardiac impulses are generated by the ventricular myocardium [13, 15]. Formation of the specialized conduction system from myocardial cells is marked by the development of the sinus and atrioventricular node during the fifth week of gestation [4, 13, 15]. This is followed by the development of the His–Purkinje system during chamber formation and septation [15, 16]. Subsequent development of insulating nonconductive tissue between the atria and ventricles, likely derived at least partially from the proepicardium, reduces the risk of rapid ventricular response [16].

Fetal Growth and Cardiac Maturation

The embryonic heart is fully formed and functional before the end of the first trimester of pregnancy. However, the fetal heart continues to grow and mature, and the neonatal heart undergoes significant changes in sarcomere composition, metabolism, and growth following birth [5]. Mechanisms of cardiac growth in utero and during the neonatal period occur secondary to cellular proliferation. Cardiac growth in the adolescent human heart occurs primarily by cell hypertrophy, however recent studies using [14] C radiolabeling suggest continued cardiomyocyte self-renewal from birth to age 50, with replacement of up to half of human cardiomyocytes [17]. These studies support the notion of persistent, although limited cardiomyocyte turnover in the human heart. Along with genetic labeling studies performed in nonhuman model systems [18], these studies provide evidence that the pathways that promote cardiomyocyte proliferation are intact in the mature heart, and suggest that they may be harnessed to enhance the endogenous repair process in response to myocardial injury.

Mouse Models of Cardiogenesis

Although many of the processes in vertebrate heart development are highly conserved, adaptations during evolution have occurred, leading to variability in the final form and function of the vertebrate heart. Cardiac development in mammalian model systems closely resembles human cardiac development and provides a rationale for the use of genetic mouse models to study cardiogenesis (Fig. 2.1).

The basic stages of cardiac development outlined for the human heart are condensed into the 21-day gestational period of the mouse. Common developmental stages conserved in mice include the specification of mesodermal cells formed dur-

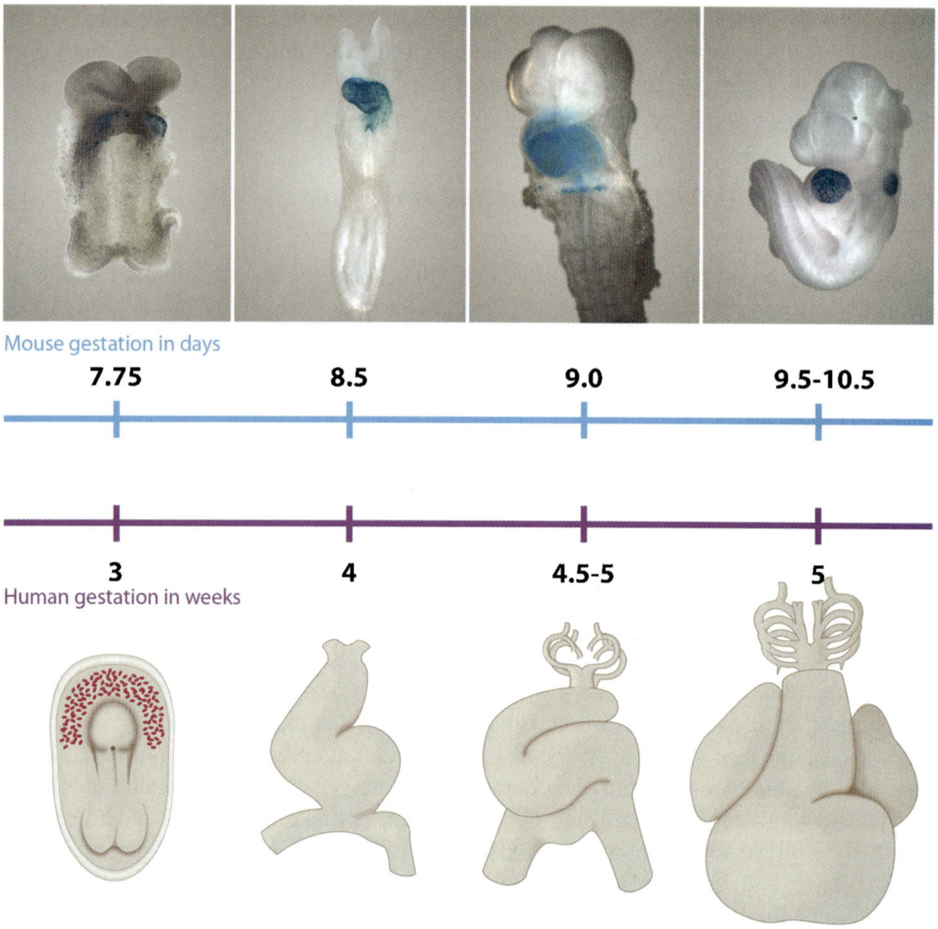

Fig. 2.1 Comparative timeline for mouse and human cardiogenesis during development. *Top*, mouse embryos at the postconception day (E) noted on the timeline. Mouse cardiac structures are marked by *LacZ* expression driven by a 6-kb cardiac enhancer region for *Nkx 2-5*. From *left* to *right*, cardiac crescent stage (E7.75), early looping heart stage (E8.5), looping and proepicardial development stage (E9.0), and late looping/early septation stage (E10.5). Septation is complete by day E14.5. Mouse gestation is 21 days. *Bottom*, graphic representations of human cardiac development at the corresponding stages. The human timeline is in weeks postconception during the 40-week human gestational period

ing gastrulation to a cardiac fate from days 6.75–7.75 postconception (E6.75–E7.75) [19, 20], formation of the symmetric cardiac crescent at E7.75, fusion to form the straight heart tube at E8.25, the onset of cardiac looping at E8.5, septal formation at E10.5, and remodeling of the cardiac outflow tract by E12.5 [20].

Tissues outside the primary heart field contribute to heart formation in mice, as in humans. The secondary heart field forms in the pharyngeal mesoderm and contributes cells to the outflow tract during looping. Neural crest cells migrate through the branchial arches and pharyngeal mesenchyme to help form the outflow tract cushions, outflow septum, and parasympathetic innervation of the heart. Furthermore, cells of the proepicardium migrate through the dorsal mesocardium over the heart to form the epicardium and coronary arteries.

Transgenic Mouse Models

The mouse model system has become the standard for studying the genetic control of cardiogenesis [21, 22]. DNA manipulation in the mouse can lead to stable overexpression of a gene, complete loss of a gene product (protein) or a "knockout," or a conditional loss of gene expression that allows temporal or spatial analysis of gene function (Fig. 2.2). Modification of gene expression in the mouse is performed using techniques of molecular cloning to identify, isolate, and manipulate DNA sequence into a construct that can be injected into a single cell.

Transgenesis can be obtained by injection of DNA into the pronucleus of a fertilized oocyte, followed by implantation of the oocyte into a female mouse to gestate [23, 24]. This method relies on random integration of the DNA into the genome, generating overexpression of the gene product throughout the mouse embryo. Alternatively, a targeted gene construct can be engineered and electroporated into embryonic stem cells. This construct is designed to have affinity for recombination events at the gene locus where homologous recombination is desired [25].

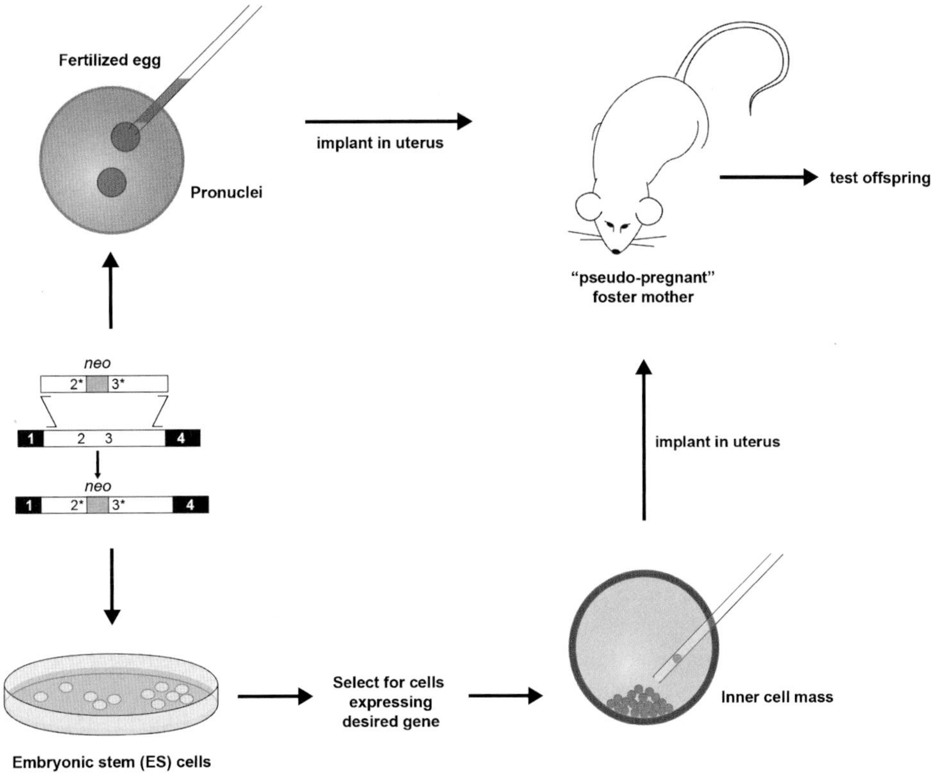

Fig. 2.2 Schematic for the generation of transgenic mice. A construct with a reporter and the gene of interest is engineered and either injected into the pronucleus of a one-cell embryo or an ES cell which is then selected for gene expression and cultured to form an embryonic blastocyst. The injected one-cell embryo or the inner cell mass from the transformed, cultured ES cells are transplanted into a pseudo-pregnant host female. After delivery, the newborn mice are genotyped. Mice that are heterozygous for the gene construct are mated, and the offspring are genotyped

Embryonic stem cells that have undergone homologous recombination are selected using antibiotic resistance or construct-mediated cell death (via thymidine kinase or sensitivity to diphtheria toxin), and the surviving embryonic stem cells are used to reconstitute an embryo that is implanted into a female mouse [26]. Mice with germline mutations are selected by breeding and mated with heterozygotes to give a complete "knockout" of gene function in 25% of the offspring. Genes inserted with promoters and no regulatory elements will be ubiquitously expressed or knocked out in the embryo, which can lead to severe early phenotypes that may preclude the definition of the functional role of the gene in the heart.

An alternative to global gene knockouts is the engineering of conditional mutants in the mouse. Conditional mutants are generated by placing the gene construct under the control of a tissue-specific or stage-specific promoter to drive expression. This strategy enables the functional role of genes to be defined during development and is invaluable if the early loss of these genes is lethal to the embryo [27]. Further regulation of cell- or tissue-specific gene activation or excision is performed using the Cre–lox system. This system utilizes phage Cre recombinase driven by a spatially or temporally restricted promoter to efficiently excise a gene inserted between two *loxP* sites. Further spatial control of this system is possible by adding an inducible promoter of expression upstream of the Cre recombinase, using a mutant estrogen receptor or a tetracycline-sensitive system. Loss of gene function can be temporally controlled in these transgenic mice by administration of tamoxifen or doxycycline [27].

Use of Mouse Embryonic Stem Cells to Study Cardiac Development

Mouse embryonic stem cells (ES cells) are derived from the inner cell mass of the preimplantation embryo. These cells have the ability to self-renew, have an unlimited proliferative capacity, and are pluripotent or able to "daughter" all cell lineages [28]. ES cells can undergo genetic manipulation as described for transgenic mice, including the integration of constructs to generate conditional or inducible gene expression. Wild-type ES cells differentiate into cardiomyocytes in vitro, and this process can be altered by gene manipulation, making the ES cell system a powerful tool for studying the genetic control of cardiac differentiation and myocyte formation [28]. In vitro differentiation of ES cells into cardiomyocytes requires formation of cellular aggregates or embryoid bodies (EBs) [28–30]. Gene expression patterns in EBs recapitulate those observed early during cardiac differentiation.

Following aggregation (day 4 of differentiation), beating cardiomyocytes can be identified between a basal layer of mesenchyme and epithelial cells. Wild-type and genetically manipulated ES cells can be assayed for gene expression patterns, single-cell electrophysiology and mechanical characteristics, and protein expression patterns to further examine the regulation of myocyte development and maturation.

Molecular Regulation of Cardiac Development

The ability to genetically manipulate mouse cardiac development in vivo has enhanced our understanding of the molecular regulation of cardiac development and differentiation. The information obtained in the mouse model system has been augmented by studies in other vertebrate and invertebrate model systems. Human genetic studies have confirmed a role for many of these genes in the etiology of CHD [31–33].

Specification of the Cardiac Mesoderm and Heart Tube Formation

The presumptive cardiac mesoderm requires expression of the helix–loop–helix transcription factors *Mesp1* and *Mesp2* to migrate to its anterior-lateral position in the embryo [34] (Fig. 2.3). Specification of early mesoderm to a cardiac cell fate occurs following migration and is regulated by inductive signals, including *BMP2*, *FGF8*, *Shh*, and *Wnt11*, from the embryonic endoderm [1, 35]. Simultaneously, signals from the midline neuroectoderm, including *Chordin*, *Noggin*, and the canonical *Wnts 1/3/8*, inhibit cardiac specification in the embryonic midline [1, 35, 36].

Cell labeling studies at the cardiac crescent stage in mice (E7.75) suggest that the anterior–posterior patterning of the primary heart field is defined by this stage, with cells in the anterior crescent mapping to the ventricles and those in the posterior crescent destined to be inflow or atrial cells in the forming heart tube [1, 37, 38]. At the crescent stage, the first cardiac-specific transcription factor, *Nkx2-5*, is expressed in the primary heart field [20, 21, 39]. *Nkx2-5* is a homologue of the *Drosophila tinman* gene, and loss of *tinman* is associated with a complete absence of cardiac structures [40]. In contrast, disruption of *Nkx2-5* expression in mice results in early heart tube formation, followed by failure of cardiac looping and embryonic death [41]. *Nkx2-5* mutations in humans are associated with conduction system abnormalities and structural heart disease, including atrial septal defect (ASD), ventricular septal defect (VSD), and tetralogy of Fallot (TOF) [31, 32], suggesting functional redundancy for this key cardiac transcriptional regulator in vertebrate evolution.

A regulatory network of transcription factors is present at the crescent stage (*Nkx2-5*, *Tbx5*, *Tbx20*, and *Gata4*) and is required for normal cardiac development [1, 35, 36]. Persistent expression of *Nkx2-5* and *Gata4* is necessary for normal formation and differentiation of the straight heart tube. Absence of *Gata4* in a mouse embryo results in cardiac bifida or failure of fusion of the bilateral heart tubes [42, 43]. *Nkx2-5* has a regulatory role during heart tube formation and is important for the differentiation of both myocardial and *ER71*-derived endocardial lineages [39] (Fig. 2.3).

During formation of the heart tube, a second heart field composed of pharyngeal mesenchyme is formed and expresses the master regulatory genes *Tbx5*, *Nkx2-5*, and *Gata4*, along with second heart field–specific genes, which include *Isl-1*, *Tbx1*, *FGF10*, and *Wnt5a* [1, 44–47]. The cells of the second heart field differentiate into myocardium and are required for normal looping, right ventricular formation, and septation of the cardiac outflow tract [1, 35, 48]. *Tbx1* expression in the second heart field requires sonic hedgehog (*Shh*) signaling [49] and is required for normal myocardial differentiation in the outflow tract [35, 46]. The *Tbx1* gene is on the 22q11 region of the human genome, and deletion of this region is responsible for the high incidence of cardiac outflow tract defects in DiGeorge syndrome [35, 46].

Cardiac Looping

The linear heart tube becomes asymmetric by E8.5, marked by a highly conserved rightward and cranial looping pattern that brings the atria posterior to the outflow tract. The process of looping requires the normal establishment and signaling of left–right asymmetry. In the mouse, the earliest demonstrated asymmetry is clockwise rotation of cilia in the embryonic node [50, 51]. This cilial motion is associated with asymmetric calcium signaling and results in activation of a left-sided signaling cascade in the lateral plate mesoderm that is highly conserved across species [50]. Conserved left-sided signaling molecules include *Nodal*, *Cripto*, and *Lefty* [52].

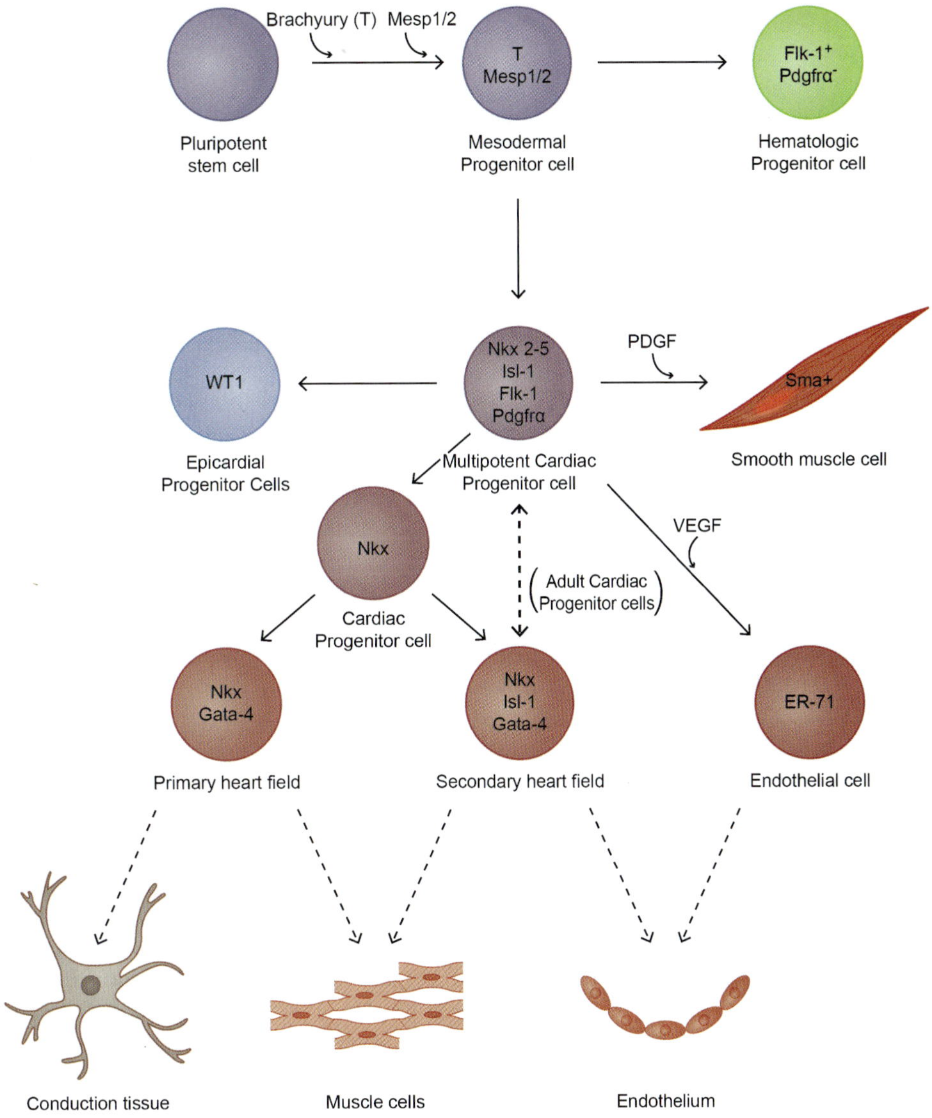

Fig. 2.3 Differentiation of mesodermal progenitor cells and multipotent cardiac progenitor cells (MCPCs) from pluripotent stem cells requires the expression of the *Brachyury (T)*, *Mesp1*, and *Mesp2* genes. Precursor cells can be differentiated by the markers Flk-1$^+$ and Pdgfr$^-$. Cardiac precursor cells are positive for both of these markers, while hematologic progenitor cells are only positive for Flk-1$^+$. MCPCs can differentiate into smooth muscle, epicardial cells, endothelial cells, cardiac muscle, or cardiac conduction tissue with the appropriate environment and molecular cues

The first reported molecular asymmetry in the heart is the left-sided expression of the transcription factor, *Pitx2*, which is required for normal heart morphogenesis [53, 54]. *Pitx2* induces cellular proliferation through the regulation of Cyclin-D2 [55] but does not drive looping morphogenesis independently [1]. Recent data suggest that molecular asymmetry begins much earlier than looping stages in the heart and may be governed by *Nkx2-5*.

Chamber Formation and Septation

Studies of transcriptional control of chamber formation have led to an understanding of a hierarchy of transcription factors that regulate cardiac differentiation. *Mef2C* expression is dependent on *Nkx2-5* and is required for normal looping morphogenesis and right ventricular formation [56]. In *Mef2c* mutants, downstream expression of *Hand2* and the cardiac muscle markers *ANF* and *myosin light chain 1A* is disrupted [56].

The hand genes, *Hand1* and *Hand2*, are further downstream in the regulatory cascade [57]. Both *Hand1* and *Hand2* are expressed in the primary and secondary heart fields; however, *Hand1* is required primarily for left ventricular formation and *Hand2* for right ventricular formation [35, 57, 58]. Overexpression of the *Hand* genes has also been shown to result in congenital heart defects, including lack of septation (VSD) and disorganization of the myocardial architecture, confirming their role in regulating cardiogenesis [59, 60].

Tbx5 is expressed in the early heart fields and persists during chamber formation and septation. *Tbx5* insufficiency and haploinsufficiency are associated with a decreased expression of *ANF* and *connexin 40* [61]. Mutations in *Tbx5* cause Holt–Oram syndrome, which is characterized by septal defects and limb defects [33, 61]. Both *Tbx5* and *Gata4* have been shown to interact with *Baf60c*, a chromatin-remodeling complex, to direct ectopic cardiomyocyte formation in mouse embryos [62]. This ability may have interesting implications for these genes in promoting cardiac regeneration. Lastly, microRNAs, small RNA molecules that regulate the translation of proteins from mRNA, have been implicated in the "fine-tuning" of the regulatory transcriptional networks involved in cardiogenesis [35, 63, 64].

Cardiac Outflow Formation

Failure of cardiac outflow tract septation accounts for about 30% of all CHD [65]. Normal cardiac outflow tract septation requires maturation and migration of the second heart field onto the outflow tract. This process is regulated by global cardiac transcription factors including *Nkx2-5*, *Gata4*, and transcription factors specific to the second heart field, including *Isl*, *Tbx1*, and *Wnt5a*. Mouse models lacking any one of these three second heart field–specific genes are associated with outflow tract defects, including subarterial VSD, TOF, and truncus arteriosus.

Normal outflow tract septation also requires the formation and migration of CNCs into the outflow tract and endocardial cushions. Neural crest cells are induced by multiple signaling pathways, including Wnt, BMP, FGF, and Notch pathways, which converge at the border of neural and non-neural ectoderm [66]. Neural crest cells are induced to form in the neural folds and migrate through the pharyngeal arches to the cardiac outflow tract. Absence of *Wnt5a* in the second heart field reduces the number of neural crest cells populating the outflow tract and results in a high incidence of failure of septation, causing persistent truncus arteriosus [47].

Formation of the Epicardium and Coronary Arteries

The proepicardium is another migratory cell population required for normal cardiac formation. The proepicardium is derived from cardiac progenitor cells that initially express *Nkx2-5* and *Isl-1* and does not form in the absence of *Gata4* [67, 68]. These cells are located near the sinus venosus, and once they begin to differentiate, they express the markers *Wilms tumor 1* (*WT1*) and *Tbx18*. As these cells mature, they migrate over the surface of the heart. Their fate is determined by the balance of other signaling pathways, including fibroblast growth factors (FGFs) and bone morphogenetic proteins (BMPs). Ultimately, they give rise to the epicardium and all cell layers of the coronary arteries, and a small number may transform into myocardial cells, making them of potential use in cardiac regeneration [7, 8, 67, 68].

Stem Cell Biology and Cardiac Repair

Intense interest has focused on the genesis of the cardiomyocyte as a means to uncover new therapies for both congenital and acquired heart disease. Multipotent cardiac progenitor cells (MCPCs) have been observed to daughter all cardiac cell lineages and have been isolated from EBs, embryos, neonatal hearts, and adult mouse hearts [69–72]. These cells are mesodermal in origin and express *Isl-1*, *Flk-1*, and *Nkx2-5*. Under appropriate conditions, they can differentiate into cardiomyocytes, vascular smooth muscle cells, and endocardial cells.

By staining sections for *Isl-1*, a population of MCPCs has been found in human fetal hearts at 11 and 18 weeks gestation [45]. These cells express markers of cardiomyocyte, smooth muscle, and endothelial lineages. Using genetic lineage labeling techniques in combination with EB formation, these human cells were shown to express markers of late cardiogenesis in a pattern that reflects known molecular regulation of cardiac development, including differentiation into an epicardial lineage [45]. These progenitor cells populate the right ventricle of human fetuses well into midgestation and postnatal development. However, their role in the causation or potential for therapy of heart disease remains unclear.

Alternative sources of progenitor cells include small populations of cells isolated from the adult heart that may have stem cell properties. These include cKit+/Lin− cells isolated from the adult mouse heart [73]. These cells give rise to cardiomyocytes, smooth muscle cells, and endothelial cells when cultured in vitro and form cardiospheres when expanded [74]. Clonal cKit+ expressing cells have been established and shown to daughter all lineages of the heart and undergo self-renewal (characteristics of stem cell populations). Interestingly, these cells improve myocardial function after an acute ischemic event [72].

Another population of stem cells that reside in the adult heart includes side population (SP) cells. These cells are rare and express a multidrug resistance protein that effluxes Hoechst 33342 dye. Using FACS analysis, the SP cells can be isolated and show increased proliferation and plasticity. Molecular techniques have further shown that oxidative stress present during myocardial injury increases Hif2a, which directly transactivates Abcg2. Increased Abcg2 serves a cytoprotective role and promotes survival of the cardiac SP cell population. This is the first example of a stem cell marker (Abcg2) that has a functional role in cellular survival [75].

Additional stem or progenitor cells being evaluated for myocardial regeneration include those expressing Sca1 and SSEA1, and mesenchymal stem cells (MSCs), skeletal myoblasts, bone marrow mononuclear cells, CD34+ cells, endothelial progenitors, and others, including small molecule cofactors [35, 76–79].

Current trials of stem cell therapy for heart repair utilize stem cells derived from the bone marrow, heart, and skeletal muscle, most often harvested from the patient receiving therapy (autologous cell therapy). While a number of phase I and II trials are underway, results to date support the safety of cell therapy for ischemic cardiomyopathy. Moreover, these initial studies support the notion that cell therapy may promote reverse remodeling (via vascular neogenesis or antiapoptosis mechanisms) to a greater extent than cardiomyocyte regeneration. Future trials aimed at delivery route, time of delivery (following myocardial injury), cellular population, number of cells delivered, and other parameters will need definition for this new field.

Cardiac progenitor cells have been derived from ES cells as well as induced pluripotent stem cells [78, 80]. ES cells with a GFP reporter targeted to the *Brachyury* (*Bry*) gene have been used to isolate Flk-1+/Bry-GFP+ cells that can give rise to cells of two distinct lineages, one hematopoietic and endothelial, and one cardiac. The ability to isolate cardiac stem cells from ES cells is promising, as these cells can be genetically engineered for isolation, proliferation, or therapeutic purposes. Unfortunately, initial trials with murine ES cells resulted in teratomas, and there are concerns about uncontrolled cell proliferation of incompletely differentiated cell types [81].

Recent studies with nonhuman, primate ES cells have been more hopeful. These progenitor cells were isolated prior to expression of *Isl-1* and differentiated into cardiomyocytes, smooth muscle cells, and endothelial cells. When transplanted into infarcted myocardium of nonhuman primates, the SSEA-1+ cells differentiated into ventricular myocytes, reconstituted 20% of the scar tissue, and did not form teratomas [81]. These studies suggest that, with more refinement, ES cells, iPS cells, MCPCs, and adult stem cells may provide options for aggressive cell therapy treatments of acquired heart disease.

Congenital Heart Disease

Incidence and Genetics

Incidence

Based on large population studies performed in the late twentieth century, CHD has an incidence of approximately 4–8/1,000 live births [10, 82, 83]. Study design can significantly affect incidence estimates, and if reporting is based on incidence of severe abnormalities requiring referral to a pediatric cardiac center, the number is reduced to only 4–5/1,000 live births. In contrast, if vigorous surveillance is performed by echocardiography in a broader age range, and if bicuspid aortic valve and silent patent ductus arteriosus are included, incidence figures can reach 12–14/1,000 [10].

Unlike some types of birth defects (e.g., neural tube defects), CHD is increasing in incidence and prevalence [83, 84], likely due to improved early detection and increased survival of CHD patients to reproductive age, increasing the risk of CHD in offspring. The outcome of many forms of CHD surgical repair is greater than 90% survival; however, survivors of complex CHD and its palliation or CHD in the setting of prematurity, genetic syndromes, or other illnesses often have an increased risk of mortality, chronic illness, or disability.

Genetics of CHD

Although the majority of CHD occurs in an otherwise healthy children, at least 25% of patients with CHD have extracardiac malformations, and 10–15% have chromosomal anomalies identifiable by karyotypic or fluorescent in situ hybridization

(FISH) analyses [85–87]. These patients are at increased risk for poor perioperative outcomes, increased need for reoperation, and long-term complications. Infants with trisomy 21 (Down syndrome) account for a large proportion of these patients and have a 40–50% risk of CHD that most commonly includes VSD or atrioventricular canal (AVC) defect, although cyanotic CHD including TOF does occur in this patient population.

Other genetic syndromes associated with a high incidence of CHD include DiGeorge syndrome (22q11 deletion syndrome), which occurs in approximately 1:4,000–1:7,000 live births [86, 88]. Up to 75–80% of patients with DiGeorge syndrome have cardiac or vascular anomalies [88]. These patients often come to medical attention in infancy because of CHD, and infants who present with classical conotruncal or outflow tract lesions, TOF, PTA, interrupted aortic arch (IAA); or CHD and other features of DiGeorge syndrome, including hypocalcemia, athymia, craniofacial abnormalities, or unusual facial features – should be screened by FISH or comparative genomic hybridization (CGH).

Other common syndromes associated with CHD at a slightly lower frequency include Noonan syndrome (characterized by septal defects, pulmonary valve dysplasia, and cardiomyopathy); Turner syndrome (XO chromosomal defect, coarctation, bicuspid aortic valve hyper tension and progressive aortic root dilation); and William's syndrome (septal defects, supravalvar aortic stenosis, and multiple arterial obstructive lesions, including pulmonary and coronary artery obstruction due to an elastin deficiency) [86]. In general, infants who present with a form of CHD classically associated with a genetic syndrome or infants who present with multiple congenital anomalies should undergo genetic evaluation.

Heredity and CHD

Isolated CHD frequently has complex multifactorial inheritance that complicates the prediction of recurrence risk. While some forms of isolated CHD are associated with single-gene defects (*Nkx2-5* and septal defects; *Notch1* and aortic valve disease) and have classical, single-gene inheritance patterns, single-gene testing in isolated CHD is rarely performed outside of the research setting. In the absence of an identified genetic cause of isolated CHD, recurrence risk is most often calculated based on population studies of all CHD grouped together and on individual family pedigree [89]. In general, the risk of CHD in the population is approximately 1% of all live births. Identification of a single, first-degree relative with CHD increases the risk for CHD in a subsequent pregnancy to approximately 3% [89]. Large, population-based studies suggest that this risk is higher if there is an affected mother rather than an affected father [89, 90]. If two first-degree relatives are affected in a family, the risk of CHD in a subsequent pregnancy increases further [90–92]. In the last decade, studies on the recurrence risk of single categories of CHD have provided information that may improve counseling for families affected by CHD [91].

Reported recurrence risks for nonsyndromic TOF have been reported to range from 3–50%, suggesting that transmission can be multifactorial, autosomal recessive, or autosomal dominant, depending on the etiology [92]. Families with a child who has hypoplastic left heart syndrome (HLHS) face an approximately 5% recurrence risk for HLHS, but the risk of any left-sided obstructive lesion, including bicuspid aortic valve, is significantly increased and has been reported to be as high as 30% [93, 94]. Given the lack of identified genetic markers for CHD risk in most of these families, prenatal echocardiographic screening (fetal echo) can be offered in the second trimester of pregnancies when there is a family history of CHD.

Congenital Heart Defects

Septal Defects/Left-to-Right Shunt Lesions

Septal defects and patent ductus arteriosus are the most common forms of CHD, with isolated VSDs affecting 2–5% of newborns [10]. The majority of isolated VSDs will close spontaneously or not require intervention [10]. VSDs can occur in the muscular septum, the membranous septum, the infundibulum (subarterial defects), or the inlet septum below the tricuspid valve. Muscular VSDs often close spontaneously while membranous VSDs can be occluded by tricuspid valve tissue. Infundibular and inlet VSDs are unlikely to close spontaneously and usually require surgical repair. Infants and children with small VSDs will present with an asymptomatic murmur, while larger VSDs can cause cardiac enlargement, congestive heart failure due to a left-to-right shunt, and, if left untreated, irreversible pulmonary hypertension. Infants with a large VSD typically present with tachypnea, poor feeding, and failure to thrive due to pulmonary overcirculation, and pallor, diaphoresis, and sinus tachycardia due to activation of the sympathetic nervous system related to decreased systemic output resulting from a large left-to-right shunt.

Surgical repair of VSDs has become a routine procedure since the closure of the first VSD using controlled cross-circulation at the University of Minnesota by C. Walton Lillehei, MD, PhD, and colleagues in 1954 [95], and the introduction of a right atrial approach to membranous VSD closure by Lillehei in 1957 [96]. Current surgical outcomes are excellent if the VSD is closed before irreversible pulmonary vascular changes occur. Closure of a membranous VSD is often associated with asymptomatic, nonprogressive right bundle branch block.

Complications after isolated VSD closure include permanent, complete heart block due to disruption of the conduction system below the atrioventricular node during repair [97] and residual VSD. A residual VSD does incur an increased risk of endocarditis over the patient's lifetime. Ventricular dysfunction and arrhythmias are rare postoperative complications. Overall life expectancy in patients with isolated VSD after early closure is approaching norms for the population [98].

Approximately half of patients who undergo operative closure of VSDs have additional cardiac defects, most commonly PDA, ASD, coarctation of the aorta, aortic valve disease, or right ventricular muscle bundles. Infundibular (subarterial) or membranous VSDs are often observed in complex or cyanotic lesions. These patients have increased operative risk and an increased incidence of postoperative complications.

Transcatheter approaches to VSD closure have been developed over the last decade. Muscular VSDs can be routinely closed by transcatheter or perventricular placement of a self-expanding device without bypass (Fig. 2.4e–h). Devices have been developed and tested for transcatheter closure of membranous VSDs; however, they are currently unavailable in the United States due to a concern about the development of late heart block [99, 100].

ASDs are less likely to be symptomatic in infancy and early childhood and may be diagnosed later in life based on the presence of a pulmonary flow murmur, a widely split and fixed second heart sound, or right ventricular enlargement. Late presentations include atrial arrhythmias or pulmonary vascular disease, which generally present after the third or fourth decade of life. ASDs can be readily closed surgically with very low mortality rates. Secundum defects of any size with adequate septal rims can be closed by a variety of catheter implantable devices safely and effectively (Fig. 2.4a–d).

The ductus arteriosus is a fetal structure that shunts blood from the pulmonary artery to the descending thoracic aorta in utero, limiting circulation to the uninflated lungs and high-resistance pulmonary vascular bed before birth. After birth, the pulmonary vascular resistance drops precipitously, and ductal shunting reverses, resulting in a transient left-to-right shunt in most infants. Spontaneous ductal closure usually occurs within the first 72 h of life but can be delayed in premature infants and infants living at high altitude, suggesting a role for ambient oxygen in ductal closure. Persistence of a patent ductus arteriosus can lead to pulmonary overcirculation, left-sided cardiac enlargement, and pulmonary hypertension, if untreated. Surgical treatment, often at the bedside in the neonatal intensive care unit, is the norm in premature infants who fail medical therapy with indocin or ibuprofen. Transcatheter options, including occluder devices and implantable coils, are safe and effective in older infants, children, and adults with normal pulmonary vascular resistance [101].

Semilunar Valve Stenosis and Coarctation of the Aorta

Isolated pulmonary valve stenosis accounts for about 6% of all CHD and can range from mild and asymptomatic to critical in the newborn period [83]. Most forms of pulmonary stenosis are characterized by thin but fused valve leaflets and are amenable to balloon dilation in the newborn, child, and adolescent. Severe valvular stenosis or atresia in the newborn, or "critical" pulmonary stenosis, is life-threatening, but stabilization of the ductus arteriosus with prostaglandin E1 (PGE1) allows resuscitation of the infant and elective catheter therapy. A small subset of patients have thickened, dysplastic pulmonary valve leaflets and require surgical valvulotomy. Both catheter balloon and surgical valvulotomy can be complicated by pulmonary insufficiency, which is well tolerated in most patients. Severe pulmonary insufficiency associated with decreased exercise tolerance or significant right ventricular enlargement is an indication for placement of a valved homograft or bioprosthetic pulmonary valve to preserve right ventricular size and function [102].

Aortic valve stenosis is less common than pulmonary valve stenosis in newborns and is more likely to present later in life. Aortic stenosis is more common in males than females [103]. Severe aortic stenosis in the newborn may present with shock and left ventricular failure and require PGE1 to maintain ductal patency and allow augmentation of systemic blood flow by the right ventricle. Balloon valvulotomy is frequently the initial mode of intervention in infancy and childhood. Residual valve stenosis and mild insufficiency are common, and valve replacement in childhood with a valved homograft or pulmonary autograft (Ross procedure) may be required. Aortic stenosis and a bicuspid aortic valve can be associated with other structural heart disease including coarctation of the aorta.

Coarctation of the aorta occurs in less than 1 in 1,000 births and is found both in isolation and in association with bicuspid aortic valve, VSD, and complex congenital heart defects. Coarctation can present in infancy with shock and left ventricular

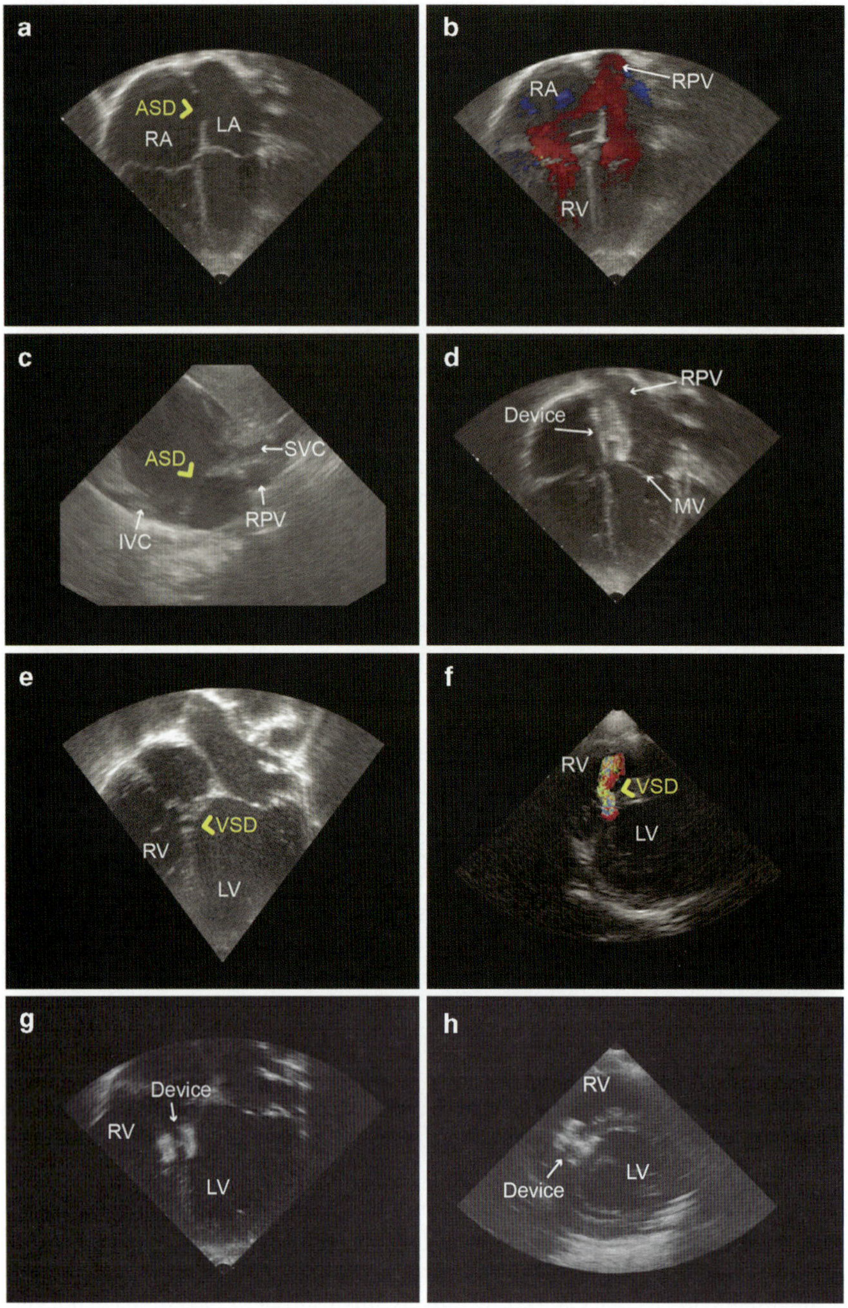

Fig. 2.4 Device closure of cardiac septal defects. Atrial septal defect (ASD) closure, (**a**) a moderate-sized secundum ASD (*yellow arrowhead*) with enlargement of the right atrium (RA) from an apical four-chamber view during preprocedure echocardiography. (**b**) Doppler color flow signal from the right pulmonary veins (RPVs) entering the left atrium and then flowing through the ASD to the enlarged RA and right ventricle (RV). (**c**) A high right parasternal view demonstrating the ASD and its relationship to the superior vena cava (SVC), inferior vena cava (IVC), and right pulmonary veins (RPVs), and the septal rims necessary for proper seating and stabilization of the device. (**d**) A postprocedure echocardiogram showing placement of an AMPLATZER® Atrial Septal Occluder device and its relationship to the RPV and mitral valve (MV). (**e–h**) A muscular ventricular septal defect (VSD) from an apical four-chamber view (**e**) (*yellow arrowhead*) with left ventricular (LV) enlargement and a short-axis view with color flow from LV to RV. (**f**) An AMPLATZER device has been placed across in the catheterization laboratory, as shown in (**g**) (four-chamber view) and (**h**) (short-axis view). "AMPLATZER" is a registered trademark of AGA Medical Corporation. EDITOR: product name from www.amplatzer.com/products/asd_devices/tabid/179/default.aspx. Trademark acknowledgement from: www.amplatzer.com/about_aga/terms_of_use/tabid/93/default.aspx

failure, or later in childhood, with hypertension. Surgical repair is usually accomplished using resection and end-to-end anastomosis of the descending thoracic aorta, although the subclavian flap repair technique has been widely used in the past. Late coarctation repair is associated with persistent hypertension, reduced survival, and morbidity due to heart failure and stroke [104]. Early repair in infancy is associated with improved blood pressure control later in life; however, there is an

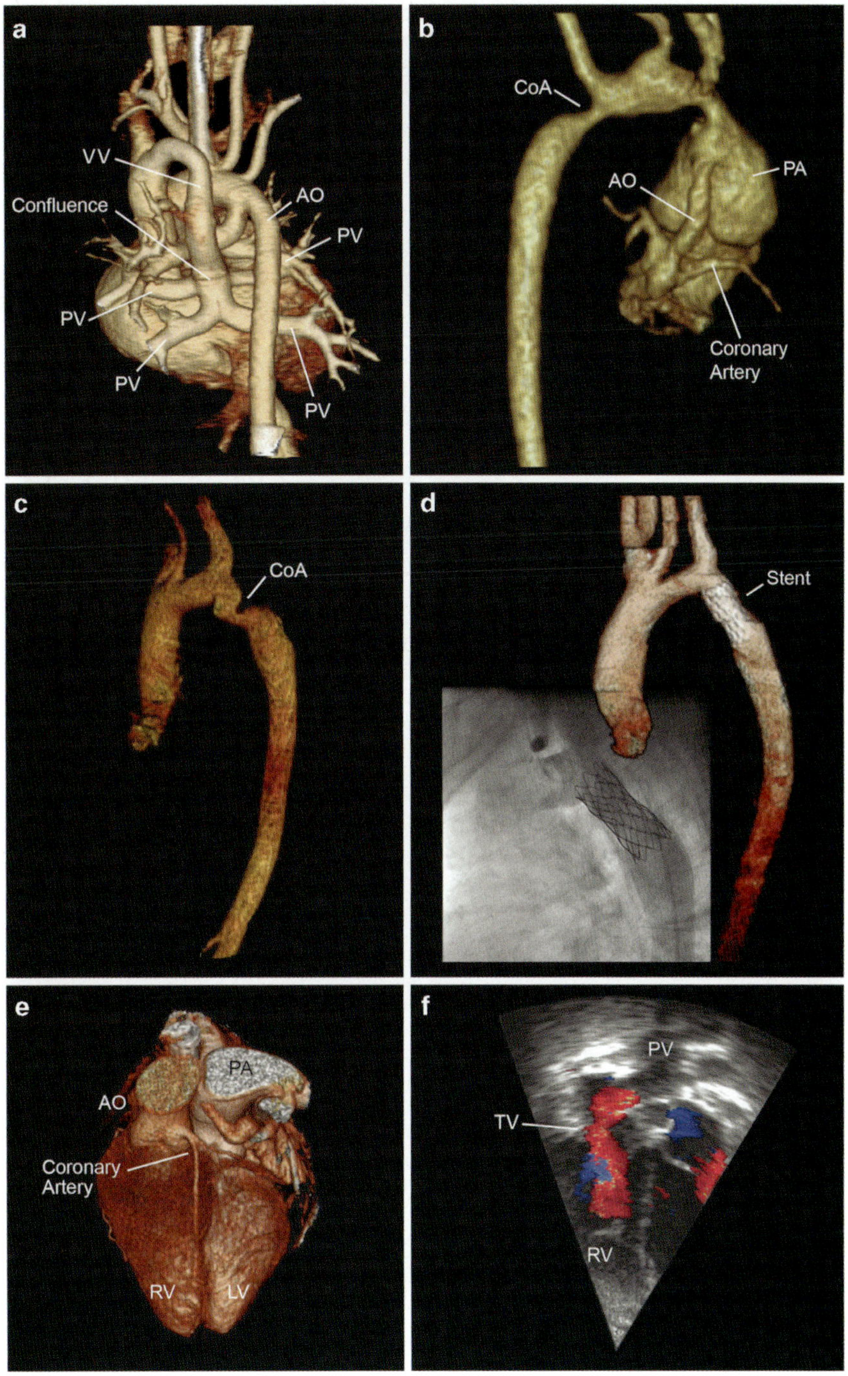

Fig. 2.5 Images of CHD. (**a**) Total anomalous pulmonary venous connection in an infant with heterotaxy syndrome and single ventricle physiology. The pulmonary veins (PVs) return to a posterior confluence and drain through a vertical vein (VV) into the superior vena cava (SVC). This is repaired by anastomosis of the confluence to the back wall of the left atrium and ligation of the vertical vein. (**b**) Hypoplastic left heart syndrome (HLHS) with hypoplastic aorta (AO) after anastomosis to pulmonary artery (PA). Note that coronary arteries (CAs) are supplied by the hypoplastic AO. There is coarctation of the aorta (CoA) distal to the left subclavian artery, also common in HLHS. (**c**, **d**) Coarctation of the aorta in an adult prior to repair (**c**) and during and after stenting (**d**). TGA after atrial baffle procedure. Note the coronary artery arising from the anterior aorta which receives oxygenated blood from the right ventricle. (**f**) An echocardiogram from the patient in (**e**), showing the baffling of pulmonary venous blood (PV) to the tricuspid valve (TV) and right ventricle (RV)

increased incidence of reoperation due to restenosis [103, 104]. Balloon dilation of native coarctation in infancy is not an effective long-term therapy; however, balloon angioplasty of recoarctation may be effective. A multicenter trial to evaluate the safety and efficacy of balloon angioplasty and stenting compared to surgery for native coarctation in older children and adolescents is currently underway (Fig. 2.5c, d).

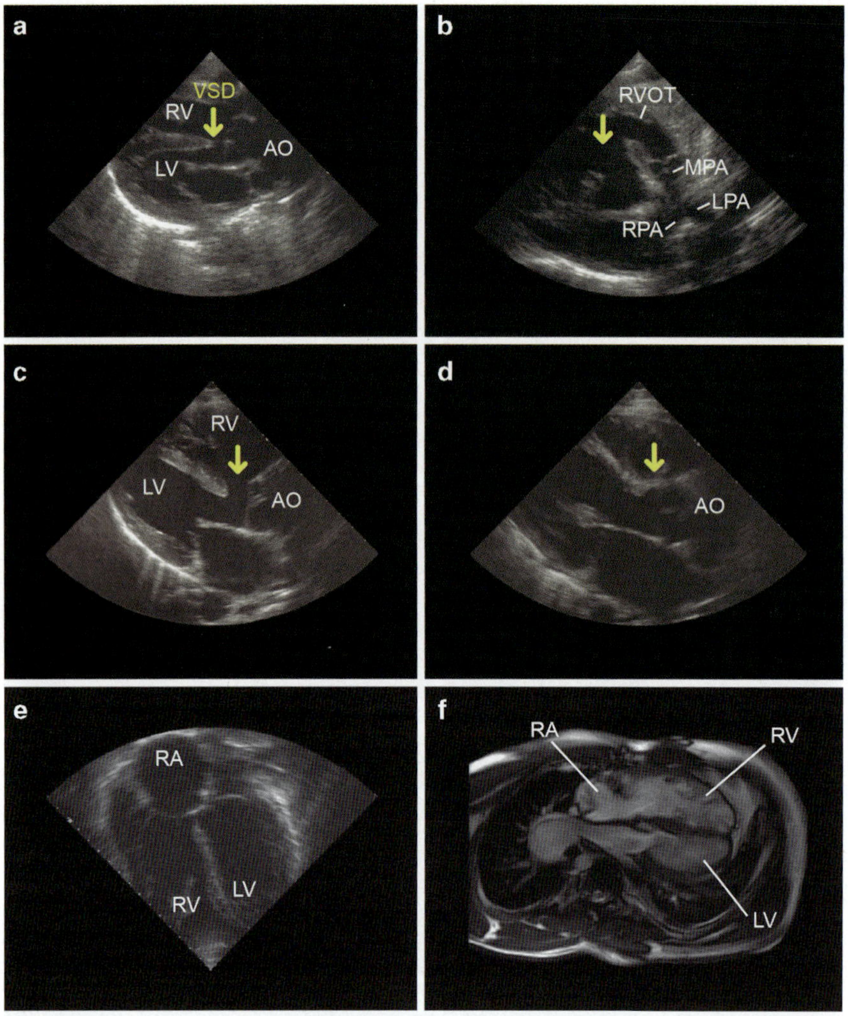

Fig. 2.6 Tetralogy of Fallot (TOF). (**a**) and (**b**) demonstrate the anatomy of TOF in an infant. (**a**) Parasternal long-axis view from a transthoracic echocardiogram that demonstrates the large subarterial VSD (*yellow arrow*) and overriding aorta (AO). The short-axis view in (**b**) demonstrates the subarterial VSD (*yellow arrow*) and the anterior displacement of the outflow tract septum with a narrowed right ventricular outflow tract (RVOT), pulmonary valve annulus, and main pulmonary artery (MPA). The right and left branch pulmonary arteries (RPAs, LPAs) are confluent and appropriately sized for an infant. (**c**) Intracardiac anatomy of TOF in an older child with the subarterial VSD (*yellow arrow*) and overriding AO, as well as enlargement and hypertrophy of the right ventricle (RV). (**d**) Same child after repair with a VSD patch (*yellow arrow*) and right ventricular outflow patch (not seen). (**e**) Right atrial and right ventricular enlargement in a teenager after TOF repair as an infant. Chronic RV volume overload due to pulmonary insufficiency after RV outflow patch causes RV enlargement (RV) and right atrial enlargement (RA) as well as flattening of the intraventricular septum. (**f**) An MRI in an adult patient with TOF after repair with chronic pulmonary insufficiency. It demonstrates significant RV enlargement and hypertrophy (RV) with an RV volume of 245 m/m^2 and right atrial enlargement (RA)

Cyanotic Lesions

The most common cyanotic congenital heart lesions are TOF and transposition of the great arteries. TOF was first described in detail in 1888 and first palliated surgically using a Blalock–Taussig shunt (subclavian artery to pulmonary artery anastomosis) in 1945. The four anatomic variations that comprise TOF are (1) a subarterial VSD; (2) overriding of the aorta above the ventricular septum due to septal malalignment; (3) right ventricular outflow tract obstruction at the subpulmonary, valvar, or supravalvar levels; and (4) right ventricular hypertrophy as a result of these lesions (Fig. 2.6).

At least 15% of TOF is associated with chromosomal abnormalities, most often DiGeorge syndrome (22q11 deletion). About 5% of TOF patients have coronary artery abnormalities. The first repair of TOF was performed at the University of Minnesota by C. Walton Lillehei, MD, PhD, and colleagues in 1954 [105]. Today, the best results are achieved with single-stage complete repair in infancy [106]. This usually involves VSD closure and placement of a right ventricular outflow tract patch that crosses the narrowed pulmonary valve annulus. Most patients require placement of a competent bioprosthetic

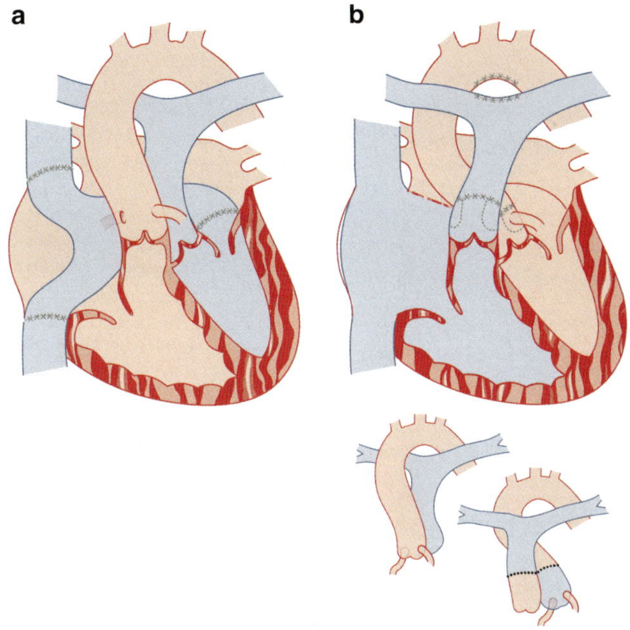

Fig. 2.7 Operative palliation or repair of transposition of the great arteries (TGA). (**a**) Graphic representation of an atrial baffle procedure. Variations include the Mustard and Senning procedures. In the uncorrected condition, the aorta is anterior to the pulmonary artery and receives deoxygenated blood from the right ventricle. To eliminate cyanosis, the systemic venous flow from the superior vena cava and inferior vena cava is baffled to the mitral valve. Pulmonary venous flow is directed around the baffle to the tricuspid valve. The right ventricle remains the systemic ventricle. (**b**) A graphic representation of the arterial switch procedure used more commonly now for repair of TGA. The pulmonary artery and aorta are transected, and the pulmonary artery is pulled forward (Lecompte maneuver) and anastomosed to the right ventricular outflow. The coronary arteries are excised from the anterior vessel with a button of tissue, mobilized, and reimplanted on the aorta posteriorly. Short- and long-term complications include stenosis at the vascular suture lines, branch pulmonary artery stenosis, coronary insufficiency, and ventricular dysfunction

pulmonary valve later in childhood, adolescence, or young adulthood to preserve right ventricular function [102, 107] (Fig. 2.6). Early survival in uncomplicated TOF is excellent, with a perioperative mortality of less than 3%. However, repair may be staged or delayed in challenging anatomic variants, and morbidity and mortality are increased.

In contrast to TOF, which is common in infants with genetic syndromes, transposition of the great arteries occurs most often in otherwise healthy newborns. It presents in the newborn nursery with profound cyanosis and comfortable tachypnea. Cardiomegaly develops rapidly as pulmonary vascular resistance drops, and acidosis can occur if intracardiac mixing is limited and oxygenation is poor.

TGA is most often an isolated defect, although it can occur with VSD, pulmonary stenosis, or complex single-ventricle defects. Stabilization of the infant with TGA includes volume resuscitation, PGE1 to rapidly improve mixing of oxygenated and deoxygenated blood at the ductus arteriosus, and, often, balloon atrial septostomy to further improve mixing and oxygenation. Historically, infants were stabilized and underwent an atrial baffle procedure (SVC and IVC baffled to mitral valve and subpulmonary left ventricle) (Figs. 2.5e, f and 2.7a) as older infants or toddlers.

Many of these patients are currently young adults, and their long-term well-being is compromised by atrial arrhythmias and failure of the systemic right ventricle requiring heart transplantation [108]. Development of the Lecompte maneuver to bring the pulmonary artery anterior to the aorta and the development of successful techniques for coronary artery transfer led to more successful use of the arterial switch procedure for repair of TGA. It has been routinely used for neonatal repair in straightforward TGA since the 1990s (Fig. 2.7b). Although early operative mortality of the arterial switch procedure is slightly higher than palliative procedures, the long-term outcome has been very good in the majority of postoperative survivors, but arterial stenosis, coronary insufficiency, ventricular dysfunction, and arrhythmias are potential long-term complications [109].

Single-Ventricle Conditions and Fontan Palliation

Hypoplastic left heart syndrome (HLHS) is defined as a diminutive left ventricle that is unable to support systemic output with underdevelopment or atresia of the mitral and aortic valves. It is most often associated with severe hypoplasia of the ascending aorta and narrowing of the transverse aortic arch. HLHS accounts for 1% of all CHD, is more common in male

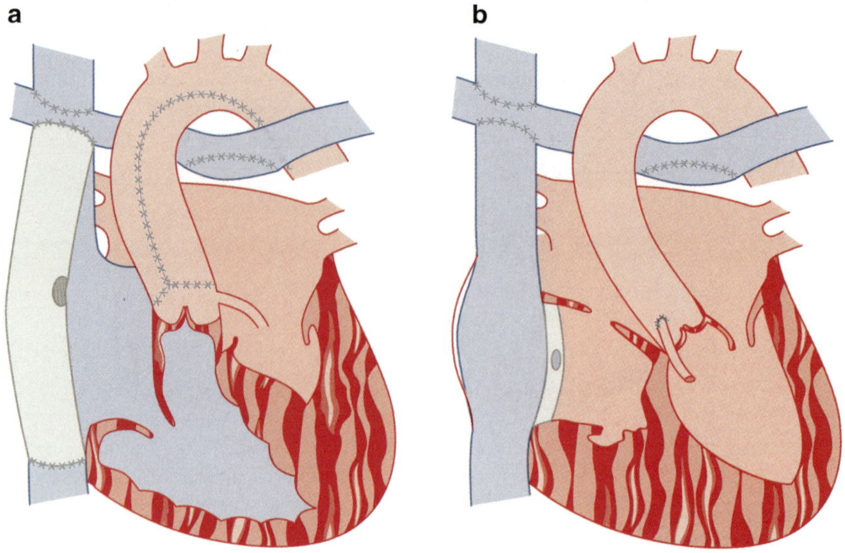

Fig. 2.8 Fontan palliation of single-ventricle physiology. The extracardiac Fontan procedure (**a**) and lateral tunnel Fontan procedure (**b**) are variations of the classic intracardiac Fontan operation that are in common use today. (**a**) Completion of an extracardiac Fontan procedure in a staged palliation of hypoplastic left heart syndrome with aortic atresia. In earlier operations for HLHS, the hypoplastic aorta was anastamosed to the pulmonary artery (Norwood procedure), and the superior vena cava was anastamosed to the right pulmonary artery (Glenn procedure). (**b**) A lateral tunnel Fontan procedure for tricuspid atresia and hypoplasia of the right ventricle. Both Fontan variations can be fenestrated to allow for communication between the venous circulation and the left atrium if pulmonary artery resistance is mildly elevated

infants (67%), and has been associated with genetic syndromes including trisomy 13 and 18, Turner syndrome (XO), and Jacobsen's syndrome, a rare chromosomal defect (11p deletion) [110, 111]. Infants with HLHS may present with pallor and tachypnea in the newborn nursery or be missed and present with complete cardiovascular collapse after closure of the ductus arteriosus, which is the only source of systemic blood flow. Stabilization of the ductus arteriosus with PGE1 is necessary for survival. Results of surgical palliation have improved since the mid-1990s, and although in most centers, the 5-year survival is 50–80%, in some centers, it approaches 95% [112].

After stabilization, infants born with HLHS typically undergo a Norwood procedure, which includes transection of the pulmonary artery and anastomosis of the proximal segment to the aorta, with a comprehensive aortic arch augmentation (Figs. 2.5b and 2.8a). Pulmonary blood flow is reestablished by an arterial to pulmonary artery shunt (modified Blalock–Taussig shunt) or a right ventricle to pulmonary artery shunt (Sano procedure) [113]. Early complications of the Norwood procedure include right ventricular failure, pulmonary venous obstruction, aortic coarctation, and pulmonary hypertension. Interstage mortality is highest between the Norwood procedure and the second stage of palliation, and there is a significant risk of cognitive disorders or global development delay in survivors.

Once the pulmonary vascular resistance has dropped and pulmonary artery pressures have normalized, a superior vena cava to pulmonary artery anastomosis (Glenn procedure) is performed to reduce the volume load on the right ventricle and provide stable pulmonary blood flow. The palliation is completed in early childhood by performing one of several variants of the Fontan operation (Fig. 2.5), which directs blood flow from the inferior vena cava to the pulmonary arteries with or without a small residual communication to the left atrium (fenestration). The Fontan procedure reduces the volume load on the single right ventricle and improves oxygenation, but results in reduced exercise tolerance. Long-term complications of palliation for HLHS include aortic arch obstruction, arrhythmias, protein-losing enteropathy, and ventricular failure.

An alternative procedure for the palliation of HLHS has been recently introduced [114]. In this "hybrid" procedure, the infant undergoes a median sternotomy in a combined operating room and catheterization laboratory or "hybrid" suite, followed by stenting of the ductus arteriosus and surgical placement of bilateral pulmonary artery bands. After recovery, a balloon atrial septostomy is performed. At age 4–6 months, a Norwood-like arch reconstruction and Glenn anastomosis are performed, and the Fontan is completed in early childhood as in the classic staged surgical palliation. Initial results suggest improved survival, especially for high-risk patients in the initial stages. There may also be improvement in neurodevelopmental outcomes; however, no long-term outcome data are available.

Many other forms of complex CHD require single ventricle palliation with the Fontan procedure. These conditions include tricuspid atresia, right ventricular hypoplasia, and heterotaxy syndromes. Tricuspid atresia has a similar strategy for palliation as HLHS, although the aorta is typically normal and, therefore, arch reconstruction is not required (Fig. 2.8b).

Long-term outcomes after Fontan are generally better for tricuspid atresia than for HLHS, likely because the single ventricle is of left ventricular morphology and adapted to support the systemic circulation. The heterotaxy syndromes are complex defects in left–right patterning of the developing organs that result in defects in every segment of heart formation from systemic and pulmonary venous inflow to the outflow tract (Fig. 2.5a). These patients often have conduction system anomalies, asplenia, intestinal malrotation, or pulmonary disease associated with severe CHD and have an increased incidence of mortality and perioperative and long-term complications despite single-ventricle palliation as described above.

Heart Transplantation and Bridging to Heart Transplantation in Children

About 7,500 pediatric heart transplants have been performed since the first successful transplant in 1984, and from 2007 to 2010, about 450 pediatric heart transplants were performed per year worldwide [115].

The indications for orthotopic cardiac transplantation in children include life-threatening, intractable heart failure and CHD not amenable to palliation; intractable, life-threatening arrhythmias not amenable to medical or device therapy; unresectable cardiac tumors; and retransplantation due to ventricular dysfunction or coronary vasculopathy [115]. Heart transplantation may also be an important therapeutic option for failed Fontan circulation with protein-losing enteropathy or exercise intolerance; CHD with progressive pulmonary hypertension that would preclude later transplantation; restrictive cardiomyopathy; and valve disease not amenable to surgical correction.

In infants under age 1, CHD remains the most frequent indication for heart transplantation (63% CHD vs. 31% cardiomyopathy), but this percentage has decreased over the last several years with improved early outcomes for surgical and hybrid palliation of HLHS. After 1 year of age, heart failure due to cardiomyopathy is the most common indication for heart transplantation, accounting for 55% of patients receiving a heart transplant from ages 1–10 and 64% of adolescents undergoing heart transplantation [115].

Wait-list mortality is a significant issue in pediatric transplantation, as 25–30% of infants listed for heart transplantation die before receiving a donor heart. Infants on extracorporeal membrane oxygenation (ECMO), ventilator support, PGE1, or with a weight less than 3 kg are at the highest risk of dying before a donor becomes available [115]. This has led to strategies for safely increasing both the waiting time and increasing the donor pool. Ventricular assist devices (VADs), including the Berlin Heart, have been sized to allow extended waiting times and have been successful in a limited number of centers [116, 117]. Alterations in donor allocation strategies, including ABO-incompatible donors, have been successful in Canada [115], and donations from sudden infant death syndrome (SIDS) victims increased availability without increasing posttransplant mortality for infants [118].

Overall, the 20-year survival for cardiac transplantation in children is 40%. One-year survival rates range from 75 to 80%, with the highest mortality in the first 6 months after transplantation, and 5-year survival rates are 65–68% in pediatric age groups. Long-term complications of cardiac transplantation in infants, children, and adolescents include growth failure, malignancies, infection, and chronic rejection (chronic allograft vasculopathy) [115].

Adult Congenital Heart Disease

Prevalence of Adult Congenital Heart Disease

Improvements in the diagnosis and treatment of children with CHD have led to an exponential growth in the population of adults with CHD [119]. In the United States and Canada, the number of adults with CHD surpasses the number of children with CHD [120, 121]. The ACC/AHA Task Force on Adult Congenital Heart Disease has predicted that in this decade, one in 150 young adults will have some form of CHD [108]. The growth in the population of adults with CHD that require specialized care has rapidly outpaced the growth in the number of health care professionals adequately trained to meet the needs of this diverse group of patients, and therefore, adults with CHD can be considered an underserved, vulnerable population [121].

Adult congenital heart disease (ACHD) patients are particularly likely to be lost to follow-up after their graduation from pediatric cardiology care. These young adults often have inadequate health insurance coverage and can be unaware of their specialized follow-up needs, long-term prognosis and risks, and how their CHD affects activity, work, and reproductive issues [108, 122]. Long periods without appropriate follow-up may result in a worsening of clinical status and a need for

Table 2.1 Common complications of repaired or palliative CHD in adults

CHD type	Surgical repair or palliation	Potential late sequelae
Atrial septal defect (ASD)	Suture repair; rare patch repair; device closure	Pulmonary artery hypertension (PAH) after late closure; sinus node dysfunction; atrial arrhythmias; mitral or tricuspid valve regurgitation; right ventricular (RV) dysfunction; pulmonary venous obstruction in sinus venosus subtypes
Ventricular septal defect (VSD)	Patch repair	Residual shunt; PAH; aortic regurgitation; outflow obstruction; ventricular dysfunction; complete heart block; endocarditis
Coarctation of the aorta	Subclavian flap repair; end-to-end anastomosis; intravascular stent placement	Hypertension; restenosis; aortic aneurysm formation; intracranial aneurysm; complications related to associated anomalies (bicuspid aortic valve, VSD, mitral stenosis)
Tetralogy of Fallot (TOF)	VSD closure; RVOT patch repair or valve sparing repair	Pulmonary regurgitation; RV dilation and dysfunction; RV outflow obstruction; RV outflow aneurysm; tricuspid valve regurgitation; aortic valve regurgitation; left ventricular dysfunction; arrhythmias (atrioventricular block, atrial tachycardia, ventricular tachycardia); sudden death
Transposition of the great arteries (TGA)	Atrial baffle procedure (Mustard or Senning)	Pulmonary venous or systemic venous baffle obstruction; baffle leak with cyanosis or paradoxical emboli; sinus bradycardia; atrial tachycardia; subpulmonary stenosis; RV dysfunction (systemic); tricuspid regurgitation
	Arterial switch procedure	Coronary insufficiency; myocardial ischemia; ventricular dysfunction; ventricular arrhythmias; arterial stenosis; aortic or pulmonary valve regurgitation
Single-ventricle physiology (hypoplastic left heart syndrome/tricuspid atresia/heterotaxy)	Fontan procedure ± fenestration Intracardiac Lateral tunnel Extracardiac	Outflow tract obstruction; atrial arrhythmias; atrioventricular block; thrombosis; air embolism (if fenestration or arteriovenous fistulas); ventricular dysfunction; valve regurgitation; hepatic congestion or cirrhosis; protein-losing enteropathy
Unrepaired or cyanotic CHD	–	PAH; polycythemia; thromboembolism; air embolism; arrhythmias; ventricular dysfunction; renal failure; gout; anemia; stroke; brain abscess; endocarditis

"emergent" intervention. It is therefore imperative that patients be transitioned from a pediatric cardiologist to both a primary care provider and an adult CHD program with a thorough understanding of their CHD diagnosis, treatment, prognosis, limitations, and recommended follow-up plan.

Care of the ACHD Patient

The American College of Cardiology/American Heart Association Task Force on Practice Guidelines for ACHD has published extensive guidelines for lesion-specific management of ACHD [108]. This document provides an algorithm for stratification of ACHD patients by level of complexity. It can be used to determine the need for ACHD expertise for routine cardiac management and noncardiac admissions for ACHD patients. In general, ACHD patients are at risk for multiple medical complications as described in the following sections and in Table 2.1.

Arrhythmias

Repaired and palliated CHD is associated with an increased incidence of arrhythmias in both pediatric and adult patients; however, adult patients may have more frequent or chronic refractory arrhythmias and are at a higher risk of sudden death [108, 123]. Strategies for arrhythmia management include optimization of hemodynamics, pharmacologic therapy, and device treatment, as indicated. An electrophysiologist with interest and expertise in CHD is an integral part of the ACHD care team.

Thrombosis and Thromboembolic Events

A subset of ACHD patients have right-to-left shunts, mixing of the venous and arterial blood at the ventricular level, atrial arrhythmias, ventricular dysfunction, or genetic or lifestyle factors that increase the risk of thromboembolism. Prophylaxis for thromboembolism should be implemented for high-risk patients, and medications or behaviors which increase risk for thrombosis should be discouraged (oral contraceptives, smoking). Postoperative thromboprophylaxis following cardiac and noncardiac surgery is required in adult patients who are not ambulatory for extended periods of time.

Anemia and Polycythemia

ACHD patients who are chronically ill, have comorbidities, poor nutritional status, or are menstruating or peripartum women are at risk for anemia. Routine surveillance of hemoglobin and iron levels should be performed in ACHD patients, and adequate iron supplementation provided. ACHD patients with cyanotic CHD may be at increased risk of stroke due to reduced distensibility of red blood cells with iron deficiency despite normal or elevated hemoglobin levels. Increased hemoglobin levels (>20 gm/dL) may be associated with headache, lethargy, fatigue, muscle weakness, lightheadedness, and visual disturbances. Dehydration should be avoided in these patients, and phlebotomy with volume replacement should be used sparingly and only in highly symptomatic cases [108].

Infective Endocarditis and Prophylaxis

Infective endocarditis accounts for a small number of admissions of ACHD patients yearly [124]. High-risk lesions include systemic to pulmonary artery shunts or arterial conduits, residual or unrepaired VSDs, bicuspid aortic valve with stenosis or insufficiency, prosthetic valves, and repaired TOF or TGA [108]. The need for regular dental care and specific recommendations for prophylaxis should be discussed at each ACHD visit. In general, ACHD patients with prosthetic valves, aortopulmonary shunts, palliated or repaired cyanotic CHD, acyanotic repaired CHD with residual shunting or hemodynamic disturbance, or previous history of endocarditis should receive prophylaxis for dental cleanings and contaminated procedures [108].

Heart Failure and Transplantation in the ACHD Patient

Patients with cardiac failure refractory to conventional medical management may benefit from placement of a ventricular assist device (VAD). Thoratec's HeartMate II® left ventricular assist system has recently been approved by the FDA not only as a bridge to transplantation but also for patients ineligible for transplantation (destination therapy). Although clinical experience in patients with two ventricles transitioning to VAD therapy is significant, little data are available on VADs and univentricular circulation. A pilot study, DEFINE (Destination Therapy Evaluation for Failing Fontan), is underway in the Pacific Northwest, with the goal of assembling a large multicenter trial to evaluate the safety of destination VAD therapy in Fontan patients who are not candidates for transplantation.

The timing of referral for VAD therapy in ACHD patients is critical to avoid significant end-organ dysfunction, including kidney and liver failure. Pulmonary vascular resistance is often initially elevated or can become elevated in heart failure. It requires serial measurement and aggressive treatment during mechanical circulatory support (i.e., bridging VAD therapy) to prevent graft failure due to pulmonary hypertension. Before VAD placement or cardiac transplantation is undertaken, an adequate social support network must be available to the patient. After cardiac transplantation, a new set of concerns focused on the cardiac graft and immunosuppression takes precedence, but preexisting issues attributable to CHD such as renal dysfunction, systemic and pulmonary hypertension, and vascular anomalies may complicate management.

Outcomes for orthotopic heart transplantation in adults with CHD are similar to those for adults transplanted without CHD and children with CHD who survive to transplant (70–80% 1-year survival; 60–69% 5-year survival) [125–127]. Single-ventricle physiology and TGA after an atrial baffle procedure were the most common diagnoses in ACHD patients undergoing transplant. A high percentage of patients require some anatomical correction at the time of transplant.

Pregnancy in the ACHD Patient

Women with repaired or unrepaired CHD should seek evaluation from an ACHD team and maternal–fetal medicine specialist prior to becoming pregnant. Women with high-risk cardiovascular conditions including cyanotic CHD, pulmonary hypertension, and significant ventricular dysfunction or reduced exercise ability may be counseled to avoid or terminate a pregnancy due to a significant risk of maternal mortality or other serious cardiac event [108, 128, 129].

Cardiovascular medications commonly used in ACHD may be detrimental to the fetus and should be stopped prior to pregnancy. These include, but are not limited to, angiotensin-converting enzyme (ACE) inhibitors and angiotensin II receptor blockers (ARBs). Use of warfarin or other medications not proven to be safe during pregnancy should be evaluated carefully. Vaginal delivery is most often tolerated in patients with CHD; however, cesarean section can be performed safely for obstetrical indications, if the mother and infant are fully anticoagulated, or if the hemodynamic changes of labor and delivery are not likely to be tolerated due to ventricular dysfunction.

Pregnancy is a prothrombotic condition associated with a 50% increase in circulating blood volume and an increase in cardiac output that peaks at the beginning of the third trimester [129]. Heart rate increases, systemic vascular resistance (SVR) drops due to the low-resistance placental bed, and hemoglobin concentration is reduced by dilution. During labor, intravascular volume abruptly increases with contractions, and SVR increases abruptly, which may precipitate ventricular failure. After delivery, intra-abdominal pressure is reduced abruptly, which can lead to hypotension and cardiovascular collapse. Women with aortic root dilation may also be at increased risk of aortic root dissection during pregnancy due to increased blood pressure and circulating hormones that may weaken the aortic wall.

Anesthetic Management for Noncardiac Procedures

Most anesthetic and analgesic agents reduce afterload and lower blood pressure. The effect is deleterious for a left-side obstructive lesion since lower blood pressure jeopardizes myocardial perfusion. Hypotension can also be detrimental if there is pulmonary hypertension. Afterload reduction is well tolerated by most individuals with ventricular dysfunction or a valvular anomaly. A number of inhalational agents have a proarrhythmic effect, so cardiac monitoring is mandatory. Careful choice of anesthetic agents and judicious use of volume expansion, especially during induction of anesthesia, allows safe management of anesthesia for most patients. Patients at high risk or with complex palliated CHD should have anesthesia administered in a monitored setting with cardiac care available. Given the risk of systemic air embolus, all cyanotic patients should have filters placed on their peripheral venous catheters. Patients who underwent an operative procedure prior to 1992 or with nontransfusion-related risk factors should also be screened for hepatitis C [108].

Quality of Life with ACHD

Adults with CHD should be part of clear and frequent conversations about exercise restrictions, vocational limitations, insurability, emotional difficulties associated with chronic disease, and reproductive concerns. Patients with CHD and chronic disease may have difficulty obtaining medical and life insurance [108] and may suffer from depression or psychoses. The ACHD team needs to be aware of the medical, social, and psychiatric conditions associated with ACHD and have the resources in place to provide care to this unique group of patients.

HeartMate II is a registered trademark of Thoratec Corporation (www.thoratec.com/medical-professionals/vad-product-information/heartmate-ll-lvad.aspx).

References

1. Brand T. Heart development: molecular insights into cardiac specification and early morphogenesis. Dev Biol. 2003;258:1–19.
2. Chinn A, Fitzsimmons J, Shepard TH, Fantel AG. Congenital heart disease among spontaneous abortuses and stillborn fetuses: prevalence and associations. Teratology. 1989;40(5):475–82.
3. Moore KL, Persaud TVN, editors. The developing human: clinically oriented embryology. In: The cardiovascular system. Philadelphia, PA: Saunders; 2008. p. 285–337.

4. Kirby ML, Waldo KL. Molecular embryogenesis of the heart. Pediatr Dev Pathol. 2002;5:516–43.
5. Martinsen BJ, Lohr JL. Cardiac development. In: Iaizzo P, editor. Handbook of cardiac anatomy, physiology and devices. New York: Springer Science; 2009. p. 23–32.
6. Manner J, Perez-Pomares JM, Macias D, Munoz-Chapuli R. The origin, formation and developmental significance of the epicardium: a review. Cells Tissues Organs. 2001;169:89–103.
7. Svensson EC. Look who's talking: FGFs and BMPs in the proepicardium. Circ Res. 2009;105:406–7.
8. Van Wijk B, van den Berg G, Abu-Issa R, et al. Epicardium and myocardium separate from a common precursor pool by crosstalk between bone morphogenetic protein and fibroblast growth factor. Circ Res. 2009;105:431–41.
9. Linask KK. Regulation of heart morphology: current molecular and cellular perspectives on the coordinated emergence of cardiac form and function. Birth Defects Res C Embryo Today. 2003;69:14–24.
10. Hoffman JIE, Kaplan S. The incidence of congenital heart disease. J Am Coll Cardiol. 2002;39(12):1890–900.
11. Martinsen BJ, Groebner NJ, Frasier AJ, Lohr JL. Expression of cardiac neural crest and heart genes isolated by modified differential display. Gene Expr Patterns. 2003;3:407–11.
12. Hildreth V, Webb S, Bradshaw L, Brown NA, Anderson RH, Henderson DJ. Cells migrating from the neural crest contribute to the innervation of the venous pole of the heart. J Anat. 2008;212:1–11.
13. Larsen W. Development of the heart. In: Schmitt WR, Otway M, Bowman-Schulman E, editors. Human embryology. New York: Churchill Livingstone; 1997. p. 151–87.
14. Combs MD, Yutzey KE. Heart valve development: regulatory networks in development and disease. Circ Res. 2009;105:408–21.
15. Moorman AFM, de Jong F, Denyn M, Lamers WH. Development of the cardiac conduction system. Circ Res. 1998;82:629–44.
16. Jongbloed MR, Mahtab EA, Blom NA, Schalij MJ, Gittenberger-de Groot AC. Development of the cardiac conduction system and the possible relation to predilection sites of arrhythmogenesis. Sci World J. 2008;8:239–69.
17. Bergmann O, Bhardwaj RD, Bernard S. et al Evidence for cardiomyocyte renewal in humans. Science. 2009;324(5923):98–102.
18. Hsieh P, Segers V, Davis ME. et al Evidence from a genetic fate-mapping study that stem cells refresh adult mammalian cardiomyocytes after injury. Nat Med. 2007;13:970–4.
19. Downs K, Davies T. Staging of gastrulating mouse embryos by morphological landmarks in the dissecting microscope. Development. 1993;118:1255–66.
20. Harvey RP. Patterning the vertebrate heart. Nat Rev Genet. 2002;3(7):544–56.
21. Moses KA, DeMayo F, Braun RM, Reecy JL, Schwartz RJ. Embryonic expression of an NKX2-5/Cre gene using Rosa26 reporter mice. Genesis. 2001;31:176–80.
22. Montoliu L, Whitelaw CBA. Using standard nomenclature to adequately name transgenes, knockout gene alleles and any mutation associated to a genetically modified mouse strain [technical report]. Transgenic Res. 2010;20(2):435–40. (doi: 10.1007/s11248-010-9428-z). www.springerlink.com/content/y50782un6vjn1673/fulltext.pdf. Accessed 3 March 2011.
23. Gordon JW, Scangos GA, Plotkin DJ, Barbosa JA, Ruddle FH. Genetic transformation of mouse embryos by microinjection of purified DNA. Proc Natl Acad Sci USA. 1980;77:7380–4.
24. Brinster RL, Chen HY, Trumbauer M, Senear AW, Warren R, Palmiter RD. Somatic expression of herpes thymidine kinase in mice following injection of a fusion gene into eggs. Cell. 1981;27:223–31.
25. Thomas KR, Folger KR, Capecchi MR. High frequency targeting of genes to specific sites in the mammalian genome. Cell. 1986;44(3):419–28.
26. Mortensen R. Production of a heterozygous mutant cell line by homologous recombination (single knockout). In: Current protocols in molecular biology. April 1, 2008 (doi: 10.1002/0471142727.mb2305s82, online ISBN: 9780471142720). 23.5.1-23.5.11. Wiley. Online access options at: http://onlinelibrary.wiley.com/book/10.1002/0471142727/homepage/Order.html. Accessed March 12, 2011.
27. Nagy A, Mar L, Watts G. Creation and use of a Cre recombinase transgenic database. In: Kuhn R, Wurst W, editors. Gene knockout protocols. 2nd ed. New York, NY: Humana Press; 2009. p. 365–78.
28. Boheler KR, Czyz J, Tweedie D, Yang HT, Anisimov SV, Wobus AM. Differentiation of pleuripotent embryonic stem cells into cardiomyocytes. Circ Res. 2002;91:189–201.
29. Ma YD, Lugus JJ, Park C, Choi K. Differentiation of mouse embryonic stem cells into blood. Current Protoc Stem Cell Biol (Published On Line). 2008; 6:1F.4.1–1F.4.19.
30. Robbins J, Doetschman T, Jones WK, Sanchez A. Embryonic stem cells as a model for cardiogenesis. Trends Cardiovasc Med. 1992;2(2): 44–50.
31. Schott JJ, Benson DW, Basson CT, et al. Congenital heart disease caused by mutations in the transcription factor NKX2-5. Science. 1998; 281(5373):108–11.
32. McElhinney DB, Geiger E, Blinder J, Benson DW, Goldmuntz E. NKX2,5 mutations in patients with congenital heart disease. J Am Coll Cardiol. 2003;42(9):1650–5.
33. Basson CT, Huang T, Lin RC, et al. Different TBX5 interactions in heart and limb defined by Holt-Oram syndrome mutations. Proc Natl Acad Sci U S A. 1999;96(6):2919–24.
34. Kitajima S, Takagi A, Inoue T, Sagay I. Mesp1 and Mesp 2 are essential for the development of cardiac mesoderm. Development. 2000;27: 3215–26.
35. Srivastava D. Making or breaking the heart: from lineage determination to morphogenesis. Cell. 2006;126:1037–48.
36. Foley A. Cardiac lineage selection: integrating biological complexity into computational models. Wiley Interdiscip Rev Syst Biol Med. 2009;1:334–47. doi:10.1002/wsbm.43.
37. Srivastava D, Olson EN. A genetic blueprint for cardiac development. Nature. 2000;407:221–6.
38. Yutzey KE, Kirby ML. Wherefore heart thou? Embryonic origins of cardiogenic mesoderm. Dev Dyn. 2002;223:307–20.
39. Ferdous A, Caprioli A, Iacovino M, et al. NKx2-5 transactivates the Ets-related protein 71 gene and specifies are endothelial.endocardial fate in the developing embryo. Proc Natl Acad Sci USA. 2009;106:814–9.
40. Bodmer R. The gene tinman is required for specification of the heart and visceral muscles in Drosophila. Development. 1993;118:719–29.
41. Lyons I, Parsons LM, Hartley L, et al. Myogenic and morphogenetic defects in heart tubes of murine embryos lacking the homeo box gene Nkx2-5. Genes Dev. 1995;9(13):1654–66.

42. Kuo CT, Morrisey EE, Anandappa R, et al. Gata4 transcription factor is required for ventral morphogenesis and heart tube formation. Genes Dev. 1997;11:1048–60.
43. Molkentin J, Lin Q, Duncan SA, Olson EN. Requirement of the transcription factor Gata 4for heart tube formation and ventral morphogenesis. Genes Dev. 1997;11:1061–72.
44. Cai CL, Liang X, Shi Y, et al. Isl1 identifies a cardiac progenitor population that proliferates prior to differentiation and contributes a majority of cells to the heart. Dev Cell. 2003;5:877–89.
45. Bu L, Jiang X, Martin-Puig S, et al. Human ISL1 heart progenitors generate diverse multipotent cardiovascular cell lineages. Nature. 2009; 460:113–7.
46. Watanabe Y, Miyagawa-Tomita S, Vinvent SD, Kelly RG, Moon AM, Buckingham ME. Role of mesodermal FGF8 and FGF10 overlaps in the development of the arterial pole of the heart and pharyngeal arch arteries. Circ Res. 2010;106:495–503.
47. Schleiffarth JR, Person AD, Martinsen BJ, et al. Wnt5a is required for cardiac outflow septation in mice. Pediatr Res. 2007;61(4):386–91.
48. Dyer LA, Kirby ML. The role of the second heart field in cardiac development. Dev Biol. 2009;336(2):137–44.
49. Garg V, Yamagishi C, Hu T, Kathiriya IS, Yamagishi H, Srivastava D. Tbx1, a DiGeorge syndrome candidate gene, is regulated by sonic hedgehog during pharyngeal arch development. Dev Biol. 2001;235(1):62–73.
50. McGrath J, Somlo S, Makova S, Tian X, Brueckner M. Two populations of node monocilia initiate left-right asymmetry in the mouse. Cell. 2003;114:61–73.
51. Raya A, Izpisua-Belmonte JC. Insights into the establishment of left-right asymmetries in vertebrates. Birth Defects Res C Embryo Today. 2008;84:81–94.
52. Levin M. Left-right asymmetry in embryonic development: a comprehensive review. Mech Dev. 2005;122:3–25.
53. Liu C, Liu W, Lu MF, Brown NA, Martin JF. Regulation of left-right asymmetry by thresholds of Pitx2c activity. Development. 2001;128: 2039–48.
54. Galli D, Dominguez JN, Zaffran S, Munk A, Brown NA, Buckingham ME. Atrial myocardium derives from the posterior region of the second heart field, which acquires left-right identity as Pitx2c is expressed. Development. 2008;135(6):1157–67.
55. Kioussi C, Briata P, Baek SH. et al Identification of a Wnt/Dvl/beta-catenin—Pitx2 pathway mediating cell-type-specific proliferation during development. Cell. 2002;111(5):673–85.
56. Lin Q, Schwarz J, Bucana C, Olson EN. Control of mouse cardiac morphogenesis and myogenesis by transcription factor MEF2C. Science. 1997;276(5317):1404–7.
57. Biben C, Harvey RP. Homeodomain factor Nkx2-5 controls left-right asymmetric expression of bHLH gene eHand during murine heart development. Genes Dev. 1997;11(11):1357–69.
58. Srivastava D, Thomas T, Lin Q, Kirby ML, Brown D, Olson EN. Regulation of cardiac mesodermal and neural crest development by the bHLH transcription factor, dHand. Nat Genet. 1997;16(2):154–60. Erratum in: Nat Genet. 1997;16(4)410.
59. Tsuchihashi T, Maeda J, Shin CH. et al Hand2 function in second heart field progenitors is essential for cardiogenesis. Dev Biol. 2010;351(1): 62–9.
60. Firulli AB, Firulli BA, Wang J, Rogers RH, Conway SJ. Gene replacement strategies to test the functional redundancy of basic helix-loop-helix transcription factor. Pediatr Cardiol. 2010;31(3):438–48.
61. Bruneau BG, Nemer G, Schmitt JP. et al A murine model of Holt-Oram syndrome defines roles of the T-box transcription factor Tbx5 in cardiogenesis and disease. Cell. 2001;106:709–21.
62. Takeuchi JK, Bruneau BG. Directed transdifferentiation of mouse mesoderm, to heart tissue by defined factors. Nature. 2009;459(7247):708–11.
63. Cordes KR, Srivastava D, Ivey KN. MicroRNAs in cardiac development. Pediatr Cardiol. 2010;31:349–56.
64. Ivey KN, Srivastava D. MicroRNAs as regulators of differentiation and cell fate decisions. Cell Stem Cell. 2010;1:36–41.
65. Epstein JA, Parmacek MS. Recent advances in cardiac development with therapeutic implications for adult cardiovascular disease. Circulation. 2005;112:592–7.
66. Basch ML, Bronner-Fraser M. Neural crest inducing signals. Adv Exp Med Biol. 2006;589:24–31.
67. Zhou B, von Gise A, Ma Q, Rivera-Feliciano J, Pu WT. Pu Wt. Nkx2-5 and Isl1-expressing cardiac progenitors contribute to proepicardium. Biochem Biophys Res Commun. 2008;375(3):450–3.
68. Watt AJ, Battle MA, Li J, Duncan SA. GATA4 is essential for the formation of the proepicardium and regulates cardiogenesis. Proc Natl Acad Sci USA. 2004;101(34):12573–8.
69. Wu SM, Fujiwara Y, Cibulsky SM, et al. Developmental origin of a bipotential myocardial and smooth muscle cell precursor in the mammalian heart. Cell. 2006;127(6):1137–50.
70. Wu SM, Chien KR, Mummery C. Origins and fates of cardiovascular progenitor cells. Cell. 2008;132:537–43.
71. Moretti A, Caron L, Nakano A, et al. Multipotent embryonic Isl1+ progenitor cells lead to cardiac, smooth muscle, and endothelial cell diversification. Cell. 2006;127:1151–65.
72. Garry DJ, Olson EN. A common progenitor at the heart of development. Cell. 2006;127:1101–4.
73. Beltrami AP, Barlucchi L, Torella D, et al. Adult cardiac stem cells are multipotent and support cardiac regeneration. Cell. 2003;114(6): 763–76.
74. Messina E, De Angelis L, Frati G, et al. Isolation and expansion of adult cardiac stem cells from human and murine heart. Circ Res. 2004;95: 911–21.
75. Martin CM, Meeson AP, Robertson SM, et al. Persistent expression of the ATP-binding cassette transporter, Abcg2, identifies cardiac SP cells in the developing and adult heart. Dev Biol. 2004;265:262–75.
76. Martin CM, Russell JL, Ferdous A, Garry DJ. Molecular signatures define myogenic stem cell populations. Stem Cell Rev. 2006;2:37–46.
77. Shi X, Garry DJ. Muscle stem cells in development, regeneration and disease. Genes Dev. 2006;20:1692–708.
78. Qian L, Srivastava D. Monkeying around with cardiac progenitors: hope for the future. J Clin Invest. 2010;120(4):1034–6.
79. Sadek H, Hannack B, Choe E, et al. Cardiogenic small molecules that enhance myocardial repair by stem cells. Proc Natl Acad Sci USA. 2009;105(16):6063–8.

80. Ieda M, Fu JD, Delgado-Olguin P, et al. Direct reprogramming of fibroblasts into functional cardiomyocytes by defined factors. Cell. 2010; 142(3):375–86.
81. Blin G, Nury D, Stefanovic S, et al. A purified population of multipotent cardiovascular progenitors derived from primate pluripotent stem cells engrafts in postmocardial infracted nonhuman primates. J Clin Invest. 2010;120(4):1125–39.
82. Ferencz C, Rubin JD, McCarter RJ, et al. Congenital heart disease: prevalence at live birth. The Baltimore-Washington Infant Study. Am J Epidemiol. 1985;121(1):31–6.
83. Hoffman JIE. Incidence, prevalence, and inheritance of congenital heart disease. In: Moller JH, Hoffman JIE, editors. Pediatric cardiovascular medicine. New York: Churchill Livingstone; 2000. p. 257–62.
84. Wren C, Richmond S, Donaldson L. Temporal variability in birth prevalence of cardiovascular malformations. Heart. 2000;83:414–9.
85. Lin AE. Chromosomal abnormality associated with congenital heart defect. Am J Med Genet. 1990;35(4):590–1.
86. Pierpont ME, Basson CT, Benson DW. et al Genetic basis for congenital heart defects: current knowledge: a scientific statement from the American Heart Association Congenital Cardiac Defects Committee, Council on Cardiovascular Disease in the Young: endorsed by the American Academy of Pediatrics. Circulation. 2007;115:3015–38.
87. Song MS, Hu A, Dyhamenahali U. et al Extracardiac lesions and chromosomal abnormalities associated with major fetal heart defects: comparison of intrauterine, postnatal and postmortem diagnosis. Ultrasound Obstet Gynecol. 2009;33:552–9.
88. Lin AE, Basson CT, Goldmuntz E, et al. Adults with genetic syndromes and cardiovascular abnormalities: clinical history and management. Genet Med. 2008;10(7):469–94.
89. Gill HK, Splitt M, Sharland GK, Simpson JM. Patterns of recurrence of congenital heart disease: an analysis of 6,640 consecutive pregnancies evaluated by detained fetal echocardiography. J Am Coll Cardiol. 2003;42(5):923–9.
90. Ferencz C, Boughman JA, Neill CA, Brenner JI, Perry LW. Congenital cardiovascular malformations: questions on inheritance. Baltimore-Washington Infant Study Group. J Am Coll Cardiol. 1989;14(3):756–63.
91. Oyen N, Poulsen G, Boyd HA, Wohlfahrt J, Jensen PKA, Melbye M. Recurrence of congenital heart defects in families. Circulation. 2009; 120:295–301.
92. Calcagni G, Digilio MC, Sarkozy A, Dallapiccola B, Marino B. Familial recurrence of congenital heart disease, a review of the literature. Eur J Pediatr. 2007;166:111–6.
93. Hinton Jr RB, Martin LJ, Tabangin ME, Mazwi ML, Cripe LH, Benson DW. Hypoplastic left heart syndrome is heritable. J Am Coll Cardiol. 2007;50(16):1590–5.
94. Cripe L, Andelfinger G, Martin LJ, Shooner K, Benson DW. Bicuspid aortic valve is heritable. J Am Coll Cardiol. 2004;44(1):138–43.
95. Moller JH, Shumway SJ, Gott VL. The first open-heart repairs using extracorporeal circulation by cross-circulation: a 53-year follow-up. Ann Thorac Surg. 2009;88(3):1044–6.
96. Stirling GR, Stanley PH, Lillehei CW. The effects of cardiac bypass and ventriculotomy upon right ventricular function with report of successful closure of ventricular septal defect by use of atriotomy. Surg Forum. 1957;8:433–8.
97. Tucker EM, Pyles LA, Bass JL, Moller JH. Permanent pacemaker for atrioventricular conduction block after operative repair of perimembranous ventricular septal defect. J Am Coll Cardiol. 2007;50(12):1196–200.
98. Roos-Hesselink JW, Meijboom FJ, Spitaels SEC, et al. Outcome of patients after surgical closure of ventricular septal defect at young age: longitudinal follow-up of 22–34 years. Eur Heart J. 2004;25:1057.
99. Hirsch R, Lorber A, Shapira Y. et al Initial experience with the Amplatzer membranous septal occluder in adults. Acute Card Care. 2007; 9(1):54–9.
100. Zuo J, Xie J, Yi W, et al. Results of transcatheter closure of perimembranous ventricular septal defect. Am J Cardiol. 2010;106(7):1034–7.
101. Forsey J, Kenny D, Morgan G, et al. Early clinical experience with the new Amplatzer Ductal Occluder II for closure of the persistent arterial duct. Catheter Cardiovasc Interv. 2009;74(4):615–23.
102. Bautista-Hernandez V, Hasan BS, Harrild DM, et al. Late pulmonary valve replacement in patients with pulmonary atresia and intact ventricular septum: a case-matched study. Ann Thorac Surg. 2011;91:555–60.
103. Keane JF, Fyler DC, editors. Aortic outflow abnormalities. In: Nadas' pediatric cardiology. Philadelphia, PA: Saunders; 2006. p. 581–602.
104. Toro-Salazar OH, Steinberger J, Thomas W, Rocchini AP, Carpenter B, Moller JH. Long-term follow-up of patients after coarctation of the aorta repair. Am J Cardiol. 2002;89(5):541–7.
105. Lillehei CW, Varco RL, Cohen M, et al. The first open heart corrections of tetralogy of Fallot. A 26–31 year follow-up of 106 patients. Ann Surg. 1986;104(4):490–502.
106. Al Habib HF, Jacobs JP, Mavroudis C, Tchervenkov CI, O'Brien SM, Mohammadi S, et al. Contemporary patterns of management of tetralogy of Fallot: data from the Society of Thoracic Surgeons Database. Ann Thorac Surg. 2010;90(3):813–9.
107. Aboulhosn J, Child JS. Management after childhood repair of tetralogy of Fallot. Curr Treat Options Cardiovasc Med. 2006;8(6):474–83.
108. Warnes CA, Williams RG, Bashore TM, et al. ACC/AHA 2008 Guidelines for the Management of Adults With Congenital Heart Disease. Circulation. 2008;118(23):e714–833.
109. Tobler D, Williams WG, Jegatheeswaran A, et al. Cardiac outcomes in young adult survivors of the arterial switch operation for transposition of the great arteries. J Am Coll Cardiol. 2010;56(1):5864.
110. Ye M, Coldren C, Liang X, et al. Deletion of ETS-1, a gene in the Jacobson syndrome critical region, causes ventricular septal defects and abnormal ventricular morphology in mice. Hum Mol Genet. 2010;19(4):648–56.
111. Grossfeld P, Ye M, Harvey R. Hypoplastic left heart syndrome: new genetic insights. J Am Coll Cardiol. 2009;53(12):1072–4.
112. Tweddell JS, Hoffman GM, Mussato KA, et al. Improved survival of patients undergoing palliation of hypoplastic left heart syndrome: lessons learned from 115 consecutive patients. Circulation. 2002;106(12 Suppl 1):I82–9.
113. Sano S, Ishino K, Kawada M, Yoshizumi K, Takeuchi M, Ohtsuki S. Experience over five years using a shunt placed between the right ventricle and the pulmonary arteries during initial reconstruction of hypoplasia of the left heart. Cardiol Young. 2004;14 suppl 3:90–5.
114. Holzer R, Marshall A, Kreutzer J, et al. Hybrid procedures: adverse events and procedural characteristics-results of a multi-institutional registry. Congenit Heart Dis. 2010;5(3):233–42.
115. Conway J, Dipchand AI. Heart transplantation in children. Pediatr Clin North Am. 2010;57:353–73.

116. Karimova A, Van Doom C, Brown K, et al. Mechanical bridging to orthotopic heart transplantation in children weighing less than 10 kg: feasibility and limitations. Eur J Cardiothorac Surg. 2011;39:304–9. doi:10.1016/j.ejcts.2010.05.015.
117. Fan Y, Weng YG, Xiao YB, et al. Outcomes of ventricular assist device support in young patients with small body surface area. Eur J Cardiothorac Surg Epub. 2011;39:699–704.
118. Silva JNA, Canter CE, Singh TP, et al. Outcomes of heart transplantation using donor hearts from infants with sudden infant death syndrome. J Heart Lung Transplant. 2010;29(11):1226–30.
119. Marelli AJ, Mackie AS, Ioneecu-Ittu R, Rahme E, Pilote L. Congenital heart disease in the general population: changing prevalence and age distribution. Circulation. 2007;115:163–72.
120. Khairy P, Ionescu-Ittu R, Mackie AS, Abrahamowicz M, Pilote L, Marelli AJ. Changing mortality in congenital heart disease. J Am Coll Cardiol. 2010;56:1149–57.
121. Patel MS, Kogon BE. Care of the adult congenital heart disease patient in the United States: a summary of the current system. Pediatr Cardiol. 2010;31(4):511–4.
122. Yeung E, Kay J, Roosevelt GE, Brandon M, Yetman AT. Lapse of care as a predictor for morbidity in adults with congenital heart disease. Int J Cardiol. 2008;125:62–5.
123. Bernier M, Marelli AJ, Pilote L, et al. Atrial arrhythmias in adult patients with right versus left sided congenital heart disease anomalies. Am J Cardiol. 2010;106(4):547–51.
124. Li W, Somerville J. Infective endocarditis in the grown-up congenital heart (GUCH) population. Eur Heart J. 1998;19(1):166–73.
125. Lamour JM, Addonizio LJ, Galantowicz ME, et al. Outcome after orthotopic cardiac transplantation in adults with congenital heart disease. Circulation. 1999;100:II200–5.
126. Jayakumar KA, Addonizio LJ, Kichuk-Chrisant MR, et al. Cardiac transplantation after Fontan or Glenn procedure. J Am Coll Cardiol. 2004;44(10):2065–72.
127. Irving C, Parry G, O'Sullivan J, et al. Cardiac transplantation in adults with congenital heart disease. Heart. 2001;96(15):1217–22.
128. Kovacs AH, Harrison JL, Colman JM. Pregnancy and contraception in congenital heart disease: what women are not told. J Am Coll Cardiol. 2008;52:577–8.
129. Balint OH, Siu SC, Mason J, et al. Cardiac outcomes after pregnancy in women with congenital heart disease. Heart. 2010;96:1656–61.

Chapter 3
Echocardiographic Evaluation of Ischemic Heart Disease

Richard W. Asinger, Fouad A. Bachour, and Gautam R. Shroff

Techniques and Indications

Techniques

State-of-the-art echo-Doppler is the most practical and useful technique for rapid, noninvasive bedside evaluation of coronary heart disease.

Since coronary artery disease typically results in regional dysfunction, A- (amplitude) and B (brightness)-mode echocardiography were of limited value in establishing the diagnosis. Representation of the A-Mode echocardiogram in real time, i.e., time motion or M-mode echocardiography, was a major breakthrough in the use of ultrasound for cardiac imaging. It provided hard copy capture of the motion of cardiac structures in time. Rapid sampling rates and high transducer frequency improved the resolution of structures during the cardiac cycle. Characteristic physiologic and pathophysiologic motion of cardiac structures soon became apparent and markedly improved the diagnostic ability to detect valvular and congenital abnormalities.

M-mode echocardiography from standard parasternal acoustic windows using cardiac landmarks allowed a noninvasive method to determine left ventricular size, wall thickness, and function. M-mode echocardiographic evaluation for many common conditions associated with coronary heart disease continued to be limited, however, because of the lack of spatial orientation. It was simply too difficult to know the exact orientation of this "ice pick" view of the heart from small, limited acoustic windows that relied on internal cardiac landmarks.

Development of real time, 2D echocardiography, was an important innovation in diagnostic ultrasound evaluation of coronary heart disease. Early use of real time mechanical and B-Mode, 2D scanners, however, continued to be limited by the small acoustic windows available.

Electronic phased array ultrasonoscopes allow a small transducer-skin interface and are the current standard for real time 2D echocardiography [1]. With this technique, tomographic images can be obtained from multiple acoustic windows, that allow spatial orientation spatial orientation and 3D reconstructions of cardiac structures in real time. Second harmonic imaging combined with echo contrast agents has enhanced definition of the endocardium and enables evaluation of left ventricular wall motion even in the most acoustically challenging patients [2].

The addition of pulsed- and continuous-wave Doppler followed by color flow imaging added the ability to detect and quantitate the velocity of blood flowing through the heart as well as the velocity and timing of motion of cardiac structures [3]. The latter has enhanced our understanding of diastolic function as well as the synchrony of left ventricular contraction and the important role it plays in determining cardiac function [4, 5].

These advances in technology are available now with portable, bedside ultrasonoscopes. When coupled with digital technology, they have raised the diagnostic capabilities of modern echo-Doppler techniques for evaluating cardiac structure and function in all clinical settings including coronary heart disease.

R.W. Asinger, MD (✉) • F.A. Bachour, MD, FSCAI • G.R. Shroff, MBBS
Department of Medicine, Hennepin County Medical Center, 701 Park Avenue South, Minneapolis, MN 55415, USA
e-mail: asing001@umn.edu

Z. Vlodaver et al. (eds.), *Coronary Heart Disease: Clinical, Pathological, Imaging, and Molecular Profiles*,
DOI 10.1007/978-1-4614-1475-9_3, © Springer Science+Business Media, LLC 2012

Indications

Chest Pain

Coronary heart disease may manifest itself clinically in a wide variety of presentations secondary to the effect of ischemia on ventricular, valvular, and electrical function. The hallmark presentation, however, is acute coronary syndrome (ACS). ACS typically results in a sudden disruption of blood flow to left ventricular myocardium resulting in rapid deterioration in diastolic followed by systolic function [6]. By the time symptoms and electrocardiographic manifestations of ischemia draw clinical attention, wall motion abnormalities are present and can be detected with transthoracic echocardiography. This provides a valuable diagnostic adjunct in the initial evaluation of patients with acute onset of chest pain.

If the acute onset of chest pain is associated with ST-segment elevation myocardial infarction (STEMI), as shown on an electrocardiogram (ECG) primary reperfusion therapy should be implemented immediately, unless a suspected mechanical complication may influence emergent treatment. When ECG findings are nondiagnostic, transthoracic echocardiography can assist diagnostically by defining left ventricular regional and global function. Detection of a regional wall motion abnormality, however, cannot determine whether or not it is acute or chronic; serial ECGs and biomarkers are still needed to establish a diagnosis of ACS. An additional benefit of echocardiography, when ECGs are nondiagnostic, is detecting other causes of acute chest pain such as pulmonary embolism, pericarditis, and aortic dissection.

Detailed echocardiographic evaluation for regional wall motion abnormalities and other causes of chest pain requires expertise in performance and interpretation which may not be immediately available in the emergency room setting. The use of digital technology to record and transmit images to an experienced echocardiographer for interpretation is available, but cannot replace the need for technical acquisition of high-quality images. This issue has been addressed in larger-volume emergency departments by trained technical staff in the multiple uses of diagnostic ultrasound.

Myocardial Infarction

Transthoracic echocardiography is a valuable tool to evaluate patients with STEMI and non ST-segment elevation myocardial infarction (NSTEMI) by determining regional and global function of the left ventricle (LV).

Echocardiography can assist diagnostically by identifying wall motion abnormalities when the ECG is nondiagnostic. This is illustrated by Case #1, a 48-year-old man with chest pain, serial elevation in troponin-I and the ECG results shown in Fig. 3.1a. An echocardiogram demonstrated a regional wall motion abnormality of the lateral wall (Fig. 3.1b). Coronary arteriography (Fig. 3.1c) showed an occluded obtuse marginal branch of the left circumflex coronary artery (CX).

In addition to assisting diagnostically, transthoracic echocardiography following acute myocardial infarction (AMI) establishes baseline regional and global function and has prognostic significance [7, 8]. The worse the left ventricular systolic performance, the worse the patient's prognosis. This information is valuable in establishing which patients require therapy to eliminate residual ischemia and/or to block neurohormonal mechanisms to promote positive remodeling of the LV.

Serial echocardiography following AMI also provides assessment of therapy. Since it is a noninvasive ultrasound technique, it is ideal for serial studies.

The desired result of acute reperfusion therapy following STEMI is recovery of regional and global function. This is demonstrated in Case #2, a 56-year-old male with acute anterior STEMI, as illustrated in his ECG (Fig. 3.2a). Coronary arteriography, Fig. 3.2b, demonstrated an occluded left anterior descending coronary artery (LAD) that underwent PCI with stent placement. Baseline postinfarct echocardiography, Fig. 3.2c, showed a large, anteroapical wall motion abnormality with decreased LV systolic performance. On subsequent study, Fig. 3.2c, the left ventricular systolic function completely normalized.

In contrast, Case #3 is a 50-year-old man who presented with several hours of waxing and waning symptoms of ACS. His first ECG showed no acute ischemic changes. A few minutes later, with worsening chest pain, a second ECG that was done (Fig. 3.3a) showed acute anterolateral STEMI. He was taken promptly to the Cath lab with a door-to-balloon time of 52 min (Fig. 3.3b). An echocardiogram on day one post-revascularization showed a large anterolateral wall motion abnormality, but in this case, serial echocardiography demonstrated progressive left ventricle dilatation and dysfunction despite the timely reperfusion therapy (Fig. 3.3c). Progressive deterioration in systolic performance following AMI predicts a poor prognosis and mandates aggressive evaluation and treatment.

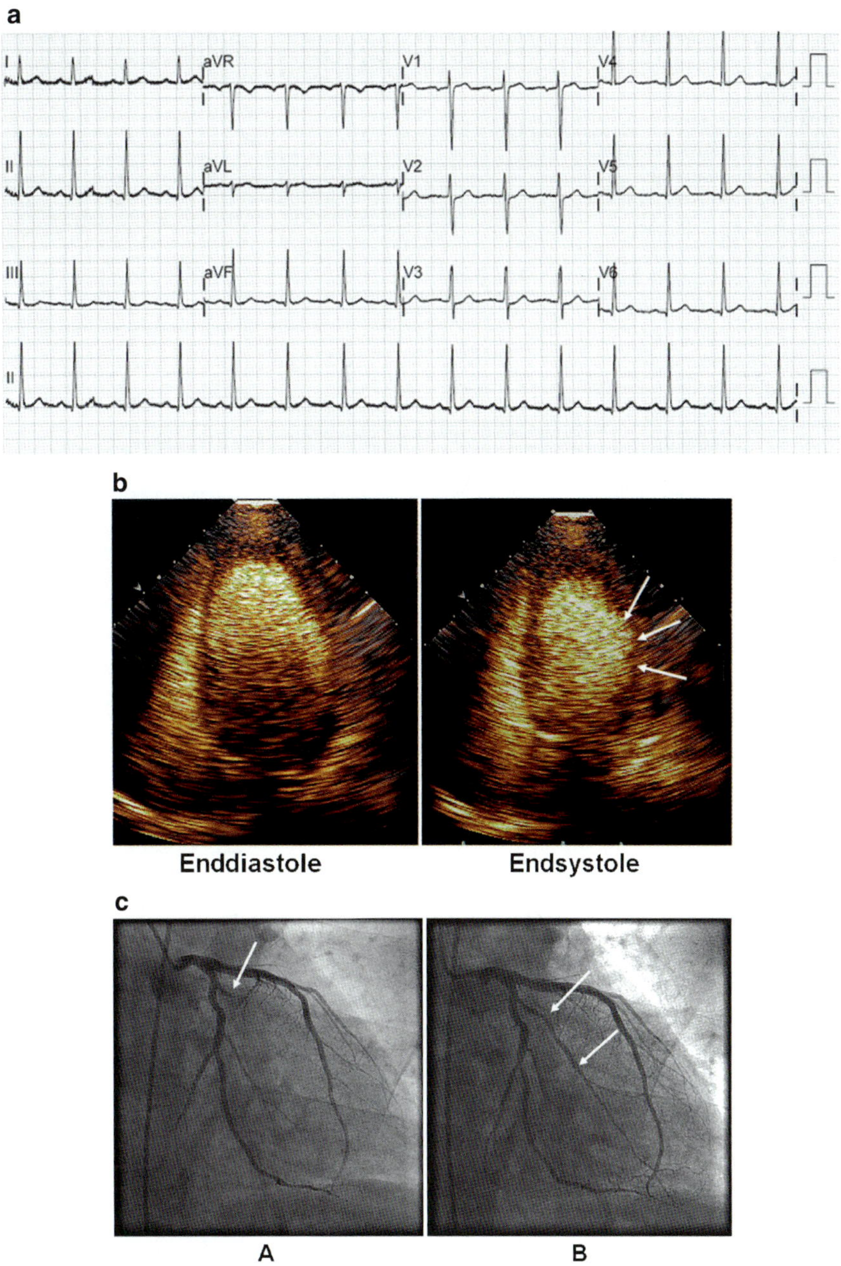

Fig. 3.1 (**a–c**) A 48-year-old man admitted with chest pain and serial elevation in troponin-1. (**a**) ECG is nondiagnostic for ischemic changes. (**b**) Echocardiogram in end diastole and systole demonstrates regional wall motion abnormality of the lateral wall (*arrows*). (**c**) *A* Left coronary arteriogram on admission showing occlusion of the obtuse marginal branch of the left circumflex artery (CX) (*arrow*). *B* Post PCI there is restoration of blood flow (*arrows*)

Hemodynamic Deterioration

A traditional indication for echocardiography in evaluating AMI is hemodynamic compromise, specifically hypotension, shock, or the development of a new murmur. In these clinical settings, echocardiography stands out since it can rapidly detect mechanical complications including rupture of the left ventricular free wall (Fig. 3.4), interventricular septum (IVS) (Fig. 3.5), and papillary muscle (Fig. 3.6a, b).

Echocardiography can also readily detect other nonmechanical clinical conditions leading to hemodynamic deterioration. Most important is global left ventricular dysfunction or new regional wall motion abnormality which may prompt other diagnostic studies and specific therapy. Echocardiography can also detect right ventricular infarction (RVI) (Fig. 3.7a–c), a complication almost exclusively seen with inferior infarction. With RVI, the systolic tricuspid insufficiency jet has a low peak velocity. This is in contrast to pulmonary embolism (PE) where the systolic tricuspid insufficiency jet will have a high peak velocity.

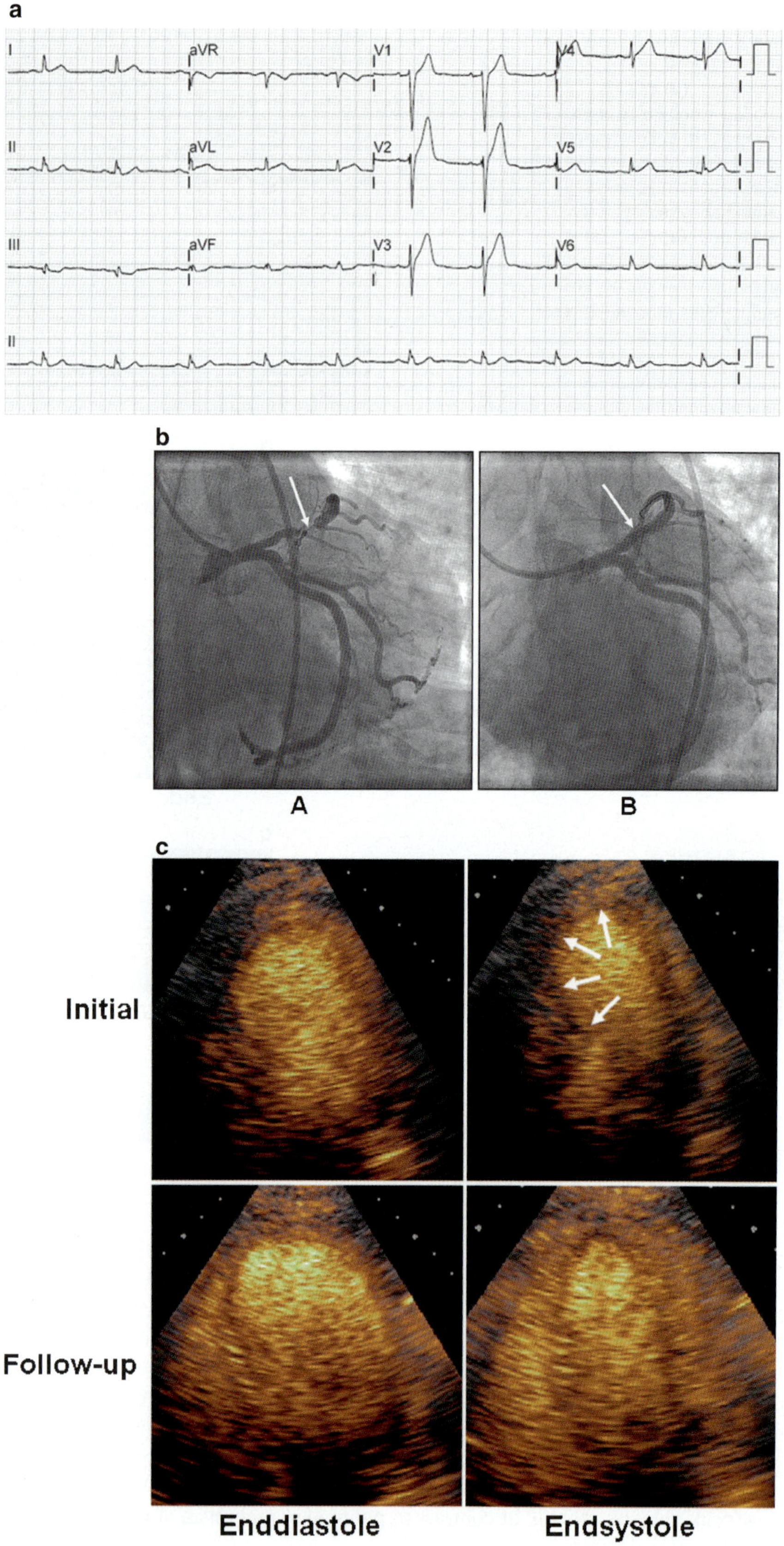

Fig. 3.2 (**a–c**) A 56-year-old male with acute STEMI. (**a**) ECG shows changes of acute anterior STEMI. (**b**) *A* Left coronary arteriogram shows sub-total occlusion left anterior descending artery (LAD) (*arrow*). *B* After PCI with stent placement (*arrow*) there is restoration of blood flow. (**c**) *A* Initial postinfarct echocardiogram shows a large anteroapical wall motion abnormality (*arrows*) and decreased ejection fraction. *B* Follow-up echocardiogram after PCI and stent placement, the left ventricular systolic function completely normalized

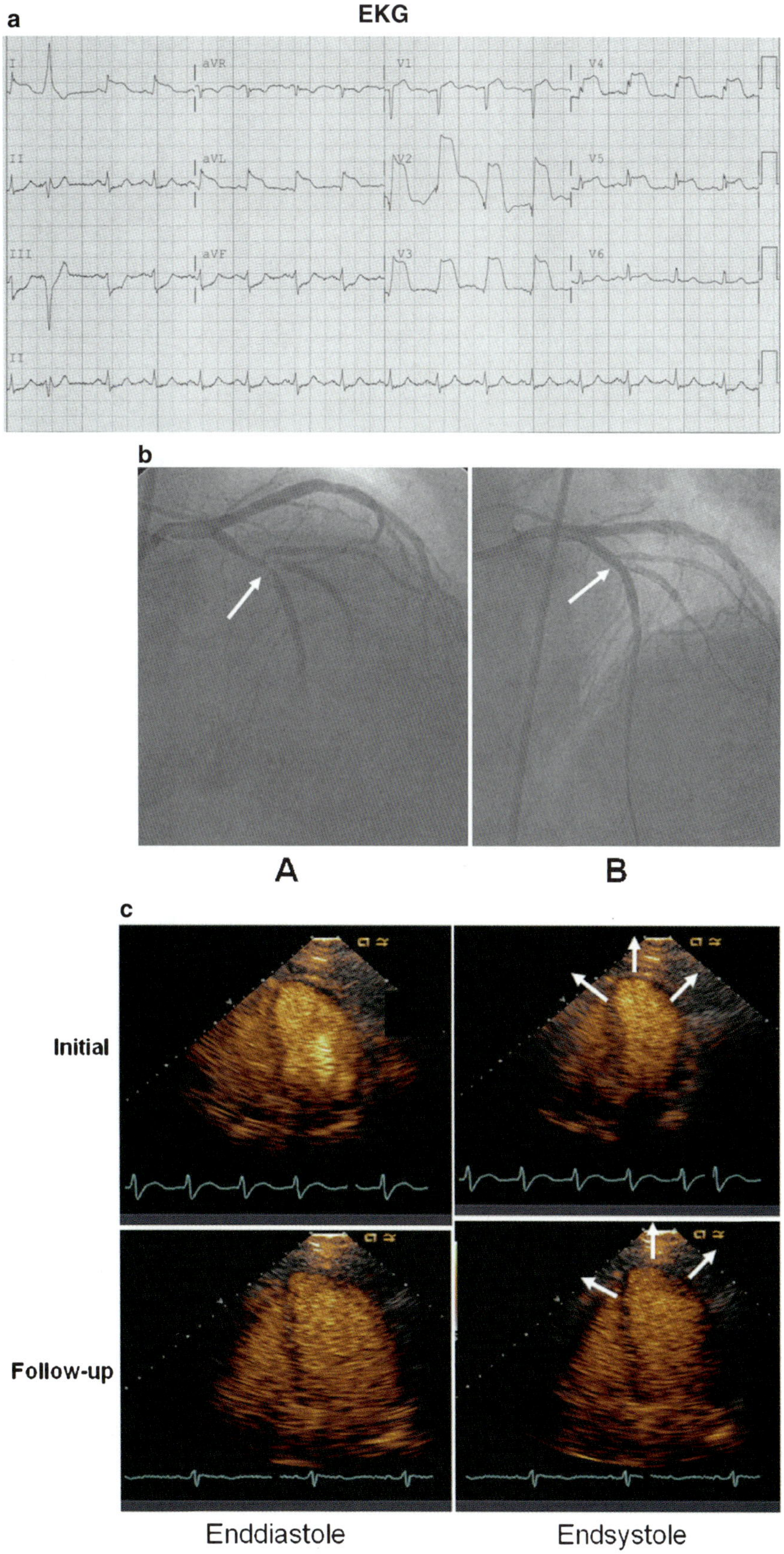

Fig. 3.3 (**a–c**) A 50-year-old man who presented with several hours of waxing and waning symptoms of ACS. (**a**) ECG shows changes of acute anterolateral STEMI. (**b**) *A* Left coronary arteriogram on admission shows sub-total occlusion of the LAD (*arrow*). *B* Post PCI shows restoration of blood flow (*arrow*). (**c**) *A* Initial echocardiogram in systole and diastole on admission demonstrates large anteroapical wall motion abnormality (*arrows*). *B* Follow-up weeks after PCI shows progressive left ventricular dilatation progress of left ventricular dilatation and LV dysfunction (*arrows*) despite timely reperfusion therapy

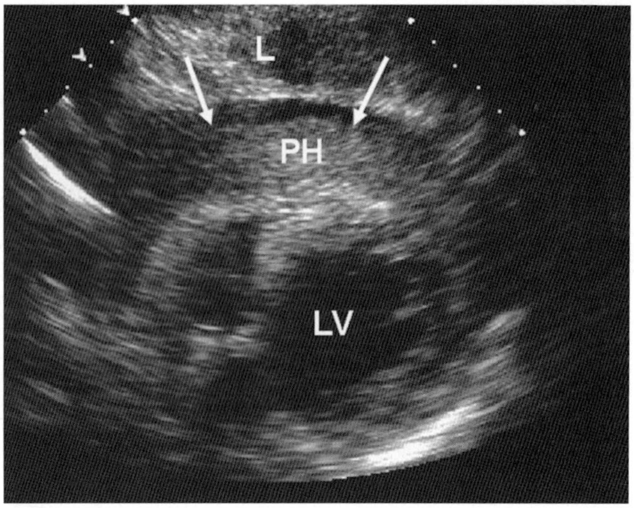

Fig. 3.4 Echocardiogram in a case of a rupture of the left ventricular free wall complicating myocardial infarction associated with hematoma within the pericardium (PH) (*arrows*)

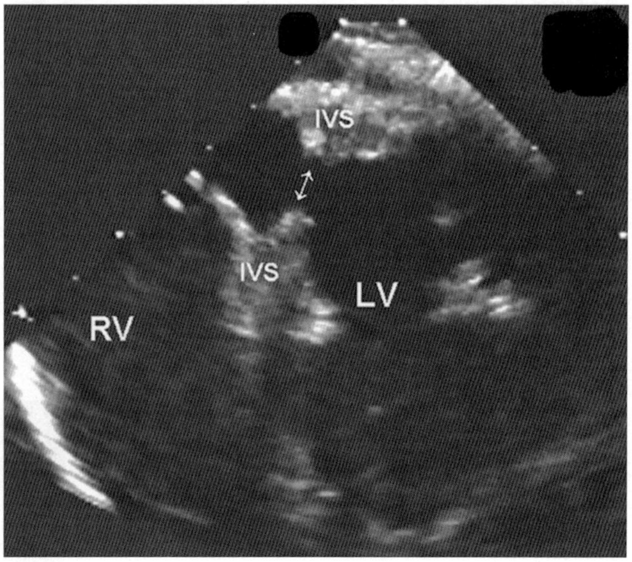

Fig. 3.5 Echocardiogram in a case of acute myocardial infarction and rupture of the interventricular septum identified by the dropout of the septum (*arrow*)

Severe mitral insufficiency independent of papillary muscle rupture may also complicate ischemia as shown in (Fig. 3.8a–c). In this case, revascularization by PCI of the two culprit lesions resulted in marked improvement in ventricular function and decrease in mitral regurgitation.

When hemodynamic compromise complicates acute infarction and the echocardiogram shows no acute mechanical problem or change in systolic performance of the left or right ventricular function, echo-Doppler evaluation can define left and right ventricular filling pressures. Left ventricular filling pressure can be estimated from assessment of mitral inflow, pulmonary venous flow, and mitral annular tissue Doppler (Fig. 3.9) [4]. Right ventricular filling pressure can be estimated from the dimensions of the inferior vena cava during the respiratory cycle [9].

Hemodynamic compromise may occur secondary to noncardiac causes and be accompanied by positive biomarkers. Figure 3.10 pertains to a 60-year-old patient with shortness of breath, hypotension, and positive troponins. An echocardiogram demonstrated features of acute cor pulmonale including dilatation of the right ventricle with decreased right ventricular function. The IVS is flat in diastole showing the typical D shape of acute pressure overload from pulmonary embolism. During systole, the circular shape of the ventricle returns. Bowing of the interatrial septum to the left also occurred, with marked dilatation of the inferior vena cava. These findings could indicate either right ventricular infarction or acute pulmonary embolus. A high peak systolic tricuspid valve insufficiency velocity would support acute cor pulmonale from pulmonary embolus rather than RVI.

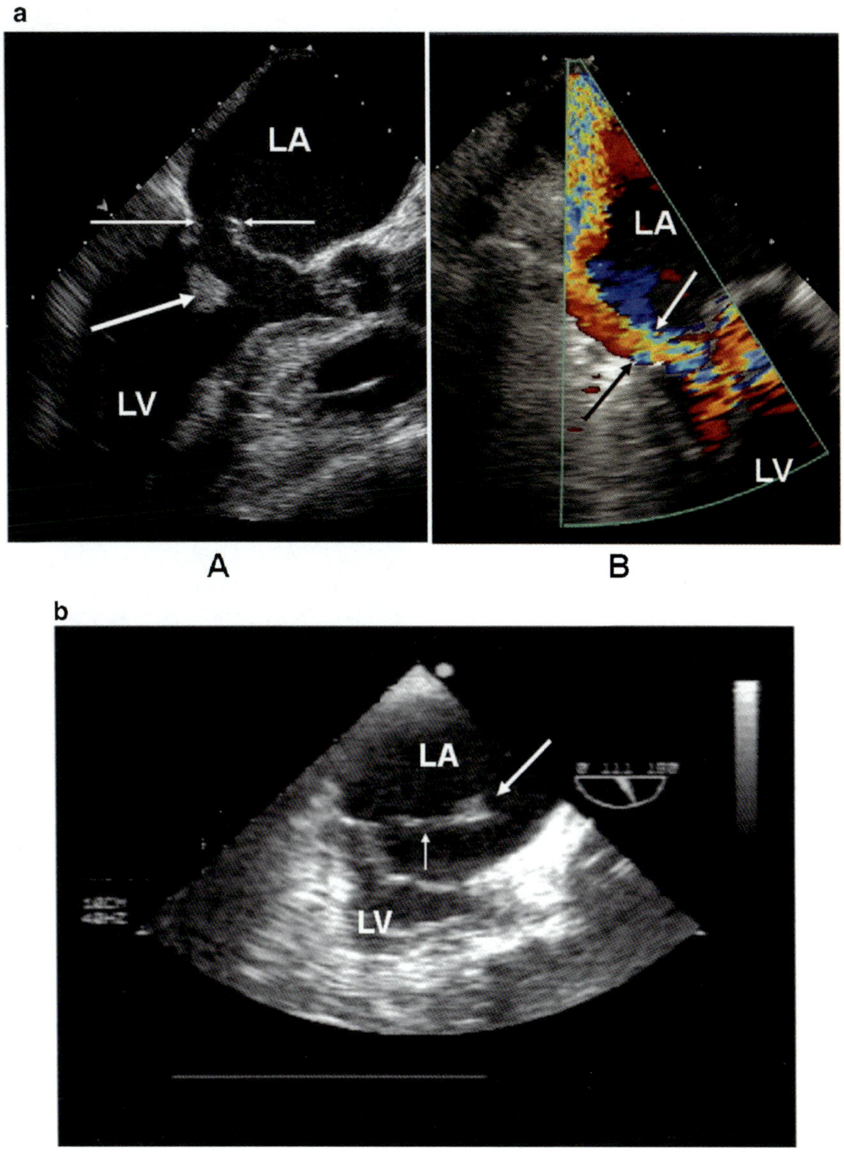

Fig. 3.6 (**a**, **b**) Transesophageal echocardiograms in a case with rupture of a papillary muscle of the mitral valve complicating myocardial infarction demonstrate. (**a**) *A* Rupture of papillary muscle (*large arrow*) and flail mitral valve (*small arrows*). (**a**) *B* Eccentric jet of severe mitral regurgitation (*arrows*). (**b**) Prolapse of ruptured papillary muscle into the left atrium (*arrows*).

Assessment of Left Ventricular Function

Global Function

Global left ventricular systolic performance is most commonly assessed by ejection fraction (EF), the percent of blood ejected from the LV with each contraction. The LVEF has the distinction of being the clinical parameter most predictive of prognosis following AMI.

Initial echocardiographic attempts to determine global function of the LV involved M-mode echocardiography [10]. Correlation with contrast angiography was reasonable in the absence of regional wall motion abnormality, but poor for patients with coronary heart disease and previous myocardial infarction.

2D echocardiography provides tomographic images of the LV and when used from multiple acoustic windows, particularly apical views, enables 3D reconstruction of the LV. Several methods have been proposed to evaluate the global function of the LV. Many assume geometric shapes and have similar limitations of M-mode echocardiography. Simpson's "poker chip" method, using apical views has good correlation with other quantitative techniques and has become the 2D echocardiography standard for determination of LVEF [11–13]. 3D echocardiography (3DE) is an obvious choice for determining LVEF but is labor intensive and time consuming which limits its clinical application.

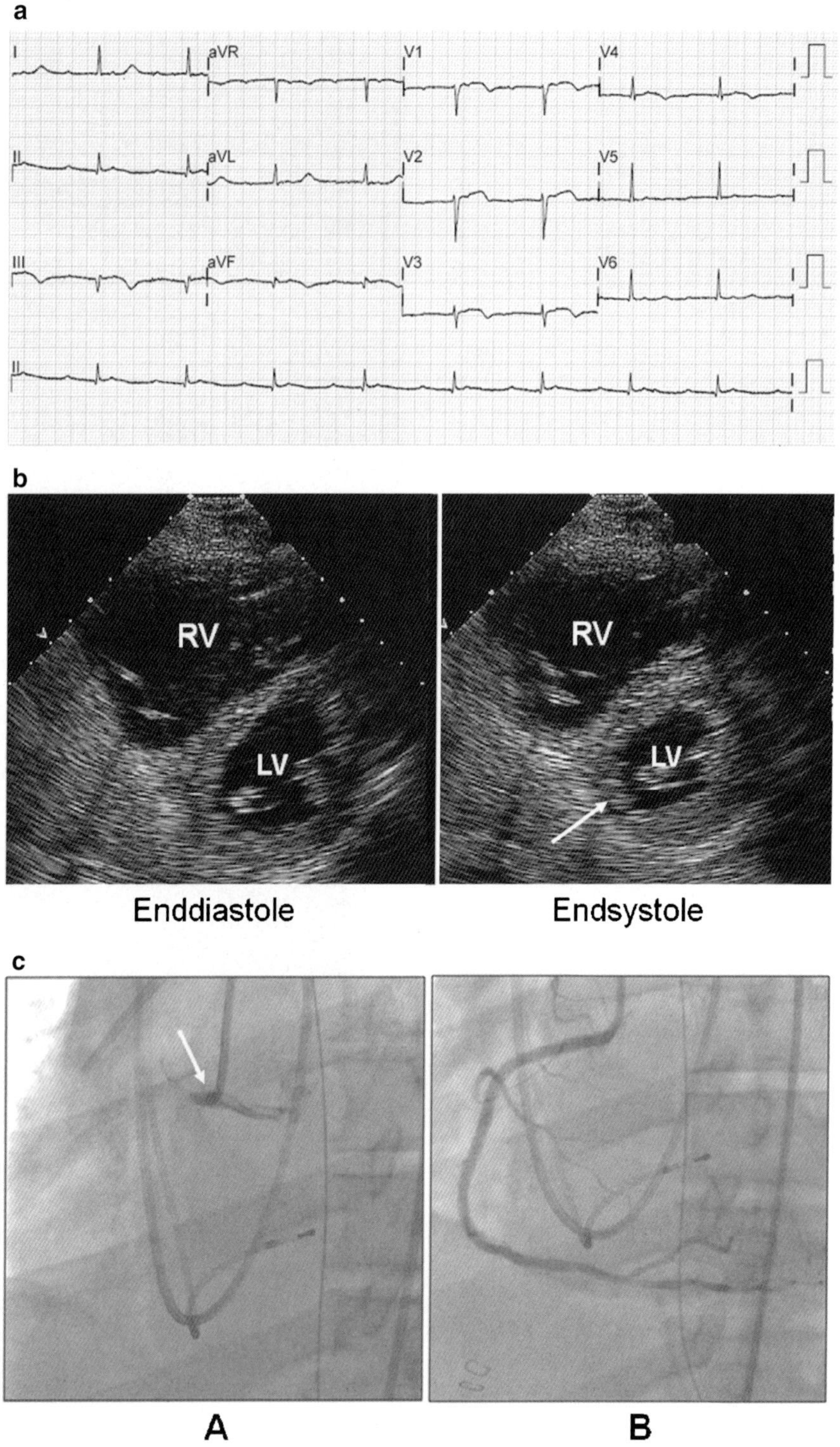

Fig. 3.7 (**a–c**) Features of right ventricular infarction, a complication seen with inferior infarction. (**a**) ECG on admission shows acute changes of inferior wall infarction. (**b**) Echocardiographic features of right ventricular infarction with dilatation of the RV, hypokinesis of the RV free wall, and left ventricular inferior wall motion abnormity (*arrow*). (**c**) *A* RC arteriogram on admission shows occluded proximal RCA (*arrow*). *B* Post PCI there is restoration of blood flow

Regional Function

The left ventricular cavity simulates a prolate ellipse of revolution, presenting a degree of symmetry in contrast to the right ventricle but its blood supply is far from symmetric. Regions of the LV affected by occlusion of a specific epicardial coronary artery do not follow a geometric distribution. This was the major factor limiting the use of M-mode echocardiography for the evaluation of regional and global function in coronary heart disease particularly from acoustic windows that do not

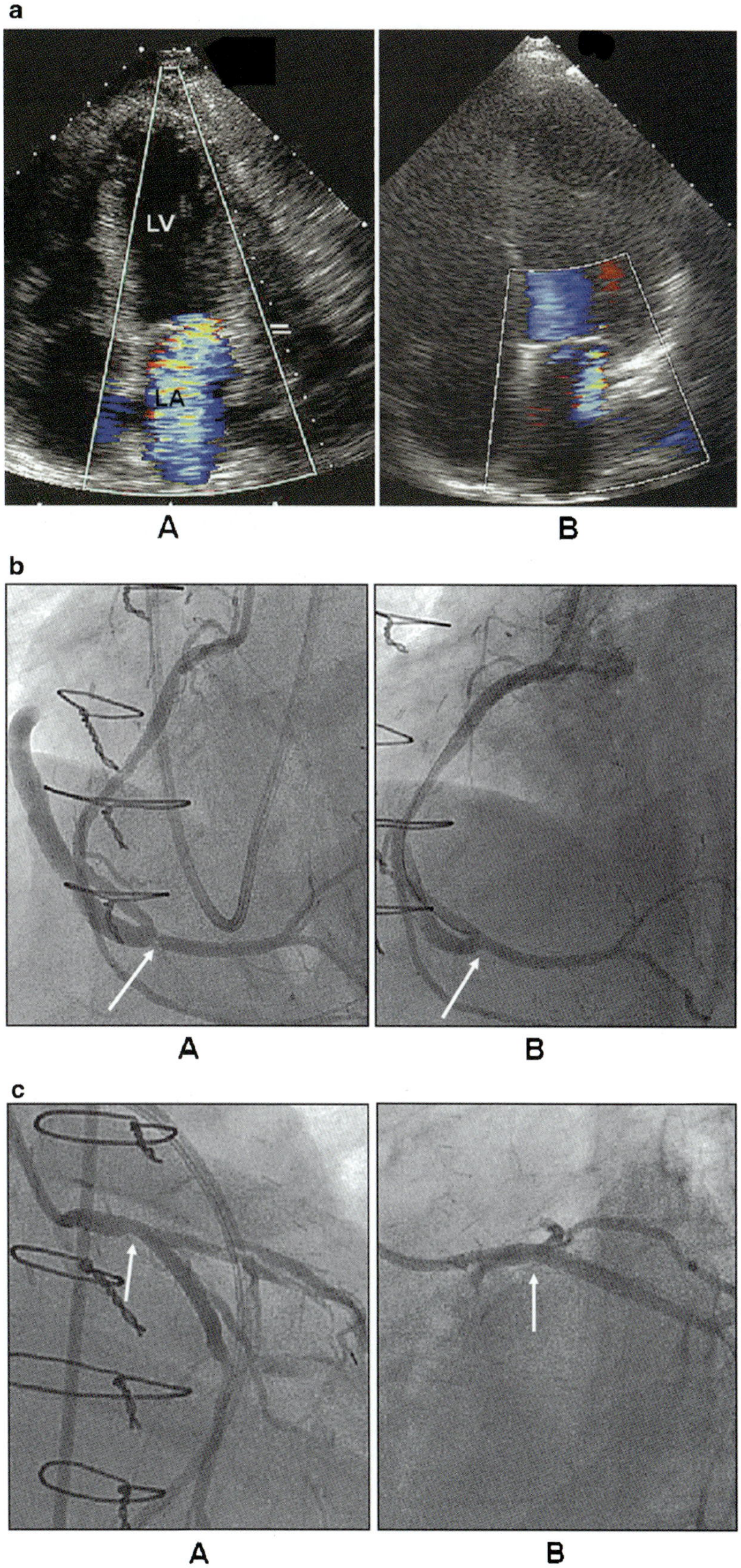

Fig. 3.8 (**a–c**) A patient with severe mitral regurgitation after myocardial infarction without papillary musclerupture. (**a**) *A* Echocardiogram shows severe mitral regurgitation. *B* Post coronary revascularization by PCI, there is improved LV systolic function and only residual mild mitral regurgitation. (**b**) Right coronary arteriorgram from the patient illustrated in Fig. 3.8a. *A* Severe stenosis of the distal RCA (*arrow*). *B* Shows restoration of blood flow post revascularization by PCI (*arrow*). (**c**) Left coronary arteriogram. *A* Severe stenosis of the left main (*arrow*) (LM). *B* Shows restoration of blood flow post PCI (*arrow*)

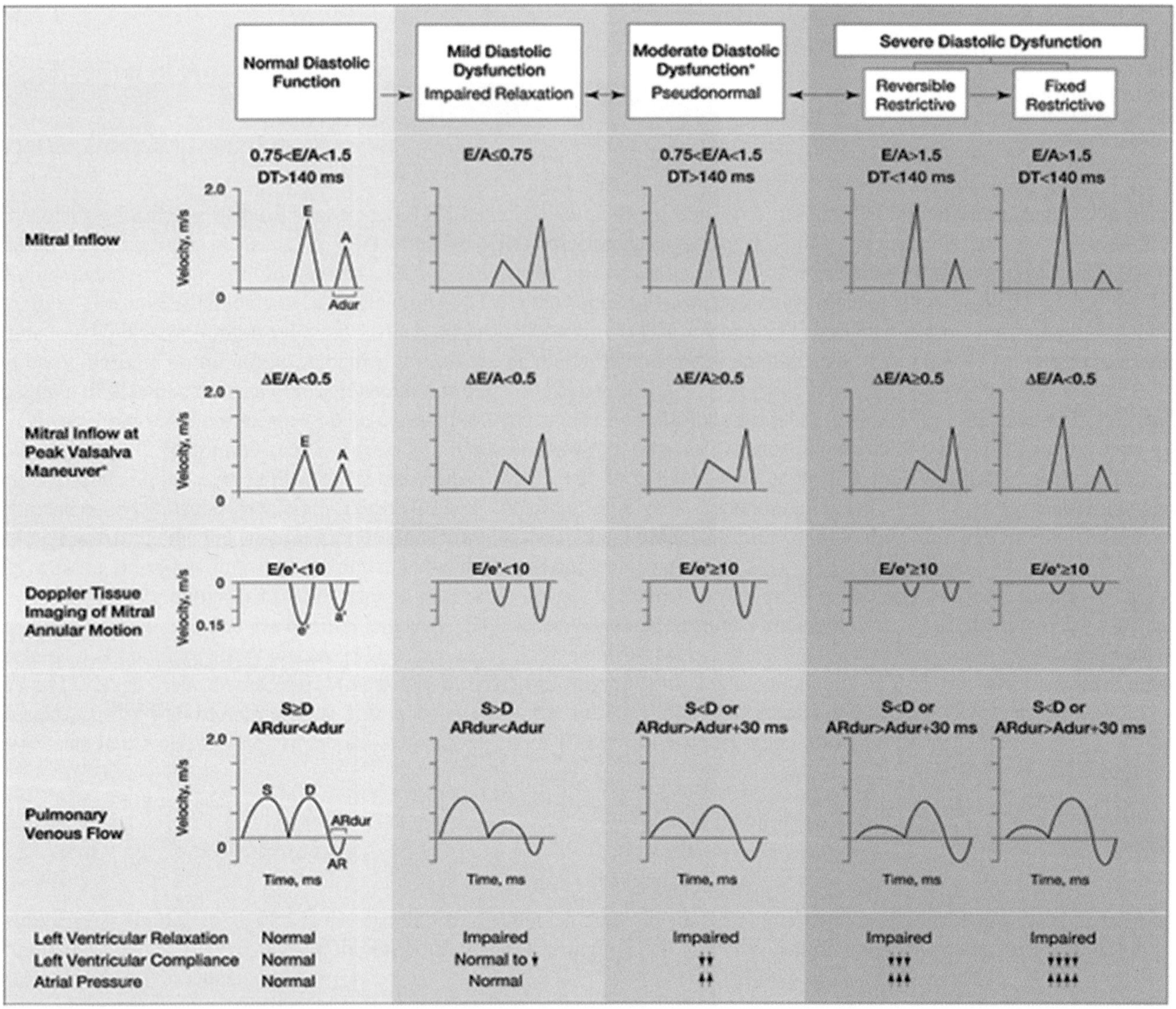

Fig. 3.9 Evaluation of left ventricular filling pressure from assessment of mitral inflow, mitral annular tissue Doppler, and pulmonary venous flow (Adapted from Nagueh et al. [4], Copyright 2009. Elsevier Publishing)

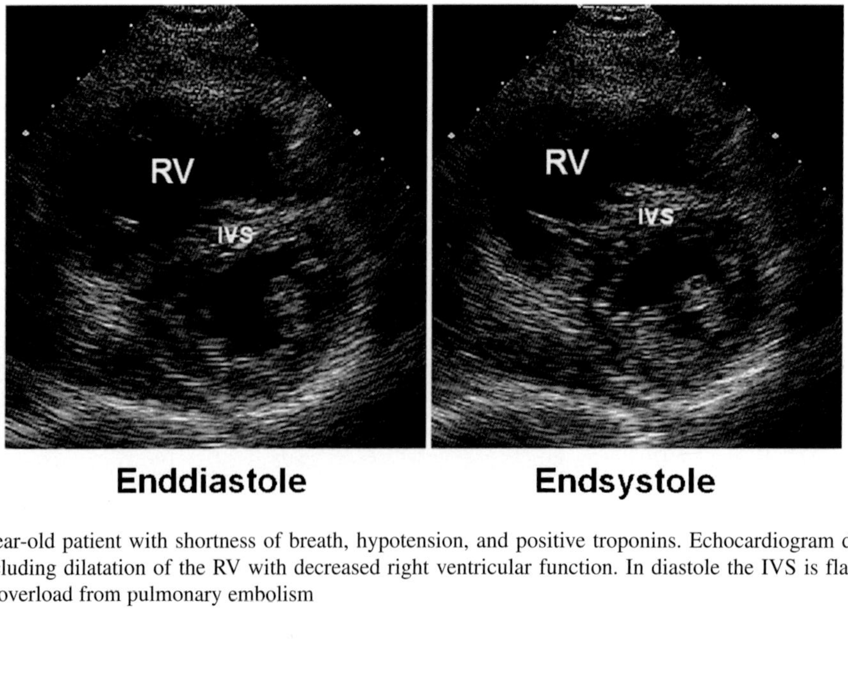

Fig. 3.10 From a 60-year-old patient with shortness of breath, hypotension, and positive troponins. Echocardiogram demonstrates features of acute cor pulmonale including dilatation of the RV with decreased right ventricular function. In diastole the IVS is flat showing the typical D shape of acute pressure overload from pulmonary embolism

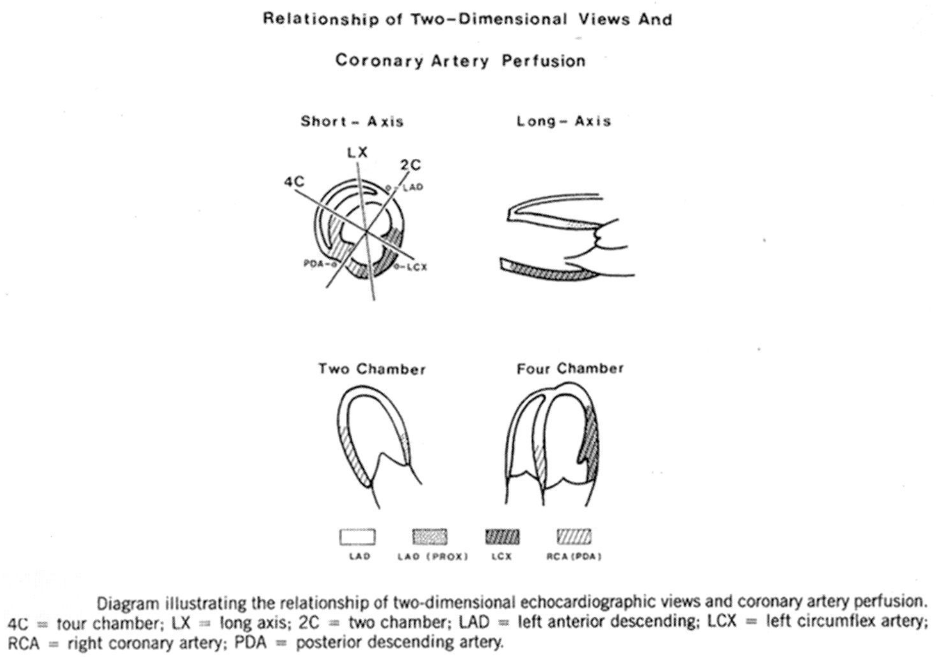

Fig. 3.11 Diagram illustrating the relationship of 2D echocardiographic views and coronary artery perfusion (Adapted from Feigenbaum et al. [14])

include structural cardiac landmarks. 2D echocardiography, however, can provide images of the entire LV, and when certain areas show dysfunction, can be predictive of specific coronary artery occlusion.

The standard views used to image the LV with 2D echocardiography include the parasternal long and short axis and the apical four- and two-chamber views. These are shown in Fig. 3.11 along with the usual coronary artery supply to each area [14]. It is important to remember that coronary artery anatomy is variable and the description of coronary artery supply to various areas of the LV is approximate.

Because the LV is basically symmetrical, one way to determine its global function involves "dividing it" into 16 geometric segments, as shown in Fig. 3.12 [15]. The sum of segmental wall motion scores for each of these 16 segments (normal = 1, hypokinetic = 2, akinetic = 3, dyskinetic = 4 and aneurysmal = 5) divided by 16, can give an assessment of global left ventricular function. Higher wall motion scores are associated with a poor prognosis.

Although ECG changes of STEMI are reasonably specific for acute thrombotic occlusion of an epicardial coronary artery, there are exceptions as illustrated in the following case. The patient was a 45-year-old female who collapsed while rushing to catch a bus. She was found to be in ventricular fibrillation and was resuscitated. An ECG on arrival in the emergency room showed anterolateral ST-segment elevation (Fig. 3.13a) but coronary arteriography at the time of the ECG showed angiographically normal coronary arteries.

An echocardiogram demonstrated a large wall motion abnormality involving the distal 75% of the LV – so called "apical ballooning" (Fig. 3.13b). This syndrome has been described variably in the literature and perhaps is most appropriately referred to as stress cardiomyopathy [16]. It is most typically seen in young women under severe emotional trauma, although we have noted it to be common in either sex with severe trauma or medical conditions. In the case described above, the cause was subarachnoid hemorrhage. In this syndrome, the ST-segment elevation is usually minor but on serial ECGs, the QT interval prolongs and there is marked T wave inversion. Serial echocardiography demonstrates progressive improvement in regional and global left ventricular function.

Although this syndrome typically involves the apex of the LV, atypical cases occur where the wall motion abnormality involves only the base- or midportions of the LV and it may even involve the right ventricle. Importantly, these wall motion abnormalities are not in a typical distribution of an epicardial coronary artery. Their detection with transthoracic echocardiography may be the first indication that the clinical problem is stress cardiomyopathy rather than ACS.

Fig. 3.12 Proposed 16-segment model for wall motion analysis (Adapted from Schiller et al. [15], Copyright 1989. Elsevier publishing)

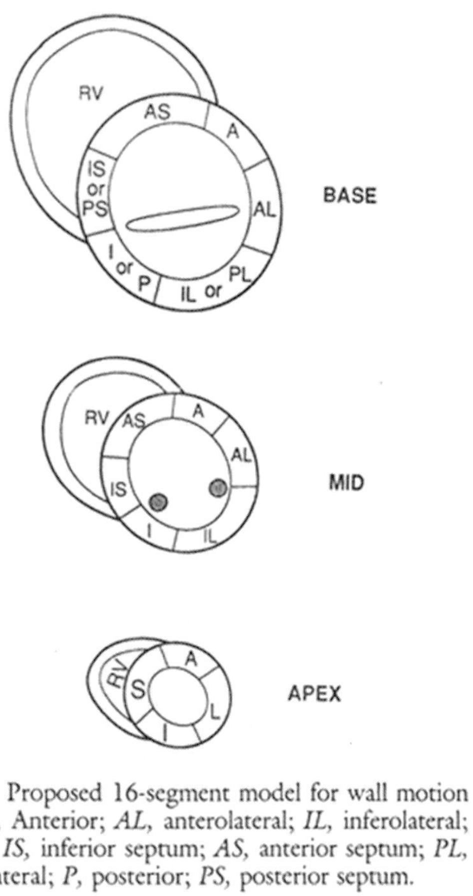

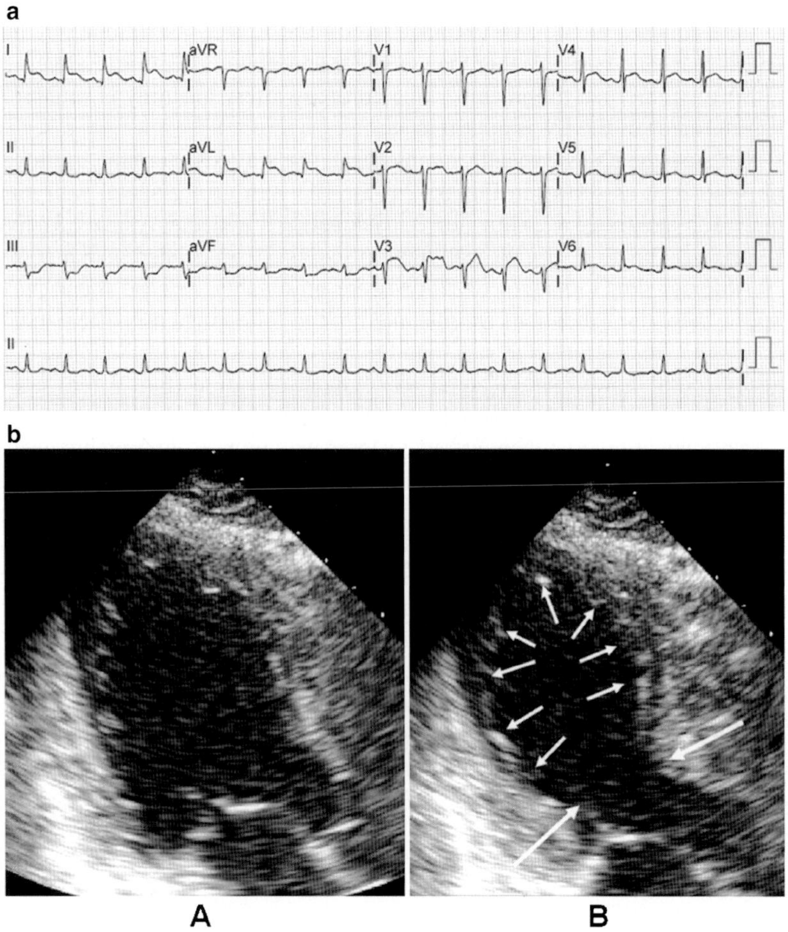

Fig. 3.13 (**a**, **b**) Echocardiographic features seen in stress cardiomyopathy from a 45-year-old female who collapsed while rushing to catch a bus. (**a**) ECG on admission shows anterolateral ST-segment elevation. (**b**) Echocardiogram in endiastole *A* and systole *B* demonstrates a large wall motion abnormality including the distal 75% of the LV called "apical balloning" (*arrows*)

Complications of Myocardial Infarction

Mechanical Complications

Mechanical complications of acute STEMI are less common in the era of primary reperfusion therapy. When the clinical status of a patient with AMI suddenly deteriorates due to shock or pulmonary edema, echocardiography can rapidly diagnose mechanical complications. Rupture of the heart is a mechanical complication that causes devastating hemodynamic compromise, and can involve the LV free wall, the IVS, or the papillary muscle.

Rupture of the Left Ventricular Free Wall

Rupture of the free wall of the LV usually leads to cardiac tamponade and instantaneous death. Occasionally, the rupture is heralded by sudden bradycardia and hypotension with recovery after several minutes [17]. These symptoms should warrant emergent echocardiography since the differential diagnosis would include myocardial rupture and pulmonary embolism.

If the free wall has ruptured, an echocardiogram will show a hematoma within the pericardial space. Although this can be seen in many standard views, it is usually easiest to spot on the subcostal view (Fig. 3.4). The mortality rate is high and emergent surgical intervention is the treatment of choice.

Rupture of the free wall is occasionally contained by accompanying pericarditis, hematoma, or thrombus. The patient may survive initially, only to succumb when the contained rupture again ruptures into the free pericardial space. Echocardiography can detect such contained ruptures and the use of echocontrast can be valuable in defining thrombus in the left ventricular that extends beyond the borders of the LV, indicating a contained rupture (Fig. 3.14a). If free wall rupture is contained, it may develop into a pseudoaneurysm of the LV after the contained thrombus lyses (Fig. 3.14b). These are also prone to rupture causing tamponade and sudden death so their detection warrants surgical intervention.

Rupture of the Interventricular Septum

Patients with rupture of the IVS usually have acute hemodynamic compromise and a new holosystolic murmur along the left sternal border. This clinical course warrants immediate transthoracic echocardiography to detect this possible mechanical complication. The mechanical rupture may be apparent by 2D imaging (Fig. 3.5) but if the rupture is small, color flow imaging showing left-to-right communication is useful to establishing the diagnosis. Surgical repair can be successful and may even be delayed pending stability of the patient.

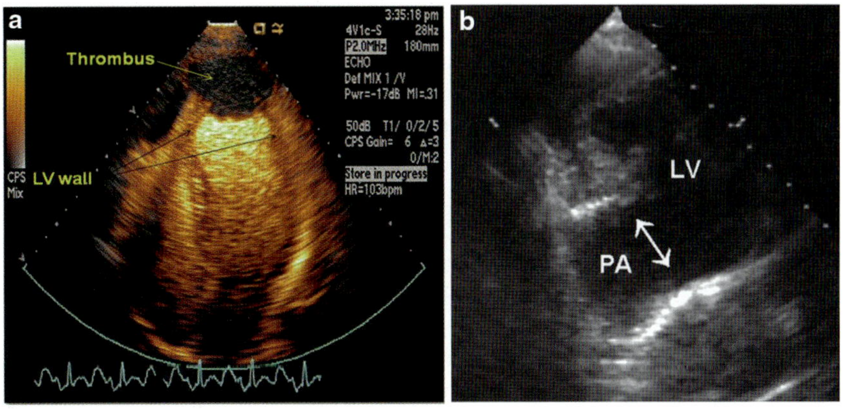

Fig. 3.14 (**a**) Contained rupture of LV apex with large thrombus following anterior infarction. Courtesy from Drs. Alok Sharma and Valerie K Ulstead, Hennepin County Medical Center, Minneapolis, MN. (**b**) Echocardiogram in rupture of the free wall of the LV. After the contained thrombus lysed, a pseudoaneurysm developed. (PA) (*arrows*)

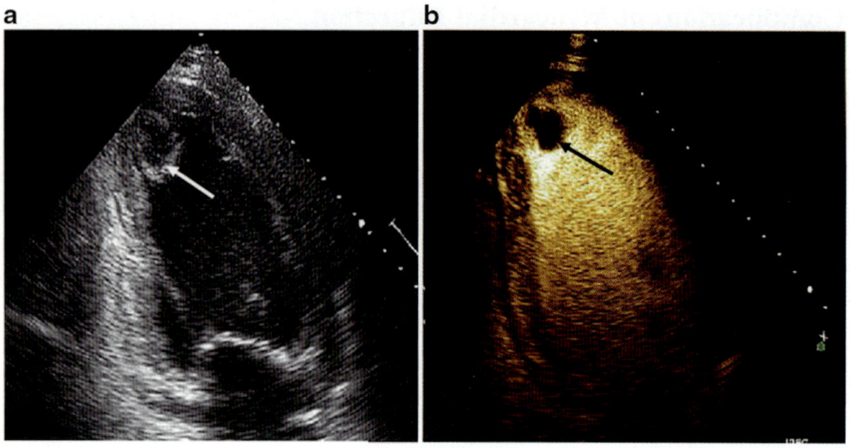

Fig. 3.15 (**a**) Echocardiogram illustrating left ventricular thrombus protruding into the left ventricular cavity (*arrow*). (**b**) The thrombus is better defined with the use of contrast agent (*arrow*)

Rupture of a Papillary Muscle

Patients may survive acute rupture of a papillary muscle, but show evidence of acute hemodynamic compromise, usually in the form of pulmonary edema and hypotension accompanied by an apical holosystolic murmur. Standard images particularly from the apical view frequently establish the diagnosis and demonstrate torrential mitral insufficiency. When the transthoracic findings are not typical or nondiagnostic, transesophageal echocardiography is most helpful in establishing anatomy of the mitral valve and its supporting structures (Fig. 3.6a, b). This diagnosis should prompt emergent surgical intervention.

Nonmechanical Complications of Acute Myocardial Infarction

Mural Thrombus

Mural thrombi can complicate AMI. The most common location for thrombi is the apex of the LV following anterior myocardial infarction [18]. Apical stasis is likely to be severe following acute anterior STEMI particularly when effective reperfusion is not achieved. In the pre-reperfusion era, as many as 30% of patients with acute anterior STEMI developed left ventricular thrombi and about 10% of these had a peripheral embolism.

Isolated infarctions in the distribution of the right or left circumflex coronary arteries usually do not cause apical stasis, and are less likely to be complicated by left ventricular thrombus and systemic embolism. There is a higher risk of embolism from left ventricular thrombus when the thrombus protrudes into the left ventricular cavity and/or exhibits independent motion (Fig. 3.15) [19]. Thrombi are less likely to embolize when they are mural or flat, and do not exhibit free intercavity motion, as illustrated in Fig. 3.16. Echo contrast agents significantly enhance the diagnostic capability of 2D echocardiography for detection of left ventricular thrombus [20, 21]. Since thrombi have no blood flow, they are echo lucent with echo contrast and easily distinguished from left ventricular blood and myocardium.

Right Ventricular Infarction

Inferior wall myocardial infarction may be complicated by right ventricular infarction [22]. This occurs with occlusion in the right coronary artery before its acute marginal branches (Fig. 3.7a–c). Right ventricular infarction is commonly associated with systemic hypotension and shock. Echocardiographic features include a dilated, poorly functioning right ventricle. When tricuspid insufficiency is present and its jet can be evaluated with Doppler, the peak velocity is low, indicating reduced contractility of the right ventricle. This contrasts with acute pulmonary embolus, where the peak flow velocity would be increased (Fig. 3.10).

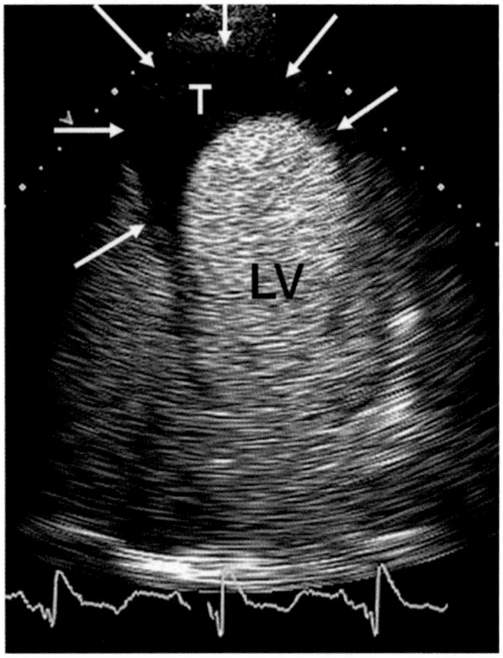

Fig. 3.16 Echocardiogram with contrast agent demonstrating a mural or flat thrombus (*arrows*)

Mitral Insufficiency

Occasionally severe mitral insufficiency develops after myocardial infarction without papillary muscle rupture. The usual causes include ischemic papillary muscle dysfunction or dilatation of the LV. Regardless of the cause, severe mitral insufficiency can be detected by color flow imaging (Fig. 3.8a). In this case, PCI of severe right (Fig. 3.8b) and left main (Fig. 3.8c) coronary lesions markedly decreased mitral insufficiency.

Pericardial Effusion

Occasionally, STEMI can be complicated by pericarditis, with free pericardial fluid but no hematoma. Postinfarction pericarditis is much less common with timely, successful reperfusion and the absence of long-term therapeutic anticoagulation.

Stress Echocardiography

Digital technology has sped and improved interpretation of stress echocardiography through side-by-side comparison of pre- and post-stress images from the same acoustic window. Contrast agents that enhance endocardial definition have also improved the ability to obtain diagnostic images from patients who are otherwise difficult to image [23, 24]. These technical advances have markedly improved the quality and diagnostic capabilities of stress echocardiography which can be done with either exercise or pharmacologic stress.

Exercise Stress

Exercise stress imaging is based on the principle that when myocardial oxygen demand exceeds supply to a segment of left ventricular wall, it decreases or stops normal thickening and motion. The earliest sign of ischemia experimentally is a decrease in diastolic performance followed by a decrease in systolic thickening and motion [6].

A reversible change in systolic thickening and motion is the echocardiographic hallmark for myocardial ischemia. Relief of ischemia reverses this process and systolic function improves before diastolic function. Since diastolic parameters recover more slowly than systolic parameters of wall thickening and motion after stress-induced ischemia, they may be obtained after acquiring systolic parameters. The combination of reduced systolic motion and wall thickening in the distribution of an epicardial coronary artery indicates ischemia and the reversibility of these findings specifically supports the diagnosis of occlusive coronary artery disease.

Bicycle

Bicycle exercise has the potential advantage of continuous monitoring of the echocardiogram to detect ischemic changes or decline in global function of the LV. However, this technique is labor intensive and, in general, has been replaced with treadmill exercise. It is used primarily to monitor hemodynamic parameters such as pulmonary artery pressure in patients being evaluated for valvular heart disease.

Treadmill

Treadmill exercise is the traditional mode of exercise for evaluating coronary artery disease. It does not allow continuous monitoring of echocardiographic images, instead relying on the rapid acquisition of images immediately after exercise. When using treadmill exercise, it is critical to obtain images within the first two minutes following exercise.

Using digital technology and large memory storage, images of each beat postexercise are routinely obtained from the four traditional acoustic windows (parasternal long and short axes and apical four and two-chamber views). A single beat from each view is chosen from rest and postexercise. With bi- or quad-screen capabilities, it is then possible to view pre- and postexercise beats side-by-side for comparison. Figure 3.17a compares pre- and postexercise echocardiograms from a patient with exertional angina. Also included is a coronary angiogram that demonstrates a subtotal occlusion of the LAD which was treated with PCI and placement of a stent (Fig. 3.17b).

Pharmacologic

Dobutamine

Dobutamine stress echocardiography is performed with constant ECG and blood pressure monitoring. Typically it is performed with the patient in the left lateral decubitus position with echocardiographic images obtained from the four standard views. Dobutamine is infused in incremental doses while evaluating the effect on heart rate and rhythm, blood pressure, and both global and regional systolic performance of the LV. Dobutamine has a positive chronotropic and ionotropic effect, increasing the contractility of the myocardium. As with treadmill exercise, the objective is to increase myocardial oxygen demand. If the heart rate does not respond, atropine is frequently used in conjunction with dobutamine to achieve 85% maximum heart rate for the patient's age. In contrast to treadmill exercise, dobutamine stress echocardiography is performed in a stationary position throughout the study optimizing image acquisition. A unique advantage of dobutamine over exercise stress echocardiography is the ability to assess for viable but hibernating myocardium [25, 26]. This is performed with relatively low doses of dobutamine while evaluating the function of a region of severe hypokinesis or akinesis of the LV. If the function of this area increases with low dose of dobutamine, viability is assumed and revascularization is likely to improve contractility. Higher doses of dobutamine may result in ischemia and the function of the affected area may decrease. This combination of improvement in regional function at low doses and deterioration in function at higher doses of dobutamine is referred to as a biphasic response.

In contrast to exercise stress echocardiography, provocable ischemia may not result in an increase in end-diastolic left ventricular volume although regional dysfunction may occur. Experience in interpretation is needed given this limitation. Further, arrhythmias occasionally occur with the use of dobutamine, including atrial fibrillation and ventricular tachycardia.

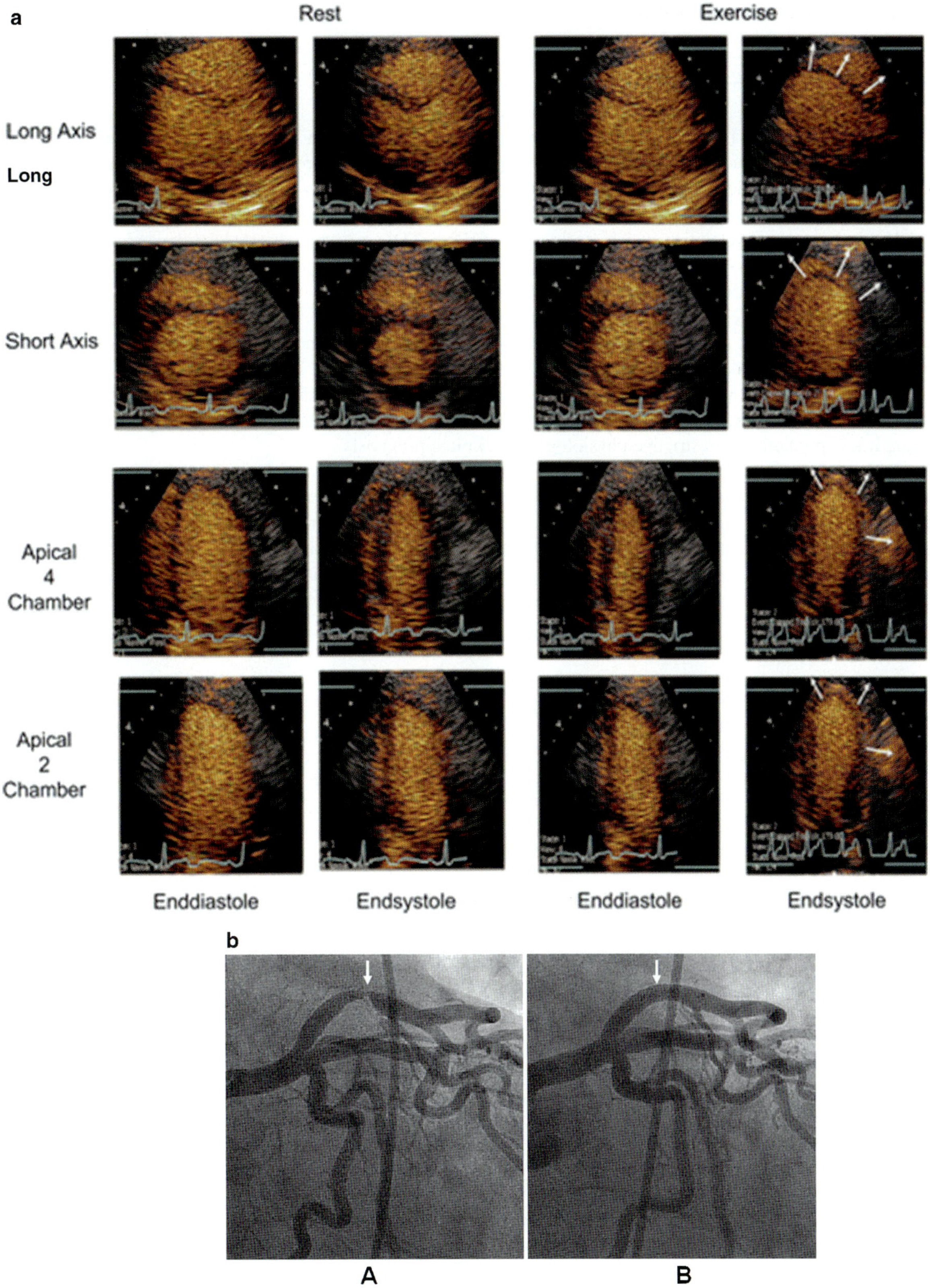

Fig. 3.17 (**a**, **b**) A patient with exertional angina. (**a**) Treadmill exercise compares pre- and postexercise echocardiogram, demonstrating apical wall motion abnormality (*arrows*) at peak exercise. (**b**) *A* Coronary angiogram demonstrates a subtotal occlusion of the LAD (*arrow*). *B* Post PCI and placement of a stent shows no residual stenosis (*arrow*)

Application of Advance Techniques

Tissue Doppler Imaging

Systolic performance of the LV has powerful prognostic value in patients with myocardial infarction or congestive heart failure. The addition of tissue Doppler imaging (TDI) to echocardiography provides considerable ancillary information complementary to LV systolic function. TDI uses Doppler principles to quantify low-velocity signals of myocardial tissue motion. The most commonly used application of TDI in the context of coronary artery disease is assessing the LV's diastolic function. Unlike transmitral velocities, which are preload sensitive, TDI assessment is less load-dependent. The combination of early diastolic mitral inflow velocities (E) and the medial or lateral mitral annular motion (e') helps characterize varying patterns of diastolic dysfunction as illustrated in Fig. 3.9 [27].

An E/e' ratio >15 correlates with an elevated left ventricular end-diastolic pressure [28] and is an independent predictor of survival [29]. Importantly, an E/e' ratio >15 has been shown to provide prognostic information beyond that provided by clinical and routine echocardiographic parameters. Moreover, in patients with acute MI, the "restrictive" filling pattern, characterized by a short deceleration time (DT), is a predictor of adverse LV remodeling and mortality [30]. One limitation of TDI is that the medial annulus motion may be abnormal in the presence of inferior infarction with wall motion abnormality, making it less predictive of restrictive physiology and clinical prognosis.

Color TDI superimposes a color map on gray scale images to indicate direction of myocardial velocity, thereby increasing image resolution. The use of color encoded TDI has been studied in patients undergoing stress echocardiography for the detection of coronary artery disease [31]. When using dobutamine stress echocardiography, peak systolic myocardial velocity and average tissue displacement (measured by TDI) were significantly lower in patients with more cardiovascular events, despite similar wall motion scores. TDI is also used in the echocardiographic assessment of LV dyssynchrony, which has relevance in the optimization of cardiac resynchronization therapy in patients with cardiomyopathy [32].

2D Strain by Speckle Tracking

The primary limitation of TDI is the inability to distinguish active myocardial contractility or thickening from passive or "tethering" myocardial motion on the basis of changes in myocardial velocity. Additionally, assessing apical function is difficult using TDI alone.

Strain rate imaging offers a more "site-specific" approach to counter these limitations. Strain measures regional deformation. It is defined as the change in length between myocardial contraction and relaxation (expressed as a percentage). Strain rate measures the velocity gradient between two points and represents rate of change of myocardial deformation [33].

This technique is also referred to as "myocardial deformation imaging" and is exemplified by "myocardial speckle tracking" using 2D echocardiography. A small myocardial area of interest with its unique speckle pattern can be tracked throughout the cardiac cycle using commercially available software. This can be performed in a multidimensional fashion in different directions, lending to the estimation of radial and circumferential strains.

Being Doppler based, the accuracy of this technique is dependent on the angle of incidence. Myocardial strain is significantly load-dependent like TDI [34]. The primary application of this technology is assessment of systolic LV function, especially regional function.

3D Echocardiography

The most obvious use of 3DE for coronary heart disease is accurate determination of left ventricular volumes to calculate LVEF. With coronary heart disease, regional variation in wall motion limits the accuracy of M-mode and 2D echocardiography for determining LV volumes. This is particularly true if the techniques make geometric assumptions about the left ventricular shape.

Simpson's biplane technique from 2D echocardiographic apical images does not assume specific geometry of the LV, but uses limited tomographic views. 3DE allows assessment of "true" LV volumes by avoiding geometric assumptions, and the potential for underestimation of volumes secondary to foreshortening.

The improved accuracy and reproducibility of this technique has also been demonstrated with real time (RT)-3DE [35]. RT-3DE has also been studied in conjunction with stress echocardiography, which is advantageous in that it provides shorter acquisition times with full volume datasets and reduced operator dependence [36]. However, the spatial resolution of the images is limited and frame rates are typically low at peak stress. Overall, this technique is time consuming, which limits its clinical use.

Myocardial Contrast Echocardiography

Myocardial contrast echocardiography (MCE) determines myocardia perfusion with continuous intravenous infusion of a contrast agent. MCE utilizes high-molecular-weight, inert gases that form microbubbles which can consistently traverse the pulmonary circulation after intravenous injection [37]. With echo contrast circulating in the myocardium, a pulse of high-energy ultrasound breaks all microbubbles instantaneously. Reperfusion of LV then occurs and its timing and intensity can characterize blood flow to specific areas of the myocardium.

With this technique's added potential for quantification, several clinical applications are possible. First, MCE can be used in the setting of chest pain to detect ACS and to assess adequacy of myocardial revascularization [38, 39]. Second, it can be used following stress echocardiography to identify myocardial ischemia, indicating obstructive coronary artery disease [40]. Third, assessing myocardial perfusion can determine whether the myocardial microcirculation is intact, differentiating viable, stunned, or hibernating myocardium from nonviable myocardium [41].

References

1. Kisslo JA, vonRamm OT, Thurstone FL. Dynamic cardiac imaging using a focused, phased-array ultrasound system. Am J Med. 1977;63(1): 61–8.
2. Tei C, Sakamaki T, Shah PM, et al. Myocardial contrast echocardiography: a reproducible technique of myocardial opacification for identifying regional perfusion deficits. Circulation. 1983;67(3):585–93.
3. Quinones MA, Otto CM, Stoddard M, Waggoner A, Zoghbi WA. Recommendations for quantification of Doppler echocardiography: a report from the Doppler Quantification Task Force of the Nomenclature and Standards Committee of the American Society of Echocardiography. J Am Soc Echocardiogr. 2002;15(2):167–84.
4. Nagueh SF, Appleton CP, Gillebert TC, et al. Recommendations for the evaluation of left ventricular diastolic function by echocardiography. J Am Soc Echocardiogr. 2009;22(2):107–33.
5. Gorcsan III J, Abraham T, Agler DA, et al. Echocardiography for cardiac resynchronization therapy: recommendations for performance and reporting–a report from the American Society of Echocardiography Dyssynchrony Writing Group endorsed by the Heart Rhythm Society. J Am Soc Echocardiogr. 2008;21(3):191–213.
6. Stewart JT, Grbic M, Sigwart U. Left atrial and left ventricular diastolic function during acute myocardial ischaemia. Br Heart J. 1992; 68(4):377–81.
7. Alpert JS. No change in post-myocardial infarction prognostic factors. Eur Heart J. 1997;18(1):11–2.
8. Touboul P, Andre-Fouet X, Leizorovicz A, et al. Risk stratification after myocardial infarction. A reappraisal in the era of thrombolysis. The Groupe d'Etude du Pronostic de l'Infarctus du Myocarde (GREPI). Eur Heart J. 1997;18(1):99–107.
9. Bendjelid K, Romand JA, Walder B, Suter PM, Fournier G. Correlation between measured inferior vena cava diameter and right atrial pressure depends on the echocardiographic method used in patients who are mechanically ventilated. J Am Soc Echocardiogr. 2002;15(9):944–9.
10. Teichholz LE, Kreulen T, Herman MV, Gorlin R. Problems in echocardiographic volume determinations: echocardiographic-angiographic correlations in the presence of absence of asynergy. Am J Cardiol. 1976;37(1):7–11.
11. Lang RM, Bierig M, Devereux RB, et al. Recommendations for chamber quantification: a report from the American Society of Echocardiography's Guidelines and Standards Committee and the Chamber Quantification Writing Group, developed in conjunction with the European Association of Echocardiography, a branch of the European Society of Cardiology. J Am Soc Echocardiogr. 2005;18(12):1440–63.
12. Gehrke J, Leeman S, Raphael M, Pridie RB. Non-invasive left ventricular volume determination by two-dimensional echocardiography. Br Heart J. 1975;37(9):911–6.
13. Goerke RJ, Carlsson E. Calculation of right and left cardiac ventricular volumes. Method using standard computer equipment and biplane angiocardiograms. Invest Radiol. 1967;2(5):360–7.
14. Feigenbaum H, Armstrong WF, Ryan TJ, editors. Feigenbaum's echocardiography, 6 edn. Philadelphia, PA: Lippincott Williams & Wilkins; 2005. p. 876.
15. Schiller NB, Shah PM, Crawford M, et al. Recommendations for quantitation of the left ventricle by two-dimensional echocardiography. American Society of Echocardiography Committee on Standards, Subcommittee on Quantitation of Two-Dimensional Echocardiograms. J Am Soc Echocardiogr. 1989;2(5):358–67.
16. Sharkey SW, Lesser JR, Zenovich AG, et al. Acute and reversible cardiomyopathy provoked by stress in women from the United States. Circulation. 2005;111(4):472–9.

17. Oliva PB, Hammill SC, Edwards WD. Cardiac rupture, a clinically predictable complication of acute myocardial infarction: report of 70 cases with clinicopathologic correlations. J Am Coll Cardiol. 1993;22(3):720–6.
18. Asinger RW, Mikell FL, Elsperger J, Hodges M. Incidence of left-ventricular thrombosis after acute transmural myocardial infarction. Serial evaluation by two-dimensional echocardiography. N Engl J Med. 1981;305(6):297–302.
19. Haugland JM, Asinger RW, Mikell FL, Elsperger J, Hodges M. Embolic potential of left ventricular thrombi detected by two-dimensional echocardiography. Circulation. 1984;70(4):588–98.
20. Mansencal N, Nasr IA, Pilliere R, et al. Usefulness of contrast echocardiography for assessment of left ventricular thrombus after acute myocardial infarction. Am J Cardiol. 2007;99(12):1667–70.
21. Thanigaraj S, Schechtman KB, Perez JE. Improved echocardiographic delineation of left ventricular thrombus with the use of intravenous second-generation contrast image enhancement. J Am Soc Echocardiogr. 1999;12(12):1022–6.
22. Cohn JN, Guiha NH, Broder MI, Limas CJ. Right ventricular infarction. Clinical and hemodynamic features. Am J Cardiol. 1974;33(2): 209–14.
23. Mulvagh SL, Rakowski H, Vannan MA, et al. American Society of Echocardiography Consensus Statement on the Clinical Applications of Ultrasonic Contrast Agents in Echocardiography. J Am Soc Echocardiogr. 2008;21(11):1179–201.
24. Timperley J, Mitchell AR, Becher H. Contrast echocardiography for left ventricular opacification. Heart. 2003;89(12):1394–7.
25. La CG, Alfieri O, Giubbini R, Gargano M, Ferrari R, Visioli O. Echocardiography during infusion of dobutamine for identification of reversibly dysfunction in patients with chronic coronary artery disease. J Am Coll Cardiol. 1994;23(3):617–26.
26. Pierard LA, De Landsheere CM, Berthe C, Rigo P, Kulbertus HE. Identification of viable myocardium by echocardiography during dobutamine infusion in patients with myocardial infarction after thrombolytic therapy: comparison with positron emission tomography. J Am Coll Cardiol. 1990;15(5):1021–31.
27. Redfield MM, Jacobsen SJ, Burnett Jr JC, Mahoney DW, Bailey KR, Rodeheffer RJ. Burden of systolic and diastolic ventricular dysfunction in the community: appreciating the scope of the heart failure epidemic. JAMA. 2003;289(2):194–202.
28. Ommen SR, Nishimura RA, Appleton CP, et al. Clinical utility of Doppler echocardiography and tissue Doppler imaging in the estimation of left ventricular filling pressures: a comparative simultaneous Doppler-catheterization study. Circulation. 2000;102(15):1788–94.
29. Hillis GS, Moller JE, Pellikka PA, et al. Noninvasive estimation of left ventricular filling pressure by E/e' is a powerful predictor of survival after acute myocardial infarction. J Am Coll Cardiol. 2004;43(3):360–7.
30. Temporelli PL, Giannuzzi P, Nicolosi GL, et al. Doppler-derived mitral deceleration time as a strong prognostic marker of left ventricular remodeling and survival after acute myocardial infarction: results of the GISSI-3 echo substudy. J Am Coll Cardiol. 2004;43(9):1646–53.
31. Marwick TH, Case C, Leano R, et al. Use of tissue Doppler imaging to facilitate the prediction of events in patients with abnormal left ventricular function by dobutamine echocardiography. Am J Cardiol. 2004;93(2):142–6.
32. Yu CM, Fung JW-H, Zhang Q, et al. Tissue Doppler imaging is superior to strain rate imaging and postsystolic shortening on the prediction of reverse remodeling in both ischemic and nonischemic heart failure after cardiac resynchronization therapy. Circulation. 2004;110(1):66–73.
33. Smiseth OA, Stoylen A, Ihlen H. Tissue Doppler imaging for the diagnosis of coronary artery disease. Curr Opin Cardiol. 2004;19(5):421–9.
34. Urheim S, Edvardsen T, Torp H, Angelsen B, Smiseth OA. Myocardial strain by Doppler echocardiography. Validation of a new method to quantify regional myocardial function. Circulation. 2000;102(10):1158–64.
35. Jenkins C, Bricknell K, Hanekom L, Marwick TH. Reproducibility and accuracy of echocardiographic measurements of left ventricular parameters using real-time three-dimensional echocardiography. J Am Coll Cardiol. 2004;44(4):878–86.
36. Takeuchi M, Lang RM. Three-dimensional stress testing: volumetric acquisitions. Cardiol Clin. 2007;25(2):267–72.
37. Sieswerda GT, Yang L, Boo MB, Kamp O. Real-time perfusion imaging: a new echocardiographic technique for simultaneous evaluation of myocardial perfusion and contraction. Echocardiography. 2003;20(6):545–55.
38. Rinkevich D, Kaul S, Wang XQ, et al. Regional left ventricular perfusion and function in patients presenting to the emergency department with chest pain and no ST-segment elevation. Eur Heart J. 2005;26(16):1606–11.
39. Biagini E, van Geuns RJ, Baks T, et al. Comparison between contrast echocardiography and magnetic resonance imaging to predict improvement of myocardial function after primary coronary intervention. Am J Cardiol. 2006;97(3):361–6.
40. Tsutsui JM, Elhendy A, Anderson JR, Xie F, McGrain AC, Porter TR. Prognostic value of dobutamine stress myocardial contrast perfusion echocardiography. Circulation. 2005;112(10):1444–50.
41. McLean DS, Anadiotis AV, Lerakis S. Role of echocardiography in the assessment of myocardial viability. Am J Med Sci. 2009;337(5): 349–54.

Chapter 4
Nuclear Imaging in Ischemic Heart Disease

Sharmila Dorbala and Marcelo F. Di Carli

Introduction

Ischemic heart disease is one of the major causes of mortality and morbidity in men and women accounting for 34.3% (1 of every 2.9) deaths in the US in 2006 [1]. Noninvasive imaging techniques of echocardiography, nuclear imaging, cardiac CT, and cardiac magnetic resonance imaging have played a major role in the evaluation and management of patients with ischemic heart disease. This chapter will focus on the role of nuclear imaging techniques in the evaluation of ischemic heart disease. We will discuss the clinical applications of the most commonly used nuclear imaging techniques of single-photon emission computed tomography (SPECT) and positron emission tomography (PET) in the evaluation of patients with known or suspected stable coronary artery disease (CAD), acute chest pain and acute coronary syndromes (ACS) (NSTEMI and STEMI), and chronic heart failure.

Stable CAD

Diagnostic Value of MPI

Conventionally, the diagnostic value of MPI in patients with stable CAD has been studied using >50% or >70% stenosis on invasive coronary angiography as a reference standard for CAD (i.e., the test was optimized for detection of obstructive epicardial CAD). However, coronary atherosclerosis is a continuum and even milder degrees of stenoses may be associated with perfusion abnormalities, particularly if associated with endothelial dysfunction. Quantitative assessment of absolute myocardial perfusion with PET MPI may be an ideal technique to assess abnormalities in myocardial perfusion related to either epicardial or microvascular dysfunction of the coronary arteries.

SPECT: The diagnostic value of SPECT MPI in the evaluation of patients with stable symptoms and suspected CAD is well known. In pooled analysis [2], SPECT MPI showed a sensitivity of 87, 89% (exercise and vasodilator SPECT MPI) and a specificity of 73, 75% (exercise and vasodilator SPECT MPI), for the detection of obstructive epicardial CAD on invasive coronary angiography. For tests that are widely used in clinical practice, the sensitivity of the test can be overinflated and the specificity artificially lowered due to posttest referral bias [3]. This is because most patients are referred to an angiogram for the evaluation of an abnormal SPECT MPI thereby increasing test sensitivity and reducing test specificity. Hence, normalcy rates (percent of normal SPECT in patients with a low pretest likelihood of CAD), has been used as a useful surrogate measure for specificity of SPECT MPI. The normalcy rate of SPECT MPI from pooled analysis is 91% [2].

The other factor that can affect test specificity of SPECT MPI is attenuation artifacts. Gated SPECT is a useful technique to discriminate real defects from artifacts. This was initially demonstrated with gated Technetium 99m imaging compared to Thallium-201 imaging [4]. Indeed, several studies have demonstrated that attenuation correction improves test

S. Dorbala, MBBS, FACC (✉)
Division of Nuclear Medicine and Molecular Imaging, Department of Radiology, Brigham and Women's Hospital, Boston, MA, USA
e-mail: sdorbala@partners.org

M.F. Di Carli, MD, FACC
Division of Nuclear Medicine and Molecular Imaging, Department of Radiology and Medicine,
Brigham and Women's Hospital, Boston, MA, USA

Z. Vlodaver et al. (eds.), *Coronary Heart Disease: Clinical, Pathological, Imaging, and Molecular Profiles*,
DOI 10.1007/978-1-4614-1475-9_4, © Springer Science+Business Media, LLC 2012

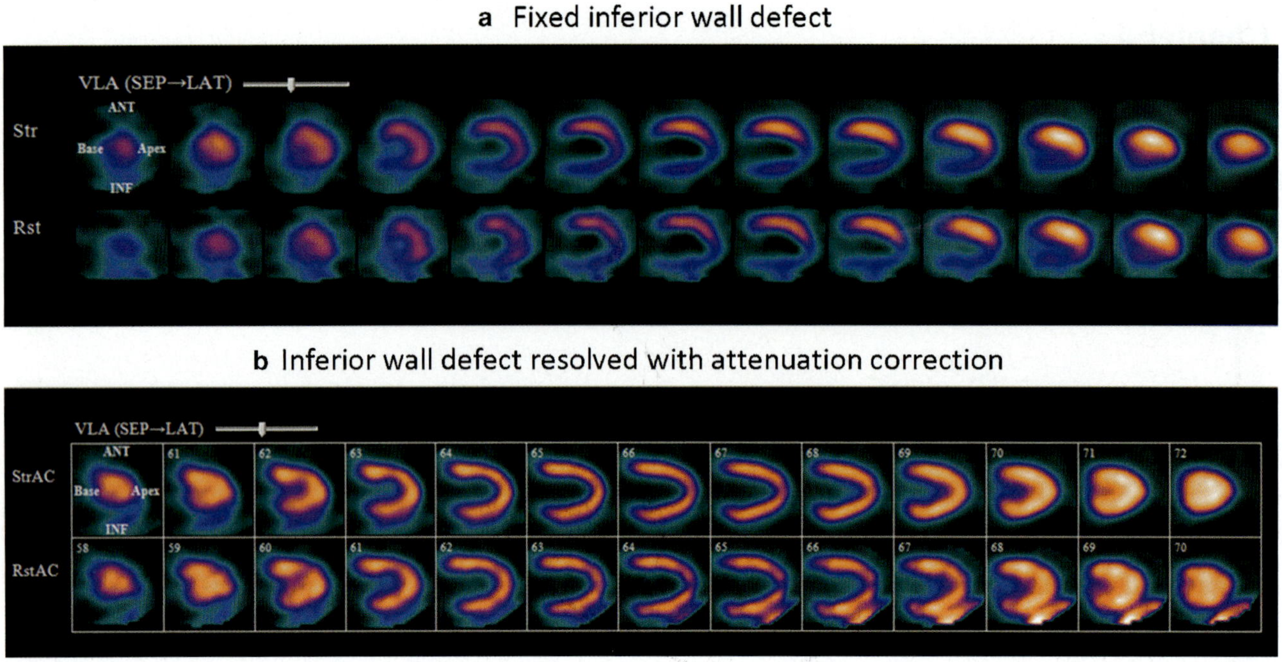

Fig. 4.1 Rest and exercise stress Tc-99m SPECT MPI images in a 58-year-old male with atypical symptoms, demonstrate a fixed inferior wall defect (**a**). The attenuation corrected images (**b**) are normal confirming that the fixed inferior wall defect was likely related to attenuation artifact

specificity while maintaining test sensitivity [5–8]. However, radionuclide attenuation correction for SPECT is not as effective as with PET and hence not widely used.

More recently, SPECT/CT scanners are becoming available. Two studies of SPECT/CT MPI demonstrated improved specificity with no significant changes in sensitivity for SPECT MPI with CT attenuation correction (Fig. 4.1) [9, 10]. Also, there has been a growth in fast SPECT scanners with Cesium Zinc Telluride (CZT, a semiconductor material) detectors. This detector material eliminates the step of scintillation, photomultiplier tubes, and the elaborate electronics required to convert the photon signal into imaging signal. These scanners are typically small foot print SPECT scanners that can complete the rest and stress imaging in 4–6 min, some of them incorporate CT attenuation correction. The CZT detectors have much higher sensitivity (count rich images) and with upright imaging have less interference with subdiaphragmatic activity, and protocols are much faster than with conventional scanners (Fig. 4.2) [11]. Diagnostic accuracy of SPECT MPI with the fast scanners in relation to angiography is not reported; yet, the perfusion images with one of the fast SPECT scanners (DSPECT) have been shown to be concordant to the images with a conventional SPECT scanner [11]. Finally, with the advances in technology and the increasing availability of CT coronary angiography (CTCA), the diagnostic accuracy of MPI is increased by additional testing with CTCA in cases of equivocal SPECT or PET MPI test results (Fig. 4.3).

Last, there has been a heightened awareness among the imaging community and the patients about radiation burden related to medical imaging [12]. Dose estimates for a single day rest and stress Technetium-99 sestamibi are about 13 mSv and for a dual isotope rest Thallium-201 and stress Tc-99m sestamibi study at 25 mSv [12]. Several centers are proposing the use of stress only MPI in low-risk subjects and thereby reduce radiation dose to the patients. Stress only perfusion imaging is also more feasible due to attenuation correction [13, 14].A study of the prognostic value of stress only MPI showed that this technique can be safely used in select patients [15, 16]. In a study of 16,854 patients with normal Tc-99m SPECT (8,034 stress only, 8,820 stress and rest SPECT), all-cause mortality after 5 years of follow-up was similar between patients who underwent stress only compared to rest and stress MPI protocols [15]. Ultra-low-dose protocols are being developed and validated with the newer generation SPECT scanners. With one of the newer generation high sensitivity SPECT scanners, studies are underway using 3 mCi of Technetium −99 m and longer duration of scan acquisition (rather than 10 mCi rest dose and a 4-min scan, use a 3 mCi rest dose and a 10-min scan).

PET: The last decade has evidenced a surge in the use of PET MPI. This is because, scanners are more widely available (for oncology applications) and a generator-produced radiotracer Rubidium-82 has made PET MPI feasible at sites without cyclotrons. PET MPI offers several advantages compared to SPECT MPI in the diagnostic evaluation of ischemic heart disease [17–20]. PET images have higher resolution (spatial and temporal) and attenuation correction is accurate. Accurate attenuation correction (Fig. 4.4) improves diagnostic accuracy (due to high specificity) and makes possible absolute quantification of myocardial blood flow, which is important for assessment of preclinical disease as well as balanced flow

a Conventional SPECT **b** Fast SPECT (DSPECT)

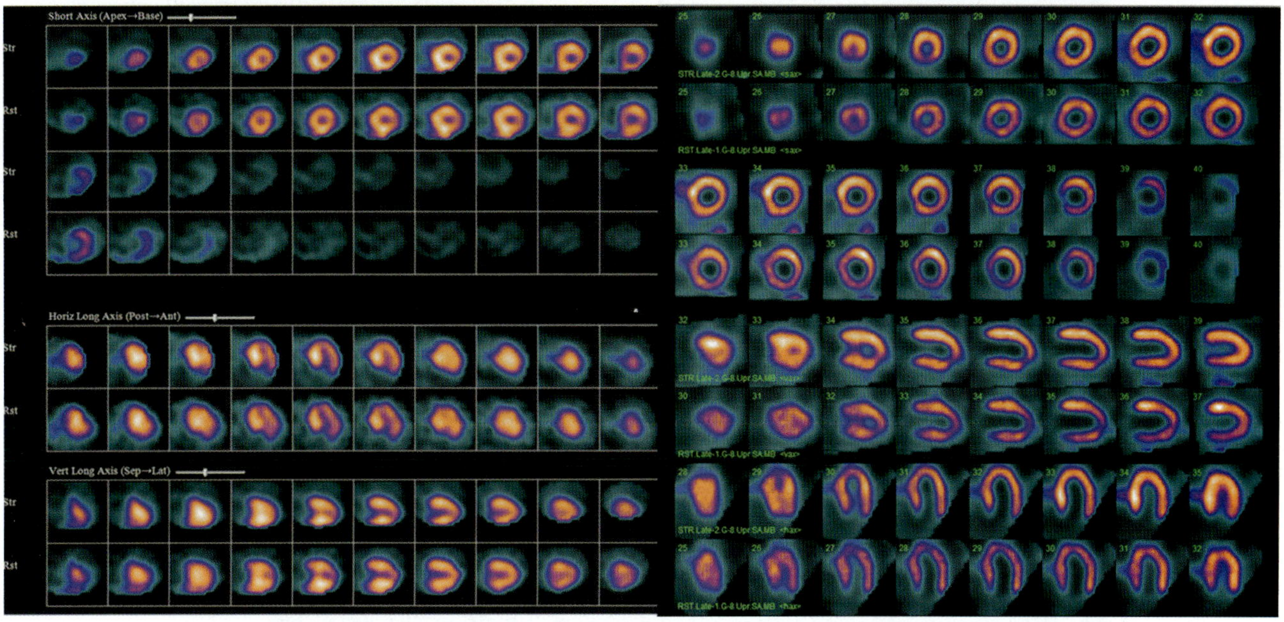

Fig. 4.2 (**a**) Rest and stress Tc99m SPECT images on a conventional dual headed SPECT scanner (rest imaging 14 min, stress imaging 12 min) with limited signal-to-noise ratio a small ventricle. (**b**) Tc99m SPECT images on the same patient imaged using a fast SPECT scanner (DSPECT, rest imaging 6 min, stress imaging 4 min) showing much better image resolution and signal-to-noise ratio

a

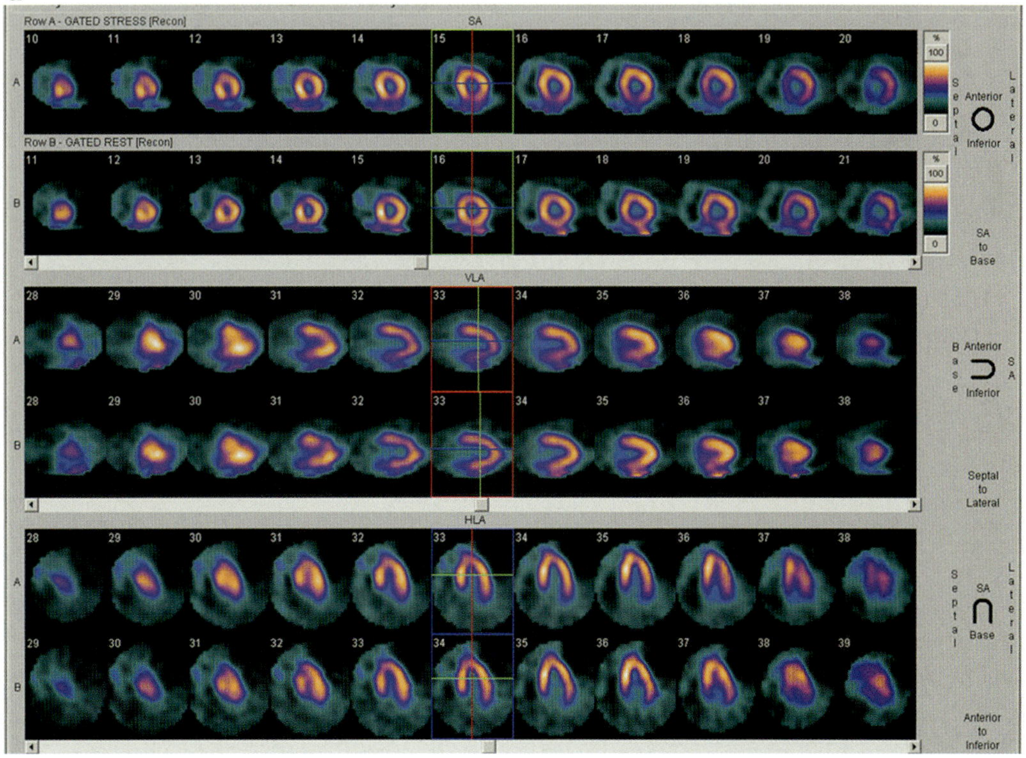

Fig. 4.3 Rest and stress Tc-99m SPECT images of a 67-year-old woman demonstrating a reversible inferior wall perfusion defect (**a**). Rest images were limited by subdiaphragmatic activity. The stress images were repeated in the prone position (**b**), with significant improvement in the inferior wall perfusion defect. The patient exercise 10 min on a standard Bruce protocol without ECG changes, but, experienced typical anginal symptoms. Hence, these findings were felt to be equivocal diagnostically and a CT coronary angiogram study was performed (**c**). These images confirmed severe stenosis in the proximal RCA that was subsequently confirmed on invasive angiography

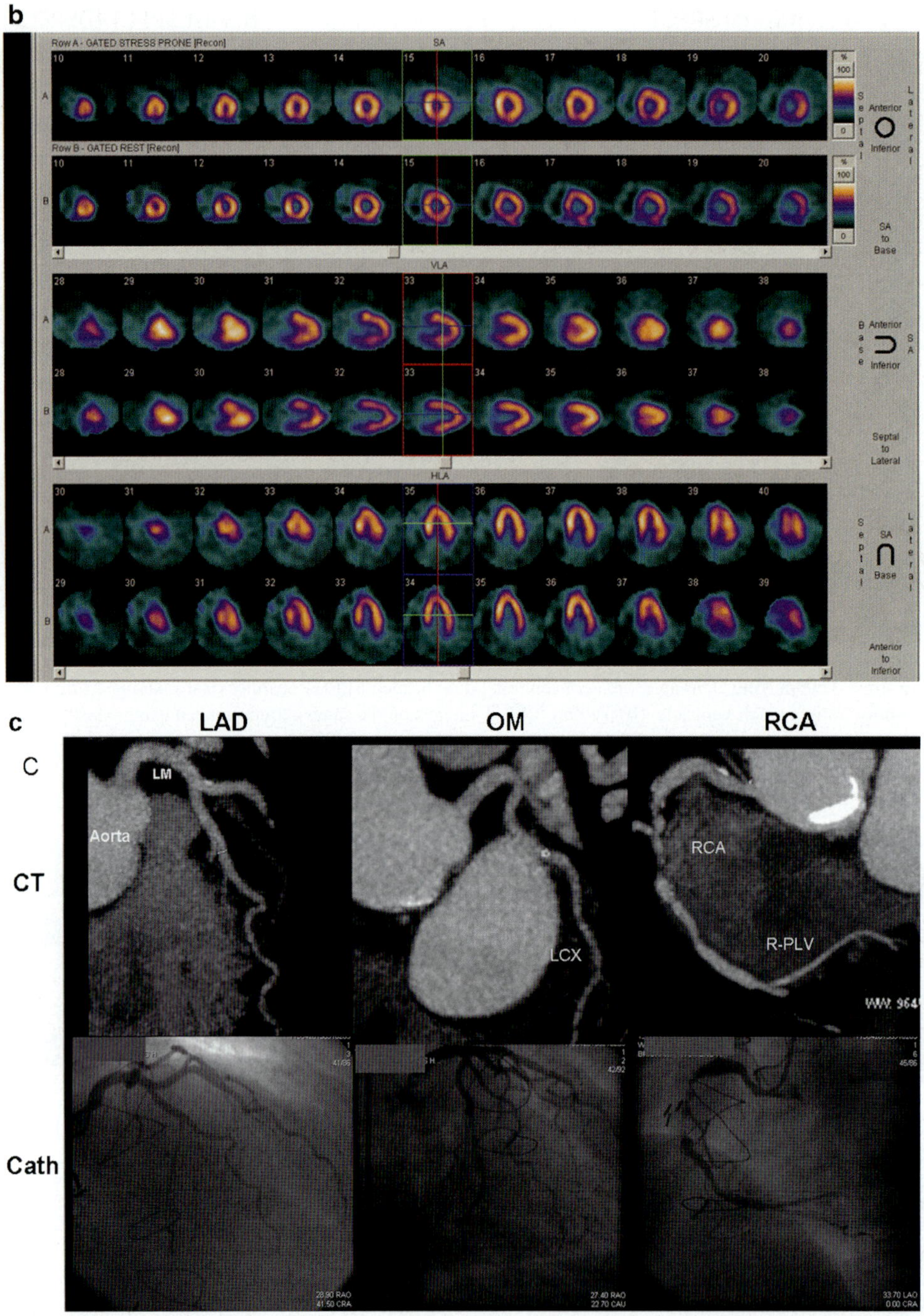

Fig. 4.3 (continued)

reduction (balanced ischemia). Also, the short half-life of the radiotracers makes possible rapid protocols with reduction in radiation dose and peak-stress gating (peak-stress ejection fraction and regional myocardial wall motion abnormalities), which is helpful to identify multivessel CAD. However, PET MPI is expensive and not widely available. Phase 2 clinical studies are underway to evaluate a new perfusion tracer F-18 BMS [21]. This agent will be available as unit doses and has the potential to make PET MPI more widely available.

In pooled analyses, relative PETMPI with N-13 ammonia or Rubidium-82 demonstrated a sensitivity and specificity of 90 and 89%, respectively, for the diagnosis of obstructive epicardial CAD (Table 4.1) [2, 19]. In a study comparing patients undergoing PET MPI with radionuclide attenuation correction with patients undergoing non-attenuation corrected SPECT, diagnostic accuracy of PET MPI was higher due to the higher specificity of PET MPI [22]. Most of the current generation PET scanners are PET/CT scanners with CT-based attenuation correction. Sampson et al. [23] demonstrated a high sensitivity (93%), specificity (83%), and normalcy rate (100%) with Rubidium-82 PET/CT MPI.

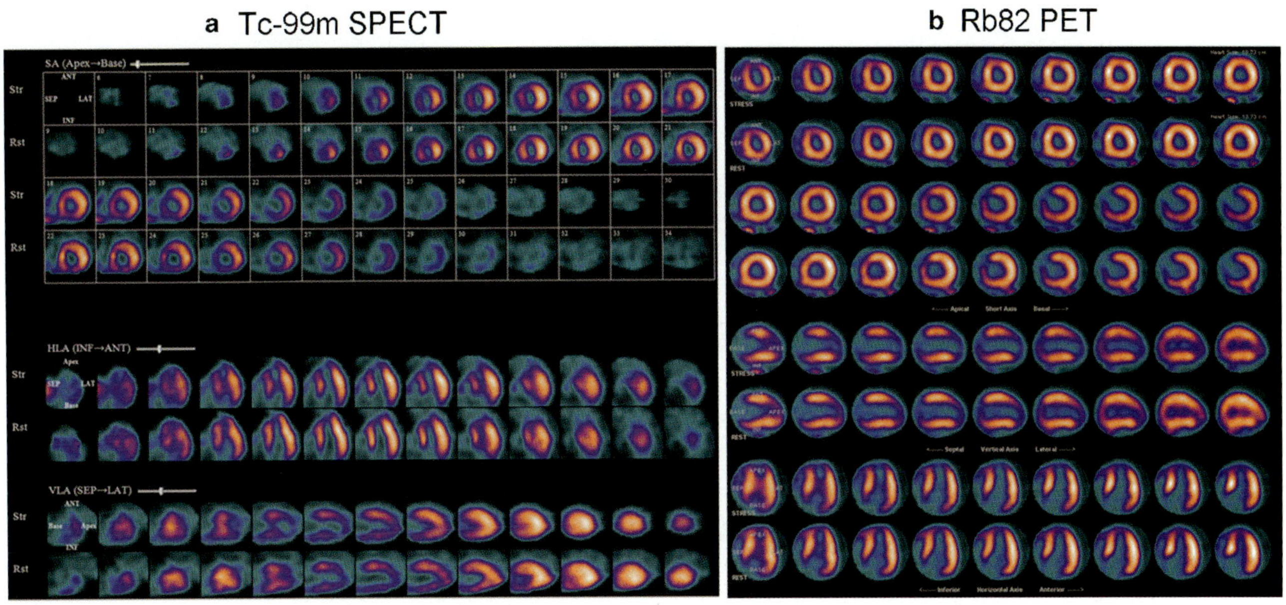

Fig. 4.4 (**a**) Rest and stress Tc99m SPECT images with limited signal-to-noise ratio and a mildly reversible perfusion defect in the mid-anterior and anteroseptal walls, the apical anterior wall, septum, inferior wall, and apex. (**b**) Rubidium-82 PET images on the same patient with a clear cut mildly reversible perfusion defect in the same segments, but with much improved images quality (better signal-to-noise ratio)

Table 4.1 Summary of published literature regarding diagnostic accuracy of PET MPI (Adapted with permission from Di Carli et al. [19])

First author	Stress agent	Patients	Women	Prior CAD	PET radiotracer	Sens	Spece	PPV	NPV	Accuracy
Sampson	Dipyridamole, Adenosine, Dobutamine	102	0.42	0	^{82}Rb	0.93	0.83	0.80	0.94	0.87
Bateman	Dipyridamole	112	0.46	0.25	^{82}Rb	0.87	0.93	0.95	0.81	0.89
Marwick	Dipyridamole + Hand grip	74	0.19	0.49	^{82}Rb	0.90	1	1	0.36	0.91
Gover-Mckay	Dipyridamole + Hand grip	31	0.01	0.13	^{82}Rb	1	0.73	0.80	1	0.87
Stewart	Dipyridamole	81	0.36	0.42	^{82}Rb	0.83	0.86	0.94	0.64	0.84
Go	Dipyridamole	202	NR	0.47	^{82}Rb	0.93	78	0.93	0.80	0.90
Demer	Dipyridamole	193	0.26	0.34	^{82}Rb/^{13}NH$_3$	83	0.95	0.98	0.60	0.85
Tamaki	Supine Bike	51	NR	0.75	^{13}NH$_3$	0.98	1	1	0.75	0.98
Gould	Dipyridamile + Hand grip	31	NR	NR	^{82}Rb/^{13}NH$_3$	0.95	1	1	0.90	0.97
Weighted summary		877	0.29	0.35		0.90	0.89	0.94	0.73	0.90

Sens Sensitivity; *Spec* Specificity; *PPV* positive predictive value; *NPV* negative predictive value; *82Rb* Rubidium 82; *13NH3* N-13 ammonia
[a] Study using PET/CT (where CT is used for attenuation correction only)

Quantitative PET MPI with N-13 ammonia or O-15 water has been used extensively in the evaluation of preclinical functional abnormalities in myocardial blood flow related to atherosclerotic heart disease and coronary risk factors. Subjects with hypertension, left ventricular hypertrophy, diabetes [24], dyslipidemia [25], or smoking [26], and women in postmenopausal state demonstrate abnormalities in stress myocardial blood flow and coronary flow reserve independent of obstructive epicardial coronary artery stenoses [27–29]. Also, subjects with nonischemic [30] and hypertrophic cardiomyopathy [31] demonstrate abnormalities in MBF, which appear to be useful for risk assessment. Indeed, quantitative PET is more sensitive than quantitative coronary angiography in following changes in MBF in response to therapeutic interventions [28].

Risk Stratification with MPI

Myocardial perfusion imaging with SPECT and PET MPI has significant prognostic value. The prognostic value of SPECT MPI has been demonstrated in well over 50,000 patients [2]. Perfusion defect size, severity, and location can be useful to determine risk of future events and therapy [32]. Likewise, the prognostic value of PET MPI has also been validated, albeit in only several thousands of patients (Table 4.2) [17]. A normal SPECT [33] or PET MPI [34] portends excellent prognosis with <1%/year rate of cardiac death or nonfatal myocardial infarction, and an abnormal study is associated with higher event rates (Fig. 4.5).

Table 4.2 Summary of studies evaluating the prognostic value of PET MPI (Reproduced with permission from Al-Mallah et al [17])

First author (Year)	Stress agent	Tracer	Patients No.	Events No.	Event type	Prior CAD%	Percent normal scans	Event/year in normal MPI (%)	Event/year in abnormal MPI
Marwick (1997)	Dipyridamole	^{82}Rb	685	81	Cardiac death	Prior MI 48%, prior revascularization 37%	24	0.9	Mild 2.6%, moderate 5.1%, severe 5.1%
Yoshinaga (2006)	Dipyridamole	^{82}Rb	367	17	Cardiac death or MI	40.3%	70.5	0.4	Mild 2.3%, moderate-severe 7.0%
Lertsburapa (2009)	Dipyridamole	^{82}RB	1,441	132	All cause mortality	53.6%	64.8	2.4	Mild 4.1%, moderate-severe 6.9%
Dorbala (2009)	Dipyridamole	^{82}Rb	1432	140	Cardiac death or MI	30.6%	54	0.7	Mild 5.5%, moderate 5%, severe 11%
Herzog (2009)	Adenosine	^{13}N ammonia	256	29	Cardiac death	66%	45	0.5	3.1%
Chow (2009)	Exercise and Dobutamine	^{82}Rb	124	16	Cardiac death, MI revascularization	MI 40% PCI 29% CABG 15%	37%	1.7%	13%

^{82}Rb = ^{82}Rubidium MI = non-fatal myocardial infarction

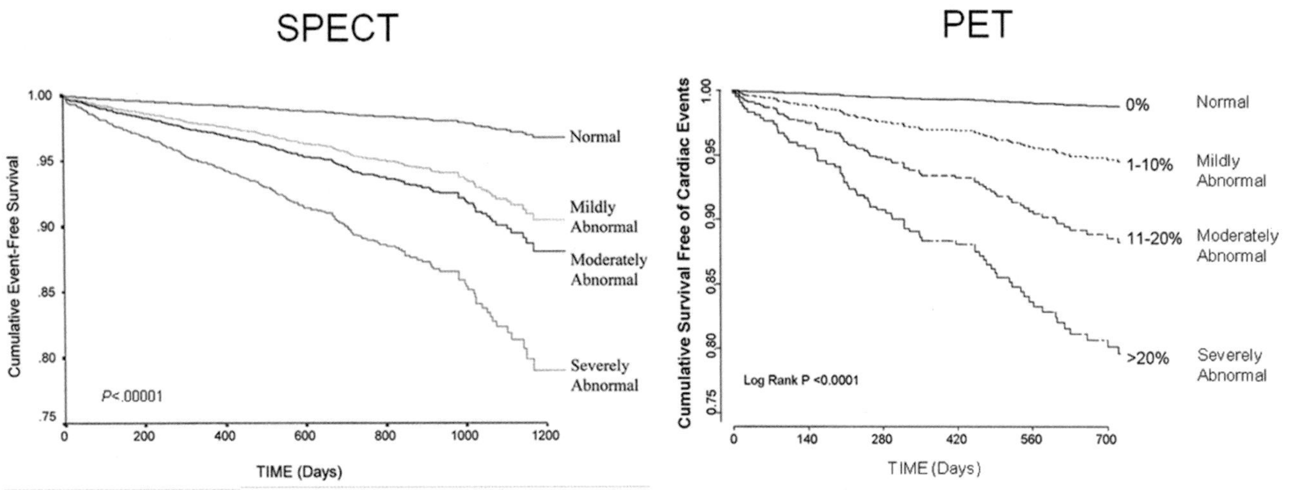

Fig. 4.5 The prognostic value of SPECT (A) and PET (B) MPI to determine survival free of cardiac death or myocardial infarction is shown (Figures adapted and reproduced with permission from Hachamovitch et al. [33] and Dorbala et al. [34])

The warranty period of a normal SPECT MPI is approximately 1–2 years, and lower in patients with diabetes (especially female diabetics), older individuals, and in those undergoing pharmacological SPECT [35]. Also, subjects with a submaximal heart rate response to exercise, known CAD, are unable to exercise and undergo pharmacological stress MPI, have diabetes, or older age may have an event rate of 1–2% despite a normal MPI. In contrast, a severely abnormal SPECT or PET MPI is associated with the worst outcomes, while those with mild and moderately abnormal SPECT or PET MPI have intermediate outcomes [17].

MPI to Guide Clinical Management

The results of SPECT or PET MPI can be used to guide patient management. For instance, patients with abnormal MPI can undergo aggressive risk factor modification or revascularization may be considered. There is evidence from large observational studies that patients with significant ischemic burden (>10%) do better with coronary revascularization than with optimal medical therapy (OMT) alone [36]. However, in the recent COURAGE study, which included select patients with stable CAD, percutaneous coronary intervention (PCI) did not reduce the risk of death, myocardial infarction, or other major cardiovascular events when added to OMT [37]. In a subset of patients that underwent SPECT MPI at baseline and at 18 months, PCI+OMT significantly reduced ischemia compared to OMT alone, with the greatest benefit in patients with at least moderate to severe baseline ischemic burden (>10% ischemic myocardium) [38]. Exploratory analyses revealed that ischemic burden of <5% at follow-up was associated with improved risk. However, larger randomized controlled studies are required to study whether reduction in ischemia to <5% with therapy translates into a prognostic benefit.

The changes in management based on scan results are more controversial in patients with normal MPI. Since perfusion defects on stress MPI detect obstructive epicardial CAD, extensive coronary atherosclerosis may exist in the absence of ischemia. Indeed, all of the existing techniques that rely on ischemia detection underestimate anatomic atherosclerosis burden. Several studies wherein patients underwent both an MPI and calcium score have underscored the diagnostic value of calcium score in identifying calcified atherosclerosis burden in patients with normal MPI [39–42]. In the presence of extensive coronary artery calcification (Agatston calcium score >400), almost 45% of the patients demonstrate ischemic MPI scans [39–42]. Furthermore, the findings of the several studies suggest that, patients with normal SPECT MPS and high calcium score (Fig. 4.6) have a low short-term risk and an intermediate long-term risk compared to patients with normal MPI and no/minimal coronary artery calcium [43, 44]. Also, several studies suggest that the presence of high coronary artery calcification may influence patient behavior [45] or physician practice with greater medication use to modify risk factors [46, 47].

Quantitative PET has been used in several research studies to evaluate progression or regression of atherosclerosis in response to therapeutic interventions [29, 48, 49] Indeed, Gould et al. [48] demonstrated that in patients with dyslipidemia treated with aggressive risk factor modification (life style changes and medications), quantitative PET is superior to quantitative coronary angiography in identifying response to therapy. This is because, small changes in atherosclerosis (not easily evident on coronary angiography) may translate into much larger changes in myocardial blood flow that is easily imaged using quantitative PET imaging.

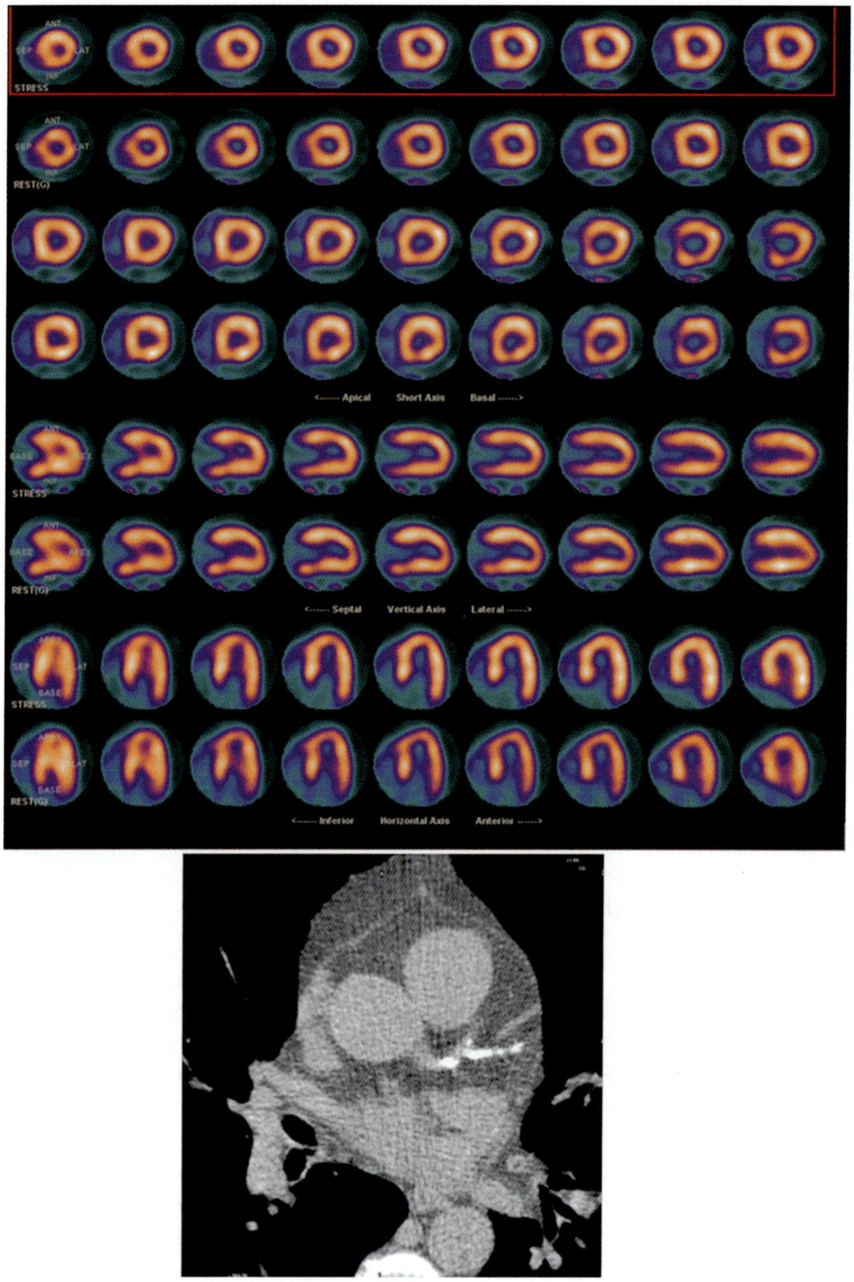

Fig. 4.6 Rest and dipyridamole stress Rubidium-82 PET images in a 52-year-old male with dyslipidemia and a family history of premature atherosclerosis. The rest and stress perfusion was normal. However, the calcium score study demonstrated extensive coronary artery calcification

Cost Effectiveness

SPECT MPI has been demonstrated to be cost effective in the evaluation of patients with chronic stable angina (Figs. 4.7a, b). In a retrospective case-controlled study from four countries (France, Germany, Italy, and the United Kingdom), the EMPIRE study found that when considering exercise ECG, MPI, and coronary angiography, a strategy including MPI was cheaper and at least as effective compared to strategies not including MPI [50]. In another study, the END study [51], 11,249 consecutive patients with stable angina patients were included and a strategy of initial medical therapy with MPI-guided coronary angiography was compared to a strategy of direct coronary angiography. The study cohorts were matched by pretest probability of CAD and diagnostic (SPECT, coronary angiography) and follow-up (late PCI and CABG) costs were evaluated. The END study established that initial diagnostic costs as well as follow-up evaluation costs are significantly lower with a strategy of initial medical therapy with MPI-guided coronary angiography compared to a strategy of direct coronary angiography, with no differences in outcomes. Patterson et al. [52] performed a cost-effectiveness decision modeling analysis of exercise ECG, SPECT MPI, PET MPI, and coronary angiography. In that study, SPECT MPI had a lower cost per unit effectiveness

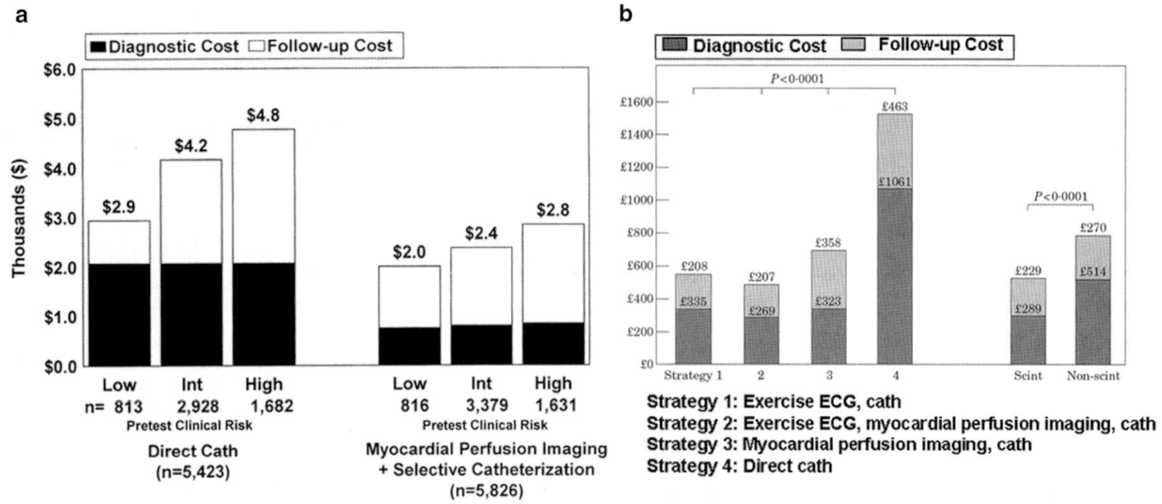

Fig. 4.7 (**a**) Results from the END study. (**b**) Results from the EMPIRE study. In both of these studies a strategy involving myocardial perfusion imaging followed by cath if necessary was less expensive than a strategy of direct cath (coronary angiography), with similar outcomes. (**b**) A strategy including imaging was cost-effective compared to a strategy of direct cath or a strategy of ECG testing and cath (Figures reproduced with permission from Shaw et al. [51] and Underwood et al. [50])

compared to exercise ECG test over a wide range of pretest probabilities of CAD. However, PET MPI had the lowest cost-per-effectiveness or cost-per-utility unit in patients with intermediate pretest likelihood of CAD (pretest likelihood of 0.70) while coronary angiography was most cost-effective in patients with >90% probability of CAD [52]. Also, in a group of intermediate risk subjects, Merhige et al. [53] showed that the downstream costs of evaluation following a PET MPI are lower than SPECT (at their institution) and lower than that reported with SPECT MPI from the END study. Coronary angiography was performed in 13% PET MPI patients vs. 31.4% of SPECT MPI patients and CABG rates were 50% lower in the PETMPI group compared to SPECT. PET MPI was cost neutral compared to SPECT MPI for diagnosis of CAD. However, costs of downstream revascularization were lower by 52 and a 30% reduction in overall costs with PET MPI with no differences in outcomes of cardiac mortality or acute MI. Last, resource utilization with various imaging tests in the contemporary era is the focus of the SPARC study [54]. The results of this study will illustrate the utility of various imaging tests (SPECT, PET, CTA, or hybrid SPECT or PET with CTA) in the evaluation of patients with intermediate pretest likelihood of CAD.

Acute Chest Pain

In this section we will evaluate the role of MPI in the evaluation of patients with suspected ACS, diagnosed ACS, and post-MI risk stratification.

Diagnostic Evaluation of Patients in the Emergency Room with Chest Pain

Several protocols have been tried to evaluate patients presenting to the emergency room for acute chest pain and ECG changes and enzymes nondiagnostic for ACS. A few of these protocols include acute chest pain injection and imaging, rest and stress imaging in patients wherein an ACS has been excluded, and more recently, the use of tracers to image myocardial ischemic memory (BMIPP). Acute chest pain injection was originally performed in 1979 using Thallium-201 [55], but, the rapid redistribution of this tracer, limited its use. Rest Technetium injection during chest pain is much more sensitive than ECG [56] and can be helpful in patients with nondiagnostic ECG's [57]. Kontos et al. [58] showed that in patients presenting to the emergency room, acute chest pain imaging is sensitive tool to identify CAD in patients with nondiagnostic ECG and more sensitive than the initial troponin value (92 vs. 39%) in predicting ACS (maximal troponin value had a sensitivity equivalent to SPECT, but at a much later time point) [59]. Indeed chest pain imaging studies have a very high negative-predictive value (>99%) for ruling out MI [60–63]. However, in patients with a negative rest/chest pain study, it may be important to perform a stress study to exclude epicardial CAD.

Chest pain imaging in the emergency room has been shown to be cost effective with similar outcomes [64] and helpful to make better triage decisions. Udelson et al. [65] studied how acute chest pain imaging would affect emergency department triage decisions when incorporated into usual care. In this study, acute Technetium-9m sestamibi imaging reduced unnecessary

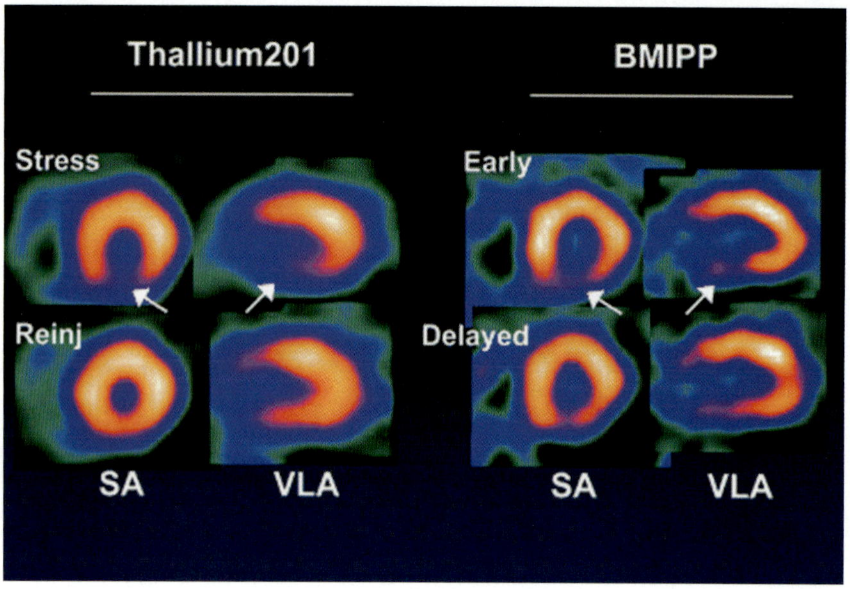

Fig. 4.8 Stress and redistribution Thallium-201 images demonstrating a reversible inferior wall perfusion defect (*left*) and the early and late BMIPP images (*right*) obtained 12 h later demonstrating a corresponding defect in myocardial fatty acid utilization (Figure reproduced with permission from Dilsizian et al. [68])

hospitalizations (52% in the usual care group vs. 42% in the acute chest pain imaging arm, $P<0.01$) among patients without acute ischemia, without reducing appropriate admission of patients with acute ischemia and improved the overall clinical effectiveness of the triage process in the emergency room. The acute chest pain protocol works well during regular hours, but can be cumbersome after hours (need an on-call technologist, injection of the radiotracer as soon as possible after the chest pain, not useful in patients with known CAD or ECG evidence of prior MI) and hence is not frequently used. A widely used strategy for ED patients with chest pain is to exclude ACS (history, ECG and troponin levels), and then perform rest stress imaging.

Lately, with the growth in CTCA, there is an interest in using CTCA for the evaluation of low-risk patients presenting to the ED with chest pain so as to make expeditious discharge decisions [66]. In the ROMICAT study, about 50% of the patients had no CAD, 31% had nonobstructive disease and 19% had inconclusive studies or severe stenosis on CTCA. In another study [67], low-risk patients presenting with chest pain to the emergency room were randomized to undergo standard of care (SOC) including SPECT MPI ($N=98$) vs. CTCA ($N=989$). Overall, 24% of the patients in the CTCA group had intermediate coronary disease or nondiagnostic scans requiring follow-up nuclear testing. In patients randomized to the CTCA arm, there were fewer direct discharges from the ED (88 vs. 97%, $P=0.03$), and greater in-hospital diagnostic catheterization (11 vs. 3%, $P=0.03$) with no significant differences in 30 days or 6 months major adverse cardiac events. However, the overall costs in the patients randomized to the CTCA arm ($1,586 (1,413–2,059)) were higher than the costs in the SOC arm ($1,872 (1,727–2,069)), $P<0.001$.

Finally, imaging of ischemic memory using 15-p-[^{123}I]iodophenyl-3-(R,S)-methylpentadecanoic acid (BMIPP) has been attempted to identify an episode of acute ischemia. BMIPP is a fatty acid analogue that provides a means of measuring myocardial fatty acid utilization in vivo. Ischemic myocardium can experience metabolic stunning and switch from fatty acid to glucose metabolism that may last upto 30 h after an ischemic insult; BMIPP imaging in this context can demonstrate corresponding metabolic defects (Fig. 4.8). Dilsizian et al. [68] studied 32 patients with exercise-induced ischemia, and found a 91% agreement between the early BMIPP and the thallium imaging for the presence or absence of a scintigraphic abnormality (95% CI, 75–98), with no significant difference between the same day or next day BMIPP imaging. There was excellent correlation between the defect size and severity in Thallium images compared to BMIPP images. These findings suggest that BMIPP can successfully image the suppression of fatty acid metabolism after exercise-induced ischemia at least up to 30 h after an ischemic episode, a distinct advantage compared to acute chest pain injection.

MPI in Patients with Acute MI

Post-MI Risk Stratification

MPI has been used widely for post-MI risk stratification prior to discharge from the hospital. The presence of reversible defects in either the infarct or non-infarct area, number of reversible defects, increased radiotracer uptake in the lung, and LVEF are known determinants of outcome following a MI and are well evaluated using an MPI study [69, 70]. The

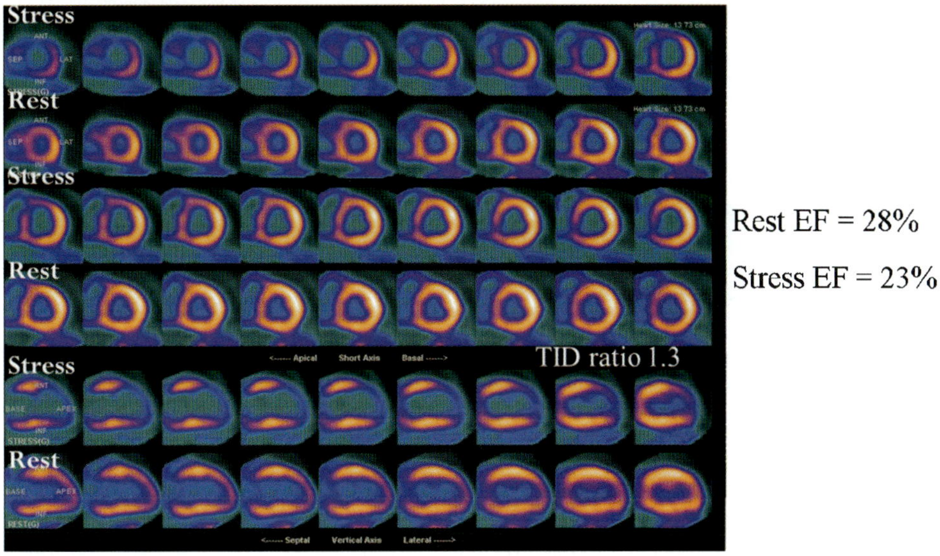

Fig. 4.9 A 72-year-old male presented with rest chest pain for 2 weeks and a troponin of 2.0. Echocardiography demonstrated akinetic anterior and septal walls and a left ventricular ejection fraction of 30%. Coronary angiography demonstrated an occluded mid-LAD artery, with severe disease in the left circumflex and the right coronary arteries. He was referred for a myocardial viability assessment prior to coronary artery bypass surgery. The rest Rubidium-82 perfusion images showed nearly normal perfusion in the entire left ventricle. A dipyridamole stress test was performed. The dipyridamole stress and rest images demonstrated significant reversibility in the entire anteroseptal wall, the mid- and apical anterior walls, the apical inferior and lateral walls, and the LV apex (mid-LAD distribution). There was transient cavity dilation of the left ventricle on the post-stress images. Resting LVEF was 28% and the EF declined to 23% on dipyridamole stress images

above features on a submaximal exercise with planar Thallium scintigraphy identified patients at high risk of future events [71].

In patients that are unable to exercise dipyridamole Thallium imaging can provide excellent risk stratification [72]. Dipyridamole SPECT MPI has been shown to be safe in individuals with an uncomplicated MI. In a multicenter study [69], 451 patients were randomized to early post-MI dipyridamole study (48–96 h later) followed by a submaximal exercise imaging study (6–12 days later) ($N=339$) or a submaximal exercise imaging study (6–12 days later) ($N=112$). This study confirmed prior observations that early post-MI dipyridamole imaging is safe and that the imaging results provide similar or improved risk stratification as compared to the predischarge submaximal exercise study.

In the current era of primary PCI, post-MI risk stratification with MPI is being used predominantly for individuals who receive thrombolytics, individuals presenting late after an MI (Fig. 4.9), those with suboptimal results of intervention of the infarct related artery or to evaluate patients with residual disease in the non-infarct related coronary artery [73]. A submaximal exercise test can be used for assessment of functional capacity following an MI. But, if the goal is to assess for ischemia in territories of residual disease or incomplete revascularization, in a post-MI patient, a vasodilator SPECT study (maximal hyperemia) is preferred.

Rest left ventricular ejection fraction [74], left ventricular end systolic volume, and infarct size are important predictors of 6-month mortality in a post-MI patient [75]. Prior to SPECT imaging, radionuclide angiography had been used in conjunction with submaximal exercise treadmill testing to assess LVEF and volumes [74, 76]. Presently, LVEF and volumes are obtained routinely on SPECT MPI study and remain valuable risk determinants in the post-MI patient.

Finally, the INSPIRE [77, 78] study included 728 patients who underwent a rest and adenosine stress MPI (1–10 days after hospitalization for an uncomplicated MI)and were then randomized to intensive medical therapy or coronary angiography with an intent to revascularization. Patients with large ischemic defects (>10% of the ventricle) and LVEF >35% on the baseline study were included in this analysis. A follow-up scan was performed after optimization of therapy (median of 62 days after initial scan).In this study, a reduction in ischemic burden was achieved in ~80% of patients (similar between the medical therapy and revascularization arms) without significant differences in 1-year outcomes between medical therapy and revascularization cohorts. Sequential adenosine sestamibi myocardial perfusion tomography effectively monitored changes in scintigraphic ischemia (LV perfusion defect size, 33.1 ± 8.9–$16.1 \pm 11\%$, $P<0.0001$). Both groups (anti-ischemic medical or coronary revascularization therapy) demonstrated comparable (-16.2 ± 10 vs.$-17.8 \pm 12\%$), but highly significant reductions in total and ischemia LV defect sizes. The authors concluded that a strategy of intensive medical therapy was comparable to coronary revascularization for suppressing ischemia in stable patients after acute infarction with preserved LV function.

Assessment of Myocardial Viability with SPECT and PET Imaging

The most common cause of left ventricular systolic dysfunction is coronary heart disease. Myocardial scarring from infarction can result in irreversible systolic dysfunction. However, in some patients with CAD, left ventricular systolic dysfunction can improve with revascularization and has been termed as hibernating myocardium. Viable myocardium can be assessed by studying myocardial perfusion, myocardial contractile reserve (in response to low dose inotropic stimulation with dobutamine), myocardial metabolism, or myocardial scar.

Myocardial Perfusion

The radiotracers used for imaging myocardial perfusion are intracellular agents and therefore, the presence of myocardial perfusion (tracer uptake) is consistent with viable myocardium. The negative predictive value of a normal resting myocardial perfusion study for excluding ischemic cardiomyopathy is high ~100% [2]. However, these patients should undergo a stress test to evaluate for ischemic burden and exclude underlying ischemia (and stunning) as a cause of their heart failure symptoms and left ventricular systolic dysfunction. In contrast, when perfusion is abnormal, the positive predictive value of an abnormal MPI to diagnose underlying ischemic cardiomyopathy is only ~40–50% [2]. This is because perfusion defects and regional wall motion abnormalities may be seen in individuals with cardiomyopathy from other etiologies, such as infiltrative heart disease, granulomatous disease, or myocarditis [2]. Also, in patients with reduced myocardial perfusion, quantitative evaluation of radiotracer uptake on myocardial perfusion images can be a useful guide for differentiating viable from nonviable myocardium. Studies have shown that segments of the myocardium with <40% peak tracer activity are unlikely to recover function, whereas the likelihood of recovery of function is higher in segments with >50% peak tracer uptake [79]. It has been shown that viability in moderate to severe myocardial perfusion defects is best evaluated by Thallium redistribution imaging or metabolic assessment [80, 81]. Some investigators have used nitroglycerin (spray or sublingually) prior to injection of rest radiotracer [82] to improve detection of viable segments, likely due to improved radiotracer delivery through collateral flow, or low dose dobutamine to improve the diagnostic accuracy of perfusion imaging [83].

Myocardial Metabolism

PET is the current gold standard test to study myocardial metabolism. Typically, myocardial metabolism images (F-18 labeled fluoro-deoxy glucose) are compared to rest myocardial perfusion. If the rest perfusion is normal, it confirms myocardial viability and an FDG study is not needed. Although not optimal, at institutions without access to PET perfusion tracers, N-13 ammonia or Rubidium-82, MPI with Technetium-99m SPECT can be compared to FDG imaging using SPECT with high energy collimation or PET.

F-18 FDG, an FDA approved PET radiotracer is used clinically for the assessment of myocardial glucose metabolism. Normal myocardium predominantly uses free fatty acids in the fasting state and glucose in the postprandial state for its metabolic needs. In contrast, ischemic/hibernating myocardium preferentially uses glucose both in the fasting and glucose loaded states. Scarred myocardium demonstrates no glucose uptake, since the myocytes are not metabolically active. Reduced blood flow with normal or increased glucose utilization (mismatch pattern), signifies viable and hibernating myocardium, and portends a high probability of improvement following revascularization (Fig. 4.10). In contrast myocardial segments with reduced blood flow and decreased glucose utilization (matched defect) are consistent with scar tissue with a low likelihood of recovery of function post-revascularization (Fig. 4.10).

Diagnostic Value of FDG PET for Viability Assessment

Myocardial perfusion abnormalities lead to abnormalities in myocardial metabolism that result in contractile dysfunction [84]. Since perfusion and metabolic abnormalities precede contractile dysfunction [84], they are more sensitive to detect viability than techniques relying on contractile reserve [85]. Using *perfusion imaging* with PET, the average positive predictive accuracy for predicting functional recovery after revascularization was 63% (range 45–78%), with an average negative predictive value of 63% (range 45–100%). FDG PET has a pooled sensitivity 88% (range 73–100%) and a pooled specificity Of 73% (range 33–100%) to identify viable myocardium [86]. Using the patterns of *perfusion metabolism mismatch and match* to indicate recovery of function or not, respectively, the average positive predictive value for predicting improvement in segmental function after revascularization was 76% (range 52–100%), whereas the average negative predictive value was 82% (range 67–100%) [86]. In contrast, low dose dobutamine echocardiography, a technique relying on assessment of contractile reserve is less sensitive and more specific than FDG PET (sensitivity 84% and specificity of 81%) [86] and low dose

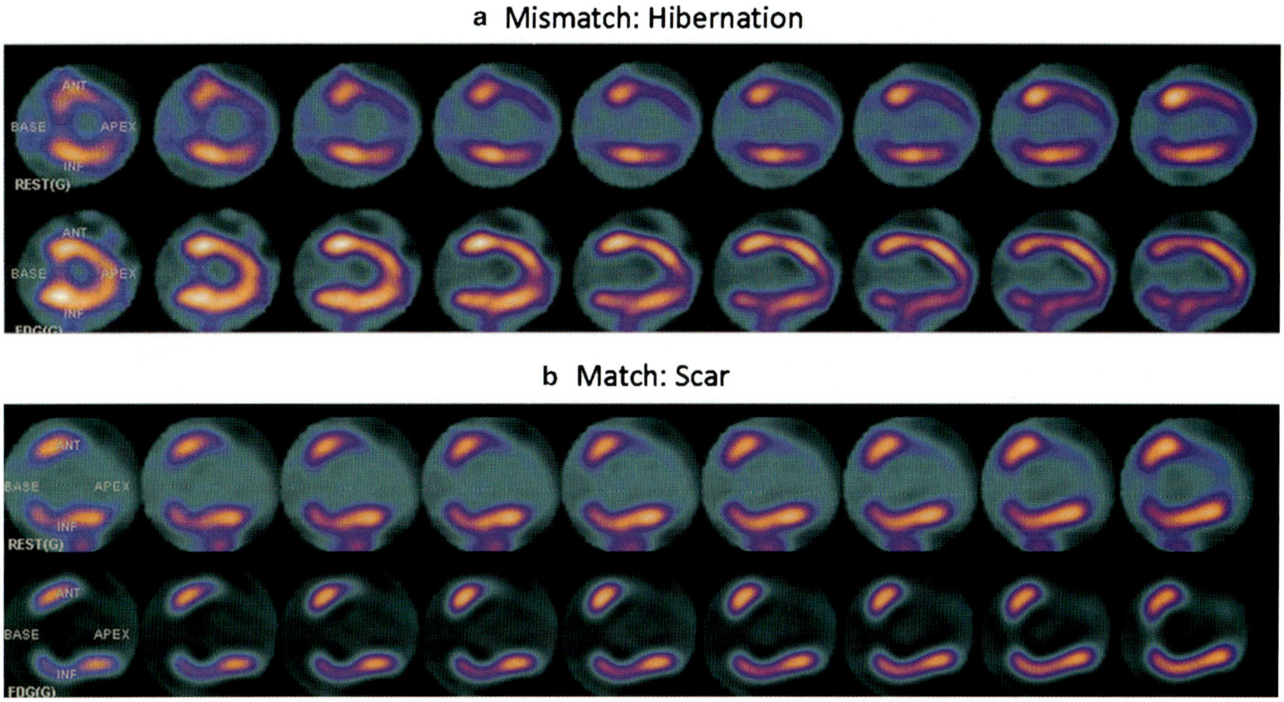

Fig. 4.10 Rest Rubidium-82 and F-18 FDG PET images of two patients with a severe resting perfusion defect in the mid- and apical anterior walls and apex are shown. Patient 1 (**a**) demonstrated significantly increased FDG uptake (mismatched defect, consistent with hibernating myocardium), in these segments, while, Patient 2 (**b**), demonstrated a matched reduction in FDG utilization (matched defect, consistent with transmural scar)

dobutamine echocardiography [85] at predicting improvement in regional function following revascularization. When compared to other techniques, overall, FDG PET appears to be slightly more accurate. Last, the predictive value of viability imaging appears to be lowest in patients with LVEF <30% [87].

Prognostic Value of FDG PET Imaging

At present we lack large randomized clinical trials evaluating the value of revascularization based on viability assessment in individuals with left ventricular systolic dysfunction. However, several studies (albeit retrospective) have demonstrated the value of FDG PET imaging in predicting improvement in left ventricular ejection fraction, heart failure symptoms, functional status, and survival following revascularization. Patients with PET mismatch pattern and subsequent revascularization had significantly lower mortality rates compared to those with nonviable or viable but non-revascularized territories [88–91].

In addition to viability, suitable coronary anatomy and good distal target vessels influence post-revascularization recovery of function. A large magnitude of viable myocardium (mismatch >17% of the left ventricle) as well as a small scar burden portend good recovery of LVEF. In contrast, extensive remodeling of the left ventricle (left ventricular end diastolic dimension >7 cm, left ventricular end systolic volume index of >100 mL/m^2) is associated with postoperative mortality and heart failure. Also, a delay is revascularization after the diagnosis of viable and hibernating myocardium was shown to be associated with a high mortality rate and absence of improvement in left ventricular function following revascularization.

Clinical Applications/Guidelines Appropriate Use Criteria

The ACC/AHA/ASNC have published guidelines for the use of radionuclide imaging in patients with suspected ACS (Table 4.3), following an STEMI (Table 4.4), following a NSTEMI or unstable angina (Table 4.5), for the assessment of myocardial viability (Table 4.6), indications for SPECT MPI (Table 4.7), and indications for PET MPI (Table 4.8). The more

Table 4.3 Recommendations for emergency department imaging for suspected ACS (Reproduced with permission from Klocke et al. [2])

Indication	Test	Class	Level of evidence
Assessment of myocardial risk in possible ACS patients with nondiagnostic ECG and initial serum markers and enzymes, if available	Rest MPI	I	A
Diagnosis of CAD in possible ACS patients with chest pain with nondiagnostic ECG and negative serum markers and enzymes or normal resting scan	Same day rest/stress perfusion imaging	I	B
Routine imaging of patients with myocardial ischemia/necrosis already documented clinically, by ECG and/or serum markers or enzymes	Rest MPI	III	C

See Figure 6 of ACC/AHA 2002 Guideline update for the management of patients with unstable angina and non-ST-segment elevation myocardial infarction at http://www.acc.org/clinical/guidelines/unstable/incorporated/figure6.htm and Figure 1 of ACC/AHA Guidelines for the Management of Patients with Acute Myocardial Infarction at www.acc.org/clinical/guidelines/nov96/1999/jac1716f01.htm

ACS indicates acute coronary syndromes; CAD, coronary artery disease; ECG, electrocardiogram; and MPI, myocardial perfusion imaging

Table 4.4 Recommendations for use of radionuclide testing in diagnosis, risk assessment, prognosis, and assessment of therapy after acute STEMI (Reproduced with permission from Klocke et al. [2])

Patient subgroup(s)	Indication	Test	Class	Level of evidence
All	Rest LV function	Rest RNA or ECG-gated SPECT	I	B
Thrombolytic therapy without catheterization	Detection of inducible ischemia and myocardium at risk	Stress MPI with ECG-gated SPECT whenever possible	I	B
Acute STEMI	Assessment of infarct size and residual viable myocardium	MPI at rest or with stress using gated SPECT	I	B
	Assessment of RV function with suspected RV infarction	Equilibrium or FPRNA	IIa	B

ECG electrocardiography; *FPRNA* first-pass radionuclide angiography; *LV* left ventricular; *MPI* myocardial perfusion imaging; *RNA* radionuclide angiography; *RV* right ventricular; *SPECT* single-photon emission computed tomography; and *STEMI* ST-segment elevation myocardial infarction

Table 4.5 Recommendations for use of radionuclide testing for risk assessment/prognosis in patients with NSTEMI and UA (Reproduced with permission from Klocke et al. [2])

Indication	Test	Class	Level of Evidence
Identification of inducible ischemia in the distribution of the "culprit lesion" or in remote areas in patients at intermediate or low risk for major adverse cardiac events	Stress MPI with ECG gating whenever possible	I	B
Identification of the severity/extent of inducible ischemia in patients whose angina is satisfactorily stabilized with medical therapy or in whom diagnosis is uncertain	Stress MPI with ECG gating whenever possible	I	A
Identification of hemodynamic significance of coronary stenosis after coronary arteriography	Stress MPI	I	B
Measurement of baseline LV function	RNA or gated SPECT	I	B
Identification of the severity/extent of disease in patients with ongoing suspected ischemia symptoms when ECG changes are not diagnostic	Rest MPI	IIa	B

ECG electrocardiography; *LV* left ventricular; *MPI* myocardial perfusion imaging; *RNA* radionuclide angiography; and *SPECT* single-photon emission computed tomography

Table 4.6 Recommendations for the use of radionuclide techniques to assess myocardial viability (Reproduced with permission from Klocke et al. [2])

Indication	Test	Class	Level of Evidence
Predicting improvement in regional and global LV function after revascularization	Stress/redistribution/reinjection ^{201}Tl	I	B
	Rest-redistribution imaging	I	B
	Perfusion plus PET FDG imaging	I	B
	Resting sestamibi imaging	I	B
	Gated SPECT sestamibi imaging	IIa	B
	Late ^{201}Tl redistribution imaging (after stress)	IIb	B
	Dobutamine RNA	IIb	C
	Postexercise RNA	IIb	C
	Postnitroglycerin RNA	IIb	C

(continued)

Table 4.6 (continued)

Indication	Test	Class	Level of Evidence
Predicting improvement in heart failure symptoms after revascularization.	Perfusion plus PET FDG imaging	IIa	B
Predicting improvement in natural history after revascularization	^{201}Tl imaging (rest-redistribution and stress/redistribution/reinjection)	I	B
	Perfusion plus PET FDG imaging	I	B

FDG flurodeoxyglucose; *PET* positron emission tomography; *RNA* radionuclide angiography; *SPECT* single-photon emission computed tomography; and *201Tl* thallium-201

Table 4.7 Indications for myocardial perfusion imaging: SPECT (Reproduced with permission from Klocke et al. [2])

Myocardial perfusion SPECT	Class	Level
Stable coronary syndromes		
Cardiac stress myocardial perfusion SPECT in patients able to exercise: Recommendations for diagnosis of patients with an intermediate likelihood of CAD and/or risk stratification of patients with an intermediate or high likelihood of CAD who are able to exercise (to at least 85% of maximal predicted heart rate)		
Exercise myocardial perfusion SPECT to identify the extent, severity, and location of ischemia in patients who do not have LBBB or an electronically paced ventricular rhythm but do have a baseline ECG abnormality that interferes with the interpretation of exercise-induced ST-segment changes (ventricular preexcitation, LVH, digoxin therapy, or more than 1-mm ST depression)	I	B
Adenosine or dipyridamole myocardial perfusion SPECT in patients with LBBB or electronically paced ventricular rhythm	I	B
Exercise myocardial perfusion SPECT to assess the functional significance of intermediate (25–75%) coronary lesions	I	B
Exercise myocardial perfusion SPECT in patients with intermediate Duke treadmill score	I	B
Repeat exercise myocardial perfusion imaging after initial perfusion imaging in patients whose symptoms have changed to redefine the risk for cardiac event	I	C
Exercise myocardial perfusion SPECT at 3–5 years after revascularization (either PCI or CABG) in selected high-risk asymptomatic patients	IIa	B
Exercise myocardial perfusion SPECT as the initial test in patients who are considered to be at high risk (patients with diabetes or patients otherwise defined as having a more than 20% 10-year risk of a coronary heart disease event)	IIa	B
Repeat exercise myocardial perfusion SPECT 1–3 years after initial perfusion imaging in patients with known or a high likelihood of CAD and stable symptoms and a predicted annual mortality of more than 1% to redefine the risk of a cardiac event	IIb	C
Repeat exercise myocardial perfusion SPECT on cardiac active medications after initial abnormal perfusion imaging to assess the efficacy of medical therapy	IIb	C
Exercise myocardial perfusion SPECT in symptomatic or asymptomatic patients who have severe coronary calcification (CT coronary calcium score more than the 75th percentile for age and sex) in the presence on the resting ECG of preexcitation (Wolff–Parkinson–White syndrome) or more than 1 mm ST-segment depression	IIb	B
Exercise myocardial perfusion SPECT in asymptomatic patients who have a high-risk occupation	IIb	B
Cardiac stress myocardial perfusion SPECT in patients unable to exercise: Recommendations for diagnosis of patients with an intermediate likelihood of CAD and/or risk stratification of patients with an intermediate or high likelihood of CAD who are unable to exercise		
Adenosine or dipyridamole myocardial perfusion SPECT to assess the functional significance of intermediate (25–75%) coronary lesions	I	B
Adenosine or dipyridamole myocardial perfusion SPECT to identify the extent, severity, and location of ischemia	I	B
Adenosine or dipyridamole myocardial perfusion SPECT after initial perfusion imaging inpatients whose symptoms have changed to redefine the risk for cardiac event	I	C
Adenosine or dipyridamole myocardial perfusion SPECT at 3–5 years after revascularization (either PCI or CABG) in selected high-risk asymptomatic patients	II	B
Adenosine or dipyridamole myocardial perfusion SPECT as the initial test in patients who are considered to be at high risk (patients with diabetes or patients otherwise defined as having a more than 20% 10-year risk of a coronary heart disease event)	II	B
Dobutamine myocardial perfusion SPECT in patients who have a contraindication to adenosine or dipyridamole	II	C
Repeat adenosine or dipyridamole myocardial perfusion imaging 1–3 years after initial perfusion imaging in patients with known or a high likelihood of CAD and stable symptoms, and a predicted annual mortality of more than1%, to redefine the risk of a cardiac event	IIb	C
Repeat adenosine or dipyridamole myocardial perfusion SPECT on cardiac active medications after initial abnormal perfusion imaging to assess the efficacy of medical therapy	IIb	C
Adenosine or dipyridamole myocardial perfusion SPECT in symptomatic or asymptomatic patients who have severe coronary calcification (CT coronary calcium score more than the 75th percentile for age and sex) in the presence on the resting ECG of LBBB or an electronically paced ventricular rhythm	IIb	B
Adenosine or dipyridamole myocardial perfusion SPECT in asymptomatic patients who have a high-risk occupation	IIb	C

Table 4.8 Indications for myocardial perfusion imaging: PET (Reproduced with permission from Klocke et al. [2])

Myocardial perfusion PET for the diagnosis of patients with an intermediate likelihood of CAD and/or risk stratification of patients with an intermediate or high likelihood of CAD	Class	Level
Adenosine or dipyridamole myocardial perfusion PET in patients in whom an appropriately indicated myocardial perfusion SPECT study has been found to be equivocal for diagnosis or risk stratification	I	B
Adenosine or dipyridamole myocardial perfusion PET for patients to identify the extent, severity, and location of ischemia as the initial diagnostic test in patients who are unable to exercise	IIa	B
Adenosine or dipyridamole myocardial perfusion PET for patients to identify the extent, severity, and location of ischemia as the initial diagnostic test in patients who are able to exercise but have a LBBB or an electronically paced rhythm	IIa	B

recent appropriate use criteria suggest that the use of radionuclide imaging (SPECT and PET) may be appropriate in specific scenarios. These documents are general guidelines and individual clinical judgment is recommended when evaluating specific patients and the appropriateness of the test used.

References

1. Lloyd-Jones D, Adams RJ, Brown TM, et al. Heart disease and stroke statistics – 2010 update: a report from the American Heart Association. Circulation. 2010;121:e46–215.
2. Klocke FJ, Baird MG, Lorell BH, et al. ACC/AHA/ASNC guidelines for the clinical use of cardiac radionuclide imaging–executive summary: a report of the American College of Cardiology/American Heart Association Task Force on Practice Guidelines (ACC/AHA/ASNC Committee to Revise the 1995 Guidelines for the Clinical Use of Cardiac Radionuclide Imaging). J Am Coll Cardiol. 2003;42:1318–33.
3. Rozanski A, Diamond GA, Berman D, Forrester JS, Morris D, Swan HJ. The declining specificity of exercise radionuclide ventriculography. N Engl J Med. 1983;309:518–22.
4. DePuey EG, Rozanski A. Using gated technetium-99m-sestamibi SPECT to characterize fixed myocardial defects as infarct or artifact. J Nucl Med. 1995;36:952–5.
5. Ficaro EP, Fessler JA, Shreve PD, Kritzman JN, Rose PA, Corbett JR. Simultaneous transmission/emission myocardial perfusion tomography. Diagnostic accuracy of attenuation-corrected 99mTc-sestamibi single-photon emission computed tomography. Circulation. 1996;93:463–73.
6. Hendel RC, Berman DS, Cullom SJ, et al. Multicenter clinical trial to evaluate the efficacy of correction for photon attenuation and scatter in SPECT myocardial perfusion imaging. Circulation. 1999;99:2742–9.
7. Kluge R, Sattler B, Seese A, Knapp WH. Attenuation correction by simultaneous emission-transmission myocardial single-photon emission tomography using a technetium-99m-labelled radiotracer: impact on diagnostic accuracy. Eur J Nucl Med. 1997;24:1107–14.
8. Links JM, DePuey EG, Taillefer R, Becker LC. Attenuation correction and gating synergistically improve the diagnostic accuracy of myocardial perfusion SPECT. J Nucl Cardiol. 2002;9:183–7.
9. Fricke E, Fricke H, Weise R, et al. Attenuation correction of myocardial SPECT perfusion images with low-dose CT: evaluation of the method by comparison with perfusion PET. J Nucl Med. 2005;46:736–44.
10. Masood Y, Liu YH, Depuey G, et al. Clinical validation of SPECT attenuation correction using x-ray computed tomography-derived attenuation maps: multicenter clinical trial with angiographic correlation. J Nucl Cardiol. 2005;12:676–86.
11. Sharir T, Slomka PJ, Hayes SW, et al. Multicenter trial of high-speed versus conventional single-photon emission computed tomography imaging: quantitative results of myocardial perfusion and left ventricular function. J Am Coll Cardiol. 2010;55:1965–74.
12. Einstein AJ, Moser KW, Thompson RC, Cerqueira MD, Henzlova MJ. Radiation dose to patients from cardiac diagnostic imaging. Circulation. 2007;116:1290–305.
13. Heller GV, Bateman TM, Johnson LL, et al. Clinical value of attenuation correction in stress-only Tc-99m sestamibi SPECT imaging. J Nucl Cardiol. 2004;11:273–81.
14. Bateman TM, Heller GV, McGhie AI, et al. Multicenter investigation comparing a highly efficient half-time stress-only attenuation correction approach against standard rest-stress Tc-99m SPECT imaging. J Nucl Cardiol. 2009;16:726–35.
15. Chang SM, Nabi F, Xu J, Raza U, Mahmarian JJ. Normal stress-only versus standard stress/rest myocardial perfusion imaging: similar patient mortality with reduced radiation exposure. J Am Coll Cardiol. 2010;55:221–30.
16. Duvall WL, Wijetunga MN, Klein TM, et al. The prognosis of a normal stress-only Tc-99m myocardial perfusion imaging study. J Nucl Cardiol. 2010;17:370–7.
17. Al-Mallah MH, Sitek A, Moore SC, Di Carli M, Dorbala S. Assessment of myocardial perfusion and function with PET and PET/CT. J Nucl Cardiol. 2010;17:498–513.
18. Di Carli MF, Dorbala S, Meserve J, El Fakhri G, Sitek A, Moore SC. Clinical myocardial perfusion PET/CT. J Nucl Med. 2007;48:783–93.
19. Di Carli MF, Hachamovitch R. New technology for noninvasive evaluation of coronary artery disease. Circulation. 2007;115:1464–80.
20. Heller GV, Calnon D, Dorbala S. Recent advances in cardiac PET and PET/CT myocardial perfusion imaging. J Nucl Cardiol. 2009;16:962–9.
21. Nekolla SG, Reder S, Saraste A, et al. Evaluation of the novel myocardial perfusion positron-emission tomography tracer 18F-BMS-747158-02: comparison to 13N-ammonia and validation with microspheres in a pig model. Circulation. 2009;119:2333–42.
22. Bateman TM, Heller GV, McGhie AI, et al. Diagnostic accuracy of rest/stress ECG-gated Rb-82 myocardial perfusion PET: comparison with ECG-gated Tc-99m sestamibi SPECT. J Nucl Cardiol. 2006;13:24–33.

23. Sampson UK, Dorbala S, Limaye A, Kwong R, Di Carli MF. Diagnostic accuracy of rubidium-82 myocardial perfusion imaging with hybrid positron emission tomography/computed tomography in the detection of coronary artery disease. J Am Coll Cardiol. 2007;49:1052–8.
24. Di Carli MF, Bianco-Batlles D, Landa ME, et al. Effects of autonomic neuropathy on coronary blood flow in patients with diabetes mellitus. Circulation. 1999;100:813–9.
25. Pitkanen OP, Raitakari OT, Niinikoski H, et al. Coronary flow reserve is impaired in young men with familial hypercholesterolemia. J Am Coll Cardiol. 1996;28:1705–11.
26. Czernin J, Sun K, Brunken R, Bottcher M, Phelps M, Schelbert H. Effect of acute and long-term smoking on myocardial blood flow and flow reserve. Circulation. 1995;91:2891–7.
27. Dayanikli F, Grambow D, Muzik O, Mosca L, Rubenfire M, Schwaiger M. Early detection of abnormal coronary flow reserve in asymptomatic men at high risk for coronary artery disease using positron emission tomography. Circulation. 1994;90:808–17.
28. Camici PG, Crea F. Coronary microvascular dysfunction. N Engl J Med. 2007;356:830–40.
29. Campisi R, Di Carli MF. Assessment of coronary flow reserve and microcirculation: a clinical perspective. J Nucl Cardiol. 2004;11:3–11.
30. Neglia D, Michelassi C, Trivieri MG, et al. Prognostic role of myocardial blood flow impairment in idiopathic left ventricular dysfunction. Circulation. 2002;105:186–93.
31. Cecchi F, Olivotto I, Gistri R, Lorenzoni R, Chiriatti G, Camici PG. Coronary microvascular dysfunction and prognosis in hypertrophic cardiomyopathy. N Engl J Med. 2003;349:1027–35.
32. Ladenheim ML, Pollock BH, Rozanski A, et al. Extent and severity of myocardial hypoperfusion as predictors of prognosis in patients with suspected coronary artery disease. J Am Coll Cardiol. 1986;7:464–71.
33. Hachamovitch R, Berman DS, Shaw LJ, et al. Incremental prognostic value of myocardial perfusion single photon emission computed tomography for the prediction of cardiac death: differential stratification for risk of cardiac death and myocardial infarction. Circulation. 1998;97:535–43.
34. Dorbala S, Hachamovitch R, Curillova Z, et al. Incremental prognostic value of gated Rb-82 positron emission tomography myocardial perfusion imaging over clinical variables and rest LVEF. JACC Cardiovasc Imaging. 2009;2:846–54.
35. Hachamovitch R, Hayes S, Friedman JD, et al. Determinants of risk and its temporal variation in patients with normal stress myocardial perfusion scans: what is the warranty period of a normal scan? J Am Coll Cardiol. 2003;41:1329–40.
36. Hachamovitch R, Hayes SW, Friedman JD, Cohen I, Berman DS. Comparison of the short-term survival benefit associated with revascularization compared with medical therapy in patients with no prior coronary artery disease undergoing stress myocardial perfusion single photon emission computed tomography. Circulation. 2003;107:2900–7.
37. Boden WE, O'Rourke RA, Teo KK, et al. Optimal medical therapy with or without PCI for stable coronary disease. N Engl J Med. 2007;356:1503–16.
38. Shaw LJ, Berman DS, Maron DJ, et al. Optimal medical therapy with or without percutaneous coronary intervention to reduce ischemic burden: results from the Clinical Outcomes Utilizing Revascularization and Aggressive Drug Evaluation (COURAGE) trial nuclear substudy. Circulation. 2008;117:1283–91.
39. Anand DV, Lim E, Hopkins D, et al. Risk stratification in uncomplicated type 2 diabetes: prospective evaluation of the combined use of coronary artery calcium imaging and selective myocardial perfusion scintigraphy. Eur Heart J. 2006;27:713–21.
40. Berman DS, Wong ND, Gransar H, et al. Relationship between stress-induced myocardial ischemia and atherosclerosis measured by coronary calcium tomography. J Am Coll Cardiol. 2004;44:923–30.
41. He ZX, Hedrick TD, Pratt CM, et al. Severity of coronary artery calcification by electron beam computed tomography predicts silent myocardial ischemia. Circulation. 2000;101:244–51.
42. Schepis T, Gaemperli O, Koepfli P, et al. Added value of coronary artery calcium score as an adjunct to gated SPECT for the evaluation of coronary artery disease in an intermediate-risk population. J Nucl Med. 2007;48:1424–30.
43. Chang SM, Nabi F, Xu J, et al. The coronary artery calcium score and stress myocardial perfusion imaging provide independent and complementary prediction of cardiac risk. J Am Coll Cardiol. 2009;54:1872–82.
44. Uebleis C, Becker A, Griesshammer I, et al. Stable coronary artery disease: prognostic value of myocardial perfusion SPECT in relation to coronary calcium scoring – long-term follow-up. Radiology. 2009;252:682–90.
45. Wong ND, Detrano RC, Diamond G, et al. Does coronary artery screening by electron beam computed tomography motivate potentially beneficial lifestyle behaviors? Am J Cardiol. 1996;78:1220–3.
46. Blankstein R, Dorbala S. Adding calcium scoring to myocardial perfusion imaging: does it alter physicians' therapeutic decision making? J Nucl Cardiol. 2010;17:168–71.
47. Bybee KA, Lee J, Markiewicz R, et al. Diagnostic and clinical benefit of combined coronary calcium and perfusion assessment in patients undergoing PET/CT myocardial perfusion stress imaging. J Nucl Cardiol. 2010;17:188–96.
48. Gould KL, Ornish D, Scherwitz L, et al. Changes in myocardial perfusion abnormalities by positron emission tomography after long-term, intense risk factor modification. JAMA. 1995;274:894–901.
49. Ornish D, Scherwitz LW, Billings JH, et al. Intensive lifestyle changes for reversal of coronary heart disease. JAMA. 1998;280:2001–7.
50. Underwood SR, Godman B, Salyani S, Ogle JR, Ell PJ. Economics of myocardial perfusion imaging in Europe – the EMPIRE Study. Eur Heart J. 1999;20:157–66.
51. Shaw LJ, Hachamovitch R, Berman DS, et al. The economic consequences of available diagnostic and prognostic strategies for the evaluation of stable angina patients: an observational assessment of the value of precatheterization ischemia. Economics of Noninvasive Diagnosis (END) Multicenter Study Group. J Am Coll Cardiol. 1999;33:661–9.
52. Patterson RE, Eisner RL, Horowitz SF. Comparison of cost-effectiveness and utility of exercise ECG, single photon emission computed tomography, positron emission tomography, and coronary angiography for diagnosis of coronary artery disease. Circulation. 1995;91:54–65.
53. Merhige ME, Breen WJ, Shelton V, Houston T, D'Arcy BJ, Perna AF. Impact of myocardial perfusion imaging with PET and (82)Rb on downstream invasive procedure utilization, costs, and outcomes in coronary disease management. J Nucl Med. 2007;48:1069–76.
54. Hachamovitch R, Johnson JR, Hlatky MA, et al. The study of myocardial perfusion and coronary anatomy imaging roles in CAD (SPARC): design, rationale, and baseline patient characteristics of a prospective, multicenter observational registry comparing PET, SPECT, and CTA for resource utilization and clinical outcomes. J Nucl Cardiol. 2009;16:935–48.

55. Wackers FJ, Lie KI, Liem KL, et al. Potential value of thallium-201 scintigraphy as a means of selecting patients for the coronary care unit. Br Heart J. 1979;41:111–7.
56. Bilodeau L, Theroux P, Gregoire J, Gagnon D, Arsenault A. Technetium-99m sestamibi tomography in patients with spontaneous chest pain: correlations with clinical, electrocardiographic and angiographic findings. J Am Coll Cardiol. 1991;18:1684–91.
57. Christian TF, Clements IP, Gibbons RJ. Noninvasive identification of myocardium at risk in patients with acute myocardial infarction and nondiagnostic electrocardiograms with technetium-99m-Sestamibi. Circulation. 1991;83:1615–20.
58. Kontos MC, Jesse RL, Schmidt KL, Ornato JP, Tatum JL. Value of acute rest sestamibi perfusion imaging for evaluation of patients admitted to the emergency department with chest pain. J Am Coll Cardiol. 1997;30:976–82.
59. Kontos MC, Jesse RL, Anderson FP, Schmidt KL, Ornato JP, Tatum JL. Comparison of myocardial perfusion imaging and cardiac troponin I in patients admitted to the emergency department with chest pain. Circulation. 1999;99:2073–8.
60. Varetto T, Cantalupi D, Altieri A, Orlandi C. Emergency room technetium-99m sestamibi imaging to rule out acute myocardial ischemic events in patients with nondiagnostic electrocardiograms. J Am Coll Cardiol. 1993;22:1804–8.
61. Hilton TC, Thompson RC, Williams HJ, Saylors R, Fulmer H, Stowers SA. Technetium-99m sestamibi myocardial perfusion imaging in the emergency room evaluation of chest pain. J Am Coll Cardiol. 1994;23:1016–22.
62. Tatum JL, Jesse RL, Kontos MC, et al. Comprehensive strategy for the evaluation and triage of the chest pain patient. Ann Emerg Med. 1997;29:116–25.
63. Heller GV, Stowers SA, Hendel RC, et al. Clinical value of acute rest technetium-99m tetrofosmin tomographic myocardial perfusion imaging in patients with acute chest pain and nondiagnostic electrocardiograms. J Am Coll Cardiol. 1998;31:1011–7.
64. Stowers SA, Eisenstein EL, Th Wackers FJ, et al. An economic analysis of an aggressive diagnostic strategy with single photon emission computed tomography myocardial perfusion imaging and early exercise stress testing in emergency department patients who present with chest pain but nondiagnostic electrocardiograms: results from a randomized trial. Ann Emerg Med. 2000;35:17–25.
65. Udelson JE, Beshansky JR, Ballin DS, et al. Myocardial perfusion imaging for evaluation and triage of patients with suspected acute cardiac ischemia: a randomized controlled trial. JAMA. 2002;288:2693–700.
66. Hoffmann U, Bamberg F, Chae CU, et al. Coronary computed tomography angiography for early triage of patients with acute chest pain: the ROMICAT (Rule Out Myocardial Infarction using Computer Assisted Tomography) trial. J Am Coll Cardiol. 2009;53:1642–50.
67. Goldstein JA, Gallagher MJ, O'Neill WW, Ross MA, O'Neil BJ, Raff GL. A randomized controlled trial of multi-slice coronary computed tomography for evaluation of acute chest pain. J Am Coll Cardiol. 2007;49:863–71.
68. Dilsizian V, Bateman TM, Bergmann SR, et al. Metabolic imaging with beta-methyl-p-[(123)I]-iodophenyl-pentadecanoic acid identifies ischemic memory after demand ischemia. Circulation. 2005;112:2169–74.
69. Brown KA, Heller GV, Landin RS, et al. Early dipyridamole (99m)Tc-sestamibi single photon emission computed tomographic imaging 2 to 4 days after acute myocardial infarction predicts in-hospital and postdischarge cardiac events: comparison with submaximal exercise imaging. Circulation. 1999;100:2060–6.
70. Verani MS. Exercise and pharmacologic stress testing for prognosis after acute myocardial infarction. J Nucl Med. 1994;35:716–20.
71. Gibson RS, Watson DD. Value of planar 201Tl imaging in risk stratification of patients recovering from acute myocardial infarction. Circulation. 1991;84:I148–62.
72. Leppo JA, O'Brien J, Rothendler JA, Getchell JD, Lee VW. Dipyridamole-thallium-201 scintigraphy in the prediction of future cardiac events after acute myocardial infarction. N Engl J Med. 1984;310:1014–8.
73. Hendel RC, Berman DS, Di Carli MF, et al. ACCF/ASNC/ACR/AHA/ASE/SCCT/SCMR/SNM 2009 appropriate use criteria for cardiac radionuclide imaging: a report of the American College of Cardiology Foundation Appropriate Use Criteria Task Force, the American Society of Nuclear Cardiology, the American College of Radiology, the American Heart Association, the American Society of Echocardiography, the Society of Cardiovascular Computed Tomography, the Society for Cardiovascular Magnetic Resonance, and the Society of Nuclear Medicine. Circulation. 2009;119:e561–87.
74. Zaret BL, Wackers FJ, Terrin ML, et al. Value of radionuclide rest and exercise left ventricular ejection fraction in assessing survival of patients after thrombolytic therapy for acute myocardial infarction: results of thrombolysis in myocardial infarction (TIMI) phase II study. The TIMI Study Group. J Am Coll Cardiol. 1995;26:73–9.
75. Burns RJ, Gibbons RJ, Yi Q, et al. The relationships of left ventricular ejection fraction, end-systolic volume index and infarct size to six-month mortality after hospital discharge following myocardial infarction treated by thrombolysis. J Am Coll Cardiol. 2002;39:30–6.
76. Corbett JR, Dehmer GJ, Lewis SE, et al. The prognostic value of submaximal exercise testing with radionuclide ventriculography before hospital discharge in patients with recent myocardial infarction. Circulation. 1981;64:535–44.
77. Mahmarian JJ, Dakik HA, Filipchuk NG, et al. An initial strategy of intensive medical therapy is comparable to that of coronary revascularization for suppression of scintigraphic ischemia in high-risk but stable survivors of acute myocardial infarction. J Am Coll Cardiol. 2006;48:2458–67.
78. Mahmarian JJ, Shaw LJ, Filipchuk NG, et al. A multinational study to establish the value of early adenosine technetium-99m sestamibi myocardial perfusion imaging in identifying a low-risk group for early hospital discharge after acute myocardial infarction. J Am Coll Cardiol. 2006;48:2448–57.
79. Udelson JE, Coleman PS, Metherall J, et al. Predicting recovery of severe regional ventricular dysfunction. Comparison of resting scintigraphy with 201Tl and 99mTc-sestamibi. Circulation. 1994;89:2552–61.
80. Bonow RO, Dilsizian V, Cuocolo A, Bacharach SL. Identification of viable myocardium in patients with chronic coronary artery disease and left ventricular dysfunction. Comparison of thallium scintigraphy with reinjection and PET imaging with 18F-fluorodeoxyglucose. Circulation. 1991;83:26–37.
81. Tamaki N, Ohtani H, Yamashita K, et al. Metabolic activity in the areas of new fill-in after thallium-201 reinjection: comparison with positron emission tomography using fluorine-18-deoxyglucose. J Nucl Med. 1991;32:673–8.
82. Sciagra R, Bisi G, Santoro GM, et al. Comparison of baseline-nitrate technetium-99m sestamibi with rest-redistribution thallium-201 tomography in detecting viable hibernating myocardium and predicting postrevascularization recovery. J Am Coll Cardiol. 1997;30:384–91.
83. Leoncini M, Marcucci G, Sciagra R, et al. Prediction of functional recovery in patients with chronic coronary artery disease and left ventricular dysfunction combining the evaluation of myocardial perfusion and of contractile reserve using nitrate-enhanced technetium-99m sestamibi gated single-photon emission computed tomography and dobutamine stress. Am J Cardiol. 2001;87:1346–50.

84. Taegtmeyer H. Tracing cardiac metabolism in vivo: one substrate at a time. J Nucl Med. 2010;51 Suppl 1:80S–7.
85. Bax JJ, Wijns W, Cornel JH, Visser FC, Boersma E, Fioretti PM. Accuracy of currently available techniques for prediction of functional recovery after revascularization in patients with left ventricular dysfunction due to chronic coronary artery disease: comparison of pooled data. J Am Coll Cardiol. 1997;30:1451–60.
86. Di Carli MF. Myocardial viability assessment with PET and PET/CT: in cardiac PET and PET/CT imaging. 1st ed. New York: Springer; 2007.
87. Di Carli MF. The quest for myocardial viability: is there a role for nitrate-enhanced imaging? J Nucl Cardiol. 2003;10:696–9.
88. Di Carli MF, Davidson M, Little R, et al. Value of metabolic imaging with positron emission tomography for evaluating prognosis in patients with coronary artery disease and left ventricular dysfunction. Am J Cardiol. 1994;73:527–33.
89. Eitzman D, al-Aouar Z, Kanter HL, et al. Clinical outcome of patients with advanced coronary artery disease after viability studies with positron emission tomography. J Am Coll Cardiol. 1992;20:559–65.
90. Lee KS, Marwick TH, Cook SA, et al. Prognosis of patients with left ventricular dysfunction, with and without viable myocardium after myocardial infarction. Relative efficacy of medical therapy and revascularization. Circulation. 1994;90:2687–94.
91. Allman KC, Shaw LJ, Hachamovitch R, Udelson JE. Myocardial viability testing and impact of revascularization on prognosis in patients with coronary artery disease and left ventricular dysfunction: a meta-analysis. J Am Coll Cardiol. 2002;39:1151–8.

Chapter 5
Noninvasive Coronary Artery Imaging with CT and MRI

Marc C. Newell, Robert S. Schwartz, and John R. Lesser

Coronary Artery Evaluation with CT Angiography

Techniques

Many technical challenges must be overcome to achieve reliable visualization of the coronary arteries. The epicardial coronary artery lumen is typically 1.5–4.5 mm in diameter, and these vessels move throughout systole and diastole.

Suspend Respiratory Motion, Gate CT Images

During CCTA, coronary motion is limited by both suspending respiratory motion and gating the CT image acquisition to the electrocardiogram (ECG). These gated CT images are acquired at prescribed time periods within the cardiac cycle. The ability of a specific CT scanner to stop coronary motion relates to its temporal resolution (TR), which is similar to the shutter speed of a camera. TR, expressed in milliseconds, is the time required to create a single image within the cardiac cycle.

Figure 5.1 shows that 165 ms is needed for a single-source, 64-slice scanner, and only 83 ms is required when using a faster, dual-source, 64-slice scanner. No current CT scanner is considered "real time" (<50 ms temporal resolution), which is necessary to capture coronary motion for an image taken any time throughout the cardiac cycle. As a result, the patient's heart rate is often slowed with beta blockers [1], and the scanner with the fastest TR is used. This improves image data by showing a relatively motionless coronary artery.

Good Spatial Resolution Needed for Small Vessels

In addition to the fastest TR, small coronary arteries require the best spatial resolution possible to discriminate between various degrees of stenosis severity and to distinguish the edge of plaque from the vessel wall. Submillimeter spatial resolution down to 0.3 mm is possible with the most advanced CT scanners [2]. This is particularly important because coronary calcium is a frequent component of coronary plaque. The CT image created of calcium "blooms" much larger than its actual dimension measured on a pathology specimen [3]. Better spatial resolution results in less "blooming" of calcium that may obscure the coronary lumen.

Data acquired with CCTA are reconstructed in a digital pixel volume with equal dimensions isovolumetric voxel. The reconstructed data are displayed with software allowing a multidimensional or multiplanar view of the coronary

M.C. Newell, MD (✉)
Minneapolis Heart Institute, Abbott Northwestern Hospital, MHI Cardiology,
800 E 28th Street, Minneapolis, MN 55407, USA
e-mail: Marc.Newell@allina.com

R.S. Schwartz, MD
Minneapolis Heart Institute, 920 E 28th Street, Minneapolis, MN 55076, USA

J.R. Lesser, MD
Minneapolis Heart Institute Foundation, 920 E. 28th Street, Minneapolis, MN 55407, USA

Z. Vlodaver et al. (eds.), *Coronary Heart Disease: Clinical, Pathological, Imaging, and Molecular Profiles*,
DOI 10.1007/978-1-4614-1475-9_5, © Springer Science+Business Media, LLC 2012

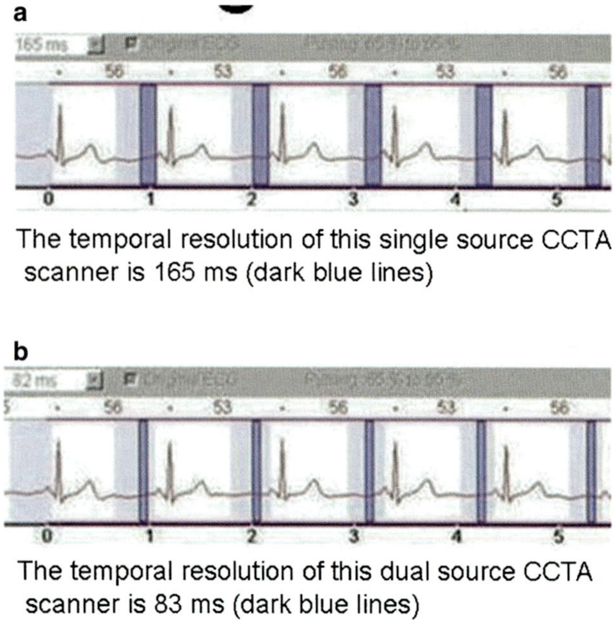

Fig. 5.1 Representative electrocardiogram (ECG) gating of a coronary computed tomography angiogram (CCTA) and comparison of single- vs. dual-source scanners. (**a**) shows the temporal resolution of a single-source CCTA scanner is 165 ms (*dark blue lines*). (**b**) shows the temporal resolution of a dual-source CCTA scanner is 83 ms (*dark blue lines*). The *dark blue vertical lines* represent the time it takes within a heartbeat to acquire data for an image. The scan in (**a**) takes twice as long as that in (**b**) to acquire data

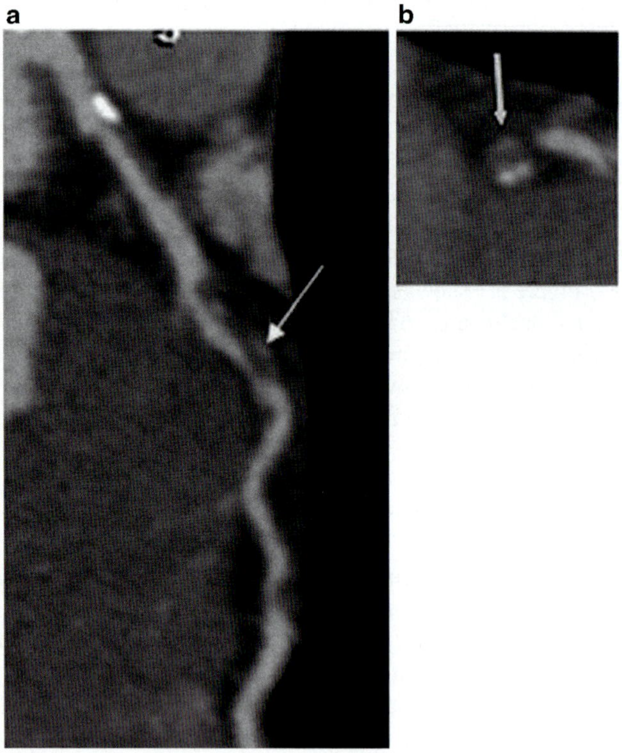

Fig. 5.2 Because CCTA data use isotropic voxels, coronary artery anatomy can be displayed in a familiar format. (**a**) shows a complex lesion in the left anterior descending artery longitudinally (*white arrow*) and (**b**) shows a lesion in the short axis (*blue arrow*)

arteries (Fig. 5.2). Better spatial resolution means smaller voxel size, but that requires more signal from intravascular contrast and/or less noise from more effective or higher radiation exposure [2, 3].

Value in Shorter Scans

It is useful to visualize the anatomy of interest – the heart – in the shortest time period possible. Shorter scans allow fewer artifacts from respiratory motion and irregular heart rhythms that interfere with coronary images. A short scan is created with either greater number of slices or faster table speeds (or higher pitch), which limit the number of heartbeats that need to be collected to fully picture the heart.

Current scanners can obtain full scans in one heartbeat. This is most important in perfusion imaging, where coverage of different locations in a similar time period is essential. The minimum technical requirements of a CT scanner capable of imaging coronary arteries include a TR of <210 ms, spatial resolution of <0.9 mm², and a scan range coverage of 32 detector rows.

Coronary CT Scan Procedure

Most coronary CT scans are performed in an outpatient setting. The experience for the patient is similar to any contrast CT scan. An intravenous, iodinated contrast dose of 60–110 mL is used. Typically, a patient will be given oral or intravenous beta-blockade to achieve a goal heart rate of <60 beats/min; an 18-gauge IV is placed in an antecubital vein. The scan time lasts from 280 ms to 6 s, requiring a breath hold from 5 to 12 s, depending on scanner and anatomical field covered.

Patient-related factors that can limit the acquisition of high-quality, interpretable scans include: irregular rhythms, fast heart rates, circumferential coronary calcium, and the inability of the patient to sustain a breath hold. (This factor is now less important with modern scanners). Obesity offers another challenge to obtaining high-quality scans, because of additional scan noise due to low X-ray photon flux. Although highly experienced centers with modern scanners can appropriately accommodate these patient-related challenges, these necessary adjustments in scan acquisition often result in higher-than-average radiation doses.

The ability of a specific CT laboratory to obtain accurate and safe coronary data is highly dependent on pretest patient preparation to limit heart rate, use of appropriate contrast injection, and scan protocols designed to answer specific clinical questions, and the ability of a trained reader to recognize artifacts and accurately interpret scans in their presence.

Diagnostic Accuracy of Coronary CT Angiography

Multiple studies have looked at the ability of cardiac CT to diagnose obstructive or clinically significant coronary artery disease. CCTA is used for two distinct clinical categories: acute chest pain in the emergency room (ER) and outpatient or chronic chest pain.

Acute Chest Pain

Patients presenting to emergency rooms with chest pain represent an important clinical and economic burden. CCTA in low- or intermediate-risk patients presenting to the emergency room has a very high negative-predictive value (NPV) and has been shown to save time and money. In one study of 368 consecutive ER patients with chest pain undergoing CCTA, 81% had no stenosis and 50% had no plaque, while 19% of the patients were identified as having significant disease, 8% of which had an acute coronary syndrome (ACS). When no plaque was seen, sensitivity and NPV were 100%. The specificity for significant stenosis was 77% [4].

In terms of time and money savings, 6 million Americans present to the ER each year with chest pain, at an estimated diagnostic cost of $10 billion. In a preliminary study of 197 ER patients, CCTA led to faster triage times and lower costs [5]. This small, single-center experience led to a similarly designed and recently completed multicenter trial (CT-STAT) that evaluated ER patients with acute chest pain. Sixteen centers enrolled 701 ER patients with chest pain and negative EKG and cardiac enzymes. They were randomized to either CCTA or nuclear perfusion imaging to diagnose the presence or absence of significant coronary disease. The primary endpoint of the trial showed that CCTA reduced time to diagnosis by 53% and reduced cost by 38% compared to nuclear perfusion imaging. No difference was seen in the incidence of ACS, angiographic procedures, or safety, as judged by a major cardiac event at 6 months [6].

Chronic Chest Pain Syndromes

Diagnostic accuracy of CCTA in chronic chest pain syndromes has been extensively studied using 64-slice scanners. As with all tests, sensitivity and specificity highly depend on the prevalence of disease in the population studied. Multiple, early, small studies showed promising results for 64-slice scanners in terms of specificity and the number of segments able to be evaluated. Early studies suggested a specificity range of 86–100% and sensitivity range of 92–99%, with most studies having a sensitivity of 95% or higher. The majority of studies also had <5% of segments that were unable to be evaluated [7–9].

CCTA vs. QCA

CCTA is excellent at ruling out significant disease when compared with invasive coronary angiography. In the most important subset of patients – those in whom CCTA finds a <50% stenosis – only 2% were found to have a significant stenosis by quantitative coronary angiography (QCA). Of those thought to have a significant lesion identified by CCTA, 50% of the lesions thought to be >70% as indicated by CCTA had a QCA >70%, while 15% of patients believed to have an intermediate lesion as indicated by CCTA (between 50 and 69% diameter stenosis) had a stenosis >70% identified by QCA [10].

When comparing CCTA with QCA using other invasive means of determining stenosis severity and physiologic significance – fractional flow reserve (FFR) and intravascular ultrasound (IVUS), the two anatomic tests were equally effective. Importantly, in a recent multicenter trial, CCTA predicted future interventions as well as diagnostic coronary angiography [11].

CCTA is most useful in patients with low- and intermediate-pretest risk of disease. A study by Meijboom and colleagues evaluated 254 symptomatic patients referred for invasive coronary angiography. Each patient had pretest risk assessed using the Duke clinical score (based on symptom characteristics and risk factors) and was placed into either a low-, intermediate-, or high-risk group for coronary artery disease. The investigators compared estimated posttest risk following CCTA with the subsequent findings of invasive qualitative coronary angiography using >50% as the threshold for lesion significance. The key findings were that in low- or intermediate-pretest risk patients, a negative CT scan resulted in a 0% posttest probability of disease. In the high pretest probability group for coronary disease, a small number of false-negative CCTA tests appeared [12].

Results From Multicenter Trials

Disease prevalence is critical to test performance in CCTA. As disease prevalence increases, fewer false-positives and more false-negatives are seen. Intermediate-risk patients typically have a pretest probability of significant CAD of 10–30% [13]. A typical outpatient CCTA population has a disease prevalence of 19% [14].

Three multicenter trials have now evaluated the diagnostic accuracy of CCTA. The first, the Accuracy trial, was a single-vendor study where CCTA was performed on outpatients referred for invasive angiography. Budoff and colleagues included 230 consecutive patients from 16 different sites. Using patient-based analysis, the sensitivity to detect a >50% stenosis with CCTA was 95% with an NPV of 99%. The rates were similar when the ability to detect a stenosis of 70% or more was assessed: a sensitivity of 94% and an NPV of 99%. The prevalence of obstructive disease in this population was 25%, consistent with an intermediate-risk patient population [15].

The second multicenter trial, CORE-64, was a single-vendor, international trial that assessed patients with both chronic and acute chest pain. A patient-based analysis in this population ($n=291$), with a very high prevalence of disease (56%), showed a sensitivity of 85% and an NPV of 83%. However, as expected, the specificity and positive predictive value (PPV) were higher (90 and 91%, respectively), given this level of disease prevalence [11].

In the only multicenter, multi-vendor, 64-slice scanner trial to date, sensitivity and NPV were very high in a large population ($n=360$, 99% sensitivity, and 97% NPV) despite a high prevalence of disease [16].

Overall, CCTA has a very high diagnostic accuracy in low- and intermediate-risk patients. Its most important attribute remains the ability to rule out significant obstructive disease as a potential cause of symptoms.

Prognosis Assessed by Coronary CT Angiography

CCTA is strongly predictive of invasive coronary angiographic results, but questions remain about its ability to assess prognosis. Many studies show that coronary calcium scoring (cardiac CT without contrast) is the best predictor of individual risk, as opposed to population-based risk scores and event prediction models.

The MESA (Multi-Ethnic Study of Atherosclerosis) study was a key coronary calcium scoring trial [17]. It used a large cohort ($n=6{,}722$) of asymptomatic patients from multiple ethnic groups who had no clinical cardiovascular disease on entry. Coronary calcium scores were obtained in addition to traditional risk factor assessment.

Calcium scoring was the strongest predictor of individual risk of a coronary event and provided risk identification beyond that of traditional risk factors in all ethnic groups. In patients with a total calcium score > 100 (compared with those with no coronary calcium), the adjusted risk of a coronary event was increased by a factor of 7.73, which jumped to 9.67 among those with an absolute score > 300. In addition, calcium scoring can reassign an individual patient's risk category from that predicted by risk factors alone [18].

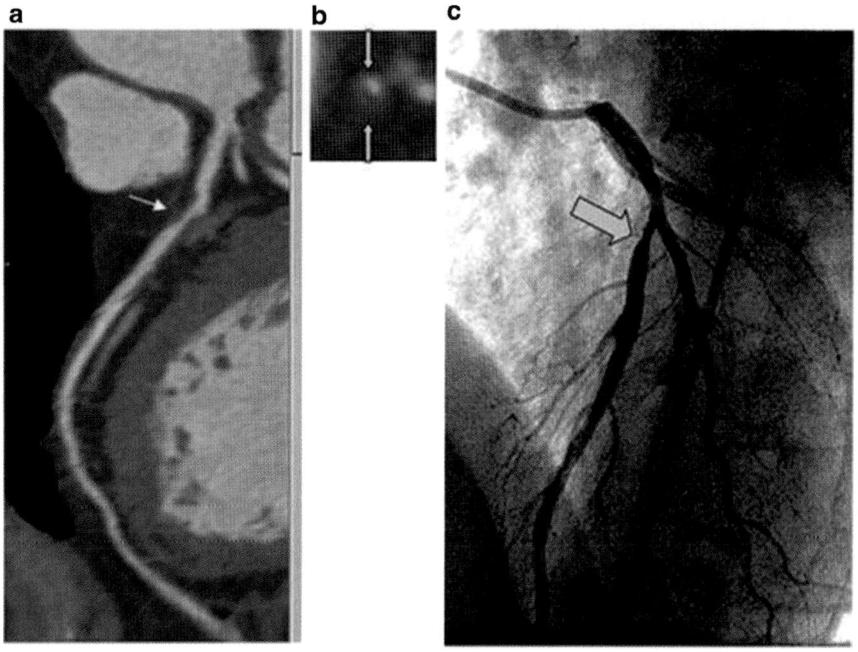

Fig. 5.3 This patient presented with transient chest pain, normal biomarkers, and a normal ECG. (**a**) shows a proximal coronary lesion (*white arrow*). (**b**) shows a short axis of the lesion with positive remodeling (*blue arrows*). (**c**) shows the lesion (*thick arrow*) from the invasive coronary angiogram. Note that positive remodeling is only seen with CCTA

CCTA also Shows Noncalcified Plaque

CCTA is a new modality that shows both coronary calcium and noncalcified plaque. Min and colleagues retrospectively evaluated 1,127 patients who underwent 16-slice CCTA. As with invasive coronary angiography, more severe and extensive coronary artery stenosis correlated with worse survival [19].

The largest study to date using CCTA for risk stratification and prognosis screened 2,538 asymptomatic patients with calcium scoring and electron-beam CT angiography (EBCTA) – e.g., a coronary CT angiogram with lower spatial resolution than multidetector CCTA – and followed them for 72 months. An individual patient's risk predicted by risk factor analysis alone was significantly improved by adding both EBCTA-diagnosed noncalcified coronary plaque and the coronary calcium score [20]. More recently, Hadamitzky and colleagues showed that 64 slice multidetector CCTA in patients who have obstructive CAD clearly identifies those at risk for a future cardiac event more accurately than from Framingham-predicted risk [21].

In addition, van Werkhoven compared the frequency of major adverse cardiac events over a 2-year period in 541 patients undergoing both CCTA and myocardial perfusion imaging (MPI). The most predictive information combined CCTA measures of both stenosis severity and the extent of noncalcified nonobstructive plaque with the physiologic-based results from MPI [22].

Clinical Indications for Coronary CT Angiography

CCTA is a new modality with emerging clinical indications. The 2006 ACC/AHA Appropriateness Criteria helped identify core indications for the technique [23].CCTA accurately defines coronary anatomy in patients following unclear physiologically based stress test results. A major clinical use of CCTA is to assess acute chest pain patients in the emergency department who have no objective evidence of an ACS (*See* Sect.5.2 and Fig. 5.3.) [12]. Many patients referred to CCTA have had either negative nuclear or echo stress tests, but do have ongoing chest pain (Fig. 5.4). Alternatively, a patient with unclear stress test results or mildly positive findings that may represent abnormalities unrelated to epicardial coronary disease, is referred to CCTA (Fig. 5.5).

In single-center studies, CCTA improved noninvasive diagnostic accuracy and resulted in fewer, subsequent invasive coronary angiograms, conferring a cost savings over the strategy of using invasive coronary angiography without the availability of CCTA [5]. Additionally, negative CCTA in this setting provides a high likelihood of freedom from symptomatic disease for years after the test [24–27].

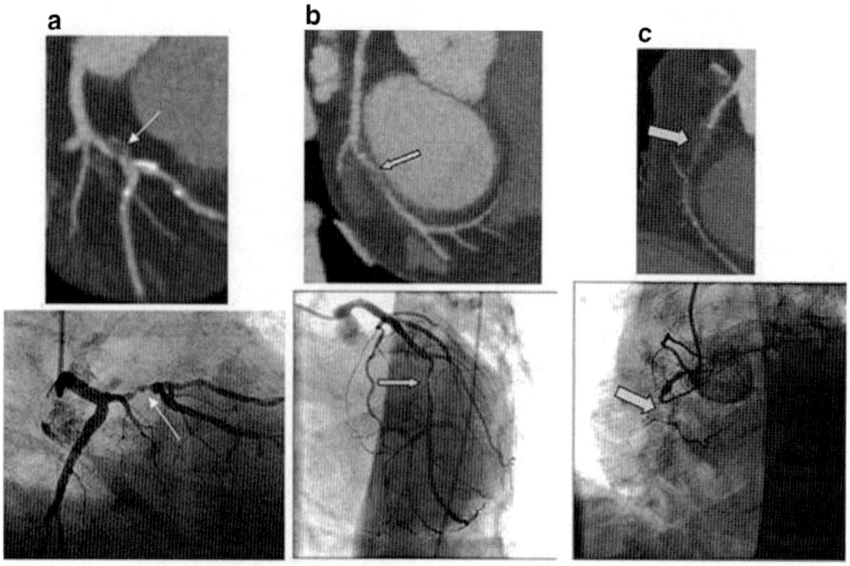

Fig. 5.4 This patient had CCTA for continuing chest pain following a normal stress test using sestamibi. CCTA images and a subsequent, invasive coronary angiogram are shown in the lower row. (**a**) (*white arrow*) demonstrates the left anterior descending (LAD) lesion, (**b**) (*thin blue arrow*) shows the circumflex lesion, and (**c**) demonstrates a totally occluded right coronary artery (*thick blue arrow*) with collaterals, as seen with CCTA

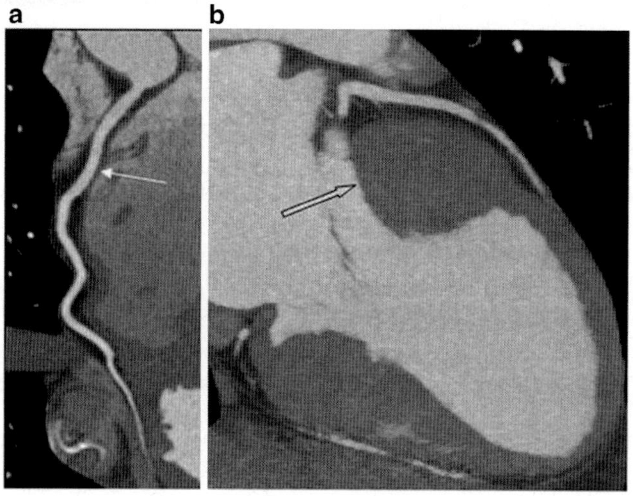

Fig. 5.5 This patient had a mildly abnormal stress test. (**a**) shows the patient had normal coronary arteries (*white arrow*). (**b**) demonstrates marked asymmetric hypertrophy (*blue arrow*), which was the likely cause of the abnormal stress test

CCTA assessment of patients with coronary artery bypass grafts is also highly accurate [28, 29]. The potential source of pain can be localized to a large bypass graft or a smaller-branch native vessel. This may help with the decision to proceed with medical therapy versus intervention without the use of invasive coronary angiography (Fig. 5.6).

Presurgical coronary assessment for noncoronary cardiac or aortic valve surgery is an excellent use of CCTA, except in those with a very high pretest probability of coronary disease [30].

Chest Pain after Stent Placement

A clinical scenario not included in the 2006 ACC/AHA Appropriateness Criteria is using CCTA in patients who have chest pain early after the placement of intracoronary stents. Current practice is to repeat invasive coronary angiography in these patients to interrogate newly placed stents for patency and thus determine whether the patient can return to full activity. Because symptomatic acute or subacute stent problems present as total occlusion, the CCTA only has to distinguish between a completely patent or occluded lumen (Fig. 5.7). However, CCTA in patients with chronic chest pain in the presence of stents has a lower PPV than CCTA of the native vessels. There remains a high NPV for CCTA if the stent size is >3 mm [31–33].

In addition, CCTA is useful in chronic total occlusion planning by demonstrating the extent of calcification and length of the occlusion site, therefore predicting the likelihood of success (Fig. 5.8) [34]. CCTA is also useful in patients with combined aortic and coronary disease [35].

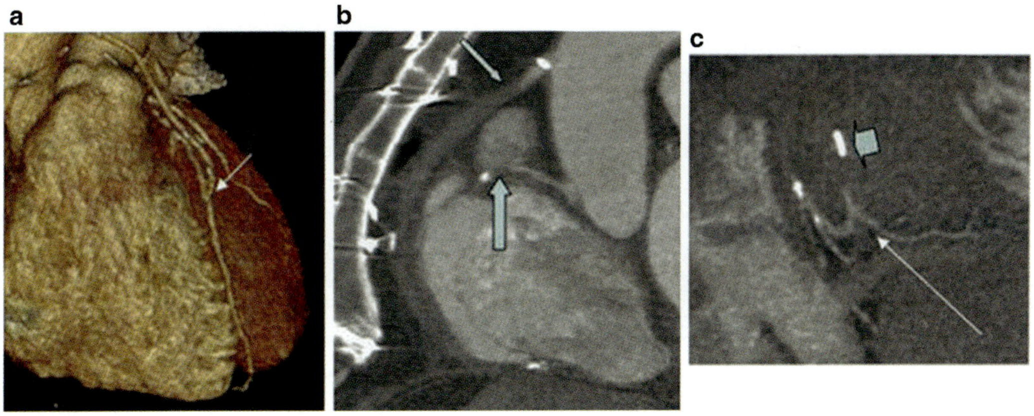

Fig. 5.6 CCTA was performed in a patient with an abnormal stress echocardiogram. (**a**) (*white arrow*) shows a patent left internal mammary artery graft to the LAD. (**b**) shows an occluded vein graft to the posterior descending artery (PDA) (*thin blue arrow*) and an occluded, native RCA (*thick blue arrow*). (**c**) shows a clip (*short arrow*) from the occluded vein graft tenting the occluded PDA filling by collaterals (*long arrow*). No invasive coronary angiogram was required

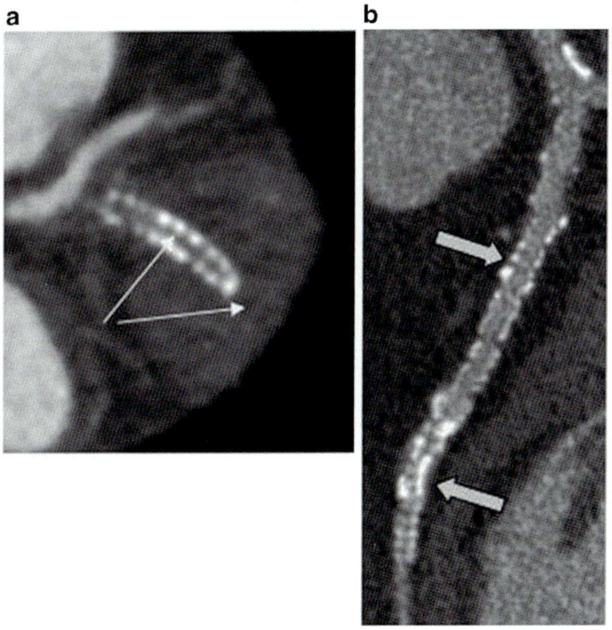

Fig. 5.7 This CCTA shows an occluded diagonal branch stent 2 weeks after its placement (*white arrows*). No contrast is noted within or distal to the stent. (**b**) shows a second patient who had a CCTA. Blue arrows show multiple patent stents in the LAD 10 days after placement

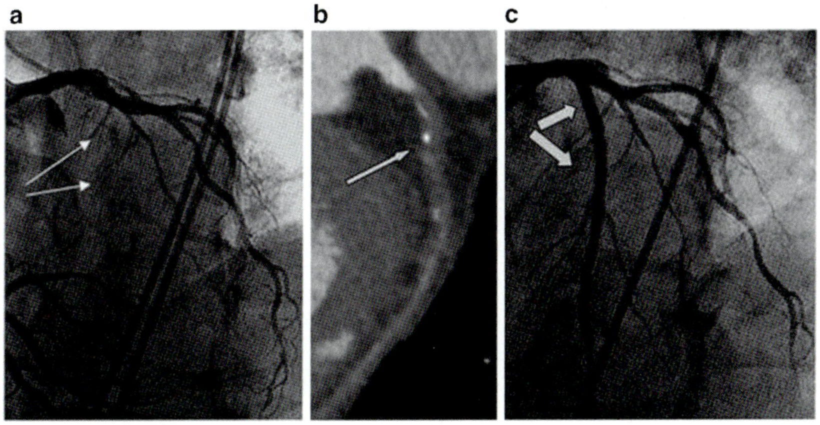

Fig. 5.8 Despite simultaneous right coronary artery and left main coronary injections (**a**), no proximal LAD lumen is seen (*white arrows*). A subsequent CCTA (**b**) showed little coronary calcium (*thin blue arrow*) and predicted a successful percutaneous intervention (**c**), as seen on the post-PCI coronary angiogram (*thick blue arrows*)

Radiation in Coronary CT Angiography

Many cardiologic and radiologic examinations require radiation exposure. A clear understanding of relative dose and how to limit exposure enables the clinician to better decide such testing's risk-benefit ratio.

A milliSievert (mSv) is the effective absorbed radiation dose equivalent. By converting ionizing radiation energies to mSv, biologic exposure can be compared when delivered from differing sources. Background radiation varies with altitude and is estimated at 3–5 mSv per year. A standard postero-anterior view (PA) and lateral chest X-ray gives 0.02 mSv. Invasive coronary angiography gives 2–7 mSv, while stress nuclear scans give different doses based on the agent used (9–11 mSv with technetium, 18–22 mSv with thallium, and as high as 26 mSv with dual-isotope studies). Chest and abdominal CT scans use 12 mSv. For repetitive screening tests such as mammography, females receive about 0.7 mSv of radiation with each exposure.

The radiation dose with CCTA is highly variable and relates to the scan operator's awareness and use of dose-sparing techniques. These techniques were evaluated in a real-world, multicenter analysis: the PROTECTION-I study [36]. Despite limited use of many of the scanning and processing techniques (which were novel at the time), the mean radiation dose across the international centers was 12 mSv, with several centers reporting doses under 5 mSv [36].

One specific technique, prospective-ECG gating, reduced radiation dose by 78%. Additionally, Raff and colleagues developed a state-wide initiative in Michigan to teach and subsequently lower radiation doses in CCTA [37]. They showed a greater than 53% decrease in radiation from the control (pre-teaching technique) to the follow-up period at all sites, with a final multicenter mean radiation dose of 10 mSv [37].

In an unpublished analysis at own, high-volume center, roughly 60% of patients had slow and stable heart rates, enabling prospective gating. Mean doses for all patients using a dual-source scanner was 3.8 mSv. Recent, dramatic improvements in scanner software and hardware, such as the use of iterative reconstruction techniques and high-pitch scanning, have allowed select CCTA scans to use under 1 mSv – equivalent to the radiation dose received with a single mammogram.

Future Directions in Coronary CT Angiography

Future applications in CCTA include plaque characterization and perfusion imaging.

Plaque Characterization

The clinical goal of plaque characterization is to identify culprit vessels as the cause of symptoms or, more importantly, to determine a patient's risk of a future cardiac event, and even an individual plaque's risk of rupture.

A small study by Motoyama involved performing CCTA in 33 patients with ACS and comparing results to those of 38 patients without an ACS, but with coronary disease. This study identified differences in plaque type between the two groups. Patients with an ACS more often had low-density plaque, presumably with a lipid-laden core, and positive vessel remodeling [38].

A larger-scale study by the same investigators followed 1,059 patients over 27 months. Patients were evaluated by CCTA for low-attenuation plaque and positive vessel remodeling. Although event rates were low, a positive correlation was found between these factors and subsequent ACS events. Patients who had plaques with both characteristics had a 22% rate of developing ACS, versus 3.7% in patients with just one factor, compared with a 0.5% rate in patients without either factor ($p<0.0001$) [39]. An example of such features is demonstrated in Fig. 5.9.

Perfusion Imaging

CTA-based stress perfusion imaging is a promising new technique [40]. CCTA protocol that provides a near-simultaneous anatomic and physiologic assessment of coronary artery disease is desirable and awaits many further refinements before it is a routine part of clinical practice.

Summary: Coronary Artery Disease Assessment by Coronary CT

CCTA as a noninvasive technique has unparalleled diagnostic accuracy, provides important prognostic information, and even the potential to determine which patients are at highest risk for future cardiac events. This now can be provided at an equivalent or lower radiation dose than other noninvasive or invasive diagnostic tests.

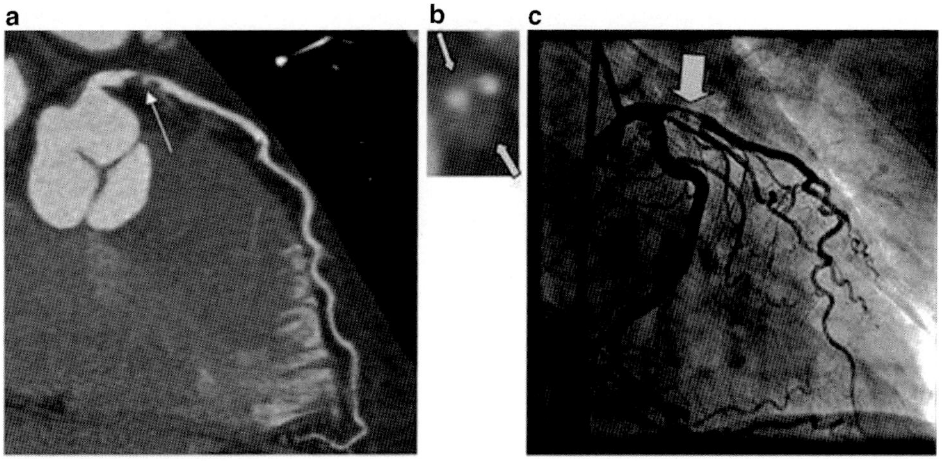

Fig. 5.9 CCTA on a patient with acute coronary syndrome who presented in the ER (**a**) shows contrast in a ruptured coronary plaque (*white arrow*). A short axis view of the lesion (**b**) demonstrates positive remodeling (*thin blue arrow*) consistent with an acute lesion. Contrast within the LAD plaque (**c**) is also seen on invasive angiography (*thick blue arrow*)

Coronary Artery Imaging with MRI

Cardiac magnetic resonance imaging (MRI) has many uses and practical applications in clinical cardiology. In this section, we review coronary artery imaging using cardiac magnetic resonance.

Cardiac MR (CMR) provides high-resolution, 3D images with intrinsic contrast, and no ionizing radiation. Additionally, CMRI enables a comprehensive cardiac assessment using multiple techniques in a single system that includes an exquisite qualitative and quantitative evaluation of myocardial function, viability, extent of fibrosis or infiltration, stress perfusion, functional importance and characteristics of pericardial disease, and valvular heart disease.

It is advisable to avoid CMR in patients with ferromagnetic devices such as certain types of cerebral aneurysm clips, inner ear and penile prostheses, and cardiac pacemaker and/or defibrillator leads (unless under a strict protocol and supervision). A high-quality study can be time-consuming and is heavily dependent on the MRI equipment as well as the experience of the technician and supervising physician.

During a magnetic resonance exam, the patient is subjected to a strong, local magnetic field – 1.5 or 3.0 T – which aligns the protons in the body. These protons are excited by a radiofrequency pulse and their decay is subsequently detected by receiver coils. Detected signals are influenced by multiple factors, including relaxation times (known as T1 and T2), proton density, motion and flow, and others. The timing of the excitation pulses and the successive magnetic field gradients determine the image contrast [41].

Noninvasive Coronary Angiography with MRI

While coronary CT angiography has garnered most of the attention in noninvasive coronary imaging, coronary MRI is useful in proximal artery coronary visualization without radiation or exogenous contrast.

Noninvasive coronary artery imaging is complicated by many factors, similar to those discussed regarding CCTA. Several similarities and differences exist between these modalities. Complicating factors in high-quality, noninvasive coronary imaging include coronary artery motion, lower spatial resolution of cardiac MRI, and small vessel sizes (most <4 mm, with percutaneous interventions being done on arteries as small as 2 mm – therefore requiring evaluation of vessels this size or smaller), and the fact that the structures surrounding the coronary arteries often have similar imaging qualities.

CMR of the coronary arteries uses specific imaging sequences and prepulses without exogenous contrast. Generally, lower resolution studies of the origin of a coronary artery to rule out a coronary anomaly may be performed quickly with breathholding and no intrinsic contrast. To assess coronary lesion severity, a higher spatial resolution technique is needed. The greater the amount of data that is incorporated in the MR imaging matrix, the higher the spatial resolution and the longer the time needed to collect the data. This has led to a novel approach which requires respiratory navigator and ECG gating (Fig. 5.10). The technique records diaphragmatic motion and only collects data when the diaphragm is at the end-expiration (the point of least respiratory motion).

In addition, a gated cineangiogram showing the mid right coronary artery allows one to choose the point in the cardiac cycle where the coronary artery is the most still. By gating MR data acquisition to both the diaphragm and electrocardiogram, the imaging matrix is theoretically filled with motionless data collected over 10–30 min. Rapid heart rates also require

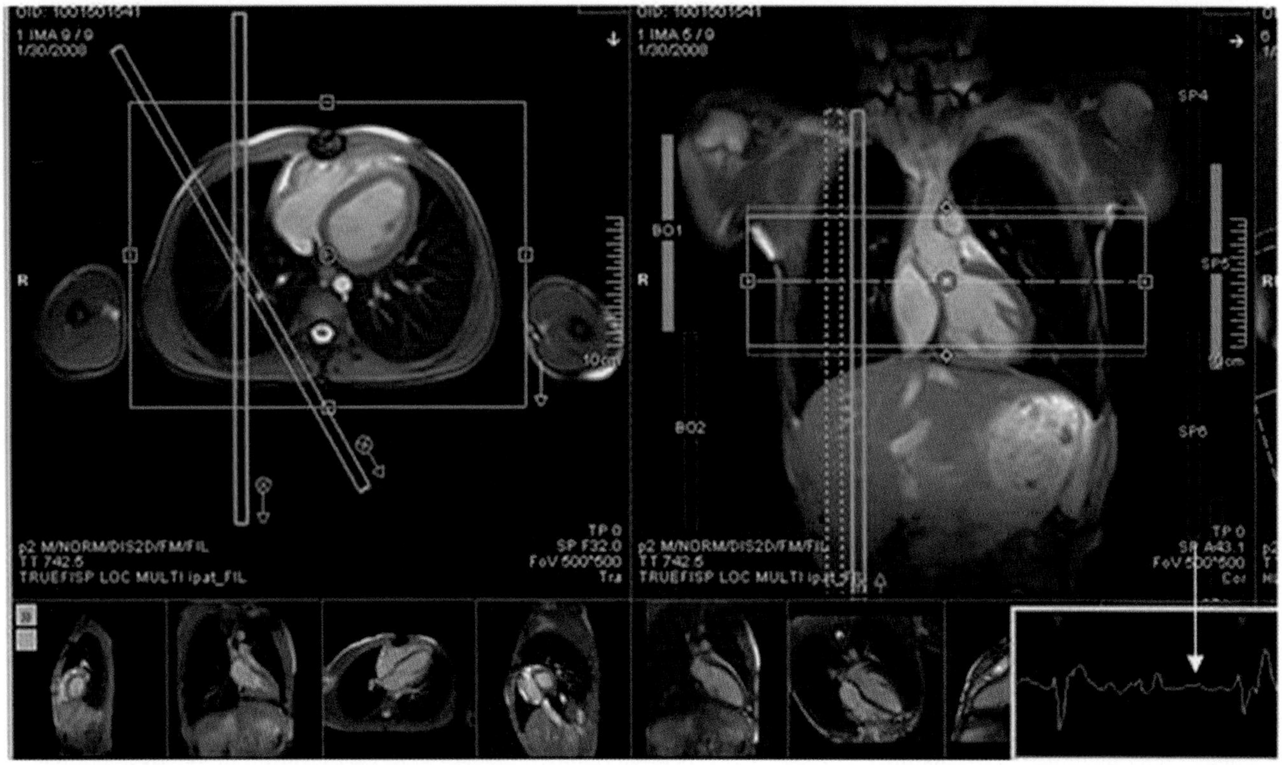

Fig. 5.10 The blue lines are for the respiratory navigator to monitor diaphragm motion. The *yellow box* contains the anatomy scanned. The *white arrow* shows the ECG-gating, allowing data to be collected in diastole and in end-expiration while free-breathing

that the temporal resolution of the acquisition technique be improved. The trade-off is a subsequent increase in the time of acquisition or a reduction in signal. Problems with ectopy or irregular breathing patterns can compromise scan quality. Although repeat scans are possible because no extrinsic contrast or radiation is used, the time of acquisition limits routine use of coronary artery imaging to assess coronary artery stenoses.

Results from Studies

Multiple studies have evaluated the feasibility of cardiac MRI for noninvasive coronary artery assessment. Studies of diagnostic accuracy have been small, but typically included patients with high prevalence of disease who were already referred for invasive coronary angiography.

A multicenter trial showed that, using CMRI, one could reasonably rule out left main and proximal three-vessel coronary disease [42]. Larger vessels such as coronary artery bypass grafts can also be visualized [43]. The difficulty of clear visualization of the smaller run-off vessels limits this clinical application of coronary MRI.

More recent data have focused on "whole-heart" coverage using steady state free processing (SSFP) and navigator diaphragmatic gating.

Jahnke et al. reported the results of 55 patients referred for coronary angiography with an average acquisition time of 18 min. When compared with invasive angiography, 83% of segments were evaluated, with reported sensitivity, specificity, and diagnostic accuracy of 78, 91, and 89%, respectively. (Disease prevalence was 50% in this study) [44].

Most recently, 3.0-T cardiac MRI has been used to improve the signal-to-noise ratio by 30% [45]. This increase in the signal-to-noise ratio can then be "traded" for improvement in temporal or spatial resolution. The largest drawback to using a 3.0 T field is that inhomogeneous artifacts are increased with stronger magnetic fields [46].

A study by Yang used 3.0 T CMRI angiography in 96 patients referred for coronary angiography. Of these, 34 patients were either ineligible for cardiac MR or unsuccessfully scanned (35%). Disease prevalence in this population was 55%.

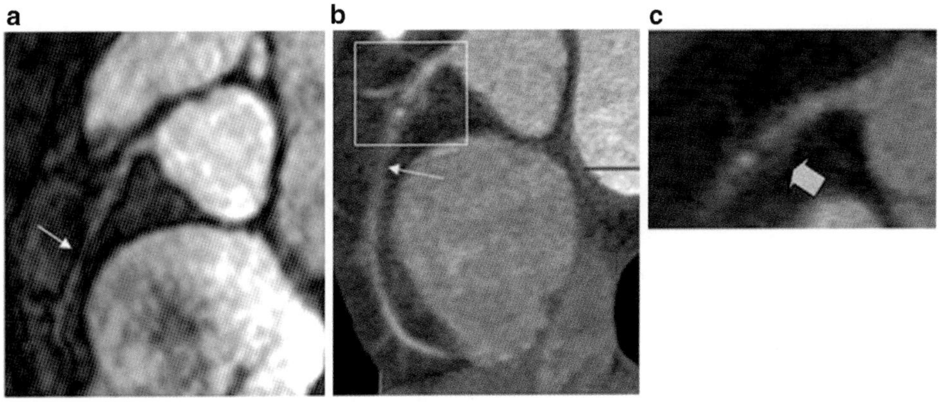

Fig. 5.11 CMRI followed by a CCTA in a 10-year-old with Kawasaki disease. Note the right coronary artery (RCA) lesion (*white arrow*) on CMR (**a**). (**b**) is the CCTA with better resolution; (**c**) shows an enlarged image of the RCA on CCTA with remodeled plaque (*thick blue arrow*) not seen on CMR

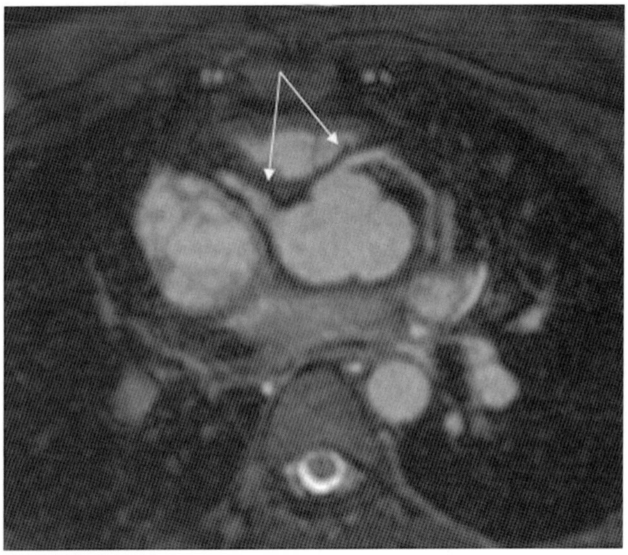

Fig. 5.12 Patent coronary artery ostia (*arrows*) are seen with CMRI following an arterial switch operation for D-transposition of the great vessels in a 9 year old

In looking at ability to detect a >50% stenosis (compared to quantitative analysis of invasive angiography), the test performed fairly well in those who could be scanned. Sensitivity was 89%; specificity, 82%; positive predictive value, 86.5%; and NPV, 92%. However, 12% of segments scanned – the smaller-caliber segments – could not be assessed [47].

When to Use CMRI

Because of multiple, possible technical problems associated with routine clinical coronary MRI use, it is best used as a substitute for coronary CT angiography in patients with the greatest radiation sensitivity such as children with Kawasaki disease [48, 49] (Fig. 5.11), visualization of coronary anomalies [50], and the assessment of post-arterial switch coronary ostia in the context of a complete pediatric CMRI exam (Fig. 5.12).

Experimentally, coronary MRI angiography has been evaluated for assessing coronary plaque and high-risk features such as positive remodeling. Using a black-blood approach, two studies showed that a difference in coronary wall thickness was a measure of plaque burden versus controls [51–53]. In addition, gadolinium uptake may be found in the coronary vessel wall, identifying a site of inflammation after an acute myocardial infarction.

Of note, 179 asymptomatic patients from the MESA study were evaluated with CMRI. Compared with calcium score (Agatston score), those patients who had subclinical atherosclerosis by calcium scoring had significantly thicker arterial walls on coronary MR angiography (>2.0 mm wall on CMR), suggesting positive remodeling could be detected with cardiac MRI [54].

Overall, coronary MRI is intriguing because of its lack of ionizing radiation and exogenous contrast. However, its current clinical application for coronary artery lesions is limited by substantial technical challenges.

References

1. Pannu HK, Alvarez W, Fishman EK. B-blockers for cardiac CT: a primer for the radiologist. Am J Roent. 2006;186:5341.
2. Nikolau K, Flohr T, Knez A, et al. Advances in cardiac CT imaging: 64-slice scanner. Intl J of Cardiovasc Imag. 2004;20:535–40.
3. Hoffman U, Ferenick M, Cury R, et al. Coronary CT Angiography J Nucl Med. 2006;47:797–806.
4. Hoffman U, Bamberg F, Chae CU, et al. Coronary computed tomography angiography for early triage of patients with acute chest pain. J Am Coll Cardiol. 2009;53:1642–50.
5. Goldstein JA, Gallagher MJ, O'Neill WW, Ross MA, O'Neil BJ, Raff GL. A randomized controlled trial of multi-slice coronary computed tomography for evaluation of acute chest pain. J Am Coll Cardiol. 2007;49:863–71.
6. Raff G, Chinnaiyan KM, Berman D, et al. Late-breaking clinical trial/science abstracts from the aha scientific sessions 2009. Circulation. 2009;120:2160.
7. Raff G, Gallagher M, O'Neill W, et al. Diagnostic accuracy of noninvasive coronary angiography using 64-slice spiral computed tomography. J Am Coll Cardiol. 2005;46(3):552–7.
8. Cademartiri F, Runza G, Mollet NR, et al. Impact of intravascular enhancement, heart rate, and calcium score on diagnostic accuracy in multislice computed tomography coronary angiography. Radiol Med. 2005;110:42–51.
9. Hausleiter J, Meyer T, Hadamitzky M, et al. Non-invasive coronary computed tomographic angiography for patients with suspected coronary artery disease: the Coronary Angiography by Computed Tomography with the Use of a Submillimeter resolution (CACTUS) trial. Eur Heart J. 2007;28(24):3034–41.
10. Cheng V, Gutstein A, Wolak A, et al. Moving beyond binary grading of coronary arterial stenoses on coronary computed tomographic angiography. Insights for the imager and referring clinician J Am Coll Cardiol Img. 2008;1:460–71.
11. Miller J, Rochitte CE, Dewey M, et al. Diagnostic performance of coronary angiography by 64-row CT. N Engl J Med. 2008;359:2324–36.
12. Meijboom WB, van Miegham CAG, Mollet NR, et al. 64-Slice computed tomography angiography in patients with high, intermediate, or low pretest probability of significant coronary artery disease. J Am Coll Cardiol. 2007;50:1469–75.
13. Budoff MJ, Copal A, Gul KM, et al. Prevalence of obstructive coronary artery disease in an outpatient cardiac CT angiography environment. Int J Cardiol. 2008;129:32–6.
14. Min JK, Shaw LJ. Noninvasive diagnostic and prognostic assessment of individuals with suspected coronary artery disease: coronary computed tomographic perspective. Circ Cardiovasc Imaging. 2008;1:270–81.
15. Budoff M, Dowe D, Jollis J, et al. Diagnostic performance of 64-multidetector row coronary computed tomographic angiography for evaluation of coronary artery stenosis in individuals without known coronary artery disease: results from the prospective multicenter ACCURACY (assessment by coronary computed tomographic angiography of individuals undergoing invasive coronary angiography) trial. J Am Coll Cardiol. 2008;52:1724–32.
16. Meijboom W, Meijs M, Schuijf J, et al. Diagnostic accuracy of 64-slice computed tomography coronary angiography. J Am Coll Cardiol. 2008;52:2135–44.
17. Detrano R, Guerci AD, Carr JJ, et al. Coronary calcium as a predictor of coronary events in four racial or ethnic groups. N Engl J Med. 2008; 358:1336–45.
18. Greenland P, LaBree L, Azen SP, Doherty TM, Detrano RC. Coronary artery calcium score combined with Framingham score for risk prediction in asymptomatic individuals. JAMA. 2004;291:210–5.
19. Min JK, Shaw LJ, Devereux RB, et al. Prognostic value of multi-detector coronary computed tomography for prediction of all-cause mortality. J Am Coll Cardiol. 2007;50:1161–70.
20. Ostrom MP, Gopal A, Ahmadi N, et al. Mortality incidence and the severity of coronary atherosclerosis assessed by computed tomography angiography. J Am Coll Cardiol. 2008;52:1335–43.
21. Hadamitzky M, Freimuth B, Meyer T, et al. Prognostic value of coronary computed tomographic angiography for prediction of cardiac events in patients with suspected coronary artery disease. JACC Img. 2009;2:404–11.
22. van Werkhoven JM, Schuijf JD, Gaemperli O, et al. Prognostic value of multi-slice computed tomography and gated single-photon emission computed tomography in patients with suspected coronary artery disease. J Am Coll Cardiol. 2009;53:623–32.
23. Hendel RC, Patel MR, Kramer CM, et al. ACCF/ACR/SCCT/SCMR/ASNC/NASCI/SCAI/SIR 2006 appropriateness criteria for cardiac computed tomography and cardiac magnetic resonance imaging. J Am Coll Cardiol. 2006;48(7):1475–97.
24. Danciu SC, Herrera CJ, Stecy PJ, Carell E, Saltiel F, Hines JL. Usefulness of multislice computed tomographic coronary angiography to identify patients with abnormal myocardial perfusion stress in whom diagnostic catheterization may be safely avoided. Am J Cardiol. 2007;100:1605–8.
25. Rubinshtein R, Halon DA, Gaspar T, et al. Impact of 64-Slice Cardiac Computed Tomography on Clinical Outcomes. Am J Cardiol. 2007; 99:925–9.
26. Menon M, Lesser JR, Hara H, et al. Multidetector CT coronary angiography for triage to invasive coronary angiography: performance and cost in ambulatory patients with equivocal or suspected inaccurate noninvasive stress tests. Cath Cardiovasc Interv. 2009;73:497–502.
27. Fazel P, Peterman MA, Schussler JM. Three year outcomes and cost analysis in patients receiving 64-slice computed tomography coronary angiography for chest pain. Am J Cardiol. 2009;104:498–500.
28. Nieman K, Pattynama PMT, Rensing BJ, et al. Evaluation of patients after coronary artery bypass surgery: angiographic assessment of grafts and coronary arteries. Radiology. 2003;229:749–56.
29. Pache G, Saueressig U, Frydrychowicz A, et al. Initial Experience with 64-slice cardiac CT: non-invasive visualization of coronary artery bypass grafts. Eur Heart J. 2006;27(8):976–80.
30. Bettencourt N, Roche J, Carvalho M, et al. Multislice computed tomography in the exclusion of coronary artery disease in patients with presurgical valve disease. Circ Cardiovasc Imaging. 2009;2:306–13.
31. Cademartiri F, Schuijf JD, Pugliesi F, et al. Usefulness of 64-slice computed tomography coronary angiography to assess in-stent restenosis. J Am Coll Cardiol. 2007;49:2204–10.
32. Rixe J, Achenbach S, Ropers D, et al. Assessment of coronary artery stent restenosis by 64-slice multi-detector computed tomography. Eur Heart J. 2006;27:2567–72.

33. Allison MA, Budoff MJ, Nasir K, et al. Ethnic specific risks for atherosclerotic calcification of the thoracic and abdominal aorta. Am J Cardiol. 2009;103:812–7.
34. Newell MC, Schwartz RS. Utility of CT Coronary Angiography for Planning CTO Intervention. March: Card Interv Today; 2009.
35. Fuechtner GM, Stolzmann P, Dichtl W, et al. Multislice computed tomography in infective endocarditis. J Am Coll Cardiol. 2009;53:436–44.
36. Hausleiter J, Meyer T, Hermann F, et al. Estimated radiation dose associated with cardiac CT angiography. JAMA. 2009;301(5):500–7.
37. Raff GL, Chinnaiyan KM, Share DA, et al. Radiation dose from cardiac computed tomography before and after implementation of radiation dose-reduction techniques. JAMA. 2009;301:2340–8.
38. Motoyama S, Kondo T, Sarai M, et al. Multislice computed tomographic characteristics of coronary lesions in acute coronary syndromes. J Am Coll Cardiol. 2007;50:319–26.
39. Motoyama S, Sarai M, Harigaya H, et al. Computed tomographic angiography characteristics of atherosclerotic plaques subsequently resulting in acute coronary syndrome. J Am Coll Cardiol. 2009;54:49–57.
40. Kitagawa K, Lardo AC, Lima JAC, et al. Prospective ECG-Gated 320 Row Detector CT: Implications for CT Angiography and Perfusion Imaging. Intl J Cardiovasc Img. 2009;53:9433–6.
41. Fayad ZA, Fuster V, Nikolaou K, Becker C. Computed tomography and magnetic resonance imaging for noninvasive coronary angiography and plaque imaging: current and potential future concepts. Circulation. 2002;106:2026–34.
42. Kim WY, Danias PG, Stuber M, et al. Coronary magnetic resonance angiography for the detection of coronary stenoses. N Engl J Med. 2001;345:1863–9.
43. Bunce N, Lorenz C, John A, et al. Coronary artery bypass graft patency: assessment with true fast imaging with steady-state precession versus gadolinium-enhanced MR angiography. Radiology. 2003;227:440–6.
44. Jahnke C, Paetsch I, Nehrke K, et al. Rapid and complete coronary arterial tree visualization with magnetic resonance imaging: feasibility and diagnostic performance. Eur Heart J. 2005;26:2313–9.
45. Sommer T, Hackenbroch M, Hofer U, et al. Coronary MR angiography at 3.0 T versus that at 1.5 T: initial results in patients suspected of having coronary artery disease. Radiology. 2005;234:718–25.
46. Wansapura K, Fleck R, Crotty W, et al. Frequency scouting for cardiac imaging with SSFP at 3 Tesla. Pediatr Radiol. 2006;36:1082–5.
47. Yang Q, Li K, Liu X, et al. Contrast-enhanced whole-heart cardiac magnetic resonance angiography at 3.0-T: a comparative study with X-ray angiography in a single center. J Am Coll Cardiol. 2009;54:69–76.
48. Greil GF, Stuber M, Botner RM, et al. Coronary magnetic resonance angiography in adolescents and young adults with Kawasaki disease. Circulation. 2002;105:908.
49. Marrogeni S, Papadopoulos G, Douskou M, et al. Spiral magnetic resonance angiography with rapid real-time localization. J Am Coll Cardiol. 2004;43(4):649–52.
50. Bunce N, Lorenz C, Keegan J, et al. Coronary artery anomalies: assessment with free-breathing three- dimensional coronary MR angiography. Radiology. 2003;227:201–8.
51. Fayad ZA, Fuster V, Fallon JT, et al. Noninvasive in vivo human coronary artery lumen and wall imaging using black-blood magnetic resonance imaging. Circulation. 2000;102:506–10.
52. BotnerBenter RM, Stuber M, Kissinger KV, et al. Noninvasive coronary vessel wall and plaque imaging with magnetic resonance imaging. Circulation. 2000;102:2582–7.
53. Ibrahim T, Makowski MR, Jankauskas A, et al. Serial contrast-enhanced cardiac magnetic resonance imaging demonstrates regression of hyperenhancement within the coronary artery wall in patients after acute myocardial infarction. JACC Cardio Img. 2009;2:580–8.
54. Miao C, Chen S, Macedo R, et al. Positive remodeling of the coronary arteries detected by magnetic resonance imaging in an asymptomatic population. J Am Coll Cardiol. 2009;53:1708–15.

Chapter 6
Catheter-Based Coronary Angiography

Robert F. Wilson and Zeev Vlodaver

Indications

The arteriogram depicts the anatomy of the coronary artery tree, demonstrates collateral channels, and provides information about small vessels and vessel segments distal to severe obstructions or occlusions that are inaccessible to other intravascular techniques.

The primary goal of coronary arteriography is the identification, localization, and assessment of stenotic lesions present within the coronary arteries to enable us to determine the pathophysiologic significance of the obstructive lesions in question (ischemia vs. nonischemia). While the arteriogram provides excellent delineation of coronary anatomy in vessel >400 μm diameter, its major deficiencies are that it shows mainly the anatomy of the arterial lumen (as opposed to the wall of the artery) and that is a 2D shadow of a 3D object.

The use of cardiac catheterization and angiography will provide significant information that is important for the management of the individual patient:

1. The extent of stenotic disease in the coronaries.
   (a) Severity of luminal narrowing
   (b) Distribution of stenotic lesions (number of vessels involved, distribution of lesions in each vessel, myocardium at risk)
   (c) Identification of acute, thrombotic lesions
2. Provide access for other studies, for example, intracoronary ultrasound, ocular coherence tomography (OCT, coronary flow reserve (CFR), and fractionated flow reserve (FFR).
3. Identify coronary arteries malformations or presence of myocardial bridges.
4. Left ventricular systolic and diastolic function, ejection fraction, and regional wall motion.
5. Myocardial perfusion, by assessing TIMI flow and TIMI blush scores.
6. Myocardial viability, by assessing TIMI blush, collaterals, improved ventricular contraction after nitrates, postextrasystolic potentiation, or dobutamine.

R.F. Wilson, MD (✉)
Division of Cardiovascular Medicine, University of Minnesota,
Minneapolis, MN, USA
e-mail: wilso008@umn.edu

Z. Vlodaver, MD
Division of Cardiovascular Medicine, University of Minnesota, Minneapolis, MN, USA

Z. Vlodaver et al. (eds.), *Coronary Heart Disease: Clinical, Pathological, Imaging, and Molecular Profiles*,
DOI 10.1007/978-1-4614-1475-9_6,

Technical Aspects

Radiographic Imaging System

Radiographic imaging of coronary arteries is demanding because they are small and move quickly with contraction of the heart. A radiographic imaging system can be divided into an X-ray tube, and an imaging chain that is composed of an imaging detector and a display (video). The general schematic is shown in Fig. 6.1.

For fluoroscopic examination, images obtained from the imaging device are displayed on a video system. The video image is composed of a pixel matrix, similar to that generated by CT imaging. Modern displays show 1,024 × 1,024 matrix of pixels per image. Recent systems use a progressive scan method where the entire image is displayed line by line every 1/60th of a second. The process permits better resolution of moving objects. It also, however, leads to additional electronic noise. Most manufacturers employ systems that pulse the X-ray exposure, which can further improve image sharpness. Radiation exposure is moderately reduced.

For cineangiography, an X-ray beam must be pulsed to provide for adequate "stop motion" imaging and to limit X-ray exposure. Thirty to sixty exposures/s are needed to give the appearance of a "live" continuous image, although 15 frames/s can produce a relatively smooth image if the software eliminates flicker and the radiation dose is reduced significantly. Some labs have reduced radiation further by reducing the frames rate to 7.5 images (X-ray pulses)/s. Nearly all newer radiographic systems incorporate digital image processing of the video pickup signal or obtain the image directly from CCD chips. A variety of pixel-processing algorithms are employed to enhance image clarity.

Display monitors should be able to show all the image detail presented by the image chain. Almost all modern monitors are flat panel LCD displays. The higher line rate provided more resolution, but also decreases the signal-to-noise ratio.

Regarding storage, digitized cineangiograms contain an enormous amount of information, typically 150 MB to 2 GB per study, making storage and computer network transfer a challenge. Nearly all digital images are stored using a DICOM (Digital Imaging and Communication in Medicine) format that permits interchange of information between different manufacturers' systems. Permanent storage is usually sent to a central PACS computer memory storage device (typically in a hospital), although storage is also done on compact disks or DVDs.

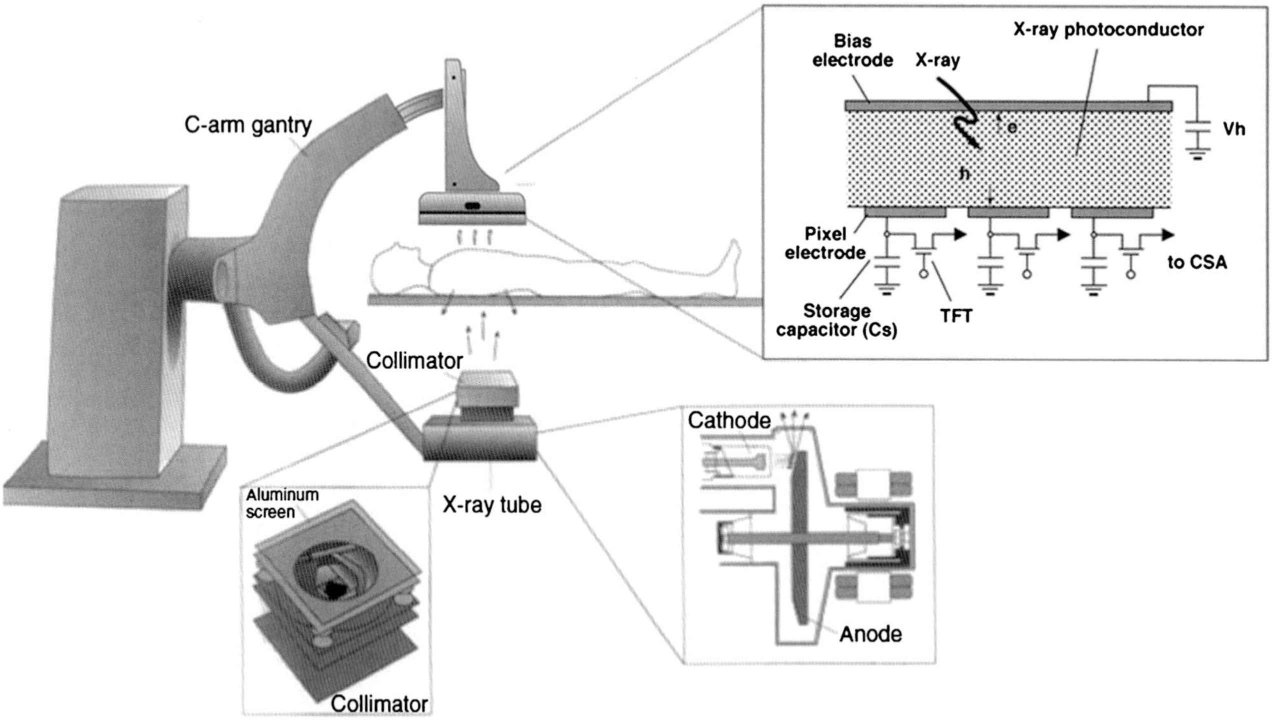

Fig. 6.1 Schematic of radiographic imaging system for cineangiography. The X-ray beam is generated by an X-ray tube (*lower right box*). The beam passes through a collimator (*lower left box*) where lead apertures form and limit the bean. On intersection with the patient, most of the beam is reflected or absorbed. The remaining photons pass through the image intensifier (*upper right box*)

History of Coronary Angiography

The first attempts to visualize the coronary arteries in living humans were published in 1945 by Radner S. [1], who used trans-sternal punctures to inject contrast material into the ascending aorta. . The complications of this method were too frequent and the results too poor; this option was abandoned.

In the late 1950s, G. Arnulf, a French researcher, made an important accidental discovery. While doing aortograms in animals, he obtained an outstanding coronary arteriorgram in a dog that had coincidentally had a cardiac arrest just before he was injected [2]. Through this observation, Arnuff described a new coronary arteriography technique to be performed during a cardiac arrest induced by the intravenous injection of a comparatively large amount of acetylcholine (3 mg/kg body weight).

A young surgeon, Dr. A. M. Bilgutay(1962), working in with Dr. C. Walton Lillehei's laboratory at the University of Minnesota, was stimulated by Arnulf's work in France. Bilgutay was able to confirm Arnulf's work in animals and achieved outstanding contrast visualization of the coronary arteries [3].

Stimulated by the pioneer work of Sones and associates, who showed that selective catheterization of the coronary arteries can be consistently carried out, selective coronary arteriography was started in the early 1960s [4]. The selective catheterization as devised by Sones introduced the catheters through the brachial cut-down technique.

In 1962, Dr Kurt Amplatz, also from the University of Minnesota, introduced a percutaneous puncture technique of the subclavian artery for selective catheterization of the coronary arteries using the Seldinger percutaneous technique [5]. Since the subclavian artery is still closer to the coronary arteries than the brachial artery, it was hoped that catheter manipulation was simplified to accomplish selective cannulation of both coronary arteries. The technique was abandoned because of several drawbacks: was difficult to achieve hemostasis with compression of the subclavian artery against the first rib; there were few cases of pneumothorax; and the catheterization of the left coronary artery was technically difficult.

With the prior introduction of the Seldinger wire cannulation method for vascular cannulation, a safer, percutaneous transfemoral catheterization technique was developed. Judkins, Amplatz, Abrams, and others invented preformed catheters that could be passed with great ease from the femoral artery to the coronary ostium. [6–8]. Since then, an explosion of catheter material and shapes has made possible nearly effortless cannulation of most coronary arteries and bypass grafts.

Patient Preparation and Vascular Access

The evaluation of patients about to undergo coronary angiography should emphasize a detailed history concerning factors that affect the approach and risks of angiography, a physical examination concentrating on the cardiovascular system, and comprehensive discussion of the procedure and its anticipated risks and benefits.

In all patients, an intravenous access line should be established prior to angiography. The infusion port should be large enough to permit a rapid infusion of fluid, should the patient develop reduced intravascular pressure (e.g., as a result of increased vagal tone or nitrate or nitrate-induced veno-relaxation). Patients with renal dysfunction, particularly those with diabetes, should be adequately hydrated before angiography. Dehydration increases the risk of contrast-induced nephropathy. In addition, several trials suggest that pretreatment with *N*-acetyl cysteine and intravenous fluids alkalinized with sodium bicardinate provide additional renal protection, although all subsequent clinical trials have not confirmed a protective effect.

Proper sedation is also important in preparation of the patient. Patients awaiting angiography are anxious, and treatment with anxiolytic drugs can improve their cooperation and reduce hypertension with the procedure.

Using the percutaneous transfemoral technique, first the skin and subcutaneous tissues about the artery are infiltrated with a local anesthetic. The common femoral artery is punctured with a thin-walled needle over the mid to lower portion of the femoral head. The position of the femoral head, which does not always correlate with the position of the inguinal crease, can be easily localized with fluoroscopy prior to the puncture.

Once the artery is punctured, a 0.035-in. flexible guidewire with a "J" tip is passed through the needle into the arterial lumen [9]. Once the guidewire is in place, an introducer sheath (a short tube with one-way valve) is advanced over the wire into the artery. The sheath size should be chosen based upon the desired diagnostic catheter used or size of the device required for any planned intervention. The angiographic catheters are advanced through hemostatic valve into the sheath and up to the ascending aorta with the aid of the J tip guidewire.

In patients with severe femoral or aortoiliac disease, radial access has been used. After performing an Allen test to ensure that the ulnar artery is patent, a small needle and guidewire is passed into the radial artery. An intravascular sheath with a

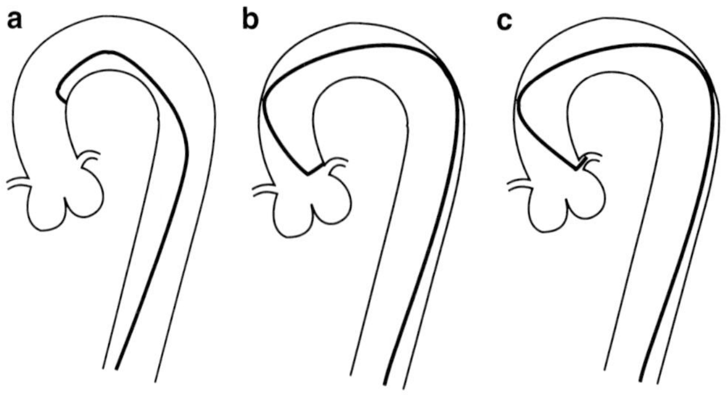

Fig. 6.2 Cannulation of the left coronary artery using a Judkins curve catheter. The catheter is passed to the proximal aorta (**a**) using a guidewire (not shown). It is then advanced to the coronary ostium while pressure is monitored from the catheter tip (**b**, **c**). The tip of the catheter should be coaxial with the artery

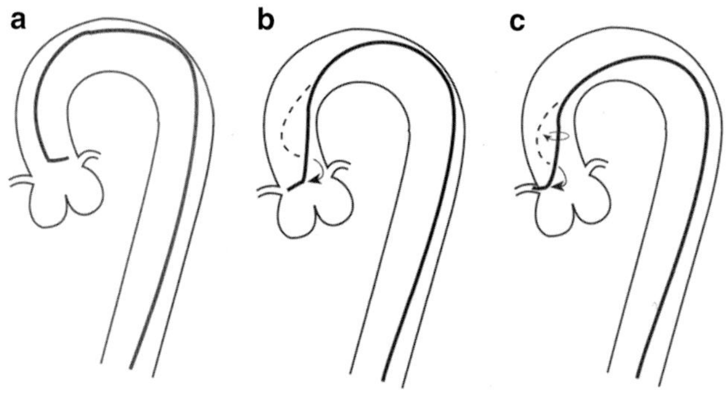

Fig. 6.3 Cannulation of the right coronary artery using Judkins curve catheter The catheter is passed to the proximal aorta (**a**) using a guidewire (not shown). It is then advanced to the level of the coronary ostium and rotated clockwise while pressure is monitored from the catheter tip (**b**, **c**) The tip should be coaxial with the artery.

hydrophilic coating is then passed into the artery. Vasospasm is common; administration of intraarterial nitroglycerin, calcium channel antagonist, and heparin is critical [10, 11].

After angiography, the extremity with the arteriotomy site should be extended and held straight. The catheter should be withdrawn from the artery, aspirating during withdrawal to help avoid extrusion of thrombus. Immediately after decannulation, the arterial puncture site should be compressed by hand or with the use of a device (e.g., Femostop). Care should be taken if a Femostop device is used as it can migrate out of position with patient movement which can result in significant bleeding complications. In addition, prolonged compression can result in a femoral neuropathy or venous thrombosis.

Several vascular closure devices have been developed; they are divided into mechanical closure devices (e.g., suture-based Perclose, or the Starclose clip) and devices that apply a hemostatic material (collagen or thrombin) to the puncture site (e.g., Angioseal). These devices allow patients to ambulate quickly, usually within an hour or less. However, caution should be exercised in using these devices in patients with significant atherosclerotic disease of the common femoral artery. In all cases, the patient should avoid actions that increase arterial pressure (e.g., coughing, sitting up).

Coronary Catheters

The essential features of a coronary angiographic catheter are an adequate lumen area, shape retention in the body, torque control, radiographic opacity, and safety. Catheters used to cannulate the coronary arteries are constructed of polymers, predominantly polyurethanes and polyethylenes that can be extruded and easily shaped. To improve shape retention and torque transmission, most manufacturers use wire braiding within the catheter wall.

Judkins and Amplatz developed a series of coronary catheters for cannulation from the femoral approach [6, 7]. Each design has a primary and secondary curve and tapers at the tip to hug the guidewire (Figs. 6.2 and 6.3).

Catheter caliber is measured in French (F) size, equal to circumference in millimeters.

In the 1990s, catheter construction improved markedly, allowing the manufacture of sizes 4–6 F, requiring a smaller arteriotomy, and reduced the time needed for hemostasis and bed rest after catheter withdrawal and may prevent peripheral complications.

Newer catheters of size 4–6 F produce acceptable angiography, particularly when used with a mechanical injector.

Cannulation and Contrast Material

Cannulation of the coronary ostium is the most important step in angiography. Catheters should be advanced to the ascending aorta root with the use of a guidewire. Inserting catheters without a guidewire can lead to retrograde peripheral arterial dissection. After aspirating the catheter to ensure that any debris or air has been removed, the catheter should be filled with contrast and connected to the pressure transducer.

Left coronary Amplatz and Judkins catheters can be advanced to the coronary ostium directly and usually require little manipulation (Fig 6.2). Right coronary Amplatz and Judkins catheters should be advanced to the aortic valve, withdrawn 1–11/2 cm and rotated clockwise until the ostium is engaged (Fig. 6.3).

After cannulation, the pressure at the catheter tip should be observed. Pressure damping implies that the catheter has burrowed into the wall of the artery wall, or that there is catheter-induced spasm, or that there is an organic ostial stenosis. If present, injection of contrast should be avoided because it could cause a coronary dissection.

Pressure damping from an improper catheter position or vasospasm is common in the right coronary artery, but in the left coronary it should alert the angiographer to the possibility of stenosis in the main left coronary artery, a particularly dangerous problem. A test injection below the artery or use of a "cusp" catheter can define the coronary ostium and permit selection of the best catheter shape. Administration of nitroglycerin can reduce the tendency for catheter-induced ostial vasospasm, although it is not always effective.

Iodine, an element that absorbs X-ray photons, is the essential constituent of angiographic contrast material. The compounds are highly water-soluble, stay within the extracellular space, and are excreted primarily by renal glomerular filtration.

Many of the unwanted effects of contrast material are related to the high osmolality of the contrast solution needed to obtain an adequate iodine concentration. "Nonionic," lower osmolality solutions have been developed, resulting in lower incidence of allergic reactions and the reduced toxic effects, mainly ventricular arrythmias, associated with the cations. Recently, a nearly iso-osmotic, nonionic contrast medium (iodixanol) has been developed. This agent appears to further reduce the risk of angiography on hemodynamics and little reflex bradycardia.

Contrast media can be injected into the coronary arteries with the use of a motorized injector or by a handheld syringe. Motorized injectors permit injection of specified amount of contrast material at a specified constant injection rate. The advantage of motorized injectors is consistency, the ability to deliver large contrast volumes at high flow rates (e.g., to hypertrophied hearts), and the ease of injection. A semiautomated injector with variable injection rate control has been developed for coronary angiography [12].

The presence of catheters within the vascular lumen causes denudation and combined with the foreign body of the catheter is a stimulus for intravascular thrombosis. Several, but not all, studies suggest that systemic anticoagulation with heparin reduces the incidence of thrombotic complications of angiography. Anticoagulation is not necessary for patients undergoing routine diagnostic angiography from the femoral approach. There is uniform agreement, however, that heparin (e.g., 2, 000 U into the artery and 3, 000 U intravenously) should be given to all patients in whom the brachial or radial approach is used.

The lumen caliber of epicardial coronary arteries measured at angiography reflects a variable degree of tone. Both atherosclerotic and normal coronary arteries dilate after nitroglycerin. Proximal vessels exhibit less dilation than distal epicardial vessels. Stenotic lesions also relax after nitroglycerin, although severely narrowed segments usually dilate little [13]. Removal of tone by nitroglycerin permits assessment of maximal coronary caliber, effectively eliminates vasospastic coronary lesions, and facilitates assessments of stenosis severity.

Complications of Coronary Angiography

Coronary arteriography is generally a safe procedure, but serious complications can occur. The overall incidence of complications and mortality increases directly with the extent of coronary artery disease, particularly left main coronary stenosis, the presence of coexistent significant valvular disease, a reduced ventricular ejection fraction, reduced functional state, and advancing age [14].

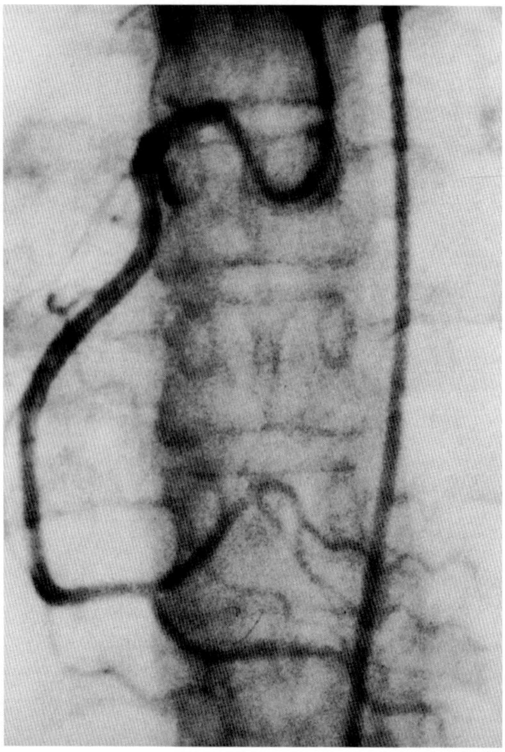

Fig. 6.4 RC arteriogram in frontal projection showing a fine line of radiolucency within the artery, suggesting a coronary arterial dissecting aneurysm (Dissect)

Arterial Dissection

Arterial cannulation performed by the Seldinger method usually causes endothelial denudation at the site of catheter or sheath insertion. During arterial puncture, the needle also may pass into through the posterior wall of the artery, and advancement of a guidewire into the posterior wall can result in arterial dissection. Fortunately, the arterial flap proceeds against the flow of blood and usually is sealed rather than propelled down the vessel by the arterial pulse. Dissection, along with endothelial injury, however, may promote local thrombosis and arterial occlusion. Perforation of peripheral arteries by a guidewire or catheter is uncommon, but probably occurs more frequently in patients with tortuous vessels and when stiff or hydrophilic wires or catheters are used.

Angiographically, the dissection can be recognized readily by demonstrating the dissected intima as a fine linear filling defect and delayed clearing of the contrast material from the false channel (Figs. 6.4 and 6.5).

Embolization

Embolization of arterial circulation can occur from injection of air, catheter-induced dislodgment of atherosclerotic plaque or vascular thrombus (e.g., clot in an abdominal aneurysm), dislodgment of left ventricular thrombus (e.g., in a ventricular aneurysm or recently infarcted ventricle), and debris or clot extruded from an improperly aspirated angiographic catheter.

Figures 6.6–6.8 are from a case with embolic occlusion of the coronary arteries. The patient was admitted for evaluation of chest pain. The coronary arteriogram showed the embolic material toward the PDA was migrating from the tip of the catheter. During the procedure, the patient was asymptomatic. The resting ECG, before the arteriogram. showed minimal aberrations. Following the study, the ECG showed nonspecific ST-T wave changes.

Catheter-induced embolization can lead to a variety of complications, depending on the target organ and makeup of the embolus [15, 16]. The sequelae of systemic embolism vary widely, from no symptoms to severe tissue necrosis. Thrombotic embolism frequently results in a loss of the peripheral pulse and occlusion of larger branch arteries that can be treated by embolectomy, anticoagulation, and in some cases, thrombolytic drugs.

Large peripheral air embolization can occur after accidental injection of air or, more commonly, from inspissation of air through a central venous access catheter in the jugular or subclavian venous system. Venous air embolisms over 50–100 mL can cause acute pulmonary hypertension and hypoxemia. Arterial air embolism can lead to profound transient tissue

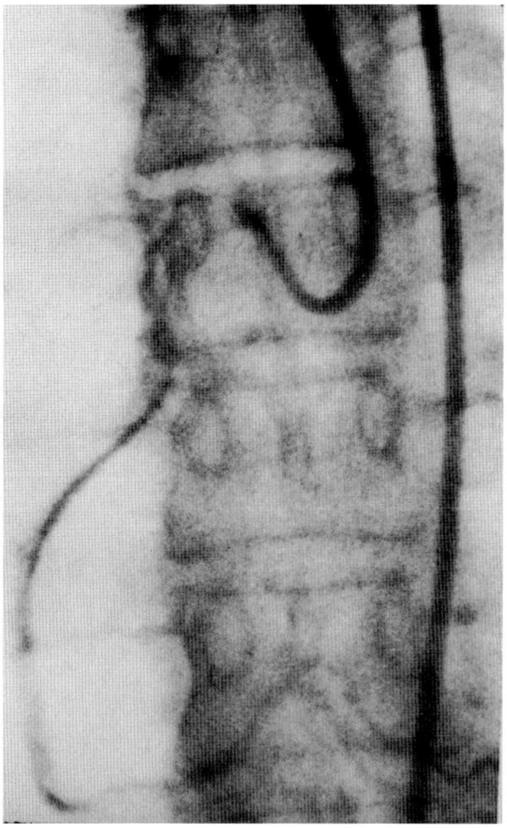

Fig. 6.5 RC arteriogram demonstrating slower flow in the false channel (Dissect) than in the principal one

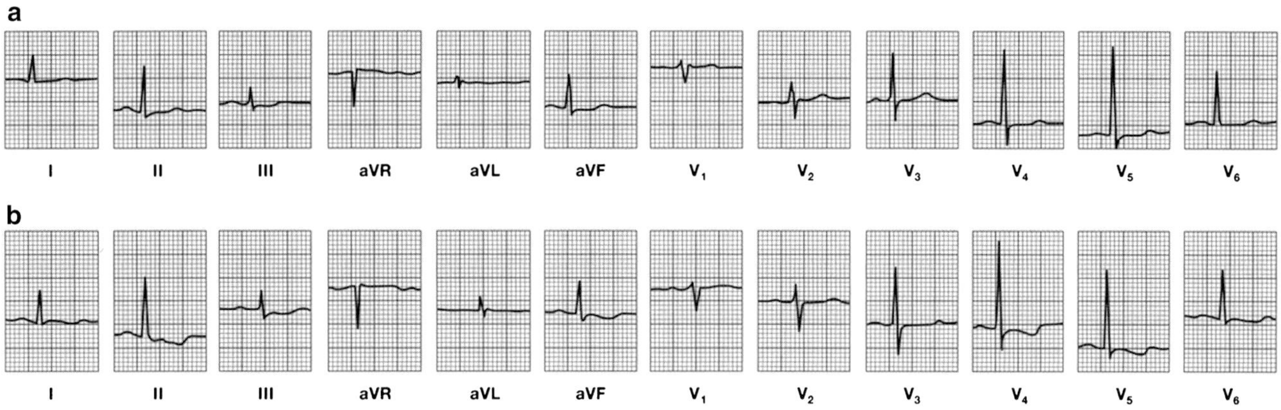

Fig. 6.6 (**a**) ECG before angiography reveals minimal aberrations, possible still within normal limits of the ST and T. There are prominent initial anterior vectors consistent with posterior lateral scarring. (**b**) ECG after angiography shows nonspecific ST-T wave changes, which, in the context of knowing that the changes have acutely occurred, are suggestive of ischemic injury without a specific location of it

ischemia, including stroke, myocardial ischemia, and cardiac arrest [17]. The immediate treatment is to tilt the patient head-down (Trendelenburg position) and on the left side to prevent air from rising to the head or passage from the venous system to the left atrium via a patent foramen ovale. Aspiration of air with a catheter in the right atrium or ventricle may be partially effective [18]. Breathing 100% oxygen may help treat hypoxemia associated with pulmonary artery flow obstruction. For larger emboli, a hyperbaric chamber may be useful if employed promptly.

Selective coronary injection of air can occur when the catheter or injection tubing is not completely flushed with fluid. Small bubbles may result in transient ischemia without consequence. (Figure 6.9) Larger selective air injections (>1–2 mL), however, often result in ventricular fibrillation and cardiovascular collapse.

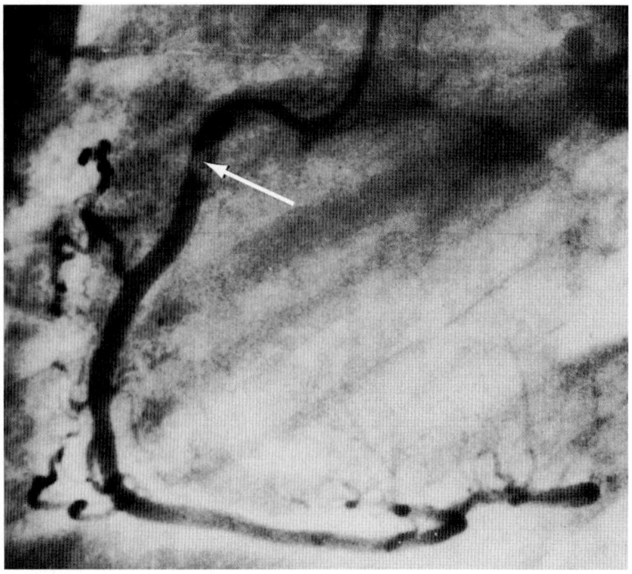

Fig. 6.7 LAO view of RC arteriogram. Evidence of embolic material probably from a catheter thrombus, or less likely, from an athero-sclerotic plaque; large RCA. Filling defect (*arrow*) can be seen clearly and was observed to migrate toward the periphery

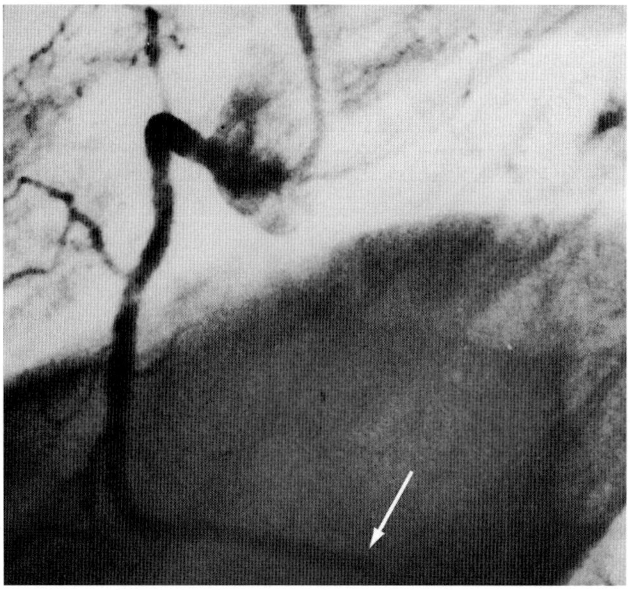

Fig. 6.8 LAO view of RC arteriogram. Repeat injection now shows occlusion (*arrow*) of the PDA

Neurologic Complications

Neurologic complications of coronary angiography include local femoral or brachial nerve injury from arterial cannulation and compression for hemostasis, ulnar nerve compression during prolonged procedures, transient ischemic attacks, and stroke. Significant neurologic events are uncommon, although they probably are underreported because the majority resolve within 24–72 h after the procedure. Most ischemic central neurologic events are embolic from the aorta and occur more often in the posterior distribution, although any territory can be affected [19].

Catheter-Induced Spasm

Spasm of the coronary arteries, particularly in the RCA, occurs mainly in the young and is more common in women than in men. This rather common localized spasm has to be differentiated from diffuse peripheral spasm at the capillary level. On rare occasions, the injection of contrast material may induce peripheral vascular spasm which is indicated by delayed

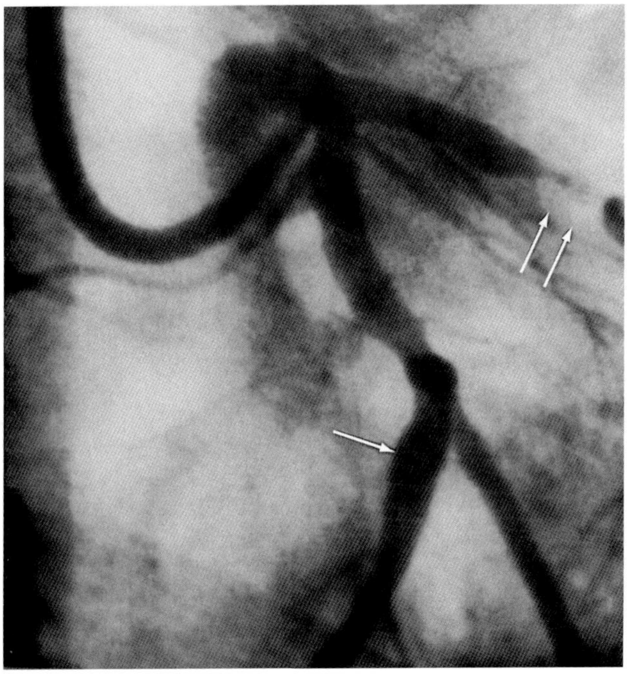

Fig. 6.9 Magnification coronary arteriography of a patient with localized stenosis of the LAD (*double arrow*). A small air bubble can be seen migrating through the Cx. The patient remained asymptomatic and no ECG changes occurred except for the transient abnormalities associated with injection of contrast material

clearing of contrast material from the coronary arteries in spite of withdrawal of the catheter. This may be associated with ECG changes, pain, and drop in blood pressure.

Since contrast material is a potent vasodilator, localized spasm is probably not produced by the contrast material itself, but by mechanical irritation of the wall of the coronary artery by the catheter tip. Therefore, the area of spasm is either at the catheter tip or in close proximity. Spasm is usually transient and disappears if the catheter is withdrawn, and the contrast material is delivered by nonselective fashion into the sinus of Valsalva (cuspogram). If narrowing persists, nitroglycerin administered sublingually may help to differentiate spasm from organic narrowing.

Angiographic features which are helpful to suggest the presence of spasm are the following: (1) The area of narrowing is smooth, concentric, and occurs usually at the catheter tip. (2) The catheter tip is seen to touch or distort the arterial wall. (3) Coronary spasm is often an isolated area of narrowing in an otherwise normal coronary arterial tree, although it may occur concomitantly with atherosclerosis. (4) The patient is a young female. (5) The narrowing disappears following nitroglycerin and withdrawal of the catheter (Fig. 6.10a, b).

Arrhythmias

Arrhythmias during angiography can occur from abrasion of the conduction system by catheters, contrast media-induced changes in repolarization, reflex-mediated changes in neural traffic to the heart, and transient myocardial ischemia from hemodynamic deterioration. The left bundle branch of the conduction system courses near the surface of the left ventricle septum and can be injured transiently during cannulation of the left ventricle [20]. The right bundle branch is located near the tricuspid annulus and can be rendered dysfunctional by a right heart catheter, particularly if the catheter is rubbed against the superior annulus repeatedly. In a patient with preexisting contralateral bundle branch block, complete heart block can occur [20]. In these patients, the immediate availability of cardiac pacing (external or by catheter) should be ascertained prior to catheterization.

Contrast media can induce sinus bradycardia, sinus node block, and atrioventricular node block by several mechanisms. The hyperosmolar and chemical properties of contrast cause activation of ventricular efferent chemoreceptors, which reflexively trigger a parasympathetic surge, reducing sinus and atrioventricular node repolarization [21]. The reflex is blocked by muscarinic receptor blockade with atropine. Iso-osmolar contrast media significantly reduce or eliminate vagally mediated bradycardia.

Prolongation of the ventricular refractory period by contrast media can initiate ventricular fibrillation. Fibrillation occurs more commonly after right compared to left coronary injection. The incidence is less with nonionic or iso-osmolar contrast material and with ionic contrast with a physiologic calcium ion content [22].

a

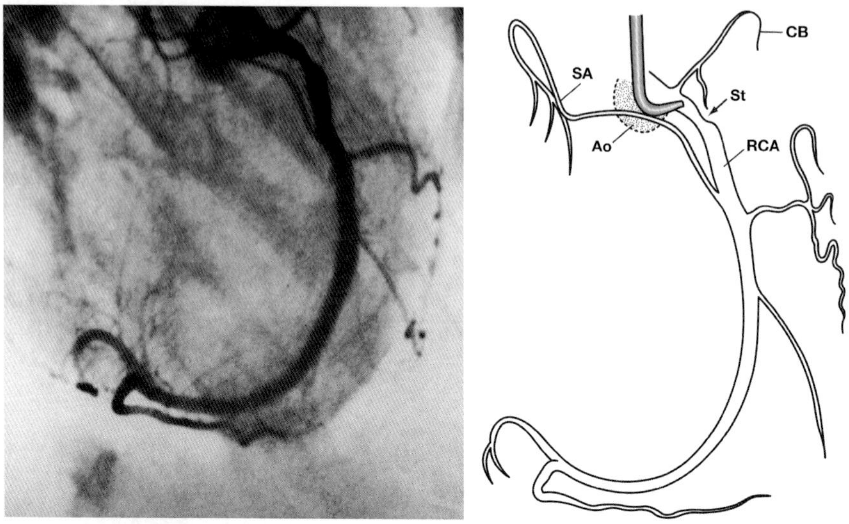

b

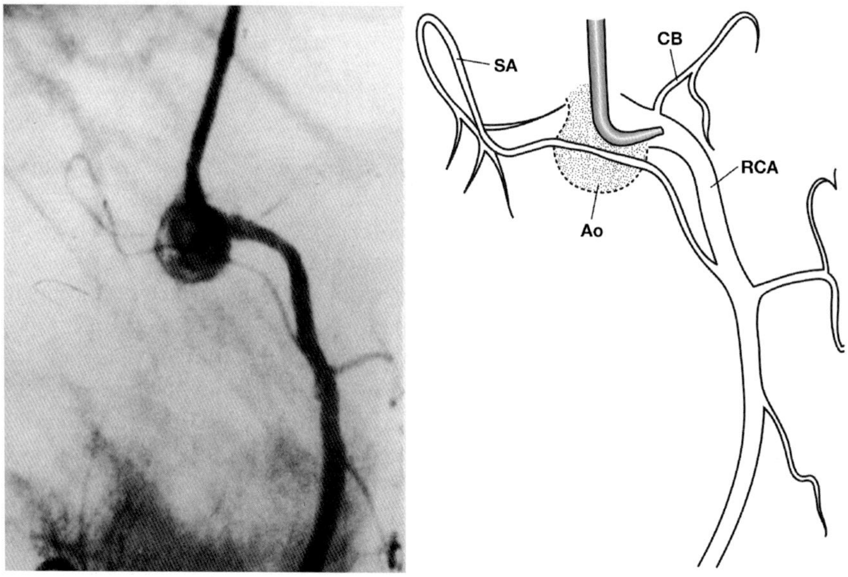

Fig. 6.10 (**a**) Localized apparent occlusion of the RCA at the catheter tip. (**b**) Following reposition of the catheter, as shown in the cuspogram, and eliminating irritation of the arterial wall by catheter tip, the spasm disappeared

Angiographic Views

Angiographic demonstration of narrowed blood vessels in various projections is of extreme importance. The maximum degree of narrowing can only be appreciated if the lesion is demonstrated in true profile. On the other hand, significant lesions may be overlooked if visualized in face. The angiographer must evaluate the entire vessel in several different views to avoid the effects of vessel foreshortening that can hide a stenotic lesion and because coronary lesions are frequently eccentric.

Since the orientation between the planes of the major cardiac grooves and septum is different from the standard anteroposterior (AP) and lateral projections utilized for chest roentgenology, oblique views must be used to obtain optical angiographic visualization of the coronary arteries.

An understanding of the orientation of the coronary arteries in the oblique positions can be facilitated using a diagram shown in Fig. 6.11 in which the eyes represent the line sight of the viewer [23]. In the LAO projection, the viewer is sighting down the interventricular and interatrial septum. All left-sided cardiac chambers appear to the viewer's right. In the LAO, the anterior and posterior descending coronary arteries are seen coursing vertically in the middle of the cardiac silhouette, following the path of the interventricular septum. In the RAO projection, the viewer's line of sight is the interventricular groove plane. In this projection, the two atria and the two ventricles are superimposed. The proximal circumflex and proximal right coronary arteries are well visualized as they follow their course in the atrioventricular groove.

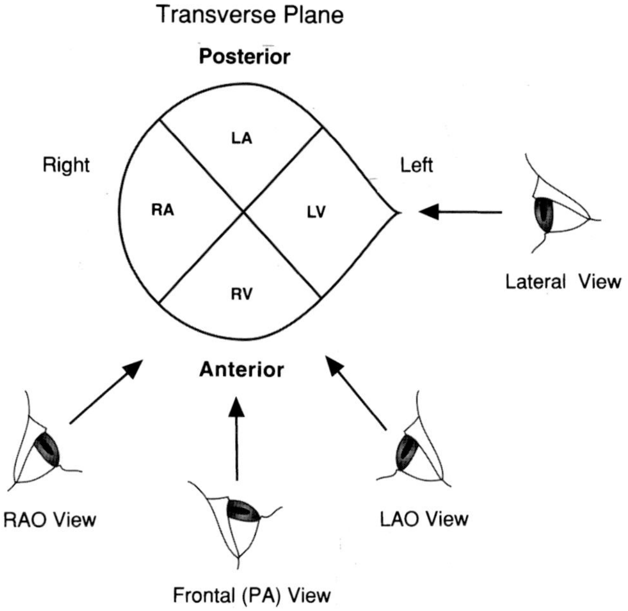

Fig. 6.11 Diagram illustrating cardiac chambers' locations as viewed in the four standard radiographic projections: frontal (posteroanterior, PA), lateral, right anterior oblique (RAO), and left anterior oblique (LAO). The eyes represent the viewer's line of sight

In 1981, Paulin [24] proposed that radiographic projections be named by following the course of the X-ray beam as it passes through the heart. The X-ray gantry can be angled in the horizontal and coronal planes. In the "cranial" view, the X-ray beam originates caudally and passes through the heart to the image intensifier, which is angled cranially. Conversely, in a caudal projection, the X-ray tube is angled cranially and projects the X-ray beam caudally to the image tube. The use of multiple oblique views in the anterolateral projections in conjunction with angulation in the caudocranial plane has greatly facilitated optimal visualization of coronary lesions and minimized the problem of foreshortening of the coronary arteries.

Optimal Projections for Left Main Coronary Artery

The left main coronary artery, which under most circumstances should be visualized first and with great care, can be seen best in the posteroanterior (PA) (Fig. 6.12a) or in a very shallow oblique projection (either RAO or LAO) so that the left main coronary is just off the spine.

Projections for the Left Anterior Descending Coronary Artery

A RAO or PA view coupled with marked cranial angulation (30°) may be helpful in delineating the course of the left anterior descending coronary artery, avoiding overlap by other branches (Fig. 6.12b).

A steep LAO view (40°) with severe cranial angulation (40°) is essential in viewing the LAD and diagonal branch bifurcation (Fig. 6.12c).

An additional LAO caudal view (LAO 40°, caudal 30°), the so-called spider view, may be used in visualizing the bifurcation of the left main, the proximal circumflex, and LAD, and at times the distal LAD (Fig. 6.12d).

Projections for the Circumflex Coronary Artery

The circumflex artery and its marginal branches can be defined in the RAO projection (20 or 30° angulation) with 20–30° of caudal angulation (Fig. 6.12).

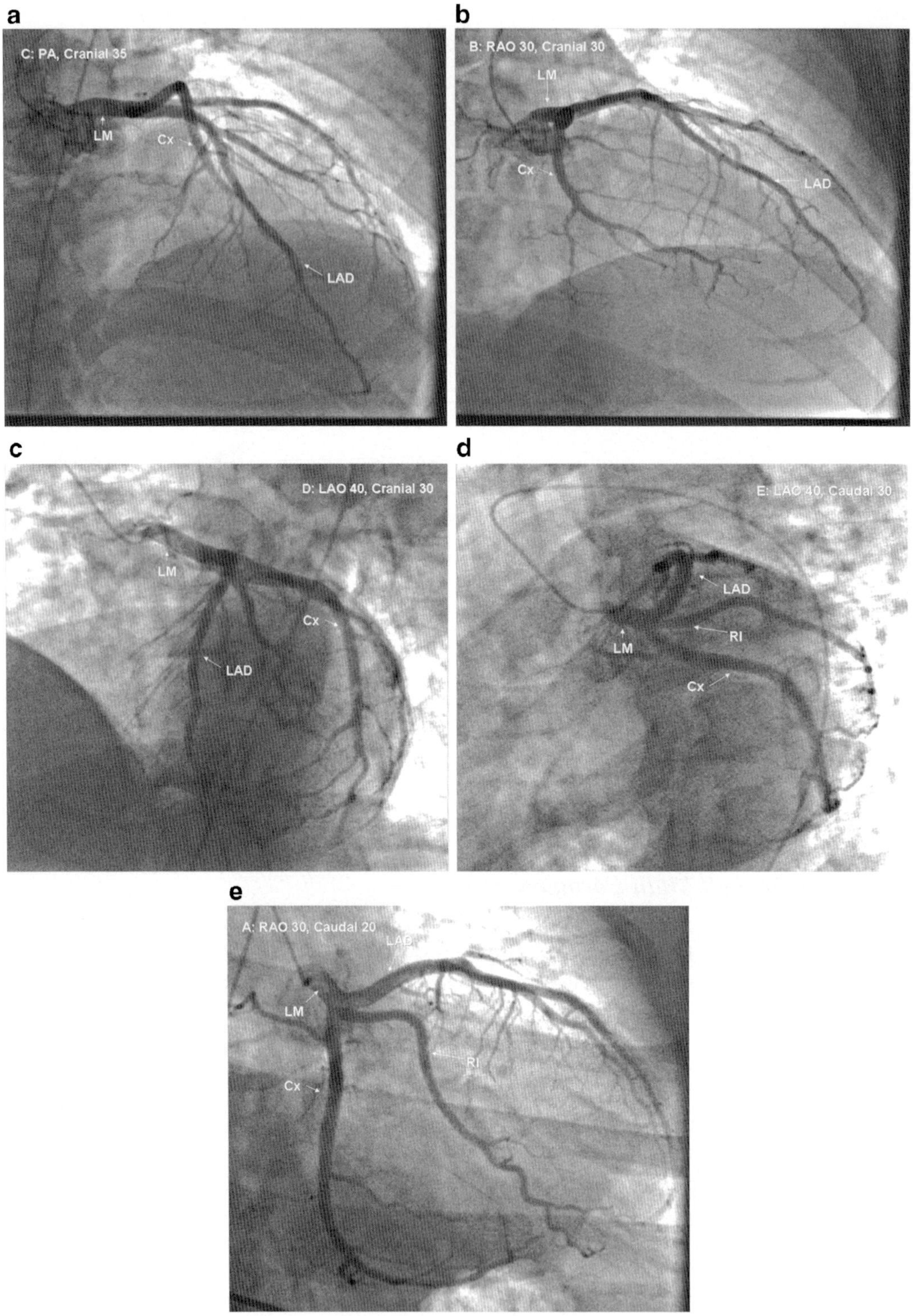

Fig. 6.12 (**a**) Normal left coronary artery viewed in the PA projection with 35° cranial angulation. (**b**) Left coronary angiogram viewed with 30° RAO and 30° cranial angulation delineating the course of the LAD. (**c**) Left coronary angiogram viewed with 40° LAO and 30° cranial angulation viewing the LAD and diagonal branch bifurcation. (**d**) LAO caudal view (LAO 40°, caudal 30°) visualizing the bifurcation of the MLC, the proximal Cx, and LAD. (**e**) Selective left coronary angiogram viewed with 30° RAO and 20° caudal angulation viewing the circumflex artery

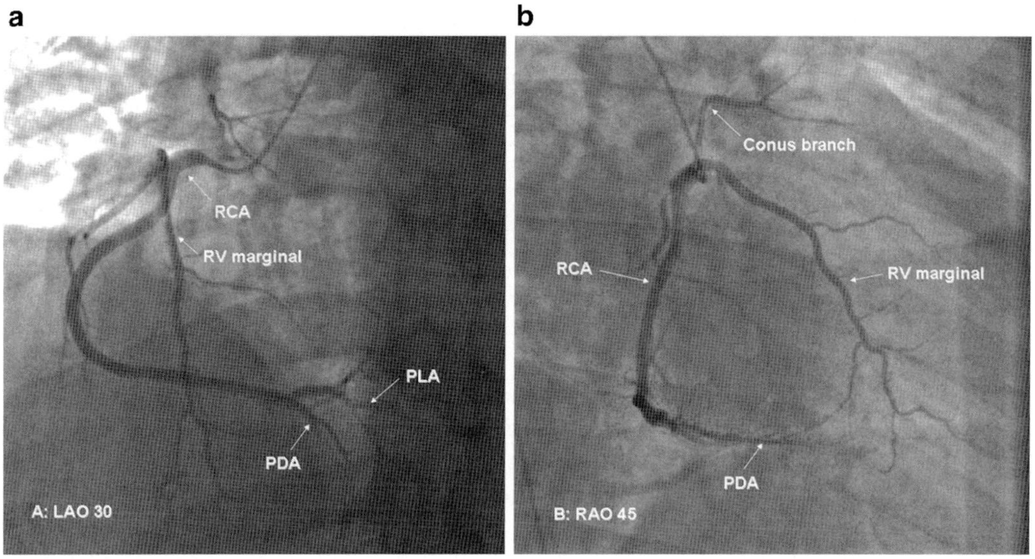

Fig. 6.13 Angiographic projections of a normal right coronary artery. (**a**) Selective right coronary angiogram viewed with 30° LAO. (**b**) Same vessel viewed with 45° RAO

Projections for the Right Coronary Artery

The proximal and mid-right coronary arteries are usually seen well in a 30–45° LAO projection. A moderate LAO view with cranial angulation (LAO 30°, cranial 20°) may be ideal for viewing the bifurcation of the distal right coronary artery into the posterior descending and posterior lateral branches (Fig. 6.13a). One view of the right coronary in the RAO view is necessary. At times, visualization of the distal right coronary is helped by adding cranial angulation (sometimes up to 60°) to the RAO view (Fig. 6.13b).

Coronary Artery Dimension

It has become recognized increasingly that measurements of coronary artery dimensions at autopsy do not correlate well with in vivo angiographic measurements of coronary diameter [25]. The importance of accurate measurements of normal coronary caliber is underscored by the understanding that coronary atherosclerosis is primarily a diffuse disease process that may be difficult to recognize angiographically [26]. Thus, without knowing the "true" caliber of an artery, it is often difficult to conclude whether a given coronary segment that appears normal angiographically is normal anatomically. The importance of recognizing diffuse coronary narrowing is underscored by studies in patients with advanced atherosclerosis showing that angiographic measurements based on lesion percent (as a fraction of the diameter of the adjacent normal segment) correlate poorly with physiologic measurements of the effect of a given focal stenosis on coronary blood flow [27]. The rationale for expressing lesion severity as percent stenosis has recently been rendered even more tenous by the findings that in atherosclerosis compensatory coronary enlargement precedes the process of luminal narrowing, and often compensates for any narrowing until this narrowing reaches 40% of the intimal lumen [28].

Dodge and coworkers used computer-based quantitation of angiograms to measure coronary lumen diameter in normal coronary arteriograms from several thousands consecutive studies. For these normal arteries, a round cross-section was assumed, and the cross-sectional area was estimated to be (coronary diameter) 2 divided by (ii.4). The summed area of the proximal right coronary, the proximal left anterior descending, and proximal circumflex arteries was called the total coronary area. In men with a large dominant right coronary distribution, the total coronary area was 32.1 ± 7.3 mm^2, with the right coronary contributing 38% of the total area, the left anterior descending 33%, and the circumflex 29%.

Multiple other physiologic and pathologic processes affect coronary caliber. Acute changes in perfusion pressure markedly alter coronary diameter by changing the distended force [29]. Increased blood flow from heightened myocardial oxygen demand (e.g., increased heart rate) or drug administration leads to coronary relaxation by endothelial-dependent mechanisms that affect coronary smooth muscle vasomotor tone [14]. The effects of intraluminal pressure endothelial-mediated dilation on coronary caliber can be altered significantly by vascular pathology. Hypertension and the wide range of conditions resulting in left ventricular hypertrophy result in marked increases in epicardial vessel size.

The evidence suggests that females have higher morbidity and mortality resulting from attempts at coronary revascularization either with angioplasty [30] or bypass surgery [31]. Speculation as to reasons for apparent differences in results has focused on differences in coronary size between men and women; the proximal coronary lumen diameter of women with normal arteries and a right-dominant coronary circulation was $9 \pm 8\%$ less than in similar men.

Quantitative Analysis of Coronary Arteriography

Since the visual interpretation of coronary angiograms is inherently flawed, numerous computer-assisted systems to aid in the geometrical assessment of epicardial coronary lesions have been developed. Although quantitation of coronary stenosis is a giant step forward (compared to visual assessment), it must be remembered that quantitative angiography is an anatomic but not a physiologic measurement tool. The coronary angiogram is a two-dimensional representation of the lumen of the artery under investigation. Changes in the size or configuration from an assumed normal vessel may not be sufficient to understand either the physiology involved or to recognize the anatomic extent of the atherosclerotic process. Despite these limitations, the development and implementation of quantitative methods for analysis of stenosis severity has improved evaluation of coronary artery lesions.

In 1977, Brown and colleagues at the University of Washington developed a quantitative coronary angiography method using the vessel edges of the lesion and the adjacent proximal and distal "normal" segments of the coronary angiogram [32]. Images obtained from standard 35-mm cine film are projected at 5× magnification onto grid. The drawn arterial outlines from two orthogonal angiographic views are manually digitized. The angiographic catheter is used as a scaling device to correct for magnification. The outlines are computer-matched at the minimum diameter or another standard point of reference visible in both views. Two orthogonal views are then combined to form a 3D representation, assuming an elliptical lumen contour.

From this composite image, lesion minimum diameter and cross-sectional area are determined in absolute (mm^2) and relative lesion percent diameter and percent area stenosis terms. This method has been used for many research applications and is highly accurate and reproducible. However, the method is time-consuming and labor-intensive. For these reason, it has not seen widespread clinical utilization.

Reiber and colleagues in 1986 developed a semiautomated method for detecting the edges of coronary artery segment of interest and of the calibrating catheter (Coronary artery analysis system (CAAS)) [33]. This and similar methods use digitized image obtained from a cineangiographic film frame or video signal. These techniques detect the arterial edge by videodensitometric methods, usually employing a weighted average of the first and second derivatives of the density change across the artery to identify the edge [34].

A number of other investigators have developed other systems for computer-assisted quantitative coronary angiography using nongeometric methods. Videodensitometry has been most commonly used. Under very carefully controlled circumstances and in a small number of patients, one videodensitometric approach appeared to correlate well with minimal luminal area measured using Brown-Dodge quantitative coronary angiography as well as measurements of CFR.

However, there are many theoretical and practical limitations to the use of videodensitometric techniques. The frequent occurrence of vessel foreshortening in many of the radiographic views results in artifactual increases in density and greatly limits the clinical utility of this technique. At present, the usual error with densitometric angiography appears between 5 and 20%, but can approach 50% [35]. For these reasons and despite initially promising results, videodensitometric approaches to lesion quantitation have not yet seen widespread application.

Although under ideal circumstances quantitative angiography can be reliable and highly accurate measurement technique, many potential pitfalls exist. Blurring of the vessel edges, the penumbra effect, and cardiac motion can lead to widened vessel edge, making edge detection less accurate. Vessel overlap and unrecognized lesion foreshortening may produce major errors because single film frames are examined.

Inaccurate calibration from the angiographic catheter can be a major problem for quantitative angiography. Reference tables for the true size of a variety of angiographic catheters, together with a comparison of their angiographic measurements as calculated by two different algorithms, are available.

For angioplasty patients populations, quantitative measurements of vessel diameters taken from only one view in which the lesion appears worst compare quiet closely with the average of two diameter measurements from nearly orthogonal views [36]. From these data, one could conclude that quantitative measurement of one view is adequate for routine clinical purposes.

However, for research purposes, orthogonal views may sometimes be required. Our experience comparing angiography to Doppler flow reserve measurements has led to the conclusion that integration of lesion diameters as seen in all views appears to relate best to physiologic measures of lesion severity.

Physiologic Assessment of Coronary Arterial Stenosis

The inaccuracies inherent in even the most sophisticated methods of anatomic assessment have led to the development of physiologically based methods to assess coronary stenosis severity. In 1939, Katz and Lindner [37] described the coronary reactive hyperemia response that has subsequently become the gold standard for the physiologic assessment of stenosis severity.

In normal coronary arteries, myocardial blood flow is primary regulated by the resistance of the arteriolar vessels (≤400/um diameter). The epicardial coronary arteries provide little resistance to coronary blood flow under physiologic circumstances. As a stenosis progresses in an epicardial vessel, a transstenotic pressure gradient develops. The microvessels dilate to compensate for the reduced distal perfusion pressure, thus maintaining normal resting flow to the myocardium.

Studies in animals have shown that resting coronary blood flow can be maintained at normal levels until more than 75% of the arterial cross-sectional area (50% of the diameter if the obstruction is concentric) is obstructed. At this point, the vasodilator reserve of the arterioles is exhausted, and further vasodilation is impossible [38]. Resting blood flow during maximal arteriolar vasodilation is termed physiologically significant (Fig. 6.14).

The ratio of maximal hyperemic blood flow (e.g., induced by coronary occlusion or drugs) to resting blood flow is termed coronary vasodilator reserve of CFR. The ratio of the intracoronary pressure distal to a stenosis to the proximal coronary or aortic pressure during conditions of maximal hyperemia is termed the fractional flow reserve. These two physiologic measurements CFR and the fractional flow reserve have provided important clinical techniques to assess limitations in hyperemic blood flow imparted by a stenosis.

Collateral Circulation

In general, the angiographic demonstration of intercoronary collateral vessels can be regarded as the hallmark of severe and extensive obstructive coronary disease. The development of coronary collaterals is based in preexistent coronary arterial anastomosis in the normal heart. Autopsy studies have shown the presence of small coronary anastomosis (native collaterals) in nearly all normal hearts.

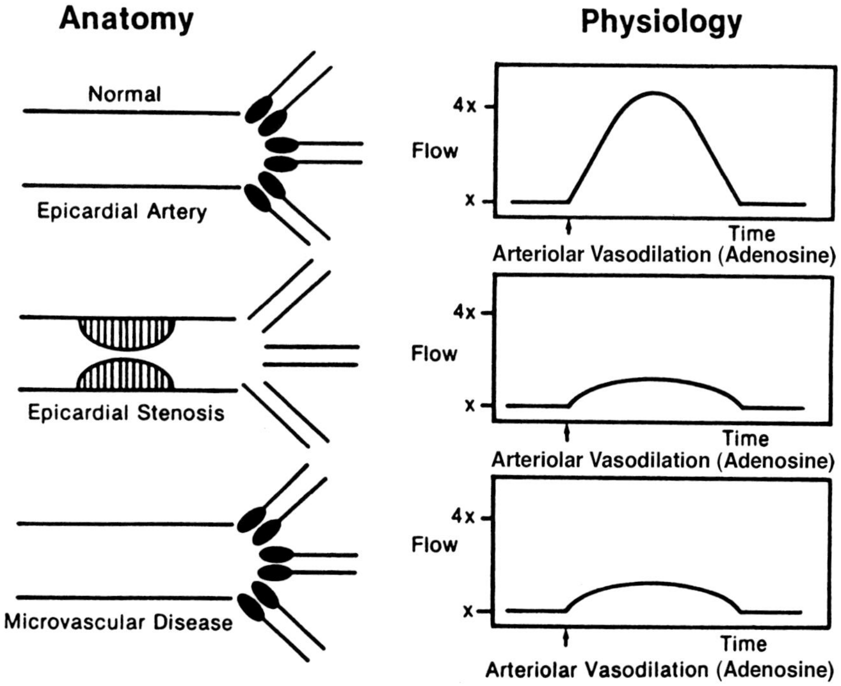

Fig. 6.14 The effects of an epicardial stenosis on coronary flow reserve (CFR). *Top*: Dilation of a normal microvasculature with adenosine causes blood flow to increase fourfold. *Middle*: An epicardial stenosis causes partial microvascular dilation, and adenosine has little additional effect. Flow reserved is reduced. *Bottom*: Microvascular disease prevents normal arteriolar dilation, reducing flow reserve

Collateral Grading
Rentrop Scale

Score	Definition
0	No collaterals
1	Fainting filling of the distal branch arteries
2	Complete filling of brach arteries
3	Collateral filling of the main artery, in addition to branches

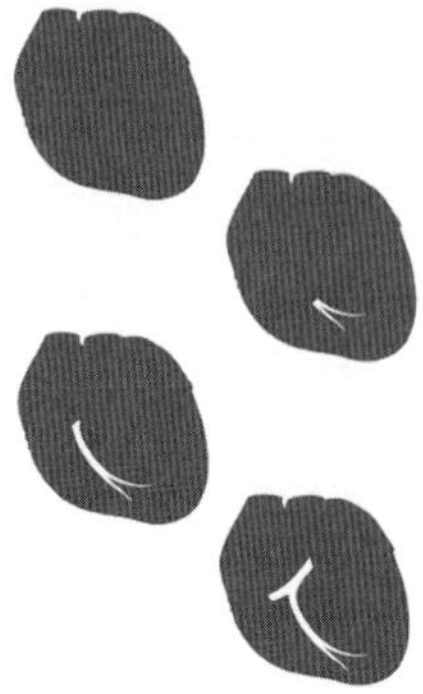

Fig. 6.15 The Rentrop semiquantitative scale for grading collateral flow to a coronary artery. Modified from Rentrop [45]

W. F. M Fulton demonstrated the existence of precapillary anastomoses in the subendocardium of the LV and septum by using the injection immersion bismuthgelatin stereodiagnostic techniques [39]. These anastomoses are not dilated capillaries. Histolologically, these vessels have an inner endothelial layer and a thin medial and adventitial layer (Vlodaver and Edwards, unpublished data).

Baroldi, Mantero, and Scomazzoni (1956) [40], among others, described 20 arterial anastomoses of 20–350 microdiameter in a group of normal hearts. The anastomoses were commonly found in the atrial and ventricular septa and the surrounding free ventricular wall, at the crux, and in the free wall of both atria.

Intermittent or gradual coronary occlusion results in the growth of coronary collaterals. This maturation process involves not only an increase in the lumen of the vessel, but also the development of new vascular smooth muscle [41]. Collateral vessels respond to several neurohormonal substances, but the response of mature coronary collaterals to several differs substantially from that of native coronary arteries and immature collateral vessels [42].

Human coronary collaterals become demonstrable by coronary angiography only when the parent vessel is subtotally or totally occluded. Unfortunately, angiographic grading of coronary collaterals based on collateral caliber is not accurate in predicting the functional ability of the collateral to provide coronary perfusion. There are several reasons for this: (1) Coronary collaterals in the 100 μm range are not angiographically visible [43]. (2) Angiographic techniques in humans for quantitating collateral function are not well validated [44]. (3) In the absence of near-total vessel occlusion, collateral vessels are not visible in the resting state (e.g., during angiography). They can, however, be rendered visible if contrast is injected into the contralateral artery during coronary spasm or during temporal balloon occlusion of the recipient artery [45]. These collaterals have been termed "recruitable" [46].

As a result of several important observations, the myocardial protective effects of collaterals are accepted widely [47]. For any given location of acute coronary occlusion, the degree of deterioration of left ventricular function is inversely related to the presence of angiographically visible coronary collaterals. In addition, the incidence of late aneurysm formation following myocardial infarction is reduced in patients with angiographically significant collateral circulation, with or without successful reperfusion [48]. The risk of hemodynamically severe consequences from acute myocardial infarction is mitigated greatly by the presence of a preexisting severe stenosis, and thus the protective effect of a developed collateral circulation. Conversely, when acute coronary occlusion occurs in the presence of mild stenosis and thus poor collateral development, it is likely to have more severe clinical consequences [49]. More recently, it has been shown that the presence of angiographically defined coronary collaterals extends the "window of time" for the beneficial effect of reperfusion therapy of myocardial infarction and results in greater improvement in cardiac function and reduction in infarction size [50].

Collateral flow can be graded using the following scale devised by Rentrop et al. [45] (Fig. 6.15):

Grade 0: No angiographically visible filling of any collateral channels.
Grade 1: Collaterals filling of the distal branches of the recipient artery, but not the epicardial portion of the artery.
Grade 2: Partial collateral filling of the recipient epicardial artery.
Grade 3: Complete collateral filling of the recipient epicardial artery.

Angiographic methods for assessing collateral flow are at best semiquantitative measures. The coronary wedge pressure (e.g., the distal coronary pressure during transient balloon occlusion at the time of angioplasty) has been used to assess more accurately collateral function. Spontaneously visible collaterals are present at angioplasty 4 times as often as recruitable collaterals. Meier et al. [46] found the coronary wedge pressure in patients with collaterals of either type is higher than in

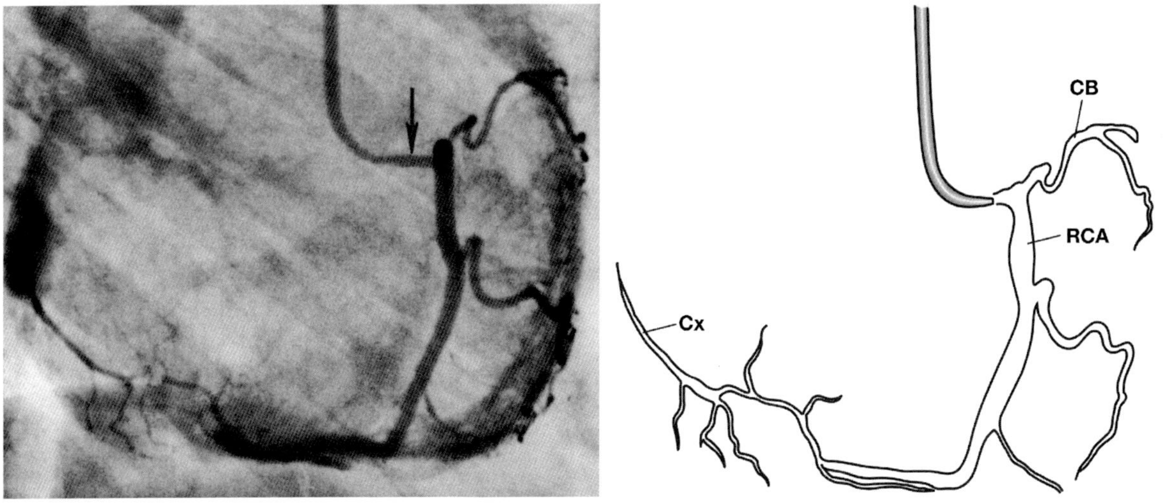

Fig. 6.16 Severe spasm of the proximal portion of RC resulting in a tight seal around the catheter tip (*arrow*). Contrast material was forced under high pressure into the coronary arteries. The RCA is normal, but there is opacification of the distal ramifications of the Cx through collateral communications

patients without collaterals. Signs and symptoms of ischemia during angioplasty balloon occlusion occur with a significantly greater frequency in patients with a low coronary wedge pressure.

Coronary arterial anastomoses may be categorized as (1) connecting branches of two different coronary arteries and (2) connections between various branches of the same artery. The latter group may be subdivided into bridging collaterals close to and across an obstructive or connecting anastomoses between distal branches of the obstructed artery.

In any given case, one or more of the foregoing types of collateral pathways may be evident. Homocoronary anastomoses are between branches of the same coronary artery. If anastomotic channels are present between two or more different coronary arteries, the term intercoronary anastomosis will be applied.

Collateral Anastomosis in the Absence of Evidenced Disease

Under unusual circumstances, anastomoses between the main coronary arteries may be shown in the absence of evidenced disease. In the arteriogram shown in Fig. 6.16, the RCA appeared to be occluded by organic disease. Later, this was shown to be arterial spasm, which occurred at the time of the initial injection of the contrast material. The spasm prevented free reflux and a wedge injection was performed, demonstrating anastomoses between the RCA and the Cx. Examination of the Cx showed no lesion. Collaterals between the RCA and the Cx were present and demonstrable by wedge injection without organic disease. This represents an unique case in which potential collaterals without obstructing disease were demonstrated in a living subject.

Figure 6.17 is an LAO view of the patient in Fig. 6.16 following injection into the LC. The entire Cx system and the previously opacified segment are now filled normally from the LC.

Bridging Anastomosis

Those are collaterals close to and across an obstructive or connecting anastomosis between distal branches of the obstructed artery (Figs. 6.18).

Kugel's Artery

In instances of RC obstruction, the distal segment of the RC may be supplied by a vessel which has coursed through the atrial septum. This is named Kugel's artery, which rarely arises from the LMC, more commonly from the Cx, and occasionally

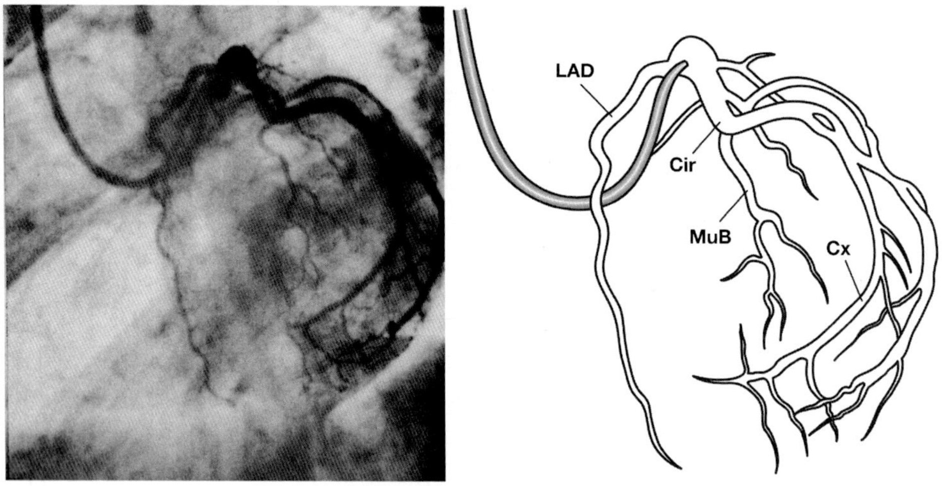

Fig. 6.17 An LAO view of the patient in Fig. 6.16 following injection into the LC

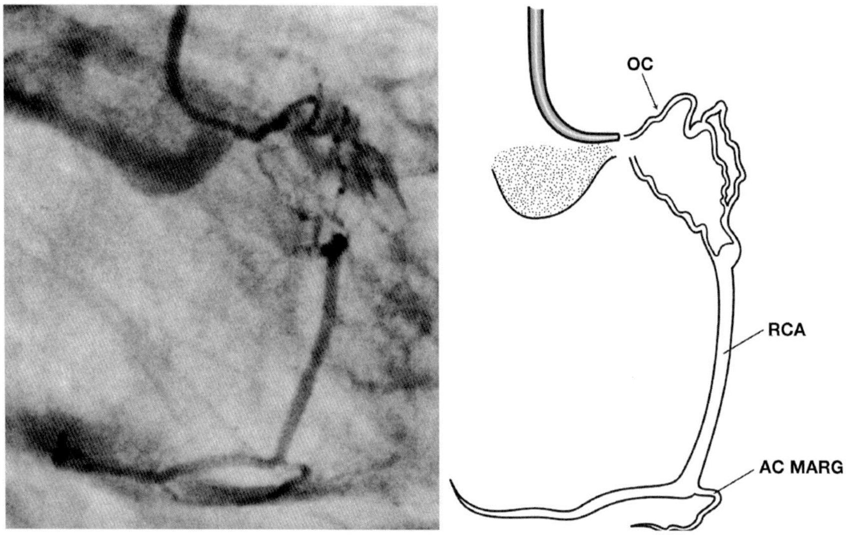

Fig. 6.18 RAO view of RC arteriogram. There is occlusion at the origin of the RCA with collaterals bridging across the site of occlusion. The distal segment of the artery is well opacified. The LC system was normal; this case also represent a good example of single-vessel disease

from the RCA. After coursing from its origin, Kugel's artery passes posteriorly in the atrial septum to supply the area of the AV node. In this general location, it may anastomose with the distal portion of the RCA, representing a collateral channel (Figs. 6.19–6.21).

Angiographic demonstration of Kugel's artery without obstruction is extremely rare. This minute branch can only be demonstrated on an excellent angiogram. On the other hand, in case of arterial obstruction there is considerable enlargement of arteria anastomatic auricularis magna, which can be readily identified. Its angiographic recognition depends on the fact that the artery remains within the confines of the heart in all projections. This anastomotic artery, which runs in the atrial septum, is often confused with LA collaterals. Although LA collaterals may simulate Kugel's artery in one projection, it will be obvious in other views that it represent a vessel running on the surface of the LA wall.

Intercoronary anastomoses with Left Anterior Descending and Posterior Descending

One of the most common intercoronary anastomoses in complete occlusion of the RCA is collateral supply from the LAD to the PDA around the apex. Often there are also interseptal collaterals demonstrable (Figs. 6.22 and 6.23).

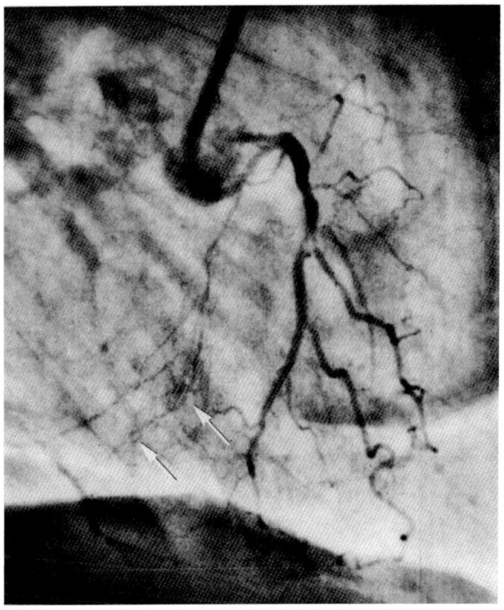

Fig. 6.19 RC arteriogram in RAO view with prominent Kugel anastomosis to the AV node artery and probably also posterior septal branches (*double arrows*). Note opacification of the PDA via these collaterals

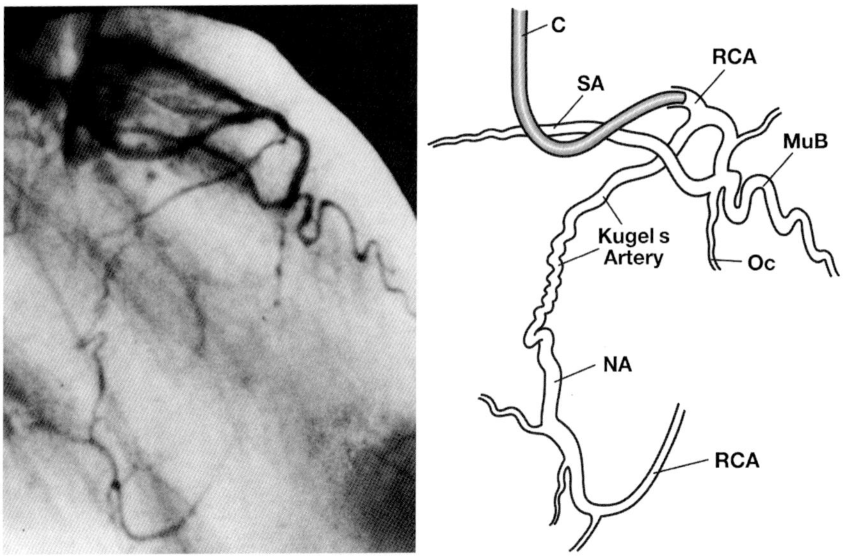

Fig. 6.20 RAO view of the RC arteriogram shows complete occlusion of the RCA and retrograde collateral flow through Kugel's artery. Note that the latter artery descends in the atrial septum from the AV node artery. Other film appear in Fig. 6.23

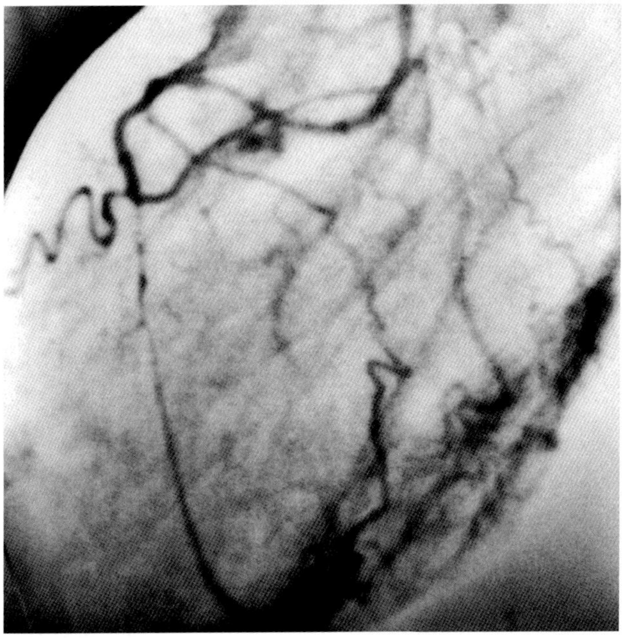

Fig. 6.21 RC arteriogram in RAO projection. The artery is completely opacified by way of collateral flow through the Kugel's artery

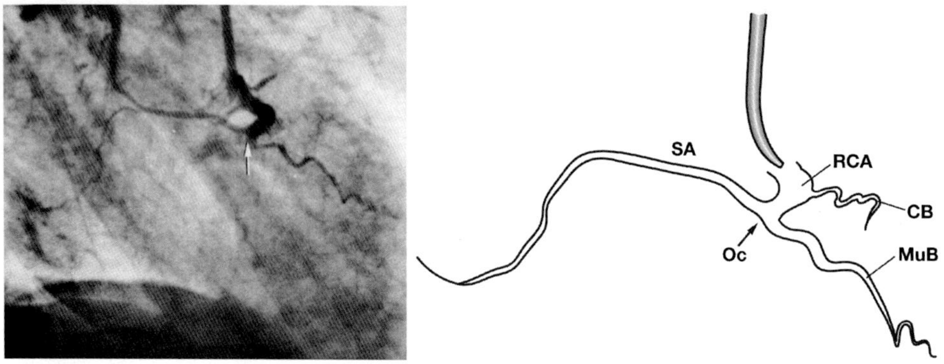

Fig. 6.22 RC arteriogram in lateral view. Complete occlusion of the RCA (*arrow*) at the origin of the muscular branch and a large sinus node artery

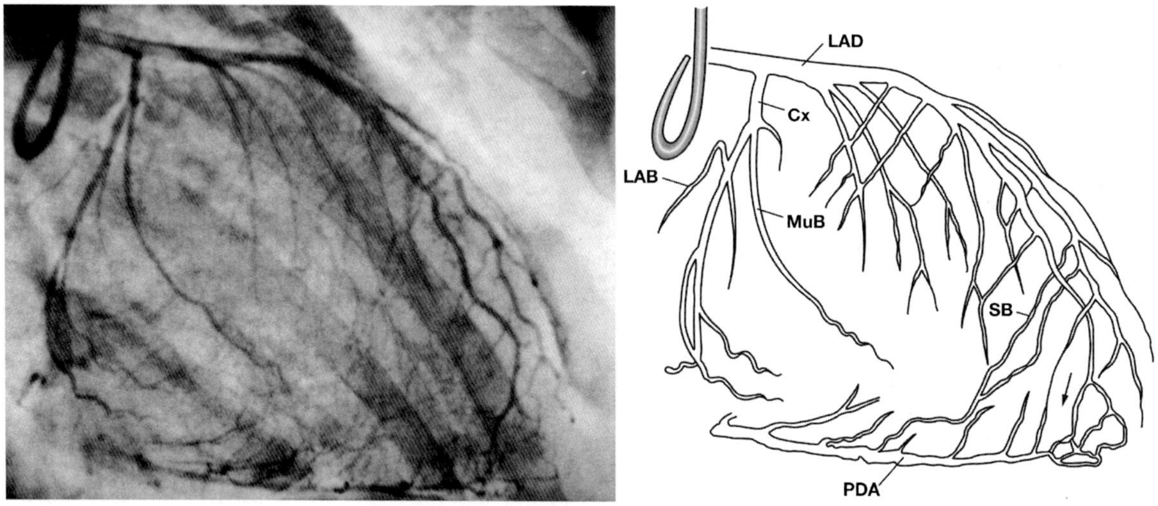

Fig. 6.23 RAO view of LC arteriogram showing septal collaterals, but the main collateralization to the RCA is around the apex from the LAD to the PDA (*arrows*). The occluded RCA is shown in Fig. 6.22

Occlusion of the Right Coronary Artery with Collaterals from the Left Anterior descending and Left Circumflex Arteries

There is a variation of collaterals pathways in patients with occlusion of the RCA, when a paired LAD supplies the distal RCA via periapical collateral channels. There opacification of the PDA also occurs (Figs. 6.24 and 6.25).

Collaterals to the Right Coronary Artery through Atrial Branches

Figure 6.26 illustrates a case of occlusion of the proximal portion of the RCA. The main collateral supply to the vessel was through the left and right atrial branches, each originating from the Cx.

Occlusion of the Left Anterior Descending Artery: Dual Collateral Supply from the Conus Artery and Muscular Branches of Right Coronary Artery. The Vieussen's Circle

Figures 6.27 and 6.28 illustrate an example in which the LAD was found to be occluded in its proximal segment in LC arteriograms. The RC arteriograms portray collateral flow into the LAD through the Mub of the RCA, as well as

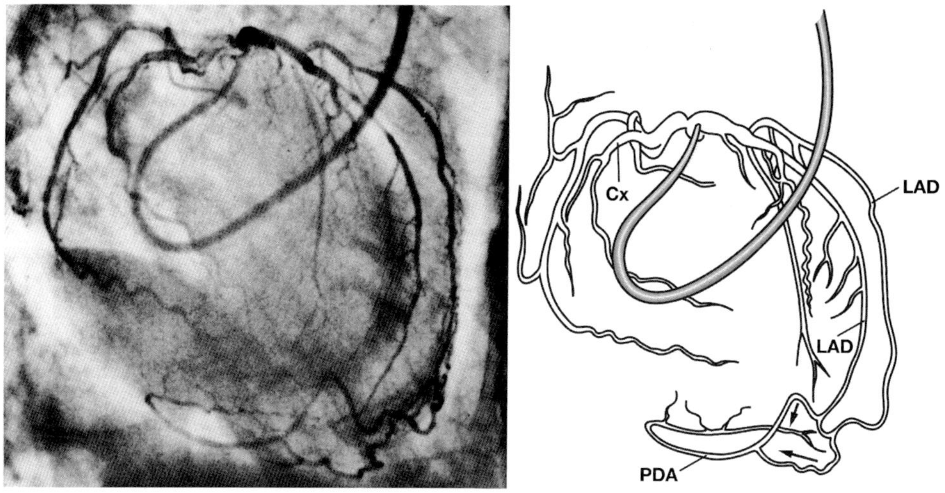

Fig. 6.24 LC arteriogram in lateral view in patient with occlusion of the RCA. The distal PDA opacifies via periapical collaterals, as well as from muscular branches from the Cx system

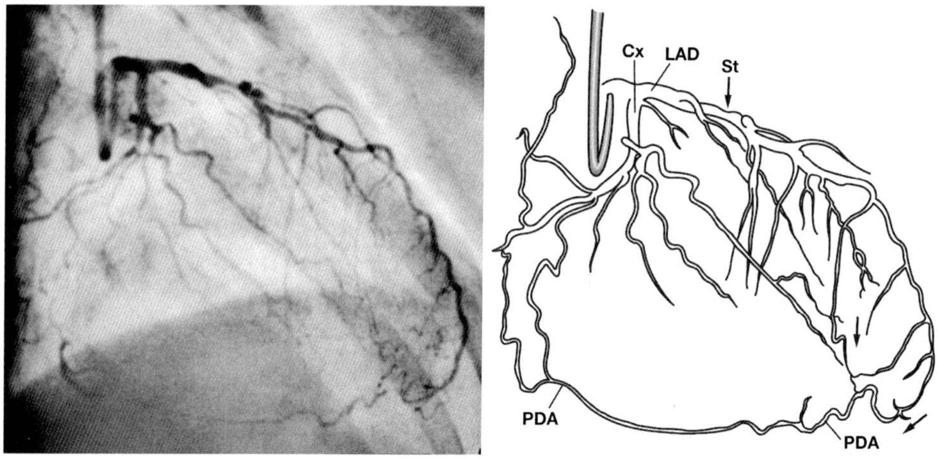

Fig. 6.25 LC arteriogram in RAO projection in case of occlusion of the RC. Collaterals to the RC come from the LAD and Cx

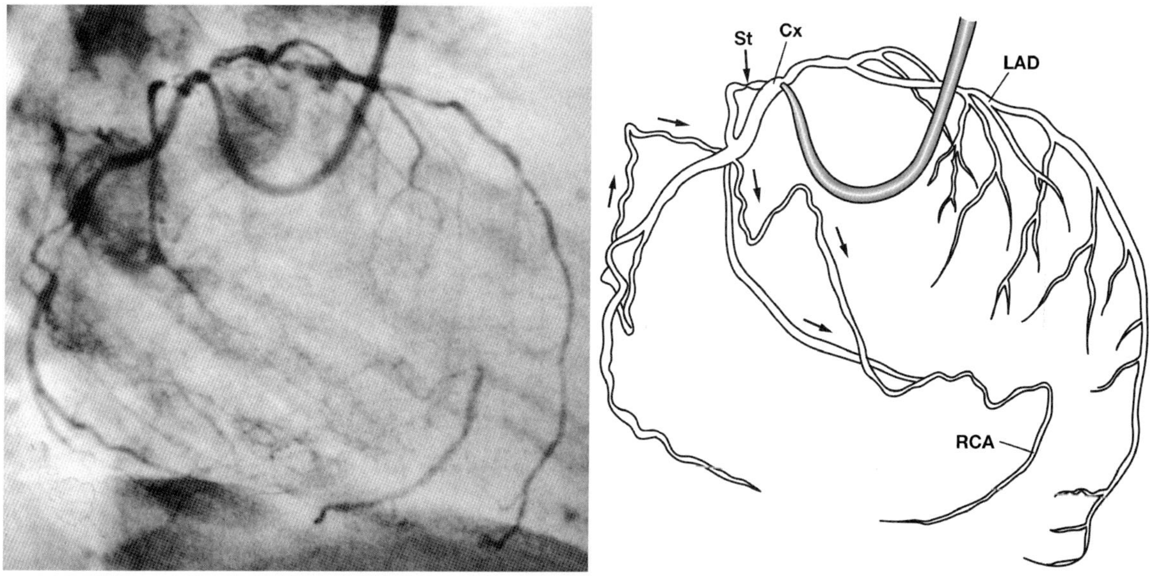

Fig. 6.26 LC arteriogram in lateral view. Atrial branches opacify segments of the RC

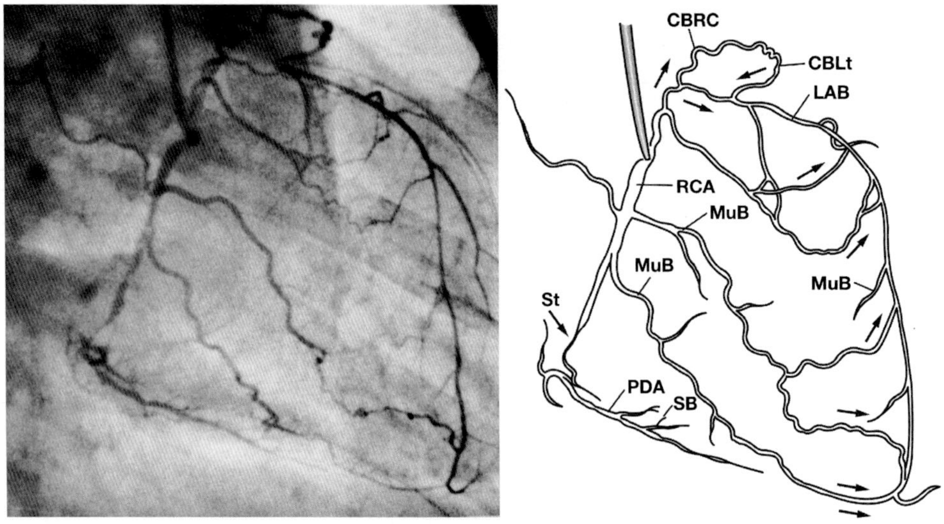

Fig. 6.27 RC arteriogram in lateral view. There is diffuse disease of the RC and collateral flow to the occluded LAD through communications between the right and left conus branches, yielding Vieussen's circle

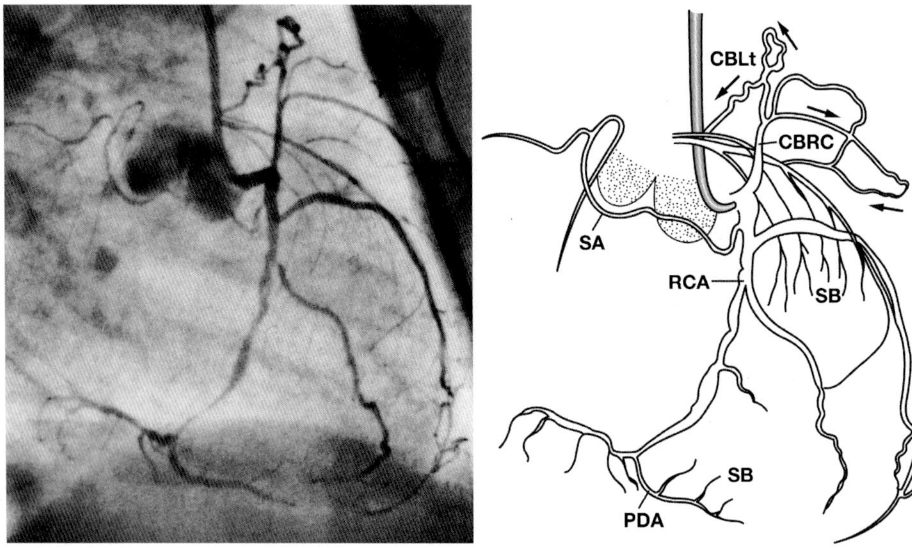

Fig. 6.28 RC arteriogram in RAO view. Coll flow into the LAD system through muscular branches and conus branches. The Vieussen's circle is prominent as a result of communications between the conus branches of the RCA and the LMC

communications between a Conus branch of the RCA and Conus branch of the LMC. The latter anastomosis yields a pattern that has been called the Vieussens circle. In Fig. 6.28, the Vieussen's circle is particularly well developed.

Collateral Flow to the Left Anterior Descending Artery through Branches of the Posterior Descending Artery Arising from the Left Circumflex

In Fig. 6.29, the proximal portion of the LAD shows major degree of obstruction. The Cx give rise to the PDA, which in turn supplies Post and Ant SBs. The Ant SBs do not opacify completely, giving the branchless tree appearance.

Collaterals from Left Circumflex to Right Coronary Artery

When occlusion of the RCA and major stenosis of the LAD occurs, the major collateral flow to the occluded vessel derived from the Cir through an atrial branch (Fig. 6.30).

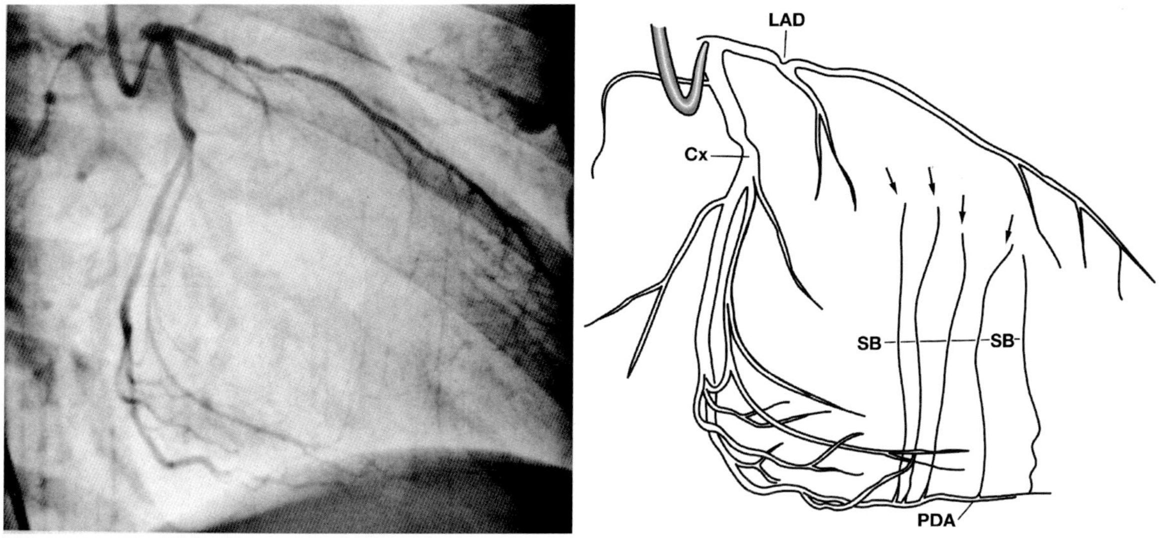

Fig. 6.29 LC arteriogram in RAO view. There is marked narrowing of the LAD (*single arrow*). Widely patent Cx opacifies septal branches which proceed toward the territory of the LAD. Note that the proximal septal branches of the LAD are not opacified, probably because of a previous infarction

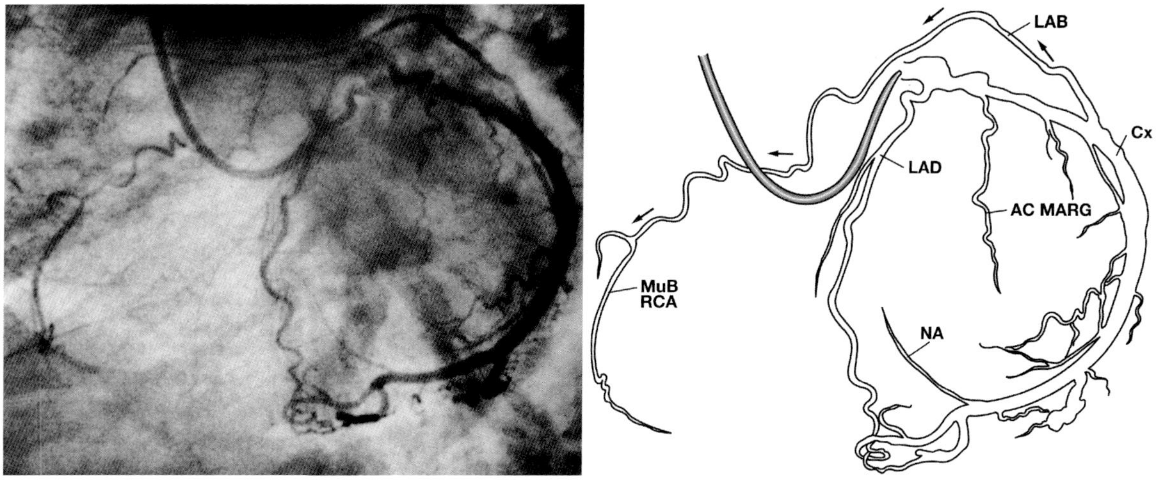

Fig. 6.30 LC arteriogram in LAO view. Minor disease of the LAD and some atherosclerotic beading of the large Cx are evident. There is an unusual collateral filling of a muscular branch of the RCA through the left atrial branch arising from the Cx, anastomosing with an RAB (*arrows*)

Muscular Branch: Source of Collaterals to Occluded Distal Right Coronary and Left Anterior Descending Arteries

Figures 6.31 and 6.32 are from a patient with an occluded LAD and distal RCA, and a large right MuB supplying the myocardium.

Myocardial Bridges

A myocardial bridge is a segment of a major coronary branch, which, for a short course, leaves the epicardium, dips through the myocardium(site of bridge), and then reappears on the myocardium. Since the obstruction occurs only during systole and blood flow occurs primarily during diastole, there usually is no impact on myocardial perfusion. The importance of this

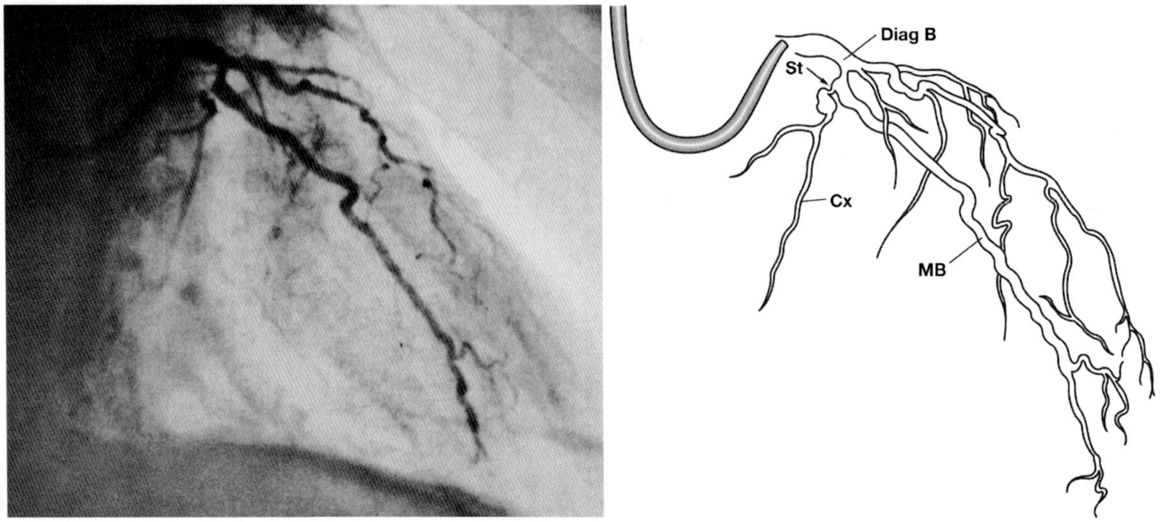

Fig. 6.31 RAO view of LC arteriogram showing occlusion of the LAD, short Cx, and a markedly stenotic diagonal branch

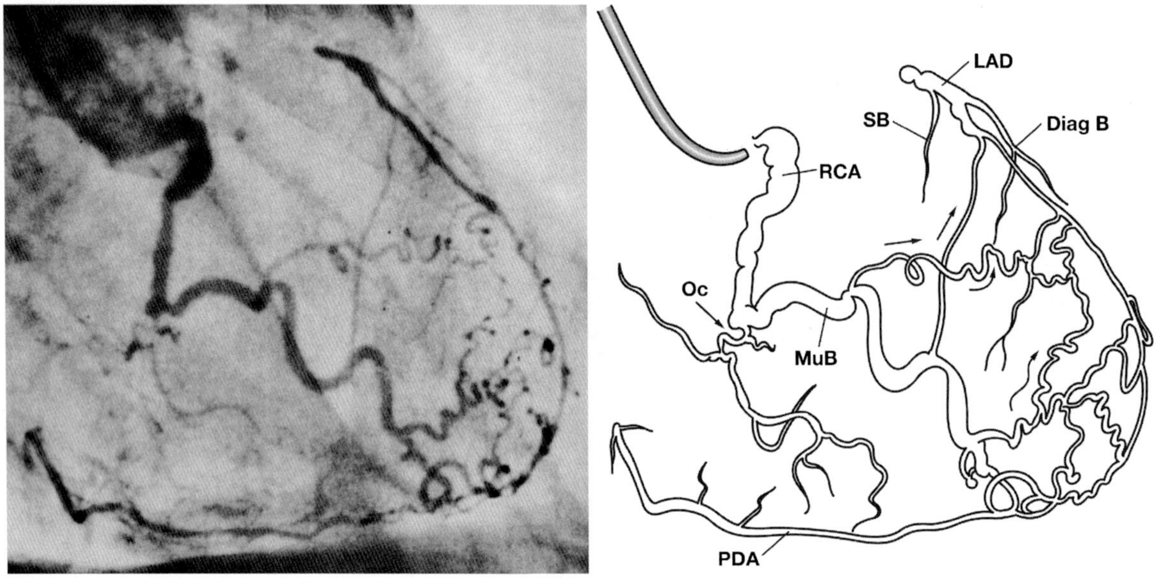

Fig. 6.32 Injection of RC in RAO position demonstrates virtual opacification of the entire heart by the RCA, primarily a huge right muscular branch. Beyond the origin of the right muscular branch, the RCA is occluded. The main collateral flow occurs through RV branches through the LAD around the apex with filling of the PDA

condition angiographically is that during ventricular systole, there appears to be an obstruction which may be confused with organic disease. Figure 6.33 shows three levels of the LAD, the middle one of which is involved in a myocardial bridge. It is of interest that the degree of atherosclerosis has been found to be more severe in those segments lying on the epicardium than in that part involved in the bridge and lying in the myocardium [51]. When myocardial bridges exist, as shown in Fig. 6.34, there may be evident obstruction of the involved segment during systole. During diastole, the obstruction disappears. Figures 6.34 and 6.35 portrays angiographic identification of myocardial bridge.

Myocardial bridge and the Effects of Nitrites

Figure 6.36 and 6.37 are LC and arteriograms in which a myocardial bridge on the proximal segment of the LAD and the effects of nitrites are seen.

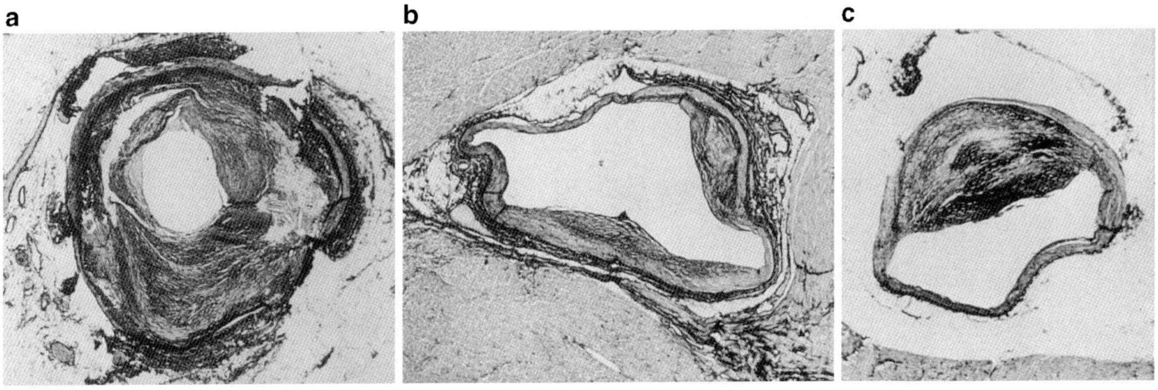

Fig. 6.33 Three levels of section of the LAD. In the upper and lower levels, the artery lies in the epicardium, while in the middle level the artery lies within the muscle. The muscle which separates the vessel from the epicardium may be considered a myocardial bridge

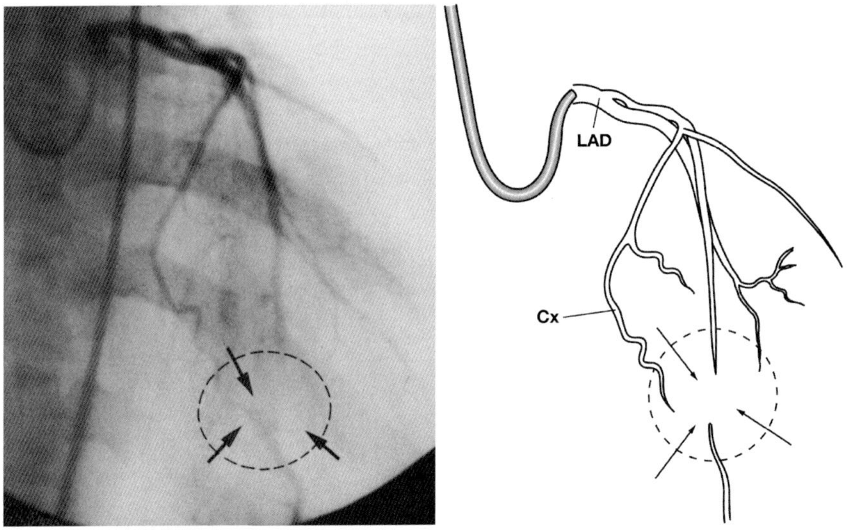

Fig. 6.34 LC arteriogram in RAO projection. During systole, the distal segment of the LAD appears occluded (*arrows*)

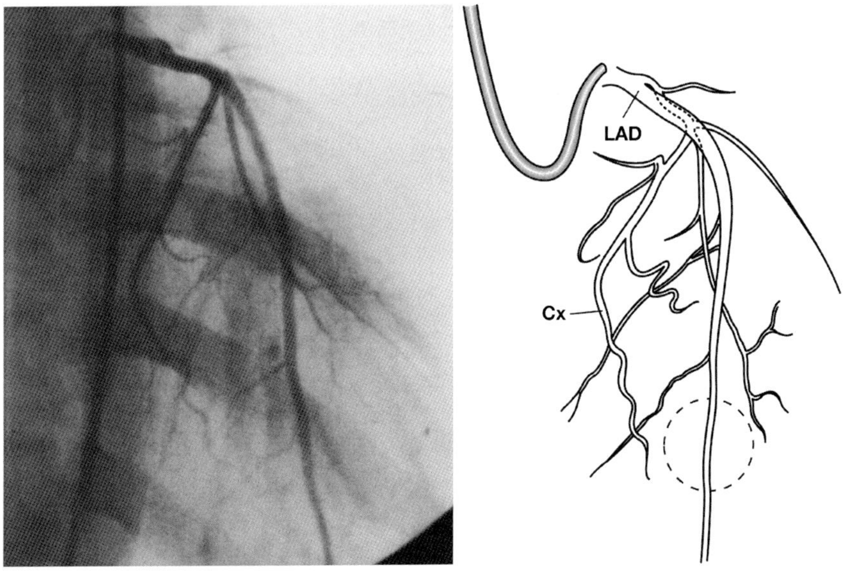

Fig. 6.35 LC arteriogram in RAO projection. During diastole, the apparent occlusion has disappeared

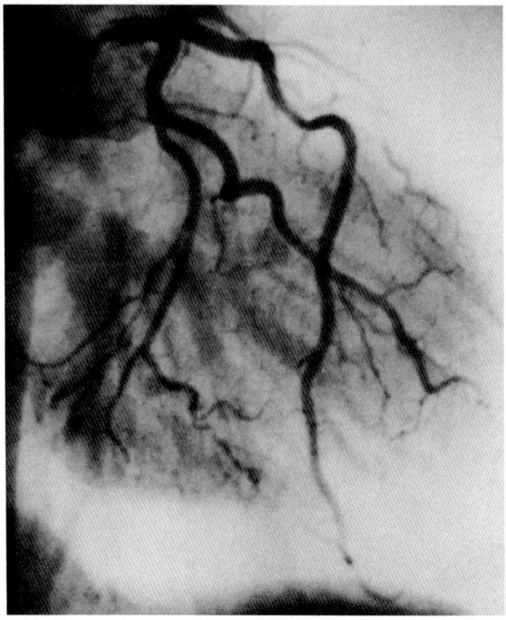

Fig. 6.36 RAO view of LC arteriogram, prenitroglycerin. A myocardial bridge over the proximal LAD can be expected because of the curvature of the LAD, but none of the films showed compression

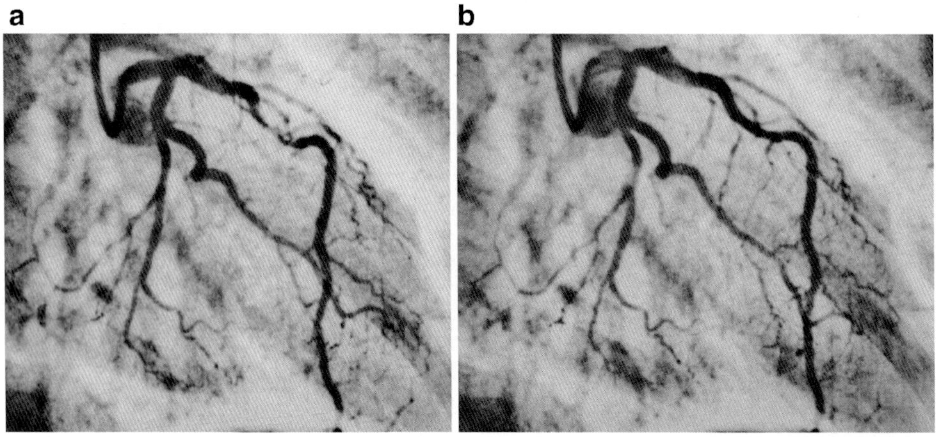

Fig. 6.37 (**a**) Systole (**b**) Diastole. Following administration of nitroglycerin, the examination in the same projection shows dilatation of the LAD and there is now intermittent compression of the proximal LAD by the myocardial bridge. Note that during systole there is also disappearance of the septal branch at the level of the myocardial bridge. This phenomenon cannot be explained at the present time. Under the relaxation effects of nitrites, the arteries may be more susceptible to myocardial compression

Limitations of Coronary Arteriography

Like any other diagnostic method, coronary arteriography has inherent limitations. It demonstrates the coronary arterial lumen, but provides no direct information about changes of the vessel wall. Depict lesions with very complex morphology, and identification of vulnerable plaques [52, 53]. In addition, uniform diffuse intimal thickening leads to a relatively uniform reduction in lumen caliber. As a result, the visual impact of focal stenotic lesions appears to be less. Conversely, diffuse abluminal dilation, common with high coronary flow states such as cardiac hypertrophy, enhances the visual impact of focal lesions, even though the minimal cross-sectional area of the stenotic lesion may provide little resistance to blood flow.

A variety of intravascular imaging techniques have been developed to compensate for the limitations of coronary arteriography. Catheter-based techniques that use intravascular ultrasound (IVUS) have been used for many years and have provided new insights into vascular biology. Optical coherence tomography (OCT) is an emerging technique that is based on the same principles as IVUS, but uses near-infrared light which provides for much greater resolution than is achievable with ultrasound and more suitable to identify unstable plaques. However, OCT has less penetrability through nontransparent tissue and image acquisition is hampered by the presence of blood [54]. Other noninvasive imaging techniques such as molecular imaging using F-FDG positron emission tomography or annexin imaging with single-photon emission computed tomography may prove to be more accurate and practical for this purpose [55].

References

1. Radner S. An attempt at the roentgenologic visualization of coronary blood vessels in man. Acta Radiol (Old Series). 1945;26:497–502.
2. De AG. l'arteriographie methodique des coronaries grace a l'Acetylcholine. Arch Mal Coeur. 1959;52:1121.
3. Bilgutay AM, Lillehei CW. Single and double contrast coronary arteriography: utilizing acetylcholine asystole with controlled return of heart rate using a cardiac pacemaker. J ThoracCardiovasc Surg. 1962;44:617.
4. Sones FM, Shirey EK. Cine coronary arteriography. Mod Concepts Cardiovascv. 1962;31:735–8.
5. Amplatz K, Harner R. A new subclavian artery catheterization technic. Preliminary report. Radiology. 1962;78:963.
6. Judkins MP. Selective coronary arteriography: part I: apercutaneurs transfemoral technic. Radiology. 1967;89:815–24.
7. Amplatz K, Formanek G, Stanger P, et al. Mechanics of selective coronary artery catheterization via femoral approach. Radiology. 1967;89: 1040–7.
8. Seldinger SI. Catheter replacement of the needle in percutaneous arteriography. Acta Radiol. 1952;39:368–76.
9. Judkins MP, Kidd HJ, Frische LH, et al. Lumen following J-guide for catheterization of tortuous vessels. Radiology. 1967;88:1127–30.
10. Archbold RA, Robinson NM, Schilling RJ. Radial artery access for coronary angiography and percutaneous coronary intervention. BMJ. 2004;329:443–6.
11. Nagai S, Abe S, Sato T, et al. Ultrasonic assessment of vascular complications in coronary arteriography and angioplasty after transradial approach. Am J Cardiol. 1999;83:180–6.
12. Goldstein JA, Kern M, Wilson R. A novel automated injection system for angiography. J Intervent Cardiol. 2001;14:147–52.
13. Feldman RL, Pepine CJ, Conti CR. Magnitude of dilatation of large and small coronary arteries by nitroglycerin. Circulation. 1981;64:324–33.
14. Wilson RF, White CW. Coronary arteriography. In: Willerson JT, Cohn JN, Wellens HJJ, Holmes DR, editors. Cardiovascular medicine. 3rd ed. London: Springer; 2007.
15. Colt HG, Begg RJ, Saporito JJ, et al. Cholesterol emboli after cardiac catheterization. Medicine. 1988;67:389–400.
16. Eggbrecht H, Oldenburg O, Dirsch O, et al. Potential embolization by atherosclerotic debris dislodged from aortic wall during cardiac catheterization: histological and clinical findings in 7621 patients. Cathet Cardiovasc Intervent. 2000;49:389–94.
17. Gottdiener JS, Papademetriou V, Notargiacomo A, et al. Incidence and cardiac effects of systemic venous air embolism: echocardiographic evidence of arterial embolization via non-cardiac shunt. Arch Intern Med. 1988;148:795–800.
18. Marco AP, Furman WR. Venous air embolism, airway difficulties, and massive transfusion. Surg Clin North Am. 1993;73:213–28.
19. Sticherling C, Berkefeld J, et al. Transient bilateral cortical blindness after coronary angiography. Lancet. 1998;351:570.
20. Gaglani RD, Turk AA, Mehra MR, et al. Ventricular standstill complicating left heart catheterization in the presence of uncomplicated right bundle brunch block. Cathet Cardiovasc Diagn. 1992;26:212–4.
21. White CW, Eckberg DL, Inasaka T, et al. Effects of angiographic contrast media on sino-atrial nodal function. Cardiovasc Res. 1976;10:214–23.
22. Ritchie JL, Nissen SE, Douglas JS, et al. American college of cardiology cardiovascular imaging committee. Use of non-ionic or low osmolar contrast agents in cardiovascular procedures. J Am Coll Cardiol. 1993;21:269–73.
23. Coleman C, Castaneda-Zuniga WR, Amplatz K. Three-dimensional teaching model for coronary angiography. Cardiovasc Intervent Radiol. 1982;5:154–6.
24. Paulin S. Terminology for radiographic projections in cardiac angiography [Letter]. Cathet Cardiovasc Diagn. 1981;7:341.
25. Marcus ML, Armstrong ML, Heistad DD, et al. A comparison of three methods of evaluation coronary obstructive lesions: Postmortem arteriography, pathological examination and measurement of regional myocardial perfusion during maximal vasodilation. Am J Cardiol. 1982;49:1699–706.
26. Johnson MR. A normal coronary artery: what size is it? Circulation. 1992;86:331–3.
27. Marcus ML, Skorton DJ, Johnson MR, et al. Visual estimates of percent diameter coronary stenosis: "A battered gold standard". J Am Coll Cardiol. 1988;11:882–5.
28. Glagov S, Weisenberg E, Zarins CK, et al. Compensatory enlargement of human atherosclerotic coronary arteries. N Engl J Med. 1987;316: 1371–5.
29. Dick C, Wyche K, Homans DC, et al. Effect of distending pressure on intravascular ultrasound measurements of lumen dimensions. Circulation. 1990;82: 459(abstr III).
30. Kalin JK, Rutherford BD, MCConobay DR, et al. Comparison of procedural results and risks of coronary angioplasty in men and women for conditions other than acute myocardial infarction. Am J Card. 1992;69:1241–2.
31. O'Connor NJ, Morton JR, Birkmeyer JD, et al. Effect of coronary artery diameter in patients undergoing coronary bypass surgery. Northern New England cardiovascular disease study group. Circulation. 1996;93(4):652–5.
32. Brown BG, Petersen RB, Pierce CD, et al. Dynamics of human coronary stenosis: interaction among stenosis flow, distending pressure and vasomotor tone. In: Santamore WP, Bove AA, editors. Coronary artery disease. Cardiac imaging. Baltimore: Urban and Schwarzenberg; 1982. p. 199.
33. Reiber JHC, Serruys PW, Kooijman CJ, Slager CJ, et al. Approaches to standardization in acquisition and quantitation of arterial dimensions from cineangiograms. In: Reiber JHL, Serruys PW, editors. State of the art in quantitative coronary arteriography. Boston: Martinus Nihoff; 1986. p. 145.
34. Reiber JHC, Serruys PW, Kooijman CJ, et al. Assessment of short-, medium-, and long-term variations in arterial dimensions from computer-assisted quantitations of coronary cineangiograms. Circulation. 1985;71:280–8.

35. Whitings JS, Pfaff JM, Eigler NL. Advantages and limitations of videodensitometry in quantitative coronary angiography. In: Reiber JHC, Serruys PW, editors. Quantitative coronary arteriography. The Netherlands: Kluwer Academic Publishers; 1988. p. 43.
36. Lesperance J, Hudon G, White CW, et al. Comparison by quantitative angiographic assessment of coronary stenosis of one view showing the severest narrowing to two orthogonal views. Am J Cardiol. 1989;64:462–5.
37. Katz LN, Lindner E. Quantitative relation between reactive hyperemia and the myocardial ischemia which it follows. Am J Physiol. 1939; 126:283.
38. Gould KL. Quantification of coronary artery stenosis in vivo. Circ Res. 1985;47:341.
39. Fulton WFM. Arterial anastomosis in the coronary circulation. II. Distribution, enumeration and measurement of coronary arterial anastomosis in health and disease. Scot Med J. 1964;8:466–74.
40. Baroldi G, Mantero O, Scomazzoni G. The collaterals of coronary arteries in normal and pathologic conditions. Circ Res. 1956;4:223–9.
41. Schaper W, Sharma HS, Quinkler W, et al. Molecular biologic concepts of coronary anastomoses. J Am Coll Cardiol. 1990;15:513–8.
42. Harrison DG, Sellke FW, Quillen JE. Neurohormonal regulation of coronary collateral vasomotor tone. Basic Res Cardiol. 1990;85 suppl 1:121–9.
43. Marcus ML. The Coronary Circulation in Health and Disease. New York: McGraw-Hill; 1983.
44. Takeshita A, Koiwaya Y, Nakamura M, et al. Immediate appearance of coronary collaterals during ergonovine-induced arterial spasm. Chest. 1982;82:319.
45. Rentrop KP, Cohen M, Blanke H, et al. Changes in collateral channel filling immediately after controlled coronary artery occlusion by angioplasty balloon in human subjects. J Am Coll Cardiol. 1985;5:587–92.
46. Meir B, Luethy P, Finci L, et al. Coronary wedge pressure in relation to spontaneously visible and recruitable collaterals. Circulation. 1987;75: 906–13.
47. Sasayama S, Fujita M. Recent insights into coronary collateral circulation. Circulation. 1992;85:1197–204.
48. Hirai T, Fujita M, Nakajima H, et al. Importance of collateral circulation for prevention of left ventricular aneurysm formation in acute myocardial infarction. Circulation. 1989;79:791–6.
49. Epstein SE. Influence of stenosis severity on coronary collateral development and importance of collaterals in maintaining left ventricular function during acute coronary occlusion. Am J Cardiol. 1988;61:866–8.
50. Topol EJ, Ellis SG. Coronary collaterals revisited: accessory pathway to myocardial preservation during infarction. Circulation. 1991;83:1084–6.
51. Bloch JH, Hurwitz MM, Edwards JE. Myocardial environment as protection against coronary atherosclerosis. Geriatrics. 1969;24:83.
52. Bruschke AVG, Sheldon WC, Shirey EK, Proudfit WL. A half century of selective coronary arteriography. J Am Coll Cardiol. 2009;54:2139–44.
53. Topol EJ, Nissen SE. Our preoccupation with coronary luminology. The dissociation between clinical and angiographic findings in ischemic heart disease. Circulation. 1995;92:2333–42.
54. Farooq MU, Khasnis A, Majid A, et al. The role of optical coherence tomography in vascular medicine. Vasc Med. 2009;14:63–71.
55. Tahara N, Imaizumi T, Virmani R, et al. Clinical feasibility of molecular imaging of plaque inflammation in atherosclerosis. J Nuc Med. 2009; 50:331–4.
56. Ovitt TW, Durst S, Moore R, Amplatz K. Guide wire thrombogenecity and its reduction. Radiology. 1974;111:43–6.

Chapter 7
Coronary Artery Anomalies

Thomas Knickelbine, Michael Bolooki, and Zeev Vlodaver

Introduction

Substantial differences exist in coronary artery anatomy. These differences vary in importance from benign alterations without clinical significance to those with a potentially lethal outcome. Anomalous coronary artery anatomy can be characterized based on abnormalities of origin, course, or termination [1]. Coronary artery anomalies (CAAs) have been reported in approximately 1% of patients undergoing invasive coronary angiography, depending on the definition of the anatomic variant [2]. More recently, advanced imaging techniques including multislice coronary computed tomography angiography (CCTA) and cardiac magnetic resonance imaging (CMRI) have been used to evaluate anomalous coronary arteries.

In our series of ambulatory patients presenting for CCTA to evaluate chest pain or abnormal stress testing, CAAs were the most common, unexpected atherosclerotic finding, noted in 8% of patients [3]. The vast majority of anomalies are associated with a benign prognosis and have no impact on the longevity of the individual. In certain instances, there may be a risk of sudden death or myocardial damage, making an accurate diagnosis imperative. In particular, those in which the origin is from the opposite sinus coursing between the aorta and pulmonary artery impose the most potential risk. In one study of young athletes treated at the Minneapolis Heart Institute, anomalous coronary artery origin from the opposite sinus was the second-leading cause of sudden death on the playing field behind hypertrophic cardiomyopathy [4].

Identifying CAAs

Identifying CAAs can be documented by autopsy, diagnostic coronary angiography, CCTA, CMRI, or echocardiography.

Coronary Angiography

Despite multiple angiographic projections and use of specialty catheters, the proximal course can be difficult to diagnose with coronary angiography due to limitations of fluoroscopy. Nearby structures cannot be assessed in relation to coronary anatomy, and the 2D nature of invasive angiography does not provide necessary spatial information.

T. Knickelbine, MD, FACC, FSCAI (✉)
Minneapolis Heart Institute, 920 E. 28th St., Minneapolis, MN 55407, USA
e-mail: thomas.knickelbine@allina.com

M. Bolooki, MD
University of Minnesota, Minneapolis, MN, USA

Z. Vlodaver, MD
Division of Cardiovascular Medicine, University of Minnesota, Minneapolis, MN, USA

Z. Vlodaver et al. (eds.), *Coronary Heart Disease: Clinical, Pathological, Imaging, and Molecular Profiles*,
DOI 10.1007/978-1-4614-1475-9_7,

Echocardiography

Echocardiography is limited to visualization of the proximal segments but is often used in the pediatric population where proximal vessel course can be readily established. More recently, CCTA and CMRI have been commonly used to further define coronary anatomy. These tools are being used with increasing frequency for the evaluation of chest pain, cardiomyopathy, and abnormal stress tests. CAAs are therefore being discovered with increased frequency, and the approach to treating these patients has become more complicated.

CCTA and CMRI

CCTA has superior spatial resolution and, when used properly in conjunction with radiation-reducing protocols, has become the preferred modality for most cases of known CAA, including the pediatric population. CCTA and CMRI also offer several additional features that cannot be judged by conventional angiography, namely the ability to define the takeoff angle acuity, the relationship to the pulmonic valve, an intraseptal course (deep within the myocardium), and the presence of associated calcified or noncalcified plaque. By visualizing nearby structures, the relationship of the anomalous coronary to the pulmonary artery, right ventricle, right ventricular outflow tract, and left and right atrium can be documented. These variations may have prognostic implications and have led to further understanding of CAAs. At many institutions, CCTA has become the gold standard for defining a CAA discovered with invasive angiography to further define the anomaly.

Benign Anomalies

Benign coronary anatomic variations are frequently well documented, but not necessarily characterized as anomalous coronary anatomy. The most common benign CAAs involve separate origins of the right coronary artery (RCA) and conus, affecting up to 50% of the population [5]. Variations in coronary artery length have been well described and similarly represent anatomic variants rather than true anomalies. These variations are discussed in Chap. 1: "Anatomy of Coronary Vessels."

Abnormal Origin of the Coronary Arteries

Variations in Level of Origin of the Coronary Arteries

Normal

The ascending aorta may be divided into two parts: the sinus or proximal portion and the tubular or distal portion. The junction between these two parts lies at the level of the free edge of the aortic cusps, commonly referred to as the sinotubular junction. Deviation of a few millimeters in the level of origin of the coronary arteries with respect to the junction is common. Figure 7.1 shows examples of normal variations in levels of origin of the coronary arteries as seen in necropsy specimens. The percentages given have been determined from an examination of 52 consecutive cases in adults [6].

Abnormal High or Low Takeoff

Congenital

When the origin is as much as 1 cm above the junction, a condition of congenital high takeoff or ectopic origin should be considered (Fig. 7.2). Instances of high takeoff of a coronary artery usually involve the RCA (Figs. 7.3 and 7.4). High takeoff may be a primary (congenital) phenomenon or acquired. While it has been suggested that congenital high takeoff of a

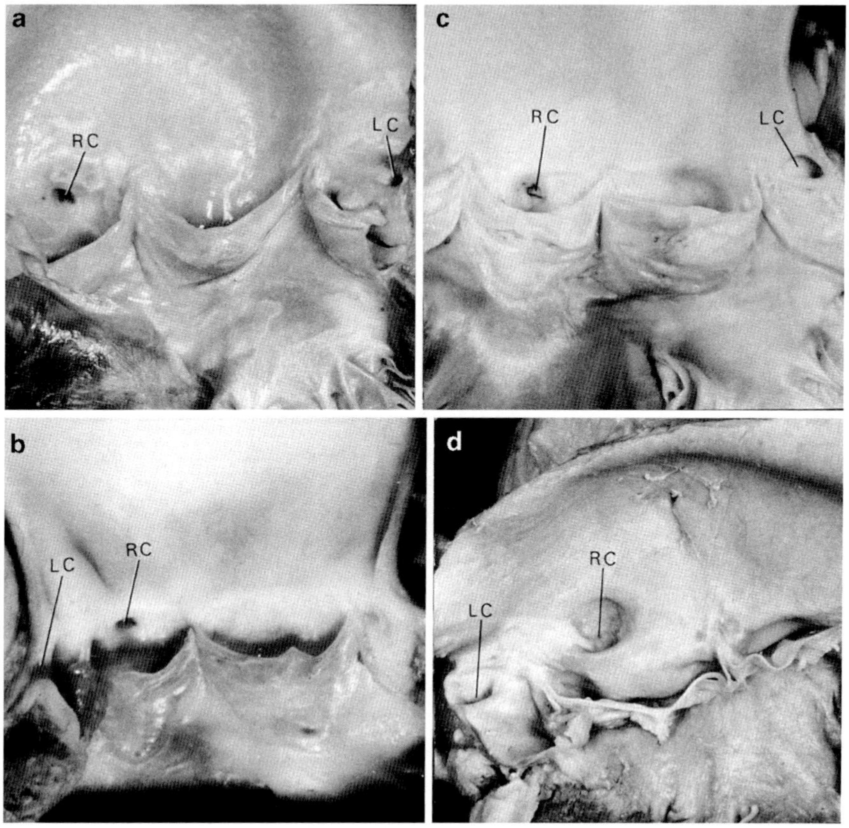

Fig. 7.1 Variations in the level of origin of the coronary arteries from an examination of 52 consecutive autopsy cases in adults. (**a**) In 56% of cases, both coronary arteries arise below the junction between the sinus and tubular portion of the aorta (Ao). (**b**) In 30% of cases, the RC ostium lies below the junction and that of the LC above the junction. (**c**) In 8% of cases, the RC ostium is above the junction and that of the LC below. (**d**) In 6% of cases, both coronary ostia lie above the junction

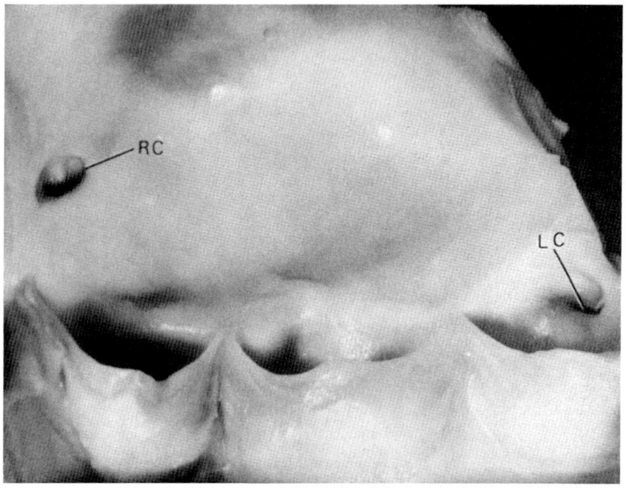

Fig. 7.2 Interior of the Ao showing the high takeoff of the RC ostium

coronary artery may predispose to premature atherosclerosis, no evidence supports this theory in our review of our autopsy series. A high takeoff of the RCA can be associated with an intramural aortic course where the proximal vessel course runs within the media of the aorta itself and may be associated with sudden death [7].

Acquired

High takeoff may also be seen as a secondary change in proximal aortic ectasia, including dilatation with cystic medial necrosis, Marfan syndrome, or a bicuspid aortic valve with associated aortic enlargement. In this situation, the high takeoff may be secondary to elongation of the aorta (Fig. 7.5). In this condition, both the left and right coronary ostia tend to be involved.

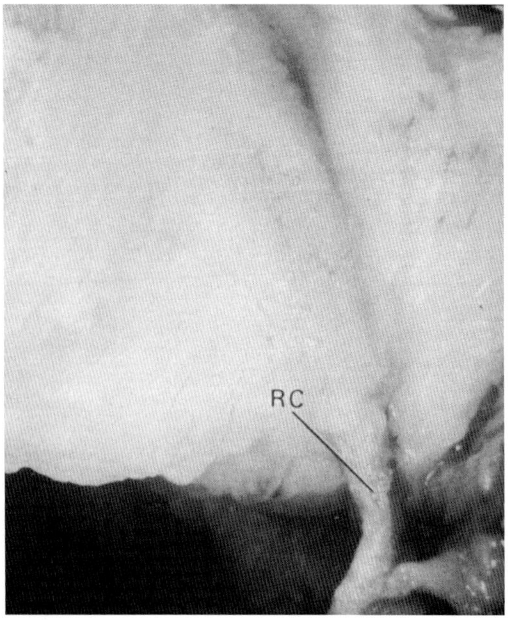

Fig. 7.3 Exterior of the Ao showing the RC, which arose at a high level and, after leaving the Ao, descended before entering the right AV sulcus

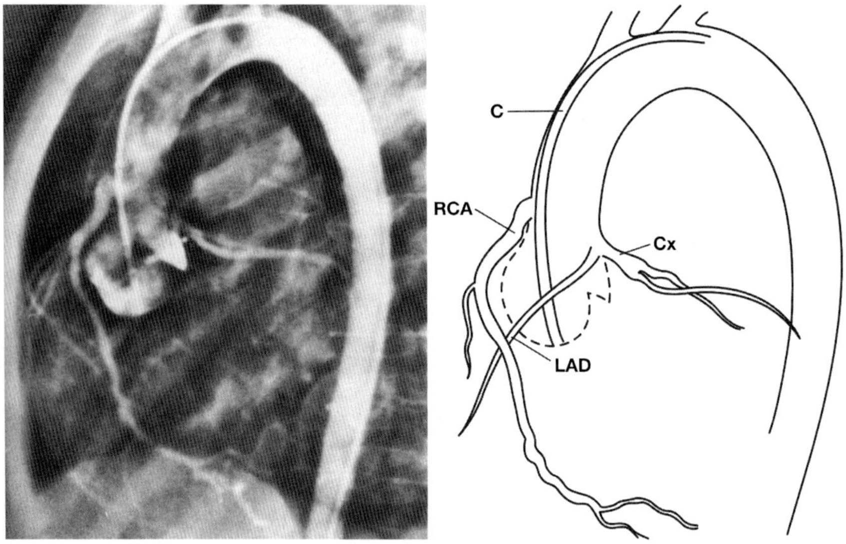

Fig. 7.4 Aortogram in lateral view showing high takeoff of the RC

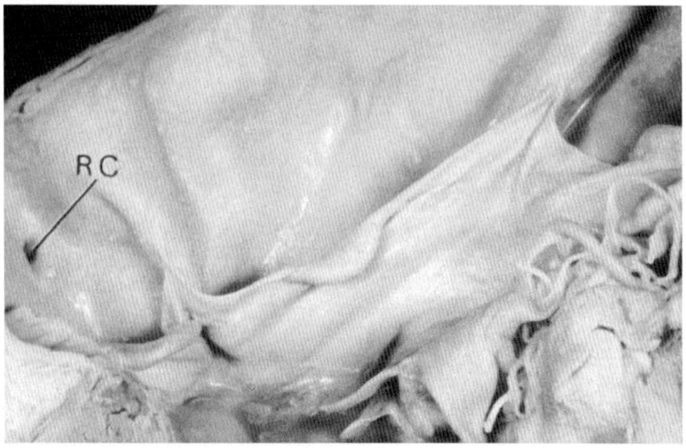

Fig. 7.5 The aortic valve and ascending Ao in an example of cystic medial necrosis of the Ao. There was dilatation of the Ao and acquired takeoff of both coronary arteries. The ostium of the RC is shown

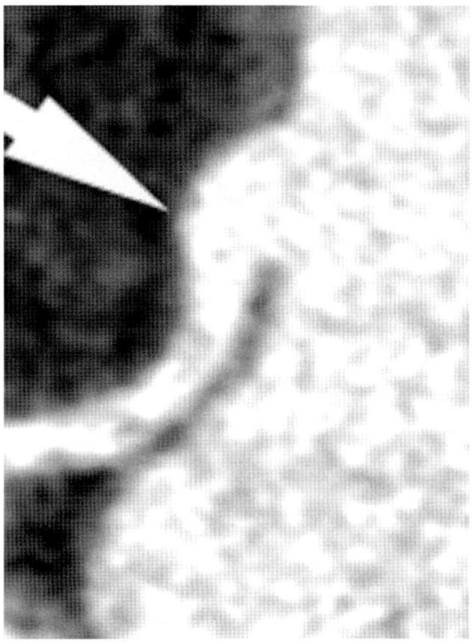

Fig. 7.6 Coronary computed tomography angiography (CCTA), multiplanar view, shows an abnormally high takeoff of the right coronary artery (RCA) well above the sinus tubular junction (*arrow*)

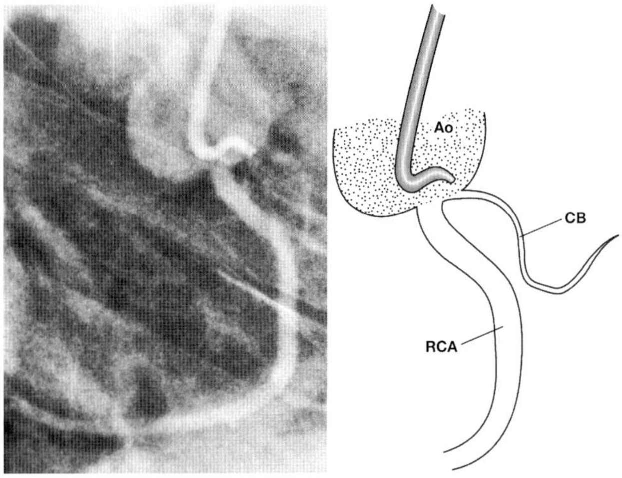

Fig. 7.7 Lateral view of right cuspogram demonstrating low origin of the RCA

As a practical point, high or very low takeoff of a coronary artery may present problems in finding the ostium during attempted coronary arteriography; CCTA or CMRI can be used to define the origin in such cases. Figure 7.6 shows CCTA findings of a high takeoff following inability to cannulate the RCA during coronary angiography.

Although uncommon, the origin of the coronary artery may lie very low in the deep part of the aortic sinus. This can have clinical importance during aortic valve replacement or repair, where the coronary ostia may require reimplantation (Fig. 7.7).

Variations in Sites of Origin of the Coronary Arteries

Single Coronary Ostium of the Aorta

When there is a single coronary arterial ostium from the aorta, two anatomic possibilities exist. The first is that the entire coronary arterial system arises from the aorta, a condition that may be termed "single coronary artery."The second possibility is that there are two coronary arteries, one arising from the aorta and the other arising from the pulmonary arterial system, usually the pulmonary trunk (PT) and rarely from one of its branches.

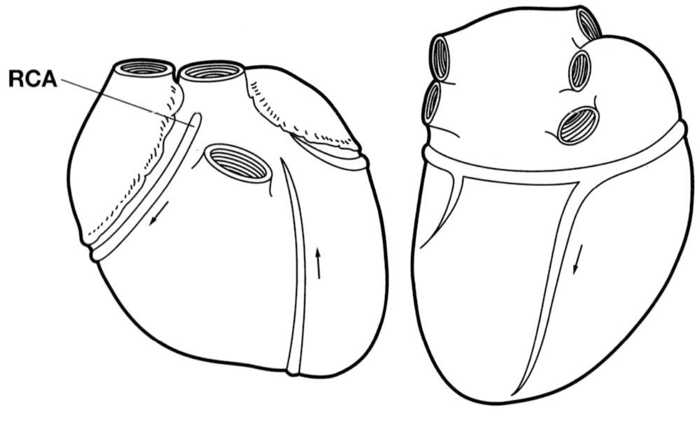

Fig. 7.8 True single coronary artery arising from the right aortic sinus. *Arrow* shows the direction of flow

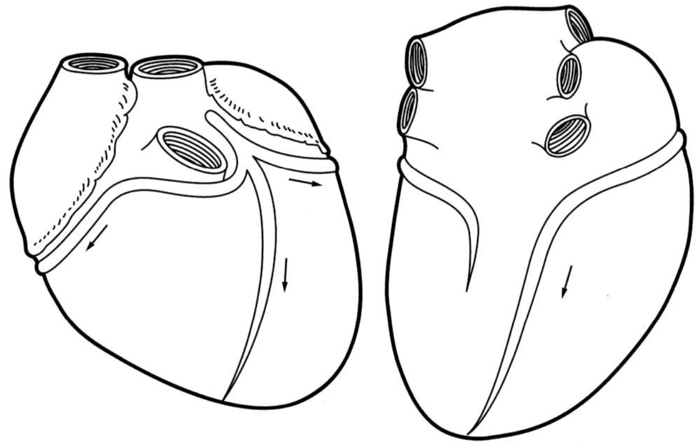

Fig. 7.9 Single coronary artery arising from left aortic sinus and dividing into RC and LC

Single Coronary Artery

Single coronary artery is a rare condition wherein only one coronary ostium is present in the aorta and one artery supplies the entire heart. While this condition is compatible with normal cardiac function, development of obstructive lesions in the vessel is more hazardous than in circumstances of separate coronary arteries.

Four types of congenital varieties of single coronary artery have been recognized:

1) The first type is a true single coronary artery characterized by a vessel originating at the usual site of either the RCA or left coronary artery (LCA), and whose terminal branches enter in the territory which would normally be supplied by the "missing" artery. Thus, such an artery may arise either from the right or left aortic sinus. In general, type 1 single coronary arteries are considered benign, although in cases of extreme physical exertion, this anomaly has been associated with sudden death [8].
2) A second type of single coronary artery is that in which the single vessel divides in such a way as to give rise to branches which simulate the arrangement of both arteries. When the single coronary artery supplies the contralateral circulation via two early-bifurcating vessels, one of those vessels may involve an interarterial course and predispose to sudden death.
3) The third type has an atypical distribution and grossly differs from the normal and is commonly associated with other cardiac malformations. Figures 7.8–7.16 show examples of types 1–3 single coronary arteries.
4) The fourth type of single coronary artery is referred to as atresia of a coronary ostium, the state in which both coronary arteries are connected to the aorta, but the ostium of one is atretic (Fig. 7.11). Atresia of the left main coronary artery is a very rare coronary anomaly. Pediatric patients are overtly symptomatic early in life. Angiographically, it may be difficult to distinguish a true single coronary artery from atresia of the coronary ostium.

The crucial point in distinction is that with a true single coronary artery, angiography shows simultaneous opacification of all major ramifications of the coronary arterial system. In contrast, atresia of a coronary ostium is characterized by early opacification of the patent vessel and late opacification of the vessel with an atretic ostium. The basis for the delay in opacification of the latter vessel is that communication between the two main coronary arterial systems depends on enlargement of the collaterals, while in a true single coronary artery, all the ramifications are fed from the primary trunk.

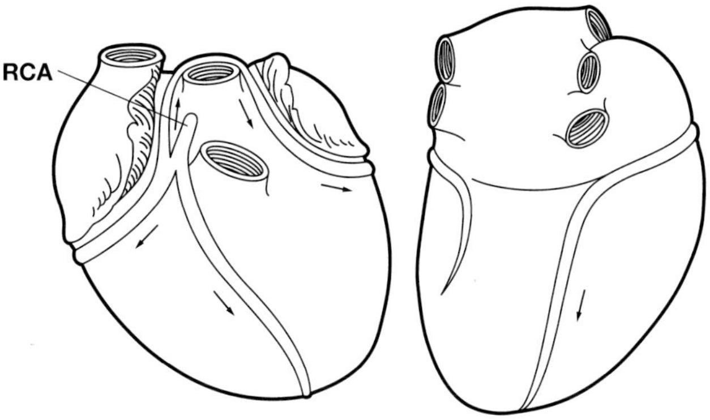

Fig. 7.10 Single RCA with atypical distribution

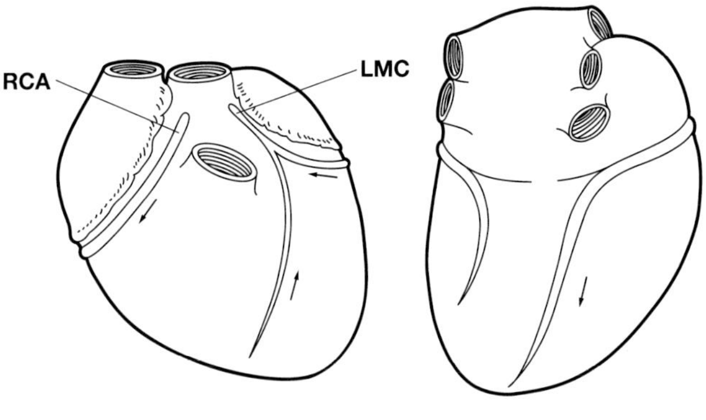

Fig. 7.11 Acquired single coronary artery resulting from atresia of ostium of LC

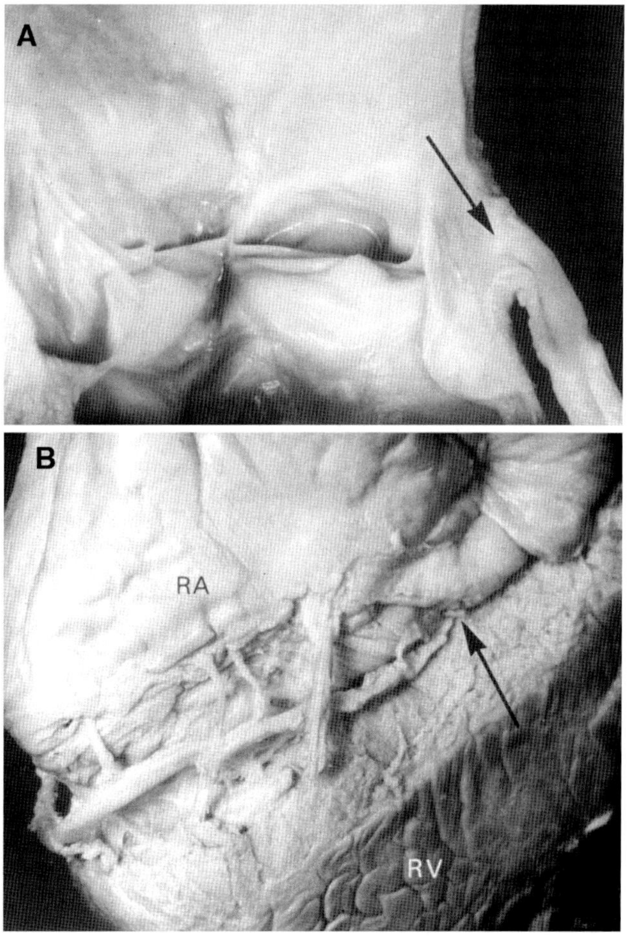

Fig. 7.12 (**a**) Opened aortic root and aortic valve. A single coronary artery arises from the left aortic sinus (*arrow*). The circumflex branch of this vessel continued across the posterior interventricular groove into the right AV sulcus and terminated anteriorly without connection to the aorta. (**b**) The right AV sulcus. The terminal part of the LC lies in the right AV sulcus and ends (*arrow*) a short distance from the aorta. Branches extend from the vessel to the RV (below) and the RA (above)

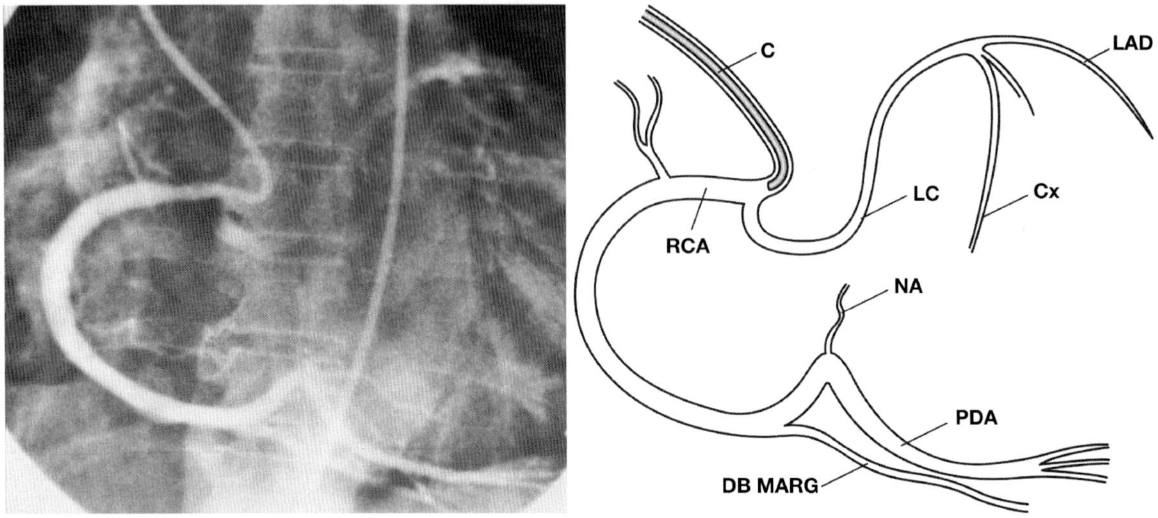

Fig. 7.13 RC coronary arteriogram in frontal view showing a large vessel arising from the right aortic sinus, which branches into the RCA and LC. The latter, after coursing around the posterior aspect of the aorta, divides into the CX and LAD branches

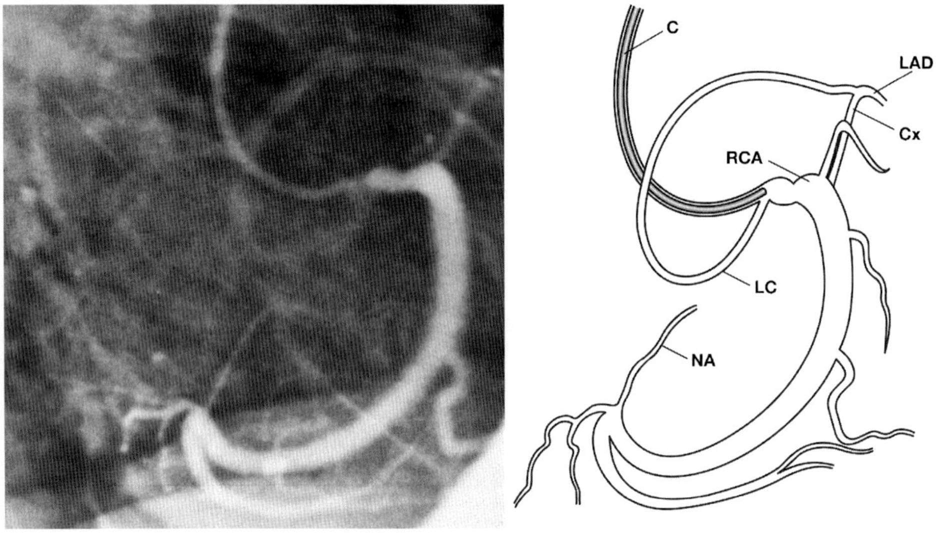

Fig. 7.14 RC arteriogram in lateral view, showing the essential features of a single coronary artery arising from the right aortic sinus and branching into the RCA and LC

Atresia of the Left Coronary Ostium

Figures 7.17–7.22 are from an infant who developed sudden symptoms of congestive heart failure at age 3 months. The ECG was typical for anterolateral myocardial infarction. A roentgenogram revealed cardiomegaly and pulmonary congestion. Aortography demonstrated a single, large RCA arising from the aorta. Following opacification of the RCA, the LCA system became partially opacified, but no evidence of opacification of the pulmonary trunk occurred. Death from congestive heart failure occurred at age 15 months. The pathological examination showed that the main LCA was a cord-like structure without a lumen connecting to the aorta.

Origin of One of Two Coronary Arteries from the Pulmonary Trunk

A situation in which both coronary arteries originate from the PT is extremely rare. It is much more common to see one coronary artery arising from the aorta and the other one from the PT. In most situations, infants present with shortness of breath, congestive heart failure (CHF), or sudden death. Rarely do patients achieve adulthood.

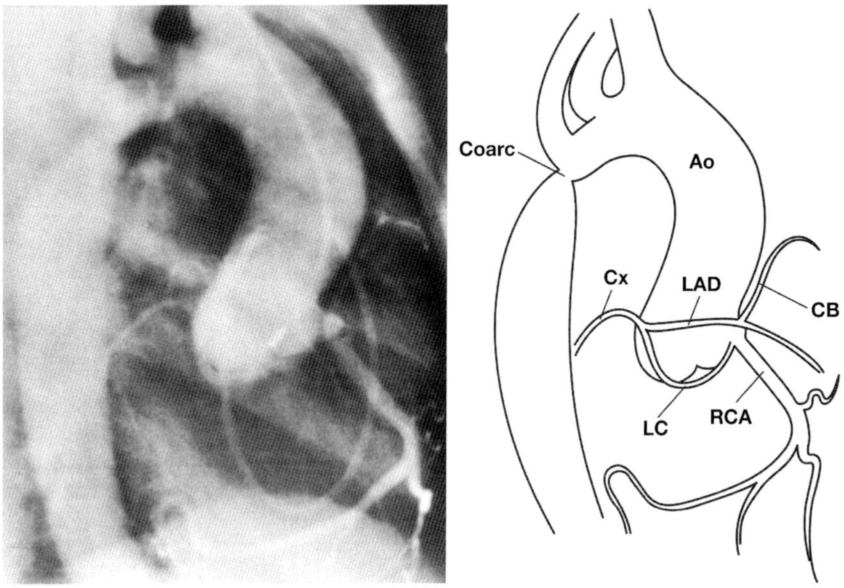

Fig. 7.15 Aortogram in lateral view. In addition to aortic coarctation, there are anomalies of the coronary arterial system. The latter are characterized by origin of a single coronary artery from the right aortic sinus. The vessel branches into the RCA and LC

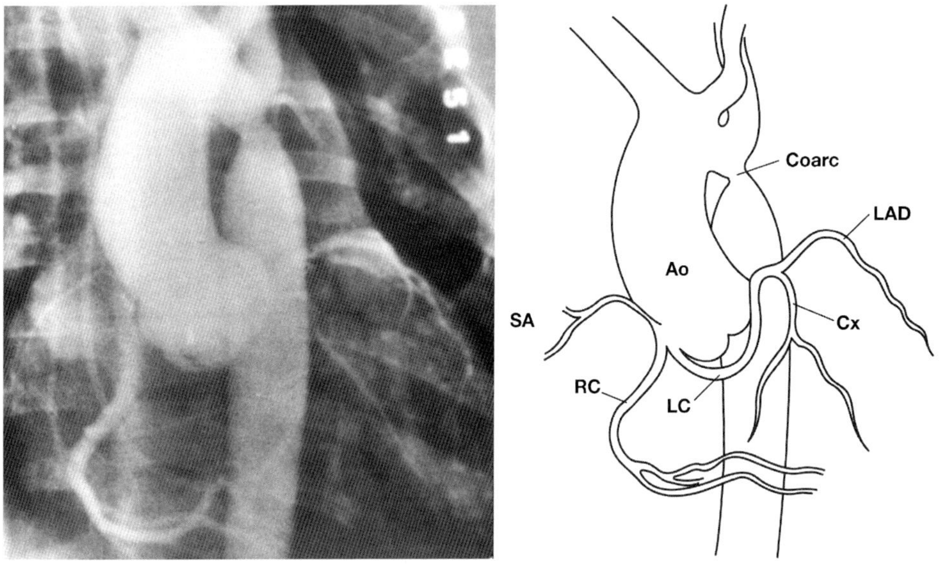

Fig. 7.16 Aortogram in frontal view showing the same features as in the lateral view (Fig. 7.15)

It is more common for the LCA than the RCA to arise anomalously. The peculiarities of the circulation are such if survival occurs, a collateral series of changes develops between branches of the aortic-arising coronary artery, on one hand, and branches of the vessel arising from the PT, on the other. As these collaterals become established, an arteriovenous, fistula-like condition develops. Aortic flow is diverted from the normal, arising coronary artery into the anomalous vessel, with the abnormal flow ultimately terminating in the PT.

The consequence of this anomalous arrangement is that the myocardium supplied by the vessel arising from the PT is deprived of blood and also of adequate perfusion pressure. This, in turn, leads to myocardial ischemia and often to infarction in the distribution of the anomalous vessel. Secondary effects include LV failure, mitral insufficiency, and sudden death. Ninety percent of these patients die in infancy and very few live to adulthood.

While anomalous origin of the RCA from the PT is sometimes a benign condition discovered at autopsy, in general, people harboring this anomaly die prematurely if untreated. If such patients receive a premortem diagnosis, surgical treatment with coronary reimplantation into the aorta is often performed.

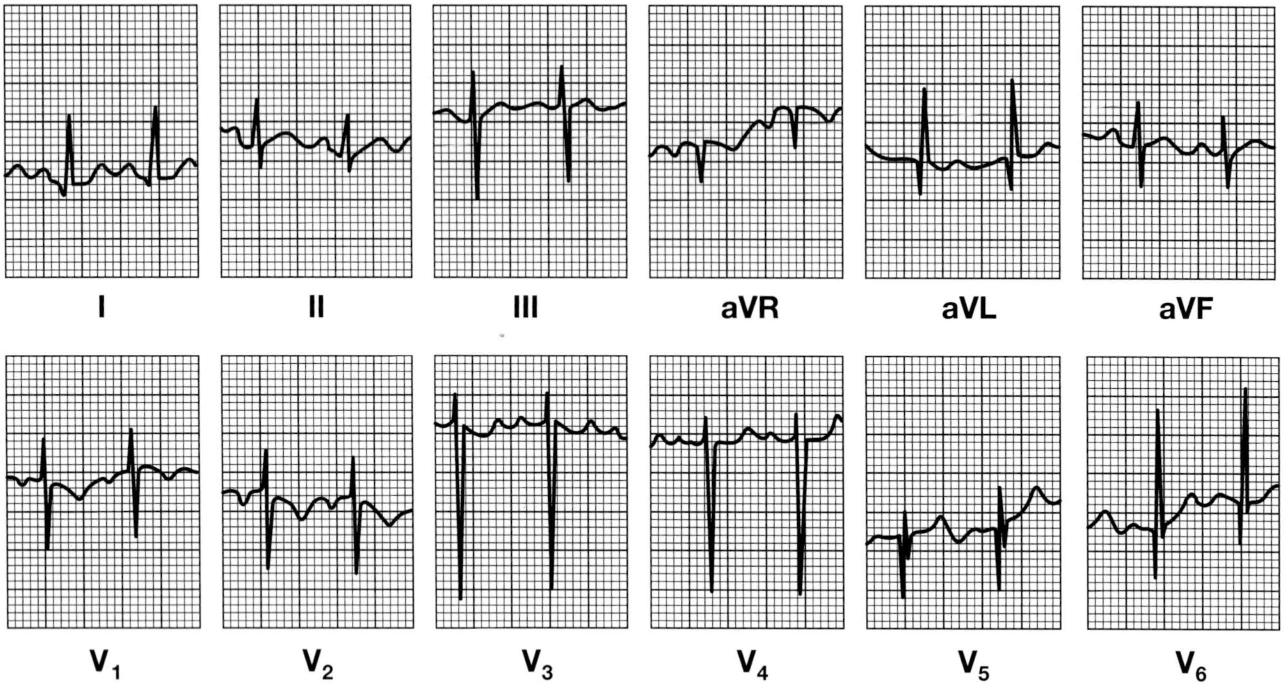

Fig. 7.17 ECG shows a left axis deviation and prominent initial vectors (Q waves in leads aVL and V5), indicating the probability of anterolateral myocardial infarction. Adapted from "Aortic dysplasia in infancy simulating anomalous origin of the left coronary artery" by Price et al. [23]. Copyright 1973 by American Heart Association

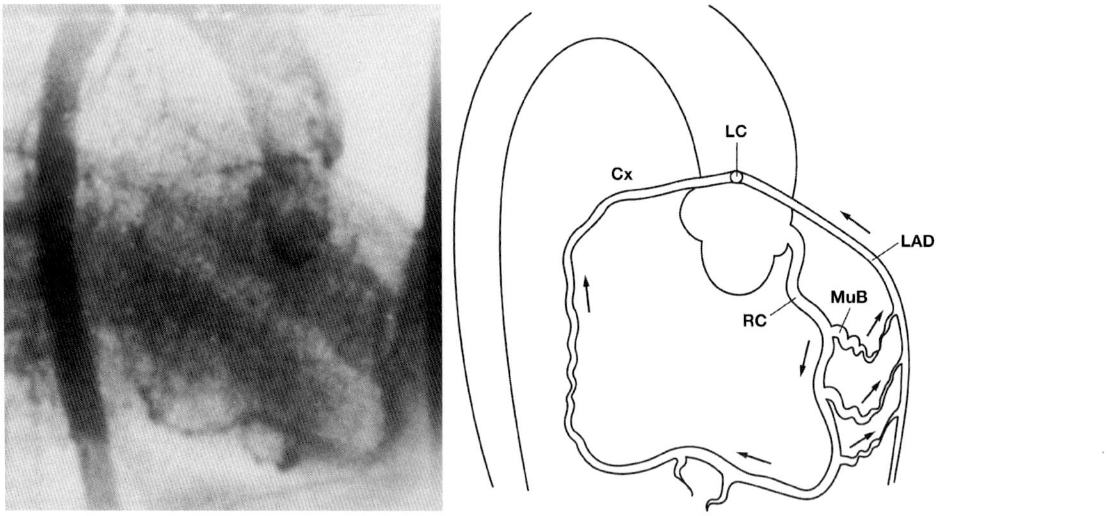

Fig. 7.18 Late stage of aortogram in lateral view. The RC is opacified, and collaterals connect this vessel to the LAD and CX. No contrast material was identified entering the pulmonic trunk. Adapted from "Aortic dysplasia in infancy simulating anomalous origin of the left coronary artery." by Price et al. [23]. Copyright 1973 by American Heart Association

The clinical diagnosis of anomalous origin of the coronary arteries from the PT depends on observing through angiography that only one coronary ostium is present in the aorta. In late stages of the angiography, the anomalous vessel becomes opacified, and ultimately, contrast material may be identified in the PT (Fig. 7.23). A coronary artery sometimes arises from a pulmonary arterial branch rather than the PT.

Fig. 7.19 (**a**) Interior of outflow tract of LV, aortic valve, and ascending aorta. The wall of the aorta is greatly thickened, and a ridge extends prominently across it at the junction of its sinus and tubular portions. The ostium of the RC is evident, while ostium of the LC is absent. (**b**) Exterior of the aorta showing the strand-like LC from which the LAD and CX branch were patent, while the main stem of the LC was not

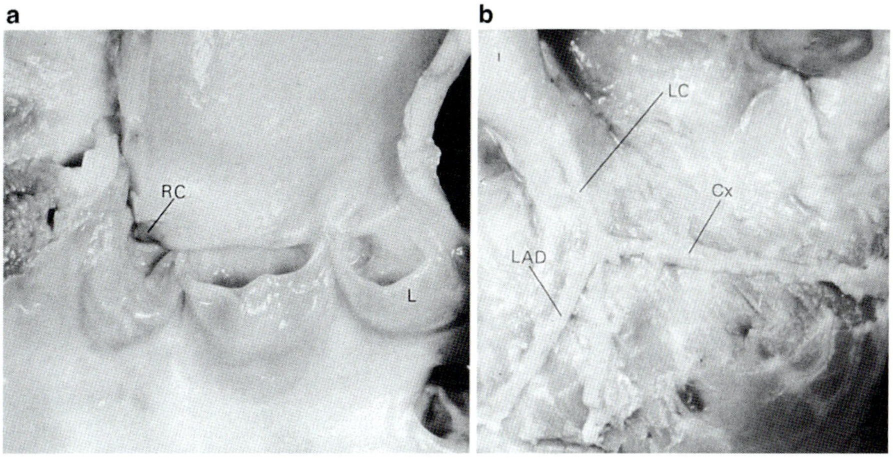

Fig. 7.20 (**a**) Diagram of the anatomic state of the coronary arteries. The shady area indicates a zone of healed myocardial infarction. RC and LC indicate right and left cusps, respectively, of aortic valve and pulmonary valve. Adapted from "Pathology of coronary disease" by Vlodaver et al. [24]. Copyright 1972 by [Elsevier]

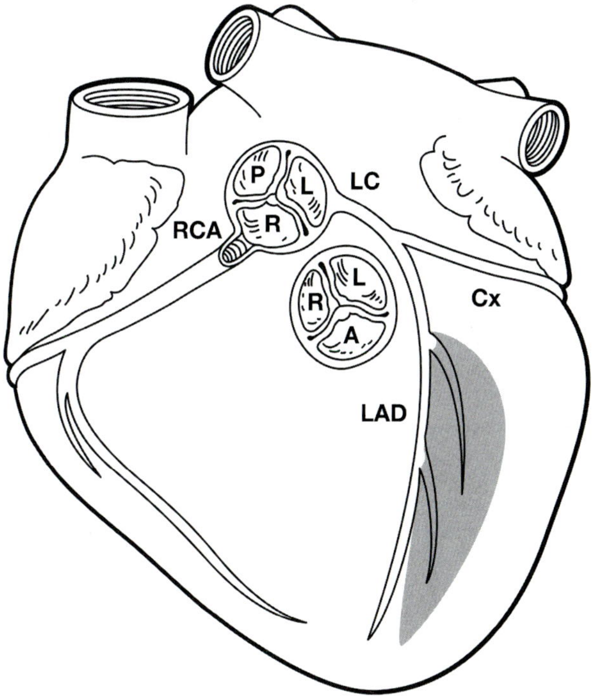

Fig. 7.21 Section through the aortic wall at the site of origin of the atretic LC shows a mosaic structure of the aorta and the small LC penetrating the aortic wall from the atretic area. Elastic tissue stain: ×15

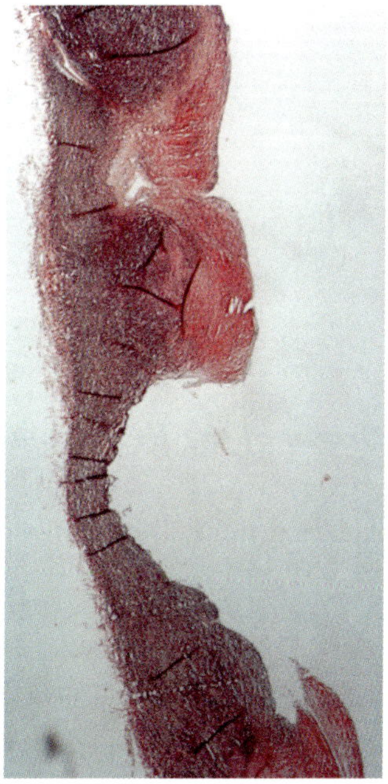

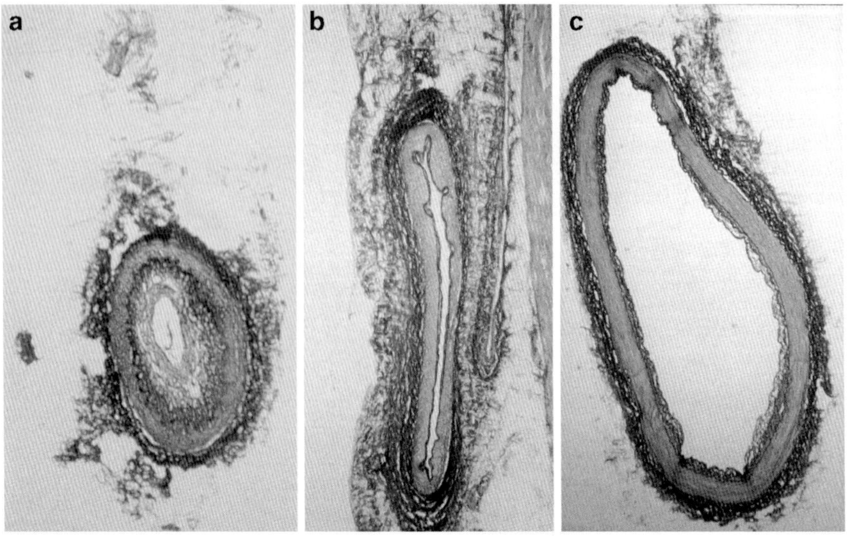

Fig. 7.22 Photomicrographs of coronary arteries. (**a**) LC: The caliber of the vessel is narrow, and in addition, the lumen is reduced by intimal fibrous thickening. (**b**) LAD near its origin. Although the vessel is collapsed, it is patent. (**c**) RC. The vessel is wide. Elastic tissue stain: ×27

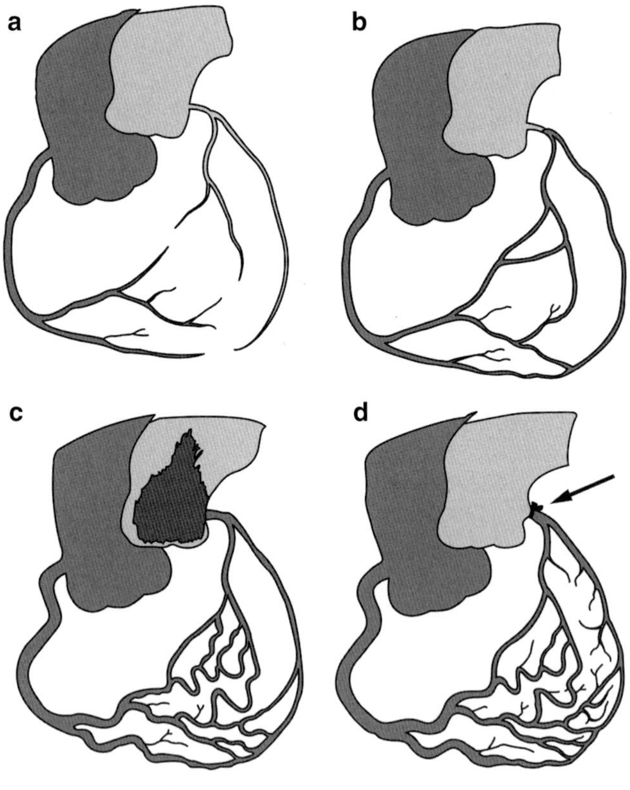

Fig. 7.23 Diagram of the angiographic features observed in the anomalous origin of the LC from the PT. (**a**) The RCA is opacified. (**b**) The collaterals show some opacification of the LC. (**c**) The collateral system is well developed and contrast material is carried into the PT. (**d**) Division of the anomalous arising LC (*arrow*) obliterates the arterial shunt to the pulmonary artery

Origin of the RCA from the Pulmonary Trunk

Arteriographic Demonstration

A 42-year-old woman had no symptoms of cardiovascular disease except for a history of cardiac murmur. Aortography revealed only a left coronary ostium. The LCA and its [ramifications] showed marked dilatation. There was late opacification of the RCA and of the PT (Figs. 7.24 and 7.25) [9].

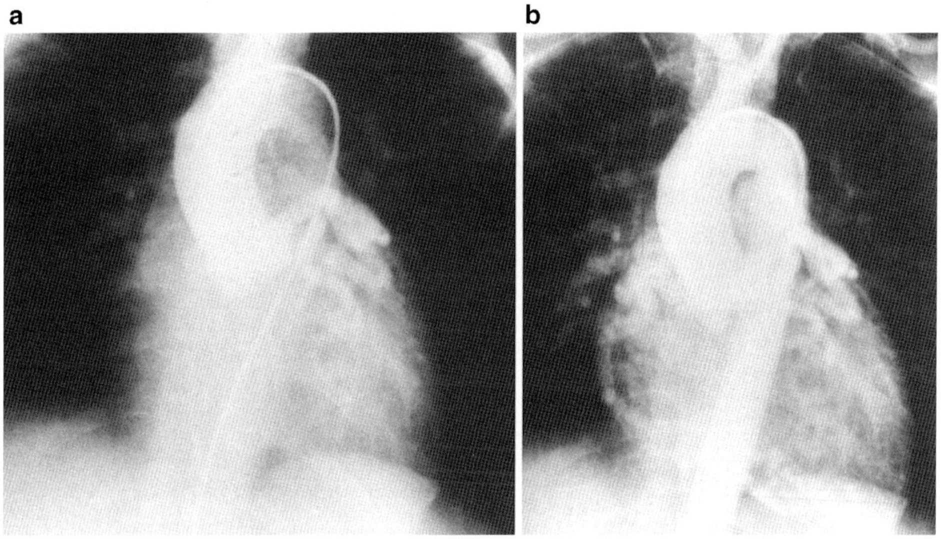

Fig. 7.24 (**a**) Aortogram in frontal view. Only the LC is opacified. This vessel and its ramifications show a wide character. (**b**) A later view of an aortogram showing opacification of the RC through collaterals. Adapted from "Anomalous origin of the RCA from the pulmonary artery," by Wald et al. [9] Copyright 1971 by [Elsevier]

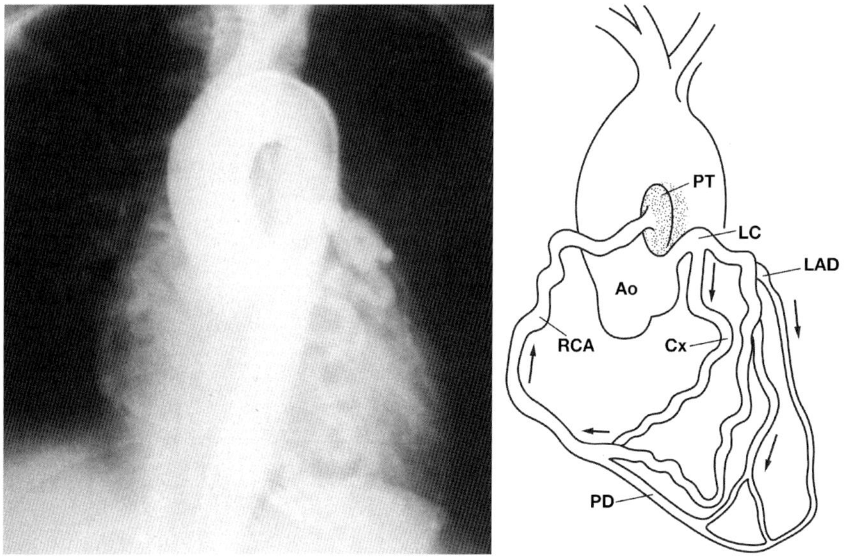

Fig. 7.25 Aortogram showing late opacification of the RCA and PT. Adapted from "Anomalous origin of the RCA from the pulmonary artery," by Wald et al. [9]. Copyright 1971 by [Elsevier]

Origin of the Left Coronary Artery from the Pulmonary Trunk

Arteriographic Demonstration

Figures 7.26 and 7.27 are examples of origin of the LCA from the PT in which the condition was demonstrated by RCA arteriography. Each shows collateral opacification of the left coronary system and ultimate opacification of the PT.

In the case of a 10-week-old infant who was observed because of poor weight gain, physical examination revealed an acyanotic, underdeveloped, female infant. A harsh, grade II, systolic murmur was heard with maximum intensity along the left sternal border and at the apex. The murmur was transmitted to the back. Hepatomegaly was present. A roentgenogram showed cardiac enlargement, and an ECG showed signs of left ventricular hypertrophy (LVH) and anterolateral myocardial infarction. The left ventriculogram showed cardiomegaly and displacement of the descending aorta to the right, considered to be a sign of left atrium (LA) enlargement. Death occurred during cardiac catheterization. Necropsy revealed origin of the left coronary artery (LCA) from the PT, while the RC arose from the aorta. The left ventricle (LV) was enlarged, and a healed myocardial infarction was evident. The observed LA enlargement was consistent with mitral insufficiency (Figs. 7.28–7.30).

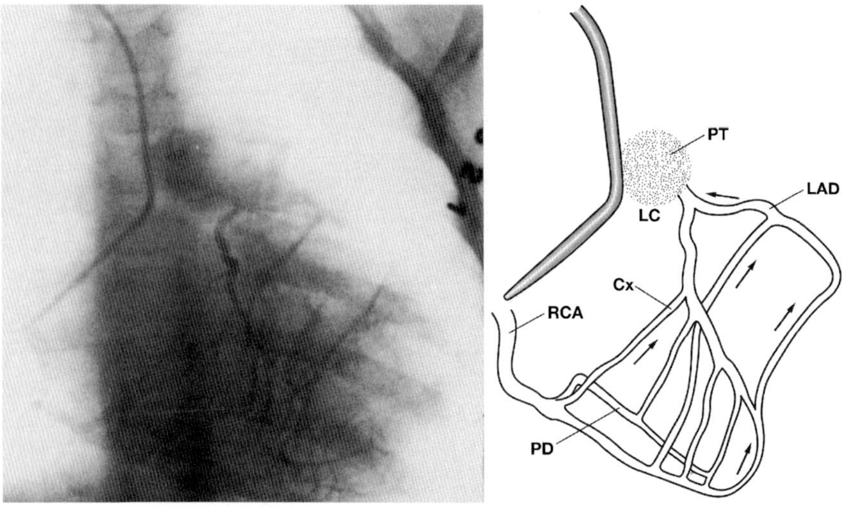

Fig. 7.26 Right coronary arteriogram in frontal view from a 2-year-old girl, with origin of the LC from the PT. Shows collateral opacification of the LC system and ultimate opacification of the PT

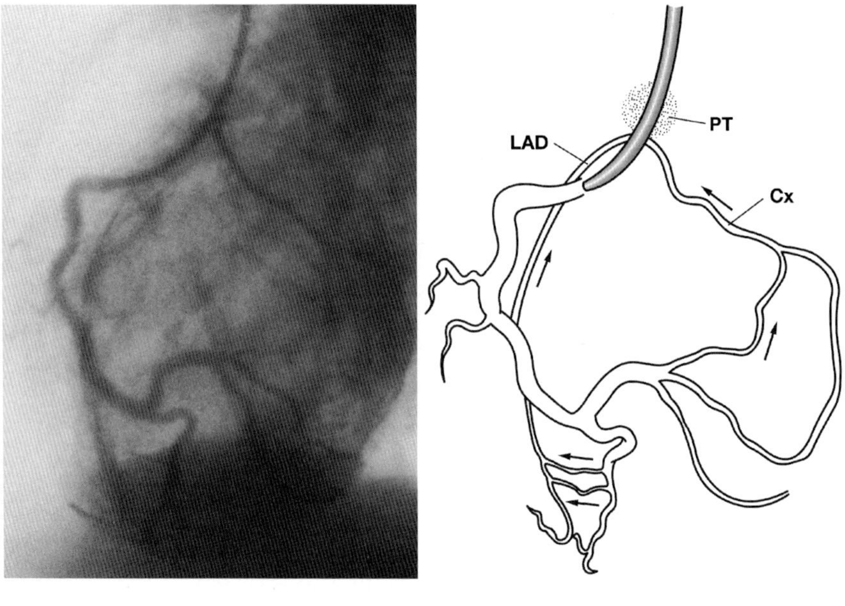

Fig. 7.27 Right coronary arteriogram in lateral view from a 9-month-old girl. Another case of origin of the LC from the PT, it shows collateral opacification of the LC system and ultimate opacification of the PT

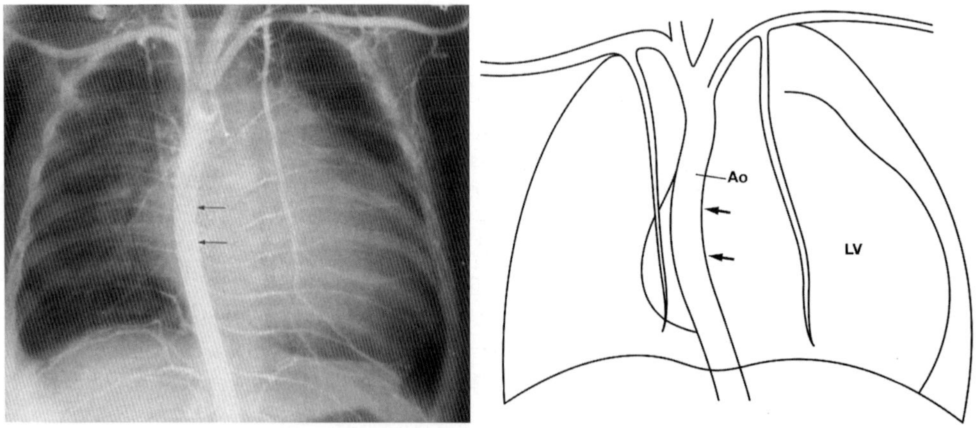

Fig. 7.28 Aortogram showing displacement of the descending aorta toward the right (*arrows*), considered to be a feature of LA enlargement secondary to mitral insufficiency

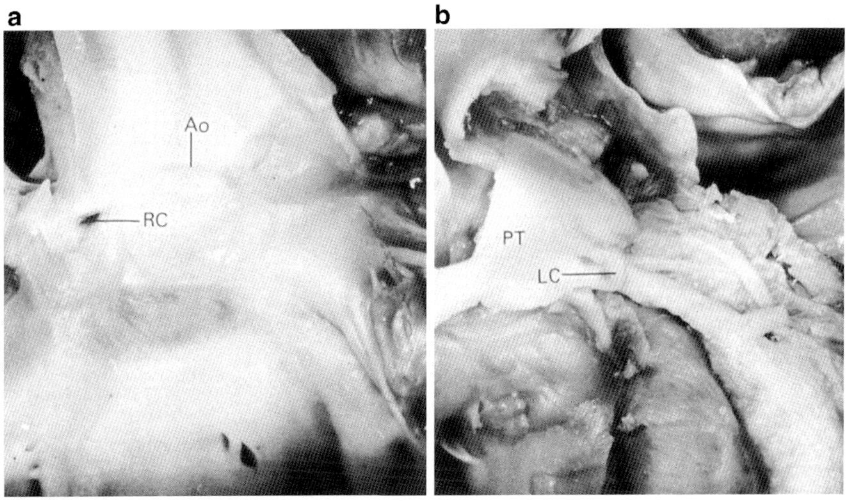

Fig. 7.29 (**a**) LV and ascending aorta. Only the RCA arises from the aorta. (**b**) PT. The LC arises from the PT

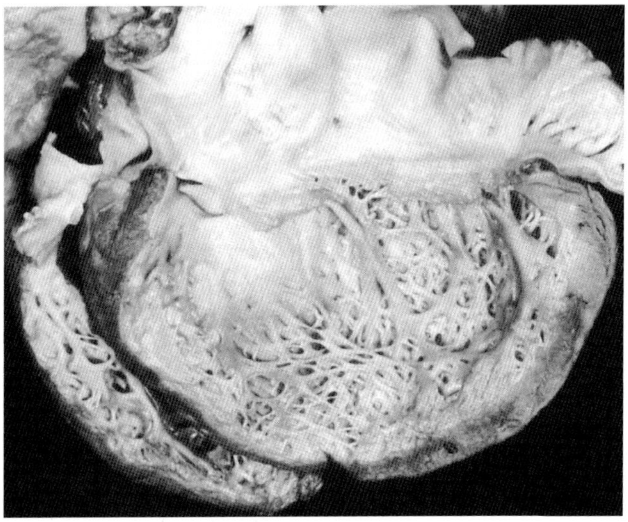

Fig. 7.30 LV and LA. LV shows dilatation, endocardial fibroelastosis, and hypertrophy. Papillary muscles are atrophic on the basis of infarction. The LA is enlarged, which is considered to be secondary to mitral insufficiency

Origin of the Left Coronary Artery from the Right Pulmonary Artery

The illustrations in Figs. 7.31 and 7.32 are from a 2-year-old girl with a ventricular septal defect (VSD) and a large left-to-right shunt, who died shortly after surgery to close the VSD. The autopsy showed that the LCA arose from the pulmonary artery rather from the PT [10].

When the ventricular septum is intact and the LCA arises from the pulmonary arterial system, a shunt from the RCA into the LCA system by virtue of the low pressure in the LCA ultimately develops.

When a large VSD is present and the pulmonary arterial pressure approximates the systemic pressure, antegrade flow through an anomalously arising coronary artery continues after birth. Blood from the PT supplies the anomalous arising coronary artery and its [ramifications]. If the VSD is closed and the pulmonary pressure falls, there is a sudden decrease in perfusion pressure into the anomalous coronary artery, and myocardial ischemia results.

Anomalous Origin of a Coronary Artery from Opposite Sinus

Cases of coronary origin with wrong sinus have been collectively termed "anomalous origin of a coronary artery from the opposite sinus" or ACAOS. These cases have special interest to the clinician as there are subvarieties which may harbor potentially lethal variants, even in the absence of symptoms. The origin may be single, as in type 2 single coronary artery,

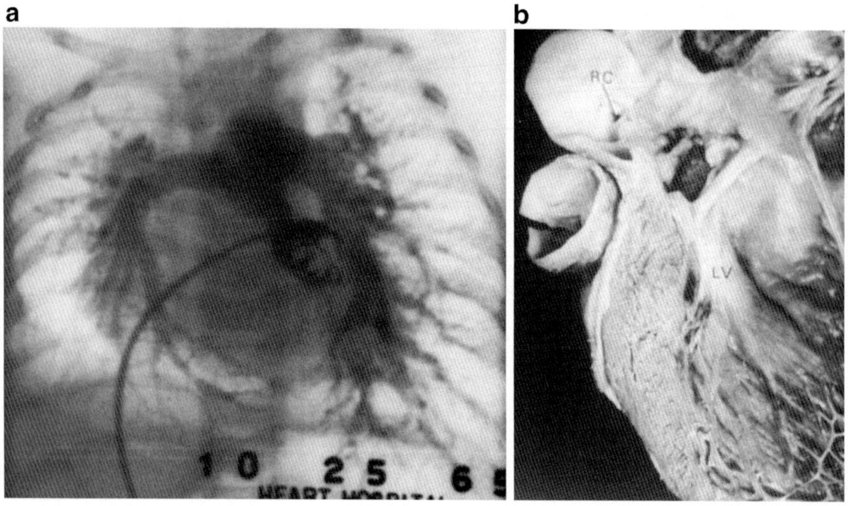

Fig. 7.31 (**a**) Front view of pulmonary arteriogram showing prominent pulmonary vascularity. Review of the films did not reveal visualization of the anomalously arising LC. (**b**) Open-end LV and proximal portion of the aorta showing surgically closed, large VSD and ostium of RC. Adapted from Rao et al. [10]. Copyright 1970 by American College of Chest Physicians

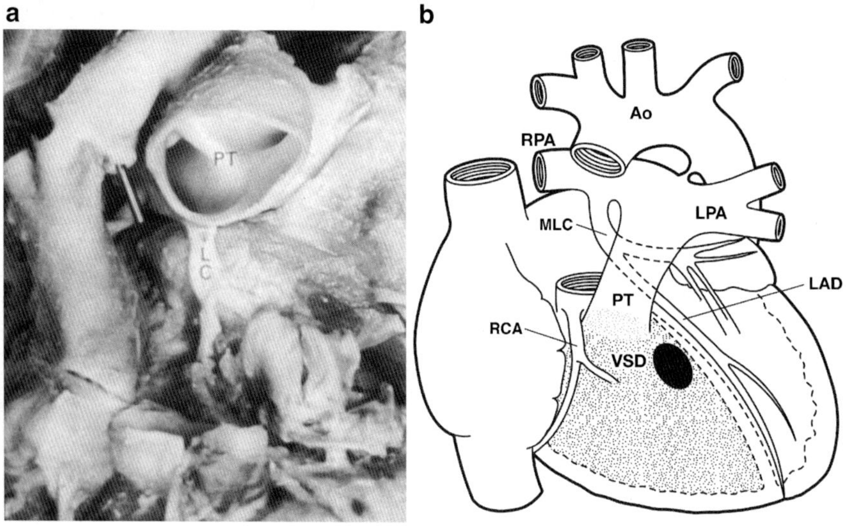

Fig. 7.32 (**a**) Transected PT showing origin of LC from proximal portion of the right pulmonary artery. Probe is in the aortic ostium of a small patent ductus arteriosus. (**b**) Diagram of the essential anomalies that were present

or frequently with separate ostia from the sinus. When an anomalous coronary artery is discovered at our institutions during invasive angiography, CCTA is performed to further characterize the origin, course, and any additional features that may help determine the best therapeutic approach. Depending on these findings, stress testing may be used to aid in management approach.

Four Courses of ACAOS

ACAOS can be characterized into one of four courses (Fig. 7.33). The anomalous origins can be readily defined by both multislice computed tomography angiography (CCTA) and CMRI but not with diagnostic angiography (Fig. 7.34):

1. A retroaortic course is associated with a benign prognosis since the artery is not compromised between the aorta and the pulmonary artery. In these cases, the artery traverses posterior to the aorta, where there is low pressure and no compromise of coronary circulation. The retroaortic course has not been associated with sudden death.
2. With a prepulmonic course, the artery course is anterior to the pulmonary artery or right ventricular tract and is associated with a benign prognosis. Again, there is no potential for compromise of the vessel.
3. An interarterial course occurs when the artery lies between the aorta and the pulmonary artery. The artery course will often be at or above the level of the pulmonic valve. There is a reported association with sudden death [11]. Sudden death

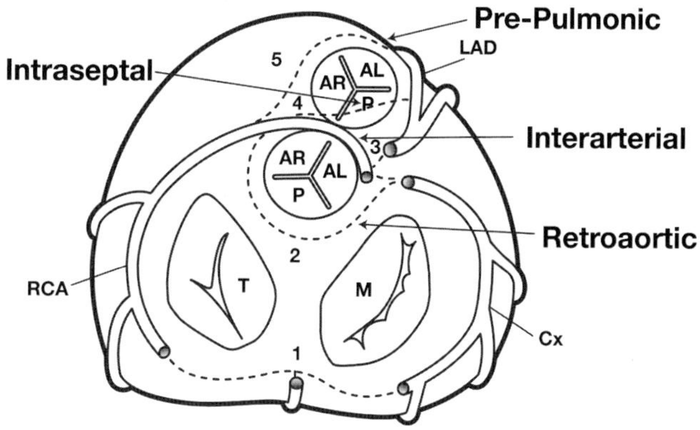

Fig. 7.33 Anatomic view, from above, outlining potential courses of anomalous coronary arteries. View is similar to axial CCTA

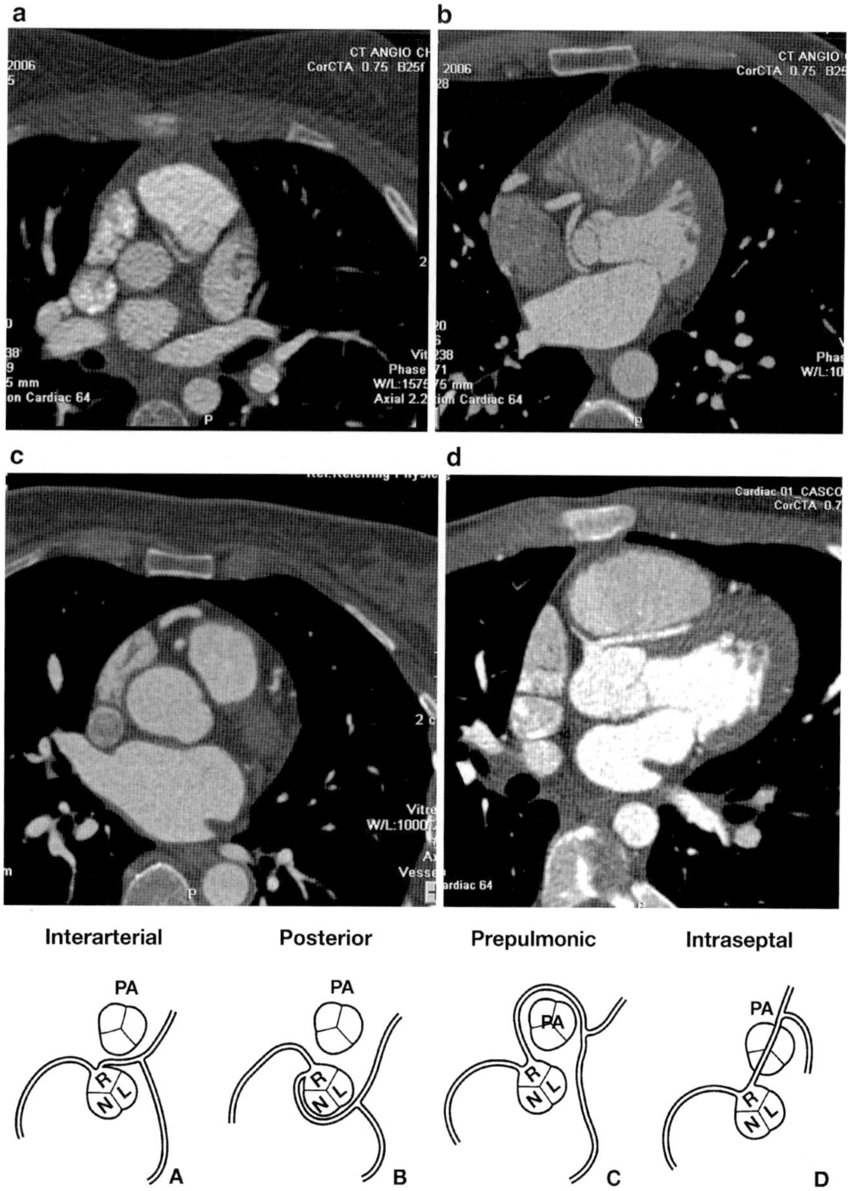

Fig. 7.34 MSCT view: Four courses of LCA from right aortic sinus. CT images showing its relationship to the pulmonary artery (PA) and myocardium: (**a**) interarterial; (**b**) posterior; (**c**) prepulmonic; (**d**) intraseptal

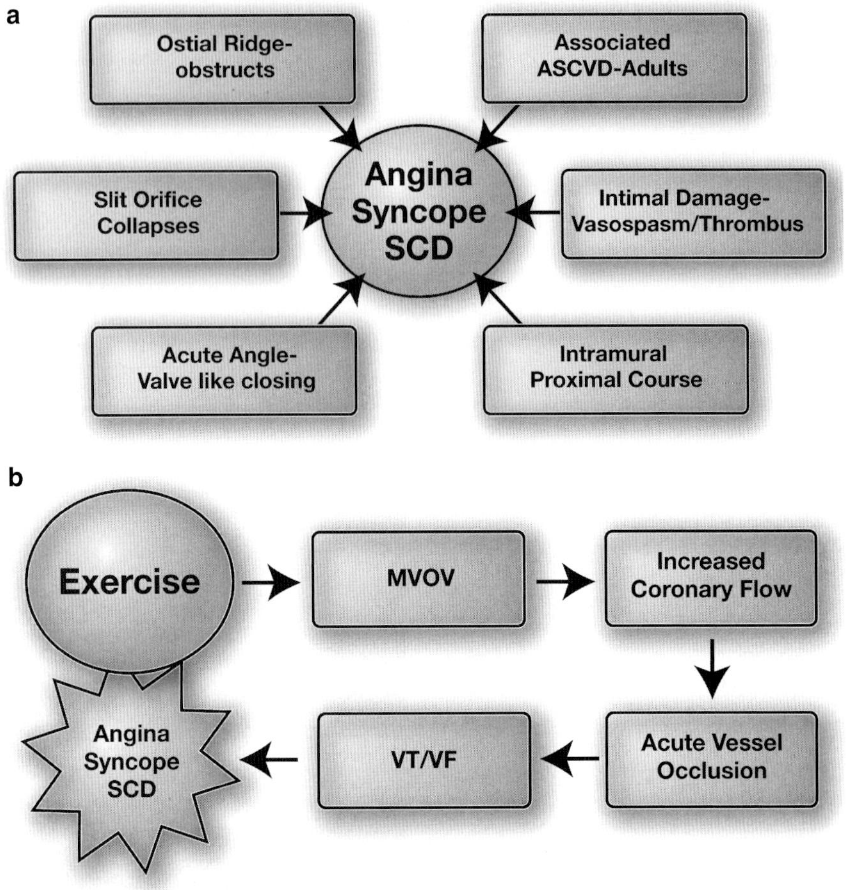

Fig. 7.35 (**a**) Proposed etiologies for the mechanism of coronary flow interruption of the interarterial course. (**b**) Potential mechanism of sudden death (SCD) in anomalous coronary arteries (ACAOS). Exercise brings increased myocardial oxygen demand (MVOV) and increased coronary flow leading to acute vessel occlusion. This will lead to angina, syncope, and cardiac arrhythmias. (VT/VF)

is most common in those under age 40 and can occur in the absence of symptoms [12]. Although the RCA originating from the left sinus is more commonly noted in symptomatic adults, the left coronary artery originating from the right sinus is more likely in cases of sudden death [13]. This may relate to the relatively larger amount of myocardium supplied by the left system compared to the right.

The mechanism of sudden occlusion of the interarterial artery course is unknown, although a number of hypotheses suggest compromise to the vessel as it leaves the aorta in the proximal segment. Figure 7.35a, b shows a summary of potential etiologies of sudden death in patients with ACAOS. Symptoms are not reliably present prior to sudden death, but when present, exertional syncope and exertional chest pain are most common.

4. Finally, with the septal or subpulmonic course, the artery travels well below the level of the pulmonic valve and is within the septal musculature. This association may protect the artery and is well below the interarterial zone. This course can be particularly difficult to distinguish from the interarterial course on invasive angiography (Fig. 7.36) [14]. Contrary to the interarterial course, the intraseptal course has not been associated with cases of sudden death.

CCTA and ACAOS

With submillimeter resolution and 3D capabilities, CCTA is well suited for assessing coronary anomalies. Advanced imaging has led to further detailed understanding of anomalous artery anatomy. Specifically, the proximal course can be evaluated for the presence of a slit-like orifice, acute angulation, and relationship to the pulmonic valve. Figure 7.37 shows two patients with ARCA (anomalous RCA), one with a slit-like orifice and one without. With further improvements in spatial resolution, it may become possible to distinguish an intramural proximal course, which may have important prognostic implications [14].

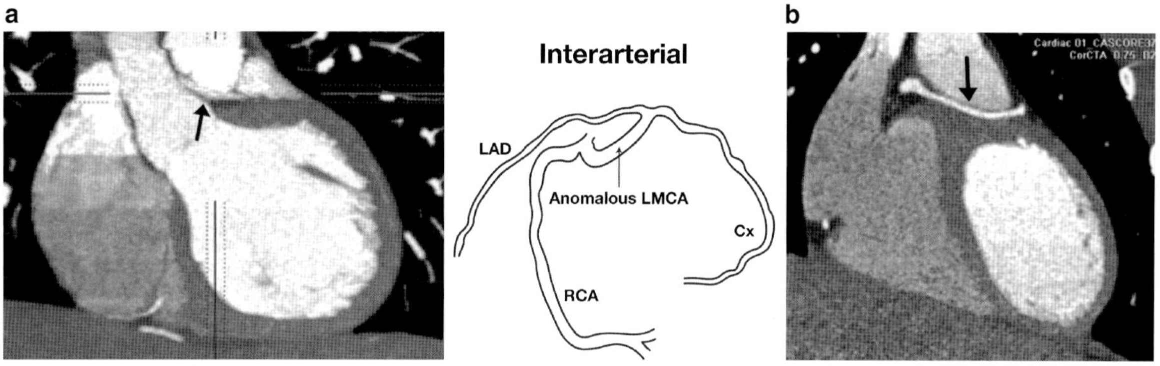

Fig. 7.36 (**a**) Interarterial course of the left main coronary artery (*arrow*). (**b**) Intraseptal course in the right (*arrow*). The intraseptal course is lower and within the myocardium. The difference is subtle but important clinically

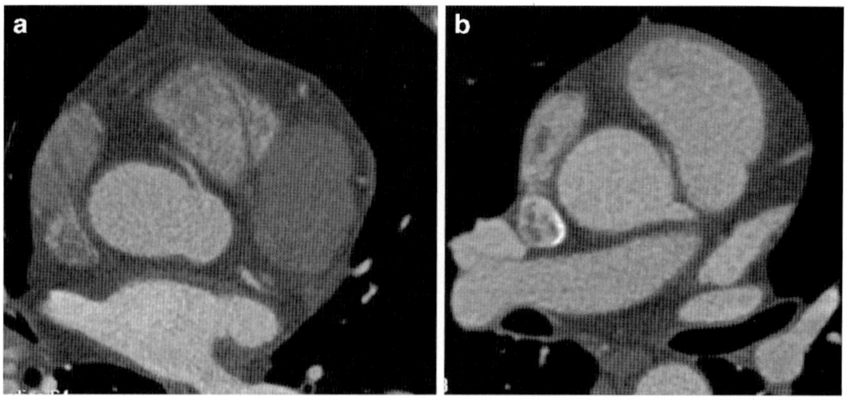

Fig. 7.37 Axial CT image. ARCA (anomalous RCA) of the left aortic sinus (*white circles*). (**a**) No slit-like orifice. (**b**) With slit orifice

Therapeutic Approach

Treatment modalities for ACAOS include activity restriction, angioplasty/stenting, and surgical intervention. Often, CCTA is performed to determine whether the patient has ARCA (anomalous RCA) or ALCA (anomalous left coronary artery), and to further define the course. In cases of ALCA with a prepulmonic, retroaortic, or intraseptal course, no further treatment is necessary as these anomalies have not been associated with a significant increased risk of sudden death. Most cases of ALCA with an interarterial course and those with high-risk ARCA are often considered for corrective surgery. The optimal approach in these patients remains controversial, with multiple strategies reported.

The most common surgical approach is the unroofing procedure, preferred with an intramural proximal segment and in children (Fig. 7.38) [15,16]. With this procedure, a new tract is created by opening the aorta along the course of the interarterial vessel and functionally creating a new coronary ostium on the correct-sided sinus. In adults with ARCA, the right internal mammary bypass, coronary reimplantation, or pulmonary artery translocation has been used [17]. Graft closure has been reported without native vessel ligation, and ligation should be performed in all cases [18]. These types of procedures are often employed in adults without an intramural proximal course. Coronary stenting may be considered in nonoperative candidates and in patients with associated CAD and acute coronary syndromes. This approach of coronary stenting is complicated by difficulty with guide catheter cannulation and the lack of long-term outcome studies. A summary of therapeutic approaches to ACAOS is shown in Fig. 7.39a, b.

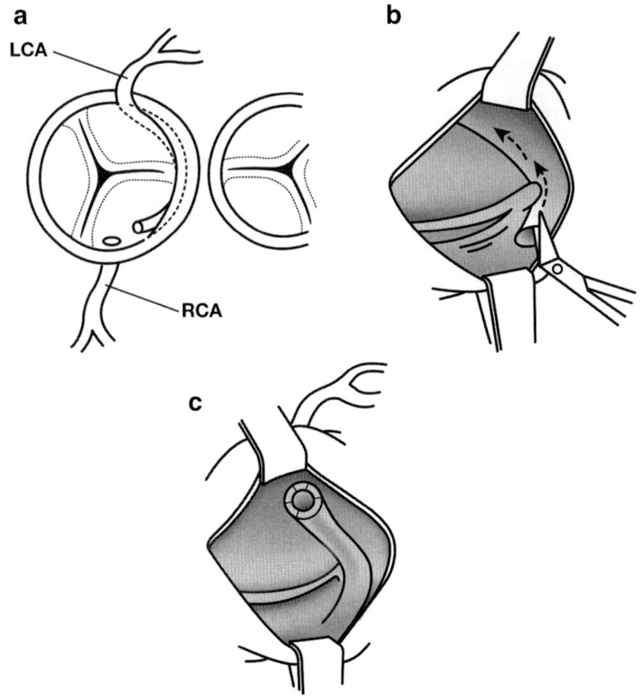

Fig. 7.38 Diagrammatic representation of unroofing surgical approach in a case with intramural RCA from the left sinus. Adapted from Jaquiss et al. [16]. Copyright 2004 by Elsevier

Case Examples: ACAOS

LCA from Right Sinus: Origin of the Left Circumflex Coronary Artery from the Right Aortic Sinus

When the left circumflex coronary artery (LCX) arises from the right aortic sinus, it may originate in or separate from the ostium of the RCA or from the beginning of the RCA itself. From either origin, the vessel proceeds around the posterior aspect of the aorta to ultimately reach the left AV sulcus (Fig. 7.40). Anomalous LCX from the right sinus is the most common coronary artery anomaly noted during invasive angiography and CCTA.

When coronary arteriography fails to show an LCX branch from the LCA, exploration in the right aortic sinus may reveal a separate origin of the LCX from the right aortic sinus (Figs. 7.41 and 7.42).

Figures 7.43 and 7.44 are from a 53-year-old man with angina pectoris. The LCA arteriogram showed only the LAD in which obstructive disease was present. The RCA arteriogram showed occlusion of the vessel. The LCX was cannulated and shown to arise from the right aortic sinus near the origin of the RCA.

Using CCTA, Fig. 7.45 shows an axial slice taken in the emergency room from a 48-year-old male with atypical CP and an anomalous LCX from the right sinus with a clear retroaortic course. The patient was discharged.

Prepulmonic LCA from Right Sinus

Figure 7.46 shows CCTA findings in a patient with chest pain. Notice the volume-rendered image clearly showing the arterial course well in front of the pulmonary outflow tract, also easily identified on the axial image. The patient was notified of the finding, and no further testing or treatment was indicated.

Intraseptal LCA from Right Sinus

The distinction of interarterial vs. intraseptal LCA from right sinus is difficult during invasive angiography. Figure 7.47 shows a case referred for CCTA following invasive angiography. Coronary angiography showed the presence of the left

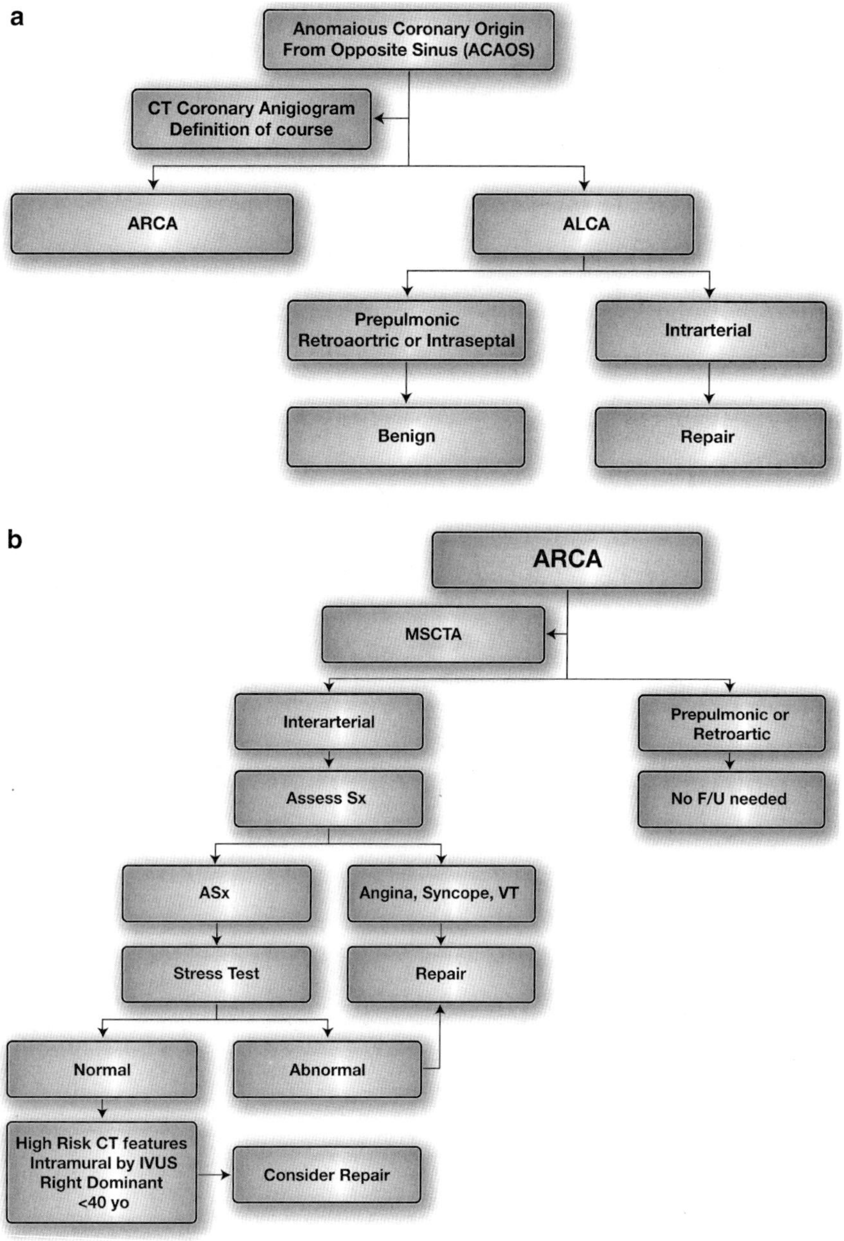

Fig. 7.39 (**a**) Therapeutic approach for patients with anomalous coronary artery origin from opposite sinus (ACAOS). ARCA: anomalous RCA. ALCA: anomalous LCA. (**b**) Therapeutic approach for patients with ARCA

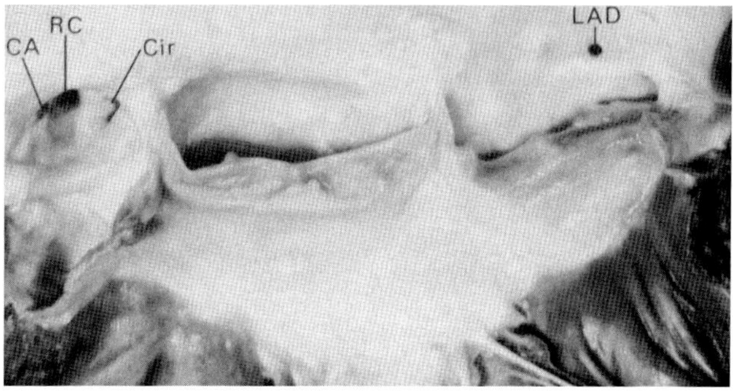

Fig. 7.40 LV and Ao. The CX arises from the right aortic sinus posterior to the origin of the RC. The LAD arose from the left aortic sinus

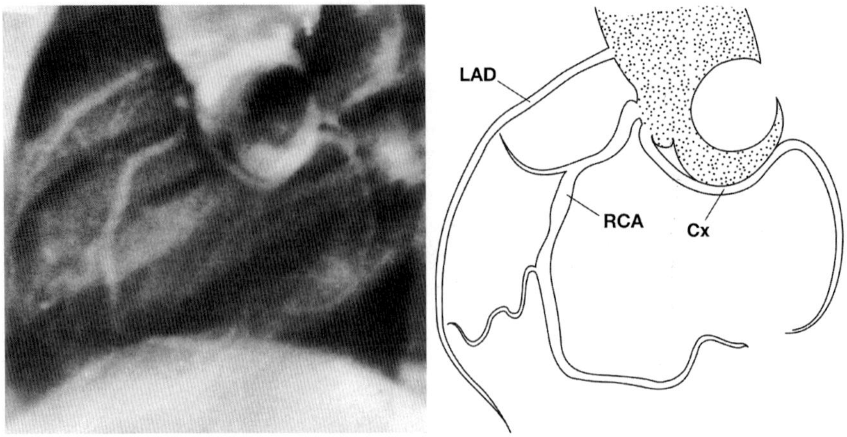

Fig. 7.41 Aortogram in lateral view shows origin of the CX from the right aortic sinus

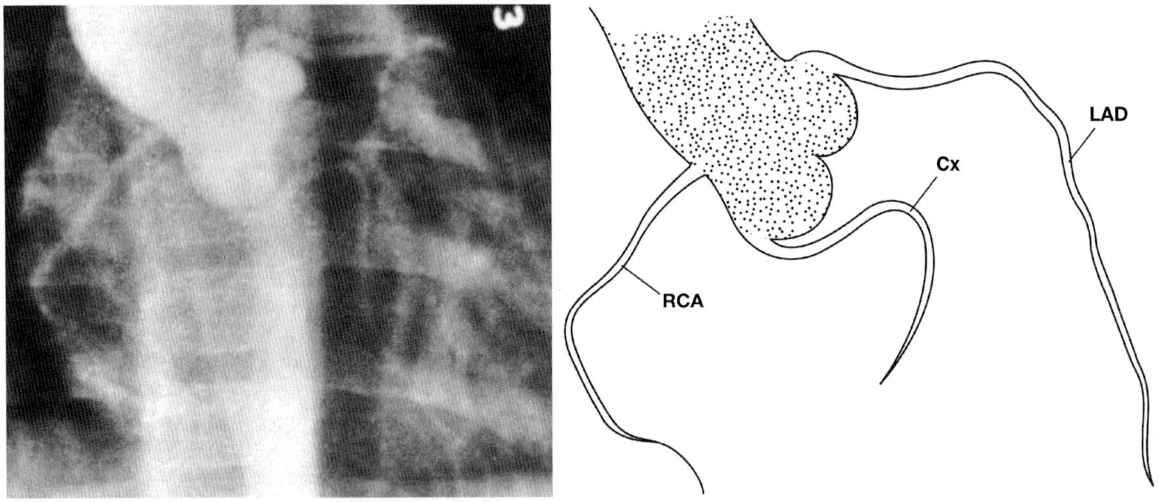

Fig. 7.42 Aortogram in frontal view showing LAD arising from the left aortic sinus. See Fig. 7.42 for another illustration

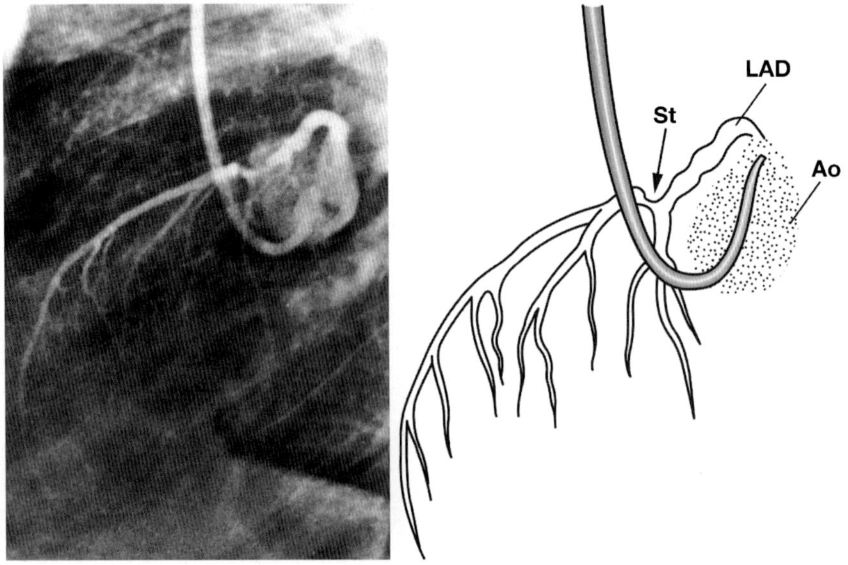

Fig. 7.43 LC arteriogram from a 53-year-old man with angina pectoris showing only the LAD in which obstructive disease was present. The CX is not opacified

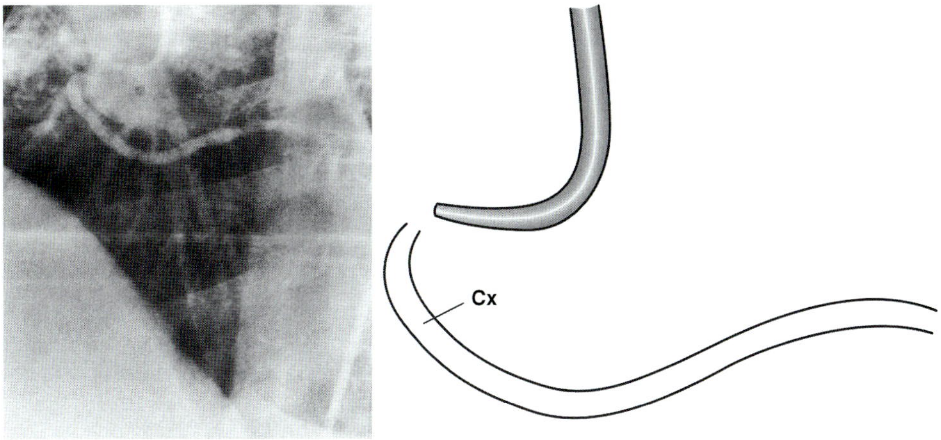

Fig. 7.44 Lateral arteriogram following cannulation of the CX as it arose from the right aortic sinus

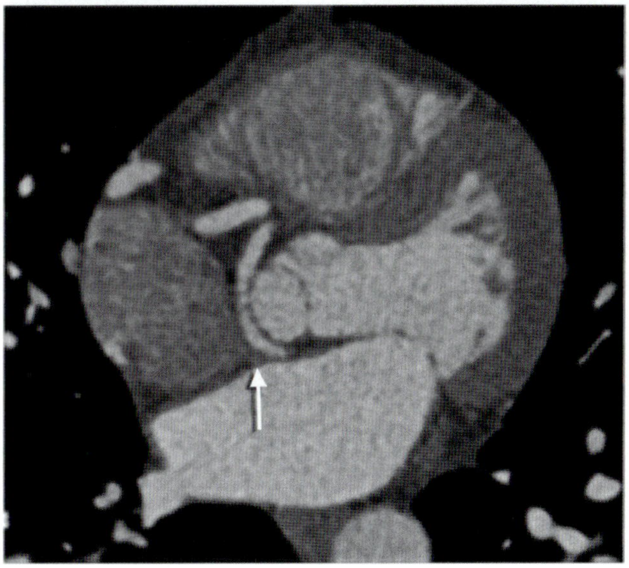

Fig. 7.45 CCTA axial view showing anomalous retroaortic LCX from the right aortic sinus (*arrow*)

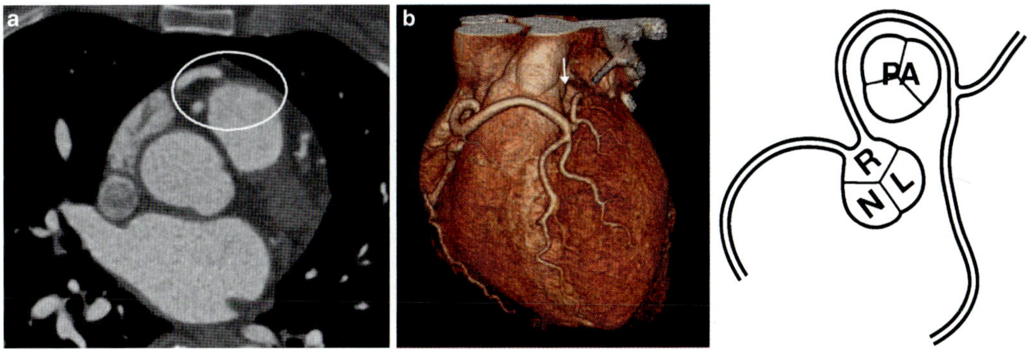

Fig. 7.46 (**a**) CCTA and (**b**) CCTA. Volume-rendered images with corresponding diagram in a patient with chest pain and a prepulmonic left coronary artery from the right coronary sinus. Notice the anterior course in front of the right ventricular outflow tract (*circle* and *arrow*)

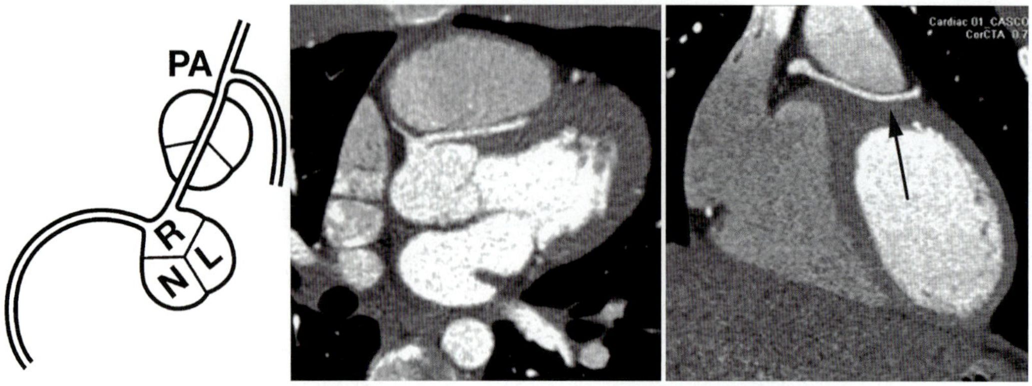

Fig. 7.47 CCTA image and corresponding diagram of an intraseptal course of LCA from right aortic sinus (*arrow*)

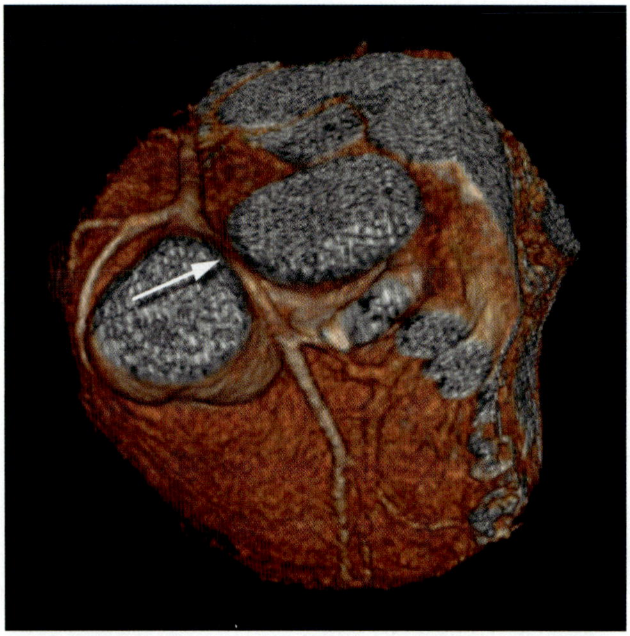

Fig. 7.48 Volume-rendered CCTA shows anomalous LCA from the right sinus with interarterial course seen from above (*arrow*)

coronary system following injection of the right sinus; however, the course could not be established. CCTA showed the presence of an intraseptal course below the level of the pulmonic valve and within the septal musculature. The patient was discharged with a good prognosis.

Interarterial LCA from Right Sinus

A 19-year-old male soccer player collapsed on the playing field, was revived by CPR, and underwent CCTA for further evaluation. Figure 7.48 shows anomalous LCA with an interarterial course between the aorta and pulmonary artery. The patient underwent surgical repair with unroofing into the left sinus position.

RCA from Left Sinus

The RCA origin from the left sinus presents a difficult challenge to the clinician. Interarterial ARCA is more common in the adult population, and when discovered, extensive counseling with the patient and family members is needed to determine the best therapeutic option. While most commonly benign, this anomaly can cause angina or sudden death [19]. If there is

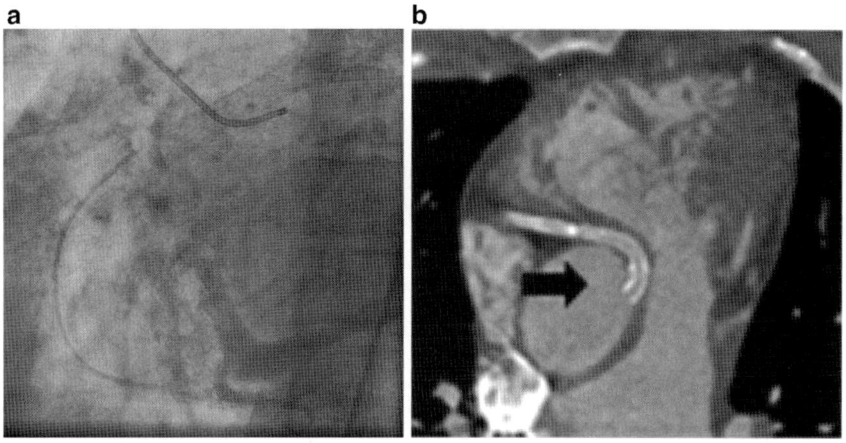

Fig. 7.49 (**a**) Right coronary invasive angiogram showing anomalous RCA from left aortic sinus and interarterial course with subtotal occlusion of the proximal segment (*arrow*). (**b**) CCTA axial dimension, poststenting, demonstrating widely patent RCA stent within the interarterial zone (*arrow*)

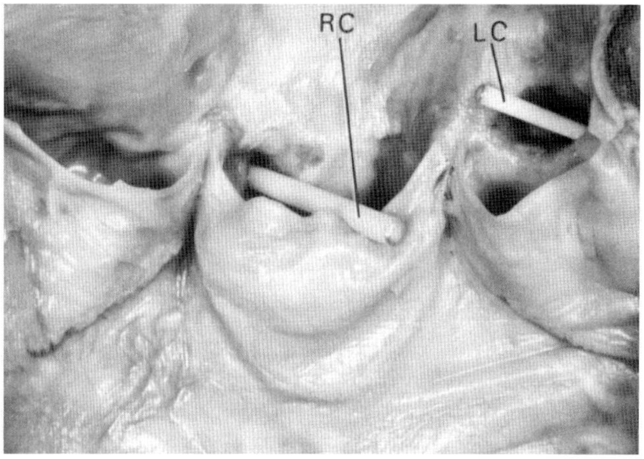

Fig. 7.50 Region of the aortic valve. The LC arises normally from the left aortic sinus, while the RCA arises from the posterior (noncoronary) aortic sinus

inducible ischemia, repair is indicated. There have been inconsistent studies attempting to correlate more malignant features to ARCA, including the presence of a slit-like orifice or a highly angulated origin. One center uses intravascular dobutamine and/or atropine to evaluate the compression effect proximally [14].

Repair is indicated if there is exertional syncope, exertional chest pain, or clear ischemia on functional stress testing. The approach to asymptomatic ARCA patients is variable, but young patients (<40 years old) with a large, dominant RCA; slit-like orifice; highly angulated origin; or an intramural proximal course are often referred for repair. ARCA has been associated with accelerated coronary artery disease [20], and patients are commonly treated with angioplasty/stenting. The long-term results are not known [21].

Figure 7.49 shows the case of a 53-year-old male presenting with acute inferior myocardial infarction (MI) with a peak creatine kinase-MB of 234. The patient was taken for emergent invasive angiography, demonstrating subtotal occlusion of the proximal RCA from the left aortic sinus with an interarterial course. Associated plaque was present, and the area was subsequently stented. A follow-up CCTA demonstrated widely patent proximal RCA stents.

Origin of the RCA from the Posterior (Noncoronary) Sinus

A coronary artery rarely arises from the posterior aortic sinus when noncongenital heart disease is present. The pathology specimen in Fig. 7.50 is from a 70-year-old man with terminal carcinoma of the prostate. The heart had no other congenital abnormalities.

Both Coronary Arteries from the Right Aortic Sinus

The cases shown in Figs. 7.51–7.54 are examples in which both coronary arteries arise from the right aortic sinus.

Figures 7.52–7.54 are coronary arteriograms from a patient in whom both main coronary arteries originated from the right aortic sinus. The patient was an adult without congenital heart disease who was studied because of atypical chest pain.

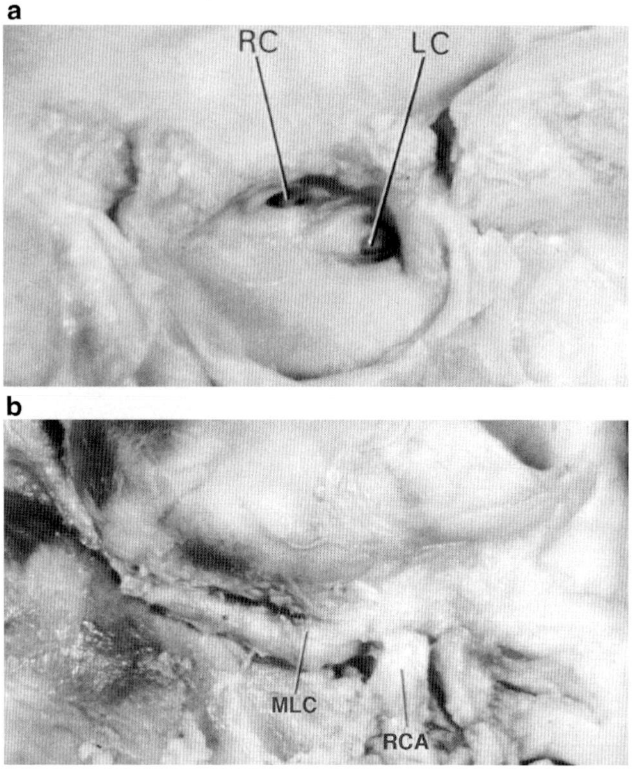

Fig. 7.51 (**a**) Interior view of the right aortic sinus showing the origins of the RC and LC from this aortic sinus. (**b**) External view of the aortic root from behind shows the proximal segments of the RCA and MLC arising from the right aortic sinus

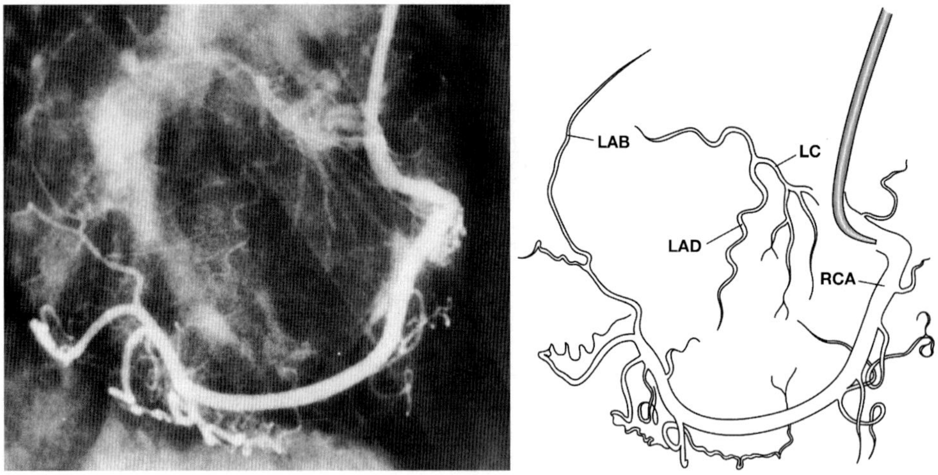

Fig. 7.52 RC arteriogram in lateral view. The pattern is not unusual

Abnormalities of Course: Myocardial Bridging

The normal coronary artery course occurs outside the epicardium within pericardial fat layers. When the artery course dips within the myocardium, the artery is called a "tunneled artery" and the muscle overlying the intramyocardial segment a "myocardial bridge." Longer, tunneled segments have been associated with myocardial ischemia. Whether the myocardial bridge is associated with sudden death or merely represents a normal, benign variation remains controversial. Myocardial bridges can be easily recognized by CCTA (Fig. 7.55).

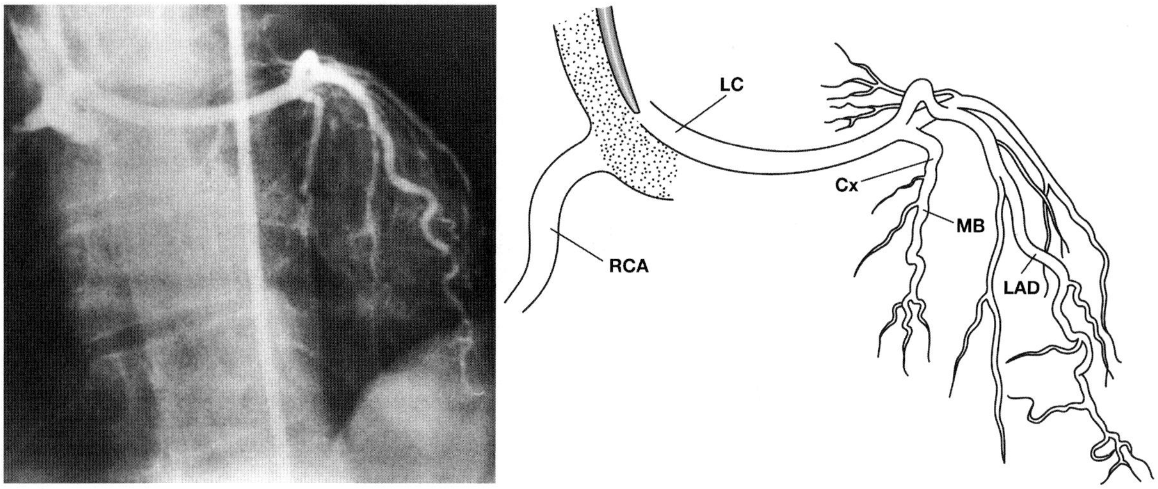

Fig. 7.53 LC arteriogram in frontal view. The LC is very long as it arises from the right aortic sinus and proceeds toward its normal position and branches. Contrast material in RC is residual from earlier RC arteriogram

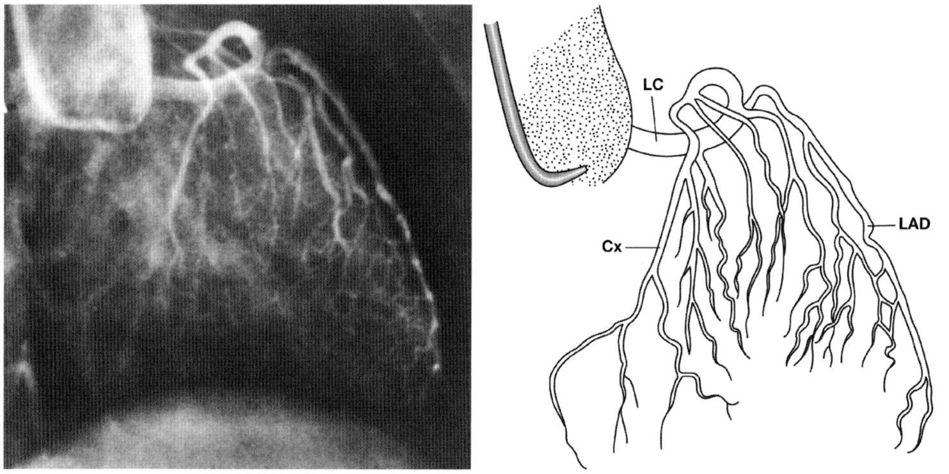

Fig. 7.54 LC in RAO projection. After a long course, the LC, which arises from the right aortic sinus, branches normally into the LAD and CX

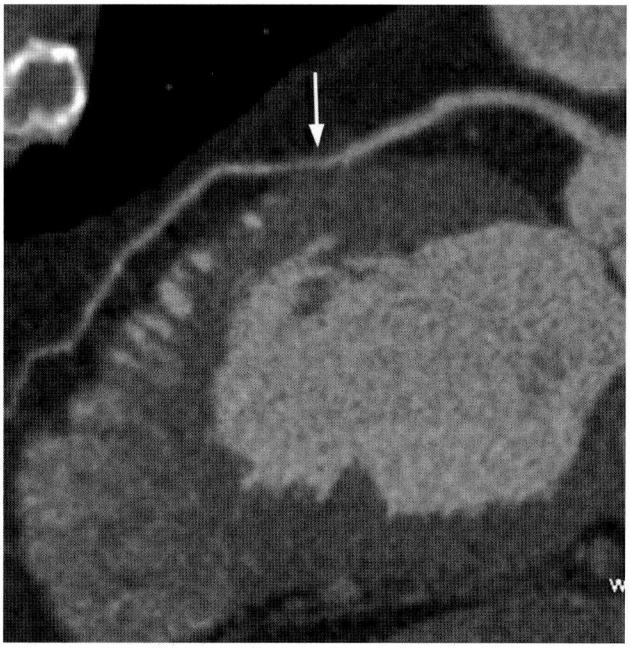

Fig. 7.55 MSCTA, MPR view of myocardial bridge. Note the midsegment of the LAD vessel with intramyocardial course, but widely patent

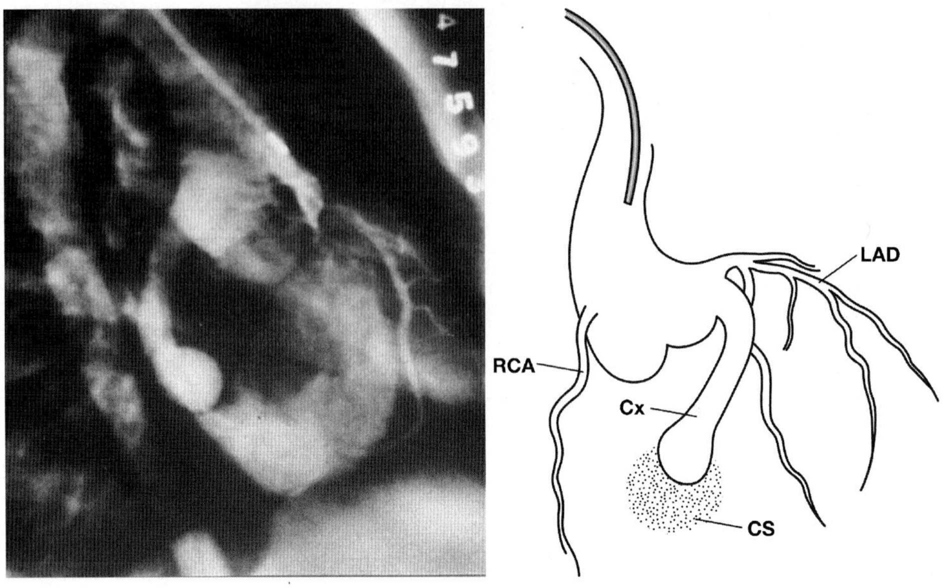

Fig. 7.56 Aortogram in lateral view showing unusually enlarged proximal CX with a small fistula into the CS

Abnormalities in the Termination of the Coronary Arteries (Coronary Fistula)

The most common CAAs are coronary fistulas. They may be single or multiple and originate from either the RCA or LCA. They can empty into any cardiac chamber (termed "coronary cameral fistula"), the superior vena cava, or the main pulmonary artery (PA), which is most common. Small, hemodynamically insignificant fistulas are most typical but, when larger, may form a significant left-to-right shunt. The RCA is more often involved in fistulas than the LCA, and about 90% connect with some element of the lesser circulation.

The coronary artery involved in the abnormal communication is usually enlarged, elongated, and tortuous and may exhibit localized saccular aneurysms. The latter are probably acquired as complications of the aorta's dilated and tortuous state.

Although the actual incidence of a congenital coronary artery fistula is unknown, it has been reported as 0.8–0.3% [22]. Frequently, the clinical differential diagnosis focuses on a continuous murmur, representing a shunt between high-pressure and low-pressure systems – for example, patent ductus arteriosus or a ruptured aortic sinus aneurysm.

The main functional disturbances of abnormal communication of a coronary artery with the lesser circulation mainly are related to coronary flow as a "steal" or runoff from the communication vessel to the low-pressure area. This may lead to ischemia, angina pectoris, or myocardial infarction, and congestive heart failure. Bacterial infection of the fistula is yet another potential complication.

Echocardiography may help identify a large fistula, but definite diagnosis is possible only with coronary angiography, CCTA, or CMRI.

Repair is recommended with symptomatic patients and is performed with surgical ligation or a percutaneous approach. If only one anomalous tract is clearly identified, ligation close to its abnormal termination should be performed. More recently, percutaneous transcatheter embolization techniques have been used. In angiomatous malformations, surgery is not recommended because the inability to locate and ligate the feeder arteries results in a serious or lethal sequelae.

Communication of the Left Circumflex Coronary Artery with the Coronary Sinus

Figures 7.56 and 7.57 show aortograms from a 6½-year-old boy in whom a continuous cardiac murmur was observed during a routine preschool physical examination. Aortography revealed the CX to be a grossly dilated vessel that terminated at the junction of the RA with the coronary sinus (CS). A saccular aneurysm involved the vessel at its termination. The LCX was surgically interrupted as it terminated in the CS. The postoperative course was uneventful.

Figure 7.58 shows the case of a 72-year-old man with chest pain who was found using CCTA to have a left circumflex artery to coronary sinus fistula. The left circumflex artery is large and dilated, and the coronary sinus is dilated. Due to the patient's multiple comorbidities, he was treated medically.

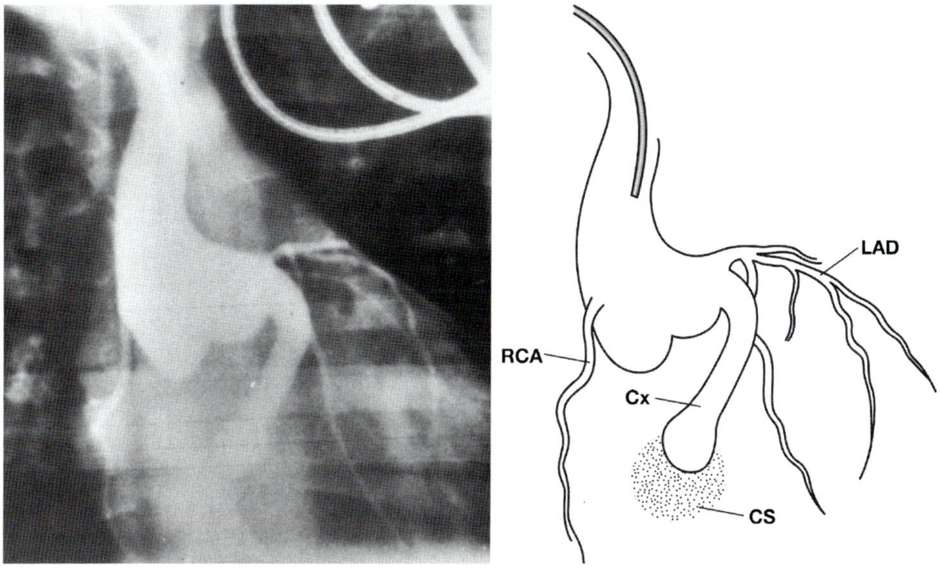

Fig. 7.57 Aortogram in frontal view, depicting similar features to those in Fig. 7.56

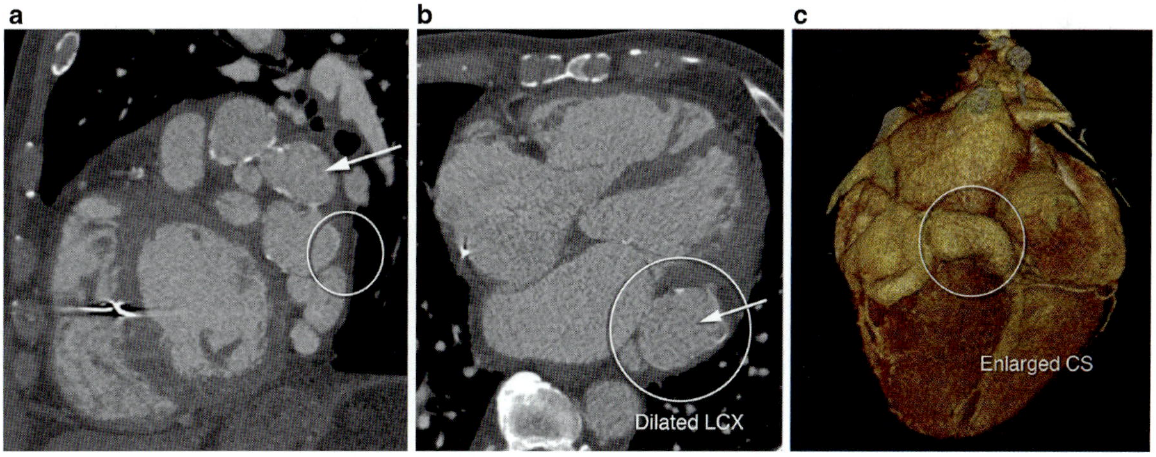

Fig. 7.58 (**a**, **b**) CCTA findings of a left circumflex coronary artery to coronary sinus fistula. The CX is markedly dilated with looping connection to the coronary sinus (*circle* and *arrow*). (**c**) CCTA volume-rendering image shows markedly enlarged coronary sinus (*circle*)

Communication of the RCA with the Right Ventricle

In a 16-year-old asymptomatic boy who was known to have a murmur since birth, physical examination revealed a continuous murmur with maximal intensity at the right lower sternal border. Blood pressure and ECG were within normal.

Cardiac catheterization showed an increase in oxygen levels in the RV. The volume of the left-to-right shunt was calculated to be 1.4 L/min. A left ventriculogram showed immediate opacification of a large vascular structure in the location of the RCA and subsequent opacification of the RV. The LCA was normal in diameter and distribution.

Aortography showed the vascular abnormality to be a markedly dilated and tortuous RCA which communicated with the RV inferiorly (Fig. 7.59). Surgical treatment consisted of double ligation of the distal RCA just proximal to its entry into the RV chamber. A follow-up report 7 years later stated that the subject was normal without any murmur.

Communication of a Single Left Coronary Artery with the Right Ventricle

Figures 7.60 and 7.61 are from a 15-year-old girl in whom a continuous, precordial murmur was heard. It was graded III/VI, and its systolic component was slightly louder than the diastolic. An ECG showed sinus rhythm, normal axis, and LVH

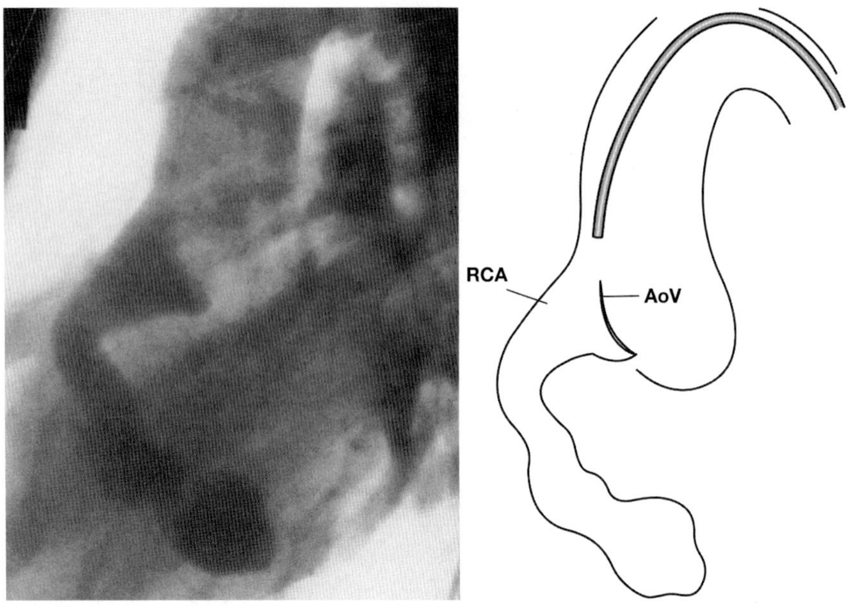

Fig. 7.59 Aortogram in left lateral view showing dilated tortuous RC and opacification of the RV

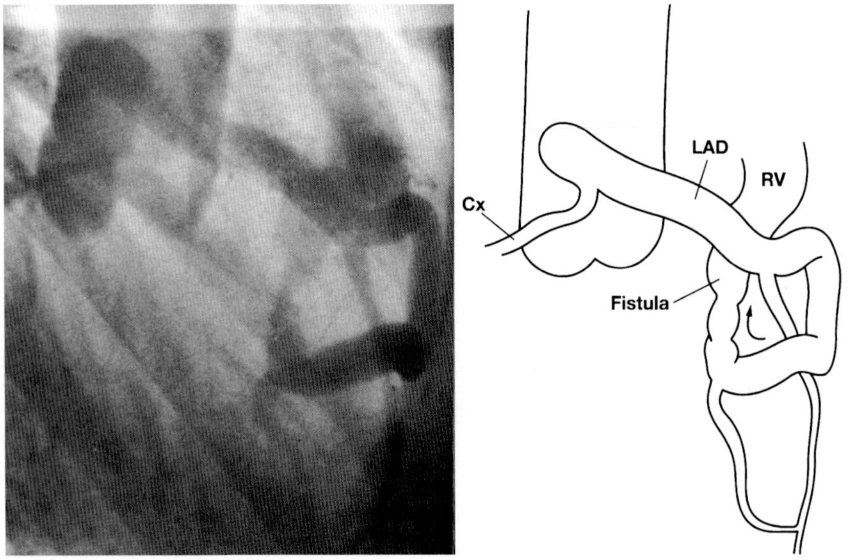

Fig. 7.60 Aortogram in right lateral view shows a huge LC and LAD from which a large branch arises and terminates in the outflow tract of the RV. The latter is also opacified

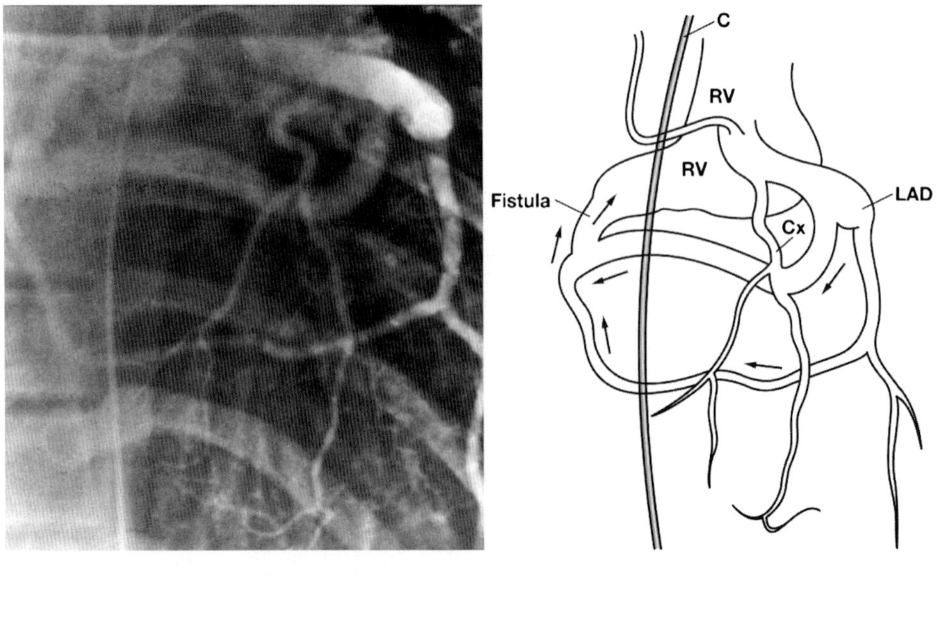

Fig. 7.61 LC arteriogram in RAO view showing a huge LC and LAD, a branch of which terminates in the outflow tract of the RV

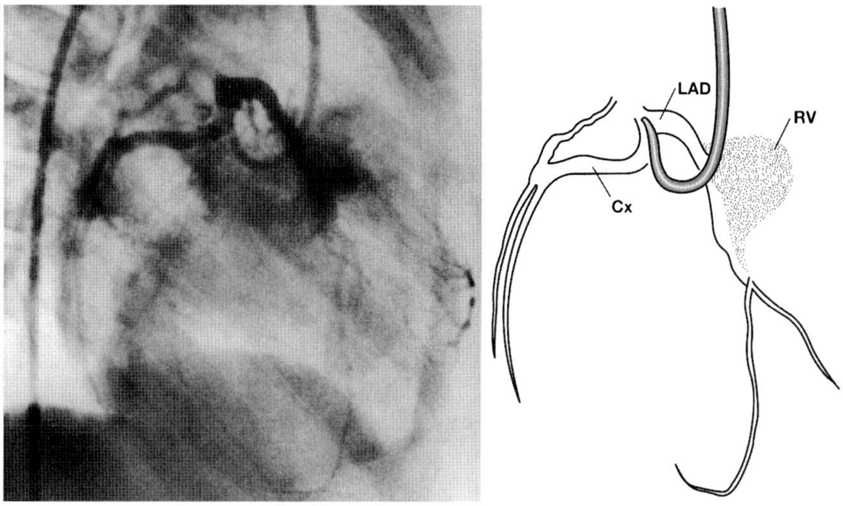

Fig. 7.62 LC arteriogram in lateral view. Both the CX and LAD branches are grossly enlarged. Diffuse angiomatous opacification of the base of the ventricular septum and of the RV infundibulum is demonstrated

with slight ST change. An LC arteriogram showed a huge LC with two branches arising from the LAD. One coursed over the basal portion of the RV and communicated with the RV outflow tract. Attempts to catheterize the RC ostium were unsuccessful.

At operation, no RCA was found. The LC had a normal origin, and it gave rise to a large branch that crossed the RV outflow tract into which it opened. At surgery, right ventriculotomy revealed that the fistulous tract entered just below the parietal limb of the crista supraventricularis. It was successfully closed.

Coronary Angiomatous Malformation Communicating with the Right Ventricle

Another case involved an asymptomatic, 7-year-old girl who presented with a grade III/IV, high-pitched, continuous murmur. An ECG showed normal axis duration and LVH.

The RC arteriogram showed a huge RC with immediate dense opacification of an angiomatous formation, which appeared to communicate through small branches with the right atrium (RA). The LC arteriogram showed enlargement of the LAD and CX, each communicating with an anterior angiomatous mass. The latter connected with the RV, which become opacified virtually simultaneously (Fig. 7.62). Surgical therapy was not believed indicated in this asymptomatic child because of the complexity of the malformation.

Communication of the LAD with the Pulmonary Trunk

A 30-year-old male complained of exertional chest pain while biking and was referred for CCTA. Findings showed an LAD coronary to PA fistula (Fig. 7.63). The patient subsequently underwent invasive studies and successful occlusion with a percutaneous coiling procedure. His symptoms resolved completely.

Communication of the Conus Branch of the Anterior Descending Artery with the Pulmonary Trunk

Figure 7.64 is from a 10-year-old asymptomatic boy with membranous subaortic stenosis (gradient 70 mmHg). Cardiac catheterization showed an increase in oxygen saturation at the pulmonary arterial level of borderline significance (5%). Selective coronary arteriography showed communication of a conus branch of the LAD with a vascular plexus which, in turn, communicated with the proximal portion of the PT.

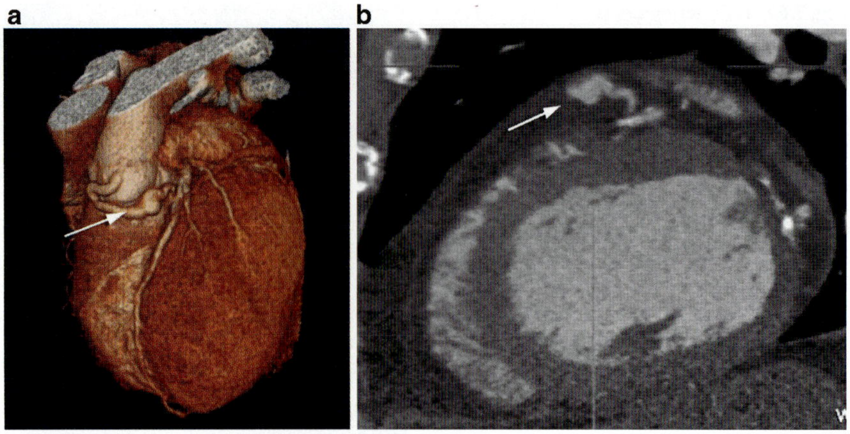

Fig. 7.63 Young male patient with exertional chest pain and communication of the LAD with the pulmonary artery. (**a**) Volume-rendering CTA image and (**b**) CTA coronal view showing fistulous connection to lower PA (*arrow*)

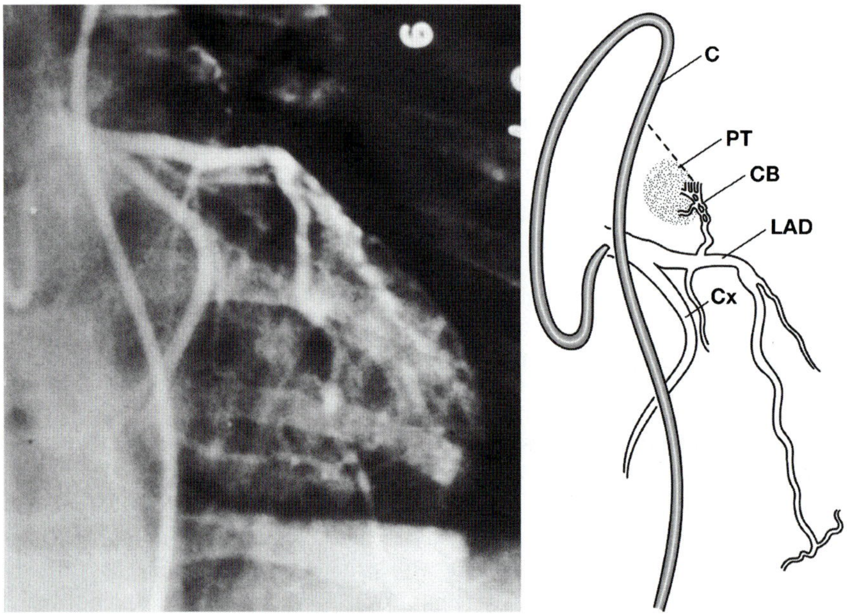

Fig. 7.64 LC arteriogram in frontal view. A conus branch of the LAD courses upward and is associated with opacification of the PT

Resection of the membranous subaortic stenosis, and division and ligation of the conus branch of the LAD that supplied the plexus communicating with the PT, was successfully performed.

Communication of the Conus Branch of the RCA with the Pulmonary Trunk

Figure 7.65 is from a 45-year-old woman who, 1 year previously, had experienced an episode of chest pain diagnosed as myocardial infarction. Recurrent chest pains believed to be atypical angina followed. The ECG displayed left bundle branch block.

An arteriogram showed mild to moderate degrees of segmental narrowing in the major coronary arteries. During RC arteriography, the conus branch of the RC proceeded toward the PT, which was lightly opacified.

Surgical therapy was debated, and the consensus favored it on the basis that the abnormal communication functioned as a "steal," limiting myocardial perfusion from the distal portion of the RC. At surgery, the conus branch of the RC proceeded upward toward the anterior wall of the PT as a single vessel and penetrated the latter artery. The vessel, 2–3 mm in diameter, was divided and ligated. The patient was asymptomatic at a follow-up evaluation.

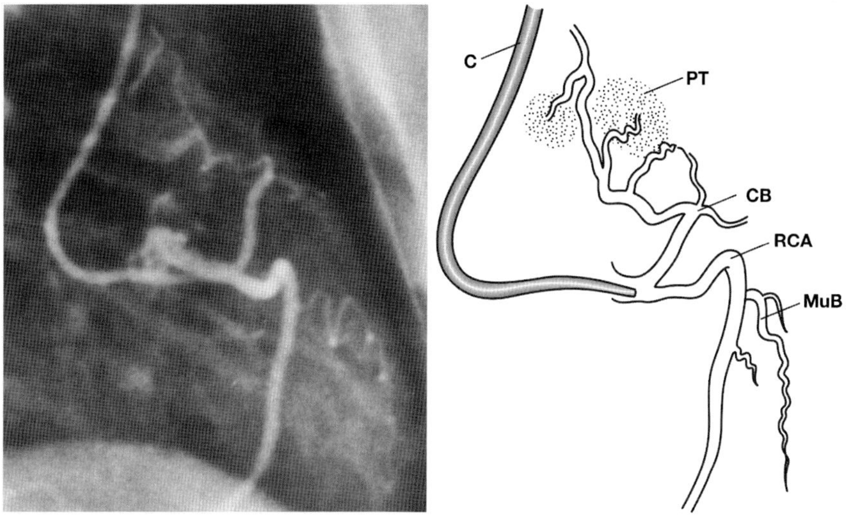

Fig. 7.65 RC arteriogram in lateral view shows opacification of the conal branch that proceeds toward the PT. The latter is somewhat opacified

References

1. Angelini P, Velasco JA, Famm S. Coronary anomalies: incidence, pathophysiology, and clinical relevance. Circulation. 2002;105:2449–54.
2. Angelini P. Coronary artery anomalies – current clinical issues: definitions, classification, incidence, clinical relevance, and treatment guidelines. Tex Heart Inst J. 2002;29(4):271–8.
3. Knickelbine T, Lesser JR, Haas TS, et al. Identification of unexpected nonatherosclerotic cardiovascular disease with coronary CT angiography. JACC Cardiovasc Imaging. 2009;2:1085–92.
4. Maron BJ. Sudden death in young athletes. N Engl J Med. 2003;349:1064–75.
5. Vlodaver Z, Neufeld HN, Edwards JE. Coronary Arterial Variations in the Normal Heart and in Congenital Heart Disease. New York, NY: Academic Press, Inc.; 1975.
6. Vlodaver Z, Amplatz K, Burchell HB, Edwards JE. Coronary heart disease. clinical angiographic and pathologic profiles. New York: Springer-Verlag; 1976.
7. Tarhan A, Kehibar T, Yilmaz M, et al. Right coronary artery with high take off. Ann Thorac Surg. 2007;83:1867–9.
8. Choi JH, Kornblum RN. Pete Maravich's incredible heart. J Forensic Sci. 1990;35(4):981.
9. Wald S, Stonecipher K, Baldwin BJ, et al. Anomalous origin of the right coronary artery from the pulmonary artery. Am J Cardiol. 1971; 27:677.
10. Rao BNS, Lucas Jr RV, Edwards JE. Anomalous origin of the left coronary artery from the right pulmonary artery. Chest. 1970;58:616.
11. Eckart RE, Scoville SL, Campbell CL, et al. Sudden death in young adults: a 25-year review of autopsies in military recruits. Ann Intern Med. 2004;141(11):829–34.
12. Maron BJ, Shirani J, Poliac LC. Sudden death in young competitive athletes. Clinical, demographic and pathological profiles. JAMA. 1996;276:199–204.
13. Maron BJ, Doerer JJ, Haas RN, Tierney DM, Mueller FO. Sudden death in young competitive athletes: analysis of 1866 deaths in the United States, 1980–2006. Circulation. 2009;119:1085–92.
14. Angelini P, Flamm S. Newer concepts for imaging anomalous aortic origin of the coronary arteries in adults. Catheter Cardiovasc Interv. 1997;69(7):942–54.
15. Davies JE, Burkhart HM, Dearani JA, et al. Surgical management of anomalous origin of a coronary artery. Ann Thorac Surg. 2009;88:844–8.
16. Jaquiss RD, Tweddell JS, Litwin SB. Surgical therapy for sudden cardiac death in children. Pediatr Clin North Am. 2004;51(5):1389–400.
17. Gulati R, Reddy VM, Curlbertson C, et al. Surgical management of coronary artery arising from the wrong coronary sinus using standard and novel approaches. J Thorac Cardiovasc Surg. 2007;134(5):1171–8.
18. Fedoruk L, Kern J, Peeler B, Kron I. Anomalous origin of the right coronary artery: right internal thoracic artery to right coronary artery bypass is not the answer. J Thorac Cardiovasc Surg. 2007;133:456–60.
19. Boissier F, Coolen N, Notaf P, et al. Sudden death related to an anomalous origin of the right coronary artery. Ann Thorac Surg. 2008;85: 1077–9.
20. Jim MH, Siu CW, Ho HH, Miu R, Lee SW. Anomalous origin of the right coronary artery from the left coronary sinus is associated with early development of coronary artery disease. J Invasive Cardiol. 2004;16:466–8.
21. Hariharan R, Kacere RD, Angelini P. Can stent-angioplasty be a valid alternative to surgery when revascularization is indicated for anomalous origination of a coronary artery from the opposite sinus? Tex Heart Inst J. 2002;29:308–13.
22. Vavurakis M, Bush CA, Boudoulas H. Coronary artery fistulas in adults: incidence and angiographic characteristics. Cathet Cardiovasc Diagn. 1995;35(2):116–20.
23. Price AC, Lee DA, Kagan KE, et al. Aortic dysplasia in infancy simulating anomalous origin of the left coronary artery. Circulation. 1973;48:434.
24. Vlodaver Z, Neufeld HN, Edwards JE. Pathology of coronary disease. Semin Roentgenol. 1972;7:376.

Chapter 8
Pathology of Chronic Obstructive Coronary Disease

Zeev Vlodaver

Lesions of the Coronary Ostia

Stenosis of the takeoff of the coronary artery from the aorta may result either from organic lesions or from spasm. Spasm of the coronary artery was discussed in detail in Chap. 6.

Coronary ostial stenosis may result entirely or in part from aortic disease. The specific lesions involved include isolated aortic atheromas, diffuse aortitis, and focal calcification of the aortic wall at the junction of its sinus and tubular portions. Other causes include compression of a coronary arterial origin by an aortic aneurysm or by extension of an aortic dissection.

Coronary Ostial Stenosis due to Aortic Atherosclerosis

The following case studies and figures cited illustrate how aortic atherosclerosis can lead to coronary ostial stenosis.

Isolated Aortic Atherosclerosis Causing Coronary Arterial Obstruction

Figure 8.1a, b illustrates stenosis of the RC ostium by a localized atheroma.

Right Coronary Ostial Stenosis Secondary to Aortic Atherosclerosis

Figures 8.2 and 8.3 illustrate stenosis of the RC ostium secondary to aortic sclerosis.

Pathologic Demonstration

A patient hospitalized for recurrent acute myocardial infarction died the day after admission. The essential findings of the autopsy included right coronary (RC) ostial stenosis associated with significant atherosclerosis of the left coronary (LC) system. Myocardial infarction in a circumferential subendocardial distribution was observed. The RC ostial stenosis resulted from atherosclerosis associated with overlying fibrous thickening (Fig. 8.2a–c).

Z. Vlodaver, MD, (✉)
Division of Cardiovascular Medicine, University of Minnesota, Minneapolis, MN, USA
e-mail: zeev.vlodaver@gmail.com

Z. Vlodaver et al. (eds.), *Coronary Heart Disease: Clinical, Pathological, Imaging, and Molecular Profiles*,
DOI 10.1007/978-1-4614-1475-9_8,

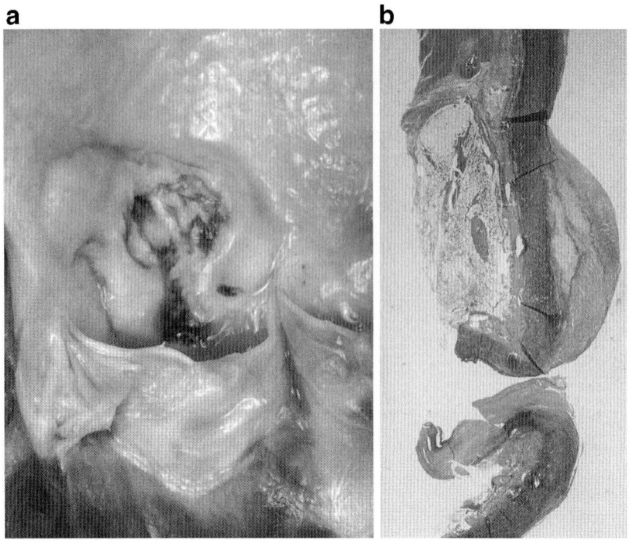

Fig. 8.1 (**a**) Gross specimen. The ostium of the right coronary artery (RCA) is related to an aortic atheroma. (**b**) Low-power photomicrograph of the junction of the Ao and RC showing stenosis of the ostium by an atheroma at the ostium. Just above the ostium lies an aortic atheroma which, in this instance, causes only minor narrowing of the ostium

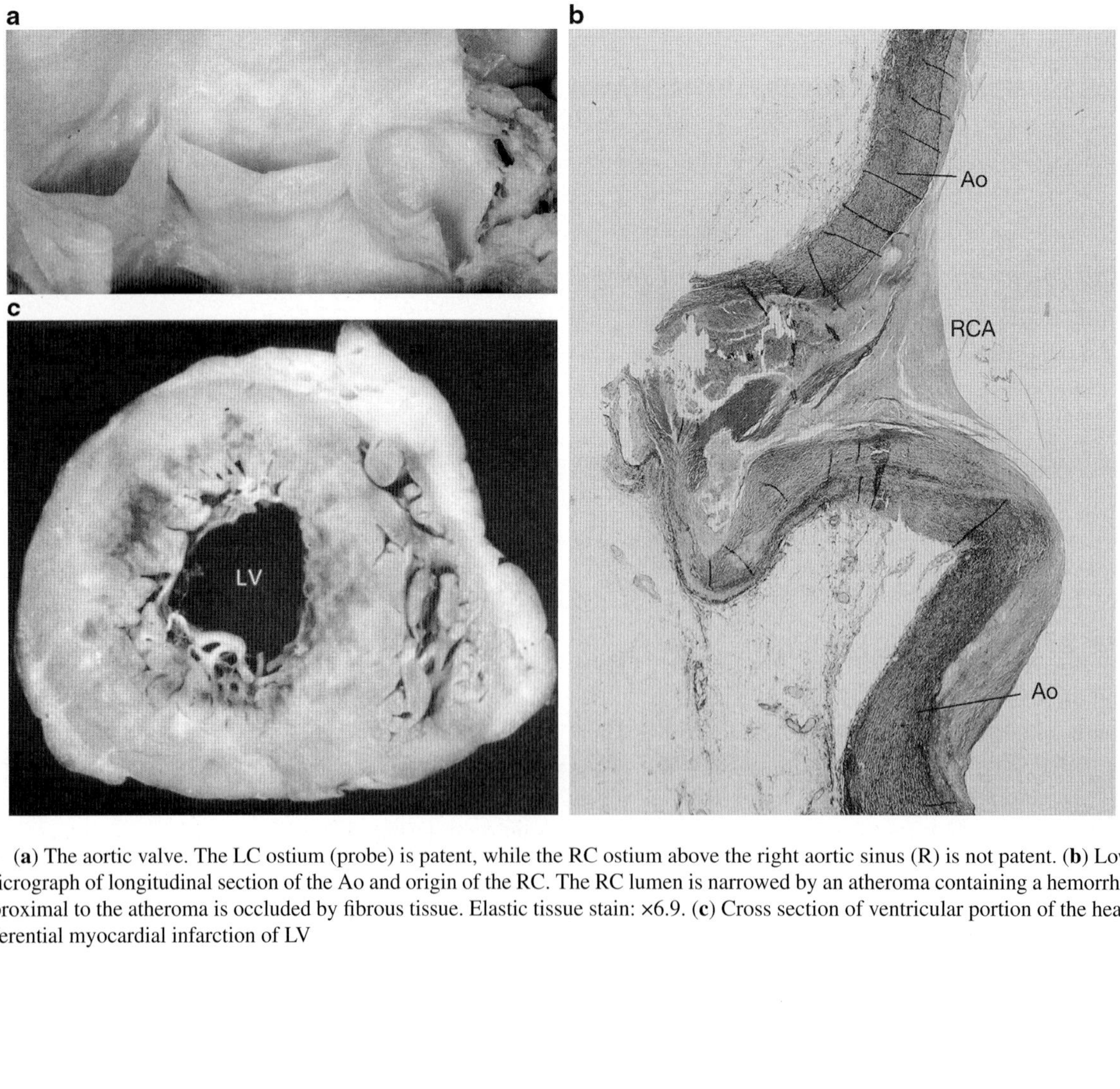

Fig. 8.2 (**a**) The aortic valve. The LC ostium (probe) is patent, while the RC ostium above the right aortic sinus (R) is not patent. (**b**) Low-power photomicrograph of longitudinal section of the Ao and origin of the RC. The RC lumen is narrowed by an atheroma containing a hemorrhage. The lumen proximal to the atheroma is occluded by fibrous tissue. Elastic tissue stain: ×6.9. (**c**) Cross section of ventricular portion of the heart shows circumferential myocardial infarction of LV

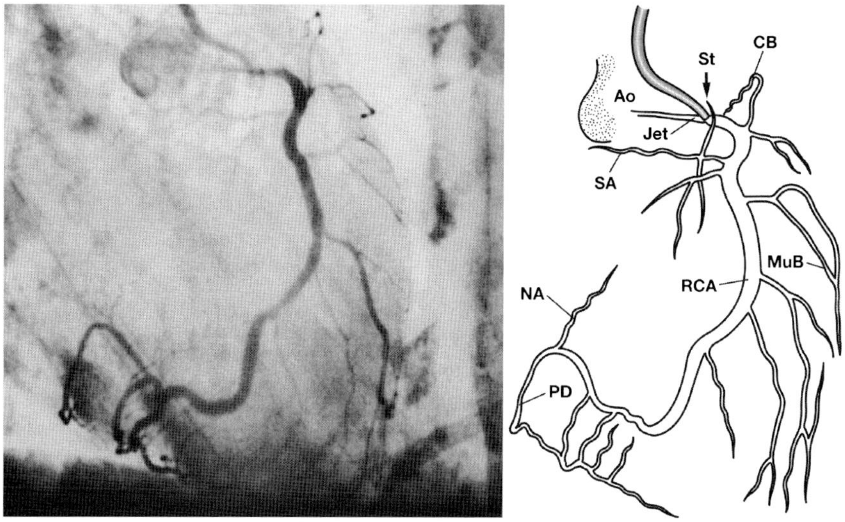

Fig. 8.3 RAO view of RCA shows catheter tip engaged in stenotic ostium. Narrow, regurgitating jet from the artery into the Ao strongly suggests coronary ostial stenosis

Angiographic Demonstration

A 47-year-old woman complained of angina for 5 years. Her treadmill exercise test was abnormal. The LC arteriogram showed 60% stenosis of the proximal left anterior descending (LAD) coronary artery. Right coronary (RC) arteriogram showed stenosis at origin of the vessel at the ostium (Fig. 8.3). An aortogram showed a narrow abdominal aorta (Ao) with atherosclerotic changes in the area just above the bifurcation, and severe stenosis (90%) at the origin of the right common iliac artery. The combination of atherosclerotic changes in the coronary arteries and in peripheral vessels is a fairly common association in women with atherosclerotic coronary disease.

Left Coronary Ostial Stenosis Secondary to Atherosclerosis

A 54-year-old man with a history of myocardial infarction 2 years previously was admitted for unstable angina. The ostium of the LC could not be engaged by a coronary arterial catheter. An autopsy showed that the LC ostium was almost totally obstructed. Histological examination of the LC showed, at its ostium, an eccentric calcified lesion which caused almost total occlusion of the artery (Fig. 8.4a–c).

Ostial Stenosis due to Calcification of the Aortic Wall

At the junction of the sinus and tubular portions of the Ao is a ridge. Calcification of the aortic media and overlying intima may occur in this area, leading to the formation of a spur. In extreme situations, the spur may encroach significantly upon a coronary ostium. Fragmentation may cause an embolism (Fig. 8.5a, b).

Coronary Ostial Stenosis due to Other Aortic Diseases

Ostial Stenosis Secondary to Syphilitic Aortitis

Figure 8.6 is an example of stenosis of the RC ostium secondary to syphilitic aortitis.

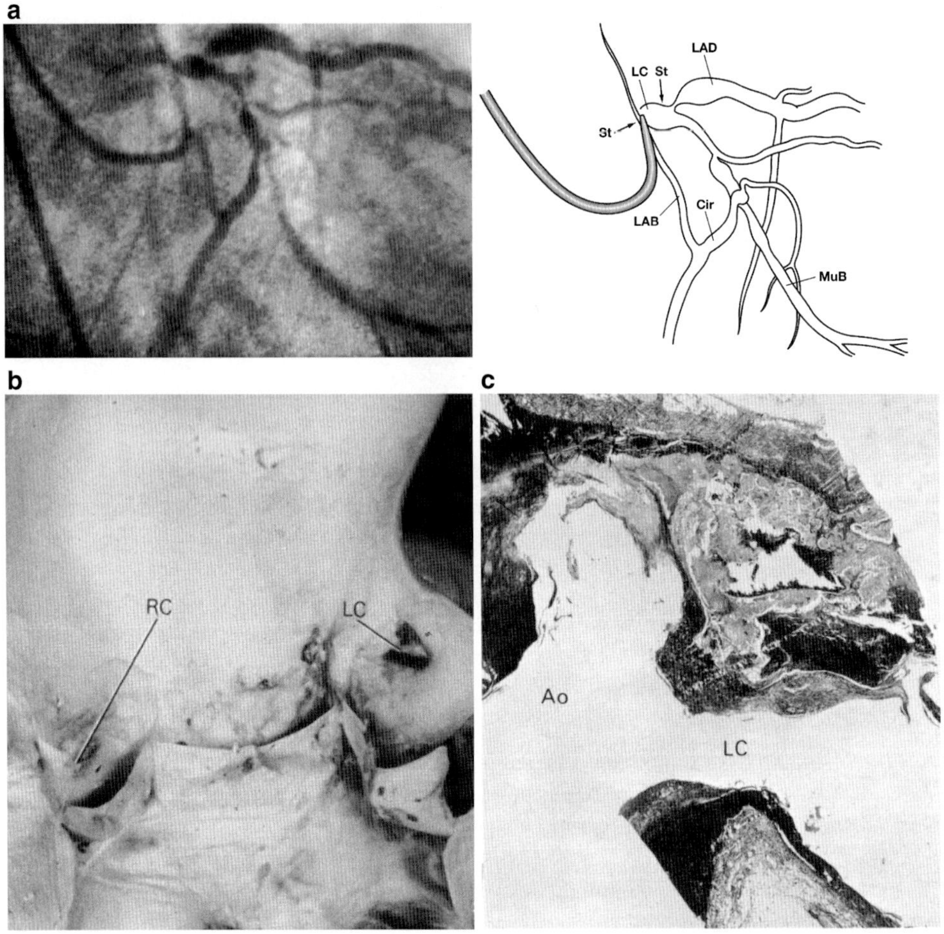

Fig. 8.4 (**a**) LC arteriogram showing severe stenosis in the LC ostium and narrowing of the LM, left anterior descending (LAD), and CX. (**b**) Specimen of ascending aorta and the region of the aortic valve. The probe is in the residual ostium of the LC. (**c**) Low-power photomicrograph of longitudinal section of origin of the LM. The lumen is narrowed by calcific mass involving the intima. Elastic tissue stain: ×8

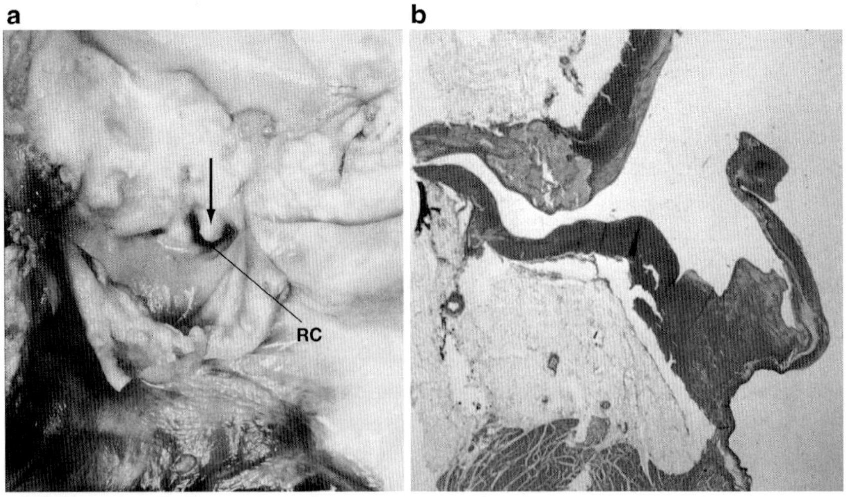

Fig. 8.5 (**a**) A spur (*arrow*), formed by a calcific lesion, at the junction of the sinus and tubular portions of the Ao. The right aortic cusp has been retracted downward. The RC is obstructed. (**b**) Low-power photomicrograph of the peripheral portion of the calcific spur shown in (**a**), as well as the right aortic sinus and cusp, and the origin of the RCA. Elastic tissue stain: ×8

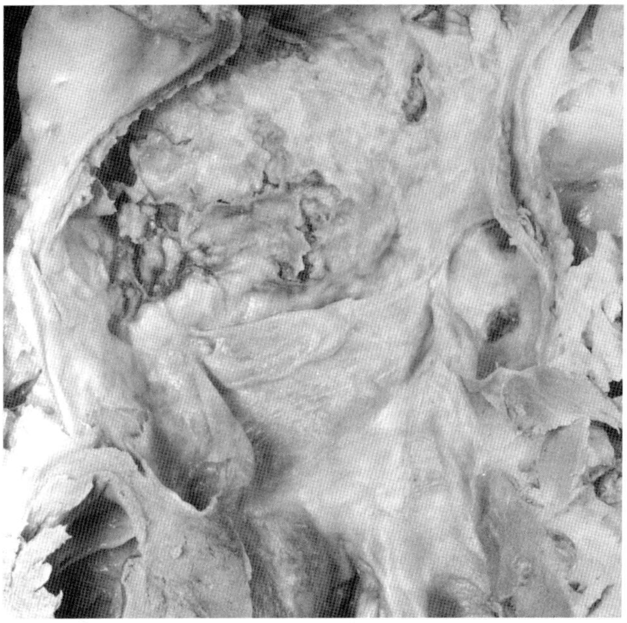

Fig. 8.6 Syphilitic aortitis. Gross specimen of aortic valve and ascending aorta. The ostium of the RCA is obscured by extensive atherosclerosis

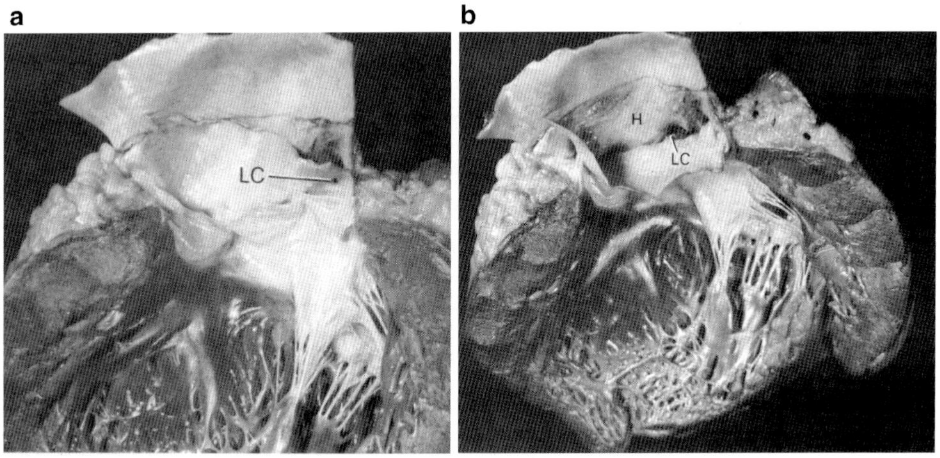

Fig. 8.7 (**a**) LV and ascending aorta from a 55-year-old hypertensive man who died suddenly. A circumferential laceration was present in the ascending aorta. (**b**) The aortic wall proximal to the site of laceration has been deflected downward. It shows the position of the false passage of the limited dissecting aneurysm. The contained hematoma (H) had extended along the aneurysm and obstructed the LC

Dissecting Aneurysm of the Aorta and Ostial Stenosis

In dissecting aneurysms of the Ao, the intramural hematoma has a strong tendency to extend into arterial branches, causing narrowing or occlusion. Either or both of the coronary arteries may be involved, but the right coronary artery is more commonly involved. Figure 8.7a, b shows a young man with a history of hypertension who died suddenly. A limited dissection of the ascending aorta caused obstruction of the left main coronary artery (LM).

Saccular Aneurysm of the Aorta and Ostial Stenosis

Saccular aneurysm of the ascending Ao may result from various causes, including congenital, inflammatory, and traumatic (including postsurgical) ones.

Saccular aneurysm of the ascending aorta, regardless of its etiology, may compress either coronary artery and cause myocardial ischemia (Fig. 8.8a–c).

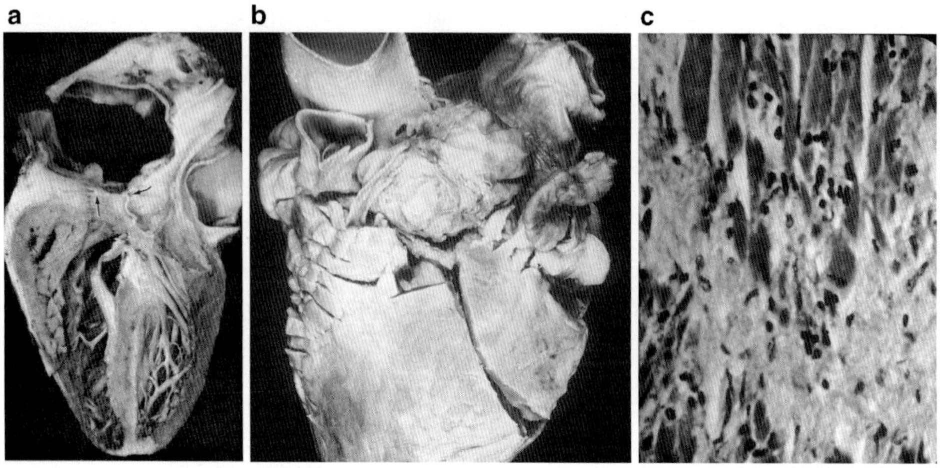

Fig. 8.8 (**a**) A 4½-year-old child developed a saccular aneurysm of the ascending aorta following repair of ventricular septal defect (VSD). The lower aspect of the aneurysm compressed the RC at its ostium (*right arrow*) and along the course (*left arrow*). (**b**) In a 54-year-old woman, a congenital aneurysm of the left aortic sinus lies beside the LC and Cir. The latter is compressed. (**c**) Photomicrograph of LV in the distribution of the Cir shows acute myocardial infarction. Coronary atherosclerosis was absent

Coronary Angiography with Ostial Stenosis

Coronary angiography in patients with ostial stenosis of the left main coronary artery is associated with significantly higher incidence of complications. Left main stenosis occurs in 2–11% of patients undergoing angiography but accounts for a significantly greater fraction of mortality associated with the procedure [1].

Myocardial infarction, persistent angina, profound hypotension, and ventricular fibrillation also occur during or immediately following angiography in patients with left main coronary stenosis. The likelihood of complications is greater in patients with angina within 24 h of catheterization. If the stenosis is in the proximal left main coronary artery, complications can be minimized by rapidly identifying the presence of LC ostial stenosis, which occurs more often in patients with widespread severe atherosclerosis and may be associated with pressure damping on left coronary cannulation.

When LC ostial stenosis is suspected, a "cusp" injection into the ostium may identify its presence and morphology. When a significant left main stenosis is present, nonionic contrast should be used, and the number of angiograms should be limited to only those views required to identify the vessels needing bypass grafts. A catheter tip shape that will not deeply cannulate the ostium should be used. If the pressure at the catheter tip damps on left main cannulation, the catheter may need to be withdrawn between injections, although repeated cannulation of a stenotic LM may increase the possibility of catheter-induced injury. If adequate filling can be obtained, a nonselective "cusp" injection should be used.

Pulmonary capillary wedge pressure monitoring during angiography can be important in patients with severe stenosis or reduced left ventricular (LV) function because contrast material may precipitously reduce LV function. If the wedge pressure rises significantly, angiography should be stopped until hemodynamics are controlled. Semi-urgent revascularization should be considered after angiography in patients with severe main LC stenosis (>90%), particularly if the lesion is in the proximal LC.

Coronary Atherosclerosis

As causes of myocardial ischemia, obstructive lesions involving the epicardial coronary arterial trunks are dominant. With few exceptions, atherosclerosis is the fundamental cause of lesions. This section will deal with atherosclerosis of coronary arteries.

Normal Structure of the Coronary Arteries

The normal coronary artery is characterized by a muscular media in which fibers are oriented in a circular manner. The intima, which is composed of delicate connective tissue with a thin layer of endothelial cells, is separated from the media by the internal elastic membrane, while the external membrane separates the media from the collagenous adventitia.

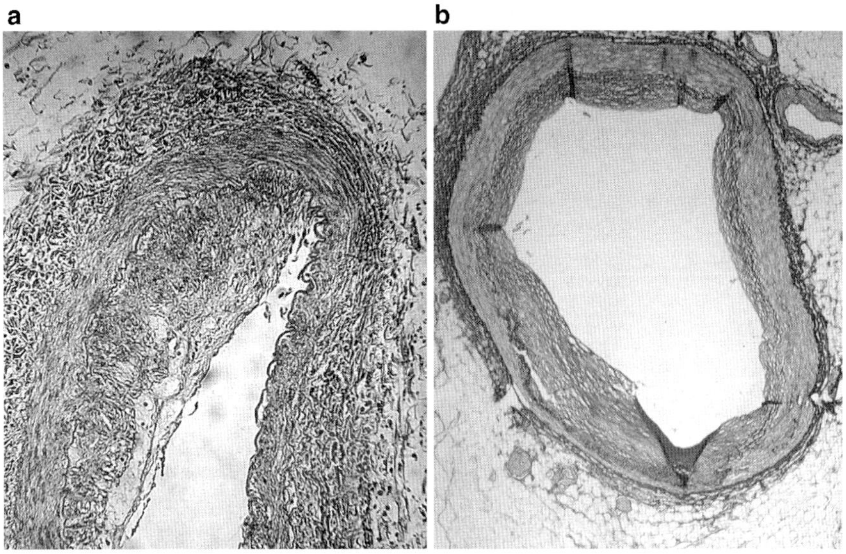

Fig. 8.9 (**a**) Coronary artery from a 2-month-old girl. The internal elastic membrane is irregular. Lying along its luminal side (upper portion of the illustration) is the musculoelastic layer. Elastic tissue stain: ×107. (**b**) Coronary artery from an 86-year-old man. The extra layer is composed of collagen and elastic fibers, which may be normal. This layer may be fibroelastic, similar to that seen in Fig. 8.9a. Elastic tissue stain: ×14

A normal variation, which may be observed even in the young, includes an extra layer between the intima and media. This is the musculoelastic layer, characterized by a focal aggregation of smooth muscle and connective tissue. Because it lies under the intima, it may be difficult to distinguish this layer from acquired disease when seen in adults (Fig. 8.9a, b).

Coronary Atherosclerosis: Primary Nature of Lesion

Atheromas occur focally along the length of the involved artery, with segments of normal artery often present between diseased segments. The focal nature of atherosclerosis is also exemplified by the histologic appearance of involved segments. Thus, one arc of the artery is very commonly uninvolved, while the remainder contains an atheroma. The result of focal distribution is that the narrowed lumen is eccentric, lying near the uninvolved arc.

In cross sections of coronary arteries afflicted with atherosclerosis, two types of lesions are identified: one is purely fibrous, and the other is a pairing of lipid pools and walling fibrous tissue.

The Fibrous Lesion

Although it is common for the plaque-like lesions of atherosclerosis to contain lipids, some atheromas are purely fibrous. Similar to lipid-containing lesions, the purely fibrous lesion involves the intimal aspect of the artery and, by virtue of its thickness, narrows the lumen (Fig. 8.10). While the pathogenesis of the purely fibrous lesion in the adult is in doubt, three possible mechanisms come to mind: (1) that the lesion is a late stage of the focal arterial thickening seen in children, (2) that the plane of section went through the peripheral part of a lesion which contains lipids at its center, or (3) that a previous rupture of the lining had allowed the lipid accumulation to be swept away, leaving only fibrous tissue.

Lightly staining areas may be found in collagen, either in instances of purely fibrous lesions or when associated with lipid accumulations. Such areas are shown to stain positively for lipids. Since the lightly staining areas are within collagen and contain lipids, Osborn has named the process "collipid," a word coined from collagen and lipid [2]. These areas are devoid of accumulations of foam cells and extracellular pools of lipid material (Fig. 8.11).

Lipid Accumulations

The most common type of atheroma represents a highly complex alteration in the intima in which collagen, lipid-containing foam cells, and interstitial accumulation of lipids (with or without crystal formation) participate. A characteristic of lipid

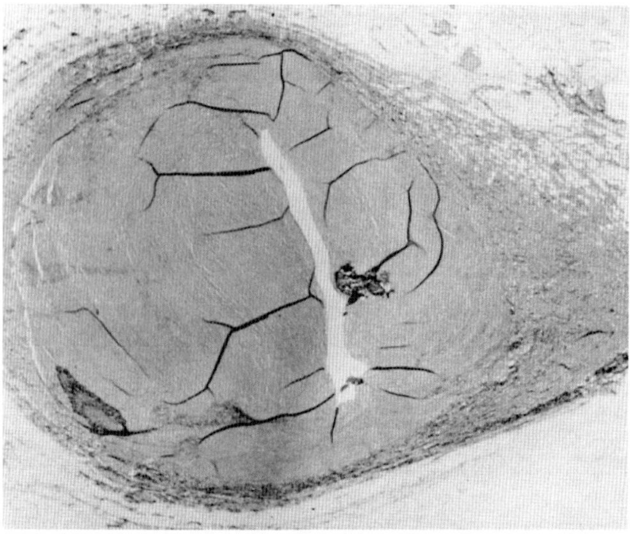

Fig. 8.10 Fibrous type of atheroma. The intima is greatly thickened by laminated fibrous tissue. No distinct accumulations of lipids are present. Two foci of calcification exist. Hematoxylin and eosin stain: ×9

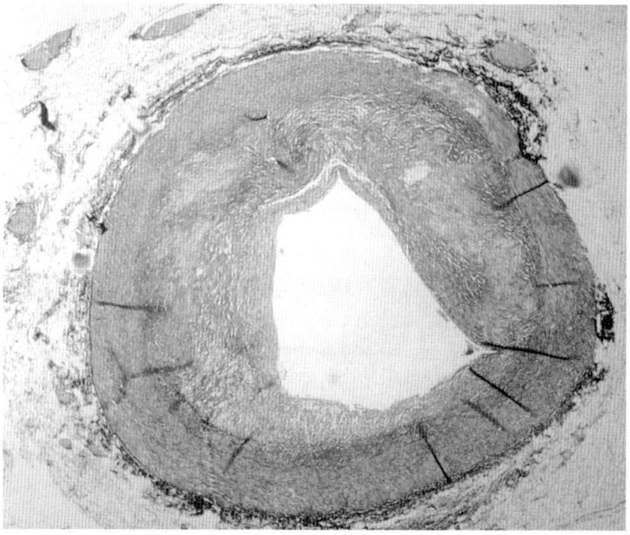

Fig. 8.11 Atheroma with lightly stained areas (left upper portion of thickened intima) represent collagen containing fatty material. Elastic tissue stain: ×15

accumulation is its association with a fibrous cap on the lumen side of the accumulation. In the minority of segments with major obstruction of the lumen, only one pair of fibrous tissue and lipoid tissue is apparent. Usually, more than one pair is present. Each pair is characterized by an accumulation of amorphous or crystalline lipids walled on the lumen side by fibrous tissue. It is significant that the amount of fibrous tissue may be greater than the accumulations of lipids. Occasional foam cells may be caught in the fibrous tissue or associated with extracellular accumulation of lipids.

In most atheromas that are significantly obstructive, a series of pairs of fibrous tissue and lipoid accumulation is more common than one pair. This suggests an episodic character to the formation of the obstructive atheroma.

Figure 8.12a–d shows photomicrographs of coronary arteries. Each shows more than one pair of fibrous tissue and lipoid accumulation, giving strong evidence for the episodic nature of ultimate narrowing of the lumen by atherosclerosis.

Angiographic Illustrative Cases of Coronary Obstruction

Normal Coronary Arteriogram

Figure 8.13a, b shows examples of normal coronary arteriograms.

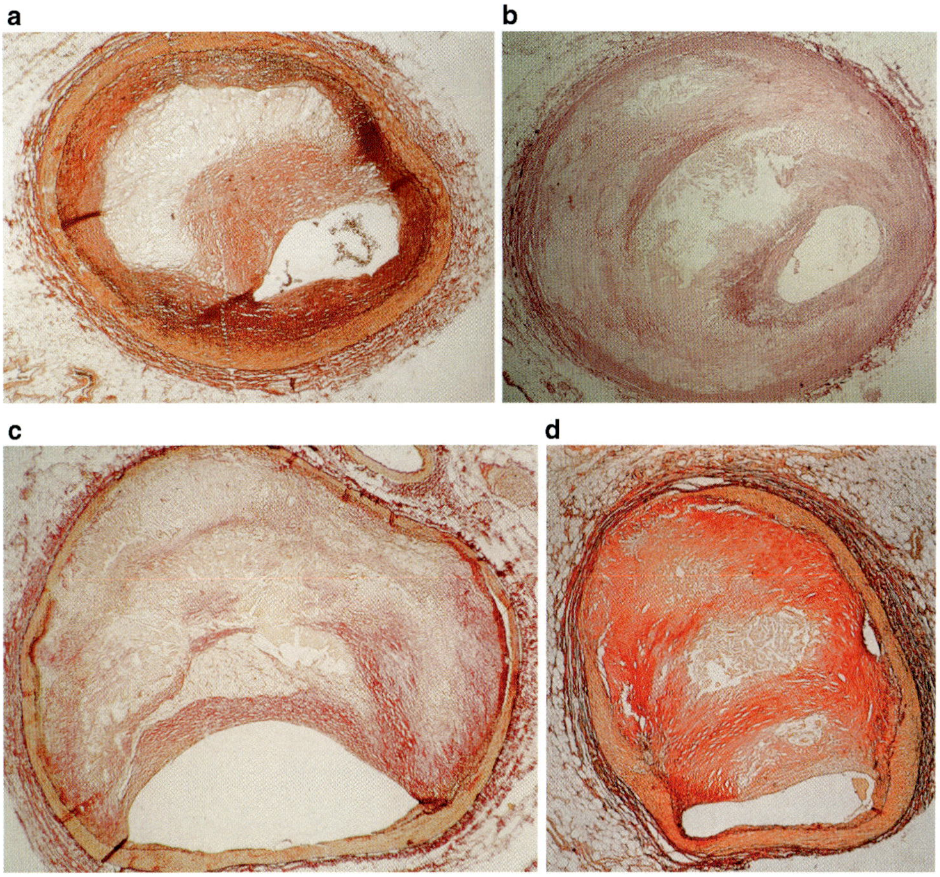

Fig. 8.12 (**a**) Photomicrograph of a coronary artery. There is one pair of complex lesion of lipoid foci in fibrous lesion involving the intima. The clear space of the lesion is composed of lipid material separated from the narrowed lumen by fibrous tissue. Elastic tissue stain: X27. (**b**) Two pairs of complex lesions are present in this coronary artery. Hematoxylin and eosin stain: x17. (**c**, **d**) Two coronary arteries, each with three pairs of complex lesions. Each elastic tissue stain: (**a**) ×19. (**b**) ×22

Minimal Obstructive Disease

Figure 8.14a, b shows examples from a young patient with hypercholesterolemia. Relatively minor obstructive lesions are visible in the LAD and right coronary artery (RCA).

Moderate Stenosis

The image shown in Fig. 8.15 belongs to a 51-year-old man; only a moderately obstructed segment was present in the LAD.

Severe Stenosis in Intermediate Segment of the Right Coronary Artery

The concept that the distal RCA is less frequently involved in severe stenosis is incorrect. As a matter of fact, the distal one third of the RCA tends to be more severely involved. Angiographically, such lesions can be missed unless a left anterior oblique (LAO) view is obtained routinely (Fig. 8.16).

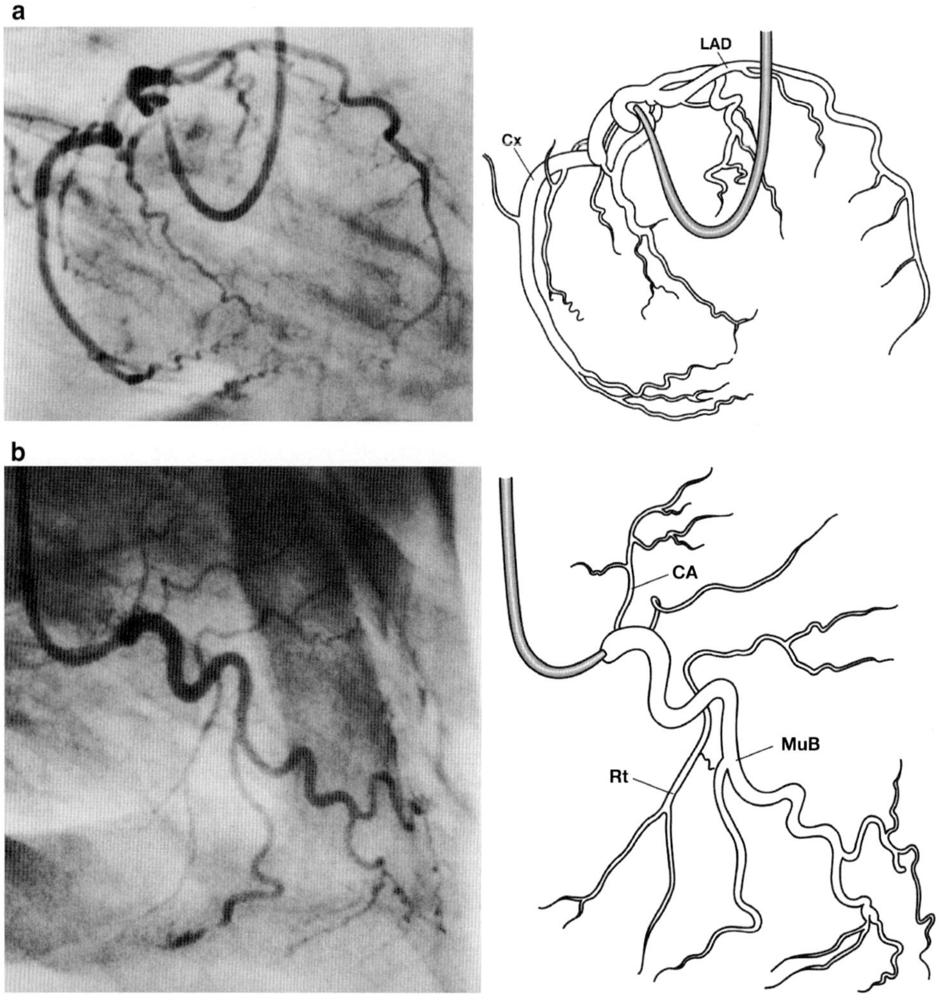

Fig. 8.13 (**a**) Normal LC arteriogram in lateral view. (**b**) Normal RC arteriogram in RAO view

Multiple Lesions in Left Coronary System

The image shown in Fig. 8.17 belongs to a 63-year-old man; the LM is markedly narrowed. The circumflex artery (CX) was totally occluded, and the LAD showed moderate stenosis.

Severe Stenosis in Small Branches

Figure 8.18a, b shows a 50-year-old woman with an episode of chest pain. A coronary arteriogram revealed a single stenotic lesion in one of the septal branches. The rest of the coronary system was normal.

Progression of Lesions

Experience has shown that patients studied angiographically over varying intervals may show progression in severity of obstructive coronary disease. In some instances, lesions considered to be progressive may, in fact, be existing lesions not identified in earlier studies. In other instances, total occlusions may result from a thrombosis in the interval between two studies, while in still other cases, progression is, in fact, the cause. Figure 8.19a, b shows results of a patient's angiographic studies performed 4 years apart. Progression in severity of disease is evident.

Fig. 8.14 (**a**) From a 35-year-old man with hypercholesterolemia. LC arteriogram in lateral view illustrating comparatively minor changes of caliber in the LAD. (**b**) RC arteriogram in lateral view showing minor atherosclerotic irregularities (between *arrows*) and general ectasia of the artery

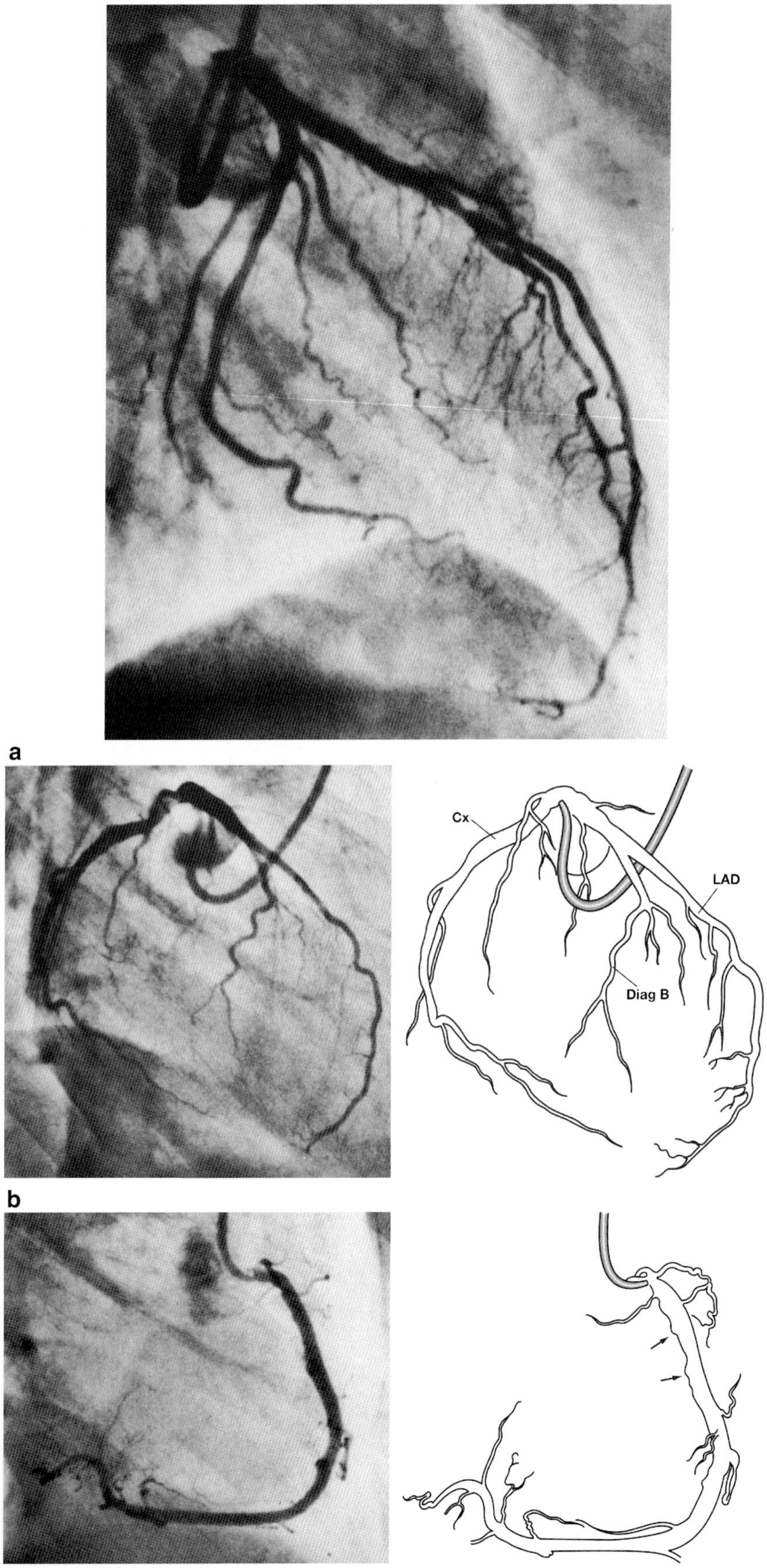

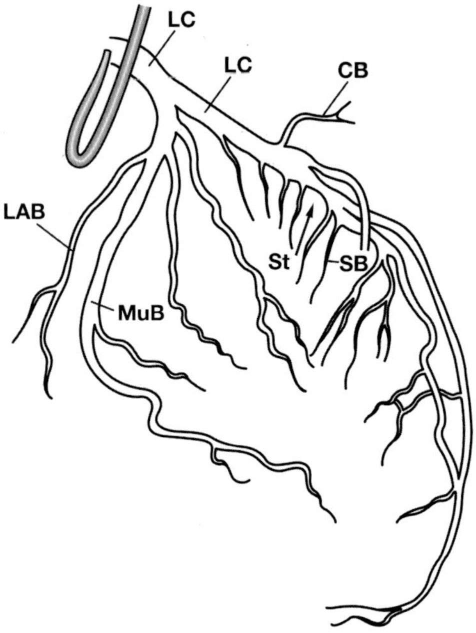

Fig. 8.15 LC arteriogram in RAO view. Focus of moderate stenosis in the LAD. The RCA was normal angiographically

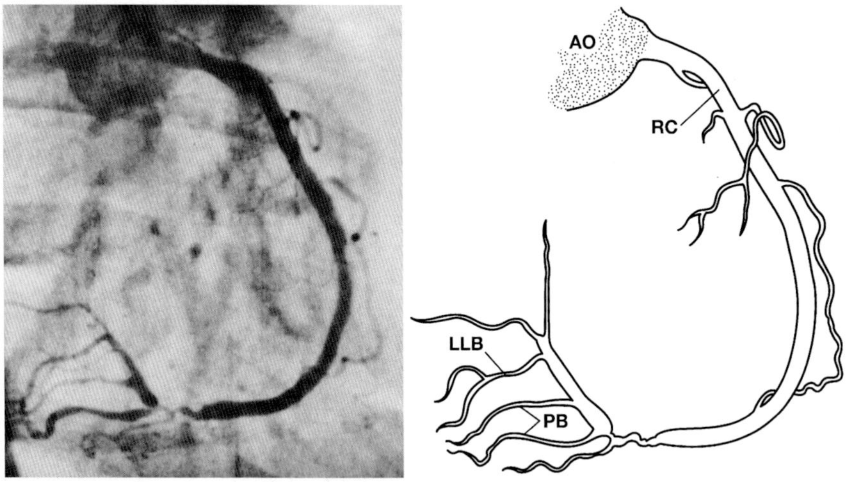

Fig. 8.16 Left anterior oblique (LAO) view of RC arteriogram demonstrating severe stenosis in the intermediate segment of the RCA

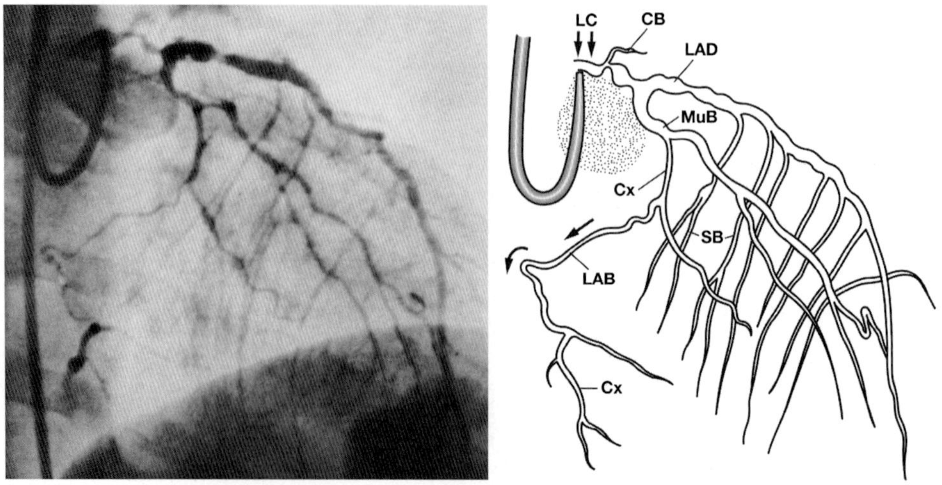

Fig. 8.17 LC arteriogram in RAO view. Almost total occlusion of LM and occlusion of the CX with collaterals from a LAB supplying the distal segment of the CX. The LAD shows a zone of moderate stenosis. There are prominent anteroposterior septal anastomoses

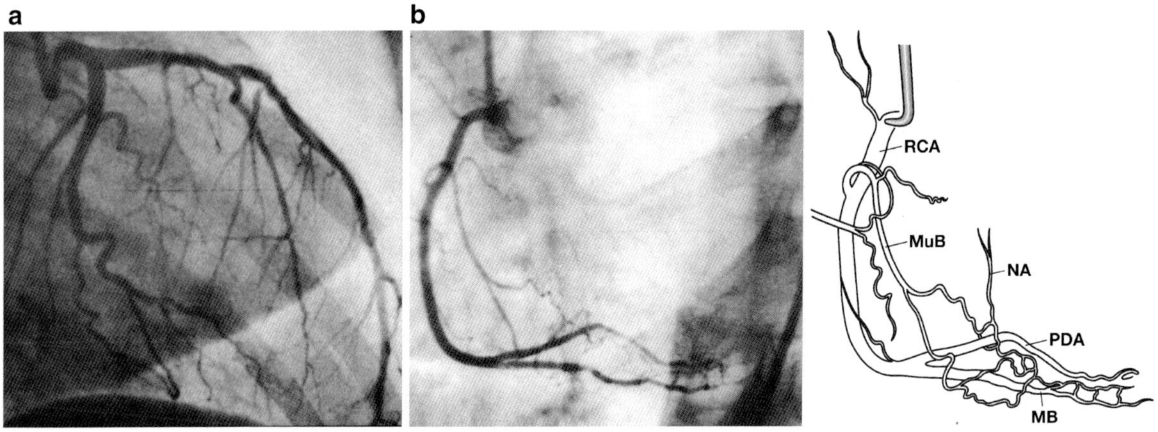

Fig. 8.18 (**a**) Lateral view of LC arteriogram. The only evident lesion is in a septal branch of the LAD. (**b**) LAO view of the RC arteriogram revealing normal coronary arteries

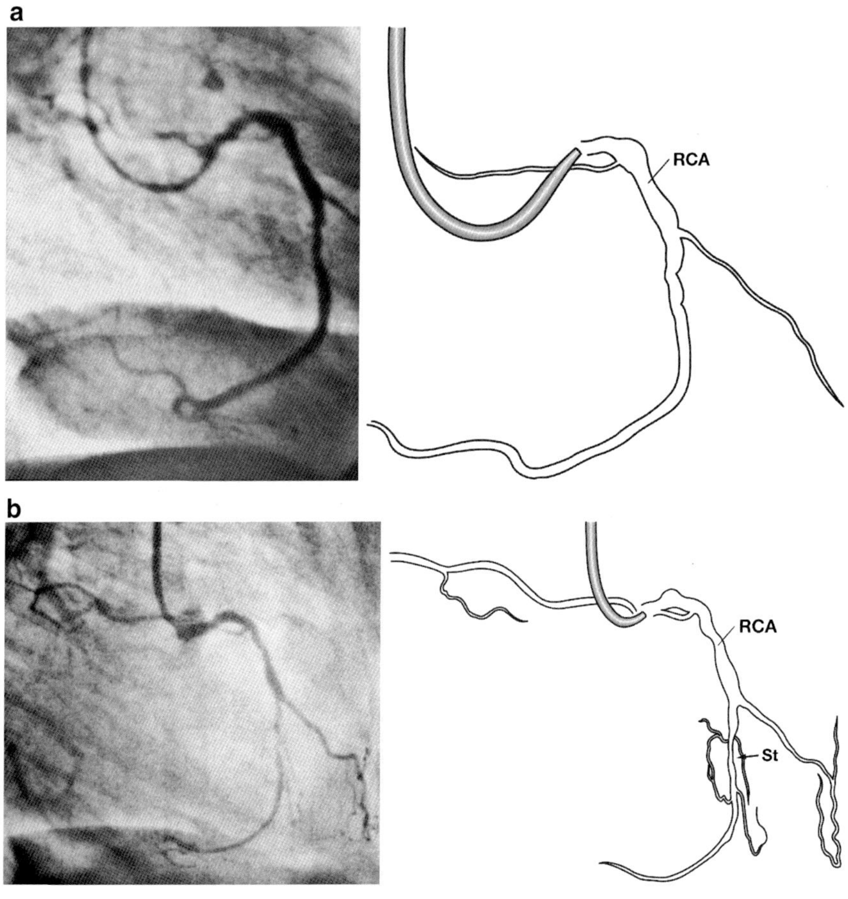

Fig. 8.19 (**a**) Lateral view of RC arteriogram shows marked diffuse disease (**b**) Lateral view of RC arteriogram 4 years later demonstrates considerable progression of narrowing of the distal part of the anterior segment

Variations in Shape of Narrowed Lumen

Depending on the distribution of atherosclerosis, a narrowed lumen may be either central (when the atheromatous process is circumferential) or, more commonly, in an eccentric position. The eccentrically located lumen may be either slit-like or vary in shape, a form referred to as "polymorphous." Usually, when the lumen is central, the degree of narrowing is less

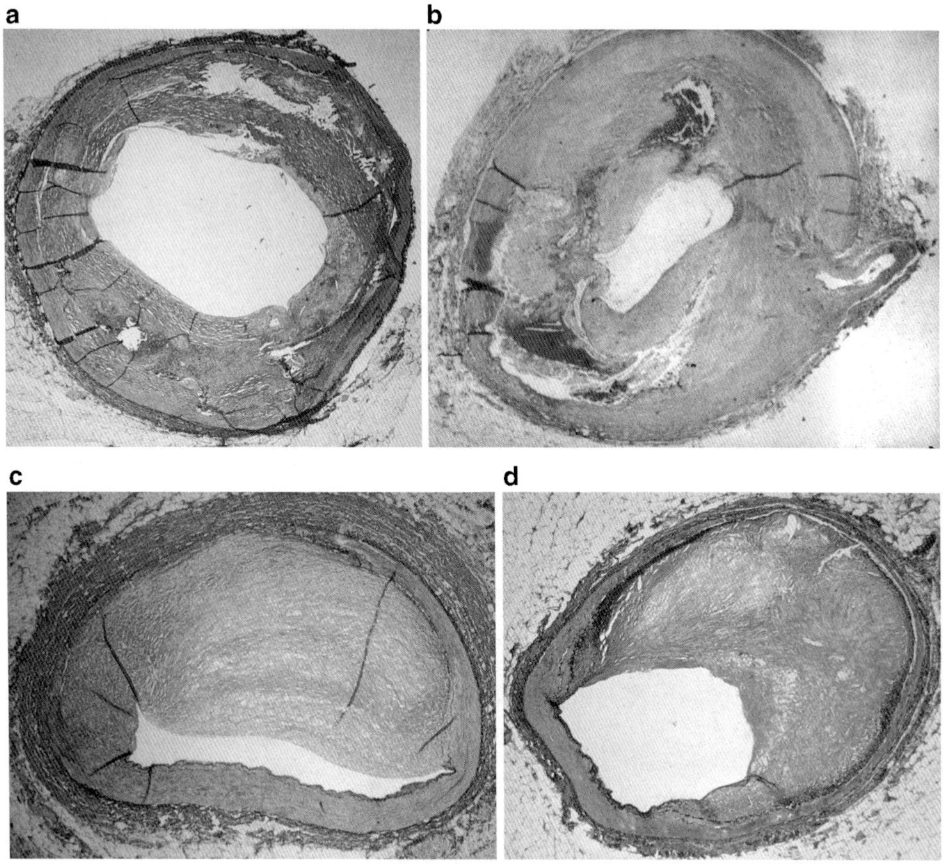

Fig. 8.20 Photomicrograph of two coronary arteries, each with a central lumen, showing different calibers of the lumens. Each elastic tissue stain: ×15. (**a**) The lumen is relatively wide. (**b**) The lumen is markedly narrowed. Two foci of hemorrhage are also present in the atheromatous intima. Two examples of eccentric lumens in coronary athero-sclerosis. (**c**) Slit-like lumen. Although narrow, the lumen has one dimension almost as wide as the original diameter of the vessel. Elastic tissue stain: ×17. (**d**) Eccentric polymorphous lumen. Elastic tissue stain: ×19

than when it is eccentric. The three types of lumens occur approximately in equal distribution among atheromatous segments of coronary arteries (Fig. 8.20a–d).

Ambrose et al [3]. developed a system for classifying coronary stenosis morphology based on its angiographic appearance (Fig. 8.21). Lesions associated with acute thrombotic syndromes (unstable angina and infarction) were usually of type II eccentric morphology, and in most thrombotic lesions, the edges of the lesion were irregular and scalloped [4].

Orientation of Atheromas

As shown in Fig. 8.22a, b atheromas tend to occur in different orientations with respect to the surface of the heart, as one traces a given vessel distally.

Distribution of Lesions

While the LAD is commonly considered to be the site of most common involvement by atheromas, experience has shown that the RCA is slightly more commonly involved by disease in patients with significant coronary atherosclerosis. In a study of coronary arteries in 50 adults whose hearts had significant coronary atherosclerosis, the intermediate segment of the RCA (the segment between the marginal and posterior descending branches) was the most common site of involvement [5]. This was followed in incidence of disease equally by the proximal half of the LAD and the anterior segment of the RCA, which lies between the origin of the vessel from the Ao and its marginal branch. Also of significance was the fact that more than 60% of patients with significant coronary atherosclerosis harbored significant lesions in the proximal half of the CX (Fig. 8.23).

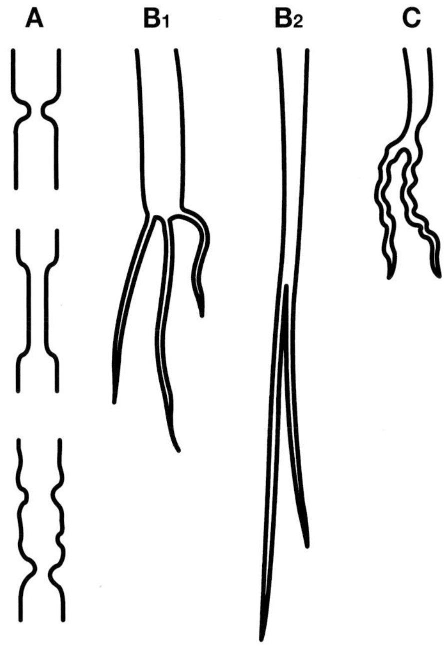

Fig. 8.21 Angiographic morphology of coronary arterial stenosis. Type A stenoses are concentric and have smooth borders. Type B lesions are eccentric and are divided into two groups. Type B1 lesions have a smooth border without overhang, while type B2 lesions have irregular borders and/or overhang. Type C lesions have multiple irregularities. Lesions associated with acute thrombotic syndromes (unstable angina and infarction) were usually type II eccentric morphology, and in most thrombotic lesions, the edges were irregular and scalloped

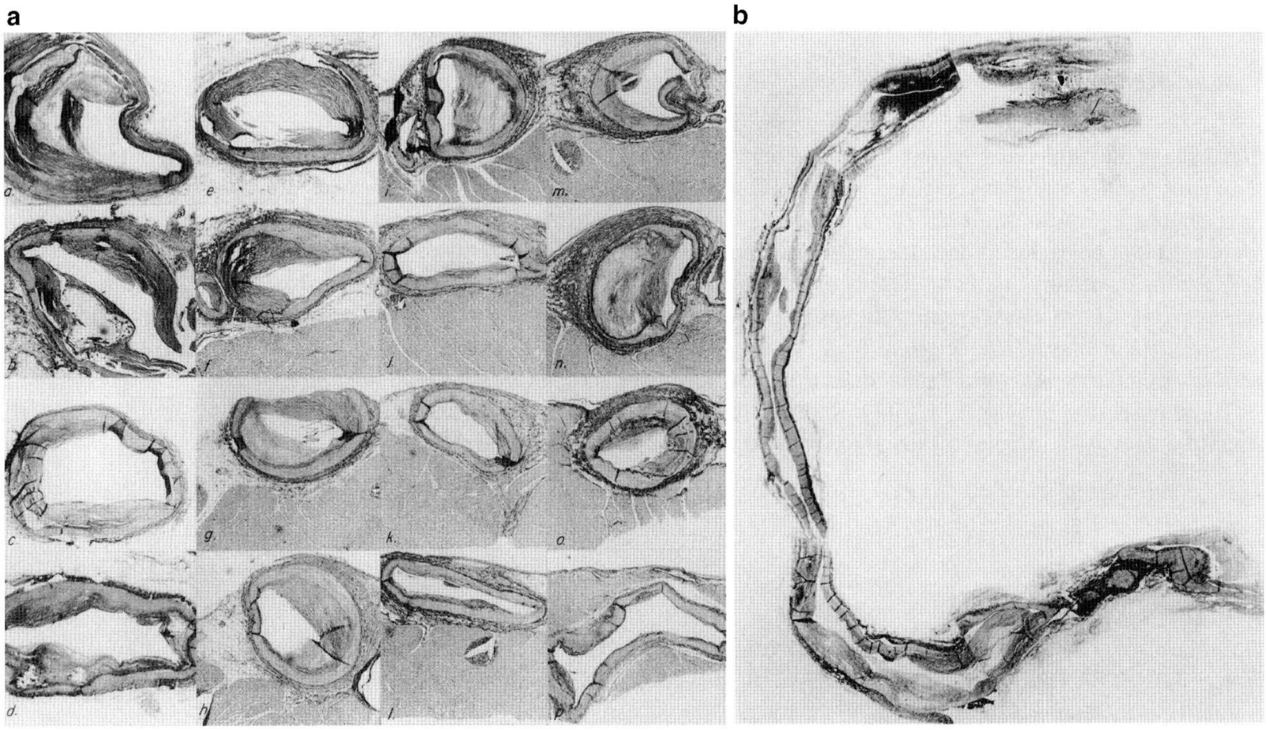

Fig. 8.22 (**a**) CX has been sectioned its entire length from its origin (A) to termination (P). Each photomicrograph is oriented in the same way with respect to the surface of the heart. The illustration shows variations in orientation of atheromas. Also, it portrays the fact that uninvolved segments may lie between segments with varying degrees of involvement by obstructive atherosclerosis. (**b**) Focal distribution of atherosclerosis. Segments of normal artery are present between segments of diseased arteries. Composite photomicrograph of longitudinal sections of the circumflex artery 2 cm from its origin

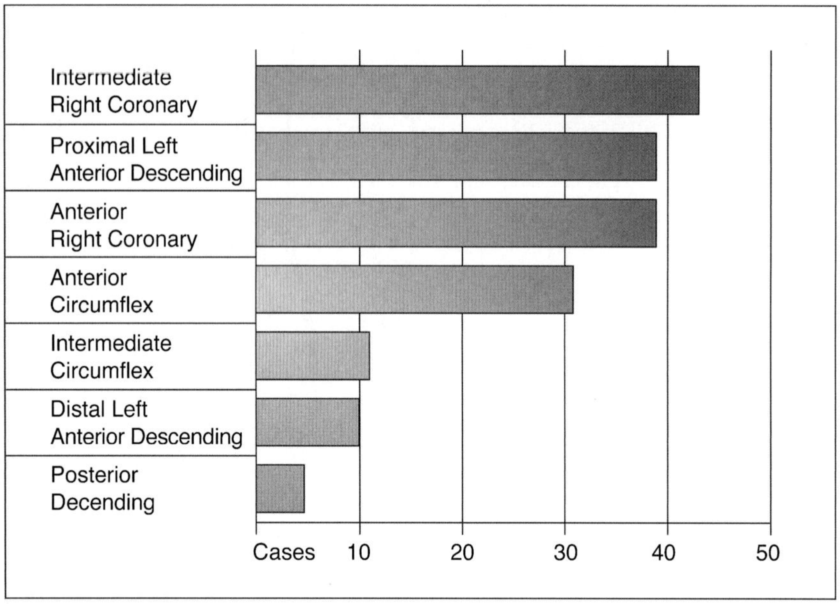

Fig. 8.23 A number of arteries with significant atherosclerosis among 50 subjects with significant coronary heart disease

Complicating Lesions

Among the complicating lesions that may occur in coronary arterial segments containing atheromas are the following: hemorrhage in the atheroma, luminal thrombosis, calcification of the atheroma, and aneurysm formation.

Plaque Hemorrhage

Hemorrhage into atheromas is a common phenomenon. Two schools of thought exist concerning its source. One is that the capillaries, which commonly appear in atheromas, rupture. The other view proposes primary fragmentation of the fibrous layer of the plaque nearest the lumen, with blood escaping from the lumen into the lipid part of the atheroma. While the first concept cannot be excluded, the latter may be demonstrated.

Fissuring or rupture of atherosclerotic plaque appears to be an inciting event in both unstable angina and acute myocardial infarction [6, 7]. Angiographic studies of coronary lesions in patients with unstable angina and plaque rupture show eccentric lesion shapes, characterized by a narrow neck and overhanging edges or scalloped borders, a high incidence of stenosis irregularity, and intraluminal defects which presumably are thrombi.

Thrombosis may appear at the site of intimal rupture. At other times, the hematoma within the atheroma may become organized, leaving a vascular plexus in the wall beside the lumen (Fig. 8.24a, b).

Thrombosis

Thrombosis may also appear at a site of plaque rupture. Plaque rupture as the nidus for subsequent thrombus formation can be seen only if the entire thrombus is examined. Serial sections frequently demonstrate that, in relation to a thrombus in a coronary artery, there has been a break in the related fibrous cap (Fig. 8.25a–c).

Pathologic and clinical evidence suggest that coronary thrombosis after plaque rupture is a dynamic process [6, 7]. The occlusive thrombus typically has a multilayered structure, suggesting that it is often formed successively over an extended period of time (days or weeks) rather than a single abrupt event. This finding fits with the often stuttering course of ischemic symptoms. In addition, clot fragmentation with distal microembolization has been identified in 73% of cases carefully studied and can be seen on the angiogram in a smaller fraction of patients [8].

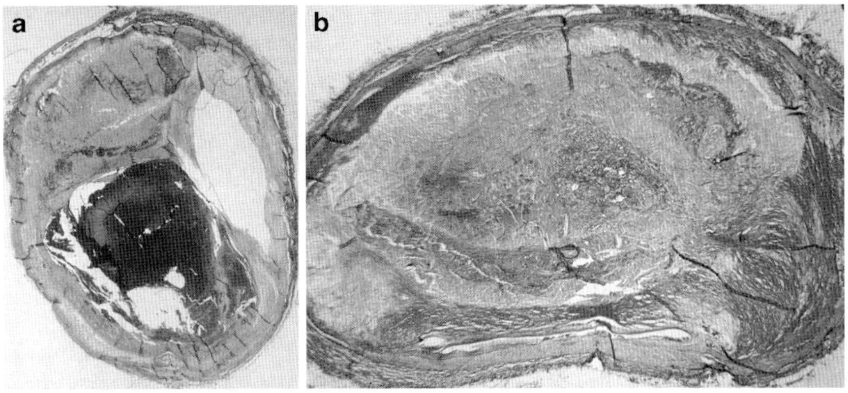

Fig. 8.24 (**a**) A large hematoma is present in atheroma, while the lumen appears not to have been disturbed. Hematoxylin and eosin stain: ×17. (**b**) Extensive hemorrhage is present in an atheroma. The lumen is at the lower portion of the illustration. It is slit-like and may have been compressed by the intimal hematoma. Hematoxylin and eosin stain: ×12

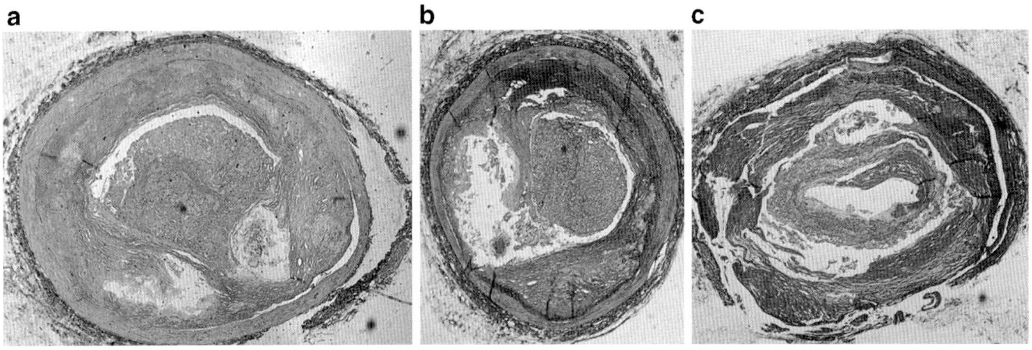

Fig. 8.25 (**a**) Segment of thrombosed coronary artery. Atherosclerosis is visible in the wall and the lumen contains a thrombus. No evidence of underlying rupture of the wall of the atheroma is evident in this plane of section. Elastic tissue stain: ×14. Two other levels of section show breaks in the covering of the atheroma: (**b**) The covering of the atheroma is broken, and the lumen contains a thrombus. Elastic tissue stain: ×18. (**c**) The intimal lining has been destroyed along its left half and intimal hemorrhage is present. Elastic tissue stain: ×17

Aggregated platelets are the major early component of the thrombus. Within one or two days, this platelet thrombus is infiltrated and consolidated, leading to a more distinct angiographic edge.

Plaque fissuring, a multilayered thrombus, and distal microembolization are also seen at postmortem examination in patients with unstable angina and in humans dying suddenly with coronary atherosclerosis and without evidence of myocardial infarction [7]. Despite clinical and angiographic evidence of plaque rupture, patients with unstable angina have a much smaller burden clot within the affected arterial segment than do patients with infarction.

Angiographically, a recent total coronary occlusion is characterized by a small remaining vessel stump that can accumulate contrast. Injection into this stump usually reveals an often "feathered" hang-up contrast with indistinct margins and slow washout.

In the usual instance of thrombosis of a coronary artery, underlying atherosclerosis of varying degrees is present. Usually, the underlying atherosclerosis reduces the lumen by more than 25% of its original caliber.

Figure 8.25a–c shows three levels of section of a thrombosed coronary artery. Without 3–5 mm serial cross sections, a chance section might have shown a simple thrombosis without a break in the fibrous covering of the atheroma.

Once formed in coronary arteries, thrombi may undergo organization. Ultimately, a thrombus is replaced by vascular connective tissue, but in the aggregate, the vessels of the organized thrombus are usually of lesser caliber than the original lumen (Fig. 8.26a–g).

Calcification

Calcification in atheromas has received considerable attention. Calcification appears to be an indication that the involved part of the lesion is old. This process occurs either in accumulations of extracellular lipid or in collagen, the sites of collipid change.

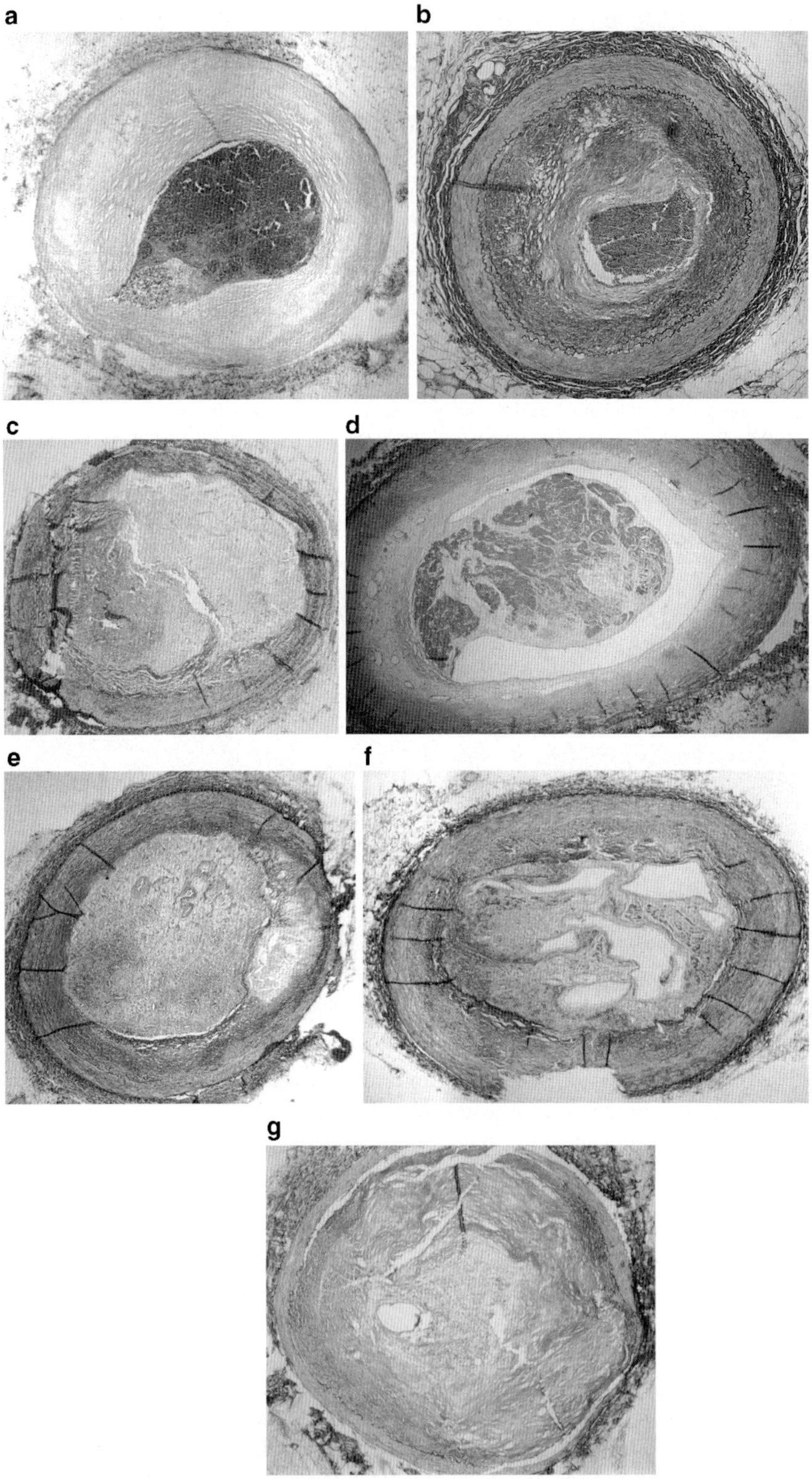

Fig. 8.26 (**a**) Recent thrombosis in a lumen that was relatively wide. Hematoxylin and eosin stain: ×18. (**b**) Recent coronary thrombosis in an artery of which the lumen is markedly narrowed by underlying atherosclerosis. No organization is yet evident. Elastic tissue stain: ×24. (**c**) Thrombosis of a coronary artery associated with a rupture of the wall of the related atheroma. Thrombus is present in the lumen, while hemorrhage is present in the atheroma. Elastic tissue stain: ×19. (**d**) Mural thrombus of a coronary artery showing encapsulation of the thrombus and the process of organization underway. Hematoxylin and eosin stain: ×18. (**e**) Thrombus occluding the lumen is being replaced by vascular granulation tissue portraying the process of early organization. Elastic tissue stain: ×19. Next are two examples of organized thrombus: (**f**) Elastic tissue stain: ×12. (**g**) Elastic tissue stain: ×27. Although the process of organization is frequently referred to as "recanalization," the aggregate diameter of the vessels of the organized thrombus characteristically is relatively narrow when compared to that of the lumen as it existed before the event of thrombosis

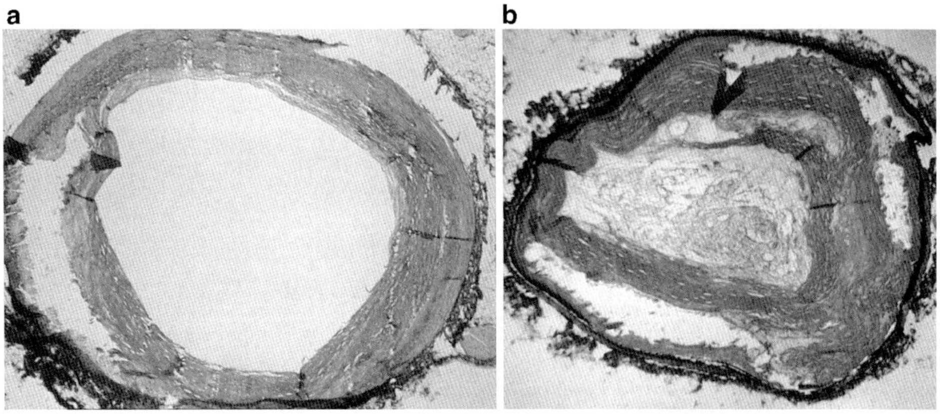

Fig. 8.27 (**a**) Calcification in atheroma associated with a lumen that is only mildly narrowed. The clear space in the wall represents calcific material which has been lost in sectioning. Hematoxylin and eosin stain: ×29. (**b**) Calcification in atheroma (clear spaces) in an artery occluded by a combination of atherosclerosis and organized thrombus. Elastic tissue stain: ×11

Foci of calcification may be seen in atheromas causing severe stenosis, as well as in those with minimal stenosis of the lumen, and are easily detectable in the coronary arteries by fluoroscopy or angiography.

Classically, the picture of calcification without significant luminal narrowing is observed in older age groups. Our interpretation of this process is that atherosclerosis had begun many years before observation, but the process failed to show a progressive character.

Recent evidence derived from electron beam computed tomography (EBCT) has challenged the old dogma that coronary plaque calcification is mainly a marker of end-stage plaque degeneration, but instead has demonstrated that intramural calcium can be observed in all degrees of atherosclerotic involvement [9].

Recent investigations have proposed using EBCT as a noninvasive screening test for coronary atherosclerosis. Regardless of gender, the prevalence and extent of coronary calcification increases with age with an epidemiologic pattern similar to that known for coronary atherosclerosis [10]. Absence of detectable coronary artery calcification on EBCT is less likely in the presence of a severe luminal coronary obstruction and has been proposed as a screening tool to identify patients at low risk (80% chance of having angiographically normal arteries) [11].

However, potentially unstable plaque characterized by high lipid content rather than calcification may make detection using the calcium score difficult. J.L. Kelly et al [12]. evaluated findings in patients with a normal calcium score undergoing coronary CT angiography and found that moderate to severe stenosis may be present in patients with no coronary calcification. Although the calcium score does add prognostic value to standard risk factors and serum markers, imaging the vessel wall directly may help identify noncalcified plaque and guide therapy.

Figure 8.27a, b shows segments of coronary arteries with calcification of atheromas. Variations in the caliber of the lumen are evident.

Aneurysm Formation

Classically, atherosclerotic aneurysms are solitary but an aneurysm involving more than one artery may occur. Thrombotic occlusion is perhaps more common in severe coronary atherosclerosis with aneurysm. Figure 8.28a–c shows a patient who had a subdiaphragmatic abscess after gastric resection. Death was sudden and unexpected. Aneurysms were present in the RCA as well as the LAD.

Angiographic Demonstration

Coronary arterial aneurysm of an atherosclerotic basis may appear angiographically either as distinct saccular dilatations or as dilatation involving a long segment of an artery, which may be termed ectasia. Determining whether an aneurysm is related to atherosclerosis or the result of some other disease is made by association with or the absence of evidence of atherosclerotic disease in the remaining portions of the coronary system (Fig. 8.29a–e).

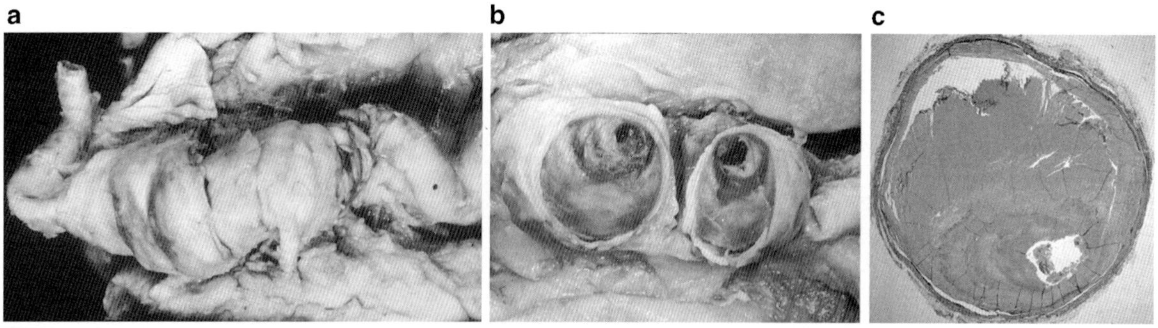

Fig. 8.28 (**a**) A 60-year-old man with sudden death. A. Gross specimen of the right coronary artery (RCA) with an unusually long aneurysm. (**b**) Cross section of the aneurysmal portion of the RCA. Although the lumen of the aneurysm is almost occluded by thrombus, there is a preserved channel (white probe). (**c**) Photomicrograph of the aneurysmal segment shows atrophy of the media as well as preservation of a lumen within the thrombus contained in the aneurysm. Elastic tissue stain: ×4

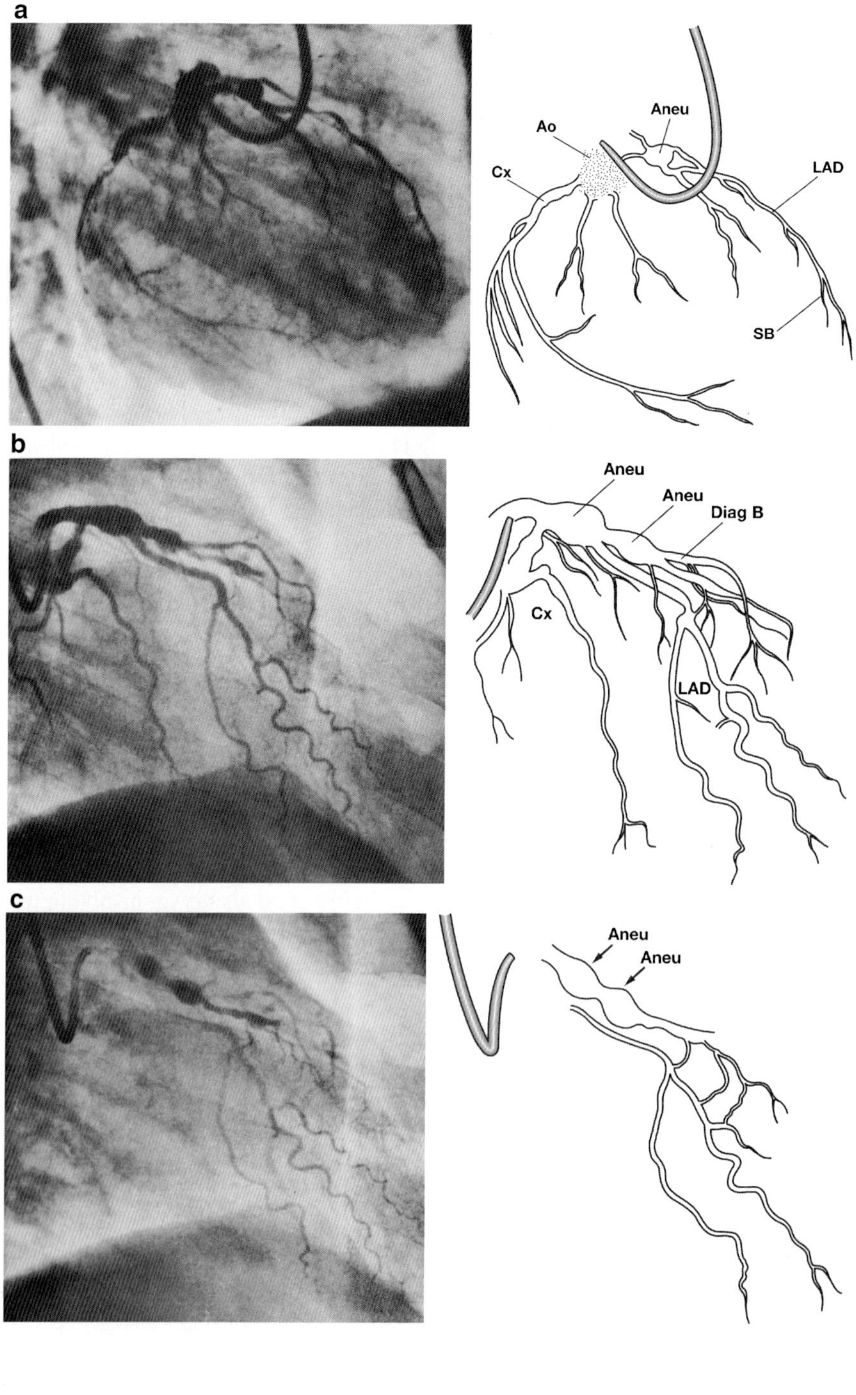

Fig. 8.29 (**a**) LC arteriogram in RAO view. Saccular aneurysm of the LAD. Signs of obstructive coronary atherosclerosis are also present in the LAD. (**b**) RAO view of LC arteriogram. Large LM with aneurysm of LAD and aneurysm of Diag B. (**c**) Late phase of coronary arteriogram shown in (b) with pooling of heavy contrast material in the aneurysm of the LAD. (**d**) RAO view of LC arteriogram showing saccular aneurysm (*arrow*) at trifurcation of the LC. (**e**) Lateral view of RC arteriogram show aneurysm and atherosclerotic ectasia of the anterior segment of the RC

Fig. 8.29 (continued)

d

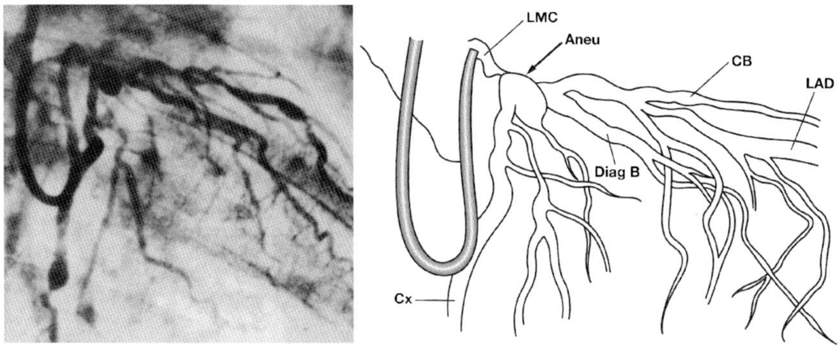

e

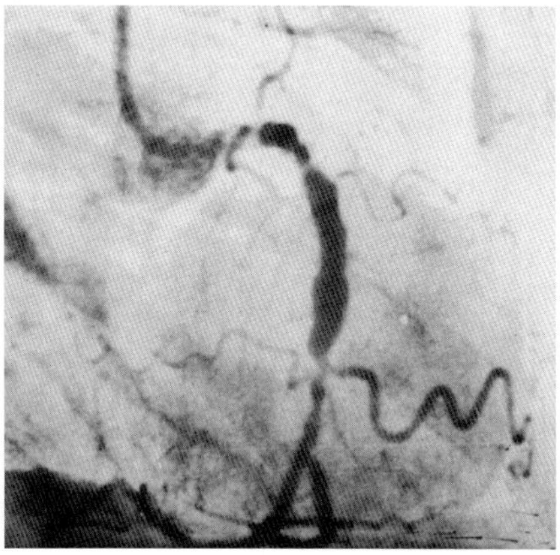

Angiographic and Pathologic Correlations

Using pressure in postmortem hearts, Glagov et al [13]. demonstrated that early in the atherosclerotic process, coronary arteries undergo a compensatory increase in outer diameter of the artery. Although various segments of the same artery may respond differently, this compensatory dilatation acts to maintain lumen caliber despite thickening of the wall. These investigators found that coronary arterial lumen encroachment does not begin until the atherosclerotic plaque occupies 40% of the original lumen area, as determined by the internal elastic membrane. Only at this point is angiography able to detect the presence of disease. This observation may explain the frequent discrepancy between pathologic and angiographic assessments of experimental atherosclerosis.

Angiographic studies of the coronary arteries show that a coronary arteriogram, in general, underestimates the degree of narrowing found at autopsy. In our experience, the segments prone to arteriographic underestimation of the degree of obstruction were the intermediate segment of the RCA, the LM, and the proximal half of the CX. The intermediate segment of the RCA, as visualized in the coronary arteriogram, is the area most frequently poorly correlated with the postmortem specimen. One possible explanation for vulnerability of the intermediate segment of the RCA and the proximal segment of the CX is that arteriographic projections ideal for visualizing the anterior segment of the RCA and the LAD are not ideal for those problematic segments.

Angiographically, false-negative readings may be recorded for segments that show only a uniform but relatively small vessel arteriographically, while pathologically, diffuse disease is demonstrated. Still another factor is comparing different degrees of stenosis. Thus, the LM and proximal segments of the CX may be subject to false-negative interpretation when adjacent segments are more severely diseased.

The presence of slit-like lumens seen pathologically in segments read as normal angiographically suggests that one may be viewing the slit on the arteriogram at its widest diameter and interpret this wide image as that of a normal segment. The lateral view is supported by our correlations of coronary arteriograms with pathologic observations [14].

In unselected sections of atherosclerotic coronary arteries, the slit-like lumen occurred in approximately 30% of sections, whereas the incidence of non-slit-like lumens (central and polymorphous lumens) was 70%. Among segments of coronary

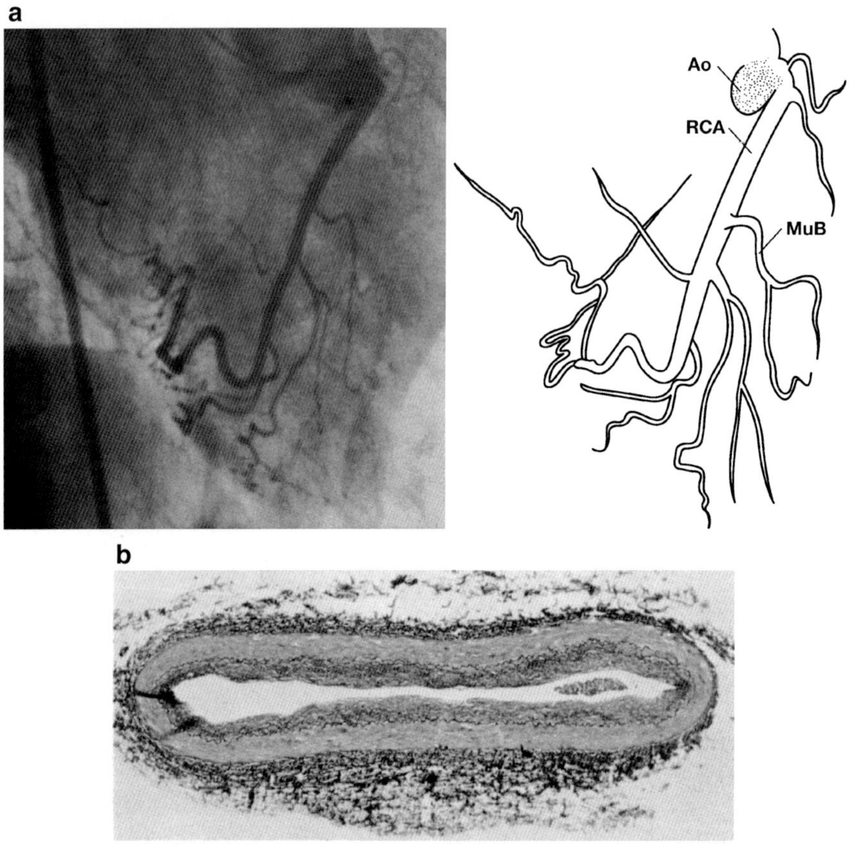

Fig. 8.30 (**a**) From a 60-year-old woman, RAO view of RC arteriogram demonstrating normal coronary arteries. (**b**) Photomicrograph of a coronary artery, representing the state of the coronary tree. Normal features are present. Elastic tissue stain: ×19

arteries with significant obstructed lumens not identified by arteriograms (false negatives), a slit-like lumen was present in 68%, while the non-slit-like lumen constituted only 32%. The varying orientation of atheromas with respect to the surface of the heart can make it more difficult to identify the lumen on arteriograms.

Confirmation of Normal

Figure 8.30a, b is of a patient with mitral stenosis and aortic stenosis who died 8 months following aortic valve replacement. Coronary arteriography before the operation showed no evidence of coronary disease. Autopsy findings were confirmatory.

False Negative: Atherosclerosis Grades II to III

Figure 8.31a–c is of a 63-year-old man with aortic insufficiency. Thoracic pain had appeared a short time before he was admitted for an operation. Coronary arteriography revealed large, normal-appearing coronary arteries. The patient died two days following aortic valve replacement. At autopsy, the coronary arteries revealed grade II to III atherosclerosis in the RCA and LAD.

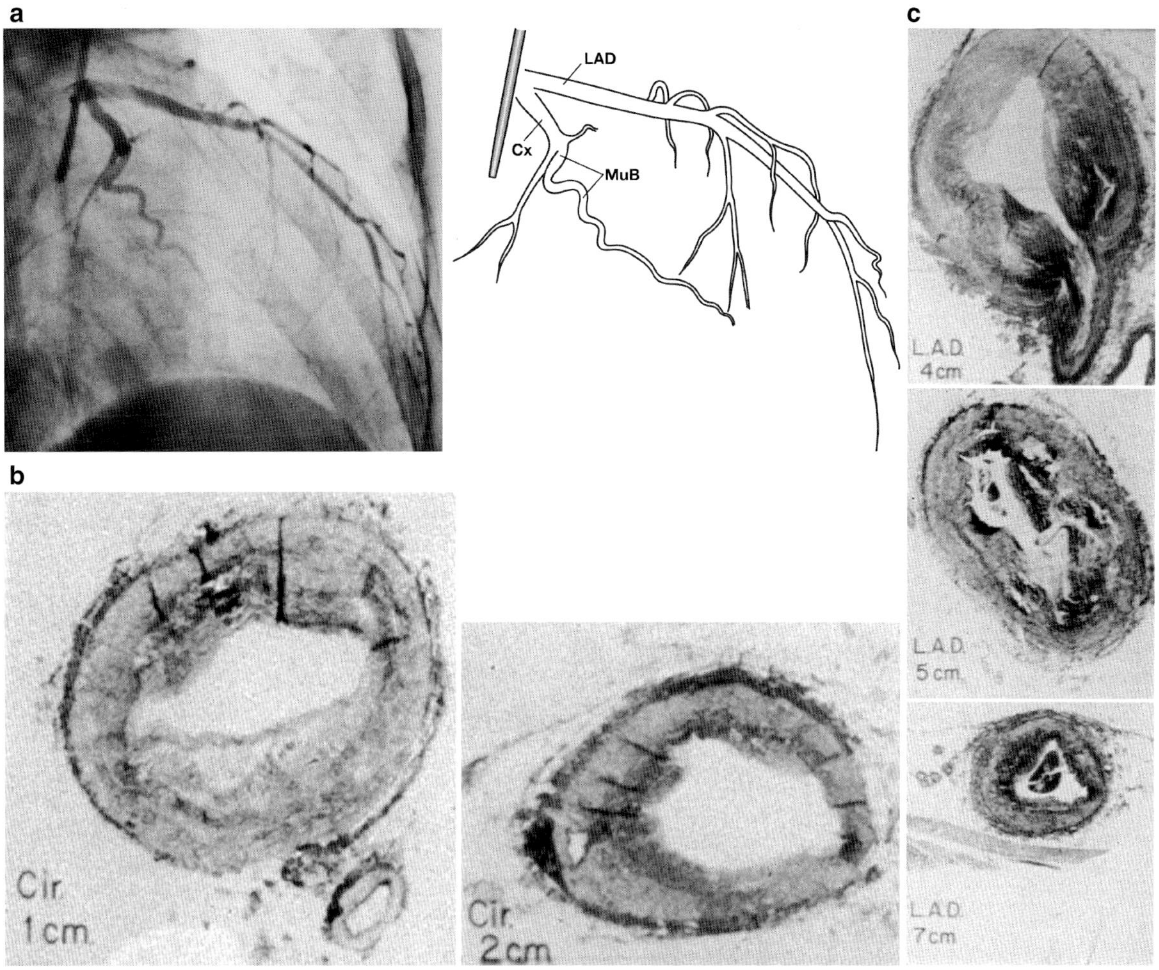

Fig. 8.31 (**a**) The arteriogram in lateral view. No evidence of lesions. (**b**) and (**c**) illustrations are photomicrographs of cross section of the ML and LAD at different levels, proceeding from origin of the vessels, as labeled. Variations in disease process are present, including grade II + atherosclerosis obstruction at several levels. Each elastic tissue stain: ×12

False Negative and Agreement

Figure 8.32a–c is of a patient with severe angina pectoris. A coronary arteriogram revealed severe obstructive disease in the anterior segment of the RCA and in the right posterior descending artery (RPDA), as well as in the left lateral branch (LLB) of the RCA. There was occlusion of the proximal LAD and CX. One week after the studies, a coronary bypass graft was inserted into the RCA. The patient did not recover from the operation.

Figure 8.33 depicts the LC arteriographic features as seen from an RC arteriogram. Visualization of the LC system through RC arteriography is correlated with the fact that LC arteriography has shown occlusion of the LAD. This was confirmed by surgical exploration and autopsy. Pathological examination showed multiple segments of either severe stenosis or occlusion by organized thrombi. The apparent continuity of the LAD is probably an illusion as a result of segmental flow into this vessel through numerous collaterals derived from the RCA.

Correlative Studies Using Longitudinal Sections

Figure 8.34a–c shows a patient with stable angina pectoris admitted for coronary bypass surgery. Two weeks before the operation, a coronary arteriogram had shown severely obstructive lesions in the anterior segment of the RCA and of its

Fig. 8.32 (**a**) From a 65-year-old man, RC arteriogram in RAO view shows severe stenosis in the PD and in the left lateral branch (LLB) of the right coronary artery (RCA). Numbers on diagram correspond to levels of section as microphotographs (**b**, **c**). (**b**) Photomicrographs of the anterior segment of the RCA and of its branches, at different levels, revealing moderate atherosclerosis correlating to the irregularities noted in the arteriogram. Each photomicrograph elastic tissue stain: ×12.5. (**c**) The severity of the lesions in the intermediate segment of the RCA at levels 8 and 9 was not apparent in the coronary arteriogram. The presence of a slit-like lumen (levels 8 and 9) suggests that, on the arteriogram, one may have viewed the slits in the widest diameter, thus interpreting this wide image as normal. There is good correlation of lesions for the PD (10) and LLB (11). Numbers correspond to those on Fig. 8.32a. Elastic tissue stain: ×12.5

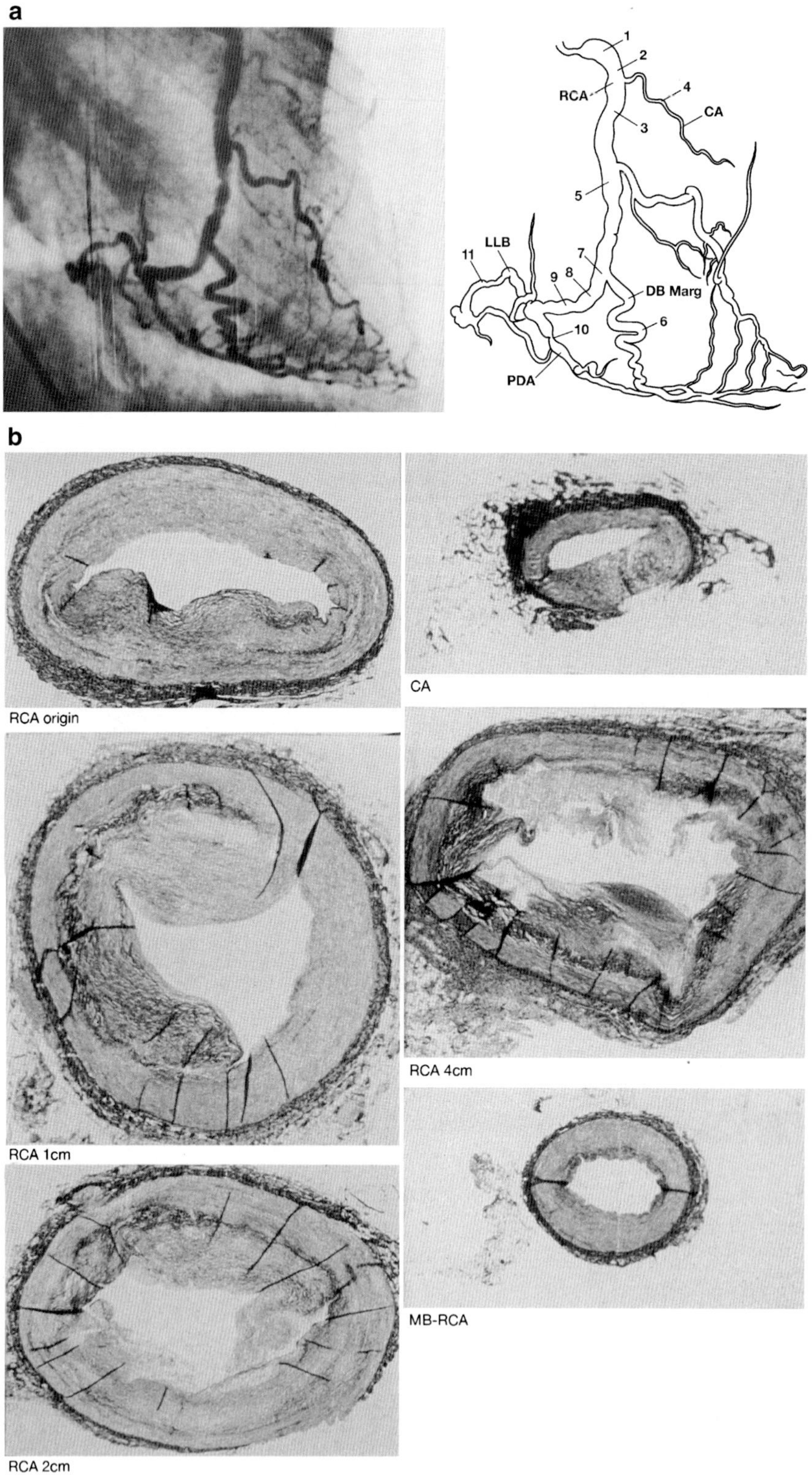

Fig. 8.32 (continued)

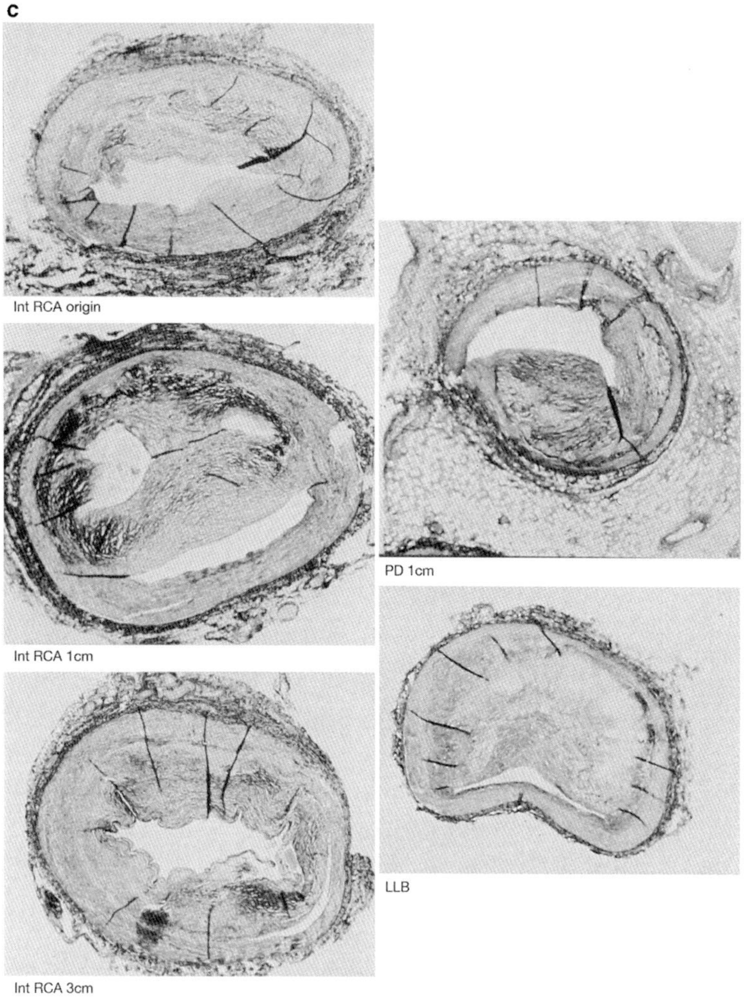

Fig. 8.33 Angiocardiogram is late phase of RC arteriogram showing opacification of the LAD. Photomicrograph shows severe segmental disease at levels indicated. Numbers on photomicrographs correspond with levels numbered on reproduction of arteriogram. Each photomicrograph elastic tissue stain: ×12.5

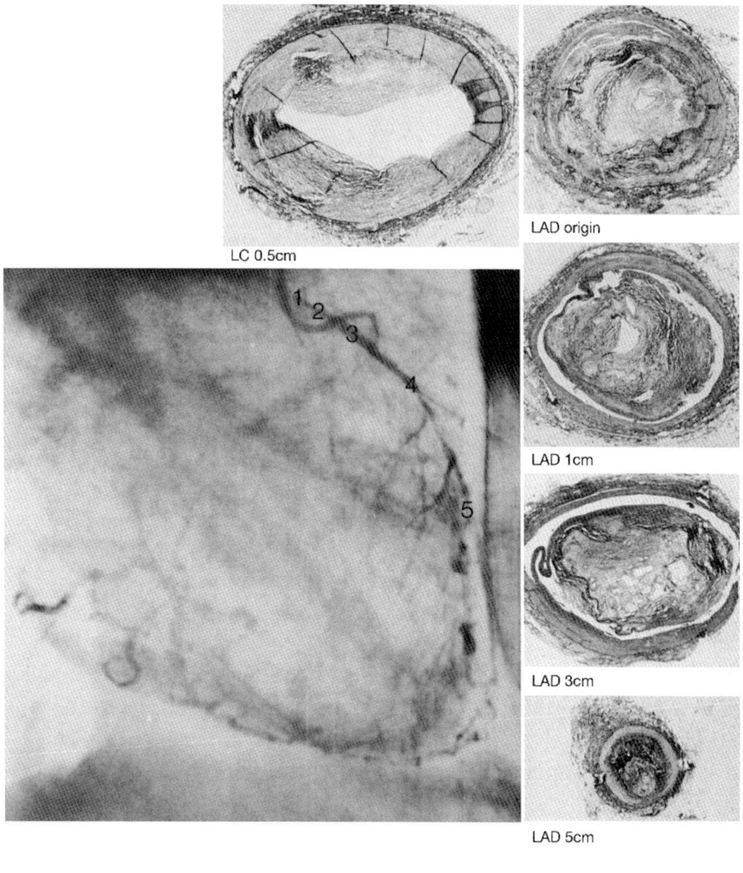

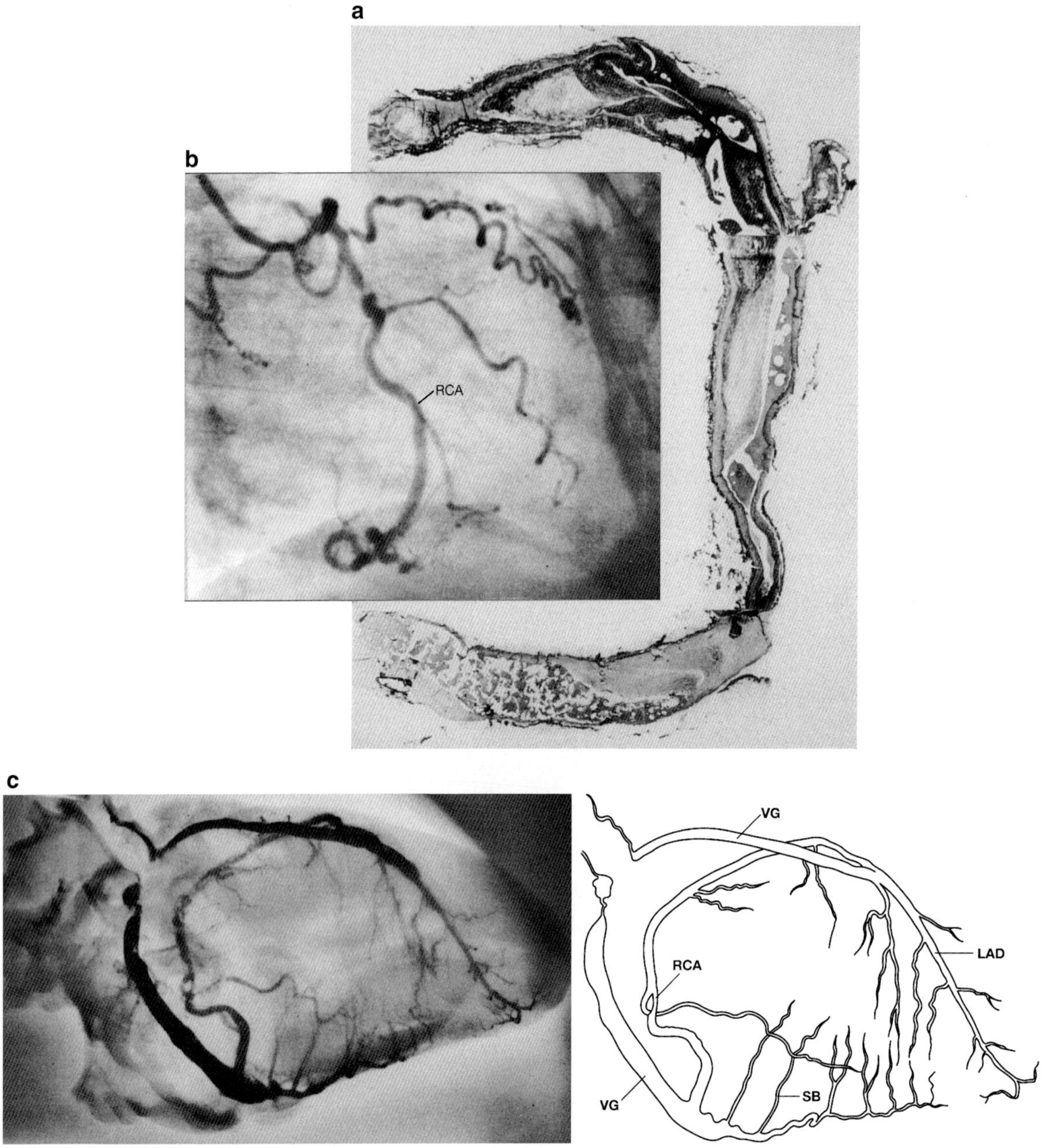

Fig. 8.34 (**a**) RAO view of the proximal RC and markedly enlarged RV branches with collateral flow to the LAD. One of the midright ventricular branches shows moderately severe disease over a long segment. (**b**) Photomicrographs are of longitudinal sections of segments of the RC. Severe atherosclerotic lesion present in the proximal portion of the anterior segment, in the intermediate segment, and the origin of the PDA. The lumen of the vessel contains opaque material injected after death. In chance longitudinal segments, the severity of disease may be exaggerated if the section is through the periphery of the lumen. In this instance, the severity of disease of the intermediate segment was supported by nearby cross sections. Each elastic tissue stain: ×3.8. (**c**) Postmortem angiography of the grafts placed into the terminal portion of the intermediate segment of the RCA and into the LAD. There is retrograde opacification of the RCA. Also, while pathologically the intermediate segment showed severe disease, neither the antemortem angiogram nor the postmortem angiogram shows this process

midright ventricular branch. The LAD revealed occlusion at its origin and was opacified from collateral originating in the RCA. Saphenous vein grafts were inserted into the distal LAD and the terminal part of the intermediate segment of the RCA. The patient did not survive the operation. Pathological examination of the coronary arteries was done by performing longitudinal sections. This approach gave an idea of the extensive distribution of disease of the arterial wall.

Pathologic-Angiographic Correlates in Acute Coronary Syndromes

Coronary angiography performed very soon after the onset of clinical symptoms of myocardial infarction usually demonstrates total occlusion of the coronary artery perusing the infarct zone. The incidence of total occlusion is nearly 90% if angiography is performed as early as 1 h after symptoms but drops to about 70% if angiography is delayed to 12–24 h [15]. Total occlusion is found less frequently (26%) in patients having angiography within 24 h of symptom onset of a non-Q-wave infarction [16]. This reduction in frequency of total coronary occlusion is probably the result of spontaneously occurring thrombolysis.

References

1. Conti CR, Selby JH, Christie LG. Left main coronary artery stenosis: clinical spectrum, pathophysiology, and management. Prog Cardiovasc Dis. 1987;22:73–105.
2. Osborn GR. The Incubation period of coronary thrombosis. London: Butterworths; 1963. p. 190.
3. Ambrose JA, Winters SL, Arora RR, et al. Coronary angiographic morphology in myocardial infarction: a link between the pathogenesis of unstable angina and myocardial infarction. J Am Coll Cardiol. 1985;6:1233–8.
4. Wilson RF, Holiday MD, White CW. Quantitative angiographic morphology of coronary stenoses leading to myocardial infarction or unstable angina. Circulation. 1986;73:286–93.
5. Vlodaver Z, Edwards JE. Pathology of coronary atherosclerosis. Prog Cardiovasc Dis. 1971;14:256–74.
6. Falk E. Thrombosis in unstable angina: pathologic aspects. Cardiovasc Clin. 1987;18(1):137–49.
7. Davies MJ, Thomas AC. Plaque fissuring - the cause of acute myocardial infarction, sudden ischemic death, and crescendo angina. Br Heart J. 1985;53:363–73.
8. Sherman CT, Litvack F, Grundfest W, et al. Coronary angioscopy in patients with unstable angina pectoris. N Engl J Med. 1986;315:913–9.
9. Rumberger JA, Sheedy II PF, Breen JF, Schwartz RS. Coronary calcium, as determined by electron beam computed tomography, and coronary disease on arteriogram: effect of patient's sex on diagnosis. Circulation. 1995;91:1363–7.
10. Rumberger JA, Simons DB, Fitzpatrick LA, Sheedy PF, Schwartz RS. Coronary artery calcium area by electron-beam computed tomography and coronary atherosclerotic plaque area: a histopathologic correlative study. Circulation. 1995;92:2157–62.
11. Schmermund A, Baumgart D, Gorge G, et al. Measuring the effect of risk factors on coronary atherosclerosis: coronary calcium score versus angiographic disease severity. J Am Coll Cardiol. 1998;31(6):1267–73.
12. Kelly JL, Thickman D, Abramson SD, et al. Coronary CT angiography findings in patients without calcification. AJR Am J Roentgenol. 2008;191:50–5.
13. Glagov S, Weisenberg E, Zarins CK, et al. Compensatory enlargement of human atherosclerotic coronary arteries. N Engl J Med. 1987; 316:1371–5.
14. Vlodaver Z, French R, Van Tassel RA, Edwards JE. Correlation of the antemortem coronary arteriogram and the postmortem specimen. Circulation. 1973;47:162–9.
15. DeWood MA, Spores J, Notske RN, et al. Prevalence of total coronary occlusion during the early hours of transmural myocardial infarction. New Engl J Med. 1980;303:897902.
16. DeWood MA, Stifter WF, Simpson CS, et al. Coronary arteriographic findings soon after non-Q-wave myocardial infarction. New Engl J Med. 1986;315:417–23.

Chapter 9
Vulnerable Plaque

Masataka Nakano, Frank D. Kolodgie, Fumiyuki Otsuka, Saami K. Yazdani, Elena R. Ladich, and Renu Virmani

The concept of atheromatous progression initially described in the early 1980s by the laboratory of Velican and colleagues focused on morphologic characterizations of coronary lesions ranging from the fatty streak to lesions with lipid-rich cores and advanced plaques complicated by hemorrhage, calcification, ulceration, and thrombosis [1–3]. Another pioneering pathologist, Michael J. Davies, devoted himself to the study of plaque rupture, describing in detail the features of plaque disruption and role of inflammation in the development of lesion instability [4, 5].

Despite these early reports, an incomplete understanding remained of the relationship between lesion progression and acute coronary syndromes. This gap was later addressed by a team led by Dr. Stary [6, 7] in the mid-1990s under the auspices of the American Heart Association (AHA) consensus group. The outcome led to two seminal reports proposing a classification scheme in which lesions were grouped in six categories:

Type I: intimal thickening
Type II: fatty streak
Type III: transitional or intermediate lesion
Type IV: advanced atheroma with well-defined region of the intima
Type V: fibroatheroma or atheroma with an overlay of new fibrous connective tissue
Type VI: complicated plaques with surface defects, and/or hematoma-hemorrhage, and/or thrombosis

Alternative mechanisms of acute coronary thrombosis were not recognized since plaque rupture was considered the sole etiology of coronary thrombosis.

Using one of the largest established autopsy registries of sudden coronary death, our laboratory recognized early on that the AHA consensus nomenclature was incomplete. We have observed other initiating factors in acute coronary thrombosis, namely plaque erosion and nodular calcification [8]. This evidence prompted us to modify the widely accepted AHA classification scheme [8] (Figs. 9.1 and 9.2, Table 9.1). Accordingly, the numerical lesions I to IV were replaced by descriptive terminology inclusive of adaptive intimal thickening, intimal xanthoma, pathologic intimal thickening (PIT), and fibroatheroma, which we have further divided into entities of early and late fibroatheroma. Reference to advanced lesions under AHA criteria fitting types V and VI was discarded mainly because these lesions did not correspond to progressive plaques accounting for all etiologies of thrombosis (rupture, erosion, and calcified nodule) nor fully explain the relationship to plaques associated with stable angina. Moreover, this terminology also fails to address healing processes, which occur subsequent to a period of lesion instability and may contribute to severe luminal narrowing or symptomatic chronic total occlusion (CTO) occurring in about 30% of sudden coronary deaths.

M. Nakano, MD • F.D. Kolodgie, PhD • F. Otsuka, MD • S.K. Yazdani, PhD
• E.R. Ladich, MD • R. Virmani, MD (✉)
CVPath Institute, 19 Firstfield Rd, Gaithersburg, MD 20878, USA
e-mail: rvirmani@cvpath.org

Z. Vlodaver et al. (eds.), *Coronary Heart Disease: Clinical, Pathological, Imaging, and Molecular Profiles*,
DOI 10.1007/978-1-4614-1475-9_9,

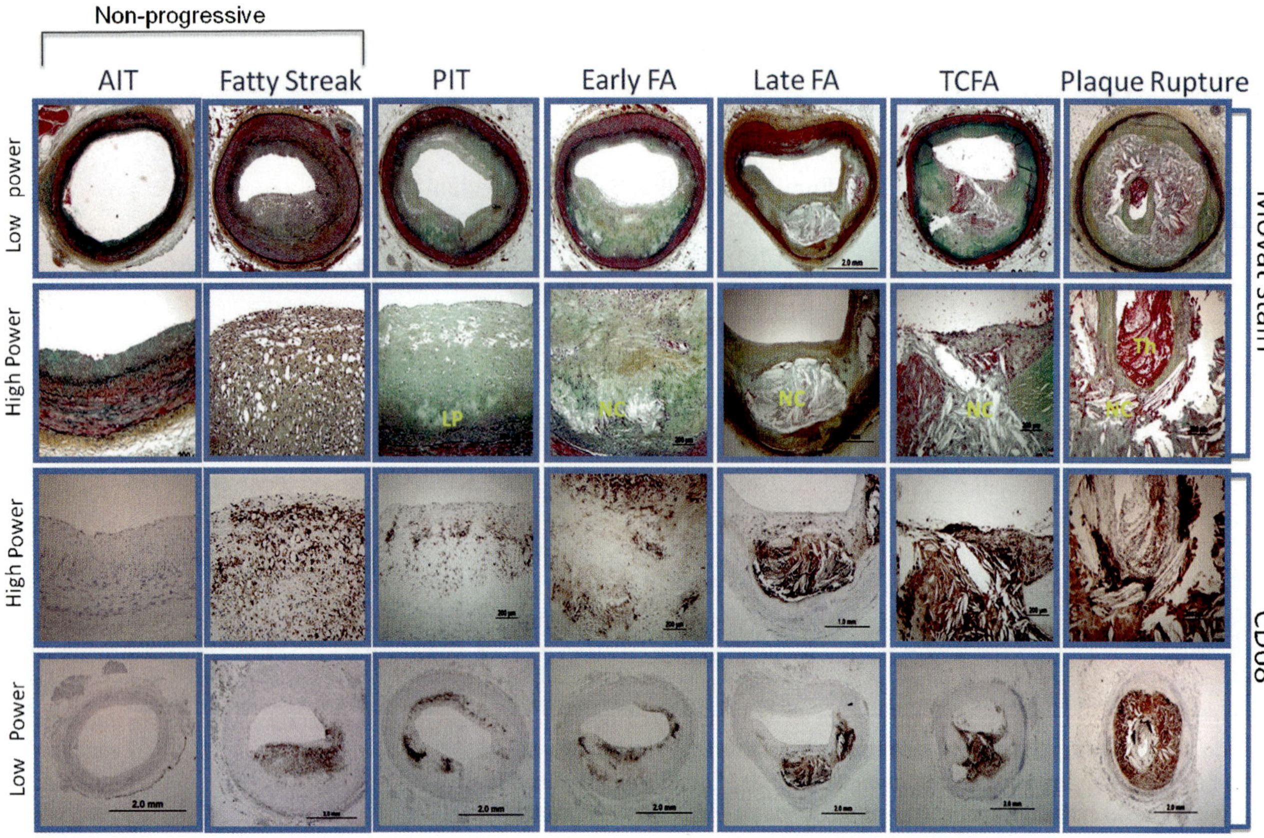

Fig. 9.1 Plaque morphologies consistent with the natural history of human coronary atherosclerosis. Upper two rows: modified Movat pentachrome staining; bottom two rows: CD68 staining as a marker of macrophage (*brown*).The two nonprogressive lesions are AIT and intimal xanthoma (foam cell collections known as fatty streaks, AHA type II). PIT (AHA type III, transitional lesions) is the first of the progressive plaques marked by an acellular lipid pool rich in proteoglycan, and inflammation, when present, is typically confined to the most luminal aspect of this plaque. Fibroatheromas (AHA type IV) are lesions with areas of necrosis characterized by cellular debris and cholesterol monohydrate. TCFA or vulnerable plaques (unrecognized by the AHA classification scheme) exhibit relatively large necrotic cores and thin fibrous caps. Plaque ruptures (AHA type IV) resemble TCFAs although differences include fibrous cap disruption and luminal thrombosis. Note that macrophages infiltrate and accumulate in lipid-rich necrotic cores as plaques progress. *PIT* pathological intimal thickening; *FA* fibroatheroma; *TCFA* thin-cap fibroatheroma; *LP* lipid pool; *NC* necrotic core; *Th* thrombus

Atheromatous Progression in Coronary Arteries (Table 9.1 and Fig. 9.1)

Intimal Thickening and Fatty Streaks

The earliest vascular change described microscopically is intimal thickening (AHA type I), which consists of layers of smooth muscle cells (SMCs) and extracellular matrix. It has been reported to occur in 35% of neonates, where the intima/media ratio at birth is 0.1 and increases progressively to 0.3 by 2 years of age [9]. Although intimal thickening is more frequent in atherosclerosis-prone arteries such as coronary, carotid, abdominal, iliac, and the descending aorta [10], the change is considered adaptive (nonatherosclerotic) because the SMCs exhibit a very low proliferative activity and show the antiapoptotic phenotype [11, 12].

The next category, termed the "intimal fatty streak" or "xanthoma" (AHA type II), includes lesions primarily composed of abundant macrophage foam cells interspersed with SMCs. Although this entity is referenced by AHA classification as the earliest of atherosclerotic lesions, from our experience and from reports of human and animal studies [13, 14], its development in the majority of cases is described as a reversible process with no progressive tendency. Many studies describe the complete regression of the intimal fatty streak [15–17]. The reasoning behind its spontaneous regression involving macrophage removal, however, remains largely uncertain.

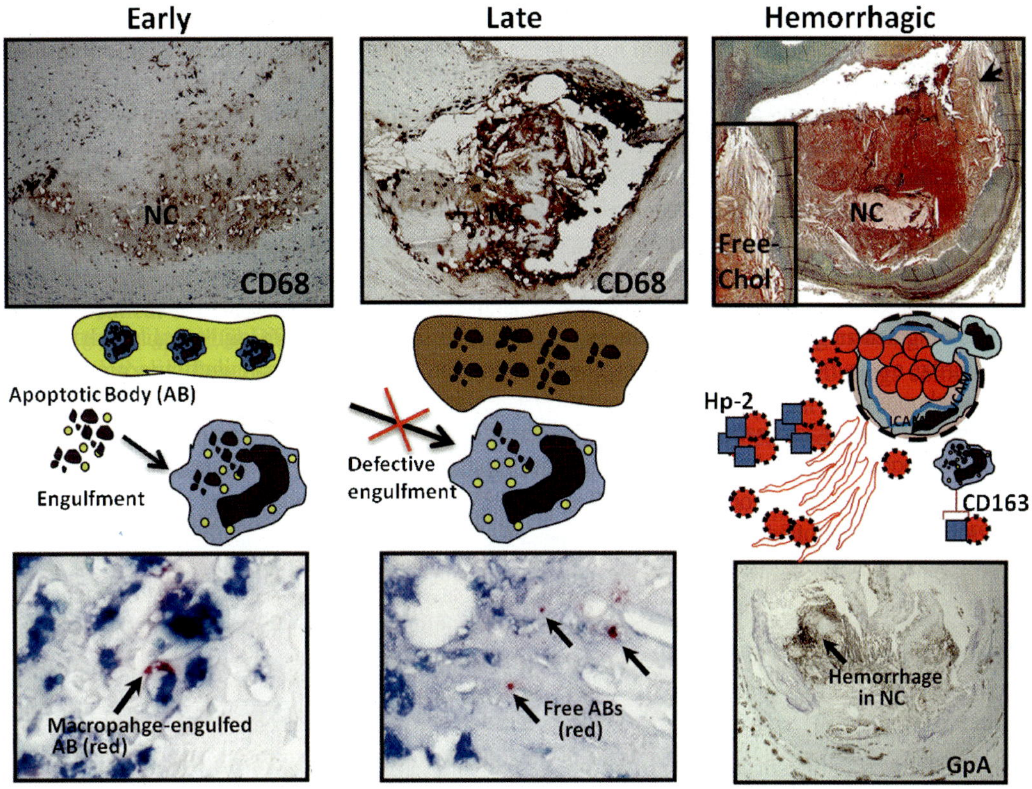

Fig. 9.2 Necrotic core expansion in human coronary plaques A lipid pool rich in proteoglycans is a hallmark that characterizes the early fibroatheroma where smooth muscle cell is generally absent (*left column*). Infiltrating macrophages engulfing apoptotic bodies (ABs) are identified within the necrotic core (NC). As the lesion advances, late necrosis is characterized by increased macrophage death and cell lysis, and loss of extracellular structure (*middle column*). In this case, free ABs are commonly observed, indicating the defective clearance (efferocytosis) by resident macrophages. Hemorrhage (*right column*) may promote the relatively rapid expansion of necrotic core where erythrocyte membranes provide free cholesterol (free-chol, *arrow*), which may cause secondary inflammation. Resident macrophages are capable of removing hemoglobin-haptoglobin complexes via the CD163 receptor, although the efficiency of this mechanism is likely compromised as well. *ER* endoplasmic reticulum; *free-chol* free cholesterol; *Hp-2* haptoglobin protein type 2 allele; *ICAM* intercellular adhesion molecule; *NC* necrotic core; *VCAM* vascular cell adhesion molecule

Pathologic Intimal Thickening

The earliest of progressive lesions recognized by our group is called PIT (AHA type III). These lesions are primarily composed of layers of SMCs aggregated near the lumen with an underlying lipid pool existing as a relatively acellular area rich in hyaluronan and proteoglycans (mainly versican) [8]. Studies have shown an affinity between the composition in the lipid pool and plasma lipoprotein, which suggests that the accumulation of extracellular lipid likely originates from the influx of plasma lipoprotein particles [18, 19]. Moreover, structural changes in the glycosaminoglycan chain of proteoglycans may represent an initial proatherogenic step that facilitates the binding and retention of atherogenic lipoproteins [20, 21].

Another important hallmark of PIT is the variable accumulation of macrophages at the adluminal aspect of the plaque (outside the lipid pool), although this does not occur in all cases. Lesions demonstrating PIT with accumulated macrophages are considered a more advanced stage as demonstrated by Nakashima et al. in their study of early plaque progression in coronary arteries near branch points [20]. The precise nature of why macrophages focally accumulate in lesions of PIT is not fully understood, although the expression of selected proteins within lipid pools may play a role.

In addition, lesions with PIT exhibit varying degrees of free cholesterol represented by empty, fine crystalline structures that accumulate within lipid pools. Although it was formerly assumed that free cholesterol was derived from dead foam cells, this is rather unlikely in the case of PIT because the majority of macrophages are confined to the more luminal aspect of the plaque. Alternatively, cholesterol monohydrate may form from the membranes of apoptotic SMCs [22], perhaps induced by the accumulation of oxidized lipids retained in the plaque. However, proof supporting this mechanism remains speculative. Apoptotic SMCs within lipid pools are recognized by membrane remnants (cages of basal lamina) and the presence of microcalcification [23, 24].

Table 9.1 Modified AHA consensus classification based on morphologic description

	Description	Thrombosis
No atherosclerotic intimal lesions		
Intimal thickening	Normal accumulation of smooth muscle cells (SMCs) in the intima in the absence of lipid or macrophage foam cells	Absent
Intimal xanthoma	Superficial accumulation of foam cells without a necrotic core or fibrous cap. Based on animal and human data, such lesions usually regress	Absent
Progressive atherosclerotic lesions		
Pathologic intimal thickening	SMC-rich plaque with proteoglycan matrix and focal accumulation of extracellular lipid	Absent
Fibrous cap atheroma	Early necrosis: focal macrophage infiltration into areas of lipid pools with an overlying fibrous cap	Absent
	Late necrosis: loss of matrix and extensive cellular debris with an overlying fibrous cap	
Thin-cap fibroatheroma	A thin fibrous cap (<65 μm) infiltrated by macrophages and lymphocytes with rare or absence of SMCs and relatively large underlying necrotic core. Intraplaque hemorrhage/fibrin may be present	Absent
Lesions with acute thrombi		
Plaque rupture	Fibroatheroma with cap disruption; the luminal thrombus communicates with the underlying necrotic core	Occlusive or nonocclusive
Plaque erosion	Plaque composition, as above; no communication of the thrombus with necrotic core. Can occur on a plaque substrate of pathologic intimal thickening or fibroatheroma	Usually nonocclusive
Calcified nodule	Eruptive (shedding) of calcified nodule with an underlying fibrocalcific plaque with minimal or absence of necrosis	Usually nonocclusive
Lesions with healed thrombi		
Fibrotic (without calcification) Fibrocalcific (±necrotic core)	Collagen-rich plaque with significant luminal stenosis. Lesions may contain large areas of calcification with few inflammatory cells and absence of necrosis. These lesions may represent healed erosions or ruptures	Absent

Adapted from "Lessons from sudden coronary death: a comprehensive morphological classification scheme for atherosclerotic lesions" by Virmani et al. [8], p. 12xx

Fibroatheroma (Fig. 9.2)

Fibroatheromas are characterized by an acellular necrotic core, which is distinguished from lipid pool lesions of PIT, and represent a further progressive stage of atherosclerotic disease (AHA type IV) [8]. Our laboratory subclassifies fibroatheromas into those with either "early" or "late" necrosis because this distinction may enable us to provide mechanistic insight into how necrotic cores evolve. Early necrosis is recognized by macrophage infiltration into lipid pools, coinciding with a substantial increase in free cholesterol and breakdown of extracellular matrix. Lesions with early necrotic cores characteristically exhibit proteoglycans versican, and biglycan and hyaluronan, which are typically absent in late necrotic cores – presumably degraded by matrix proteases produced by macrophage. Notably, the majority of macrophages within the areas of necrotic core display features consistent with apoptotic cell death, although autophagic processes may also play a role [25].

The presence of free cholesterol is another discriminating feature of the late necrotic core and is partially attributed to apoptotic cell death of macrophages, in part regulated by *acyl-coenzyme A*: *cholesterol acyltransferase inhibitor* (ACATI) [26]. The death of macrophages in the setting of defective phagocytic clearance of apoptotic cells is thought to contribute to the further development of plaque necrosis [26, 27].

The contents of the necrotic core are contained by an overlying layer of fibrous tissue forming a distinct entity referred to as the "fibrous cap." The fibrous cap is critical to maintaining the integrity of the lesion and is subject to thinning prior to the onset of rupture as further discussed below.

Contribution of Intraplaque Hemorrhage

It is generally accepted that apoptotic macrophages contribute to the accumulation of free cholesterol in plaques [28]; however, it is entirely feasible that free cholesterol could be derived from other sources. Studies from our sudden cardiac death (SCD) registry show that hemorrhage into a plaque is commonly observed in cases of plaque rupture or severe coronary artery disease. Particularly in advanced, unstable plaques, red blood cell (RBC) membranes (recognized by the RBC-specific anion transporter, glycophorin A) are associated with accumulated free cholesterol, necrotic core enlargement, and secondary macrophage infiltration [29]. The membranes of red blood cells are enriched with lipid, constituting 40% of their weight and a free cholesterol content exceeding that of all other cell types [30]. Excess membrane cholesterol can phase separate and form immiscible membrane domains consisting of pure cholesterol arranged in a tail-to-tail orientation favoring crystal formation [31]. Presumably, the extent of accumulated erythrocytes incorporated into the plaque and abundant lipids, together with impaired phagocytic efficiency of macrophages, to effectively clean up red blood cells and other debris [32] would influence both the biochemical composition and size of the necrotic core.

Heme Toxicity and Subsequent Inflammation

Extravasated red blood cells could potentially serve as a potent proinflammatory stimulus capable of recruiting monocytes/macrophages into the plaque. The precise signaling pathways for the migration of inflammatory cells are not fully understood, but proteins in coagulated blood could contribute to inflammatory cell activation [33, 34]. Alternatively, the migration of macrophages may be promoted by yet-to-be-identified receptors on erythrocyte membranes, which can bind a wide array of chemokines in the blood, including monocyte chemotactic peptide-1 [35].

Hemorrhage into a plaque may result from leaky microvessels; surrounding macrophages transform into activated foam cells producing ceroid pigment and iron as a result of erythrocyte phagocytosis [36]. The inefficient clearance of erythrocytes following a hemorrhagic event may lead to oxidative damage and continued inflammation through the availability of excess free hemoglobin (Hb) [37]. Free Hb can also bind and inactivate nitric oxide (NO), a potent mediator of vascular homeostasis, through a deoxygenation reaction. Oxygenated hemoglobin and NO form methemoglobin and nitrate. A major defense mechanism against Hb toxicity is mediated by haptoglobin (Hp), an abundant serum protein whose major function is to bind excess Hb, which attenuates its oxidative and inflammatory potential [38]. In atherosclerotic plaques, the primary route for clearing the Hb-Hp complex involves the CD163 receptor expressed on immunosuppressive macrophages with M2 polarized phenotype [39, 40]. The amount and function of CD163 positive macrophages are likely related to the process of atherosclerotic progression and plaque vulnerability.

Vulnerable Plaque, Thrombosis (Fig. 9.3)

Thin-Cap Fibroatheroma

Thin-cap fibroatheromas (TCFAs), traditionally referred to as vulnerable plaques, morphologically resemble ruptured plaque, although they are discriminated by the lack of a luminal thrombus and disrupted fibrous cap [8]. TCFAs generally exhibit large necrotic cores with overlying thin, intact fibrous caps infiltrated by macrophages. Typically, few or no SMCs are present within a fibrous cap. The fibrous cap thickness as a measure of plaque vulnerability is pathologically defined to be ≤ 65 μm since mean measurement in the thinnest part of remnant cap from a relatively large series of ruptured plaques was 23 ± 19 μm, with 95% of the caps measuring <65 μm [41].

Despite similarities with rupture, TCFAs exhibit a trend toward smaller necrotic cores and, overall, less calcification. Cross-sectional luminal narrowing is also typically less in TCFAs while ruptures with occlusive thrombi generally show greater underlying stenosis than for lesions with nonocclusive thrombi [42]. Significant differences in cellular infiltration between TCFAs and ruptures include fewer cap macrophages and less accumulation of hemosiderin and prior intraplaque hemorrhage [43].

Plaque Rupture

The hallmark of plaque rupture is focal discontinuity of the overlying thin fibrous cap (mean thickness, 23 ± 19 μm) with a relatively large necrotic core and superimposed thrombus. The fibrous cap consists mainly of type I collagen with varying degrees of macrophages and lymphocytes, and very few, if any, alpha-actin-positive SMCs. The luminal thrombus often is platelet rich near the actual rupture site, giving a white appearance (white thrombus). In contrast, near the rupture site and at sites of propagation, the luminal thrombus is composed of layers of fibrin and red blood cells (red thrombus) seen at the proximal and distal ends of the thrombus.

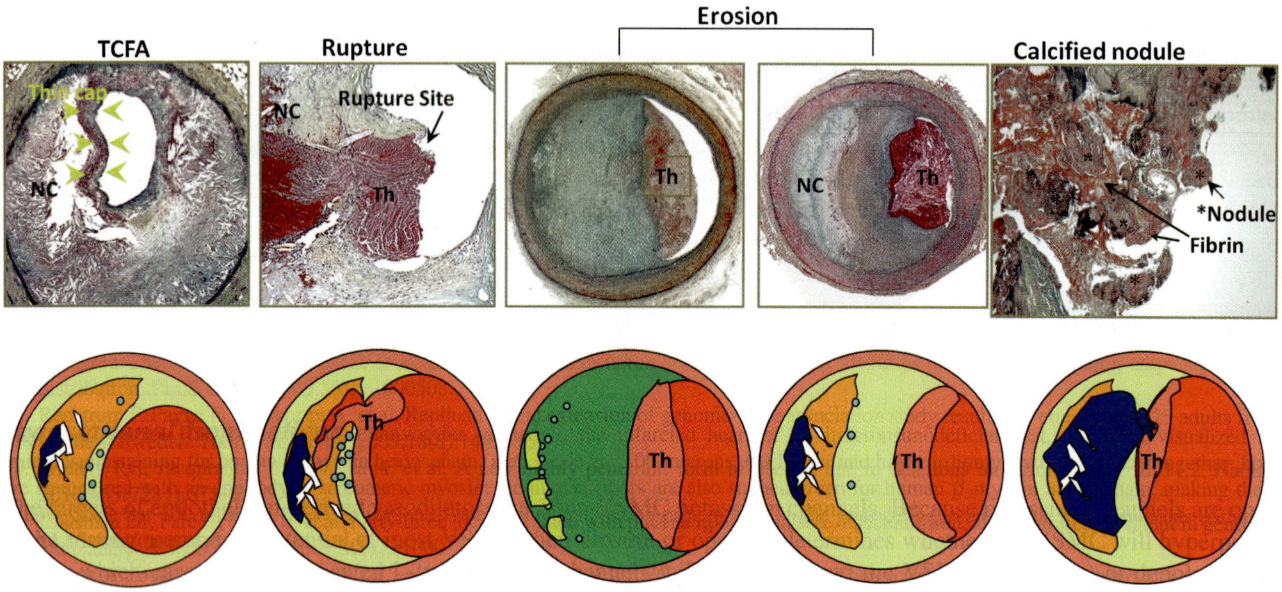

Fig. 9.3 Causative substrates of coronary thrombosis TCFAs are considered precursors to plaque rupture, the predominant substrate of coronary artery luminal thrombosis. Essentially missing from the AHA consensus classification are two alternative entities that give rise to coronary thrombosis, namely erosion and the calcified nodule. Erosions can occur on a substrate of PIT or FA while calcified nodules (a minor but viable mechanism of thrombosis) are eruptive fragments of calcium that protrude into the lumen causing a thrombotic event. *TCFA* thin-cap fibroatheroma; *PIT* pathological intimal thickening; *FA* fibroatheroma; *NC* necrotic core; *Th* thrombus

It is widely accepted that rupture occurs at a fibrous cap's weakest point, often near shoulder regions. In our experience, this is not always the case. We have seen an equal number of arteries (using serially cut sections) with ruptures at the mid-portion of the fibrous cap.

Although the underlying mechanisms of plaque rupture are poorly understood, several critical processes including matrix degradation by matrix metalloproteinases (MMPs) [44], high shear stress regions [45], stress branch points, macrophage death [46], and microcalcification and iron accumulation within the fibrous cap [47] are thought to play a role. Recent data is also revealing differentially expressed genes in stable and unstable atherosclerotic plaques. In a study by Papaspyridonos et al., transcriptional analysis revealed the differential expression of 18 genes associated with lesion instability inclusive of the metalloproteinase (ADAMDEC1), retinoic acid receptor responser-1, and cysteine protease legumain (a potential activator of MMPs and cathepsins) [48]. Moreover, Trp719Arg SNP allele in kinesin-like protein 6 (KIF6), a member of molecular motors involved in intracellular transport, showed a definite association with greater risk of coronary event and greater benefit from statin therapy in some recent clinical studies [49, 50]. Currently, several potential genes related to coronary events are being investigated by other groups, underscoring the clinical importance of deriving a comprehensive molecular model in the genesis and progression of unstable plaques [51, 52].

Plaque Erosion

Rupture of an atherosclerotic plaque had been uniformly accepted as the primary causative event in sudden coronary death [53]. This widely held paradigm was predicated on morphologic data from autopsy as well as angiographic studies in which the presence of surface irregularities was interpreted as plaque rupture [4, 54]. Meanwhile, in the mid-1990s, our laboratory described the occurrence of coronary thrombosis in the absence of rupture, but in the presence of plaque erosion. In a series of 20 patients who died with acute myocardial infarction, van der Wal et al. found plaque ruptures in 60% of lesions with thrombi, while the remaining 40% showed "superficial erosion." [55] In our series, reported by Farb et al., 50 consecutive cases of sudden death due to coronary artery thrombosis were studied by histology and immunohistochemistry; plaque rupture of a fibrous cap with communication of the thrombus with a lipid core was identified in 28 cases, while thrombi without rupture were present in 22 cases. All had superficial erosion of a proteoglycan-rich plaque [56]. In more recent studies, plaque erosion is identified as an important substrate for coronary thrombosis in patients dying from sudden death or acute myocardial infarctions (AMIs), with the occurrence being more frequent in women than men [57, 58].

Serial sectioning confirms that, with plaque erosion, the thrombus is confined to the luminal plaque surface with an absence of fissures or communication with an underlying necrotic core, as confirmed by serial sectioning. The term "erosion" is used because the luminal surface beneath the thrombus lacks endothelial cells. Other morphologic differences are clearly apparent between ruptures and erosion. Unlike the prominent fibrous cap inflammation described in ruptures, eroded surfaces contain fewer macrophages (rupture, 100%, vs. erosion, 50%; $p<0.0001$) and T lymphocytes (rupture, 75%, vs. erosion, 32%; $p<0.004$) [56, 59]. Cell activation, indicated by HLA-DR staining, was identified in macrophages and T cells in 25 (89%) plaque ruptures and in eight (36%) plaque erosions ($p=0.0002$). In addition, eroded plaques tend to be focal eccentric lesions rich in SMCs and proteoglycans, and unlike ruptures, the medial wall is generally intact. These distinctions show the need to reconsider the mechanistic differences of thrombosis between erosion and rupture, and perhaps requiring different strategies to diagnose and treat these lesions.

Calcified Nodule

Calcified nodules, the least frequent lesion associated with coronary thrombi, resemble mostly fibrotic plaques characterized by sheets of calcification that have fragmented into smaller amorphous nodules with surrounding fibrin. When present, the necrotic core is small in comparison to other atherogenic lesions. Resembling the tip of an iceberg, an eruptive nodule (often multiple and some with bone formation) is observed protruding into the lumen, accompanied by a nonocclusive platelet-rich thrombus. Deeper in the plaque, fibrin is often present between the bony spiculae, along with osteoblasts, osteoclasts, and inflammatory cells [8]. Lesions with nodular calcification and thrombosis are more common in older individuals, more likely seen in males, and are preferentially found in the middle right coronary or left anterior descending coronary arteries. They also appear to be more prevalent in the carotid arteries than coronary arteries, which may relate to a greater frequency of intraplaque hemorrhage in carotid disease.

End-Stage Lesions

Healed Plaque Rupture (Fig. 9.4)

The prevalence of silent ruptures in the clinical setting remains unknown to date; as few angiographic studies have demonstrated plaque progression, short-term studies have suggested that thrombosis is the likely cause. Autopsy studies, however, provide evidence that plaque progression beyond 40–50% cross-sectional luminal narrowing occurs secondary to repeat ruptures. Ruptured lesions with healed repair sites, designated as the healed plaque rupture (HPR) as shown by Davies et al., are easily detected microscopically by identifying breaks in the fibrous cap with an overlying repair reaction consisting of SMCs surrounded by proteoglycans and/or a collagen-rich matrix depending on the phase of healing [60]. Early healing following a coronary event is characterized by proteoglycans, along with type III collagen, which is eventually replaced by type I collagen. Davies showed that the frequency of HPRs increases in proportion with luminal narrowing [60].

Morphologic studies suggest that the incidence of HPRs is dependent on the underlying stenosis, such that approximately 8% of lesions with less than 20% diameter stenosis show HPRs with an increase in frequency to 19% for lesions with 21–50% luminal stenosis, and a further increase to 73% frequency for plaques with >50% stenosis. In our experience, approximately 61% of hearts from SCD victims show HPRs. The incidence is greater for deaths attributed to stable plaques with severe stenosis (80%), followed by acute plaque rupture (75%), and least for plaque erosions (9%) [61]. Overall, lesions with pathologic evidence of healed repair sites characterized by tissue layering were more common in arterial segments with acute and healed ruptures. In addition, the percent of cross-sectional luminal narrowing was dependent on the number of healed repair sites.

Incidence of Vulnerable Plaque in Sudden Coronary Death Victims

Among clinical parameters, the number of vulnerable plaques correlates with both high total cholesterol (TC) and the TC/high-density lipoprotein (HDL) cholesterol ratio [41]. In deaths attributed to plaque rupture, approximately 70% of cases show the presence of TCFAs remote from the actual rupture site. In contrast, the incidence of TCFAs is markedly less (30%) when deaths are associated with erosions or flow-limiting stenosis.

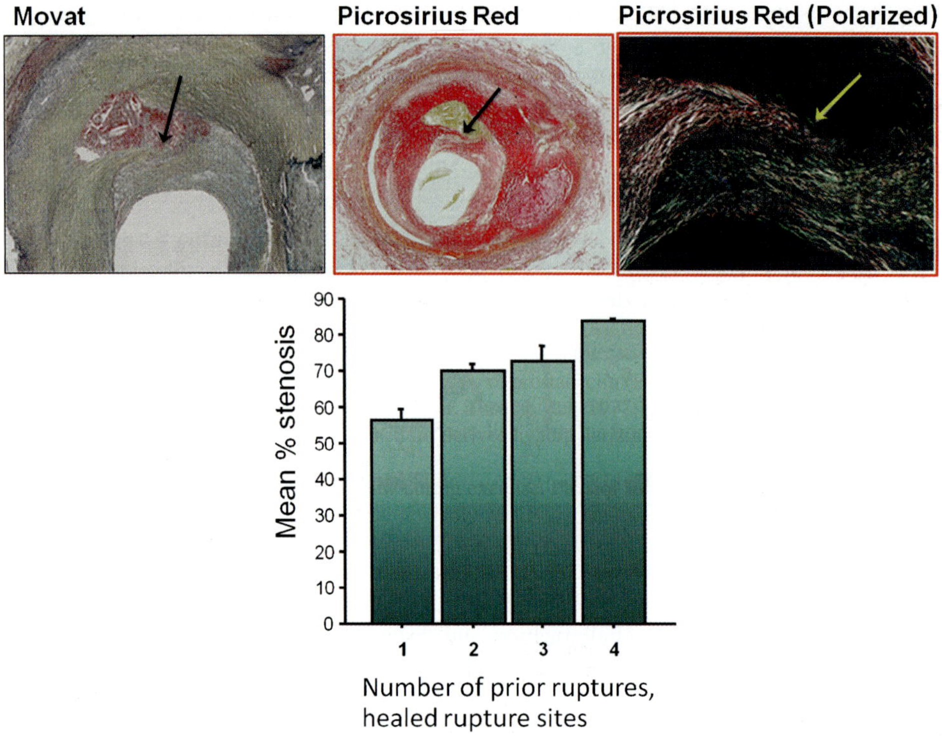

Fig. 9.4 Healed plaque rupture lesion with severe luminal narrowing (*upper-left column*) demonstrates areas of intraintimal, lipid-rich core with hemorrhage and cholesterol clefts, showing a relatively bland layer of collagenous, proteoglycan-rich neointima overlying on old disrupted fibrous cap (*arrow*). In the upper-middle column, collagen staining by picrosirius red illustrates an area of dark-red collagen (type I) surrounding lipid hemorrhagic cores seen in corresponding view in the left column. Image taken with polarized light (*upper-right column*) clearly delineates newer greenish collagen (type III) covering lighter reddish-yellow fibrous cap disruption (type I collagen). Bar graph at bottom shows that the lumen area narrows as the ruptured lesion heals. Adapted from "Healed plaque ruptures and sudden coronary death: evidence that subclinical rupture has a role in plaque progression" by Burke et al. [61], p. 9xx

The mere existence of TCFAs does not necessarily imply that plaque rupture is imminent. Yet it is essential to define the critical surrogates of lesion instability to help identify patients at the highest risk of rupture and future coronary events. In an analysis of vulnerable lesions from SCDs, the mean luminal stenosis was least for TCFAs (59.6% cross-sectional narrowing), intermediate for lesions with hemorrhage into a plaque (68.8%), and greatest for acute plaque or HPRs (~73%). Overall, nearly 75% of TCFAs showed <75% cross-sectional luminal narrowing (or <50% diameter stenosis), which may be a useful indicator of vulnerable plaque [62].

Moreover, the geographic location in the coronary vasculature is also important; about 50% of the TCFAs occur in the proximal segment of major coronary arteries in a distribution of LAD > LCx > RCA, with another one third occurring in the midportion and the remaining few distally [42]. Notably, a similar regional distribution of TCFAs is found for acute plaque rupture and HPRs. Clinical studies in acute myocardial infarction patients also confirm that the proximal portions of all three major coronary arteries are the most common location for thrombotic occlusion [63]. Positive remodeling represents another indicator of lesion vulnerability. In this regard, plaque ruptures had the highest remodeling index followed by lesions with hemorrhage, TCFAs, HPRs, and fibroatheromas, in order of descending incidence. Conversely, lesions of total occlusion or erosion exhibited negative remodeling [64].

Morphological Predictors of Vulnerable Plaque

In a more recent morphometric examination of TCFAs and ruptures based on luminal narrowing (<50, 50–75%, and >75%, Fig. 9.5), the incidence of TCFAs exhibiting underlying severe stenosis (>75% cross-sectional luminal narrowing) was 38%, while 51% exhibited a moderate stenosis (50–75% narrowing) and 11% showed mild narrowing (<50%). In contrast, the majority of ruptures, at 67%, showed severe stenosis (>75% cross-sectional luminal narrowing), 25% had moderate stenosis (50–75% narrowing), and 6% demonstrated mild narrowing (>50%). Regardless of the morphology, in a clinical setting,

a

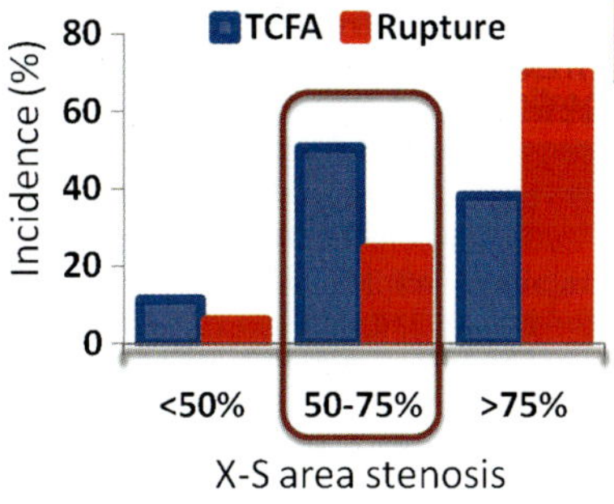

b

50-75% X-S stenosis group	Rupture (n=25)	TCFA (n=45)	P value
EEL, mm²	16.0 ± 5.9	13.8 ± 6.1	0.15
IEL, mm²	14.2 ± 5.6	12.2 ± 5.5	0.15
Lumen, mm²	5.0 ± 2.3	4.3 ± 2.1	0.22
Plaque Area, mm²	9.2 ± 3.6	7.9 ± 3.7	0.14
%Necrotic core	36 ± 22	21 ± 14	0.0007
%Calcified area	6 ± 10	4 ± 7	0.42
%Macrophages	8 ± 6	4 ± 4	0.010
Cap thickness, μm	25 ± 14	37 ± 19	0.0049

c

50-75% X-S stenosis group	P Value	Odds Ratio*	95% CI
Cap thickness	0.005	0.35	0.16 – 0.69
%Necrotic core	0.02	2.0	1.1 – 3.7
%Macrophages	0.052	1.8	0.99 – 3.2

*Adjusted by standard deviations

Fig. 9.5 Histomorphologic comparison of plaque rupture vs. thin-cap fibroatheroma (TCFA). (**a**) The frequency of plaque ruptures and TCFAs is stratified according to cross-sectional (X-S) luminal-area stenosis where TCFAs with 50–75% X-S stenosis account for 52% of lesions compared to only 25% of ruptures. (**b**) Morphometric parameters of plaque rupture and TCFA subgrouped by lesions with 50–75% stenosis. For the most part, morphologic parameters for TCFAs were similar to rupture; however, significant differences were noted for the necrotic core area (%) and fibrous cap thickness, while macrophage infiltration was of borderline significance. (**c**) Multivariate logistic regression analysis of histological measurements confirmed fibrous cap thickness as the best indicator of rupture, followed by percent of necrotic core area, and least for macrophages. *EEL* external elastic lumina; *IEL* internal elastic lumina; *CI* confidence interval

patients with plaques with >75% stenosis will likely present with symptoms or be treated by invasive procedures, thereby removing the potential risk for rupture. Moreover, TCFAs with <50% stenosis generally have less necrotic contents and are remotely considered to be responsible for clinical events, even if they were to rupture. Therefore, these results suggest that many TCFAs potentially amenable to preventive treatment are in the target stenosis range of 50–75%.

In select TCFAs and ruptures with 50–75% cross-sectional luminal narrowing, multivariate analysis showed fibrous cap thickness (odds ratio [OR] 0.35, $p=0.005$) and necrotic core (%) (OR 2.0, $p=0.02$) to be independent surrogates of rupture, while macrophage infiltration (%) was of borderline significance (OR 1.8, $p=0.052$). Other morphologic parameters such as area measurements (EEL, IEL, lumen, plaque) or calcification (%) did not achieve statistical significance. Thus, it is important to not only identify lesions with <75% narrowing but also recognize those with thinner fibrous caps, relatively large necrotic cores, and macrophage infiltration as these likely represent the highest risk for impending rupture. This strategy needs to be pursued in a clinical-based study of ACS patients using more sensitive imaging modalities such as optical coherent tomography (OCT) and/or assessment of lipid core burden using near-infrared spectroscopy (NIRS).

Summary and Perspectives

Plaque rupture is established as the primary cause of luminal thrombosis and sudden coronary death, although other important etiologies include erosion and eruptive nodular calcification. The detection of precursor lesions with the potential to rupture, including "vulnerable" plaques or even less-advanced fibroatheromatous lesions, represents an appropriate risk assessment for patients at risk for future coronary events. Morphologic and biologic processes critical to identifying vulnerable plaques have been described in this chapter, with some of these elements already proven applicable in the clinical setting.

To date, however, no clinical trials have confirmed the successful treatment of vulnerable plaque and reduction in cardiovascular mortality and morbidity. Progress will require refinements to current therapies or newer strategies with strict monitoring of all aspects of this epidemic disease. The pathophysiological features of progressive atherosclerosis as presented in this chapter are meant to guide future clinical trials focused on lesion vulnerability and risk for acute coronary syndrome.

References

1. Velican C, Velican D. Discrepancies between data on atherosclerotic involvement of human coronary arteries furnished by gross inspection and by light microscopy. Atherosclerosis. 1982;43:39–49.
2. Velican D, Velican C. Atherosclerotic involvement of the coronary arteries of adolescents. Atherosclerosis. 1982;43:39–49.
3. Velican D, Velican C. Atherosclerotic involvement of the coronary arteries of adolescents and young adults. Atherosclerosis. 1980;36:449–60.
4. Davies MJ, Thomas A. Thrombosis and acute coronary-artery lesions in sudden cardiac ischemic death. N Engl J Med. 1984;310:1137–40.
5. Davies MJ. Stability and instability: two faces of coronary atherosclerosis. The Paul Dudley White Lecture 1995. Circulation. 1996;94:2013–20.
6. Stary HC, Blankenhorn DH, Chandler AB, et al. A definition of the intima of human arteries and of its atherosclerosis-prone regions. A report from the Committee on Vascular Lesions of the Council on Arteriosclerosis, American Heart Association. Arterioscler Thromb. 1992;12:120–34.
7. Stary HC, Chandler AB, Dinsmore RE, et al. A definition of advanced types of atherosclerotic lesions and a histological classification of atherosclerosis. A report from the Committee on Vascular Lesions of the Council on Arteriosclerosis, American Heart Association. Arterioscler Thromb Vasc Biol. 1995;15:1512–31.
8. Virmani R, Kolodgie FD, Burke AP, Farb A, Schwartz SM. Lessons from sudden coronary death: a comprehensive morphological classification scheme for atherosclerotic lesions. Arterioscler Thromb Vasc Biol. 2000;20:1262–75.
9. Ikari Y, McManus BM, Kenyon J, Schwartz SM. Neonatal intima formation in the human coronary artery. Arterioscler Thromb Vasc Biol. 1999;19:2036–40.
10. Nakashima Y, Chen YX, Kinukawa N, Sueishi K. Distributions of diffuse intimal thickening in human arteries: preferential expression in atherosclerosis-prone arteries from an early age. Virchows Arch. 2002;441:279–88.
11. Orekhov AN, Andreeva ER, Mikhailova IA, Gordon D. Cell proliferation in normal and atherosclerotic human aorta: proliferative splash in lipid-rich lesions. Atherosclerosis. 1998;139:41–8.
12. Imanishi T, McBride J, Ho Q, O'Brien KD, Schwartz SM, Han DK. Expression of cellular FLICE-inhibitory protein in human coronary arteries and in a rat vascular injury model. Am J Pathol. 2000;156:125–37.
13. Fan J, Watanabe T. Inflammatory reactions in the pathogenesis of atherosclerosis. J Atheroscler Thromb. 2003;10:63–71.
14. Aikawa M, Rabkin E, Okada Y, et al. Lipid lowering by diet reduces matrix metalloproteinase activity and increases collagen content of rabbit atheroma: a potential mechanism of lesion stabilization. Circulation. 1998;97:2433–44.
15. Velican C. Relationship between regional aortic susceptibility to atherosclerosis and macromolecular structural stability. J Atheroscler Res. 1969;9:193–201.
16. Velican C. A dissecting view on the role of the fatty streak in the pathogenesis of human atherosclerosis: culprit or bystander? Med Interne. 1981;19:321–37.
17. McGill Jr HC, McMahan CA, Herderick EE, et al. Effects of coronary heart disease risk factors on atherosclerosis of selected regions of the aorta and right coronary artery. PDAY Research Group. Pathobiological Determinants of Atherosclerosis in Youth. Arterioscler Thromb Vasc Biol. 2000;20:836–45.
18. Hoff HF, Bradley WA, Heideman CL, Gaubatz JW, Karagas MD, Gotto Jr AM. Characterization of low density lipoprotein-like particle in the human aorta from grossly normal and atherosclerotic regions. Biochim Biophys Acta. 1979;573:361–74.
19. Smith EB, Slater RS. The microdissection of large atherosclerotic plaques to give morphologically and topographically defined fractions for analysis. 1. The lipids in the isolated fractions. Atherosclerosis. 1972;15:37–56.
20. Nakashima Y, Fujii H, Sumiyoshi S, Wight TN, Sueishi K. Early human atherosclerosis: accumulation of lipid and proteoglycans in intimal thickenings followed by macrophage infiltration. Arterioscler Thromb Vasc Biol. 2007;27:1159–65.
21. Nakashima Y, Wight TN, Sueishi K. Early atherosclerosis in humans: role of diffuse intimal thickening and extracellular matrix proteoglycans. Cardiovasc Res. 2008;79:14–23.
22. Preston MR, Tulenko TN, Jacob RF. Direct evidence for cholesterol crystalline domains in biological membranes: role in human pathobiology. Biochim Biophys Acta. 2003;1610:198–207.
23. Kockx MM, De Meyer GR, Muhring J, Jacob W, Bult H, Herman AG. Apoptosis and related proteins in different stages of human atherosclerotic plaques. Circulation. 1998;97:2307–15.
24. Kolodgie FD, Burke AP, Nakazawa G, Virmani R. Is pathologic intimal thickening the key to understanding early plaque progression in human atherosclerotic disease? Arterioscler Thromb Vasc Biol. 2007;27:986–9.
25. Bao L, Li Y, Deng SX, Landry D, Tabas I. Sitosterol-containing lipoproteins trigger free sterol-induced caspase-independent death in ACAT-competent macrophages. J Biol Chem. 2006;281:33635–49.
26. Tabas I. Cholesterol and phospholipid metabolism in macrophages. Biochim Biophys Acta. 2000;1529:164–74.
27. Tabas I, Marathe S, Keesler GA, Beatini N, Shiratori Y. Evidence that the initial up-regulation of phosphatidylcholine biosynthesis in free cholesterol-loaded macrophages is an adaptive response that prevents cholesterol-induced cellular necrosis. Proposed role of an eventual failure of this response in foam cell necrosis in advanced atherosclerosis. J Biol Chem. 1996;271:22773–81.
28. Tabas I. Consequences of cellular cholesterol accumulation: basic concepts and physiological implications. J Clin Invest. 2002;110:905–11.
29. Kolodgie FD, Gold HK, Burke AP, et al. Intraplaque hemorrhage and progression of coronary atheroma. N Engl J Med. 2003;349:2316–25.
30. Yeagle PL. Cholesterol and the cell membrane. Biochim Biophys Acta. 1985;822:267–87.
31. Tulenko TN, Chen M, Mason PE, Mason RP. Physical effects of cholesterol on arterial smooth muscle membranes: evidence of immiscible cholesterol domains and alterations in bilayer width during atherogenesis. J Lipid Res. 1998;39:947–56.
32. Tabas I. Consequences and therapeutic implications of macrophage apoptosis in atherosclerosis: the importance of lesion stage and phagocytic efficiency. Arterioscler Thromb Vasc Biol. 2005;25:2255–64.
33. Davis GE. The Mac-1 and p150,95 beta 2 integrins bind denatured proteins to mediate leukocyte cell-substrate adhesion. Exp Cell Res. 1992;200:242–52.
34. Hynes RO. Integrins: versatility, modulation, and signaling in cell adhesion. Cell. 1992;69:11–25.

35. Darbonne WC, Rice GC, Mohler MA, et al. Red blood cells are a sink for interleukin 8, a leukocyte chemotaxin. J Clin Invest. 1991;88: 1362–9.
36. Kockx MM, Cromheeke KM, Knaapen MW, et al. Phagocytosis and macrophage activation associated with hemorrhagic microvessels in human atherosclerosis. Arterioscler Thromb Vasc Biol. 2003;23:440–6.
37. Kim-Shapiro DB, Schechter AN, Gladwin MT. Unraveling the reactions of nitric oxide, nitrite, and hemoglobin in physiology and therapeutics. Arterioscler Thromb Vasc Biol. 2006;26:697–705.
38. Graversen JH, Madsen M, Moestrup SK. CD163: a signal receptor scavenging haptoglobin-hemoglobin complexes from plasma. Int J Biochem Cell Biol. 2002;34:309–14.
39. Van den Heuvel MM, Tensen CP, van As JH, et al. Regulation of CD 163 on human macrophages: cross-linking of CD163 induces signaling and activation. J Leukoc Biol. 1999;66:858–66.
40. Boyle JJ, Harrington HA, Piper E, et al. Coronary intraplaque hemorrhage evokes a novel atheroprotective macrophage phenotype. Am J Pathol. 2009;174:1097–108.
41. Burke AP, Farb A, Malcom GT, Liang YH, Smialek J, Virmani R. Coronary risk factors and plaque morphology in men with coronary disease who died suddenly. N Engl J Med. 1997;336:1276–82.
42. Kolodgie FD, Burke AP, Farb A, et al. The thin-cap fibroatheroma: a type of vulnerable plaque: the major precursor lesion to acute coronary syndromes. Curr Opin Cardiol. 2001;16:285–92.
43. Arbustini E, Morbini P, D'Armini AM, et al. Plaque composition in plexogenic and thromboembolic pulmonary hypertension: the critical role of thrombotic material in pultaceous core formation. Heart. 2002;88:177–82.
44. Sukhova GK, Schonbeck U, Rabkin E, et al. Evidence for increased collagenolysis by interstitial collagenases-1 and –3 in vulnerable human atheromatous plaques. Circulation. 1999;99:2503–9.
45. Gijsen FJ, Wentzel JJ, Thury A, et al. Strain distribution over plaques in human coronary arteries relates to shear stress. Am J Physiol Heart Circ Physiol. 2008;295:H1608–14.
46. Kolodgie FD, Narula J, Burke AP, et al. Localization of apoptotic macrophages at the site of plaque rupture in sudden coronary death. Am J Pathol. 2000;157:1259–68.
47. Vengrenyuk Y, Carlier S, Xanthos S, et al. A hypothesis for vulnerable plaque rupture due to stress-induced debonding around cellular microcalcifications in thin fibrous caps. Proc Natl Acad Sci USA. 2006;103:14678–83.
48. Papaspyridonos M, Smith A, Burnand KG, et al. Novel candidate genes in unstable areas of human atherosclerotic plaques. Arterioscler Thromb Vasc Biol. 2006;26:1837–44.
49. Iakoubova OA, Sabatine MS, Rowland CM, et al. Polymorphism in KIF6 gene and benefit from statins after acute coronary syndromes: results from the PROVE IT-TIMI 22 study. J Am Coll Cardiol. 2008;51:449–55.
50. Iakoubova OA, Tong CH, Rowland CM, et al. Association of the Trp719Arg polymorphism in kinesin-like protein 6 with myocardial infarction and coronary heart disease in 2 prospective trials: the CARE and WOSCOPS trials. J Am Coll Cardiol. 2008;51:435–43.
51. Koch W, Schrempf M, Erl A, et al. 4G/5G polymorphism and haplotypes of SERPINE1 inatherosclerotic diseases of coronary arteries. Thromb Haemost. 2010;103:1170–80.
52. Doosti M, Najafi M, Reza JZ, Nikzamir A. The role of ATP-binding-cassette-transporter-A1 (ABCA1) gene polymorphism on coronary artery disease risk. Transl Res. 2010;155:185–90.
53. Falk E, Shah PK, Fuster V. Coronary plaque disruption. Circulation. 1995;92:657–71.
54. Ambrose JA, Winters SL, Stern A, et al. Angiographic morphology and the pathogenesis of unstable angina pectoris. J Am Coll Cardiol. 1985;5:609–16.
55. van der Wal AC, Becker AE, van der Loos CM, Das PK. Site of intimal rupture or erosion of thrombosed coronary atherosclerotic plaques is characterized by an inflammatory process irrespective of the dominant plaque morphology. Circulation. 1994;89:36–44.
56. Farb A, Burke AP, Tang AL, et al. Coronary plaque erosion without rupture into a lipid core. A frequent cause of coronary thrombosis in sudden coronary death. Circulation. 1996;93:1354–63.
57. Arbustini E, Dal Bello B, Morbini P, et al. Plaque erosion is a major substrate for coronary thrombosis in acute myocardial infarction. Heart. 1999;82:269–72.
58. Kramer MC, van der Wal AC, Koch KT, et al. Histopathological features of aspirated thrombi after primary percutaneous coronary intervention in patients with ST-elevation myocardial infarction. PLoS One. 2009;4:e5817.
59. Kolodgie FD, Burke AP, Farb A, et al. Differential accumulation of proteoglycans and hyaluronan in culprit lesions: insights into plaque erosion. Arterioscler Thromb Vasc Biol. 2002;22:1642–8.
60. Mann J, Davies MJ. Mechanisms of progression in native coronary artery disease: role of healed plaque disruption. Heart. 1999;82:265–8.
61. Burke AP, Kolodgie FD, Farb A, et al. Healed plaque ruptures and sudden coronary death: evidence that subclinical rupture has a role in plaque progression. Circulation. 2001;103:934–40.
62. Kolodgie FD, Virmani R, Burke AP, et al. Pathologic assessment of the vulnerable human coronary plaque. Heart. 2004;90:1385–91.
63. Wang JC, Normand SL, Mauri L, Kuntz RE. Coronary artery spatial distribution of acute myocardial infarction occlusions. Circulation. 2004; 110:278–84.
64. Burke AP, Kolodgie FD, Farb A, Weber D, Virmani R. Morphological predictors of arterial remodeling in coronary atherosclerosis. Circulation. 2002;105:297–303.

Chapter 10
Genetics and Coronary Heart Disease

Jennifer L. Hall, Ryan J. Palacio, and Eric M. Meslin

Coronary Heart Disease

The prevalence of coronary heart disease (CHD) in the USA is estimated at 16.8 million or approximately 5.5% of the population. The lifetime risk of developing CHD after age 40 is about 49% for men and 32% for women [2]. In 2009, it was estimated that 1.26 million Americans would have a coronary event that year, 785,000 individuals would experience their first heart attack, and 470,000 would develop a recurrent attack [1].

The National Center for Health Statistics determined that the average life expectancy for individuals would increase by almost 7 years if all forms of major cardiovascular disease (CVD) were eliminated [1]. In comparison, if all major forms of cancer were eliminated, the gain is estimated to be 3 years [1].

Table 10.1 lists the risks for CHD relative to risk of other CVD as well as other diseases in general. The lifetime risk of atrial fibrillation (AF), for example, is one in four for both men and women. The lifetime risk of developing hypertension – a risk factor for CVD – is 9 in 10 for men and women. By contrast, the lifetime risk of hip fracture is 1 in 20 for men and 1 in 6 for women.

Significance of Family History

A family history of premature parental CHD has been shown to be associated with a twofold increased risk of CVD – independent of other risk factors [3, 4]. Additionally, while traditional risk factors are important, rare and common genetic variations have been estimated to account for more than 50% of a patient's susceptibility to CAD [5].

Evidence supporting a role for family history in premature parental CHD is shown in Table 10.2. This table illustrates the odds ratios for offspring cardiovascular events over 8 years associated with premature parental CVD, using data from the Framingham Heart Study (FHS) [3] (premature CVD was defined as an event prior to age 55 in men and age 65 in women [3]). Attributable risk percentages for premature parental CVD were estimated at 29.0 and 20.6% in men and women, respectively [3]. Additional evidence supporting a role for family history as a risk factor for CVD is strong [6–23].

Translating this knowledge into better patient care involves understanding the variability in patients' accurate assessment of their family history. In 1999, Bensen et al. surveyed more than 3,000 middle-aged Americans from four US communities [24]. These probands were asked to report on disease presence, including CHD, diabetes, hypertension, and asthma in more than 10,000 living family relatives (parents, siblings, and spouses) [24]. Using surveys completed by relatives about their own history of disease as standards, the proband sensitivity of disease knowledge was calculated. The probands had at least 81% accuracy in reporting a family history of CHD but were much less accurate (77–39%) in reporting the presence of

J.L. Hall, PhD (✉)
Department of Medicine, Lillehei Heart Institute, University of Minnesota, Minneapolis, MN, USA
e-mail: jlhall@umn.edu

R.J. Palacio, BA
Department of Anesthesiology, University of Minnesota Medical School, Minneapolis, MN, USA

E.M. Meslin, PhD
Indiana University School of Medicine, Indianapolis, IN, USA

Z. Vlodaver et al. (eds.), *Coronary Heart Disease: Clinical, Pathological, Imaging, and Molecular Profiles*,
DOI 10.1007/978-1-4614-1475-9_10, © Springer Science+Business Media, LLC 2012

Table 10.1 Risks for coronary heart disease relative to cardiovascular diseases and any other disease among men and women free of disease at 40 and 70 years of age

	Remaining lifetime risk at age 40		Remaining lifetime risk at age 70	
Diseases	Men	Women	Men	Women
Any CVD[a]	2 in 3	>1 in 2	>1 in 2	1 in 2
CHD [45]	1 in 2	1 in 3	1 in 3	1 in 4
AF [46]	1 in 4	1 in 4	1 in 4	1 in 4
CHF [47]	1 in 5	1 in 5	1 in 5	1 in 5
Stroke [48]	1 in 6[b]	1 in 5[b]	1 in 6	1 in 5
Dementia [48]	…	…	1 in 7	1 in 5
Hip fracture [58]	1 in 20	1 in 6	…	…
Breast cancer [59, 61]	1 in 1,000	1 in 8	…	1 in 14
Prostate cancer [59]	1 in 6	…	…	…
Lung cancer [59]	1 in 12	1 in 17	…	…
Colon cancer [59]	1 in 16	1 in 17	…	…
Diabetes [62]	1 in 3	1 in 3	1 in 9	1 in 7
Hypertension [63]	9 in 10[b]	9 in 10[b]	9 in 10[c]	9 in 10[c]
Obesity [64]	1 in 3	1 in 3	…	…

… indicate not estimated; *AF* atrial fibrillation

Adapted from Lloyd-Jones et al. [55], p. e24. Copyright 2010 by American Heart Association

[a]Personal communication from Donald Lloyd-Jones, based on FHS data

[b]Age 55

[c]Age 65

Table 10.2 Risks for cardiovascular disease in offspring over an 8-year period as defined by the presence of parental cardiovascular disease

Model adjustment	None	Paternal CVD	Material CVD	Both	1 or both parents
Risk for offspring male					
Unadjusted	1.0	3.0 (1.7–5.0)	3.4 (2.1–5.6)	3.3 (1.2–9.0)	3.2 (2.1–5.0)
Age adjusted	1.0	2.7 (1.6–4.7)	2.4 (1.5–4.0)	3.1 (1.1–8.3)	2.6 (1.7–4.1)
Age and SBP and anthperensive therapy	1.0	2.5 (1.4–4.3)	2.2 (1.3–3.7)	2.7 (1.0–7.6)	2.4 (1.5–3.8)
Age and total/HDL cholesterol ratio	1.0	2.8 (1.6–4.9)	2.1 (1.2–3.4)	2.9 (1.1–8.1)	2.3 (1.5–3.7)
Age and smoking	1.0	2.4 (1.4–4.1)	2.2 (1.4–3.7)	2.8 (1.0–7.5)	2.4 (1.5–3.8)
Age and diabetes and body mass index	1.0	2.5 (1.4–4.3)	2.2 (1.3–3.7)	2.7 (1.0–7.5)	2.4 (1.5–3.8)
Multivariable-adjusted[a]	1.0	2.2 (1.2–3.9)	1.7 (1.0–2.9)	2.4 (0.9–6.8)	2.0 (1.2–3.1)
Risk for offspring male					
Unadjusted	1.0	2.7 (1.3–5.8)	3.2 (1.7–6.0)	4.3 (1.2–15)	2.9 (1.6–5.3)
Age adjusted	1.0	2.8 (1.3–6.1)	2.3 (1.2–4.5)	4.1 (1.1–15)	2.3 (1.3–4.3)
Age and SBP and anthperensive therapy	1.0	2.3 (1.1–5.1)	1.9 (0.9–3.7)	3.1 (0.8–12)	1.9 (1.0–3.6)
Age and total/HDL cholesterol ratio	1.0	1.9 (0.8–4.3)	2.0 (1.0–3.9)	3.8 (1.1–14)	1.9 (1.0–3.6)
Age and smoking	1.0	2.8 (1.3–6.0)	2.3 (1.2–4.4)	4.5 (1.2–17)	2.3 (1.2–4.2)
Age and diabetes and body mass index	1.0	2.4 (1.1–5.3)	2.2 (1.1–4.3)	3.5 (1.0–13)	2.2 (1.2–4.1)
Multivariable-adjusted[a]	1.0	1.7 (0.7–3.9)	1.7 (0.8–3.4)	2.8 (0.7–11)	1.7 (0.9–3.1)

CI confidence interval; *CVD* cardovascular disease; *HDL* high-density ipoprotein; *OR* odds ratio; *SBP* systollic blood pressure

Adapted from Lloyd-Jones et al. [3]. Copyright 2004 by the American Medical Association

[a]Adjusted for age, total: HDL cholesterol ratio, SBP, antihypertensive therapy, diabetes body mass index and current smoking

diabetes, hypertension, and asthma [24]. Of note, with variation of proband age, gender, and disease status, these individuals were able to easily identify disease in spouses but were unable to articulate the same in parents and siblings [24].

An analysis in 2004 found conflicting results with Bensen et al.'s, concluding that few individuals in the USA are aware of specific health information needed to complete a family history [25]. Thus, whether or not patients are accurately reporting family history is still debatable. Whether or not clinicians are including family history as part of the equation in treating patients is also debatable.

The inability of some patients to properly assess family disease history illustrates an all-too-common problem in medicine and other disciplines; important advances in research are not translated to practice. www.hhh.umn.edu/people/bcrosby/pdf/cv.pdf (p. 7): "Rethinking Leadership," with Robert Terry, in *Common Good: Ideas from the Humphrey Institute,* (John Brandl, ed. Minneapolis: Hubert H. Humphrey Institute of Public Affairs, 2006.). In policymaking – in essence, the relationship between health-care provider and patient – it is essential to devise arrangements for the involved parties to do whatever it takes to manage responsibilities and accomplish desired goals. When the goal is to reduce CHD, a patient may simply not understand or know his/her family history, and thus, providers lose a large and potentially valuable clinical tool.

Genetics and CHD

Genetics may provide an unbiased approach to fill this gap in family history and provide more information for both doctors and patients. Utilizing genetics shifts the emphasis from reaction to prevention. Genetic tests in the clinic in the setting of CHD also raise new ethical concerns.

How does the field of genetics impact our current understanding of CHD? The genetic code was discovered in 1967. The Human Genome Project began in 1989 to map what was then thought to be 100,000 genes of the human genome on individual chromosomes. The first drafts of the human genome were published in 2001 [26–28].

This project and similar large, collaborative efforts have resulted in continued evolution and advancement of the field while reducing the costs to sequence DNA. This led to genome-wide analysis of large numbers of individuals with CHD compared to individuals without disease. The studies involved isolating and hybridizing DNA to a chip or array platform to identify differences within the DNA that were associated with CHD. A limited number of variants in genes associated with increased risk of CHD have been identified and replicated to date. The human genome project has also increased our understanding of how genetics alters the efficacy of anticoagulant therapy and platelet inhibitors in individuals.

In contrast to genome-wide association studies (GWAS), more recent studies have focused on DNA sequencing of individual patient genomes. A recent foray into individual DNA sequencing was published about a 40-year-old man with a family history of coronary artery disease and sudden death [29]. After blood was collected, DNA was isolated from cells and sequenced [29]. This technology is different from a chip platform in that every individual base pair is identified along the length of the input material. Analysis of this sequence data revealed 2.6 million single nucleotide polymorphisms (SNPs) and 752 copy number variations (CNVs) [29]. Data analysis was divided into four areas: (1) variants associated with genes for mendelian disease, (2) novel mutations, (3) variants known to modulate response to pharmacotherapy, and (4) SNPs previously associated with complex disease.

Next, a medically relevant posttest probability of disease was calculated. From this, clinical risk of major diseases was calculated, as shown in Fig. 10.1 [29]. Three rare variants specific to CVD were identified and verified. Sixty-three clinically relevant pharmacogenomic variants were identified, and an assessment of SNPs previously associated with complex diseases

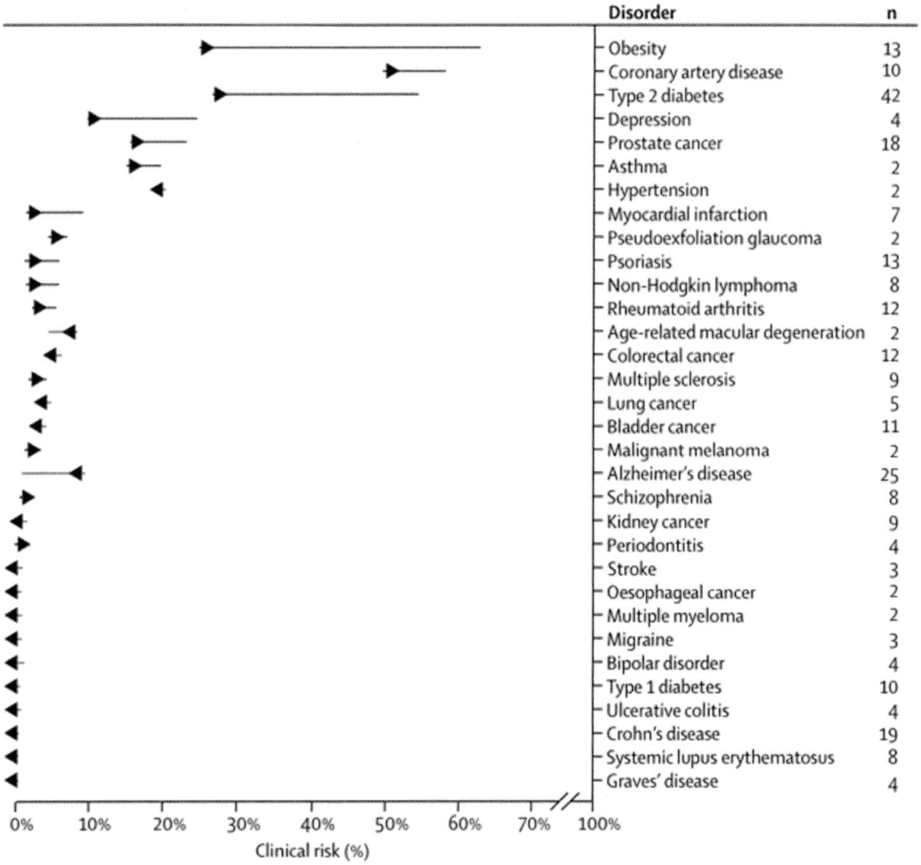

Fig. 10.1 Clinical risk incorporating genetic risk-estimates for major diseases. Adapted from Ashley et al. [29]. Copyright 2010 by [Elsevier Limited – ?]. FYI: Copyright holder based on: http://www.thelancet.com/popup?fileName=footer-terms

was analyzed and a posttest probability calculated. Overall, this approach integrated new ways to approach disease risk in a clinically relevant context to deliver to the patient. As noted below, a comprehensive database of rare mutations would be a helpful resource.

In summary, a patient's family history of CHD has been shown to be a major contributing risk factor to CVD independent of other risk factors. Unfortunately, many patients are unaware of familial disease history, and as a result, clinicians make health-care decisions without family history information. As the field of genetics continues to evolve and advance, and as the cost of individual genetic analysis continues to decrease [30] – with individual analysis perhaps becoming commonplace – genetics may provide an unbiased approach to fill a gap in family history and provide more information for both doctors and patients.

There is a critical difference between using genetics as a tool to provide increased information for diagnosing disease, and as a tool for predicting disease. Growing evidence shows that genetic testing in the clinic for identifying underlying causes of disease has been useful, especially to identify both novel, common, and rare variants associated with disease. Examples include DNA variants in genes associated with sudden cardiac death [31, 32].

By contrast, the use of genetics as a reliable predictor of common complex diseases has yet to be completely proven. Most associations between DNA variants and common diseases are weak and provide limited predictive power. Even if all genetic loci for a common disease were identified, it is believed that their predictive power would still be inadequate [29]. A recent study found that adding known genetic markers did not increase the ability to predict CVD in a prospective cohort of ~19,000 white women in the Nurses' Health Study [33]. Thus, current claims for the ability of genetics to be used for prediction of common diseases such as CHD are not proven and can be misleading to the general public. This difference is significant for another reason. By blurring this distinction, the hype of raised expectations threatens to skew conversations between clinicians and patients [34, 35].

Loci Associated with CHD

9p21.3

Independent of any standard risk factors, variations at the chromosome 9p21.3 have been shown to be associated with coronary artery disease [36–39]. Variants of 9p21.3 have not been shown to predict extent of coronary artery disease or myocardial infarction [39]. Nearly 25% of the population carries two copies of the risk alleles leading to an increased risk of early-onset coronary artery disease that is 2 times as high as the risk among persons who do not carry these alleles [5]. McPhearson et al. found numerous SNPs at the 9p21 locus, most of which were found within 58kB of 9p21.3, and were shown to increase risk of CAD 15–20% for 50% of Caucasian individuals heterozygous for the allele, and increase risk 30–40% in the 25% of individuals homozygous for the allele [37].

The ADVANCE study expanded these findings beyond US Caucasians and analyzed the role of three SNPs (rs10757274, rs2383206, and rs10757278) in CAD in US Caucasians, US East Asians, US Hispanics, and US African-Americans [40]. Although the study is underpowered to detect differences in African-Americans (with only one SNP with a statistically significant p value of 0.04), it provides an early sense of genetic variations within diverse ethnic groups (Table 10.3) [40].

Baudhuin observed the presence of seven SNPs in a 76-kb region around 9p21 that had $p<10^{-5}$ for major CHD and/or major CVD [41]. Abdullah et al. demonstrated that four SNPs within the 9p21 region were significantly ($p=6.61\times10^{-7}$ to 1.87×10^{-8}) associated with premature and familial myocardial infarction and CAD (average age of onset 40.3 ± 5.1 years) [42]. Samani et al. analyzed two GWAS while Schunkert et al. undertook a meta-analysis with seven case control studies and found that SNP rs1333049 was uniformly associated with CAD with an increased OR of approximately 1.20 and 1.24, respectively [38, 43]. Leander found that when 9p21 is combined with other loci, including 1p13.3, 2q36.3, and 10q11.21, these loci have a cumulative effect of increasing coronary artery disease by 15% [13].

Although the exact mechanisms through which 9p21.3 influences biological effects is unknown, Hannon and Beach revealed that the 3′ end of *CDKN2B* (9p21.3) encodes the cyclin-dependent kinase inhibitor p15INK4B. This particular tumor suppressor is a dependent kinase involved in cell cycle regulation and cell cycle arrest [44]. Another gene encoding a large antisense noncoding RNA (*ANRIL*) suggests that transcription of the cyclin-dependent kinase genes may be regulated, at least in part, by *ANRIL*, establishing another possible link of the functions of 9p21 to cell cycle regulation and arrest [45].

In summary, the data indicate a clear link between DNA variants of 9p21.3 and CHD. At this juncture however, the use of genetic testing for 9p21 in the clinic to improve medical decision-making is limited. It is unclear how one's genetic makeup at this locus can best be used to determine disease risk or change in treatment. Participants in the Women's Genome

Table 10.3 Risk of developing clinical coronary heart disease in carriers of high-risk alleles in 9p21 locus, compared with noncarriers in the ADVANCE study, as stratified by race/ethnicity

	Young		Older		Young and older combined					
	OR[a]	CI	OR[a]	CI	OR[a, b]	CI	OR[c] AG vs. AA	CI	OR[c] GG vs. AA	CI
White										
rs10757274	1.29*	1.02–1.65	1.27**	1.10–1.47	1.28***	1.13–1.45	1.23	0.99–1.52	1.72***	1.35–1.20
rs2383206	1.26	0.99–1.61	1.27**	1.10–1.47	1.27***	1.12–1.44	1.25*	1.00–1.56	1.69***	1.32–2.16
rs10757278	1.28	0.99–1.61	1.29**	1.12–1.49	1.28***	1.13–1.45	1.24**	1.01–1.53	1.72***	1.35–2.20
Black										
rs10757274	1.04	0.62–1.70	0.94	0.48–1.83	1.00	0.67–1.49	1.10	0.66–1.83	1.22	0.48–3.11
rs2383206	0.96	0.60–1.51	0.94	0.66–2.05	1.03	0.72–1.47	0.98	0.57–1.69	1.17	0.59–2.32
rs10757278	1.13	0.67–1.88	1.22	0.62–2.41	1.17	0.77–1.75	1.21	0.73–2.00	1.78	0.66–4.81
Hispanic										
rs10757274	1.31	0.55–3.22	1.95*	1.10–3.60	1.73*	1.07–2.85	2.02	0.92–4.42	2.70*	1.09–6.66
rs2383206	1.84	0.78–4.62	2.27*	1.27–4.22	2.12*	1.31–3.53	2.88*	0.22–6.77	3.96*	1.49–10.5
rs10757278	1.86	0.80–4.65	2.02*	1.15–3.66	1.97*	1.23–3.22	2.58*	1.18–5.62	3.04*	1.22–7.53
East Asian										
rs10757274	1.46	0.79–2.88	1.50	0.89–2.57	1.50*	1.0–2.26	1.66	0.80–3.44	2.57*	1.12–5.86
rs2383206	1.59	0.84–3.13	1.52	0.90–2.61	1.55*	1.03–2.35	1.69	0.81–3.51	2.80*	1.23–6.41
rs10757278	1.55	0.83–2.99	1.34	0.78–2.30	1.42	0.95–2.16	1.62	0.79–3.32	2.21	0.97–5.07
Admixed nonblack										
rs10757274	1.78*	1.05–3.10	0.97	0.61–1.55	1.27	0.89–1.8	1.78*	1.02–3.11	1.54[d]	0.80–2.95
rs2383206	1.49	0.84–2.60	0.86	0.54–1.38	1.08	0.75–1.54	1.24	0.68–2.27	1.26	0.64–2.47
rs10757278	1.81*	1.05–3.20	0.94	0.59–1.50	1.23	0.87–1.76	1.74	1.01–3.01	1.36	0.71–2.58
Admixed black[c]										
rs10757274	–	–	1.22	0.63–2.44	–	–	1.43[d]	0.66–3.10	0.44	0.13–1.51
rs2383206	–	–	1.28	0.68–2.44	–	–	1.79	0.77–4.15	0.88	0.32–2.41
rs10757278	–	–	1.70	0.82–3.78	–	–	1.35	0.63–2.89	0.98	0.24–4.10

Adapted from Assimes et al. [40]. Copyright 2008 by Oxford University Press
[a] Mean and standard deviation are presented
[b] Median and range presented, for all other variables counts and percentage are presented
[c] The age cutoff for a 'young case' was not the same for men (45 years) and women (55 years)
[d] Young cases may have had their qualifying coronary event as 1 January 1999, whereas all older cases had their qualifying coronary event after the start of recruitment in October 2001
[e] At event for cases, at study visit date for controls

Health Study with 9p21.3 variation did not have a modified, predicated risk when such a mutation was added to traditional risk factors [33].

Studies to date have not found genetic testing for 9p21 useful for predicting CHD. However, understanding the biological mechanism of 9p21.3 may enable the establishment of clinically useful tests that will provide better diagnostics and/or treatment options.

12p24, 3q22

High levels of white blood cells have been identified as independent risk factors for CHD and myocardial infarction [46–48]. Recent genetic studies have identified DNA variants that are risk factors for CHD and myocardial infarction, in particular the link to chromosome 12q24 – specifically, SNPs rs11066301 and rs11065987 [49]. Although the etiology is not well understood, the variants associated with 12q24 are responsible for regulating mean platelet volume and platelet count [49]. An additional hematological, chromosomal locus variation associated with increased CHD can be found on 3q22.3 MRAS [50]. Again, although the etiology is not well understood, the loci associated with 3p22 have a potential role in the processes of atherosclerosis.

As clinical indicators of heart care, measurements of white blood cells, red blood cells, and platelets continue to be used by physicians as clinical indicators for cancer and immune-related disorders. The HaemGen and Cohorts for Heart and Aging Research in Genome Epidemiology (CHARGE) consortia searched for genetic loci contributing to variation in hematological parameters, and to assess if these parameters are linked with disease outcomes [49, 51]. The approaches used by these consortia differed.

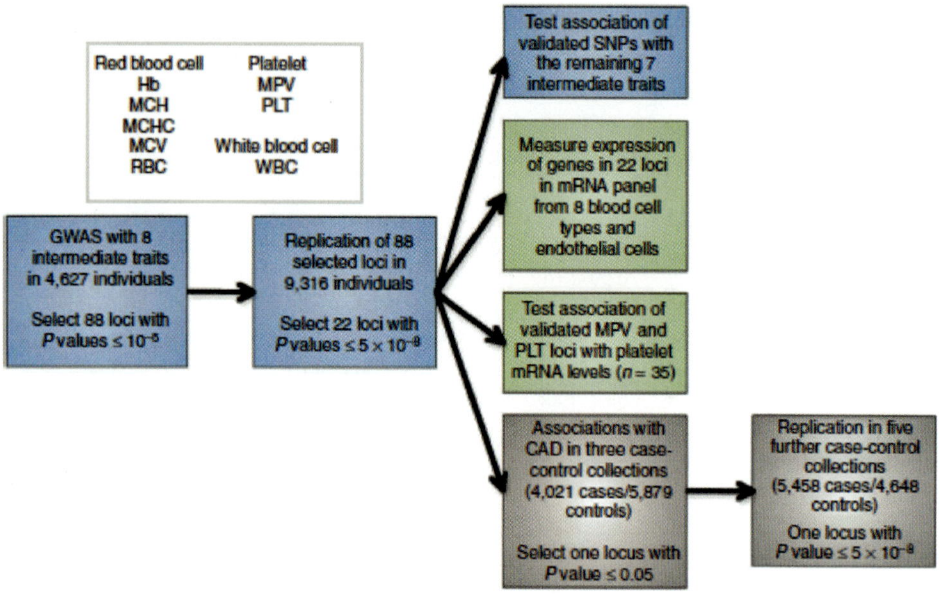

Fig. 10.2 Summary and overview of Soranzo et al. study design. Adapted from Soranzo et al. [49]. Copyright 2009 by [Nature Publishing Group – ?]. FYI: Presumed copyright holder is from: http://www.nature.com/reprints/index.html

The HaemGen consortium used one of the many next-generation strategies employed in the post-GWA era, which is illustrated in Fig. 10.2 [49]. The strategy included: (1) genomewide association (GWA) using multiple intermediate phenotypes (see white box in Fig. 10.2 for a table of intermediate phenotypes), (2) replication of selected loci, (3) testing association of validated SNPs with additional intermediate traits, (4) RNA analysis in blood cells and endothelial cells, (5) association with CHD, and (6) replication in five additional cohorts. The strengths of this approach are the power of a large consortium such as HaemGen and the multidimensional strategy described above. The outcome was the discovery of a long-range haplotype at 12q24 associated with CHD. This haplotype also contains known risk loci for type 1 diabetes, hypertension, and celiac disease.

Thus, the use of intermediate phenotypes led to successful identification of a region on chromosome 12q24 associated with CHD. Two SNPs were located ~800 kb apart and found to be high in LD in this region. (An overview of this region is shown in Fig. 10.3). This region contains 15 genes. An analysis of the mRNA expression data performed did not provide sufficient evidence to limit the pool of targets (Fig. 10.4).

The region covered by the haplotype includes other genes not assessed in this study which may play a causative role. Much remains to be explored. Previous work summarized in the literature showed that increased mean platelet volume is an independent predictor of postevent outcome in CAD [38, 49, 52–54]. These studies now move closer to defining mechanisms through which platelet volume may be unique in different individuals.

The CHARGE consortium used a more standard approach to identify DNA variants associated with erythrocyte phenotypes [51]. The consortium included five cohort studies, all of European ancestry. The SNPs identified in this first analysis were then brought forward for replication in the HaemGen consortium. The overlap of genes near the loci associated with the erythrocyte trait is shown in Fig. 10.5. The 12q24 region identified as being associated with CAD [50] was replicated in the study by Ganesh [51].

The associations of these SNPs were then tested for associations with systolic blood pressure (SBP), diastolic blood pressure, and hypertension. Analysis identified the previous associations on 12q24.1, with the nearest candidate gene being SH2B3 as the most significant. It also identified the association between the region on chromosome 7q36.1 with the nearest candidate gene being PPKAG2.

One locus on chromosome 3q22.3 has been implicated as having an association with CHD. SNP rs9818870 is found in the 3′ UTR of the MRAS gene [50]. The five exons in this region are responsible for coding the M-ras protein, a GTP binding protein, widely expressed in coronary vasculature.

In summary, studies have established a link between the immunologic system, hematologic system, and an increased risk of CHD. Specifically, mutations on or near loci 12q24 that regulate mean platelet volume and platelet count, as well as loci near 3q24, have a potential role in atherosclerosis. Although the genes and biology are not completely understood, further studies are needed for guiding treatment in a subset of patients.

Loci Associated with Modifiable Risk Factors for CHD

In the last 40 years, a shift has occurred in modifiable risk factors for CHD in the general population [55]. The prevalence of tobacco use has decreased, but high cholesterol and high blood pressure in the population have increased [55]. In addition, an increasing trend has been seen for obesity, type 2 diabetes, and high blood pressure in children [55]. How these changes

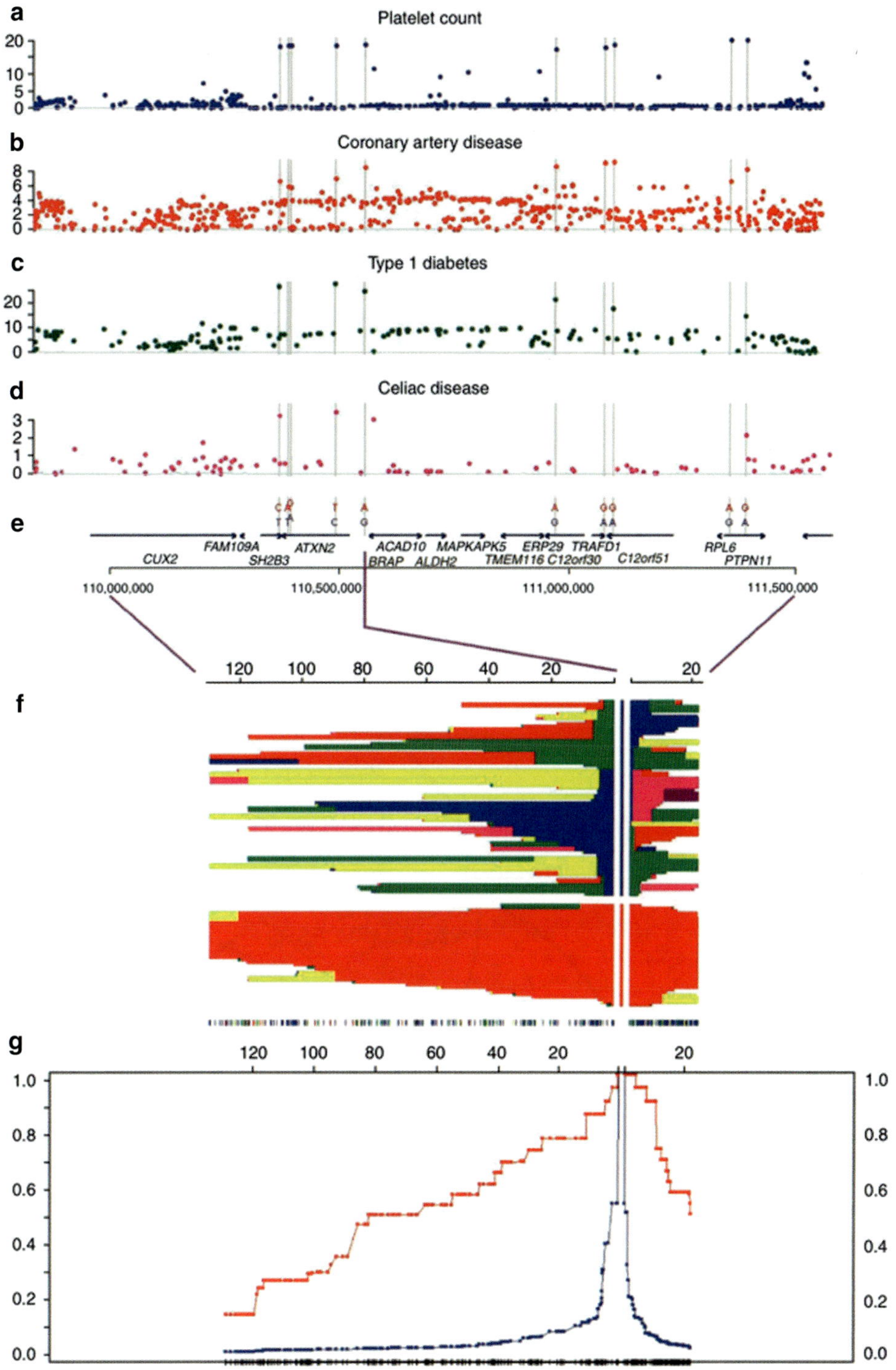

Fig. 10.3 Overview of the 12q24 region. (**a–d**) The $-\log_{10} P$ value for associations with plateiet counts (**a**), coronary artery disease (**b**), type 1 diabetes (**c**) and celiac disease (**d**) are shown for two consecutive recombination intervals in a 1.6-MB region on chromosome 12 (Build 36 pos 109,896,664–111,516,664). (**e**) The position of the 10 SNPs forming a high-frequency (MAF 40%) haplotype is highlighted by gray bars; this also displays the evolutionarly ancestral (*blue*) and derived (*red*) alleies at the 10 SNPs. (**f,g**) Signatures of positive selection obtained form Haplotter, including a graphical display of haplotypes at different distances form the lead SNP rs11065987 (**f**) and a plot marking the decay of extended haplotype homozygosity at different distances form SNP rs11065987 (**g**)

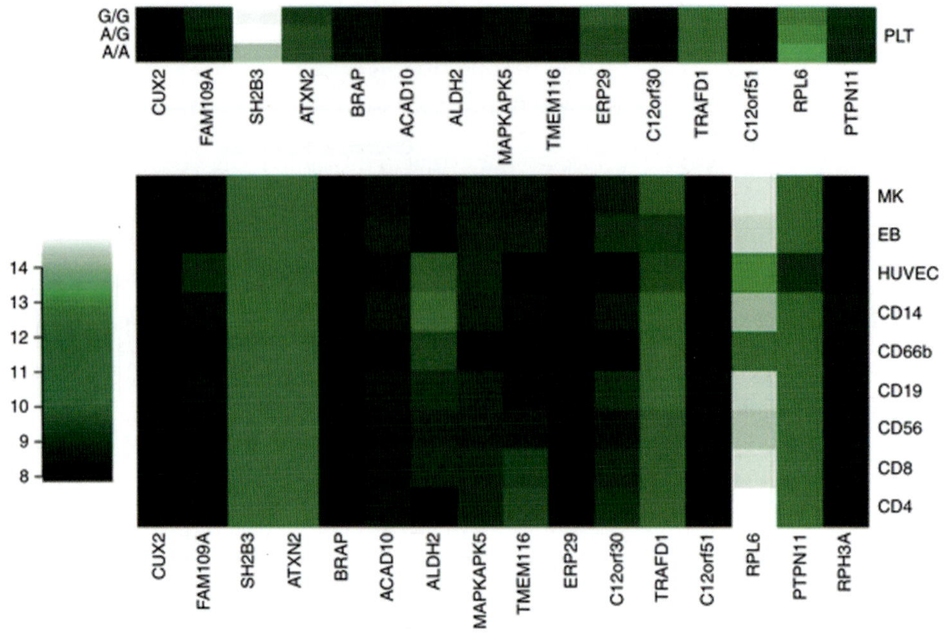

Fig. 10.4 Heat map of mRNA expression in the 12q24 region. Adapted from Soranzo et al. [49]. Copyright 2009 by Nature Publishing Group

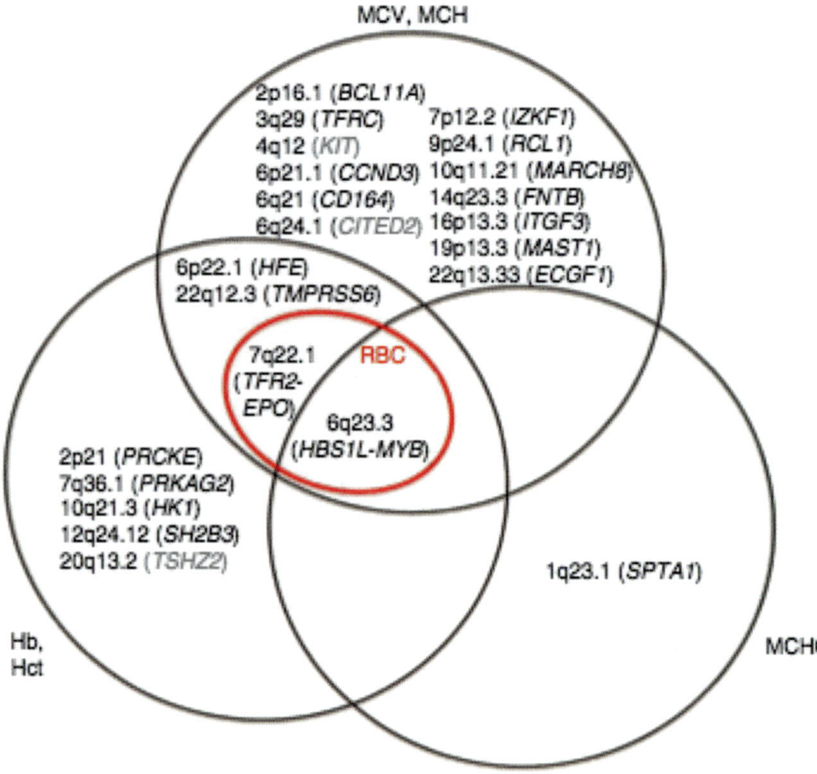

Fig. 10.5 Results of the CHARGE meta-analysis organized into a Venn diagram, demonstrating an overlap of loci meeting a genome-wide significance threshold of $p<5\times10^{-8}$. Adapted from Ganesh et al. [51]. Copyright 2009 by Nature Publishing Group

will alter the prevalence, onset, and treatment of CHD in the next 50 years remains unclear. These modifiable risk factors will also likely influence the underlying DNA. For example, if a child harbored a mutation in 9p21, and this child's diet resulted in obesity at a young age, this may modify the interaction of the mutation on CHD.

The American Heart Association's "Strategic Impact Goal through 2020 and Beyond" includes a construct for ideal cardiovascular health [55] (see Table 10.4). This construct lists seven components: smoking status, body mass index, physical activity, healthy diet score, total cholesterol, blood pressure, and fasting plasma glucose [55]. Four of these seven factors are hereditary: body mass index [55–58], total cholesterol [59–63], blood pressure [51, 64–66], and fasting plasma glucose [67]. A list of the loci identified to date that are associated with fasting plasma glucose, cholesterol and lipids, blood pressure, and BMI is listed in Table 10.5. This list is not meant to be exhaustive, but to highlight many of the major DNA variants identified to date in replicated studies with large cohorts.

Table 10.4 Definitions of poor, intermediate, and ideal cardiovascular health for each metric, along with NHANES 2005–2006 unadjusted prevalence estimates for the American Heart Association's goals for 2020

	Poor health		Intermediate health		Ideal health	
Goal/metric	Definition	Prevalence,%	Definition	Prevalence,%	Definition	Prevalence,%
Current smoking						
Adults >20 year of age	Yes	24	Former ≤12 month	3	Never or quit >12 month	73 (51 never; 22 former >12 month)
Children 12–19 year of age	Tried prior 30days	17			Never tried; never smoked whole cigarette	83
Body mass index						
Adults >20 year of age	≥30 kg/m^2	34	25–29 kg/m^2	33	<25 kg/m^2	33
Children 2–19 year of age	>95th percentile	17	85th–95th	15	<85th percentile	69
Physical activity						
Adults >20 year of age	None	32	1–149 min/week moderate intensity or 1–74 min/week vigoruos	24	≥150 min/week moderate intensity or ≥75 min/week vigorous intensity or ≥150 min/week	45
Children 12–19 year of age	None	10	>0 and <60 min of moderate of vigorous activity every day	46	≥60 min of moderate or vigorous activity every day	44
Healthy diet score						
Adults >20 year of age	0–1 components	76	2–3 components	24	4–5 components	<0.5
Children 5–19 year of age	0–1 components	91	2–3 components	9	4–5 components	<0.5
Total cholesterol						
Adults >20 year of age	≥240 mg/dL	16	200–239 mg/dL or treated to goal	38 (27; 12 treated to goal)	<200 mg/dL	45
Children 6–19 year of age	≥200 mg/dL	9	170–199 mg/dL	25	<170 mg/dL	67
Blood pressure						
Adults >20 year of age	SBP ≥140 or DBP ≥90 mmHg	17	SBP 120–139 or DBP 80–89 mmHg or treated to goal	41 (28; 13 treated to goal)	<120/<80 mmHg	42
Children 8–19 year of age	>95th percentile	5	90th–95th percentile or SBP ≥120 or DBP ≥80 mmHg	13	<90th percentile	82
Fasting plasma glucose						
Adults >20 year of age	≥126 mg/dL	8	100–125 mg/dL or treated to goal	34 (32; 3treated to goal)	<100 mg/dL	58
Children 12–19 year of age	≥126 mg/dL	0.5*	100–125 mg/dL	18	<100 mg/dL	81

Adapted from Lloyd-Jones et al. [55]. Copyright 2010 by American Heart Association
*Estimate not reliable.
SBP indicates systolic blood pressure; DBP indicated diastolic blood pressure
Some percentages do not add up because of rounding

Table 10.5 SNP, nearest gene, trait, and study for DNA variants associated with heredity risk factors associated with CHD

SNP	Nearest gene	Trait	Study
rs560887	G6PC2	Fasting glucose	Dupuis et al. [1] Sabatti et al. [2]
rs10830963	MTNR1B	Fasting glucose	Dupuis et al. [1]
rs1447352	MTNR1B	Fasting glucose	Sabatti et al. [2]
rs7121092	MTNR1B	Fasting glucose	Sabatti et al. [2]
rs4607517	GCK	Fasting glucose	Dupuis et al. [1]
rs2191349	DGKB-TMEM195	Fasting glucose	Dupuis et al. [1]
rs780094	GCKR	Fasting glucose	Dupuis et al. [1]
rs11708067	ADCY5	Fasting glucose	Dupuis et al. [1]
rs7944584	MADD	Fasting glucose	Dupuis et al. [1]
rs10885122	ADRA2A	Fasting glucose	Dupuis et al. [1]
rs174550	FADS1	Fasting glucose	Dupuis et al. [1]
rs11605924	CRY2	Fasting glucose	Dupuis et al. [1]
rs11920090	SLC2A2	Fasting glucose	Dupuis et al. [1]
rs7034200	GLIS3	Fasting glucose	Dupuis et al. [1]
rs6544713	ABCG8	LDL	Kathiresan et al. [3]
rs1501908	TIMD4-HAVCR1	LDL	Kathiresan et al. [3]
rs6102059	MAFB	LDL	Kathiresan et al. [3]
rs2650000	HNF1A	LDL	Kathiresan et al. [3]
rs4844614	CR1L	LDL	Sabatti et al. [3]
rs5031002	AR	LDL	Sabatti et al. [2]
rs174547	FADS1,2,3	HDL	Kathiresan et al. [3]
rs2271293	LCAT	HDL	Kathiresan et al. [3]
rs471364	TTC39B	HDL	Kathiresan et al. [3]
rs1800961	HNF4A	HDL	Kathiresan et al. [3]
rs7679	PLTP	HDL	Kathiresan et al. [3]
rs2967605	ANGPTL4	HDL	Kathiresan et al. [3]
rs174547	FADS1,2,3	TG	Kathiresan et al. [3]
rs7679	PLTP	TG	Kathiresan et al. [3]
rs7819412	XKR6-AMACIL2	TG	Kathiresan et al. [3]
rs12740374	CELSR2,PSRC1,SORT1	LDL	Kathiresan et al. [3]
rs515135	APOB	LDL	Kathiresan et al. [3]
rs4420638	APOE-APOC1,C4,C2	LDL	Kathiresan et al. [3]
rs6511720	LDLR	LDL	Kathiresan et al. [3]
rs3846663	HMGCR	LDL	Kathiresan et al. [3]
rs10401969	NCAN,CILP2, PBX4	LDL	Kathiresan et al. [3]
rs11206510	PCSK9	LDL	Cohen et al. [4], Kathiresan et al. [3]
rs173539	CETP	HDL	Kathiresan et al. [3]
rs12678919	LPL	HDL	Kathiresan et al. [3]
rs10468017	LIPC	HDL	Kathiresan et al. [3]
rs4939883	LIPG	HDL	Kathiresan et al. [3]
rs964184	APOA1, APOC3, A4, A5,	HDL	Kathiresan et al. [3]
rs2338104	MMAB, MVK	HDL	Kathiresan et al. [3]
rs1883025	ABCA1	HDL	Kathiresan et al. [3]
rs4846914	GALNT2	HDL	Kathiresan et al. [3]
rs964184	APOA1, APOC3, A4, A5,	TG	Kathiresan et al. [3]
rs12678919	LPL	TG	Kathiresan et al. [3]
rs1260326	GCKR	TG	Kathiresan et al. [3]
rs2954029	TRIB1	TG	Kathiresan et al. [3]
rs714052	MLX1PL	TG	Kathiresan et al. [3]
rs7557067	APOB	TG	Kathiresan et al. [3]
rs17216525	NCAN, CILP2,PBX4	TG	Kathiresan et al. [3]
rs10889353	ANGPTL3	TG	Kathiresan et al. [3]
rs10455872	Lp(a)	Lp(a)/CAD	Clarke et al. [5]
rs3798220	Lp(a)	Lp(a)/CAD	Clarke et al. [5]
rs1004467	CYP17A1	SBP	Levy et al. [6]
rs381815	PLEKHA7	SBP	Levy et al. [6]

(continued)

Table 10.5 (continued)

SNP	Nearest gene	Trait	Study
rs2681492	ATP2B1	SBP	Levy et al. [6]
rs17249754	ATP2B1	SBP/DBP	Cho et al. [7]
rs3184504	SH2B3	SBP	Levy et al. [6]
rs5068	NPPA/NPPB	SBP/DBP	Newton-Cheh et al. [8]
rs198358	NPPA/NPP	SBP/DBP	Newton-Cheh et al. [8]
rs17367504	MTHFR	SBP	Newton-Cheh et al. [9]
rs11191548	CYP17A1	SPB	Newton-Cheh et al. [9]
rs12946454	PLCD3	SBP	Newton-Cheh et al. [9]
rs16998073	PRDM8/FGF5/C4orf22	DBP	Newton-Cheh et al. [9]
rs1530440	c10orf107	DBP	Newton-Cheh et al. [9]
rs653178	SH2B3/ATXN2	DBP	Newton-Cheh et al. [9]
rs137842	CYP1A1/CYP1A2/CSK	DBP	Newton-Cheh et al. [9]
rs16948048	ZNF652	DBP	Newton-Cheh et al. [9]
rs9815354	ULK4	DBP	Levy et al. [6]
rs11014166	CACNB2	DBP	Levy et al. [6]
rs2681472	ATP2B1	DBP	Levy et al. [6]
rs3184504	SH2B3	DBP	Levy et al. [6]
rs2384550	TBX3-TBX5	DBP	Levy et al. [6]
rs6495122	CSK-ULK3	DBP	Levy et al. [6]
rs2681472	ATP2B1	Hypertension	Levy et al. [6]
rs9939609	FTO	BMI	Frayling et al. [10]
rs9930506	FTO	BMI	Scuteri et al. [11]
rs1421085	FTO	BMI	Dina et al. [12]
rs17817449	FTO	BMI	Dina et al. [12]
rs1421085	FTO	Obesity	Dina et al. [12]
rs17817449	FTO	Obesity	Dina et al. [12]
rs17782313	MC4R	BMI	Loos et al. [13]
rs10146997	NRXN3	BMI/obesity	Heard-Costa et al. [14]

LDL Cholesterol

Elevated low-density lipoprotein (LDL) cholesterol is associated with death from CHD. Recent GWAS have identified a number of DNA variants associated with changes in LDL, high-density lipoprotein (HDL), and triglycerides (Table 10.5). Recent work has found a significant association between two Lp(a) lipoprotein variants, increased Lp(a) levels, and CHD (Fig. 10.6) [68]. Figure 10.6 shows a linear relationship between the odds ratio increasing for CHD with each copy of the risk allele, as well as an increase in the Lp(a) lipoprotein levels. The LPA locus is on chromosome 6. The rare alleles of SNPs in Lp(a) correlate with a smaller isoform size of the apolipoprotein (a) and a lower copy number [68]. Remarkably, these two variants describe 36% of the total variation in Lp(a) lipoprotein levels [68]. The biological mechanism(s) whereby increased levels of Lp(a) increase risk for CHD is not well understood. More studies will be needed in this area.

A recent analysis by Kathiresan et al. of data from second- and third-generation family members of FHS participants confirmed that eight of the hypothesized SNPs associated with increased lipid levels were in fact expressed and resulted in increased lipid levels in these populations [61, 63, 68, 69] The SNP associated with LDL cholesterol is in/near SORT1 [70]. A recent study further defining the biological mechanism through which this variant alters LDL cholesterol through the expression of SORT1 in the liver has been published (Musunuru, Natum, 2010).

SNPs in genes associated with MMAB/MVK and GALNT were replicated for HDL cholesterol [68]. The minor allele (G) for this SNP (rs2338104) was associated with a decrease in transcript level of MMAB in the liver and an increase in HDL cholesterol [68]. No association was identified between transcript expression levels in the liver of GALNT and the associated SNP in this gene. The confirmed SNPs for triglycerides were in/near the following genes: GCLR, TRIB1, MLXIPL, NCAN, and ANGPTL3. The risk allele associated with SNP rs10889353 in ANGPTL3 was associated with an increase in expression of ANGPTL3 in the liver and a decrease in circulating triglycerides.

Rare mutations in PCSK9 (proprotein convertase subtilisin/kexin type 9 serine protease gene), a glycoprotein found in the liver, kidney, and intestine, were originally identified and associated with high LDL cholesterol [70]. Additional sequencing

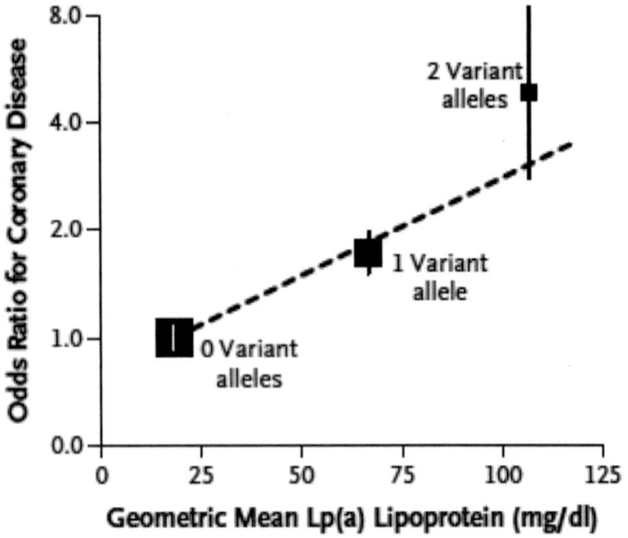

Fig. 10.6 This graph shows the significant association between three Lp(a) lipoprotein variants, increased lipoprotein (a) levels, and odds ratio for coronary heart disease. Adapted from Clarke et al. [68]. Copyright 2009 by Massachusetts Medical Society

of PCSK9 has revealed additional mutations that contribute to plasma LDL cholesterol levels (Kotowoski). A separate and distinct nonsense mutation in PCSK9 was found in African-Americans and was associated with a reduction in LDL cholesterol as well as a reduction in the risk of CHD [60, 62].

BMI

Very few identified loci have been reproducibly associated with body mass index (BMI), a risk factor for CHD (Table 10.5) [71]. The first loci identified was FTO (fat mass- and obesity-associated) on chromosome 16q12.2 [52, 53] (Fig. 10.7). SNPs in FTO in European cohorts have been associated with both increases in BMI and obesity in children and adults [52–54]. FTO was replicated in a large GWAS of Asian populations [64]. In addition to FTO and MC4R, variants in NRXN3 have also recently been associated with obesity, waist circumference, and high BMI [72].

Deletions on chromosome 16p11.2 were also recently associated with obesity [58]. In this study by Walters, Jacquemont, and colleagues, an alternative approach identifies variants associated with obesity [58]. The design was implemented in response to data from GWAS identifying numerous variants associated with obesity, but only accounting for a small fraction of the underlying heritability [58]. The hypothesis was that cohorts with extreme phenotypes that include obesity may be enriched for rare but potent risk variants [58]. To test this hypothesis, the authors tested a cohort with obesity as well as developmental delay and/or congenital malformations from three centers in the UK and France [58]. This resulted in identifying a region of heterozygous deletion on 16p11.2 in 9 individuals out of 312 (2.9%) [58]. Testing additional cases and included controls verified the association of this heterozygous deletion on 16p11.2 in additional cohorts and increased the significance to $p < 10^{-9}$ [58].

To date, no published studies have identified direct associations between risk loci and any gene associated with BMI or obesity and coronary artery disease in large cohorts with replication.

Blood Pressure

Heredity is a component of blood pressure. However, the effect size of individual common allelic variants on systolic and diastolic blood pressure remain small – ~1 mmHg for systolic and about 0.5 mmHg for diastolic blood pressure [73].

Levy et al. have recently analyzed blood pressure data from the CHARGE consortium [73], which includes more than 29,000 individuals of European ancestry from six separate studies, including Atherosclerosis Risk in Communities Study,

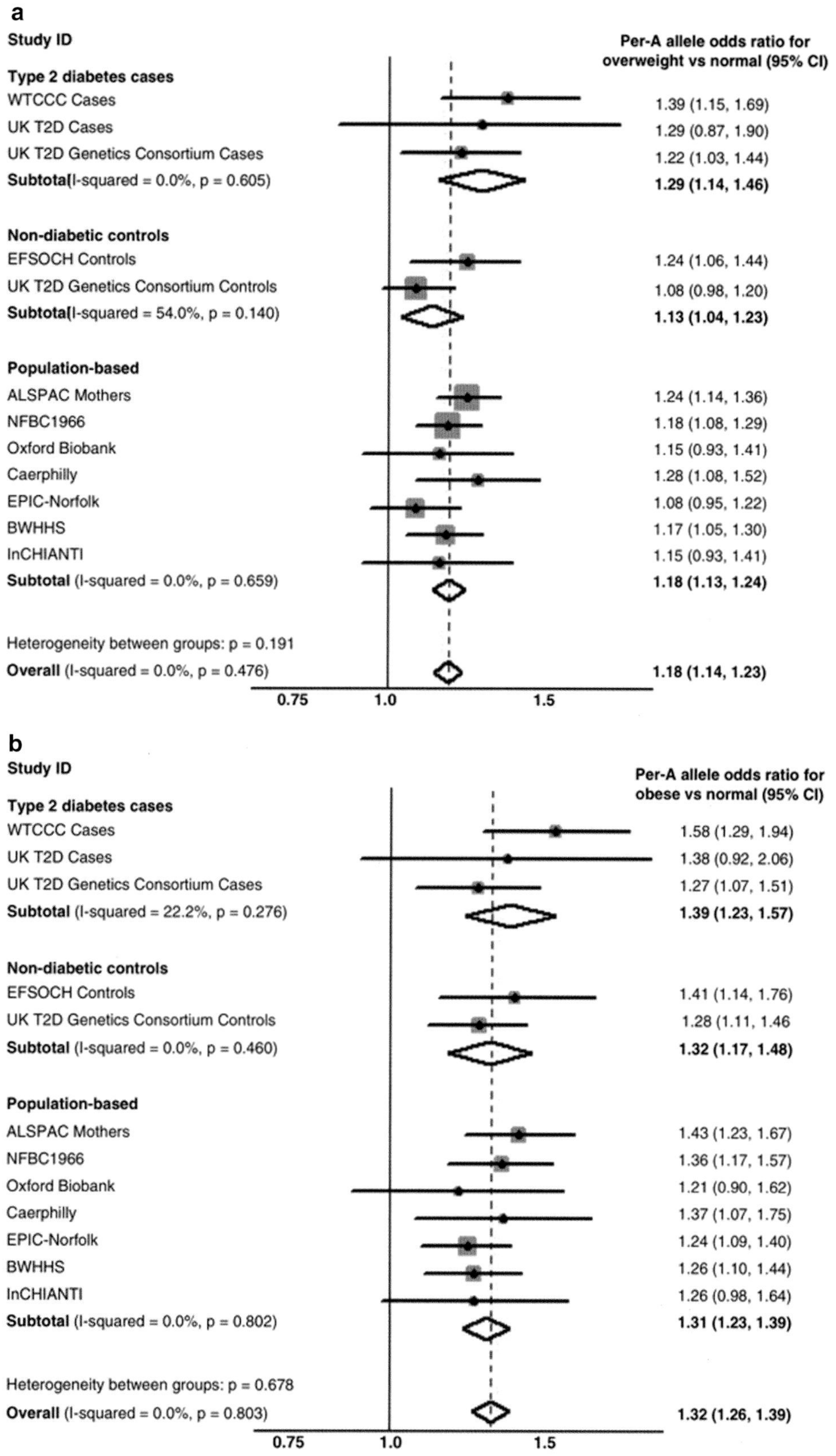

Fig. 10.7 (**a**, **b**) Meta-analysis polts for odds of (**a**) overweight and (**b**) obesity compared with normal weight in adults for each copy of the A allele of rs9939609 carried. Bar charts depicting (**c**) DEXA-measured fat mass in 9-year-old children and (**d**) DEXA-measured lean mass in older children – both from the ALSPAC study. Error bars represent 95% confidence intervals. Adapted from Frayling et al. [53]. Copyright 2007 by the American Association for the Advancement of Science. FYI: Copyright info for Science from http://www.sciencemag.org/about/copyright.dtl

Fig. 10.7 (continued)

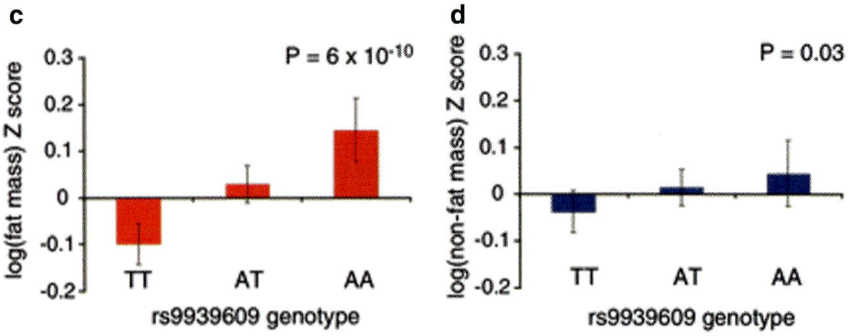

the Age, Gene/Environment Susceptibility Reykjavik Study (AGES), Cardiovascular Health Study (CHS), FHS, Rotterdam Study (RS), and the Rotterdam Extension Study (RES). The top loci for SBP is on chromosome 12q21.23, rs2681492, in the gene *ATP2B1* (Table 10.5) [43]. *ATP2B1* was also associated with hypertension and diastolic blood pressure (DBP) [43]. *ATP2B1* is a member of a family of ATPases that regulate calcium homeostasis. ATP2B1 mRNA is expressed in most tissues. (The Web site www.genecards.org includes figures and tables of expression levels and updated publications).

The region containing SH2B3/ATXN2 was also identified by Newton-Cheh et al. in the Global BPgen consortia, which included 17 cohorts of European ancestry [74]. Participants' mean age ranged from 38 years (Framingham Heart Study) to 72 years (CHS).

Identifying mutations of genome-wide significance associated with blood pressure has appeared more difficult. The reasons are not fully understood, but may in part rest on the variability in measuring blood pressure. Thus, additional approaches have been adapted to move this field forward. One approach incorporated the use of an intermediate phenotype: circulating ANP/BNP. The loci associated with blood pressure include the well-known natriuretic peptides ANP and BNP. In a cohort of ~29,000 individuals of European descent, Newton-Cheh described a significant association between SNPs in both ANP and BNP with increased circulating levels of both neuropeptides and decreased systolic and diastolic blood pressure [75]. A major difference in this study over prior studies was that an intermediate phenotype was used – circulating ANP/BNP – to preselect a collection of SNPs to carry forward for testing for associations with blood pressure. This distinction enhanced the power of the analysis.

In summary, a number of mutations have been associated with both systolic and diastolic blood pressure (Table 10.5). This list of genes includes signaling molecules, transcription factors that regulate neurogenesis, calcium-handling genes, and regulators of metabolism. Further studies are needed to determine the role of each of these mutations and genes in regulating blood pressure. The use of these mutations known to be associated with blood pressure in the clinic is not readily adaptable, given that they may alter blood pressure by only 1–2 mmHg.

Fasting Blood Glucose

Unregulated variations in fasting plasma glucose have been shown to be a modifiable risk factor for development of CVD. Adults with diabetes have heart disease death rates about 2–4 times higher than adults without diabetes. In 2004, heart disease was noted on 68% of diabetes-related death certificates among people aged 65 years or older [76]. The number of people with diabetes in the world is projected to rise from 171 million to an estimated 366 million by 2030 [76].

To further elicit the genetic underpinnings of diabetes, Dupuis et al. performed a meta-analysis of 21 GWAS involving insulin and glucose as well as indices of beta-cell function (HOMA-B) and insulin resistance. Of 25 loci studied in the 76,558 subjects, 16 were associated with fasting glucose. This suggests that mutations in these genes may increase risk for altering blood glucose level. The role of many of these genes in regulating blood glucose is not well understood and will require a series of studies to determine the cells/tissues in which they are expressing, how they are regulated, and how mutations in these genes regulate blood glucose levels (Table 10.5).

In summary, a number of loci have been associated with LDL cholesterol, BMI, fasting blood glucose, and blood pressure. A critical question is how much of the heritability in these modifiable risk factors do genetic loci contribute? Very little at this point. However, if identifying these loci opens up new pathways toward drug discovery and cardiovascular health, then the area of genetics has served a worthy end.

Pharmacogenomics/Tailored Therapeutics

The president and CEO of Eli Lilly and Company, John C. Lechleiter, PhD, recently stated (Personalized Medicine Coalition, Executive Director's Report, 2010):

> The power in tailored therapeutics is for us to say more clearly to payers, providers, and patients, 'This drug is not for everyone, but it is for you.'

Lechleiter was voicing one compelling argument for both conducting research on the relationship between medicines and individual response – pharmacogenomics – and about the emerging philosophy underlying the research and development strategy for pharmaceutical development [77, 78]. The Food and Drug Administration lists pharmacogenomic information on approximately 10% of approved drug labels [79].

Of particular interest regarding the relationship of pharmacogenomics and CHD are two drugs commonly used to treat patients with CHD. Coumadin (warfarin) is the most widely prescribed oral anticoagulant in North America [80]. In 2007, clopidogrel, a platelet aggregation inhibitor, was the sixth-most-commonly-prescribed medication in America [81] and the second best-selling drug worldwide [82]. In 2008, clopidogrel had US sales of $3.8 billion.

Cytochrome p450 enzymes are responsible for about 75% of the Phase 1 metabolism of clinical drugs [83]. DNA variation within the individual cytochrome P450 genes affects the ability of these enzymes to metabolize drugs, as do disease and environment.

Interest in the field of pharmacogenomics has led to the development of different gene chips and platforms in the clinical setting as "an aid in determining treatment choice and individualizing treatment dose for therapeutics that are metabolized primarily by the specific enzyme about which the system provides genotypic information" (FDA classification 21 CFR 862.3360). In the research setting, these gene chips and platforms are used to determine how the genotypic footprint affects the metabolism of different drugs.

Two cytochrome P450 genes present on the clinical chips are CYP2C19, CYP2D6, and CYP2C9. CYP2C19 is one of the cytochrome P450 genes that metabolizes the antiplatelet drug clopidogrel. Drugs metabolized by CYP2C19 include celecoxib, codeine, diazepam, esomeprazole, nelfinavir, omeprazole, pantoprazole, rabeprazole, and voriconazole. Known drugs metabolized by CYP2D6 include the cardiovascular drugs carvedilol, metoprolol, and propranolol, as well as acetaminophen, aripiprazole, atomexetine, cevimeline hydrochloride, clozapine, fluoxetine HCl, olanzapine, propafenone, protriptyline HCl, risperidone, tamoxifen, terbinafine, thioridazine, timolol maleate, tiotropium bromide inhalation powder, tolterodine tartrate, tramadol, and venlafaxine.

The individual response of subjects receiving Coumadin have been shown to vary significantly based on genotype of CYP2C9 (CYP2C9*2 or CYP2C9*3), CYP4F2 (V433M), and VKORC1 (−1639 G>A allele). VKORC1 (responsible for vitamin K epoxide reductase and rate-limiting enzyme in the warfarin-sensitive vitamin K-dependent gamma carboxylation) CYP2C9, and CYP4F2 have polymorphism variability that, when present, leads to increased, active warfarin metabolites and decreases the warfarin doses necessary to research therapeutic treatment levels [29, 80, 84–87].

The effect of genotype on clopidogrel dose is mainly dependent on CYP2C19; however, CYP1A2, CYP2B6, CYP2B6, CYP2C9, and CYP3A4 also may play roles. The major enzyme CYP2C19, playing a role in both steps of drug metabolism, has been shown to have more than 25 polymorphisms [88], the most common of which accounts for ~15–30% of the allelic frequency variation, and significantly decreases the metabolism of the drug, thus leading to decreased circulation levels and decreased therapeutic effects [88].

Other polymorphic variations including CYP2C19*17 (allelic frequency 4–18%) have been shown to be so-called "ultrametabolizers," increasing the amount of clopidogrel metabolite in the patient's circulation. This increases the platelet inhibition beyond therapeutic levels, potentially causing increased risk of bleeding [88]. Additionally, other genes and allelic variations have been found to alter other complements of clopidogrel absorption (ABCB1) and biologic activity (P2RY12 and ITGB3) [89].

Clearly, individual genetic variations must be considered as we prescribe anticoagulant or antiplatelet treatments for patients with CHD. As Health and Human Services Secretary Kathleen Sebelius stated in testimony during her Senate confirmation hearings in 2009:

> Today, it is common for a medical product to be fully effective for only about 60% of those who use it. As the medical community is now learning, this in part reflects biological variation among individuals that affects the clinical response to medical interventions.

Challenges remain in sequencing the genome of every individual patient, but in doing so, we are provided very useful clinical information that often guides individually tailored medical therapeutics.

Ethical, Legal, and Policy Considerations

Performing genetic, diagnostic testing in individuals at risk for coronary artery disease is a relatively new idea that is being implemented at select clinics and medical centers in the USA CAD and other countries to provide additional risk information. Understanding the impact and ramifications this testing will have on patient care, health-care decision-making, and research regulations has been a challenge for many years, and remains a complex problem [90, 91].

For example, results from studies designed to assess the early impact of genetic diagnostics are highly encouraging, but determining whether a newly identified biomarker will be clinically useful as a genetic test for an individual requires that many conditions be met. At the very minimum, one is statistical significance. Second, as pointed out by Hlatky and colleagues, the new risk marker must improve risk prediction beyond what is currently available with known approaches, as is the population prevalence of the risk marker [92].

We know, however, that while availability of highly sensitive and specific tests is the goal of the "genomic revolution" – particularly, readily accessible and affordable tests – many factors are at play that may inhibit the speedy translation, from discoveries at the bench to treatments at the bedside, and then to availability in the community. Some of these factors are:

- *Managing patient expectations*. When scientific discoveries are incompletely presented, the public is often at risk of the hype and hyperbole of science [35, 93].
- *Impact of health reform*. While the USA is further along in guaranteeing access to more people to basic health care as a result of recent health reform, the implications for affordable access to potentially diagnostic biomarkers is less assured.
- *Clinical genetics literacy*. It is one thing to develop diagnostic biomarkers to discover mutations associated with disease, but another for clinicians to effectively and appropriately use these in daily clinical practice.

Summary and Conclusions

The impact of the human genome project on our understanding of the genetic basis of CHD has just begun to unfold. Questions have been voiced by patients, health-care workers, and insurance companies. Discussions are needed for scientific discoveries to be translated into clinical practice. Thus, progress is being made.

Family history remains a stronger factor than individual genetic information for specific genes associated with CHD. Identifying rare variants associated with CHD is in early stages. The advent of the technology and the systematic decrease in the cost of sequencing the human genome have led to the human exome project and a redesign and rethinking of original strategies – away from a focus on common variants and a shift to rare variants.

As a result of the human genome project, new, basic mechanisms of CHD will likely be identified in the next 10 years. Genetics will most likely play a role in helping to direct therapy for individuals.

References

1. Lloyd-Jones D, Adams R, Carnethon M, et al. Heart disease and stroke statistics – 2009 update: a report from the American Heart Association Statistics Committee and Stroke Statistics Subcommittee. Circulation. 2009;119(3):e21–181.
2. Lloyd-Jones DM, Larson MG, Beiser A, Levy D. Lifetime risk of developing coronary heart disease. Lancet. 1999;353(9147):89–92.
3. Lloyd-Jones DM, Nam BH, D'Agostino Sr RB, et al. Parental cardiovascular disease as a risk factor for cardiovascular disease in middle-aged adults: a prospective study of parents and offspring. JAMA. 2004;291(18):2204–11.
4. Murabito JM, Nam BH, Pencina MJ, et al. Sibling cardiovascular disease as a risk factor for cardiovascular disease in middle-aged adults. JAMA. 2005;294(24):3117–23.
5. McPherson R. Chromosome 9p21 and coronary artery disease. N Engl J Med. 2010;362(18):1736–7.
6. Barrett-Connor E, Khaw K. Family history of heart attack as an independent predictor of death due to cardiovascular disease. Circulation. 1984;69(6):1065–9.
7. Colditz GA, Rimm EB, Giovannucci E, et al. A prospective study of parental history of myocardial infarction and coronary artery disease in men. Am J Cardiol. 1991;67(11):933–8.
8. Colditz GA, Stampfer MJ, Willett WC, et al. A prospective study of parental history of myocardial infarction and coronary heart disease in women. Am J Epidemiol. 1986;123(1):48–58.
9. Friedlander Y, Kark JD, Stein Y. Family history of myocardial infarction as an independent risk factor for coronary heart disease. Br Heart J. 1985;53(4):382–7.
10. Friedlander Y, Kark JD, Stein Y. Family history as a risk factor for primary cardiac arrest. Circulation. 1998;97(2):155–60.

11. Jousilahti P, Puska P, Vartiainen E, Pekkanen J, Tuomilehto J. Parental history of premature coronary heart disease: an independent risk factor of myocardial infarction. J Clin Epidemiol. 1996;49(5):497–503.
12. Khaw KT, Barrett-Connor E. Family history of stroke as an independent predictor of ischemic heart disease in men and stroke in women. Am J Epidemiol. 1986;123(1):59–66.
13. Leander K, Hallqvist J, Reuterwall C, Ahlbom A, de Faire U. Family history of coronary heart disease, a strong risk factor for myocardial infarction interacting with other cardiovascular risk factors: results from the Stockholm Heart Epidemiology Program (SHEEP). Epidemiology. 2001;12(2):215–21.
14. Myers RH, Kiely DK, Cupples LA, Kannel W. Parental history is an independent risk factor for coronary artery disease: the Framingham Study. Am Heart J. 1990;120(4):963–9.
15. Phillips AN, Shaper AG, Pocock SJ, Walker M. Parental death from heart disease and the risk of heart attack. Eur Heart J. 1988;9(3): 243–51.
16. Pohjola-Sintonen S, Rissanen A, Liskola P, Luomanmaki K. Family history as a risk factor of coronary heart disease in patients under 60 years of age. Eur Heart J. 1998;19(2):235–9.
17. Roncaglioni MC, Santoro L, D'Avanzo B, et al. Role of family history in patients with myocardial infarction. An Italian case-control study. GISSI-EFRIM Investigators. Circulation. 1992;85(6):2065–72.
18. Sesso HD, Lee IM, Gaziano JM, Rexrode KM, Glynn RJ, Buring JE. Maternal and paternal history of myocardial infarction and risk of cardiovascular disease in men and women. Circulation. 2001;104(4):393–8.
19. Shea S, Ottman R, Gabrieli C, Stein Z, Nichols A. Family history as an independent risk factor for coronary artery disease. J Am Coll Cardiol. 1984;4(4):793–801.
20. Sholtz RI, Rosenman RH, Brand RJ. The relationship of reported parental history to the incidence of coronary heart disease in the Western Collaborative Group Study. Am J Epidemiol. 1975;102(4):350–6.
21. Silberberg JS, Wlodarczyk J, Fryer J, Robertson R, Hensley MJ. Risk associated with various definitions of family history of coronary heart disease. The Newcastle Family History Study II. Am J Epidemiol. 1998;147(12):1133–9.
22. Thelle DS, Forde OH. The cardiovascular study in Finnmark county: coronary risk factors and the occurrence of myocardial infarction in first degree relatives and in subjects of different ethnic origin. Am J Epidemiol. 1979;110(6):708–15.
23. Williams RR, Hunt SC, Heiss G, et al. Usefulness of cardiovascular family history data for population-based preventive medicine and medical research (the Health Family Tree Study and the NHLBI Family Heart Study). Am J Cardiol. 2001;87(2):129–35.
24. Bensen JT, Liese AD, Rushing JT, et al. Accuracy of proband reported family history: the NHLBI Family Heart Study (FHS). Genet Epidemiol. 1999;17(2):141–50.
25. Centers for Disease Control and Prevention (CDC). Awareness of family health history as a risk factor for disease – United States, 2004. MMWR Morb Mortal Wkly Rep. 2004;53(44):1044–7.
26. Collins FS, Morgan M, Patrinos A. The Human Genome Project: lessons from large-scale biology. Science. 2003;300(5617):286–90.
27. Lander ES, Linton LM, Birren B, et al. Initial sequencing and analysis of the human genome. Nature. 2001;409(6822):860–921.
28. Venter JC, Adams MD, Myers EW, et al. The sequence of the human genome. Science. 2001;291(5507):1304–51.
29. Ashley EA, Butte AJ, Wheeler MT, et al. Clinical assessment incorporating a personal genome. Lancet. 2010;375(9725):1525–35.
30. The human genome at ten [editorial]. Nature. 2010;464:649–50.
31. Postema PG, Wolpert C, Amin AS, et al. Drugs and Brugada syndrome patients: review of the literature, recommendations, and an up-to-date website (www.brugadadrugs.org). Heart Rhythm. 2009;6(9):1335–41.
32. Ryden L, Standl E, Bartnik M, et al. Guidelines for the management of patients with ventricular arrhythmias and the prevention of sudden cardiac death–executive summary. Rev Port Cardiol. 2007;26(11):1213–74.
33. Paynter NP, Chasman DI, Buring JE, Shiffman D, Cook NR, Ridker PM. Cardiovascular disease risk prediction with and without knowledge of genetic variation at chromosome 9p21.3. Ann Intern Med. 2009;150(2):65–72.
34. Evans JP. Recreational genomics; what's in it for you? Genet Med. 2008;10(10):709–10.
35. Caulfield T. Underwhelmed: hyperbole, regulatory policy, and the genetic revolution. McGill LJ. 2000;45:437.
36. Helgadottir A, Thorleifsson G, Manolescu A, et al. A common variant on chromosome 9p21 affects the risk of myocardial infarction. Science. 2007;316(5830):1491–3.
37. McPherson R, Pertsemlidis A, Kavasla N, et al. A common allele on chromosome 9 associated with coronary heart disease. Science. 2007; 316(5830):1488–91.
38. Schunkert H, Gotz A, Braund P, et al. Repeated replication and a prospective meta-analysis of the association between chromosome 9p21.3 and coronary artery disease. Circulation. 2008;117(13):1675–84.
39. Anderson JL, Horne BD, Kolek MJ, et al. Genetic variation at the 9p21 locus predicts angiographic coronary artery disease prevalence but not extent and has clinical utility. Am Heart J. 2008;156(6):1155–62. e2.
40. Assimes TL, Knowles JW, Basu A, et al. Susceptibility locus for clinical and subclinical coronary artery disease at chromosome 9p21 in the multi-ethnic ADVANCE study. Hum Mol Genet. 2008;17(15):2320–8.
41. Baudhuin LM. Genetics of coronary artery disease: focus on genome-wide association studies. Am J Transl Res. 2009;1(3):221–34.
42. Abdullah KG, Li L, Shen GQ, et al. Four SNPS on chromosome 9p21 confer risk to premature, familial CAD and MI in an American Caucasian population (GeneQuest). Ann Hum Genet. 2008;72(Pt 5):654–7.
43. Samani NJ, Deloukas P, Erdmann J, et al. Large scale association analysis of novel genetic loci for coronary artery disease. Arterioscler Thromb Vasc Biol. 2009;29(5):774–80.
44. Samani NJ, Erdmann J, Hall AS, et al. Genomewide association analysis of coronary artery disease. N Engl J Med. 2007;357(5):443–53.
45. Holdt LM, Beutner F, Scholz M, et al. ANRIL expression is associated with atherosclerosis risk at chromosome 9p21. Arterioscler Thromb Vasc Biol. 2010;30(3):620–7.
46. Ensrud K, Grimm Jr RH. The white blood cell count and risk for coronary heart disease. Am Heart J. 1992;124(1):207–13.
47. Danesh J, Collins R, Appleby P, Peto R. Association of fibrinogen, C-reactive protein, albumin, or leukocyte count with coronary heart disease: meta-analyses of prospective studies. JAMA. 1998;279(18):1477–82.
48. Hoffman M, Blum A, Baruch R, Kaplan E, Benjamin M. Leukocytes and coronary heart disease. Atherosclerosis. 2004;172(1):1–6.

49. Soranzo N, Spector TD, Mangino M, et al. A genome-wide meta-analysis identifies 22 loci associated with eight hematological parameters in the HaemGen consortium. Nat Genet. 2009;41(11):1182–90.
50. Erdmann J, Grosshennig A, Braund PS, et al. New susceptibility locus for coronary artery disease on chromosome 3q22.3. Nat Genet. 2009; 41(3):280–2.
51. Ganesh SK, Zakai NA, van Rooij FJ, et al. Multiple loci influence erythrocyte phenotypes in the CHARGE Consortium. Nat Genet. 2009;41(11): 1191–8.
52. Dina C, Meyre D, Gallina S, et al. Variation in FTO contributes to childhood obesity and severe adult obesity. Nat Genet. 2007;39(6):724–6.
53. Frayling TM, Timpson NJ, Weedon MN, et al. A common variant in the FTO gene is associated with body mass index and predisposes to childhood and adult obesity. Science. 2007;316(5826):889–94.
54. Scuteri A, Sanna S, Chen WM, et al. Genome-wide association scan shows genetic variants in the FTO gene are associated with obesity-related traits. PLoS Genet. 2007;3(7):e115.
55. Lloyd-Jones DM, Hong Y, Labarthe D, et al. Defining and setting national goals for cardiovascular health promotion and disease reduction: the American Heart Association's strategic impact goal through 2020 and beyond. Circulation. 2010;121(4):586–613.
56. Lindgren CM, Heid IM, Randall JC, et al. Genome-wide association scan meta-analysis identifies three loci influencing adiposity and fat distribution. PLoS Genet. 2009;5(6):e1000508.
57. Renstrom F, Payne F, Nordstrom A, et al. Replication and extension of genome-wide association study results for obesity in 4923 adults from northern Sweden. Hum Mol Genet. 2009;18(8):1489–96.
58. Walters RG, Jacquemont S, Valsesia A, et al. A new highly penetrant form of obesity due to deletions on chromosome 16p11.2. Nature. 2010;463(7281):671–5.
59. Chasman DI, Pare G, Mora S, et al. Forty-three loci associated with plasma lipoprotein size, concentration, and cholesterol content in genome-wide analysis. PLoS Genet. 2009;5(11):e1000730.
60. Cohen JC, Boerwinkle E, Mosley Jr TH, et al. Sequence variations in PCSK9, low LDL, and protection against coronary heart disease. N Engl J Med. 2006;354(12):1264–72.
61. Kathiresan S, Melander O, Anevski D, et al. Polymorphisms associated with cholesterol and risk of cardiovascular events. N Engl J Med. 2008;358(12):1240–9.
62. Kathiresan S, Melander O, Guiducci C, et al. Six new loci associated with blood low-density lipoprotein cholesterol, high-density lipoprotein cholesterol or triglycerides in humans. Nat Genet. 2008;40(2):189–97.
63. Kathiresan S, Willer CJ, Peloso GM, et al. Common variants at 30 loci contribute to polygenic dyslipidemia. Nat Genet. 2009;41(1):56–65.
64. Cho YS, Go MJ, Kim YJ, et al. A large-scale genome-wide association study of Asian populations uncovers genetic factors influencing eight quantitative traits. Nat Genet. 2009;41(5):527–34.
65. Org E, Eyheramendy S, Juhanson P, et al. Genome-wide scan identifies CDH13 as a novel susceptibility locus contributing to blood pressure determination in two European populations. Hum Mol Genet. 2009;18(12):2288–96.
66. Sabatti C, Service SK, Hartikainen AL, et al. Genome-wide association analysis of metabolic traits in a birth cohort from a founder population. Nat Genet. 2009;41(1):35–46.
67. Dupuis J, Langenberg C, Prokopenko I, et al. New genetic loci implicated in fasting glucose homeostasis and their impact on type 2 diabetes risk. Nat Genet. 2010;42(2):105–16.
68. Clarke R, Peden JF, Hopewell JC, et al. Genetic variants associated with Lp(a) lipoprotein level and coronary disease. N Engl J Med. 2009;361(26):2518–28.
69. Saxena R, Voight BF, Lyssenko V, et al. Genome-wide association analysis identifies loci for type 2 diabetes and triglyceride levels. Science. 2007;316(5829):1331–6.
70. Abifadel M, Varret M, Rabes JP, et al. Mutations in PCSK9 cause autosomal dominant hypercholesterolemia. Nat Genet. 2003;34(2):154–6.
71. Walley AJ, Asher JE, Froguel P. The genetic contribution to non-syndromic human obesity. Nat Rev Genet. 2009;10(7):431–42.
72. Heard-Costa NL, Zillikens MC, Monda KL, et al. NRXN3 is a novel locus for waist circumference: a genome-wide association study from the CHARGE Consortium. PLoS Genet. 2009;5(6):e1000539.
73. Levy D, Ehret GB, Rice K, et al. Genome-wide association study of blood pressure and hypertension. Nat Genet. 2009;41:677–87.
74. Cohen J, Pertsemlidis A, Kotowski IK, et al. Low LDL cholesterol in individuals of African descent resulting from frequent nonsense mutations in PCSK9. Nat Genet. 2005;37(2):161–5.
75. Newton-Cheh C, Johnson T, Gateva V, et al. Genome-wide association study identifies eight loci associated with blood pressure. Nat Genet. 2009;41:666–76.
76. American Diabetes Association. Diabetes statistics (data from the 2007 National Diabetes Fact Sheet). http://www.diabetes.org/diabetes-basics/diabetes-statistics. Accessed 19 July 2010.
77. Evans BJ. What will it take to reap the clinical benefits of pharmacogenomics? Food Drug Law J. 2006;61(4):753–94.
78. Evans BJ, Flockhart DA, Meslin EM. Creating incentives for genomic research to improve targeting of therapies. Nat Med. 2004;10(12): 1289–91.
79. Food and Drug Administration. Table of valid genomic biomarkers in the context of approved drug labels. http://www.fda.gov/Drugs/ScienceResearch/ResearchAreas/Pharmacogenetics/ucm083378.htm. Accessed 22 July 2010.
80. Holbrook AM, Pereira JA, Labiris R, et al. Systematic overview of warfarin and its drug and food interactions. Arch Intern Med. 2005;165(10): 1095–6.
81. IMS Health. Top 10 Global Products – 2007. http://www.imshealth.com/imshealth/Global/Content/StaticFile/Top_Line_Data/Top10GlobalProducts.pdf. Published 26 Feb 2008. Accessed 22 July 2010.
82. RxList, Inc. Top 200 Drugs – US Only. http://www.rxlist.com/script/main/hp.asp. Accessed 19 July 2010.
83. Ingelman-Sundberg M, Sim SC. Pharmacogenetic biomarkers as tools for improved drug therapy; emphasis on the cytochrome P450 system. Biochem Biophys Res Commun. 2010;396(1):90–4.
84. Caldwell MD, Awad T, Johnson JA, et al. CYP4F2 genetic variant alters required warfarin dose. Blood. 2008;111(8):4106–12.
85. Klein TE, Altman RB, Ericksson N, et al. Estimation of the warfarin dose with clinical and pharmacogenetic data. N Engl J Med. 2009; 360(8):753–64.

86. Nademanee K, Schwab MC, Kosar EM, et al. Clinical outcomes of catheter substrate ablation for high-risk patients with atrial fibrillation. J Am Coll Cardiol. 2008;51(8):843–9.
87. Rieder MJ, Reiner AP, Gage BF, et al. Effect of VKORC1 haplotypes on transcriptional regulation and warfarin dose. N Engl J Med. 2005;352(22):2285–93.
88. Steinhubl SR. Genotyping, clopidogrel metabolism, and the search for the therapeutic window of thienopyridines. Circulation. 2010;121(4): 481–3.
89. Simon T, Verstuyft C, Mary-Krause M, et al. Genetic determinants of response to clopidogrel and cardiovascular events. N Engl J Med. 2009; 360(4):363–75.
90. Evans BJ, Flockhart DA. The unfinished business of U.S. drug safety regulation. Food Drug Law J. 2006;61(1):45–63.
91. Evans BJ. Seven pillars of a new evidentiary paradigm: the Food, Drug, and Cosmetic Act enters the genomic era. Notre Dame L Rev. 2009;85:2419–524.
92. Hlatky MA, Greenland P, Arnett DK, et al. Criteria for evaluation of novel markers of cardiovascular risk: a scientific statement from the American Heart Association. Circulation. 2009;119(17):2408–16.
93. Caulfield T. Popular media, biotechnology, and the cycle of hype. Hous J Health L & Pol'y. 2004;5:213.

Chapter 11
Endothelium Biology

Michael Sean McMurtry and Evangelos D. Michelakis

The endothelium is a cell layer that lines the blood vessels of the entire vascular tree, including arteries, veins, and lymphatics [1]. Originally understood as an inert barrier, the endothelium is now appreciated as an organ that is distributed throughout all tissues with multiple important functions [2]. These functions include control of vascular tone, transport of cells and nutrients from the blood compartment to tissues, hemostasis, vascular repair after injury, and innate and adaptive immunity [3]. In addition to its role in health, the endothelium is also involved in the pathogenesis of a diverse set of diseases, including atherosclerosis [4], congestive heart failure [5], valvular heart diseases [6], pulmonary arterial hypertension [7], erectile dysfunction [8], sepsis [9], and cancer [10].

Understanding endothelial functions depends on discoveries over centuries, including William Harvey's description of blood circulation between arteries and veins in 1628, the discovery of capillaries by Marcello Malpighi in 1661, the coining of the term "endothelium" by Wilhelm His in 1865, and the description of endothelial ultrastructure based on electron microscopy by Palade in the 1950s [2, 3, 11].

With the exception of capillaries, all blood vessels comprise three layers: the tunica adventitia, composed mainly of connective tissue such as collagen and elastin; the tunica media, composed mainly of circumferentially oriented smooth muscle cells; and the tunica intima, formed by the endothelium and supporting connective tissue [12]. Muscular arteries are additionally characterized by lamina of elastic fibers: the external elastic lamina between the tunica adventitia and tunica media, and the internal elastic lamina between the tunica media and tunica intima. Veins are also characterized by the presence of valves, which extend into the lumen to prevent retrograde blood flow.

Capillaries lack adventitia and media, including vascular smooth muscle cells (VSMCs), but do have supporting cells called pericytes [13]. The endothelium is a cellular monolayer that lines arteries, veins, capillaries, and lymphatics, and represents the cellular interface between the blood and underlying tissues [14].

Embryology

The endothelium forms early during development from primordial mesoderm with formation of nascent capillaries and appears even before the first heartbeat [15]. The development of the functioning cardiovascular system, including the heart, blood, and blood vessels, facilitates organogenesis [16, 17] and the development of other organs, including the lungs [18] and nervous system [19]. A mesodermally derived precursor cell called the hemangioblast, with its ability to produce both blood cell lineages and angioblasts, is believed to be the source of fetal vascular endothelial cells [20, 21].

In a process called vasculogenesis, in which de novo tubes are formed, angioblasts of the peripheral blood islands, head mesenchyme, and posterior lateral plate mesoderm connect to form a network of vessels and become endothelial cells [22] (Fig. 11.1a). Endothelial cells, derived from paraxial mesoderm, migrate to form vessels of the kidney, limbs, and dorsal aorta. Endothelial cells from splanchnopleural mesoderm yield vessels of the solid organs and gut [23].

Proper vasculogenesis depends on close proximity of endoderm to nascent endothelial cells [24]. Several signaling molecules important for vasculogenesis have been described, including fibroblast growth factor-2 (FGF-2) [25], vascular endothelial growth factor-A (VEGF-A) [26, 27], angiopoietin receptors Tie-1 and Tie-2 [28, 29], neuropilins 1 and 2 [30],

M.S. McMurtry, BASc, MD, PhD (✉) • E.D. Michelakis, MD, PhD
Department of Medicine, University of Alberta Hospital, Edmonton, AB, Canada
e-mail: mcmurtry@ualberta.ca

Z. Vlodaver et al. (eds.), *Coronary Heart Disease: Clinical, Pathological, Imaging, and Molecular Profiles*,
DOI 10.1007/978-1-4614-1475-9_11,

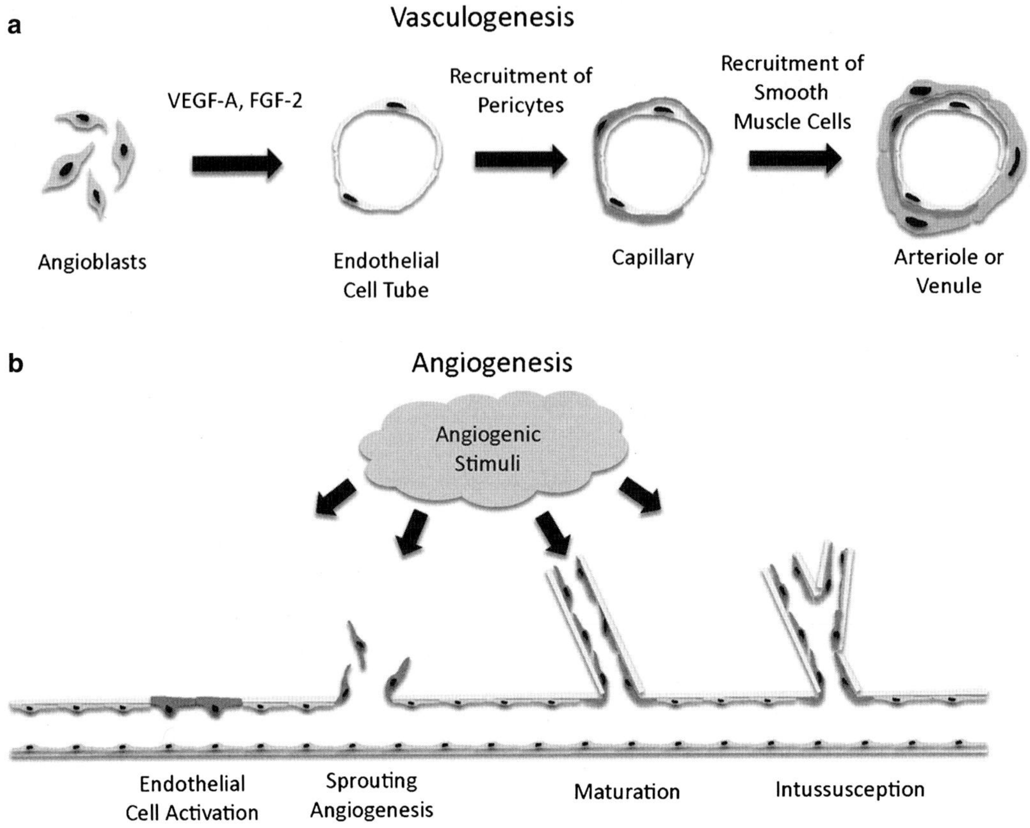

Fig. 11.1 The coronary tree forms by the processes of vasculogenesis and angiogenesis. In vasculogenesis (**a**), de novo blood vessels are formed by the coalescence of angioblasts into tubules of endothelial cells. These tubules recruit pericytes, forming nascent capillaries. Investment of the capillaries with smooth muscle cells and connective tissue leads to formation of arterioles and veins. In angiogenesis (**b**), angiogenic stimuli activate endothelial cells of existing blood vessels, causing sprouting and development of new vessels directed at the angiogenic stimuli. In a complex process, these vessels mature into networks attached to the circulation. New vessels can also be formed by intussusception, in which one capillary divides into two

and hedgehog [31], as well as signals derived from extracellular matrix [32]. Subsequent capillary formation occurs by angiogenesis, i.e., new capillary formation, and is initiated by existing capillaries [33]. This proceeds by either *sprouting angiogenesis*, in which new capillaries branch off existing ones, or *intussusceptive angiogenesis*, in which a capillary can subdivide into two capillaries [34] (Fig. 11.1b).

Angiogenesis and blood vessel maturation are complex and depend on recruitment of mural cells such as pericytes [35] to capillaries, and VSMCs [36] to arteries and veins, as well as numerous signaling molecules such as transforming growth factor-β1 [37], platelet-derived growth factor-B [38], and the angiopoietin receptors [39]. Under the control of a series of signaling molecules, including hedgehog, VEGF-A, and Notch, an arterial as opposed to venous or lymphatic endothelial cell phenotype may be favored [16, 40].

The processes of vasculogenesis and angiogenesis are augmented by branching [41, 42], pruning [22, 33], and remodeling [43], including arteriogenesis [44], to dynamically tailor the microcirculation to the physiology of the host organ, responding to local changes in flow [22], oxygen tension [45, 46], and paracrine signals from surrounding tissues [40, 43, 47]. The major epicardial coronary arteries do not form as outgrowths of the aorta, but instead form by vasculogenesis [48]. They connect to the aorta via selective apoptosis within the wall of the aorta [49], allowing coalescence of penetrating capillaries [50].

Translational Implications

The coordination and timing of the complex factors required to promote angiogenesis or vasculogenesis needs to be fully defined before clinical translation is attempted. For example, the view that supplementing a single factor like VEGF-A may promote angiogenesis in an ischemic organ quickly led to the realization that this may result in an increase in abnormal vessels. One example is "leaky" vessels that might cause adverse clinical outcomes. This "single-agent" approach favored by the industry supporting clinical trials of a patented single agent often ignores the complexity that developmental biology reveals.

Another important parameter often ignored in clinical translation is the regional metabolic and redox environment. This environment varies significantly from organ to organ and is intimately associated with the biology of the respective vascular beds. For example, the endothelium of the resistance pulmonary arteries is exposed to a PO_2 of >120 mmHg, the endothelium of the proximal aorta is exposed to a PO_2 of ~100 mmHg, and the microvascular endothelium of a systemic organ like the heart or kidney is exposed to a PO_2 of <50 mmHg.

These differences in PO_2 translate to significant differences in oxidative stress. For example, a high oxidative stress (i.e., a result of the high levels of oxygen), which is normal for a resistance pulmonary artery or an aorta endothelial cell, may not be tolerated by the endothelium of a coronary or peripheral organ microvessel. Strategies using aorta endothelial cells or human umbilical vein endothelial cells studied in "normal" in vitro conditions may fail if they are extrapolated to different organs and under very different conditions in disease states.

Endothelium of the Heart and Coronary Tree

Within the heart are five distinct types of endothelial cells, including endocardial, coronary arterial, venous, capillary, and lymphatic [51]. The endocardial endothelial cells originate in the heart field mesoderm of the primitive streak along with cardiomyocytes [52, 53]. These endocardial endothelial cells are not contiguous with other endothelial cell types, separating the cardiac chambers from the coronary circulation. Epicardial coronary arteries do not form as outgrowths of the aorta, but instead, these vessels, including endothelial cells, fibroblasts, and VSMCs, are derived from an extracardiac mesoderm called the proepicardium [54–58].

While lymph vessels appear alongside coronary arteries and veins, the cardiac lymphatics do not appear to be derived from the proepicardium [59]. Whether bone marrow–derived stem cells contribute to the development of normal coronary circulation is unclear [51, 60, 61]. These epicardial coronary arteries also connect to small muscular arteries that penetrate the myocardium, linking to the capillary bed formed in part from primitive blood islands (hemangioblasts) [62, 63]. The myocardial capillary endothelial cells invest the cardiomyocytes and outnumber them 3:1 [64]. As in other vascular beds, vasculogenesis, angiogenesis, and remodeling into arteries, capillaries, or veins are under the influence of stimuli such as hypoxia, shear stress, and growth factors, including various members of the VEGF family, members of the FGF family, the hedgehog system, the angiopoietins, and transforming growth factor (TGF)-β [65, 66].

Translational Implications

The different embryological origin of the endothelial cells of the epicardial coronary arteries and the coronary microcirculation is an important potential source for diversity in function between these two sites of the coronary tree. Endothelial function at one site may not reflect endothelial function at the other. Embryological differences may contribute to why diseases, such as atherosclerosis, preferentially affect certain segments of the vasculature.

Markers of vessel type–specific endothelial cells need to be discovered before animal or human tissue immunohistochemistry data can be interpreted appropriately. For example, an endothelium marker like von Willebrand factor (vWF) will stain arteries, veins, and lymphatics – vessels that operate under very different metabolic environments and have different physiologic regulatory mechanisms. Thus, a measure of a nonspecific endothelial marker as an index of angiogenesis in the arterial circulation of an ischemic organ is too superficial and of unclear physiologic significance by itself.

Endothelial Diversity

A central feature of the endothelium is diversity, both in structure and function [3, 67]. Endothelial cells are diverse in size and range in thickness from 0.1 μm in capillaries to 1 μm in the aorta [68]. In a study of rat blood vessels, aortic endothelial cells were long and narrow, measuring 55×10 μm, while those of the pulmonary artery were broader and shorter, measuring 30×14 μm [69]. In rat capillaries, the average endothelial cell thickness ranges from 0.1 to 0.3 μm, with the average lengths

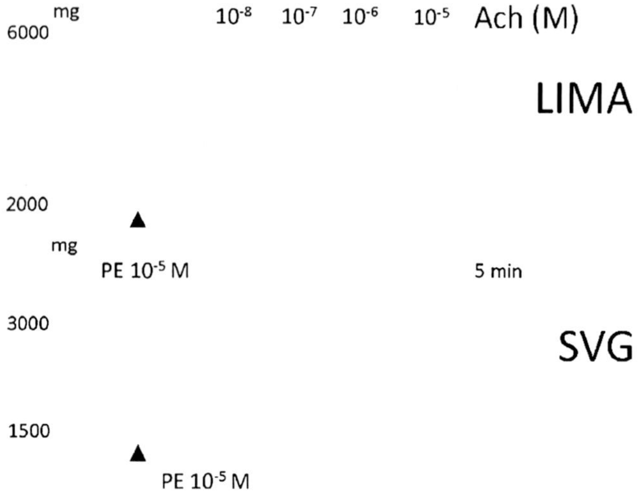

Fig. 11.2 Endothelium-dependent vasodilation is reduced in human saphenous vein grafts compared to human left internal mammary arteries. Endothelial cell diversity may explain differential capacities of different vascular beds

and widths ranging from approximately 10 to 22 μm and 8 to 19 μm, respectively [70]. The endothelial cells of various vascular beds are diverse in shape: typically flat and aligned with the direction of flow in arteries [71], while endothelial cells of postcapillary venules in lymphoid tissue are plump and cuboidal [72].

Other structural differences of endothelial cells across vascular beds include various structures that facilitate endothelial permeability, including clathrin-coated pits and vesicles that facilitate endocytosis [73] and membrane-bound vesicles called *caveolae* that participate in transcytosis [74]. Additional evidence of diversity includes differences in fenestrae [70], which are transcellular pores ~70 nm in diameter that span the endothelial cell, with diaphragms across the pore entrance; and whether or not the endothelial layer is continuous or discontinuous [3]. For example, endothelium of the liver sinusoids is discontinuous, with large fenestrations of up to 200 nm in diameter that lack a diaphragm [75], while the endothelium of the myocardium is nonfenestrated [70]. Lumenal glycocalyx varies in thickness across the endothelium [76], as does the amount of surrounding supporting cells such as pericytes or smooth muscle cells [3].

Endothelial cells are also diverse in terms of gene expression [77] and endothelial cell surface markers [78]. For example, arterial and venous endothelial cells express different sets of molecular markers [12, 79], which are different again from lymphatic endothelial cells [80]. Expression of vWF also varies across vascular beds in different organs and appears to be controlled by the endothelial local microenvironment [81]. Similarly, in pulmonary circulation, both constitutive expression and induced expression of tissue plasminogen activator appear confined to a subset of endothelial cells of intermediate-size arteries [82].

The broad array of endothelial cells' structural differences facilitates various functions of the endothelium. So diverse are endothelial cells that one investigator has argued that "it is not a stretch to imagine that each one of our approximately 60 trillion ECs is phenotypically distinct [3]."

One feature of this diversity is that endothelial cells appear to be "plastic" regarding phenotype and able to adapt to local changes in humoral and biochemical stimuli [83]. For example, cell culture conditions can dramatically alter endothelial phenotype in vitro [84]. In addition, although human saphenous vein bypass grafts have different endothelium than internal mammary arteries, characterized by reduced endothelium-dependent vasodilation but similar response to vasoconstrictors (Fig. 11.2), vein graft segments exposed to the arterial circulation can change phenotypically, or "arterialize [85]."

The sources of endothelial diversity have been reviewed [86] and include the influence of epigenetic programming of endothelial cells of a specific vascular bed to behave in certain ways [77], as well as local signals from the extracellular environment, including blood shear stress and strain, pH, oxygenation, growth factors, cytokines, chemokines, hormones, serine proteases, lipoproteins, sphingolipids, nucleosides, complements, and components of the extracellular matrix [86].

Translational Implications

A major feature of endothelial diversity is that the surface markers of endothelial cells differ across the vascular bed. For example, lectins, which are proteins that bind highly selectively to particular carbohydrate moiety, can be used to selectively bind to and target endothelial cells from particular segments of a vascular bed [87]. This technology can be used for molecular imaging, but in theory could also be used to target pharmacotherapy to particular segments of the coronary tree.

Normal Endothelial Function

Endothelial cells have many functions, although most are not universally shared. Instead, they are performed by specific subsets in particular vascular beds or organs. These functions include physiologic permeability, leukocyte trafficking, hemostasis, vascular tone, angiogenesis, and innate and acquired immunity [3, 79, 88].

The endothelium forms a physical barrier that separates blood from tissue [89] but also is responsible for transcytosis, or transport across the endothelium in discrete membrane-bound vesicles, facilitating communication between the circulating blood and tissues [70]. Endothelial cells regulate leukocyte trafficking, matching vascular injury with inflammatory response [90]; this process has significant implications for atherosclerosis [91]. In arteries, including the coronary tree, a major function of the healthy endothelium is maintaining vascular tone in order to match blood flow with local metabolic requirements. Furchgott and colleagues first observed that the endothelium has an obligatory role in the vasodilation of isolated arteries in response to acetylcholine [92].

Subsequent investigators identified an endothelium-derived relaxing factor (EDRF) [93] as nitric oxide [94], which is produced within endothelial cells, hyperpolarizes adjacent smooth muscle cells in a paracrine manner, and induces blood vessel relaxation [95]. In addition to nitric oxide, vasodilating prostaglandins, such as prostacyclin, are also produced by endothelial cells [96, 97].

In addition, various other mechanisms, collectively known as endothelium-derived hyperpolarizing factors, have been described in various vascular beds, including hydrogen peroxide, epoxyeicosatrienoic acids (EETs), potassium ions, and electrical communications through gap junctions [98]. These vasodilating substances, together with secretion of vasoconstricting substances such as endothelins, maintain vascular tone under basal circumstances and in response to stimuli, such as hypoxia or exercise [95, 98, 99].

Nitric oxide, prostacyclin, and other endothelium-derived hyperpolarizing factors cause VSMC hyperpolarization by opening potassium channels in the VSMC plasma membrane (Fig. 11.3a), decreasing VSMC intracellular calcium by closing voltage-sensitive calcium channels, and depriving actin-myosin complexes of calcium [99]. Nitric oxide binds with soluble guanylate cyclase within VSMCs and increases cyclic guanosine monophosphate (cGMP) levels, which activates

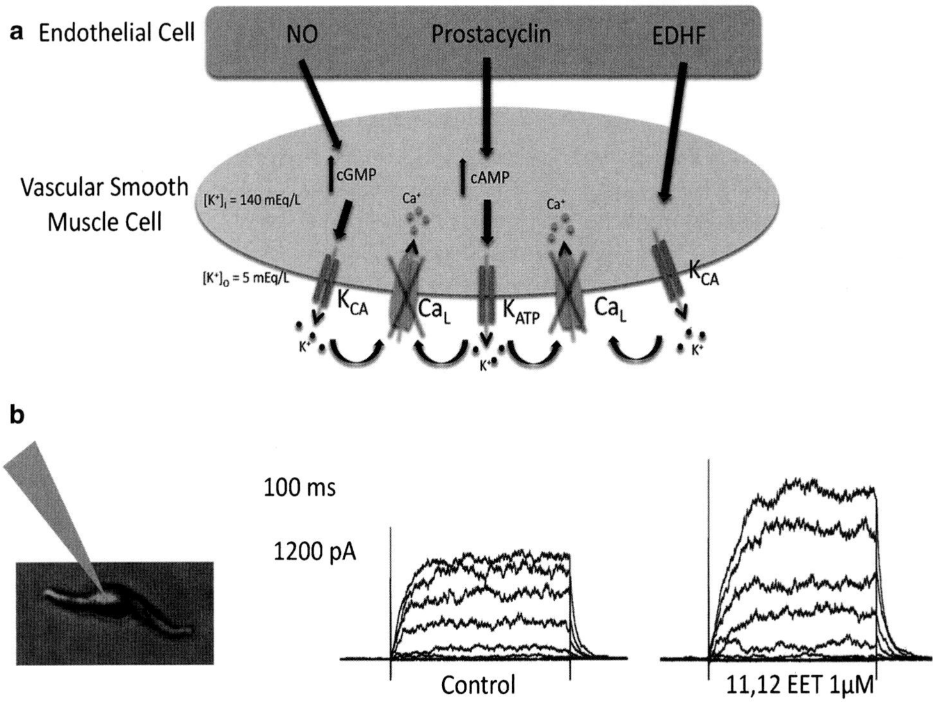

Fig. 11.3 Endothelium-dependent vasodilation involves signaling pathways that culminate in hyperpolarization of adjacent vascular smooth muscle cells (VSMCs), closure of L-type voltage-sensitive calcium channels, decreased levels of intracellular calcium, and relaxation (**a**). Nitric oxide interacts with soluble guanylate cyclase, increasing cyclic GMP levels and activating calcium-sensitive potassium channels (K_{Ca}). Similarly, prostacyclin increases cyclic AMP levels, activating ATP-sensitive potassium channels (K_{ATP}). There are several, putative "endothelium-dependent" hyperpolarizing factors, but ultimately, they all lead to VSMC hyperpolarization. For example, the molecule 11,12-epoxyeicosatrienoic acid is a putative endothelium-derived hyperpolarizing factor (**b**) [102]

calcium-activated potassium channels (K_{Ca}) in the VSMC plasma membrane, inducing VSMC hyperpolarization [100]. Similarly, prostacyclin increases cyclic adenosine monophosphate (cAMP) levels within VSMCs, activating adenosine triphosphate-sensitive potassium channels (K_{ATP}) and hyperpolarizing the VSMCs [101].

Other endothelium-derived hyperpolarizing factors directly activate VSMC potassium channels; for example, 11,12-epoxyeicosatrienoic acid directly activates the large-conductance, calcium-sensitive potassium channel (BK_{Ca}; Fig. 11.3b) [102]. These endothelium-based signaling pathways have been the target of a large number of routinely used cardiovascular vasoactive drugs, including nitrates, phosphodiesterase inhibitors, endothelin antagonists, and prostacyclin analogues. In the context of atherosclerotic coronary artery disease, endothelium-dependent vasodilation in response to stress or exercise may be insufficient to increase blood flow to meet metabolic demands because of a proximal stenosis, leading to ischemia.

Translational Implications

The targets of endothelium-derived vasodilators are often VSMC potassium channels. Because potassium channels are open at the resting membrane potential of most VSMC, their closure or opening determines whether the VSMC will hyperpolarize (in which case the voltage-gated L-type calcium channels will be closed and the VSMC will relax) or depolarize (in which case the calcium channels will open, calcium will influx because there is a 10,000 fold increase in the extracellular vs. intracellular calcium), and the VSMC will contract. Potassium channels are very dynamically expressed proteins that can be altered by the activation of several transcription factors important in vascular disease, such as the nuclear factor of activated T cells (NFAT).

This important fact needs to be kept in mind when interpreting the response of vessels to endothelium-based vasodilators. For example, insufficient vasodilatation in response to pharmacologic or physiologic stimuli may be due to a downregulation or abnormality of VSMC potassium channels, and not necessarily a problem with endothelial signaling.

Endothelial Dysfunction and Activation

Although the term "endothelial dysfunction" was coined in 1980 to describe hyperadhesiveness of endothelium to platelets [14], human in vivo studies of acetylcholine-induced vasoconstriction of coronary arteries suggested a defect in the endothelium-dependent vasomotor function [103]. This is the most common understanding of the term endothelial dysfunction, which usually refers to reduced endothelium-dependent relaxation of a blood vessel.

The term "endothelial activation" stems from in vitro studies that showed that certain stimuli, such as interleukin-1 or TNF-α, could induce the expression of antigens on the surface of endothelial cells, such as E-selectin. These changes are observed in humans in vivo [104] and are associated with a procoagulant phenotype [14, 105]. Endothelial activation may also occur in response to shear stress, pressure, and hypoxia [106].

This concept has led to an understanding that activated endothelial cells respond to a potentially injurious stimulus and have a procoagulant, proadhesive, and vasoconstricting phenotype, which is in turn implicated in atherogenesis [107]. Endothelial activation with proadhesive and procoagulant effects may be a later stage of endothelial disease that is first expressed as a relative imbalance of endothelium-derived vasodilators vs. vasoconstrictors. In other words, the ability to detect endothelium dysfunction based on vascular tone abnormalities, either by history or simple diagnostic tests, may be a powerful predictor of impending, severe, vascular disease.

Translational Implications

Because endothelial dysfunction could represent or evolve into a systemic disease, early diagnosis may predict the imminent expression of atherosclerotic disease. Similarly, recognizing signs of endothelial dysfunction in one vascular bed may predict the presence of vascular disease in other vascular beds. For example, erectile dysfunction is a well-known result of abnormal endothelium-derived vasodilation in penile circulation. Defective nitric oxide–dependent vasodilation in penile arteries results in inability to increase the blood input to the penis and thus inability to achieve or maintain erection. This common problem can be detected with simple history taking, but is now known to strongly predict the coexistence of coronary artery disease or diffuse atherosclerosis, and may facilitate early diagnosis of atherosclerotic vascular disease.

Assaying Endothelial Function in the Clinic

Ross proposed that endothelial injury led to smooth muscle cell proliferation, in turn leading to the arterial lesions of atherosclerosis [108]. Systemic endothelial dysfunction is a key parameter associated with the pathogenesis [109] and complications of atherosclerosis [4]. Endothelial dysfunction correlates with traditional risk factors, including hypertension [11], hypercholesterolemia [110, 111], diabetes [112, 113], smoking [114], and age [115], and it may precede overt atherosclerotic plaques [116]. When identifying patients with subclinical atherosclerosis or at risk for future complications of atherosclerosis, the term endothelial dysfunction primarily refers to loss of normal endothelium-dependent vasodilation [90]. It may also include aspects of endothelial activation [14], including proinflammatory and procoagulant changes of the endothelium that promote atherosclerosis [107].

Atherosclerotic coronary arteries fail to dilate during exercise [117], and paradoxically constrict in response to acetylcholine [103], contributing to impaired myocardial blood flow [118]. The degree of loss of endothelium-mediated vasodilation correlates with the amount of coronary atherosclerosis [119]. Endothelial dysfunction, as well as atherosclerosis itself, is a systemic process [120], and peripheral arterial vasomotor responses strongly predict coronary arterial vasomotor responses [121].

Several techniques to evaluate endothelial function in humans have been developed, including intracoronary assessment of acetylcholine-induced vasomotion [103]; assessment of myocardial blood flow in response to dipyridamole (coronary flow reserve) using positron emission tomography [122]; impedance plethysmography [123, 124]; ultrasound measurements of brachial artery flow-mediated vasodilation (FMD) [110]; assessment of arterial stiffness [125], including arterial pulse wave velocity (PWV); arterial compliance and analyses of arterial pulse waveforms; and laser Doppler flowmetry. Typically, these techniques involve comparing an index of endothelium-dependent vasodilation to an index of endothelium-independent vasodilation.

For example, with brachial artery FMD, the diameter of the brachial artery is measured in response to increased flow due to 5 min of ischemia caused by blood pressure cuff occlusion (endothelium-dependent vasodilation). This measurement is compared with the diameter of the same brachial artery segment after 0.4 mg SL of nitroglycerin, which directly dilates the arterial smooth muscle independent of the endothelium (endothelium-independent vasodilation). Many of these techniques have been shown to complement traditional risk factor assessment in identifying subjects at risk for atherosclerotic events.

Intracoronary Assessment

The gold standard for coronary artery endothelial dysfunction testing is arguably intracoronary assessment [107], in which coronary artery diameter is measured in response to stimuli such as infusion of acetylcholine, cold pressor testing (an extremity exposed to ice-cold water), increased blood flow, or nitroglycerine [103, 119]. Normal coronary artery endothelium responds to intracoronary acetylcholine by releasing nitric oxide [94], which diffuses to adjacent smooth muscle cells, stimulates soluble guanylate cyclases, causing increased levels of cGMP. The cGMP induces relaxation of the smooth muscle cell by activating potassium channels in the plasma membrane, leading to hyperpolarization, decreased calcium entry into the cell, and relaxation, as well as stimulating a cGMP-dependent protein kinase that activates myosin light chain phosphatase, also leading to relaxation [103, 126].

Nitroglycerin (an NO donor) infusion bypasses the endothelium and induces smooth muscle cells to relax directly. In vessels with dysfunctional endothelium, this endothelium-dependent relaxation in response to acetylcholine is absent, but smooth muscle cell receptors for acetylcholine induce paradoxical vasoconstriction (Fig. 11.4a) [103]. In addition to angiographic assessments of coronary diameter, blood flow can also be evaluated concomitantly using Doppler flow wires [127, 128] (Fig. 11.4b).

In a cohort of 147 patients with coronary artery disease, abnormal coronary artery vasodilation predicted symptomatic cardiovascular events over a follow-up period of 7.7 years independently of other risk factors [129]. Similarly, in a cohort of 308 patients, including 132 with coronary artery disease and 176 without coronary artery disease, coronary artery endothelial dysfunction predicted cardiovascular events independently of other risk factors [130].

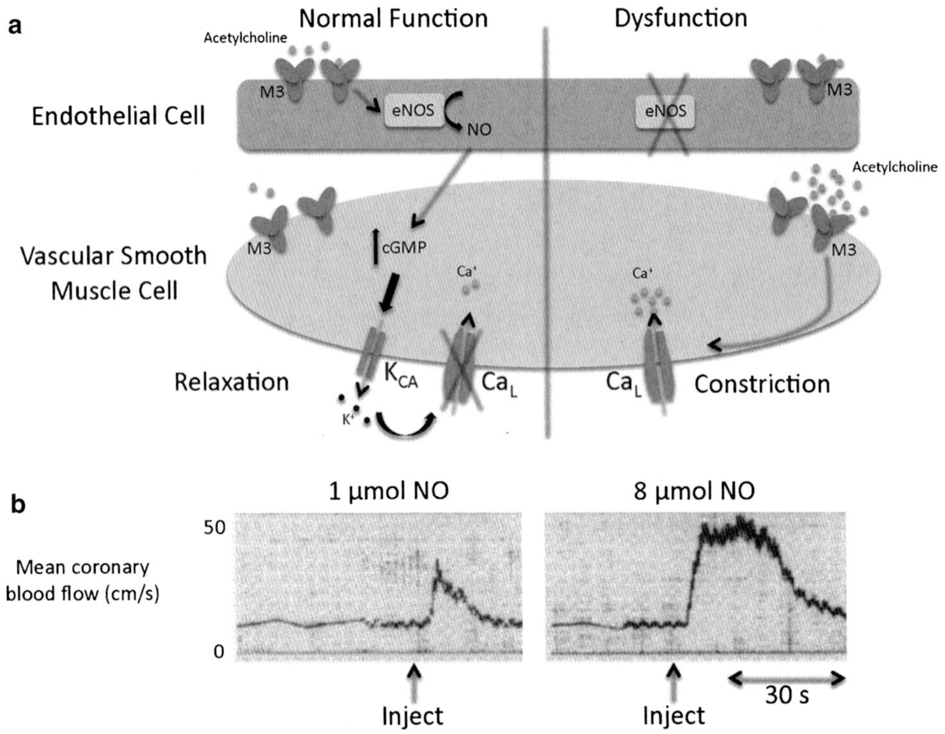

Fig. 11.4 Acetylcholine can be used to identify endothelial dysfunction in humans in vivo (**a**). In normal coronary arteries, acetylcholine activates the M3 muscarinic receptor on endothelial cells and activates endothelial nitric oxide synthase (eNOS), inducing nitric oxide (NO) production, VSMC hyperpolarization, and relaxation. In dysfunctional endothelial cells, nitric oxide production is deficient. At higher concentrations of acetylcholine, the muscarinic receptors on the VSMCs are activated, leading to opening of L-type calcium channels and constriction. Changes in tone can be detected angiographically or using Doppler wires. (**b**) Coronary artery mean blood flow is measured in response to low- and high-dose nitric oxide with a Doppler wire. (**b**) Adapted from Chambers et al. [127]. Copyright 1996 by American Physiological Society

Impedance Plethysmography

In 1975, Hokanson and colleagues described impedance plethysmography as a technique for measuring limb blood flow [123]. It involves measuring small changes in electrical resistance (impedance) of the limb that correspond to changes in blood flow. When a blood pressure cuff prevents venous return but not arterial inflow, the rate of increase in volume of the limb is proportional to arterial inflow.

In subjects not exposed for at least 12 h to substances that might affect endothelial function, including food, cigarette smoke, and vasoactive drugs, a brachial artery line is inserted for blood pressure measurement and infusion of drugs. A venous occlusion plethysmograph, calibrated in milliliter per 100 mL of tissue per minute, is applied to the limb. After steady-state heart rate and blood pressure is reached, each arm is supported above the heart level, and venous occlusion is achieved using a blood pressure cuff (approximately 35 mmHg). Blood flow is recorded at baseline and in response to intra-arterial infusions of vasoactive drugs [124]. Endothelial function can be assayed using this technique, with intra-arterial challenges of methacholine or acetylcholine [124, 131] or reactive hyperemia [132]. Endothelial dysfunction assayed by this technique has been demonstrated to predict cardiovascular complications in small cohorts [133–136].

Brachial Artery FMD

Arguably the most common in vivo measurement of endothelial function in humans, ultrasound measurements of brachial artery FMD were initially described by Celemajer and colleagues in 1992 [110]. In essence, the diameter of the brachial artery is measured before and after peripheral ischemia induced by blood pressure cuff occlusion distal to the site of measurement (FMD) or oral nitroglycerin (pharmacologic vasodilation). This technique has been standardized, and guidelines [137] exist to

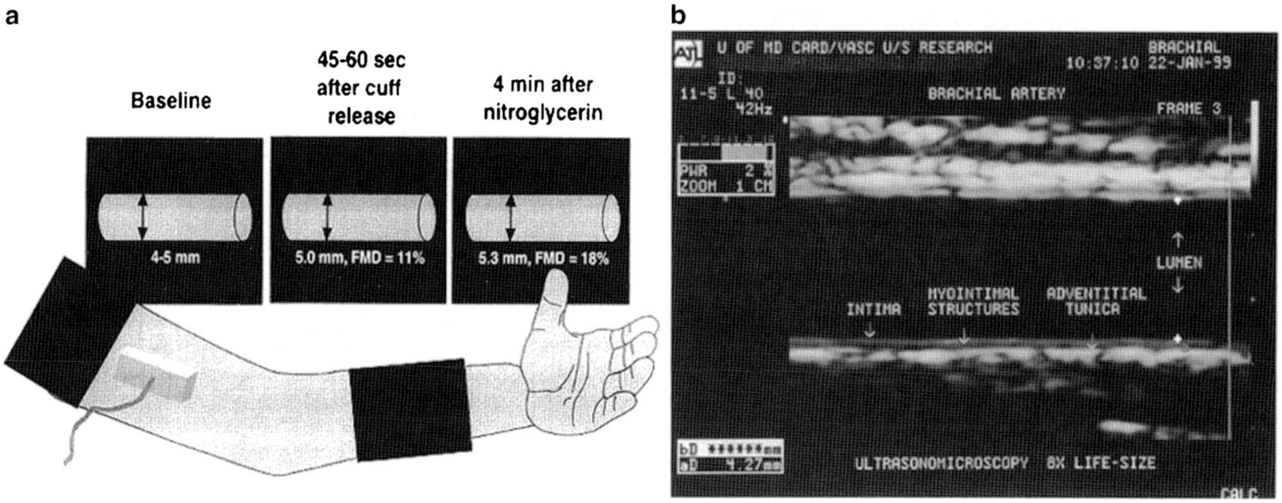

Fig. 11.5 A ratio of ultrasound measurements of the brachial artery before and after either 5 min of cuff-induced ischemia or 4 min of nitroglycerin 0.4 mg SL yields the brachial artery flow-mediated vasodilation (FMD), a common index of endothelial dysfunction. The brachial artery is imaged with a high-frequency linear array ultrasound probe, and typically, the blood pressure cuff is placed distal to the brachial artery (**a**). The brachial artery diameter is measured from the lumen-intima interface at the same point of the cardiac cycle (**b**). After hyperemic stimulus or nitroglycerin, the brachial artery diameter increases. Adapted from Corretti et al. [137]. Copyright 2002 by American College of Cardiology Foundation

assist laboratories implement standard protocols. Occlusion proximal to the site of measurement is avoided in order to prevent any effect of ischemia on the vessel itself [138].

As with impedance plethysmography, the patient is prepared by fasting and avoiding substances that affect endothelial function for at least 12 h [137]. Studies should be performed in a dimly lit, temperature-controlled, quiet room. The patient is positioned supine, and the brachial artery is imaged in the antecubital fossa using a high-frequency, linear ultrasound array. A segment with clearly visible anterior and posterior intimal surfaces is selected for continuous imaging; usually 2D imaging is used, as opposed to M-mode imaging. A blood pressure cuff occludes arterial blood flow in the forearm distal to the imaging site, and the limb is made ischemic for at least 5 min. Brachial artery diameter is measured offline either with electronic calipers or edge-detection software. Maximal change in brachial artery diameter is usually observed 45–60 s after release of the cuff.

When response to 0.4 mg sublingual nitroglycerin is measured, measurements are made 3–4 min after the dose is given (Fig. 11.5). This technique is able to measure interventions that either decrease or improve endothelial function in a noninvasive, sensitive, and immediate way. For example, improvements in endothelial function can be measured within minutes of ingesting dark chocolate [139] while worsening of endothelial function can be documented even after brief inhalation of secondhand tobacco smoke (Fig. 11.6).

The ease and sensitivity of this method make it very attractive for use in either the outpatient clinical or in research protocols, although the technique still suffers from reproducibility. Several cohort studies have demonstrated a significant association between ultrasound-demonstrated endothelial dysfunction and cardiovascular events [140–145].

Arterial Stiffness (Applanation Tonometry and Pulse Waveform Analysis)

Epidemiological evidence linking hemodynamic evidence of arterial stiffness, or wide pulse pressure, with adverse cardiovascular outcomes [146] has led to the development of several techniques to measure arterial stiffness noninvasively [125]. Although arterial stiffness is a complex property that depends in part on arterial wall collagen, elastin, and smooth muscle bulk and tone [147], endothelium-derived relaxation is an important regulator of arterial distensibility [148]. Arterial stiffness may be considered an analogue of endothelial dysfunction.

Methods to measure arterial stiffness fall into three general groups: (1) measuring PWV, (2) relating intra-arterial pressure changes to artery dimension changes (diameter or area), and (3) evaluating arterial pressure waveforms [125]. PWV, or the velocity of arterial wave propagation, correlates with arterial stiffness and can be measured using several techniques,

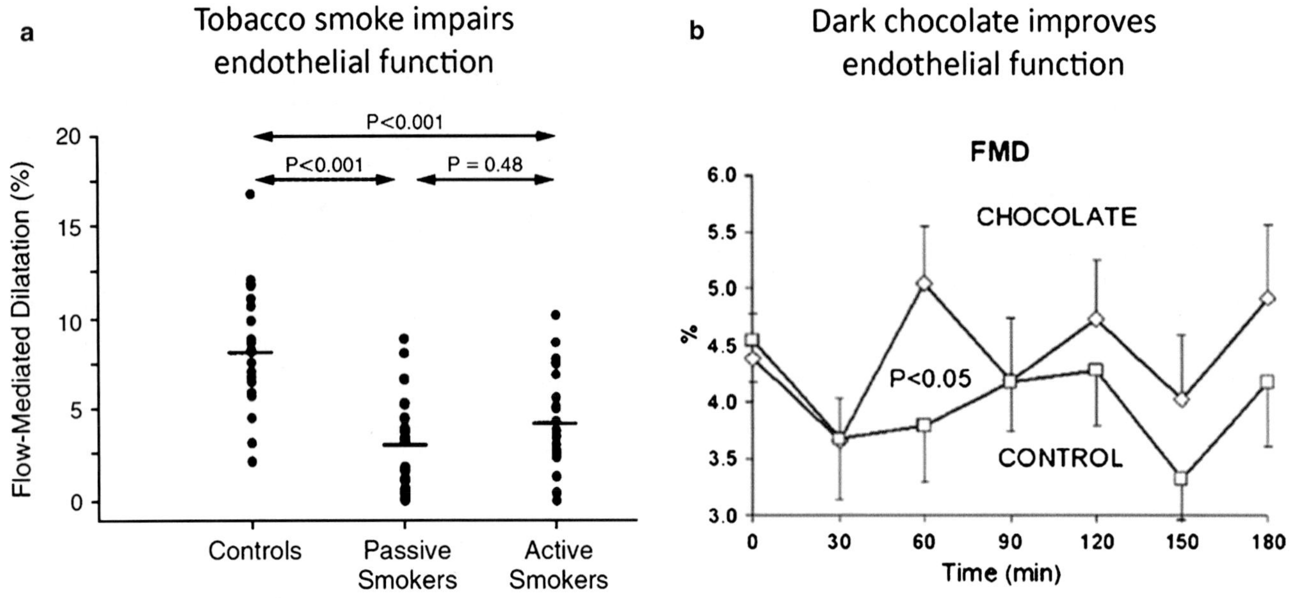

Fig. 11.6 Ultrasound measurements of brachial artery FMD is a sensitive technique to measure endothelial function in humans. Exposure to tobacco smoke, whether through active smoking or passive exposure, reduces brachial artery FMD ((**a**) endothelium-dependent vasodilation), while the ability of the brachial artery to dilate in response to nitroglycerin is unchanged. Ingestion of dark chocolate can improve brachial artery FMD ((**b**) endothelium-dependent vasodilation). Brachial artery FMD is a useful, noninvasive technique for assaying positive or negative changes in endothelial function. (**a**) Adapted from Celermajer et al. [220]. Copyright 1996 by Massachusetts Medical Society. (**b**) Adapted from Vlachopoulos et al. [139]. Copyright 2005 by Nature Publishing Group

including pressure transducers [149], Doppler ultrasound [150], applanation tonometry [151], and magnetic resonance imaging [152]. Arterial PWV increases with standard cardiovascular risk factors [125], and increased PWV predicts cardiovascular events independently of traditional cardiovascular risk factors [153].

Arterial distensibility curves, relating artery dimension to artery pressure, can be generated using blood pressure measurements and imaging (usually with ultrasound [125]), obtained either noninvasively [154] or invasively [155]. Although arterial distensibility has not been evaluated in large cohorts as a predictor of cardiovascular risk, it can predict mortality in patients with advanced renal failure [156, 157].

Arterial pulse waveforms can be measured both invasively with intra-arterial catheter and noninvasively, usually with applanation tonometry [125]. Systolic pulse contour analysis uses a transfer function to calculate central aortic waveforms based on those from a more distal artery, usually the radial artery [158]. From the central waveform, an augmentation index is calculated as the portion of central pulse pressure that results from arterial wave reflection, and is interpreted as an index of arterial stiffness [159]. In diastolic pulse contour analysis, the circulation is modeled as a modified windkessel, and compliance of large and small artery beds is calculated [160, 161].

As an alternative to measuring pulse waveforms in more proximal arteries, digital arterial pressure and volume waveforms are easily measurable. "Transfer functions" exist that relate digital waveforms to central waveforms [162] and therefore arterial stiffness [163]. Digital pulse amplitude, measured using digital artery tonometry, correlates with cardiovascular risk factors [164].

Digital Thermal Monitoring

Endothelial function can also be noninvasively assessed by measuring temperature changes digitally in response to reactive hyperemia due to 5 min of ischemia caused by cuff occlusion of an upper extremity [165]. Abnormal endothelial function detected using this technique correlates with extent of atherosclerosis [166] and other measures of cardiovascular risk, including Framingham risk scores and coronary calcium scores [167].

Biomarkers

Although endothelial dysfunction usually implies impaired endothelium-dependent relaxation, activated endothelium may change the rate of release of certain molecules. Altered levels of these molecules may be detected in the serum, facilitating early diagnosis of endothelial activation and subclinical atherosclerosis. The vWF, soluble thrombomodulin, adhesion molecules (including ICAM-1, VCAM-1, E-selectin, P-selection, soluble CD40 ligand), cytokines (including interleukins 6, TNF-α, and hsCRP), and circulating progenitor cells have all been proposed as markers of endothelial dysfunction [168–170]. Of these, hsCRP arguably has been studied the most; increased levels of hsCRP are associated with higher rates of incident cardiovascular events [171]. While novel biomarkers and cardiovascular risk factors are a hot topic of research, so far, the contribution of biomarkers to predicting cardiovascular outcomes beyond standard risk factor assessment has been small.

Imaging

While not strictly measures of endothelial function, other methods of atherosclerosis imaging have come to complement standard risk factor assessment and measurement of endothelial dysfunction to predict cardiovascular risk. These techniques include carotid ultrasound measurements of intima-medial thickness (IMT), computed tomography coronary calcium scores, and other forms of noninvasive imaging of atherosclerotic plaques [172]. Of these, carotid ultrasound assessments of IMT [173] and plaque [174], as well as computed tomographic imaging of coronary calcium [175], enhance cardiovascular risk prediction beyond traditional risk factor assessment [176, 177]. Imaging techniques may complement measures of endothelial dysfunction in identifying patients at risk of complications [178].

Limitations

Several of the listed techniques for measuring endothelial dysfunction in humans have limitations. Intracoronary techniques are invasive, expensive, and involve risk of significant complications, disqualifying them from routine use in ambulatory care. Similarly, impedance plethysmography involving brachial artery cannulation has attendant risks and arguably little utility beyond research laboratories.

Variability is a key limitation of all techniques of endothelial vasomotor response [107]. For example, despite rigorous attention to method and protocol, brachial artery ultrasound flow-mediated dilatation (FMD) assessments of endothelial function can vary by up to 25% from day to day [107]. Similarly, day-to-day variability limits the use of impedance plethysmography [179]. Compounding intralaboratory or intrasubject laboratory variability, differences in technical aspects of measurement implemented by different laboratories can result in marked differences across the published literature [180]. With respect to biomarkers, endothelial cell diversity, both across time and vascular beds, may limit the utility of global serum markers of endothelial dysfunction or activation [14].

Finally, and perhaps most importantly, while there are data from large randomized controlled trials of therapies for established cardiovascular risk factors, such as statins for dyslipidemia or angiotensin-converting enzyme inhibitors for hypertension, that demonstrate an association between improved endothelial function and lowered cardiovascular risk, it is unclear whether improved endothelial function is causal in reductions in atherosclerotic complications, or a by-product of less atherosclerosis, and whether endothelial function should be a pharmacologic target per se. Despite these limitations, measuring endothelial function in humans is an important clinical and research tool. Of the techniques listed above, brachial artery FMD is the most commonly used.

Translational Implications

A comprehensive, university-based vascular medicine clinic should provide a comprehensive set of services to deliver excellent clinical care and perform patient-centered translational research. These clinics should be prepared to evaluate and treat a diverse set of cardiovascular disorders, including atherosclerotic cardiovascular disease in any territory, venous thromboembolism, pulmonary hypertension, erectile dysfunction, aneurismal disorders, and vasculidities, as well as provide early disease detection and primary prevention. This care may cross traditional medical subspecialty boundaries, with access to many medical specialties and nonphysician providers (nurses, pharmacists, and dieticians). Coordination between medical specialists, imaging specialists, endovascular specialists, and surgeons is essential.

In addition, noninvasive vascular testing, including vascular ultrasound, segmental Doppler, ankle and toe pressure measurements, are required to evaluate the presence of vascular disease at the bedside. Access to more advanced imaging, including computed tomography and magnetic resonance angiography of the vasculature, is needed, as well as invasive angiography and endovascular therapies.

In order to facilitate early disease detection, an endothelial function assay is also required. Of the techniques available, brachial artery FMD is the most widely used and validated.

Facilities to obtain, process, and store human blood and tissue samples must be located in close proximity to clinical space to facilitate research. And a database is needed to log the clinical experience for research purposes.

Medical Therapy for Endothelial Dysfunction

Several interventions are known to enhance endothelial function, and many of these are associated with reductions in subsequent cardiovascular events [4, 107, 132]. Therapeutic lifestyle changes, including smoking cessation [114, 181], exercise [182], and a low-cholesterol diet [183, 184], improve both endothelial function and rates of cardiovascular outcomes. Antihypertensive therapy, in particular, inhibition of the angiotensin-converting enzyme or angiotensin receptor, is associated with both improved endothelial function [140, 185, 186] and better cardiovascular outcomes [187, 188]. Similarly, lipid lowering with statins improves endothelial function [189, 190] and cardiovascular outcomes [191]. Therapy with aspirin is similarly beneficial [192, 193].

Not all interventions that improve endothelial function are associated with improvements in cardiovascular outcomes. For example, both estrogen [194] and antioxidant vitamins [183, 195] appear to enhance endothelial function, but neither has been demonstrated to improve cardiovascular outcomes in clinical trials [196, 197]. Supplementation with L-arginine [198], a substrate of nitric oxide synthase, also improves endothelial function.

Endothelial Progenitor Cells

Endothelial progenitor cells (EPCs) were first described in 1997, when Asahara and colleagues isolated cells from the human peripheral circulation using antigen-coated magnetic beads that had the potential to differentiate into endothelial cells in vitro and contribute to angiogenesis in animal models of ischemia [199]. Subsequent experiments demonstrated that these cells are derived from bone marrow and that postnatal neovascularization may rely in part on circulating EPCs incorporating into new blood vessel structures, as opposed to angiogenesis from preexisting capillaries only [200]. With the half-life of an adult endothelial cell estimated at about 3 years [201], these EPCs may be an important mechanism for vascular maintenance and repair [202].

Many antigenic markers have been used to identify EPCs, including CD34, CD133, CD45, VEGFR-s, CD133, CXC chemokine receptor 4, CD14, and CD31 [203], but there is no consensus that a single marker or set of markers definitively identifies EPCs [204]; this is an area of controversy and intense research. Understanding master transcription factors, such as Nkx2-5, may help elucidate how particular EPCs ultimately become functional endothelium [205]. Consensus parameters that will help identify putative EPCs include the capacity to mobilize from niches in response to vascular injury, and participation in neovessel formation [203].

Despite the controversy of identity of EPCs, circulating (CD34/KDR–positive) EPCs are reduced in patients with CAD compared to controls [206], and EPCs from subjects with risk factors have an impaired migratory response [207]. Major risk factors for atherosclerosis, including smoking [208], hypertension [207], dyslipidemia [209], and diabetes [210], are all associated with reduced EPC numbers or function, and EPC levels predict cardiovascular outcomes [211]. Defective EPC capacity can be considered a biomarker or an extension of endothelial dysfunction.

In addition to use as a biomarker to identify cardiovascular disease, EPCs may have promise as therapy [212–214]. Although initially thought to engraft into forming or healing blood vessels, more recent studies attribute a substantive portion of the therapeutic effect of EPCs on paracrine enhancement of angiogenesis and vascular repair [215–217]. In this contemporary paradigm, bone marrow–derived EPCs, monocytic cells, and mature endothelial cells work together to effect blood vessel healing (Fig. 11.7) [218].

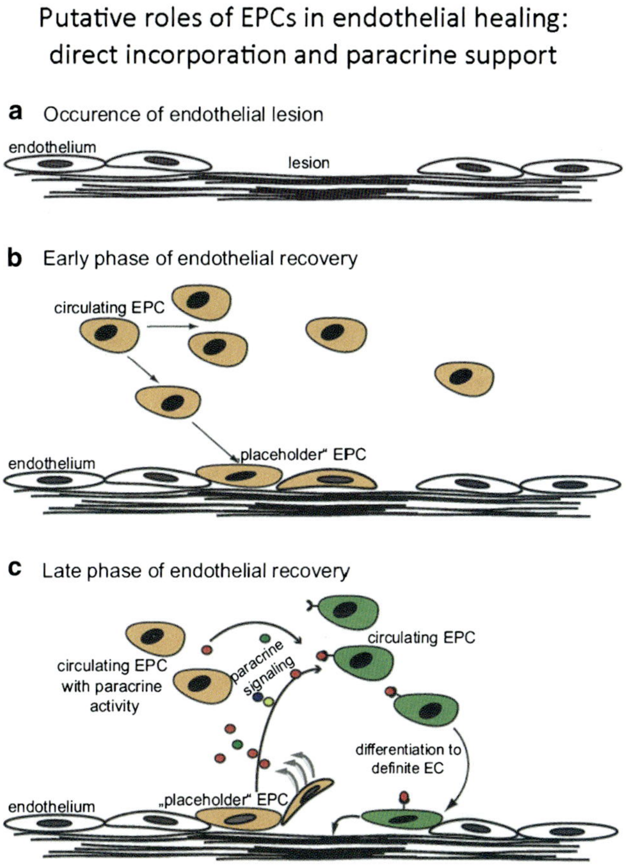

Fig. 11.7 Putative roles of EPCs in endothelial healing. In the early stage, circulating EPCs adhere to lesion sites (**a**) to begin the healing process (**b**). In the later phase, circulating and "place-holding" EPCs may support the healing process in a paracrine manner (**c**). Figures reproduced with permission from Steinmetz et al. [221]. Copyright 2010 by American Heart Association

In the early stage, circulating EPCs, perhaps monocyte-derived, adhere to lesion sites and initiate repair [218]. In the later phase, other circulating and "place-holding" EPCs within the vascular wall may support adhesion of EPCs and repair in a paracrine manner [218]. The details of these processes are areas of intense current research. While the potential of EPCs as therapy has yet to be realized, accomplishments such as the development of functional in vitro blood vessels attest to the great promise of progenitor cells [219].

Future Directions

Despite advances in cardiovascular science and clinical care, cardiovascular diseases, including atherosclerotic coronary artery disease, remain an important source of morbidity and mortality worldwide. Improved understanding of endothelial biology may lead to better understanding of the role of the endothelium in the pathogenesis of coronary artery disease as well as significant improvements in cardiovascular care in the future.

Priorities for translational cardiovascular medicine include: (1) determining the therapeutic potential, if any, of endothelial precursor cells; (2) better understanding the fundamentals of endothelial developmental biology and applying them to repairing vascular injury in vivo or ex vivo (i.e., artificial blood vessels and organs); and (3) taking advantage of endothelial diversity to develop novel imaging modalities to track response to therapy within a specific vascular bed or guide selective molecular therapies to a specific vascular bed.

References

1. Jaffe EA. Cell biology of endothelial cells. Hum Pathol. 1987;18(3):234–9.
2. Fishman AP. Endothelium: a distributed organ of diverse capabilities. Ann N Y Acad Sci. 1982;401:1–8.
3. Aird WC. Phenotypic heterogeneity of the endothelium: I. Structure, function, and mechanisms. Circ Res. 2007;100(2):158–73.

4. Bonetti PO, Lerman LO, Lerman A. Endothelial dysfunction: a marker of atherosclerotic risk. Arterioscler Thromb Vasc Biol. 2003;23(2):168–75.
5. Ferrari R, Bachetti T, Agnoletti L, Comini L, Curello S. Endothelial function and dysfunction in heart failure. Eur Heart J. 1998;19(Suppl G):G41–7.
6. Leask RL, Jain N, Butany J. Endothelium and valvular diseases of the heart. Microsc Res Tech. 2003;60(2):129–37.
7. Morrell NW, Adnot S, Archer SL, et al. Cellular and molecular basis of pulmonary arterial hypertension. J Am Coll Cardiol. 2009;54(1 Suppl):S20–31.
8. Solomon H, Man JW, Jackson G. Erectile dysfunction and the cardiovascular patient: endothelial dysfunction is the common denominator. Heart. 2003;89(3):251–3.
9. Schouten M, Wiersinga WJ, Levi M, van der Poll T. Inflammation, endothelium, and coagulation in sepsis. J Leukoc Biol. 2008;83(3):536–45.
10. Nikitenko LL. Vascular endothelium in cancer. Cell Tissue Res. 2009;335(1):223–40.
11. Palade GE. Blood capillaries of the heart and other organs. Circulation. 1961;24:368–88.
12. dela Paz NG, D'Amore PA. Arterial versus venous endothelial cells. Cell Tissue Res. 2009;335(1):5–16.
13. Kutcher ME, Herman IM. The pericyte: cellular regulator of microvascular blood flow. Microvasc Res. 2009;77(3):235–46.
14. Aird WC. Spatial and temporal dynamics of the endothelium. J Thromb Haemost. 2005;3(7):1392–406.
15. Risau W, Flamme I. Vasculogenesis. Annu Rev Cell Dev Biol. 1995;11:73–91.
16. Swift MR, Weinstein BM. Arterial-venous specification during development. Circ Res. 2009;104(5):576–88.
17. Crivellato E, Nico B, Ribatti D. Contribution of endothelial cells to organogenesis: a modern reappraisal of an old Aristotelian concept. J Anat. 2007;211(4):415–27.
18. deMello DE, Reid LM. Embryonic and early fetal development of human lung vasculature and its functional implications. Pediatr Dev Pathol. 2000;3(5):439–49.
19. Larrivee B, Freitas C, Suchting S, Brunet I, Eichmann A. Guidance of vascular development: lessons from the nervous system. Circ Res. 2009;104(4):428–41.
20. Vogeli KM, Jin SW, Martin GR, Stainier DY. A common progenitor for haematopoietic and endothelial lineages in the zebrafish gastrula. Nature. 2006;443(7109):337–9.
21. Choi K, Kennedy M, Kazarov A, Papadimitriou JC, Keller G. A common precursor for hematopoietic and endothelial cells. Development. 1998;125(4):725–32.
22. Ribatti D, Nico B, Crivellato E. Morphological and molecular aspects of physiological vascular morphogenesis. Angiogenesis. 2009;12(2):101–11.
23. Pardanaud L, Luton D, Prigent M, Bourcheix LM, Catala M, Dieterlen-Lievre F. Two distinct endothelial lineages in ontogeny, one of them related to hemopoiesis. Development. 1996;122(5):1363–71.
24. Vokes SA, Krieg PA. Endoderm is required for vascular endothelial tube formation, but not for angioblast specification. Development. 2002;129(3):775–85.
25. Flamme I, Frolich T, Risau W. Molecular mechanisms of vasculogenesis and embryonic angiogenesis. J Cell Physiol. 1997;173(2):206–10.
26. Carmeliet P, Ferreira V, Breier G, et al. Abnormal blood vessel development and lethality in embryos lacking a single VEGF allele. Nature. 1996;380(6573):435–9.
27. Ferrara N, Carver-Moore K, Chen H, et al. Heterozygous embryonic lethality induced by targeted inactivation of the VEGF gene. Nature. 1996;380(6573):439–42.
28. Suri C, Jones PF, Patan S, et al. Requisite role of angiopoietin-1, a ligand for the TIE2 receptor, during embryonic angiogenesis. Cell. 1996;87(7):1171–80.
29. Puri MC, Partanen J, Rossant J, Bernstein A. Interaction of the TEK and TIE receptor tyrosine kinases during cardiovascular development. Development. 1999;126(20):4569–80.
30. Takashima S, Kitakaze M, Asakura M, et al. Targeting of both mouse neuropilin-1 and neuropilin-2 genes severely impairs developmental yolk sac and embryonic angiogenesis. Proc Natl Acad Sci U S A. 2002;99(6):3657–62.
31. Byrd N, Grabel L. Hedgehog signaling in murine vasculogenesis and angiogenesis. Trends Cardiovasc Med. 2004;14(8):308–13.
32. Risau W, Lemmon V. Changes in the vascular extracellular matrix during embryonic vasculogenesis and angiogenesis. Dev Biol. 1988;125(2):441–50.
33. Carmeliet P. Angiogenesis in life, disease and medicine. Nature. 2005;438(7070):932–6.
34. Makanya AN, Hlushchuk R, Djonov VG. Intussusceptive angiogenesis and its role in vascular morphogenesis, patterning, and remodeling. Angiogenesis. 2009;12(2):113–23.
35. Sims DE. The pericyte – a review. Tissue Cell. 1986;18(2):153–74.
36. Hirschi KK, Rohovsky SA, D'Amore PA. PDGF, TGF-beta, and heterotypic cell-cell interactions mediate endothelial cell-induced recruitment of 10T1/2 cells and their differentiation to a smooth muscle fate. J Cell biol. 1998;141(3):805–14.
37. Dickson MC, Martin JS, Cousins FM, Kulkarni AB, Karlsson S, Akhurst RJ. Defective haematopoiesis and vasculogenesis in transforming growth factor-beta 1 knock out mice. Development. 1995;121(6):1845–54.
38. Hellstrom M, Kalen M, Lindahl P, Abramsson A, Betsholtz C. Role of PDGF-B and PDGFR-beta in recruitment of vascular smooth muscle cells and pericytes during embryonic blood vessel formation in the mouse. Development. 1999;126(14):3047–55.
39. Sato TN, Tozawa Y, Deutsch U, et al. Distinct roles of the receptor tyrosine kinases Tie-1 and Tie-2 in blood vessel formation. Nature. 1995;376(6535):70–4.
40. Rocha SF, Adams RH. Molecular differentiation and specialization of vascular beds. Angiogenesis. 2009;12(2):139–47.
41. Horowitz A, Simons M. Branching morphogenesis. Circ Res. 2008;103(8):784–95.
42. Djonov VG, Kurz H, Burri PH. Optimality in the developing vascular system: branching remodeling by means of intussusception as an efficient adaptation mechanism. Dev Dyn. 2002;224(4):391–402.
43. Risau W. Differentiation of endothelium. Faseb J. 1995;9(10):926–33.
44. Schaper W. Collateral circulation: past and present. Basic Res Cardiol. 2009;104(1):5–21.
45. Hoper J, Jahn H. Influence of environmental oxygen concentration on growth and vascular density of the area vasculosa in chick embryos. Int J Microcirc Clin Exp. 1995;15(4):186–92.

46. Semenza GL, Agani F, Iyer N, et al. Regulation of cardiovascular development and physiology by hypoxia-inducible factor 1. Ann N Y Acad Sci. 1999;874:262–8.
47. Cleaver O, Melton DA. Endothelial signaling during development. Nat Med. 2003;9(6):661–8.
48. Bogers AJ, Gittenberger-de Groot AC, Poelmann RE, Peault BM, Huysmans HA. Development of the origin of the coronary arteries, a matter of ingrowth or outgrowth? Anat Embryol. 1989;180(5):437–41.
49. Velkey JM, Bernanke DH. Apoptosis during coronary artery orifice development in the chick embryo. Anat Rec. 2001;262(3):310–7.
50. Ando K, Nakajima Y, Yamagishi T, Yamamoto S, Nakamura H. Development of proximal coronary arteries in quail embryonic heart: multiple capillaries penetrating the aortic sinus fuse to form main coronary trunk. Circ Res. 2004;94(3):346–52.
51. Ishii Y, Langberg J, Rosborough K, Mikawa T. Endothelial cell lineages of the heart. Cell Tissue Res. 2009;335(1):67–73.
52. Garcia-Martinez V, Schoenwolf GC. Primitive-streak origin of the cardiovascular system in avian embryos. Dev Biol. 1993;159(2):706–19.
53. Linask KK, Lash JW. Early heart development: dynamics of endocardial cell sorting suggests a common origin with cardiomyocytes. Dev Dyn. 1993;196(1):62–9.
54. Manner J, Perez-Pomares JM, Macias D, Munoz-Chapuli R. The origin, formation and developmental significance of the epicardium: a review. Cells Tissues Organs. 2001;169(2):89–103.
55. Nahirney PC, Mikawa T, Fischman DA. Evidence for an extracellular matrix bridge guiding proepicardial cell migration to the myocardium of chick embryos. Dev Dyn. 2003;227(4):511–23.
56. Mikawa T, Fischman DA. Retroviral analysis of cardiac morphogenesis: discontinuous formation of coronary vessels. Proc Natl Acad Sci U S A. 1992;89(20):9504–8.
57. Mikawa T, Gourdie RG. Pericardial mesoderm generates a population of coronary smooth muscle cells migrating into the heart along with ingrowth of the epicardial organ. Dev Biol. 1996;174(2):221–32.
58. Wessels A, Perez-Pomares JM. The epicardium and epicardially derived cells (EPDCs) as cardiac stem cells. Anat Rec. 2004;276(1):43–57.
59. Wilting J, Buttler K, Schulte I, Papoutsi M, Schweigerer L, Manner J. The proepicardium delivers hemangioblasts but not lymphangioblasts to the developing heart. Dev Biol. 2007;305(2):451–9.
60. Torella D, Ellison GM, Karakikes I, Nadal-Ginard B. Resident cardiac stem cells. Cell Mol Life Sci. 2007;64(6):661–73.
61. Asahara T, Isner JM. Endothelial progenitor cells for vascular regeneration. J Hematother Stem Cell Res. 2002;11(2):171–8.
62. Ratajska A, Czarnowska E, Ciszek B. Embryonic development of the proepicardium and coronary vessels. Int J Dev Biol. 2008;52(2–3):229–36.
63. Reese DE, Mikawa T, Bader DM. Development of the coronary vessel system. Circ Res. 2002;91(9):761–8.
64. Hsieh PC, Davis ME, Lisowski LK, Lee RT. Endothelial-cardiomyocyte interactions in cardiac development and repair. Annu Rev Physiol. 2006;68:51–66.
65. Tomanek RJ. Formation of the coronary vasculature during development. Angiogenesis. 2005;8(3):273–84.
66. Lavine KJ, Ornitz DM. Shared circuitry: developmental signaling cascades regulate both embryonic and adult coronary vasculature. Circ Res. 2009;104(2):159–69.
67. Gerritsen ME. Functional heterogeneity of vascular endothelial cells. Biochem Pharmacol. 1987;36(17):2701–11.
68. Florey L. The endothelial cell. Br Med J. 1966;2(5512):487–90.
69. Sumagin R, Sarelius IH. TNF-alpha activation of arterioles and venules alters distribution and levels of ICAM-1 and affects leukocyte-endothelial cell interactions. Am J Physiol Heart Circ Physiol. 2006;291(5):H2116–25.
70. Simionescu M, Simionescu N, Palade GE. Morphometric data on the endothelium of blood capillaries. J Cell Biol. 1974;60(1):128–52.
71. Flaherty JT, Pierce JE, Ferrans VJ, Patel DJ, Tucker WK, Fry DL. Endothelial nuclear patterns in the canine arterial tree with particular reference to hemodynamic events. Circ Res. 1972;30(1):23–33.
72. Girard JP, Springer TA. High endothelial venules (HEVs): specialized endothelium for lymphocyte migration. Immunol Today. 1995;16(9):449–57.
73. Muro S, Koval M, Muzykantov V. Endothelial endocytic pathways: gates for vascular drug delivery. Curr Vasc Pharmacol. 2004;2(3):281–99.
74. Bendayan M. Morphological and cytochemical aspects of capillary permeability. Microsc Res Tech. 2002;57(5):327–49.
75. Wisse E. An electron microscopic study of the fenestrated endothelial lining of rat liver sinusoids. J Ultrastruct Res. 1970;31(1):125–50.
76. van den Berg BM, Vink H, Spaan JA. The endothelial glycocalyx protects against myocardial edema. Circ Res. 2003;92(6):592–4.
77. Chi JT, Chang HY, Haraldsen G, et al. Endothelial cell diversity revealed by global expression profiling. Proc Natl Acad Sci U S A. 2003;100(19):10623–8.
78. Arap W, Kolonin MG, Trepel M, et al. Steps toward mapping the human vasculature by phage display. Nat Med. 2002;8(2):121–7.
79. Aird WC. Phenotypic heterogeneity of the endothelium: II. Representative vascular beds. Circ Res. 2007;100(2):174–90.
80. Jurisic G, Detmar M. Lymphatic endothelium in health and disease. Cell Tissue Res. 2009;335(1):97–108.
81. Aird WC, Edelberg JM, Weiler-Guettler H, Simmons WW, Smith TW, Rosenberg RD. Vascular bed-specific expression of an endothelial cell gene is programmed by the tissue microenvironment. J Cell Biol. 1997;138(5):1117–24.
82. Levin EG, Santell L, Osborn KG. The expression of endothelial tissue plasminogen activator in vivo: a function defined by vessel size and anatomic location. J Cell Sci. 1997;110(Pt 2):139–48.
83. Garcia-Cardena G, Gimbrone Jr MA. Biomechanical modulation of endothelial phenotype: implications for health and disease. Handb Exp Pharmacol. 2006;176(Pt 2):79–95.
84. Durr E, Yu J, Krasinska KM, et al. Direct proteomic mapping of the lung microvascular endothelial cell surface in vivo and in cell culture. Nat Biotechnol. 2004;22(8):985–92.
85. Kwei S, Stavrakis G, Takahas M, et al. Early adaptive responses of the vascular wall during venous arterialization in mice. Am J Pathol. 2004;164(1):81–9.
86. Aird WC. Mechanisms of endothelial cell heterogeneity in health and disease. Circ Res. 2006;98(2):159–62.
87. King J, Hamil T, Creighton J, et al. Structural and functional characteristics of lung macro- and microvascular endothelial cell phenotypes. Microvasc Res. 2004;67(2):139–51.
88. Cines DB, Pollak ES, Buck CA, et al. Endothelial cells in physiology and in the pathophysiology of vascular disorders. Blood. 1998;91(10):3527–61.

89. Stevens T, Garcia JG, Shasby DM, Bhattacharya J, Malik AB. Mechanisms regulating endothelial cell barrier function. Am J Physiol Lung Cell Mol Physiol. 2000;279(3):L419–22.
90. Luscinskas FW, Gimbrone Jr MA. Endothelial-dependent mechanisms in chronic inflammatory leukocyte recruitment. Annu Rev Medicine. 1996;47:413–21.
91. Sima AV, Stancu CS, Simionescu M. Vascular endothelium in atherosclerosis. Cell Tissue Research. 2009;335(1):191–203.
92. Furchgott RF, Zawadzki JV. The obligatory role of endothelial cells in the relaxation of arterial smooth muscle by acetylcholine. Nature. 1980;288(5789):373–6.
93. Feletou M, Vanhoutte PM. Endothelium-dependent hyperpolarization of canine coronary smooth muscle. Br J Pharmacol. 1988;93(3): 515–24.
94. Ignarro LJ, Buga GM, Wood KS, Byrns RE, Chaudhuri G. Endothelium-derived relaxing factor produced and released from artery and vein is nitric oxide. Proc Natl Acad Sci U S A. 1987;84(24):9265–9.
95. Vanhoutte PM, Mombouli JV. Vascular endothelium: vasoactive mediators. Prog Cardiovasc Dis. 1996;39(3):229–38.
96. Moncada S, Gryglewski R, Bunting S, Vane JR. An enzyme isolated from arteries transforms prostaglandin endoperoxides to an unstable substance that inhibits platelet aggregation. Nature. 1976;263(5579):663–5.
97. Moncada S, Herman AG, Higgs EA, Vane JR. Differential formation of prostacyclin (PGX or PGI2) by layers of the arterial wall. An explanation for the anti-thrombotic properties of vascular endothelium. Thromb Res. 1977;11(3):323–44.
98. Bellien J, Thuillez C, Joannides R. Contribution of endothelium-derived hyperpolarizing factors to the regulation of vascular tone in humans. Fundam Clin Pharmacol. 2008;22(4):363–77.
99. Duncker DJ, Bache RJ. Regulation of coronary blood flow during exercise. Physiol Rev. 2008;88(3):1009–86.
100. Quayle JM, Nelson MT, Standen NB. ATP-sensitive and inwardly rectifying potassium channels in smooth muscle. Physiol Rev. 1997; 77(4):1165–232.
101. Lamontagne D, Konig A, Bassenge E, Busse R. Prostacyclin and nitric oxide contribute to the vasodilator action of acetylcholine and bradykinin in the intact rabbit coronary bed. J Cardiovasc Pharmacol. 1992;20(4):652–7.
102. Archer SL, Gragasin FS, Wu X, et al. Endothelium-derived hyperpolarizing factor in human internal mammary artery is 11,12-epoxyeicosatrienoic acid and causes relaxation by activating smooth muscle BK(Ca) channels. Circulation. 2003;107(5):769–76.
103. Ludmer PL, Selwyn AP, Shook TL, et al. Paradoxical vasoconstriction induced by acetylcholine in atherosclerotic coronary arteries. N Engl J Med. 1986;315(17):1046–51.
104. Cotran RS, Gimbrone Jr MA, Bevilacqua MP, Mendrick DL, Pober JS. Induction and detection of a human endothelial activation antigen in vivo. J Exp Med. 1986;164(2):661–6.
105. Cybulsky MI, Gimbrone Jr MA. Endothelial expression of a mononuclear leukocyte adhesion molecule during atherogenesis. Science. 1991;251(4995):788–91.
106. Bassenge E, Heusch G. Endothelial and neuro-humoral control of coronary blood flow in health and disease. Rev Physiol Biochem Pharmacol. 1990;116:77–165.
107. Anderson TJ. Assessment and treatment of endothelial dysfunction in humans. J Am Coll Cardiol. 1999;34(3):631–8.
108. Ross R, Glomset JA. Atherosclerosis and the arterial smooth muscle cell: proliferation of smooth muscle is a key event in the genesis of the lesions of atherosclerosis. Science. 1973;180(93):1332–9.
109. Ross R. The pathogenesis of atherosclerosis: a perspective for the 1990s. Nature. 1993;362(6423):801–9.
110. Celermajer DS, Sorensen KE, Gooch VM, et al. Non-invasive detection of endothelial dysfunction in children and adults at risk of atherosclerosis. Lancet. 1992;340(8828):1111–5.
111. Chowienczyk PJ, Watts GF, Cockcroft JR, Ritter JM. Impaired endothelium-dependent vasodilation of forearm resistance vessels in hypercholesterolaemia. Lancet. 1992;340(8833):1430–2.
112. De Angelis L, Marfella MA, Siniscalchi M, et al. Erectile and endothelial dysfunction in type II diabetes: a possible link. Diabetologia. 2001;44(9):1155–60.
113. Bhargava K, Hansa G, Bansal M, Tandon S, Kasliwal RR. Endothelium-dependent brachial artery flow mediated vasodilatation in patients with diabetes mellitus with and without coronary artery disease. J Assoc Physicians India. 2003;51:355–8.
114. Celermajer DS, Sorensen KE, Georgakopoulos D, Bull C, Thomas O, Robinson J, et al. Cigarette smoking is associated with dose-related and potentially reversible impairment of endothelium-dependent dilation in healthy young adults. Circulation. 1993;88(5 Pt 1):2149–55.
115. Celermajer DS, Sorensen KE, Bull C, Robinson J, Deanfield JE. Endothelium-dependent dilation in the systemic arteries of asymptomatic subjects relates to coronary risk factors and their interaction. J Am Coll Cardiol. 1994;24(6):1468–74.
116. Reddy KG, Nair RN, Sheehan HM, Hodgson JM. Evidence that selective endothelial dysfunction may occur in the absence of angiographic or ultrasound atherosclerosis in patients with risk factors for atherosclerosis. J Am Coll Cardiol. 1994;23(4):833–43.
117. Gordon JB, Ganz P, Nabel EG, et al. Atherosclerosis influences the vasomotor response of epicardial coronary arteries to exercise. J Clin Invest. 1989;83(6):1946–52.
118. Zeiher AM, Drexler H, Wollschlager H, Just H. Endothelial dysfunction of the coronary microvasculature is associated with coronary blood flow regulation in patients with early atherosclerosis. Circulation. 1991;84(5):1984–92.
119. Zeiher AM, Drexler H, Wollschlager H, Just H. Modulation of coronary vasomotor tone in humans. Progressive endothelial dysfunction with different early stages of coronary atherosclerosis. Circulation. 1991;83(2):391–401.
120. Anderson TJ, Gerhard MD, Meredith IT, et al. Systemic nature of endothelial dysfunction in atherosclerosis. Am J Cardiol. 1995;75(6):71B–4.
121. Anderson TJ, Uehata A, Gerhard MD, et al. Close relation of endothelial function in the human coronary and peripheral circulations. J Am Coll Cardiol. 1995;26(5):1235–41.
122. Uren NG, Crake T, Lefroy DC, de Silva R, Davies GJ, Maseri A. Delayed recovery of coronary resistive vessel function after coronary angioplasty. J Am Coll Cardiol. 1993;21(3):612–21.
123. Hokanson DE, Sumner DS, Strandness Jr DE. An electrically calibrated plethysmograph for direct measurement of limb blood flow. IEEE Trans Biomed Eng. 1975;22(1):25–9.
124. Creager MA, Cooke JP, Mendelsohn ME, et al. Impaired vasodilation of forearm resistance vessels in hypercholesterolemic humans. J Clin Invest. 1990;86(1):228–34.

125. Oliver JJ, Webb DJ. Noninvasive assessment of arterial stiffness and risk of atherosclerotic events. Arterioscler Thromb Vasc Biol. 2003;23(4):554–66.
126. Birschmann I, Walter U. Physiology and pathophysiology of vascular signaling controlled by guanosine 3',5'-cyclic monophosphate-dependent protein kinase. Acta Biochim Pol. 2004;51(2):397–404.
127. Chambers JW, Voss GS, Snider JR, Meyer SM, Cartland JL, Wilson RF. Direct in vivo effects of nitric oxide on the coronary circulation. Am J Physiol. 1996;271(4 Pt 2):H1584–93.
128. Doucette JW, Corl PD, Payne HM, et al. Validation of a Doppler guide wire for intravascular measurement of coronary artery flow velocity. Circulation. 1992;85(5):1899–911.
129. Schachinger V, Britten MB, Zeiher AM. Prognostic impact of coronary vasodilator dysfunction on adverse long-term outcome of coronary heart disease. Circulation. 2000;101(16):1899–906.
130. Halcox JP, Schenke WH, Zalos G, et al. Prognostic value of coronary vascular endothelial dysfunction. Circulation. 2002;106(6):653–8.
131. Panza JA, Quyyumi AA, Brush Jr JE, Epstein SE. Abnormal endothelium-dependent vascular relaxation in patients with essential hypertension. N Engl J Med. 1990;323(1):22–7.
132. Schwartz BG, Economides C, Mayeda GS, Burstein S, Kloner RA. The endothelial cell in health and disease: its function, dysfunction, measurement and therapy. Int J Impot Res. 2010;22(2):77–90.
133. Perticone F, Ceravolo R, Pujia A, et al. Prognostic significance of endothelial dysfunction in hypertensive patients. Circulation. 2001;104(2):191–6.
134. Heitzer T, Baldus S, von Kodolitsch Y, Rudolph V, Meinertz T. Systemic endothelial dysfunction as an early predictor of adverse outcome in heart failure. Arterioscler Thromb Vasc Biol. 2005;25(6):1174–9.
135. Heitzer T, Schlinzig T, Krohn K, Meinertz T, Munzel T. Endothelial dysfunction, oxidative stress, and risk of cardiovascular events in patients with coronary artery disease. Circulation. 2001;104(22):2673–8.
136. Fichtlscherer S, Breuer S, Zeiher AM. Prognostic value of systemic endothelial dysfunction in patients with acute coronary syndromes: further evidence for the existence of the "vulnerable" patient. Circulation. 2004;110(14):1926–32.
137. Corretti MC, Anderson TJ, Benjamin EJ, et al. Guidelines for the ultrasound assessment of endothelial-dependent flow-mediated vasodilation of the brachial artery: a report of the International Brachial Artery Reactivity Task Force. J Am Coll Cardiol. 2002;39(2):257–65.
138. Guthikonda S, Sinkey CA, Haynes WG. What is the most appropriate methodology for detection of conduit artery endothelial dysfunction? Arterioscler Thromb Vasc Biology. 2007;27(5):1172–6.
139. Vlachopoulos C, Aznaouridis K, Alexopoulos N, Economou E, Andreadou I, Stefanadis C. Effect of dark chocolate on arterial function in healthy individuals. Am J Hypertens. 2005;18(6):785–91.
140. Modena MG, Bonetti L, Coppi F, Bursi F, Rossi R. Prognostic role of reversible endothelial dysfunction in hypertensive postmenopausal women. J Am Coll Cardiol. 2002;40(3):505–10.
141. Neunteufl T, Heher S, Katzenschlager R, et al. Late prognostic value of flow-mediated dilation in the brachial artery of patients with chest pain. Am J Cardiol. 2000;86(2):207–10.
142. Schroeder S, Enderle MD, Ossen R, et al. Noninvasive determination of endothelium-mediated vasodilation as a screening test for coronary artery disease: pilot study to assess the predictive value in comparison with angina pectoris, exercise electrocardiography, and myocardial perfusion imaging. Am Heart J. 1999;138(4 Pt 1):731–9.
143. Gokce N, Keaney Jr JF, Hunter LM, Watkins MT, Menzoian JO, Vita JA. Risk stratification for postoperative cardiovascular events via noninvasive assessment of endothelial function: a prospective study. Circulation. 2002;105(13):1567–72.
144. Gokce N, Keaney Jr JF, Hunter LM, et al. Predictive value of noninvasively determined endothelial dysfunction for long-term cardiovascular events in patients with peripheral vascular disease. J Am Coll Cardiol. 2003;41(10):1769–75.
145. Brevetti G, Silvestro A, Schiano V, Chiariello M. Endothelial dysfunction and cardiovascular risk prediction in peripheral arterial disease: additive value of flow-mediated dilation [dilatation?] to ankle-brachial pressure index. Circulation. 2003;108(17):2093–8.
146. Franklin SS, Khan SA, Wong ND, Larson MG, Levy D. Is pulse pressure useful in predicting risk for coronary heart disease? The Framingham heart study. Circulation. 1999;100(4):354–60.
147. Bank AJ, Wang H, Holte JE, Mullen K, Shammas R, Kubo SH. Contribution of collagen, elastin, and smooth muscle to in vivo human brachial artery wall stress and elastic modulus. Circulation. 1996;94(12):3263–70.
148. Kinlay S, Creager MA, Fukumoto M, et al. Endothelium-derived nitric oxide regulates arterial elasticity in human arteries in vivo. Hypertension. 2001;38(5):1049–53.
149. Asmar R, Benetos A, Topouchian J, et al. Assessment of arterial distensibility by automatic pulse wave velocity measurement. Validation and clinical application studies. Hypertension. 1995;26(3):485–90.
150. Sutton-Tyrrell K, Mackey RH, Holubkov R, Vaitkevicius PV, Spurgeon HA, Lakatta EG. Measurement variation of aortic pulse wave velocity in the elderly. Am J Hypertens. 2001;14(5 Pt 1):463–8.
151. Wilkinson IB, Fuchs SA, Jansen IM, et al. Reproducibility of pulse wave velocity and augmentation index measured by pulse wave analysis. J Hypertens. 1998;16(12 Pt 2):2079–84.
152. Mohiaddin RH, Firmin DN, Longmore DB. Age-related changes of human aortic flow wave velocity measured noninvasively by magnetic resonance imaging. J Appl Physiol. 1993;74(1):492–7.
153. Boutouyrie P, Tropeano AI, Asmar R, et al. Aortic stiffness is an independent predictor of primary coronary events in hypertensive patients: a longitudinal study. Hypertension. 2002;39(1):10–5.
154. van Popele NM, Grobbee DE, Bots ML, et al. Association between arterial stiffness and atherosclerosis: the Rotterdam Study. Stroke. 2001;32(2):454–60.
155. Stefanadis C, Stratos C, Vlachopoulos C, et al. Pressure-diameter relation of the human aorta. A new method of determination by the application of a special ultrasonic dimension catheter. Circulation. 1995;92(8):2210–9.
156. Blacher J, Pannier B, Guerin AP, Marchais SJ, Safar ME, London GM. Carotid arterial stiffness as a predictor of cardiovascular and all-cause mortality in end-stage renal disease. Hypertension. 1998;32(3):570–4.
157. Blacher J, Guerin AP, Pannier B, Marchais SJ, London GM. Arterial calcifications, arterial stiffness, and cardiovascular risk in end-stage renal disease. Hypertension. 2001;38(4):938–42.

158. Karamanoglu M, O'Rourke MF, Avolio AP, Kelly RP. An analysis of the relationship between central aortic and peripheral upper limb pressure waves in man. Eur Heart J. 1993;14(2):160–7.
159. Kelly RP, Millasseau SC, Ritter JM, Chowienczyk PJ. Vasoactive drugs influence aortic augmentation index independently of pulse-wave velocity in healthy men. Hypertension. 2001;37(6):1429–33.
160. Watt Jr TB, Burrus CS. Arterial pressure contour analysis for estimating human vascular properties. J Appl Physiol. 1976;40(2):171–6.
161. Cohn JN, Finkelstein S, McVeigh G, et al. Noninvasive pulse wave analysis for the early detection of vascular disease. Hypertension. 1995;26(3):503–8.
162. Millasseau SC, Guigui FG, Kelly RP, et al. Noninvasive assessment of the digital volume pulse. Comparison with the peripheral pressure pulse. Hypertension. 2000;36(6):952–6.
163. Chowienczyk PJ, Kelly RP, MacCallum H, et al. Photoplethysmographic assessment of pulse wave reflection: blunted response to endothelium-dependent beta2-adrenergic vasodilation in type II diabetes mellitus. Am Coll Cardiol. 1999;34(7):2007–14.
164. Hamburg NM, Keyes MJ, Larson MG, et al. Cross-sectional relations of digital vascular function to cardiovascular risk factors in the Framingham Heart Study. Circulation. 2008;117(19):2467–74.
165. Gul KM, Ahmadi N, Wang Z, et al. Digital thermal monitoring of vascular function: a novel tool to improve cardiovascular risk assessment. Vasc Med. 2009;14(2):143–8.
166. Ahmadi N, Nabavi V, Nuguri V, et al. Low fingertip temperature rebound measured by digital thermal monitoring strongly correlates with the presence and extent of coronary artery disease diagnosed by 64-slice multi-detector computed tomography. Int J Cardiovasc Imaging. 2009;25(7):725–38.
167. Ahmadi N, Hajsadeghi F, Gul K, et al. Relations between digital thermal monitoring of vascular function, the Framingham risk score, and coronary artery calcium score. J Cardiovasc Comput Tomogr. 2008;2(6):382–8.
168. Constans J, Conri C. Circulating markers of endothelial function in cardiovascular disease. Clin Chim Acta. 2006;368(1–2):33–47.
169. Brunner H, Cockcroft JR, Deanfield J, et al. Endothelial function and dysfunction. Part II: association with cardiovascular risk factors and diseases. A statement by the Working Group on Endothelins and Endothelial Factors of the European Society of Hypertension. J Hypertens. 2005;23(2):233–46.
170. Deanfield J, Donald A, Ferri C, et al. Endothelial function and dysfunction. Part I: methodological issues for assessment in the different vascular beds: a statement by the Working Group on Endothelin and Endothelial Factors of the European Society of Hypertension. J Hypertens. 2005;23(1):7–17.
171. Buckley DI, Fu R, Freeman M, Rogers K, Helfand M. C-reactive protein as a risk factor for coronary heart disease: a systematic review and meta-analyses for the U.S. Preventive Services Task Force. Ann Intern Med. 2009;151(7):483–95.
172. Rivera JJ, Nasir K, Cox PR, et al. Association of traditional cardiovascular risk factors with coronary plaque sub-types assessed by 64-slice computed tomography angiography in a large cohort of asymptomatic subjects. Atherosclerosis. 2009;206(2):451–7.
173. Lorenz MW, Markus HS, Bots ML, Rosvall M, Sitzer M. Prediction of clinical cardiovascular events with carotid intima-media thickness: a systematic review and meta-analysis. Circulation. 2007;115(4):459–67.
174. Johnsen SH, Mathiesen EB. Carotid plaque compared with intima-media thickness as a predictor of coronary and cerebrovascular disease. Curr Cardiol Rep. 2009;11(1):21–7.
175. Chang SM, Nabi F, Xu J, et al. The coronary artery calcium score and stress myocardial perfusion imaging provide independent and complementary prediction of cardiac risk. J Am Coll Cardiol. 2009;54(20):1872–82.
176. Simon A, Chironi G, Levenson J. Comparative performance of subclinical atherosclerosis tests in predicting coronary heart disease in asymptomatic individuals. Eur Heart J. 2007;28(24):2967–71.
177. Novo S, Carita P, Corrado E, et al. Preclinical carotid atherosclerosis enhances the global cardiovascular risk and increases the rate of cerebro- and cardiovascular events in a five-year follow-up. Atherosclerosis. 2010;211:287–90.
178. Corrado E, Rizzo M, Coppola G, Muratori I, Carella M, Novo S. Endothelial dysfunction and carotid lesions are strong predictors of clinical events in patients with early stages of atherosclerosis: a 24-month follow-up study. Coron Artery Dis. 2008;19(3):139–44.
179. Benjamin N, Calver A, Collier J, Robinson B, Vallance P, Webb D. Measuring forearm blood flow and interpreting the responses to drugs and mediators. Hypertension. 1995;25(5):918–23.
180. Bots ML, Westerink J, Rabelink TJ, de Koning EJ. Assessment of flow-mediated vasodilatation (FMD) of the brachial artery: effects of technical aspects of the FMD measurement on the FMD response. Eur Heart J. 2005;26(4):363–8.
181. Ockene JK, Kuller LH, Svendsen KH, Meilahn E. The relationship of smoking cessation to coronary heart disease and lung cancer in the Multiple Risk Factor Intervention Trial (MRFIT). Am J Public Health. 1990;80(8):954–8.
182. Hambrecht R, Wolf A, Gielen S, et al. Effect of exercise on coronary endothelial function in patients with coronary artery disease. N Engl J Med. 2000;342(7):454–60.
183. Plotnick GD, Corretti MC, Vogel RA. Effect of antioxidant vitamins on the transient impairment of endothelium-dependent brachial artery vasoactivity following a single high-fat meal. JAMA. 1997;278(20):1682–6.
184. Executive Summary of The Third Report of The National Cholesterol Education Program (NCEP) Expert Panel on Detection, Evaluation, and Treatment of High Blood Cholesterol in Adults (Adult Treatment Panel III). JAMA. 2001;285(19):2486–97.
185. Mancini GB, Henry GC, Macaya C, et al. Angiotensin-converting enzyme inhibition with quinapril improves endothelial vasomotor dysfunction in patients with coronary artery disease. The TREND (Trial on Reversing ENdothelial Dysfunction) Study. Circulation. 1996;94(3):258–65.
186. Ghiadoni L, Virdis A, Magagna A, Taddei S, Salvetti A. Effect of the angiotensin II type 1 receptor blocker candesartan on endothelial function in patients with essential hypertension. Hypertension. 2000;35(1 Pt 2):501–6.
187. Law MR, Morris JK, Wald NJ. Use of blood pressure lowering drugs in the prevention of cardiovascular disease: meta-analysis of 147 randomised trials in the context of expectations from prospective epidemiological studies. Br Med J (Clin Res Ed). 2009;338:b1665.
188. Turnbull F. Effects of different blood-pressure-lowering regimens on major cardiovascular events: results of prospectively-designed overviews of randomised trials. Lancet. 2003;362(9395):1527–35.
189. Treasure CB, Klein JL, Weintraub WS, et al. Beneficial effects of cholesterol-lowering therapy on the coronary endothelium in patients with coronary artery disease. N Engl J Med. 1995;332(8):481–7.

190. Mercuro G, Zoncu S, Saiu F, Sarais C, Rosano GM. Effect of atorvastatin on endothelium-dependent vasodilation in postmenopausal women with average serum cholesterol levels. Am J Cardiol. 2002;90(7):747–50.
191. Baigent C, Keech A, Kearney PM, et al. Efficacy and safety of cholesterol-lowering treatment: prospective meta-analysis of data from 90,056 participants in 14 randomised trials of statins. Lancet. 2005;366(9493):1267–78.
192. Husain S, Andrews NP, Mulcahy D, Panza JA, Quyyumi AA. Aspirin improves endothelial dysfunction in atherosclerosis. Circulation. 1998;97(8):716–20.
193. Baigent C, Blackwell L, Collins R, et al. Aspirin in the primary and secondary prevention of vascular disease: collaborative meta-analysis of individual participant data from randomised trials. Lancet. 2009;373(9678):1849–60.
194. Lieberman EH, Gerhard MD, Uehata A, et al. Estrogen improves endothelium-dependent, flow-mediated vasodilation in postmenopausal women. Ann Intern Med. 1994;121(12):936–41.
195. Levine GN, Frei B, Koulouris SN, Gerhard MD, Keaney Jr JF, Vita JA. Ascorbic acid reverses endothelial vasomotor dysfunction in patients with coronary artery disease. Circulation. 1996;93(6):1107–13.
196. Nelson HD, Humphrey LL, Nygren P, Teutsch SM, Allan JD. Postmenopausal hormone replacement therapy: scientific review. JAMA. 2002;288(7):872–81.
197. Yusuf S, Dagenais G, Pogue J, Bosch J, Sleight P. Vitamin E supplementation and cardiovascular events in high-risk patients. The Heart Outcomes Prevention Evaluation Study Investigators. N Engl J Med. 2000;342(3):154–60.
198. Bai Y, Sun L, Yang T, Sun K, Chen J, Hui R. Increase in fasting vascular endothelial function after short-term oral L-arginine is effective when baseline flow-mediated dilation is low: a meta-analysis of randomized controlled trials. Am J Clin Nutr. 2009;89(1):77–84.
199. Asahara T, Murohara T, Sullivan A, et al. Isolation of putative progenitor endothelial cells for angiogenesis. Science. 1997;275(5302):964–7.
200. Asahara T, Masuda H, Takahashi T, et al. Bone marrow origin of endothelial progenitor cells responsible for postnatal vasculogenesis in physiological and pathological neovascularization. Circ Res. 1999;85(3):221–8.
201. Schwartz SM, Benditt EP. Clustering of replicating cells in aortic endothelium. Proc Natl Acad Sci USA. 1976;73(2):651–3.
202. Crosby JR, Kaminski WE, Schatteman G, et al. Endothelial cells of hematopoietic origin make a significant contribution to adult blood vessel formation. Circ Res. 2000;87(9):728–30.
203. Jarajapu YP, Grant MB. The promise of cell-based therapies for diabetic complications: challenges and solutions. Circ Res. 2010;106(5): 854–69.
204. Yoder MC. Defining human endothelial progenitor cells. J Thromb Haemost. 2009;7 Suppl 1:49–52.
205. Ferdous A, Caprioli A, Iacovino M, et al. Nkx2-5 transactivates the Ets-related protein 71 gene and specifies an endothelial/endocardial fate in the developing embryo. Proc Natl Acad Sci USA. 2009;106(3):814–9.
206. Hill JM, Zalos G, Halcox JP, et al. Circulating endothelial progenitor cells, vascular function, and cardiovascular risk. N Engl J Med. 2003; 348(7):593–600.
207. Vasa M, Fichtlscherer S, Aicher A, et al. Number and migratory activity of circulating endothelial progenitor cells inversely correlate with risk factors for coronary artery disease. Circ Res. 2001;89(1):E1–7.
208. Kondo T, Hayashi M, Takeshita K, et al. Smoking cessation rapidly increases circulating progenitor cells in peripheral blood in chronic smokers. Arterioscler Thromb Vasc Biol. 2004;24(8):1442–7.
209. Chen JZ, Zhang FR, Tao QM, Wang XX, Zhu JH. Number and activity of endothelial progenitor cells from peripheral blood in patients with hypercholesterolaemia. Clin Sci (Lond). 2004;107(3):273–80.
210. Krankel N, Adams V, Linke A, et al. Hyperglycemia reduces survival and impairs function of circulating blood-derived progenitor cells. Arterioscler Thrombosis Vasc Biol. 2005;25(4):698–703.
211. Werner N, Kosiol S, Schiegl T, et al. Circulating endothelial progenitor cells and cardiovascular outcomes. N Engl J Med. 2005;353(10): 999–1007.
212. Ward MR, Stewart DJ, Kutryk MJ. Endothelial progenitor cell therapy for the treatment of coronary disease, acute MI, and pulmonary arterial hypertension: current perspectives. Catheter Cardiovasc Interv. 2007;70(7):983–98.
213. Sekiguchi H, Ii M, Losordo DW. The relative potency and safety of endothelial progenitor cells and unselected mononuclear cells for recovery from myocardial infarction and ischemia. J Cell Physiol. 2009;219(2):235–42.
214. Krenning G, van Luyn MJ, Harmsen MC. Endothelial progenitor cell-based neovascularization: implications for therapy. Trends Mol Med. 2009;15(4):180–9.
215. He T, Peterson TE, Katusic ZS. Paracrine mitogenic effect of human endothelial progenitor cells: role of interleukin-8. Am J Physiol Heart Circ Physiol. 2005;289(2):H968–72.
216. He T, Lu T, d'Uscio LV, Lam CF, Lee HC, Katusic ZS. Angiogenic function of prostacyclin biosynthesis in human endothelial progenitor cells. Circ Res. 2008;103(1):80–8.
217. Santhanam AV, Smith LA, He T, Nath KA, Katusic ZS. Endothelial progenitor cells stimulate cerebrovascular production of prostacyclin by paracrine activation of cyclooxygenase-2. Circ Res. 2007;100(9):1379–88.
218. Steinmetz M, Nickenig G, Werner N. Endothelial-regenerating cells: an expanding universe. Hypertension. 2010;55(3):593–9.
219. Ross JJ, Hong Z, Willenbring B, et al. Cytokine-induced differentiation of multipotent adult progenitor cells into functional smooth muscle cells. J Clin Invest. 2006;116(12):3139–49.
220. Celermajer DS, Adams MR, Clarkson P, et al. Passive smoking and impaired endothelium-dependent arterial dilatation in healthy young adults. N Engl J Med. 1996;334(3):150–4.
221. Steinmetz M, Nickenig G, Werner N. Endothelial-regenerating cells: an expanding universe. Hypertension. 2010;55:593–9.

Chapter 12
Stem Cells and Atherosclerosis

Jay H. Traverse

Introduction

Atherosclerosis is a complex, inflammatory disease involving medium and large arteries [1]. Beginning early in life as a benign fatty streak, it may progress over decades to become obstructive atheromatous plaque, culminating in acute myocardial infarction (AMI) or stroke as a result of plaque rupture or erosion. A variety of mechanisms contributes to the development and progression of atherosclerosis including genetic and immunologic mechanisms, hemodynamic effects, and risk factors both known and unknown. However, a principal initiator of atherosclerosis appears to be the development of endothelial dysfunction following arterial injury.

Circulating stem cells and progenitor cells derived from the bone marrow and vasculature play critical roles in vascular repair and homeostasis and may serve to counteract the development of atherosclerosis following vessel injury [2]. Since the initial observation that circulating human $CD34^+/KDR^+$ mononuclear cells assume an endothelial phenotype in culture and incorporate into newly formed vasculature in the ischemic hind limb [3], a new paradigm for postnatal vasculogenesis was discovered. Multiple studies have since confirmed the importance of these putative endothelial progenitor cells (EPCs) and other bone-marrow-derived cells in promoting vascular health. This is supported, in part, by the relationship in many studies between the number of circulating EPCs and the development of atherosclerosis [4].

Paradoxically, stem cells and progenitor cells may also contribute to the progression of atherosclerosis. The development of transgenic animals that develop atherosclerosis – apolipoprotein E knockout ($ApoE^{-/-}$) mice – or express markers on bone-marrow-derived cells – green fluorescent protein (GFP) – has provided new insight into how vascular and bone-marrow-derived stem cells and progenitor cells are involved in the biology of atherosclerosis.

Recent investigation has demonstrated that bone-marrow-derived EPCs and smooth muscle progenitor cells (SPCs) may play important roles in the biology of atherosclerosis and plaque rupture. EPCs may increase vascularization of the plaque that may increase the likelihood of plaque rupture [5], while SPCs may increase plaque stability [6]. These seemingly contradictory roles of stem and progenitor cells in atherosclerosis are the subject of ongoing investigation.

Endothelial and Smooth Muscle Progenitor Cells

A prevailing dogma in vascular biology was that vasculogenesis was confined to the early embryonic period and that postnatal vasculogenesis did not occur in the adult mammal. In 1997, Asahara et al. [3] identified a mononuclear cell population in the circulating blood of humans that carried the hematopoietic stem cell marker CD34 and/or the vascular endothelial growth factor (VEGF) receptor KDR (Fig. 12.1). In culture, these cells developed an endothelial phenotype, including uptake of acetylated low-density lipoprotein (AcLDL) in addition to expression of CD31 and endothelial nitric oxide synthase (eNOS). These cells were referred to as putative EPCs.

J.H. Traverse, MD (✉)
Department of Cardiology, University of Minnesota Medical School, Minneapolis Heart Institute at Abbott Northwestern Hospital, Minneapolis, MN, USA
e-mail: trave004@umn.edu

Z. Vlodaver et al. (eds.), *Coronary Heart Disease: Clinical, Pathological, Imaging, and Molecular Profiles*,
DOI 10.1007/978-1-4614-1475-9_12,

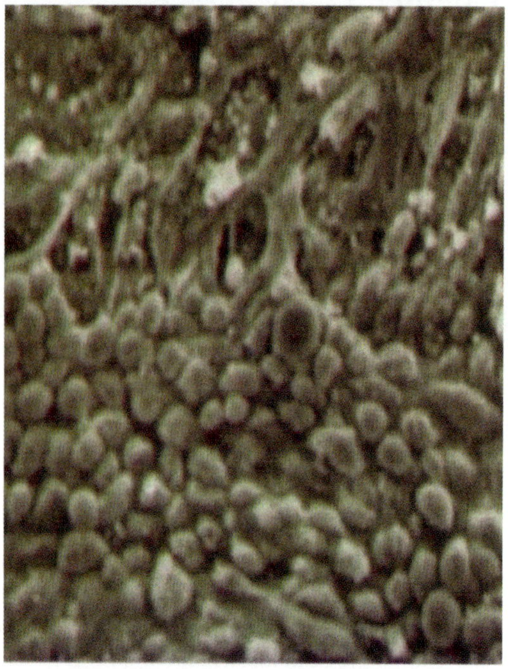

Fig. 12.1 Scanning electron microscopy of rat carotid artery treated with localized VEGF gene therapy 3 days following balloon injury. The lower section, treated with VEGF, shows accumulation of putative EPCs contributing to restoration of endothelium. Photograph courtesy of Takayuki Asahara

Injection of these human cells into the ischemic hind limb of athymic nude mice resulted in augmented neovascularization in the ischemic region with incorporation of these cells into newly formed capillaries by 6 weeks. The origin of these cells from the bone marrow was confirmed in a canine bone marrow transplant model by Shi et al. [7] who demonstrated that circulating $CD34^+$ progenitor cells become endothelial cells in vitro and coat the luminal surface of an implanted prosthetic aortic graft.

Importantly, neither of these studies was able to directly demonstrate that the cells they identified in vitro were the identical cells that participated in the neovascularization process or colonization of the prosthetic graft. This distinction continues to be a source of controversy in EPC biology – that cells displaying the purported EPC phenotype do not necessarily have the actual vasculogenic properties that arise during culture. As a result, the identification of true EPCs in circulating blood has proven to be elusive despite their reported identification in multiple studies. Currently, no specific markers exist to identify authentic EPCs, and multiple cell types including hematopoietic precursors (macrophages) may express identical surface markers [8].

Despite these limitations, it is widely believed that these cells likely play a significant participatory role in neovascularization. However, the current inability to identify true EPCs may partially obscure their functional role in the biology of atherosclerosis.

SPCs represent a second class of progenitor cells involved in vascular repair that may have important biological effects in atherosclerosis. SPCs are found in circulating blood [9], and their derivation from bone marrow has been confirmed in six mismatched bone marrow transplant studies [10] (Fig. 12.2).

Human SPCs grown in culture appear to be principally derived from mononuclear (myeloid) cells and are characterized in culture by a variety of mesenchymal or smooth muscle markers including calponin, smooth muscle myosin heavy chain (MHC), and α-smooth muscle actin (SMA) [11]. Currently, it is unclear how SPCs fully participate in vascular repair, although it is speculated that monocytes may initially adhere to injured or denuded endothelium, and acquire a smooth muscle phenotype in response to local cytokines and growth factors [11].

Atherosclerosis: Potential Role of Endothelial and Smooth Muscle Progenitor Cell

In the vast majority of cases, AMI is precipitated by plaque rupture [5]. Although a variety of factors contributes to plaque rupture, common features include a thin, fibrous cap overlying a large, lipid-rich core that contains an increased density of microvessels [12]. These immature capillary structures are subject to intraplaque hemorrhage where the accumulation of red

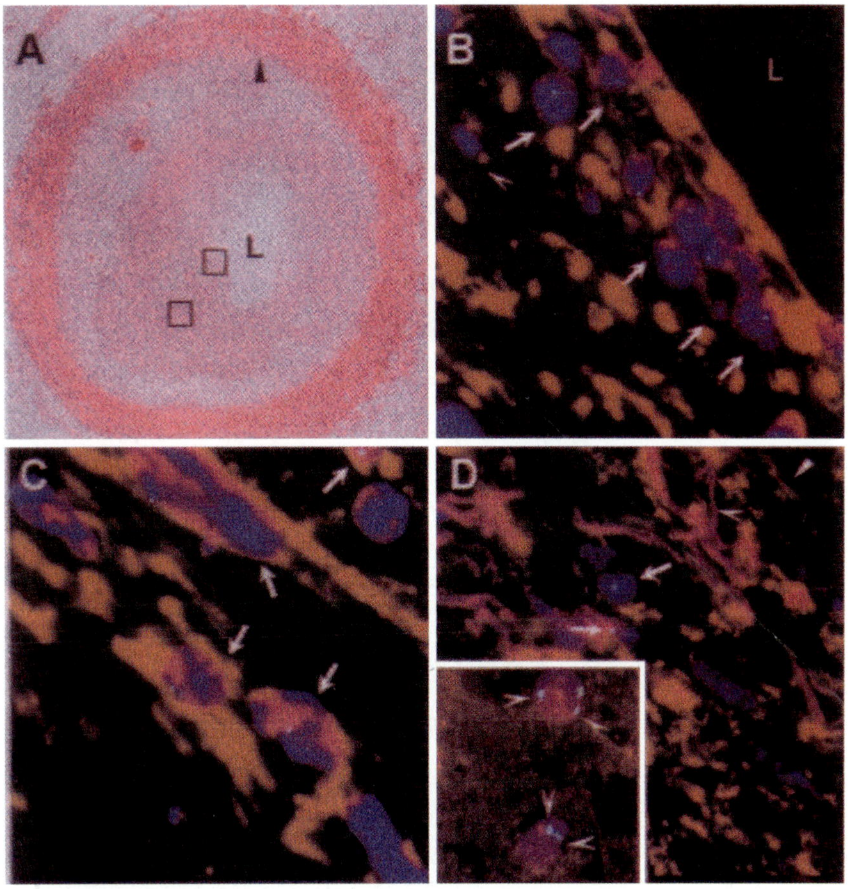

Fig. 12.2 (**a**) Hematoxylin and eosin staining of atherosclerotic plaque in coronary artery from female patient who received a male bone marrow transplant. L, lumen; *filled arrowhead*, internal elastic lamina. The *two boxes* indicate subendothelial intima and deep intima shown in (**b**, **c**). (**b**) Combined immunostaining for α-smooth muscle actin (SMA) and FISH for Y chromosome showing clusters of male cells (blue DAPI-stained nuclei with green dot) surrounded by positive α-SMA staining (red Cy-3 stain surrounding male nuclei, *white arrows*) in the subendothelial intima. (**c**) Male smooth muscle cells deeper within intima of plaque colabeling for α-SMA and Y chromosome (*white arrows*). (**d**) Male smooth muscle cells in the media of coronary artery showing combined labeling for α-SMA and Y chromosome. Inset: chromosomal multiploidy analysis of male donor smooth muscle cells in female coronary artery showing diploid nature and lack of cell fusion. Shown are two separate nuclei showing single X chromosome (large red dot) and Y chromosome (green dot). Adapted from Caplice et al. [10], p. 475x. Copyright 2003 by the National Academy of Sciences

blood cells may adversely affect plaque stability [5]. Intimal microvessels predominantly arise from the adventitia, develop with progressive luminal stenosis [13], and are highly correlated with aortic plaque progression [14].

The predominant mechanism of microvessel formation likely occurs via angiogenesis, although its regulation in atherosclerosis is not fully understood. Inhibitors of angiogenesis such as angiostatin have been shown to reduce atherosclerotic progression in ApoE mice and inhibit macrophage accumulation in the plaque [15]. An important stimulant of angiogenesis is thought to be hypoxia-induced activation of HIF-1α that arises from luminal diffusion limitations of oxygen through the thickening vessel wall [16].

The complex role of stem and progenitor cells in atherosclerosis' neovascularization process is not completely known. However, reports that infusions of EPCs and bone marrow mononuclear cells (BMCs) increase atherosclerotic plaque size suggest a possible role for EPCs in plaque neovascularization [17, 18]. In patients undergoing coronary bypass surgery, proximal aortic segments with early atherosclerosis were analyzed using immunofluroescence for the presence of progenitor cells [19] CD34, VEGF2R, Sca-1, c-kit, and CD133. Although these cells were not common (<1% of total), the majority of progenitor cells in fatty streaks and adventitia expressed $CD34^+$ and VEGF2R. Smaller contributions of $Sca\text{-}1^+$ and $c\text{-}kit^+$ cells were also observed with the complete absence of CD133, a marker lost upon EPC differentiation into mature endothelial cells.

In normal arterial segments (internal mammary) harvested from the same patients, far fewer cells displayed progenitor cell markers. Although the source of these cells was not determined, these findings demonstrated for the first time the presence of progenitor cells in human atherosclerotic plaques and adventitia that could serve as a source for SMCs and endothelial cells.

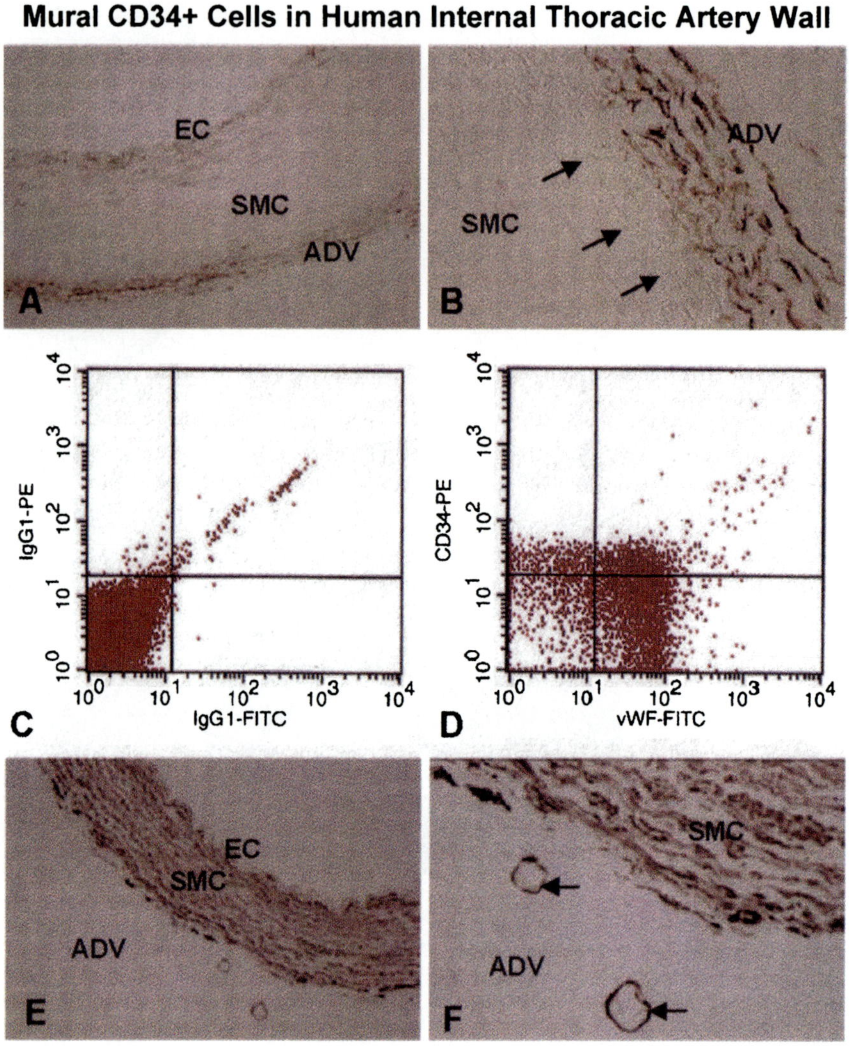

Fig. 12.3 (**a**) Localization of $CD34^+/CD31^-$ cells in the transition area from smooth muscle to adventitia in human internal thoracic artery vessels. (**b**) Higher magnification demonstrating proximity of $CD34^+$ cells to external elastic membrane (*arrows*). (**c**, **d**) FACS analysis demonstrating $CD34^+$ cells partially positive for von Willebrand factor. (**e**, **f**) Negative immunostaining for α-SMA in the $CD34^+$ zone in the artery wall and vaso vasorum (*arrows*). Adapted from Zengin et al. [20]. Copyright [see http://dev.biologists.org/site/misc/rights_permissions.xhtml]

Zengin et al. [20] identified a zone in the vessel wall of human internal thoracic artery segments between the smooth muscle and adventitial layer that served as a niche for EPCs (Fig. 12.3). These cells were $CD34^+/CD31^-$, which expressed VEGFR2 and TIE2, and formed capillary sprouts in culture. In vessel rings, these cells migrate through the vessel wall to the intima, forming capillary channels throughout the vessel. These findings support the earlier study of Ingram et al. [21] who described a complete hierarchy of EPC-like cells in human umbilical artery and vein segments.

Rauscher et al. [22] hypothesized that the progression of atherosclerosis over time is related to an age-related decline in progenitor cells. Enriched hematopoietic and stromal cells from bone marrow of nonatherosclerotic young (4 weeks) and severely atherosclerotic old (6 months) $ApoE^{-/-}$ mice were transplanted into $ApoE^{-/-}$ mice fed a high-fat diet beginning at 3 weeks of age. By 14 weeks, there was a marked reduction in atherosclerosis development in the recipients of young, but not old bone marrow. Rauscher et al. further observed a marked reduction of vascular progenitor cells ($CD31^+/CD45^-$) from older mice, suggesting that vascular progenitor cells from young donors help repair areas of endothelial senescence as assessed by reduced telomere length.

George et al. [17] observed that infusion of spleen-derived EPCs or bone marrow mononuclear cells (BMCs) to $ApoE^{-/-}$ mice resulted in a 34–54% increase in aortic plaque area with localization of the infused cells in the atherosclerotic lesions. EPC infusion resulted in smaller fibrous caps and increased lipid cores, consistent with an increase in plaque vulnerability, while BMC infusion resulted in decreased interleukin-10 (IL-10) levels and increased levels of IL-6 and monocyte chemotactic protein-1 (MCP-1), consistent with increased inflammation. Additionally, the EPC group was associated with increased levels of oxidized LDL, suggesting an elevation in oxidative stress.

SMCs also constitute an important component of atherosclerotic plaques that were assumed to be exclusively derived from the media of the vessel. In a mouse model of atherosclerosis, lethally irradiated $ApoE^{-/-}$ mice that undergo bone marrow transplantation from GFP mice develop significant accumulation of GFP^+ cells in aortic atherosclerotic plaques [23]. The majority of these cells express α-SMA consistent with smooth muscle cells, while many cells also expressed MOMA-2, a macrophage marker.

These findings challenged the prevailing assumption at the time that SMCs in atherosclerotic plaques were exclusively derived from the outer medial layer. However, more recent studies have suggested that the homing of bone-marrow-derived cells to the intima only occurs over the first few days following arterial injury, are predominantly of monocyte/macrophage etiology, and are replaced by SMCs from the media [24]. In $ApoE^{-/-}$ mice, Hu et al. [25] observed that the aortic root is enriched in progenitor cells not derived from bone marrow, and display the markers $Sca\text{-}1^+$, $c\text{-}kit^+$, and $CD34^+$. When $Sca\text{-}1^+$ cells carrying the LacZ gene were applied to the adventitia of a transplanted, irradiated vein graft anastomosed to the carotid artery, significant accumulation of $\beta\text{-}gal^+$ cells of a SMC phenotype were located within the atherosclerotic plaques. Although the possibility of cell fusion with intima SMCs could not be ruled out, these findings demonstrate that SMC progenitor cells derived from the adventitia can migrate across the media or circulate in blood, contributing to the development of atherosclerosis.

Metharom et al. [11] identified smooth muscle outgrowth cells from circulating human peripheral mononuclear cells. They noted that these cultured cells shared distinct myeloid markers (CD68 and CD14) of smooth muscle cells involved in developing microvessels (vasculogenesis) of the intima and adventitia of transplant gender-mismatched atherosclerotic vessels. Their findings are consistent with the hypothesis that circulating mononuclear cells "home" to areas of vascular injury and differentiate into smooth muscle cells in response to local expression of cytokines and growth factors.

Smooth muscle cells also constitute an important component of the atherosclerotic cap, which has a direct bearing on plaque rupture. Human $CD34^+$ cells enriched from cord blood and cultured into two distinct populations characteristic of EPCs and SPCs were serially injected into immunodeficient $ApoE^{-/-}$ $RAG2^{-/-}$ mice fed a high-fat diet [6]. In mice that received SPCs, the aortic plaque area decreased by 42% compared to control, accompanied by a marked increase in collagen and SMC content, and a decrease in macrophage infiltration. No change was noted in those mice that received EPCs. These findings suggest that SPCs contribute to plaque stabilization either directly or indirectly through paracrine and anti-inflammatory mechanisms.

Relationship Between EPCs and Coronary Artery Disease

Several clinical studies have investigated the role of circulating EPCs and their relationship to coronary artery disease (CAD), given their known beneficial effects on vascular repair and homeostasis. In general, the majority of these studies have observed that a person's number of circulating EPCs carries an inverse correlation with their risk of cardiovascular events, and that the presence of CAD is associated with a reduced number of circulating EPCs.

Vasa et al. [26] demonstrated that patients with CAD had reduced numbers of circulating EPCs and that their migratory capacity in response to VEGF was reduced compared to controls. Kunz et al. [27] measured EPC colony-forming unit (CFU) counts in 122 patients undergoing diagnostic coronary angiography and observed a significant decline in EPC counts with increasing CAD severity. Hill et al. [4] measured CFU levels of EPCs in peripheral blood and endothelial function in 45 healthy men free of overt cardiovascular disease. They observed that CFU levels were significantly reduced with increasing Framingham risk score and that endothelial function as measured by flow-mediated brachial artery reactivity strongly correlated with the number of endothelial CFUs.

Werner et al. [28] measured EPCs in arterial blood at the time of angiography in 519 consecutive patients with CAD. EPCs were defined as mononuclear cells staining positive for $CD34^+$ and KDR^+ using flow cytometry. The patients were stratified into low, medium, and high EPC levels. At 12-month follow-up, they observed that increasing EPC number was highly correlated with freedom from cardiovascular events, including death and revascularization (Fig. 12.4). Furthermore, the functional status of EPCs as assessed by CFU also correlated with EPC numbers in a subgroup of 203 patients. These findings suggest that EPC levels may be an important parameter in cardiovascular risk assessment.

In a cardiovascular screening study, Xiao et al. [29] measured EPCs and CFU in 574 northern Italians. Mononuclear cells from venous blood were counted as EPCs if they took up both acetylated LDL and lectin following 5 days of culture; no antibody analysis was performed. They observed an age-related decline in EPC number and a reduced EPC count in postmenopausal women compared to age-matched males. The authors noted the positive influence of medications such as statins, hormone replacement therapy, and ACEI/ARBs on EPC numbers. In contrast to the study by Hill et al. [4], Xiao et al. found a positive correlation between EPC numbers and Framingham risk score, and noted no relationship between EPC numbers and the presence of CAD, although this may have been affected by their limited methods of EPC identification. Importantly, they noted a significant, 40–50% diurnal variation in circulating EPCs, suggesting that the timing of EPC collection is important.

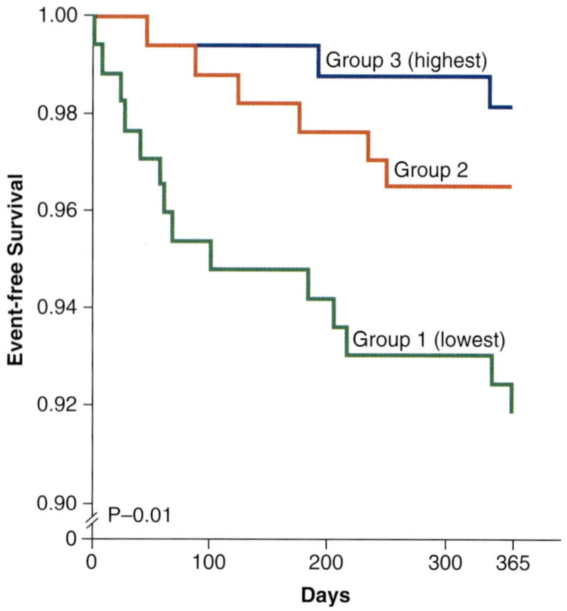

No. at Risk					
Group 1	168	160	158	156	77
Group 2	172	170	168	166	83
Group 3	167	166	165	165	82
Total	507	496	491	487	242

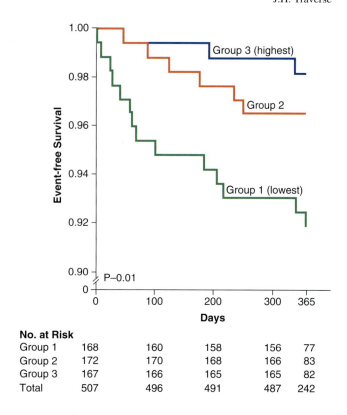

Fig. 12.4 Cumulative event-free survival in an analysis of death from cardiovascular causes at 12 months, according to levels of circulating CD34$^+$/KDR$^+$ endothelial progenitor cells (EPCs) at the time of enrollment. Adapted from Werner et al. [28]. Copyright 2005 by the Massachusetts Medical Society

Guven et al. [30] measured EPC numbers in 48 patients with CAD referred for coronary angiography. Importantly, they performed extensive culturing and labeling of circulating mononuclear cells in order to differentiate true, circulating EPCs, described as late-outgrowth cells (14–28 days of culture), vs. early outgrowth cells (7–12 days of culture) described as circulating angiogenic cells (CAC). EPCs had abundant expression of CD34$^+$ and CD31$^+$, but not CD45$^+$, and were much rarer than CACs. In contrast to previous studies, EPCs were observed to increase with CAD severity evaluated by angiography, with the highest EPC numbers being in those patients referred for revascularization.

These results, which are in contrast to Werner et al. [28] and others [26, 27], are likely because of many patients having ongoing ischemia, a known stimulus for EPC mobilization [31], and their more precise determination of an EPC-like cell. It is likely that many of the EPC determinations in previous studies were more representative of CAC cells described by Guven [30], and not EPCs. Although the inconsistent findings in some of these studies reflect different patient populations and heterogeneity of EPC measurements, it highlights the critical need for the development of standards of EPC identification.

Much less information is known regarding the relationship between circulating SPC levels and atherosclerosis. In a clinical study [6] of patients presenting with acute coronary syndromes (ACS), it was observed that patients with stable CAD compared to patients with ACS had a significant decrease in the number of circulating progenitor cells with an SPC phenotype. These findings suggest that SPCs, in addition to EPCs, may have a clinical role in cardiovascular events.

Does Administration of Stem and Progenitor Cells Increase the Progression of Atherosclerosis in Patients?

Stem cells and progenitor cells secrete a variety of angiogenic cytokines such as VEGF that could promote neovascularization and plaque rupture. Administration of VEGF to ApoE$^{-/-}$/ApoB100$^{-/-}$ mice or rabbits fed a high-cholesterol diet results in a significant increase in atherosclerotic plaque area containing increased macrophage and endothelial cell content [32]. Infusion of unfractionated BMCs from wild-type mice into ApoE$^{-/-}$ mice with hind limb ischemia improves neovascularization and perfusion [18] at the expense of significant increases in aortic atherosclerotic plaque area.

The use of stem cells in clinical trials involving patients with AMI and chronic ischemia is increasing throughout the world. To date, more than 2,000 patients with CAD have participated in cell therapy trials involving a variety of cell types, including mesenchymal stem cells (MSCs), EPC-like cells including CD34$^+$ and CD133$^+$ cells, and unfractionated BMCs.

The vast majority of these patients have received intracoronary BMCs following AMI at a mean dose range of 68×10^6 to 246×10^7 million cells.

Because BMCs contain small fractions of $CD34^+$ cells (<2.0% of the total cell count), $CD133^+$, and MSCs, these angiogenic cells have the potential to accelerate atherosclerosis (target vessel revascularization (TVR)) as observed in animal models. Follow-up is now available from several large, randomized trials providing the opportunity to examine if this occurs in a clinical setting. Fortunately, the 1- and 2-year follow-up data from randomized trials using unfractionated intracoronary BMCs have found no increase in the incidence of TVR or myocardial infarction secondary to plaque rupture.

The largest of these trials, REPAIR-AMI [33], observed that target (16 vs. 26) and nontarget (7 vs. 16) revascularization and recurrent MI (0 vs. 6) were significantly reduced at 1 year in 204 patients randomized to intracoronary BMCs, compared to patients receiving placebo, suggesting that cell therapy conferred a vasculoprotective effect [34]. This is supported by a substudy demonstrating that BMCs improved the coronary flow reserve to adenosine compared to placebo, consistent with BMCs improving endothelial function [35].

Results from the BOOST trial [36] showed no significant difference in TVR or AMI at 18 months of follow-up in 60 patients. Similar findings were reported by the ASTAMI investigators in 100 patients at 1 year of follow-up [37]. These findings demonstrate that intracoronary infusion of unfractionated BMC is safe and does not appear to accelerate atherosclerosis or plaque rupture.

In hypercholesterolemic rabbits, intravenous infusion of MSCs (5×10^7) resulted in an increase in atherosclerotic plaque size and vasa vasorum vascularity of the aortic sinus [38]. However, in the OSIRIS trial [39], 48 patients with AMI were randomized to intravenous allogeneic MSCs at a dose of $1–5 \times 10^6$/kg vs. placebo. No increase in TVR or myocardial infarction was noted. In the ACT34 trial, 167 patients with refractory angina due to chronic ischemia were administered $CD34^+$ progenitor cells ($1–5 \times 10^5$/kg) or placebo by intramyocardial injections [40]. The investigators noted that TVR and AMI were reduced in the cell therapy group compared to placebo. Although both of these studies used an enriched cell population, they were not delivered by an intracoronary route so their effects on atherosclerosis and plaque rupture may have been mitigated.

In contrast, several studies illustrate the potential vascular complications that may arise when an enriched cell population of angiogenic cells is administered by an intracoronary route. The MAGIC trial [41] investigated the intracoronary infusion of peripheral blood mononuclear cells enriched with $CD34^+$ cells following G-CSF administration (10 μg/kg × 4 days) vs. G-CSF therapy alone after stenting for AMI. At 6-month follow-up, quantitative coronary angiography (QCA) demonstrated a marked increase in in-stent restenosis in both groups of patients (7 of 10) compared to a control group.

Bartunek et al. [42] infused high-dose $CD133^+$ cells (1.5 to 33.6×10^6) by an intracoronary route in 19 patients following PCI for AMI. By 4 months of follow-up, 2 patients had stent thrombosis, 7 patients had significant in-stent restenosis, and 2 patients developed new coronary stenosis distal to the stent, requiring revascularization. In a control group of 16 patients, only 4 had developed restenosis, likely secondary to the use of bare-metal stents. Importantly, analysis by QCA demonstrated significant late loss in the stented segments where the cells were infused but not in the contralateral vessels [43]. In a subset of patients who underwent intravascular ultrasound, a significant dose-related increase in the plaque burden was shown in those patients who received enriched $CD133^+$ cells. This increased plaque burden was associated with higher plasma levels of VEGF-A and lower levels of IL-10 compared to those patients without vascular complications. This important study and its follow-up highlight the pernicious vascular, biologic effects of delivering enriched angiogenic cells in the setting of atherosclerosis.

Conclusions

The role of stem and progenitor cells in the biology of atherosclerosis is evolving. Much of the hypotheses derived to date rely on transgenic models of hyperlipidemia that may differ from the human condition. Furthermore, bone marrow transplantation of labeled cells following whole body radiation may produce deleterious effects on resident progenitor cells in the recipient's vasculature that could make them more reliant on bone-marrow-derived progenitor cells.

Many clinical studies reveal an inverse association between number of circulating EPC-like cells and severity of CAD or associative risk factors. However, because no true EPC marker has been identified, these studies show marked heterogeneity in the measurement and identification of EPCs. To date, the use of unfractionated BMCs containing small fractions of stem and progenitor cells in patients with CAD appears safe and is not associated with accelerated atherosclerosis or myocardial infarction. However, intracoronary administration of enriched progenitor cell populations may be associated with late lumen loss and increased target vessel revascularization.

References

1. Ross R. Atherosclerosis – an inflammatory disease. NEJM. 1995;340:115–26.
2. Goldschmidt-Clermont PJ, Creager MA, Losordo DW, et al. Atherosclerosis 2005: recent discoveries and novel hypotheses. Circulation. 2005;112:3341.
3. Asahara T, Murohara T, Sullivan A, et al. Isolation of putative progenitor endothelial cells for angiogenesis. Science. 1997;275:964–7.
4. Hill JM, Zalos G, Halcox JPJ, et al. Circulating endothelial progenitor cells, vascular function, and cardiovascular risk. N Engl J Med. 2003;348:593–600.
5. Virmani R, Kolodgie FD, Burke AP, et al. Atherosclerotic plaque progression and vulnerability to rupture. Angiogenesis as a source of intraplaque hemorrhage. Arterioscler Thromb Vasc Biol. 2005;25:2054–61.
6. Zoll J, Fontaine V, Gourdy P, et al. Role of human smooth muscle cell progenitors in atherosclerotic plaque development and composition. Cardiovasc Res. 2008;77:471–80.
7. Shi Q, Rafii S, Wu MH-D, et al. Evidence for circulating bone marrow-derived endothelial cells. Blood. 1998;92:362–7.
8. Hirschi KK, Ingram DA, Yoder MC. Assessing identity, phenotype, and fate of endothelial progenitor cells. Arterioscler Thromb Vasc Biol. 2008;28:1584–95.
9. Simper D, Stalboerger PG, Panetta CJ, et al. Smooth muscle progenitor cells in human blood. Circulation. 2002;106:1199–204.
10. Caplice NM, Bunch TJ, Stalboerger PG, et al. Smooth muscle cells in human coronary atherosclerosis can originate from cells administered at marrow transplantation. Proc Natl Acad Sci USA. 2003;100:4754–9.
11. Metharom P, Liu C, Wang S, et al. Myeloid lineage of high proliferative potential human smooth muscle outgrowth cells in circulating in blood and vasculogenic smooth muscle-like cells *in vivo*. Atherosclerosis. 2008;198:29–38.
12. Moreno PR, Purushothaman R, Fuster V, et al. Plaque neovascularization is increased in ruptured atherosclerotic lesions of human aorta. Implications for plaque vulnerability. Circulation. 2004;110:2032–8.
13. Zhang Y, Cliff WJ, Schoefl GI, et al. Immunohistochemical study of intimal microvessels in coronary atherosclerosis. Am J Pathol. 1993;143:164–72.
14. Langheinrich AC, Michniewicz A, Sedding DG, et al. Correlation of vaso vasorum neovascularization and plaque progression in aortas of apolipoprotein $E^{-/-}$/low-density lipoprotein$^{-/-}$ double knockout mice. Arterioscler Thromb Vasc Biol. 2006;26:347–52.
15. Moulton KS, Vakili K, Zurakowski D, et al. Inhibition of plaque neovascularization reduces macrophage accumulation and progression of advanced atherosclerosis. Proc Natl Acad Sci USA. 2003;100:4736–41.
16. Moreno PR, Purushothaman KR, Zias E, et al. Neovascularization in human atherosclerosis. Curr Mole Med. 2006;6:457–77.
17. George J, Afek A, Abashidze A, et al. Transfer of endothelial progenitor and bone marrow cells influence atherosclerotic plaque size and composition in apolipoprotein E knockout mice. Arterioscler Thromb Vasc Biol. 2005;25:2636–41.
18. Silvestre J-S, Gojova A, Brun V, et al. Transplantation of bone marrow-derived mononuclear cells in ischemic apolipoprotein E-knockout mice accelerates atherosclerosis without altering plaque composition. Circulation. 2003;108:2839–42.
19. Torsney E, Mandal K, Halliday A, et al. Characterization of progenitor cells in human atherosclerotic vessels. Atherosclerosis. 2007;191:259–64.
20. Zengin E, Chalajour F, Gehling UM, et al. Vascular wall resident progenitor cells: a source for postnatal vasculogenesis. Development. 2006;133:1543–51.
21. Ingram DA, Mead LE, Moore DB, et al. Vessel wall-derived endothelial cells rapidly proliferate because they contain a complete hierarchy of endothelial progenitor cells. Blood. 2005;105:2783–6.
22. Rauscher FM, Goldschmidt-Clermont PJ, Davis BH, et al. Aging, progenitor cell exhaustion, and atherosclerosis. Circulation. 2003;108:457–63.
23. Sata M, Saiura A, Kunisato A, et al. Hematopoietic stem cells differentiate into vascular cells that participate in the pathogenesis of atherosclerosis. Nat Med. 2002;8:403–9.
24. Daniel JM, Tillmanns H, Sedding DG. Time course analysis of bone marrow-derived progenitor cell transdifferentiation during neointima formation. Circulation. 2009;120:S1130.
25. Hu Y, Zhang Z, Torsney E, et al. Abundant progenitor cells in the adventitia contribute to atherosclerosis of vein grafts in ApoE-deficient mice. JCI. 2004;113:1258–65.
26. Vasa M, Fichtlscherer S, Aicher A, et al. Number and migratory activity of circulating endothelial progenitor cells inversely correlate with risk factors for coronary artery disease. Circ Res. 2001;89:E1–7.
27. Kunz GA, Liang G, Cuculi F, et al. Circulating endothelial progenitor cells predict coronary artery disease severity. Heart. 2006;152:109–95.
28. Werner N, Kosiol S, Schiegl T, et al. Circulating endothelial progenitor cells and cardiovascular outcomes. N Engl J Med. 2005;353:999–1007.
29. Xiao Q, Kiechl S, Patel S, et al. Endothelial progenitor cells, cardiovascular risk factors, cytokine levels and atherosclerosis-results from a large population-based study. PLoS One. 2007;2:e975.
30. Guven H, Shepherd RM, Bach RG, et al. The number of endothelial progenitor cell colonies in the blood is increased in patients with angiographically significant coronary artery disease. J Am Coll Cardiol. 2006;48:1579–87.
31. George J, Goldstein E, Abashidze S, et al. Circulating endothelial progenitor cells in patients with unstable angina: association with systemic inflammation. Eur Heart J. 2004;25:1003–8.
32. Celletti FL, Waugh JM, Amabile PG, et al. Vascular endothelial growth factor enhances atherosclerotic plaque progression. Nat Med. 2001;7:425–33.
33. Schachinger V, Erbs S, Elasser A, et al. Intracoronary bone marrow-derived progenitor cells in acute myocardial infarction. N Engl J Med. 2006;355:1210–21.
34. Schachunger V, Erbs S, Elasser A, et al. Improved clinical outcome after intracoronary administration of bone-marrow-derived progenitor cells in acute myocardial infarction: final 1-year results of the REPAIR-AMI trial. Eur Heart J. 2006;27:2775–83.
35. Erbs S, Linke A, Schachinger V, et al. Restoration of microvascular function in the infarct-related artery by intracoronary transplantation of bone marrow progenitor cells in patients with acute myocardial infarction. Circulation. 2007;116:366–74.

36. Meyer GP, Wollert KC, Lotz J, et al. Intracoronary bone marrow cell transfer after myocardial infarction – eighteen months' follow-up data from randomized, controlled BOOST (bone marrow transfer to enhance ST-elevation infarct regeneration) trial. Circulation. 2006;113:1287–94.
37. Lunde K, Solheim S, Forfang K, et al. Anterior myocardial infarction with acute percutaneous coronary intervention and intracoronary injection of autologous mononuclear bone marrow cells. Safety, clinical outcome, and serial changes in left-ventricular function during 12-months' follow-up. J Am Coil Cardiol. 2008;51:674–6.
38. Liu PX, Zhang L, Liao WB, et al. Transfusion of allogeneic mesenchymal stem cells promotes progression of atherosclerotic plaque in rabbits. Zhongguo Shi Yan Xue Ye Xue ZaZhi. 2009;17:700–5.
39. Hare JM, Traverse JH, Henry TD, et al. A randomized, double-blind, placebo-controlled, dose escalation study of intravenous adult human mesenchymal stem cells (Prochymal) after acute myocardial infarction. J Am Coll Cardiol. 2009;54:2277–86.
40. Losordo DW, Henry TD, Schatz RA, et al. Autologous CD34+ cell therapy for refractory angina: 12 month results of the phase II ACT34-CMI study. Circulation. 2009;120:S1132.
41. Kang HJ, Kim HS, Zhang SY, et al. Effects of intracoronary infusion of peripheral blood stem cells mobilized with granulocyte-colony stimulating factor on left-ventricular systolic function and restenosis after coronary stenting in myocardial infarction: the MAGIC cell randomized clinical trial. Lancet. 2004;363:751–6.
42. Bartunek J, Vanderheyden M, Vandekerckhove B, et al. Intracoronary infusion of CD133+ enriched bone marrow progenitors promotes cardiac recovery after recent myocardial infarction. Feasibility and safety. Circulation. 2005;112:I178–83.
43. Mansour S, Vanderheyden M, De Bruyne B, et al. Intracoronary delivery of hematopoietic bone marrow stem cells and luminal loss of the infarct-related artery in patients with recent myocardial infarction. J Am Coll Cardiol. 2006;47:1727–30.

Chapter 13
Induced Pluripotential Stem Cells and the Prospects for Cardiac Cell Therapy

Jonathan M.W. Slack and James R. Dutton

Embryonic Stem Cells

Embryonic stem (ES) cells are grown in culture from the inner cell mass (ICM) of blastocyst-stage embryos (Fig. 13.1). These small cells grow as tight, refractile colonies. ES cells are usually cultured on a feeder layer of mitotically inactive fibroblasts, which supply the cells with necessary growth factors and extracellular matrix support. Feeder cell-free cultivation is also possible. Mouse ES cells were first isolated in 1981 [1, 2] and human ES cells in 1998 [3].

Much debate has ensued about whether the phenotype of ES cells is closer to the ICM or the embryonic epiblast, and whether these are in fact the same cell type [4]. Various behavioral differences exist between mouse and human ES cells, and some believe the latter are closer to the epiblast phenotype [5, 6]. However, transcriptional profiling does show considerable affinity between human and mouse ES cells [7]. Ironically, whichever cell type is the true in vivo counterpart of the ES cell, it clearly does not function in a stem cell-like manner in vivo. Both the ICM, the epiblast, and all other early cell populations in the embryo are quite short-lived and soon develop into other cell types committed to form specific body parts or tissue types. So in this sense, ES cells are an in vitro artifact. However, this fact does not detract from their great importance for various applications.

In the appropriate media, mouse ES cells can be cultivated without limit. Differentiation can be prevented either by the feeder cells or by maintaining the cells in the presence of inhibitors of the FGF and Wnt signal transduction pathways [8]. When their feeder cells, or inhibitors, are withdrawn, ES cells are capable of differentiation into a wide range of cell types, representing most cell types of the normal mammalian body.Early on, mouse ES cells were shown to integrate into the ICM of a host embryo and form germ-line chimeras [9]. This property means that it is possible to carry out genetic manipulations on the cells in vitro, reintroduce the cells into mouse blastocysts, grow the embryos to maturity in a foster mother, and then recover mice with the altered genetic constitution. In this way, ES cells have been enormously important in enabling the process of targeted mutagenesis [10]. This has made possible the study of the developmental role of many genes by production of loss-of-function mutants. It has also enabled the creation of a wide range of mouse models for human diseases.

The discovery of human ES cells created huge interest in the potential applications that they offered. Four distinct areas are currently envisioned:

1. First is the investigation of normal development. The availability of cells that will carry out some developmental steps in vitro offers a method of investigating certain aspects of normal human development which would not otherwise be accessible.
2. Second is the study of cellular pathology for those human genetic diseases where the relevant cells can be obtained in vitro. While tissue samples may sometimes be obtained from affected individuals, ES cells of the appropriate genotype give access to embryonic and immature cell populations whose function may be compromised by the disease.
3. Third is the possibility of obtaining normal or genetically abnormal human cells for drug screening. Some cell types, such as cardiomyocytes, are normally very difficult to obtain. Even human hepatocytes are in very short supply.

J.M.W. Slack, MA, PhD (✉) • J.R. Dutton, BSc, PhD
Stem Cell Institute, University of Minnesota, Minneapolis, MN, USA
e-mail: slack017@umn.edu

Z. Vlodaver et al. (eds.), *Coronary Heart Disease: Clinical, Pathological, Imaging, and Molecular Profiles*, DOI 10.1007/978-1-4614-1475-9_13, © Springer Science+Business Media, LLC 2012

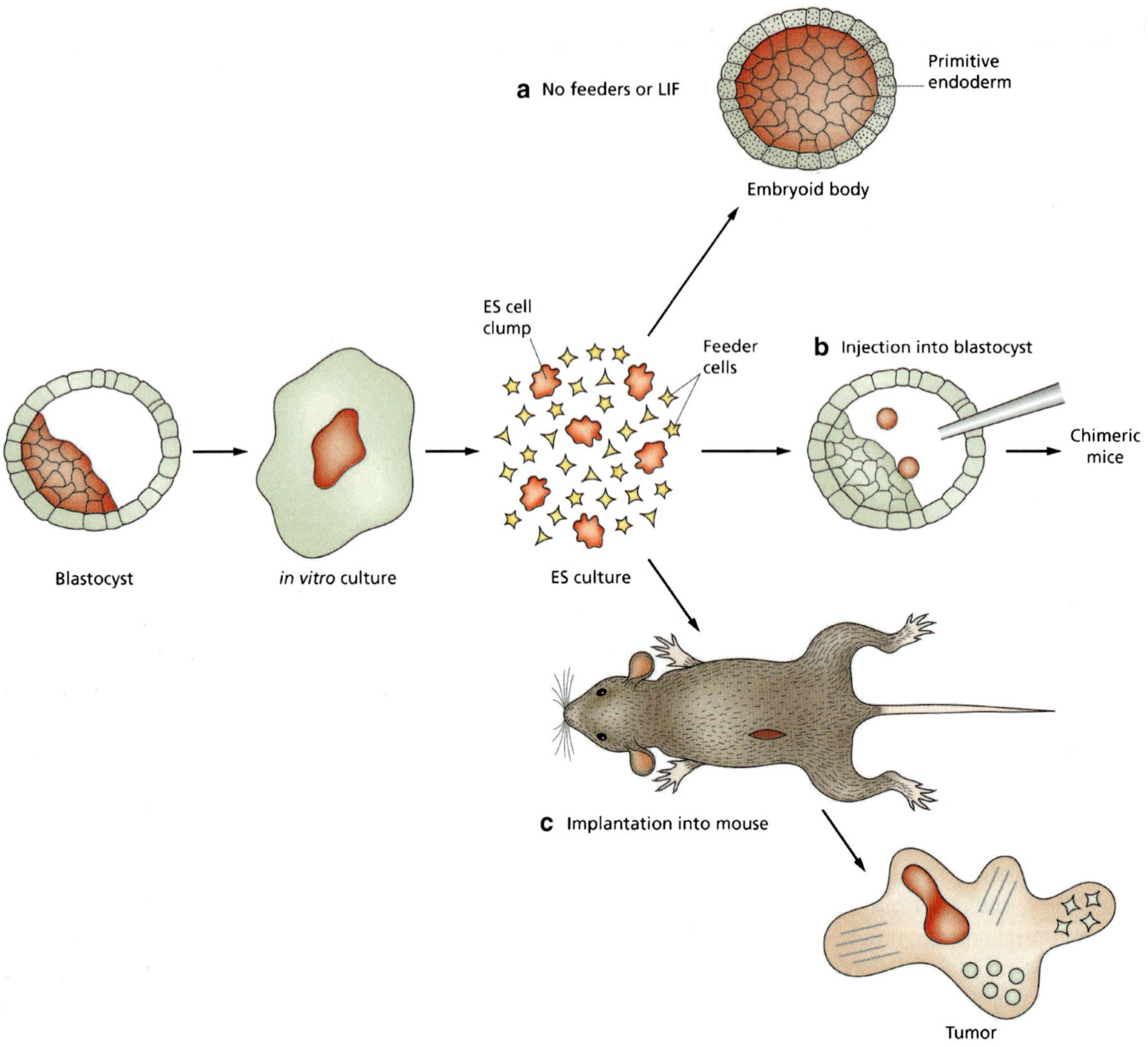

Fig. 13.1 Properties of mouse embryonic stem cells (ES cells). The cells originate from in vitro culture of the inner cell mass (ICM) of preimplantation embryos, and can be expanded in pluripotent form. They will also differentiate in vitro, contribute to all tissues of developing mouse embryos, and form multitissue tumors (teratomas) as grafts in adult mice (Adapted from Slack) [86]

4. Finally, and the most publicized in the general media, is the possibility of making differentiated cell populations for transplantation therapy [11]. Most of the common degenerative diseases that afflict the western world involve the loss of or damage to certain specific cell populations. ES cells offer a source of healthy cells that could potentially be transplanted to repair damaged tissues or organs.

When plated without feeders in nonadhesive dishes, mouse ES cells will form embryoid bodies which, in some ways, resemble normal mouse embryos [12]. However, they are not quite the same as embryos. First, they are not enveloped by trophectoderm. The trophectoderm is the outer layer of the blastocyst and the first component of the future placenta to develop. Although mouse ES cells can form trophectoderm under some circumstances [13], they do not normally do so. For this reason, they are described as "pluripotent" rather than "totipotent."

Embryoid bodies have a certain internal structure, including a Wnt signaling center at one end of the cell mass [14]. However, they develop in a range of sizes. The different surface-volume ratios and spatial relationships between parts mean that the embryoid bodies in one dish can be quite diverse in structure and composition [15]. Over 2–3 weeks, embryoid bodies normally generate cell populations representing many of the major body parts, tissue types, and cell types formed in a normal embryo. However, the spatial pattern is variable and abnormal, and certain tissue types, such as skeletal muscle, are not normally formed. Embryoid body-like development can also occur in cell monolayer on adhesive plastic dishes. Human ES cells can form similar embryoid bodies [16] although in this case, trophectoderm usually is generated.

When implanted into an immunocompatible adult animal, both mouse and human ES cells will form a type of tumor called a teratoma [3, 17]. It contains proliferating nests of cells similar to the original ES cells. The teratoma also contains zones of differentiation into many body parts and tissue types. Arrangement of the zones is generally highly chaotic and varies from one tumor to the next. Since it is impossible to implant human ES cells into human embryos in order to test their pluripotency, the teratoma assay is particularly important. The assay is usually performed by implanting ES cells into immunocompromised mice such as NOD-SCIDs. The ES cells being tested are presumed to be pluripotent if the resultant teratomas form tissues characteristically derived from all three embryonic germ layers: ectoderm, mesoderm, and endoderm.

The pluripotent character of ES cells is maintained by a network of transcription factors. Three critical factors are Oct4, Sox2, and Nanog [18, 19]. The factors upregulate each other and a whole range of target genes, resulting in a reasonably stable pluripotent state. Many of the developmental control genes required for formation of body parts and tissue types in an embryo are not active in ES cells. Instead, they are maintained in a state of competence by a "bivalent mark," namely the presence of antagonistic pairs of modified histones that can activate or repress activity of the associated genes. For example, bivalent domains with histone methylation at both H3K27 and H3K4 have been described on many genes [20]. Bivalent chromatin domains are not, however, unique to ES cells.

Induced Pluripotent Stem Cells

A remarkable discovery concerning the biology of pluripotency was first published in 2006 by Yamanaka [21]. He showed that it was possible to make cells resembling ES cells by introducing four pluripotency genes into normal fibroblasts. He called these cells "induced pluripotent stem cells" or "induced pluripotential stem cells (iPS cells)." Although these initial iPS cells were probably not fully reprogrammed to an ES-like state, this work set off an explosion of activity around the world, and the technology of preparing iPS cells has since advanced very rapidly (Figs. 13.2 and 13.3). Human iPS cells were reported in 2007 [22–25]. Mouse iPS cells were soon shown to be capable of contributing to all tissues in mouse embryos, including the germ line. Thus, they really do resemble ES cells in this crucial respect. Mouse iPS cells also have ES-like patterns of DNA methylation and histone modifications [26, 27]. iPS cells can be made from cell types other than fibroblasts [28–30]. Undifferentiated cells, such as tissue-specific stem cells, tend to give higher efficiencies of iPS colony formation, perhaps because of their more open chromatin state.

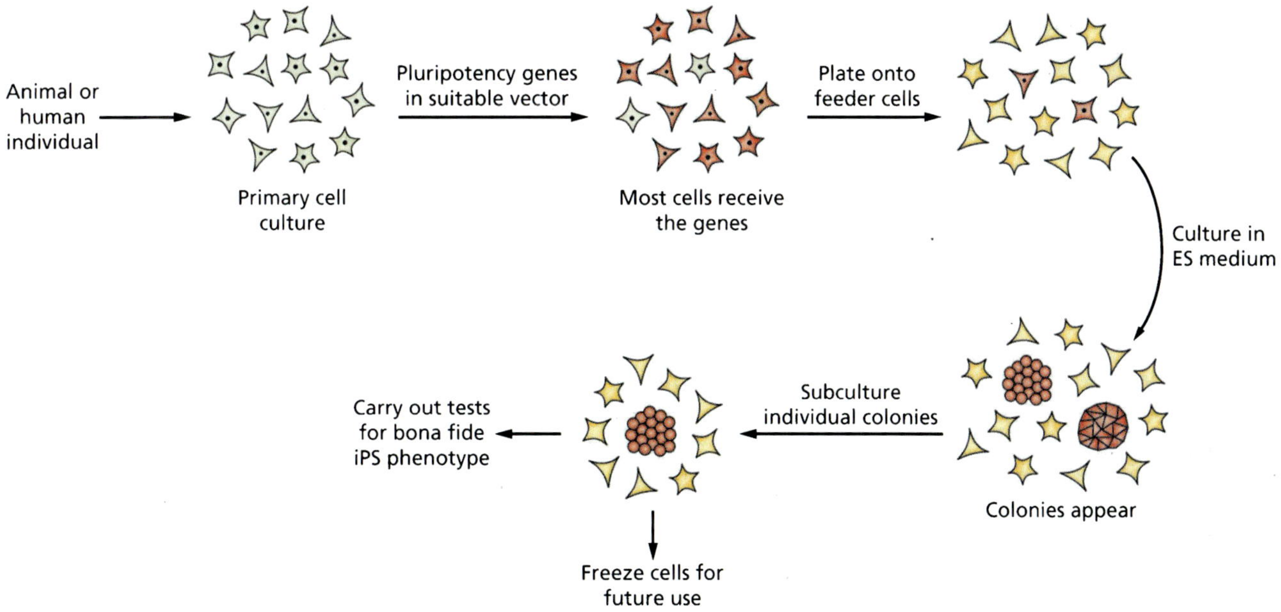

Fig. 13.2 Method for preparation of induced pluripotent stem cells (iPS cells). Not all colonies that develop are genuine iPS cells, so careful characterization is necessary

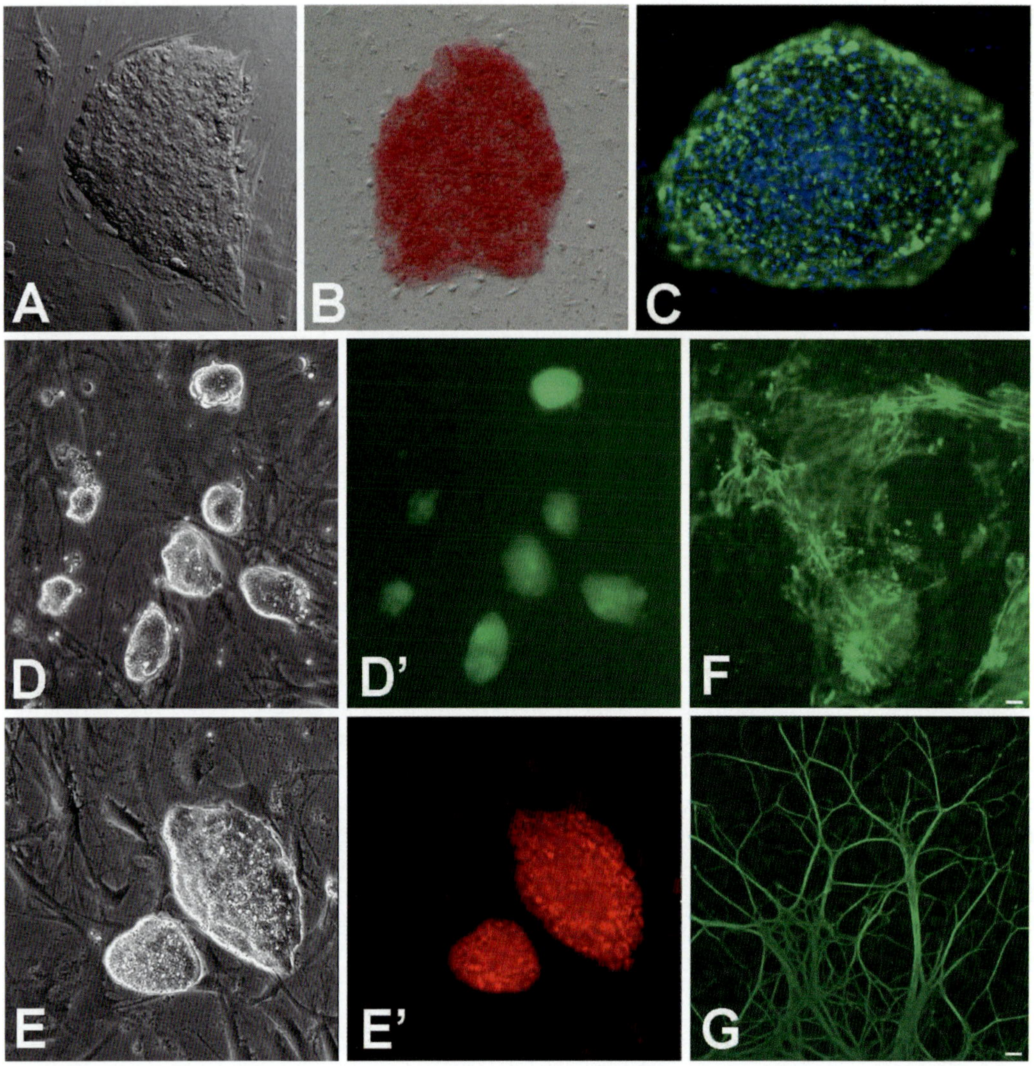

Fig. 13.3 iPS cells prepared by Dr. James Dutton, Stem Cell Institute, University of Minnesota. (**a–c**) Human iPS cell colonies. (**a**) Interference contrast. (**b**) Alkaline phosphatase histochemistry. (**c**) TRA 1-81 surface antigen stain (*green*) with DAPI (*blue*). (**d–g**) Mouse iPS cells. (**d, d'**) iPS colonies made from *Oct4-GFP* mice: Green colonies are *Oct4* positive. (**e, e'**) Expression of Nanog (*red*) in mouse iPS colonies. (**f**) Extensive differentiation of cardiomyocytes visualized by troponin T immunostaining (*green*). This monolayer culture showed spontaneous beating. (**g**) Differentiation of neurons visualized by neurofilament 200 immunostaining (*green*). Scale bar 50 mm

Genes used to initiate iPS cell formation include representatives of those encoding the core group of pluripotency-regulating transcription factors active in ES cells: Oct4, Sox2, and Nanog. In addition, genes whose function is less clear, but which in some way improve the efficiency of the process, are usually included. These include genes encoding c-Myc, Klf4, and Lin28. Genes are delivered using retroviral vectors that insert their DNA into the genome of the cells. The usual procedure is infecting the target cells with all four retroviruses, then waiting a few days, and plating the cells onto feeders in ES culture medium. Under these conditions, ES-like cells will grow, but the parent fibroblasts will not.

Various selective systems can be used with mouse cells to ensure that ES-like cells will grow. One example is using mice with an antibiotic-resistance gene driven by one of the pluripotency gene promoters. Once iPS cell colonies have appeared, those resembling ES cells by morphology are picked and subcultured on fresh feeder cells. The efficiency of generating iPS cells is very low. Even among cells that express all four viral-encoded genes, only a small proportion will establish iPS colonies. The critical event is establishing a stable web of activation of a set of pluripotency genes whose activity is mutually maintained and no longer dependent on the expression of viral transgenes. Many other types of colonies may develop, especially when the transforming oncogene *c-Myc* is included in the cocktail. So it is important to characterize iPS lines very carefully to make sure that they really do closely resemble ES cells, rather than being some sort of transformed colony with only superficial ES characteristics.

Testing iPS Characteristics

Tests normally carried out to characterize iPS cell lines are

1. Morphology: Genuine iPS cell colonies are refractile with a clearly defined edge. The cells have a large nucleus with prominent nucleoli and little cytoplasm. Human iPS cell colonies are flatter than murine ones.
2. Genuine iPS cells exhibit ES cell-like growth characteristics, proliferating as undifferentiated cells without passage limit.
3. Expression of a range of pluripotency factors, including the endogenous counterparts of the genes used to induce the transformation.
4. Expression of characteristic cell surface antigens (SSEA1 for mouse, and SSEA3 and 4, TRA 1-60, and 1-81 for human).
5. An ES-like pattern of minimal DNA methylation in promoter regions of genes involved in maintaining the pluripotent state.
6. A normal karyotype.
7. Ability to form embryoid bodies in which the cells differentiate and produce tissues characteristically derived from all three embryonic germ layers.

In addition, mouse iPS cells should be able to form chimeras when injected into mouse embryos. Ideally, these should be germline chimeras – i.e., the resulting mice should be capable of reproducing and generating offspring of the iPS cell genotype. Even more demanding is the tetraploid rescue test [31] where the host embryo becomes tetraploid by electrofusion of the two cells of the two-cell stage into a single tetraploid cell. Tetraploid cells cannot contribute to the fetus, although they can still form extraembryonic structures. When good quality ES cells are injected into a tetraploid host embryo, they can form the entire fetus with no significant contribution from host cells. This has also been achieved with iPS cells, showing that it is possible to achieve complete pluripotency [32, 33].

It is *not* possible to inject human iPS cells into embryos, so the standard approach is the teratoma assay. iPS cells are injected into an immunocompatible host, usually to a subcutaneous or intramuscular location [3, 17]. If the resulting tumors contain tissues characteristically derived from all three embryonic germ layers, then the cells are presumed to be pluripotent in character.

Patient-Specific iPS Cell Lines

Good quality iPS cells are virtually identical in their properties to ES cells. But the technology to create iPS cells has an important practical attribute that ES cells do not share. This is the ability to establish new cell lines from specific individuals. Speculation has been raised for years about the possibility of creating patient-specific ES cell lines. But this relied on the hope that somatic cell nuclear transfer of patient cell nuclei could be performed into donor oocytes to create preimplantation embryos of a genotype identical to the patient. This would be followed by derivation of an ES line from the embryos thus created [34]. This procedure has never actually been successfully achieved using human cells, although it is probably feasible because it has been achieved in rhesus monkeys [35]. The main, practical problem is the low efficiency of cloning coupled with the extreme difficulty of obtaining sufficient human oocytes to make the experiments feasible. There are also ethical problems. The somatic cell nuclear transfer procedure is a form of whole organism cloning, and this provokes more ethical objections than the use of surplus human embryos to derive ES lines. Moreover, the procurement of human oocytes involves additional ethical problems due to issues of informed consent and payment of donors.

In contrast to the difficulties surrounding somatic cell nuclear cloning, many patient-specific iPS lines have already been made. These include cell lines from several patients with specific genetic diseases [36–41]. The technology appears robust and has been used in many different laboratories. The attraction of a patient-specific cell line, of course, is that any differentiated cells made from it will be a perfect, immunological match to the patient and, therefore, could potentially be grafted safely and without the use of immunosuppressive drugs.

Improved Methods of iPS Generation

In order to make patient-specific iPS preparation a reality, the efficiency of the process needs to improve. Moreover, the potential use of iPS cells for therapeutic transplantation has meant there is a great desire to find a routine way to make them without the use of insertional viruses. It is known that insertional viruses can create mutations during the integration process.

Moreover, silenced genes may become reactivated at low frequency and cause formation of tumors. This has happened frequently in mice grown from iPS cells [27]. So the ideal is to improve efficiency of generation from 10^{-4} to 10^{-5} up to about 10^{-3}, and to do so using nonintegrating delivery vectors.

Because the critical processes occur in a small number of cells that cannot be identified until they form colonies, the early mechanisms of iPS cell formation are still obscure [42]. But some information has been obtained using cells from mice containing doxycycline-inducible copies of the four genes. This enables synchronous and uniform induction of the genes at a dose known to induce the iPS state. When cells from such mice are cloned, all clones can generate iPS cells, so the low efficiency of the process seems to be caused by unknown stochastic effects, rather than the presence of a small minority of susceptible cells in the animal [43]. iPS cell colonies from those mice do not become established unless the transgenes are active for about 8–12 days. Oddly, it seems that markers of the ES state, including alkaline phosphatase and SSEA1, are activated before Oct4 and Nanog, and before the iPS state is irreversibly established [44]. The genes introduced by the retroviruses became silenced in correctly reprogrammed iPS cell lines [27]. It has been established that the integration sites are not the same in different cell lines. These various pieces of information indicate that a high-level expression of the transgenes is required for about 12 days, after which, it should be completely shut off.

For the iPS cell phenotype to become established, the introduced gene products must locate their own binding domains in the DNA and activate the set of genes required to establish a stable pluripotency program. Some of the additional genes in the gene sets used (*c-Myc, Lin28, Klf4*) may have rather nonspecific functions regarding general opening of chromatin to make gene targets more accessible. In addition, they may promote cell division, which is favorable for iPS cell generation, perhaps because genes become accessible during DNA replication. Certain small molecules that serve to open chromatin – for example, those inhibiting histone deacetylases – have also helped increase efficiency of iPS generation [45].

Some researchers believe that all four genes used to generate iPS cells could be replaced by a judicious choice of small molecules. However, while a small molecule might increase efficiency by opening chromatin, it seems unlikely that it could fully mimic the effects of a transcription factor such as Oct4, with its sequence-specific binding both to DNA and to a variety of partner proteins.

Despite a strong desire to do so, it has proved difficult to make iPS cells using methods that do not involve genomic integration. The most efficient approach is to allow integration, but then excise the transgenes after they have had their effect [46, 47]. This is likely to prove difficult for routine applications, as guaranteeing complete excision requires knowledge of the sequence of the original integration sites. Methods involving the use of plasmids or nonintegrating viruses have been shown to work occasionally, but with significantly lower efficiencies than integrating viruses [48, 49]. Some limited success has also been reported using proteins equipped with cell-penetrating transduction domains but, presently, this also shows very low efficiency [50, 51].

Fusaki, Ban, Nishiyama, Saeki, and Hasegawa described the successful use of Sendai virus vector [52]. This ribonucleic acid (RNA) virus undergoes RNA replication in the cytoplasm, and thus may be able to avoid the effects of dilution of the exogenous factors during cell division.

The need for continued expression of the transgenes during the prolonged period when prospective iPS cells are being reprogrammed, and before the iPS cell state is endogenously stable, suggests that this requirement may not be genomic integration per se. Instead, it may be maintenance of high transgene expression for the necessary period of time. In the future, a combination of nonintegrating gene delivery and chemical enhancement of reprogramming efficiency will probably allow routine generation of iPS cells in the absence of any gene integration.

Cardiomyocyte Differentiation Methods

The formation of cardiomyocytes and other cell types contributing to the structure of the heart has been a major research objective with ES cells for years. Lessons learned are now being applied to iPS cells.

Two strategies are used to control differentiation of ES cells:

1. One is to force development by introducing developmental control genes at an appropriate developmental stage. This has been done, for example, to promote the development of skeletal muscle from mouse ES cells, which is difficult to achieve by other means [53]. The use of inserted transgenes is discouraged for potential therapeutic applications, however, for the same reasons as their use to make iPS cells. These reasons are the risks of insertional mutagenesis or inappropriate reactivation of a potential oncogene following transplantation.
2. The second and generally more practiced method attempts to recapitulate the normal steps in embryonic development by exposing the cells to a succession of embryonic-inducing factors such as FGFs, Wnts, activins, and BMPs, as well as a judicious selection of media and extracellular matrix components [11].

The earliest stages of heart development have been studied most thoroughly in chicks and mice [54–56]. Fate mapping shows that the cardiogenic mesoderm originates in the epiblast lateral to the node. During gastrulation, it passes through the anterior third of the primitive streak, forming lateral territories which then move anteriorly to form two elongated strips on either side of the embryonic axis. Various transcription factors become expressed in an anterior crescent region, including Nkx2.5, GATA4-6, MEF2, Hand1, and Tbx5. From this stage on, the microsurgical interchange of regions or removal of explants in the chick blastoderm causes heart defects, so the appearance of the anterior crescent probably corresponds to the time of initial specification of the heart.

As the head lifts off the blastoderm surface, the heart rudiments move underneath it toward the midline. The two rudiments fuse to form a single tube which has four layers: the endocardium; a layer of extracellular matrix called the cardiac jelly; the myocardium, which forms the actual cardiac muscle; and the pericardium, which becomes the thin, outer connective tissue sheath. Cre-lox labeling in mouse embryos, using the *Nkx2.5* promoter to drive the *Cre* recombinase, shows that all heart tube layers are formed from cells that formerly had the *Nkx2.5* promoter active. However, the cardiogenic cells begin to segregate into endocardial and myocardial populations during the migration phase.

The initially linear heart tube forms the two atria and the left ventricle, and as its regionalization and looping proceeds, a further recruitment of cells takes place into its anterior end. These cells come from what is now called the secondary heart field, which initially lies within the pharyngeal mesenchyme, and later anterior to the crescent region expressing the cardiac transcription factors. The secondary heart field is characterized by expression of the transcription factors Islet-1 and Hand2, and largely forms the right ventricle and outflow tract. In addition, neural crest cells migrate to the outflow tract and form the septum dividing the future pulmonary and aortic circulations.

This brief description indicates that even normal development of heart tissue is quite complex. Three regions of the embryo contribute to the heart: the anterior crescent, the secondary heart field, and the cardiac neural crest. During early heart development, the cells acquire a regional identity (ventricle, atrium, outflow tract), an inside-outside identity (endo-, meso-, pericardium), and a cell-type identity (cardiomyocytes, conduction system, smooth muscle, endothelium, septa). In view of this complexity, generating a complete heart from ES or iPS cells is unlikely. However, every possibility exists of generating quantities of cardiac tissue. In fact, cardiac tissue often develops spontaneously in embryoid bodies, or the equivalent monolayer cultures, to which no specific inducing factors have been applied.

ES and iPS cell differentiation studies have focused on the formation of cardiomyocytes. Results from clinical cell therapy trials (see below) have suggested that improvements in function may equally depend on improved angiogenesis, which may require an augmented supply of smooth muscle cells and endothelial cells. The exact specification state of cells at each stage of development, and in each position within the developing heart, is not well understood. Evidence does show the existence of progenitors that can form all three of the major cell types: cardiomyocytes, smooth muscle, and endothelium. In addition, clonal cultures of Isl1-positive cells from embryos will form all three cell types [57]. It is likely that Nkx2.5-positive cells are also pluripotent to this degree [58].

Generating Cardiomyocytes

Protocols for generating cardiomyocytes from human ES cells have been refined over the last few years. Mature organs do not contain the inducing factors required to drive ES cells through a sequential, multistep pathway of differentiation. For cardiac tissues, this sequence comprises ES cell to mesoderm, to anterior mesoderm, to primary or secondary heart field, to heart tube, and to specific cell types. If undifferentiated ES cells are grafted into the heart, they do not undergo this complex pathway of development, but simply form teratomas [59]. In contrast, multiple developmental stages seem to be achieved when ES cells are allowed to form embryoid bodies. Some spontaneously beating cardiomyocytes develop simply on embryoid body differentiation without additional treatments [60, 61]. The yield can be increased by various manipulations of conditions, such as reducing the concentration of serum [62], adding TNFα [63], or inhibiting p38 MAP kinase [64].

An enrichment method favored in ES differentiation studies is selecting the population of cells required. For human ES-derived cardiomyocytes, one published method is to incorporate a lentiviral reporter consisting of eGFP driven by the myosin light chain 2V promoter [65]. More recent protocols seek a closer match to events of normal development and involve an initial treatment with Wnt, activin, and BMP to induce mesoderm formation. This is followed by inhibition of Wnt signaling to bias cells toward the anteroventral-type mesoderm [66]. In this study, cardiomyocytes from human ES cells were grafted into infarcted rat hearts (Fig. 13.4). This showed some survival of donor cardiomyocytes and a small improvement in cardiac function, although interspecies grafts like this are compromised by the large difference in normal heart rate between rat (450 beats/min) and human (70 beats/min).

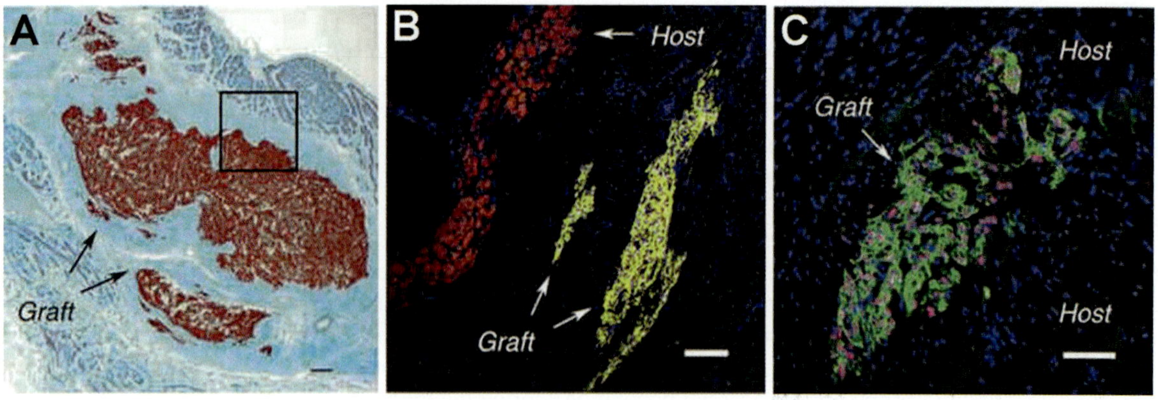

Fig. 13.4 Human ES cell-derived cardiomyocytes grafted to the infarcted heart of an imicronsunodeficient rat. (**a**) Graft visualized by imicronsunostaining for human β-myosin heavy chain (*red*). Scale bar 100 microns. (**b**) Donor and host cardiomyocytes visualized together: both are stained red with an antibody to sarcomeric myosin; the human fibers are also stained green for human β-myosin heavy chain, making them yellow. Scale bar 100 microns. (**c**) Visualization of nuclear human Nkx2.5 protein (*red*) in the graft cells (*green*). Scale bar 50 microns (Adapted from Laflamicronse et al.) [66]

Recently published studies show that cardiomyocytes can also be made from iPS cells. Similar protocols were employed as previously used for ES cells. Success was initially achieved with mouse iPS cells [67, 68], followed soon after by human iPS cells [69–71]. We can certainly expect more publications in the near future describing grafts of these cells to small and large animal models with studies of cell survival, cell differentiation, and host cardiac function. In addition, cardiomyocytes derived from iPS cells are likely to be important for physiological studies in vitro, especially studies of response to various drugs, and the effects of human genetic variation on these responses [69].

Clinical Applications

The work described above with ES and iPS cells is devoted to creating cardiac tissues with a possible future application in clinical transplantation. But technical and regulatory issues will delay any use of ES- or iPS-derived cells for some years to come. Meanwhile, a substantial industry using clinical stem cell therapy of the heart has already become established. These therapies mostly involve the use of autologous bone marrow cells. The original rationale was based on studies indicating that bone marrow grafts between animals could populate the heart muscle and other nonhematopoietic-derived structures of the hosts [72–74]. These studies have mostly proved irreproducible, and such positive results as could be reproduced are now ascribed to cell fusion [75]. So the original rationale for the clinical work has disappeared.

The clinical trials did produce abundant data indicating small but real, beneficial effects of autologous bone marrow grafts on cardiac performance [76–78]. Given the source of the cells, and the results from similar grafts in animal models, it is unlikely that any graft cells actually become cardiomyocytes, but it is quite possible that the grafts contain endothelial and smooth muscle progenitors. They may also release substances which have a beneficial effect on recovery from ischemic attack. The current consensus is that the modest beneficial effects arise from some combination of reduced inflammation, immune modulation, and improved angiogenesis.

There are various important ways that ES or iPS cells might add to what has so far been achieved in the clinical domain. First is the potential to create genuine cardiomyocytes which could replace those that have been lost. These might be delivered by cell injection into the damaged region of the heart wall, or by catheter via coronary vessels, or be introduced into patches of extracellular material and used to make physical grafts to replace areas of damaged tissue. The utility of such patch grafts has been demonstrated in animal experiments [79]. Very sophisticated patches may be made using a decellularization–recellularization procedure [80]:

1. It is now possible to remove all the cells from an animal heart – for example, that of a pig – and reintroduce human cells. These need not be cardiomyocytes. They could be smooth muscle and endothelial cells to line the blood vessels, which are still present and patent, or cardiac progenitor cells which have the potency to form all three major cell types and to undergo some self-organization on a suitable extracellular support. While it may be difficult to reconstruct a whole functioning heart by this method, it certainly has potential for producing "patches" with an appropriate structure and vascular supply.

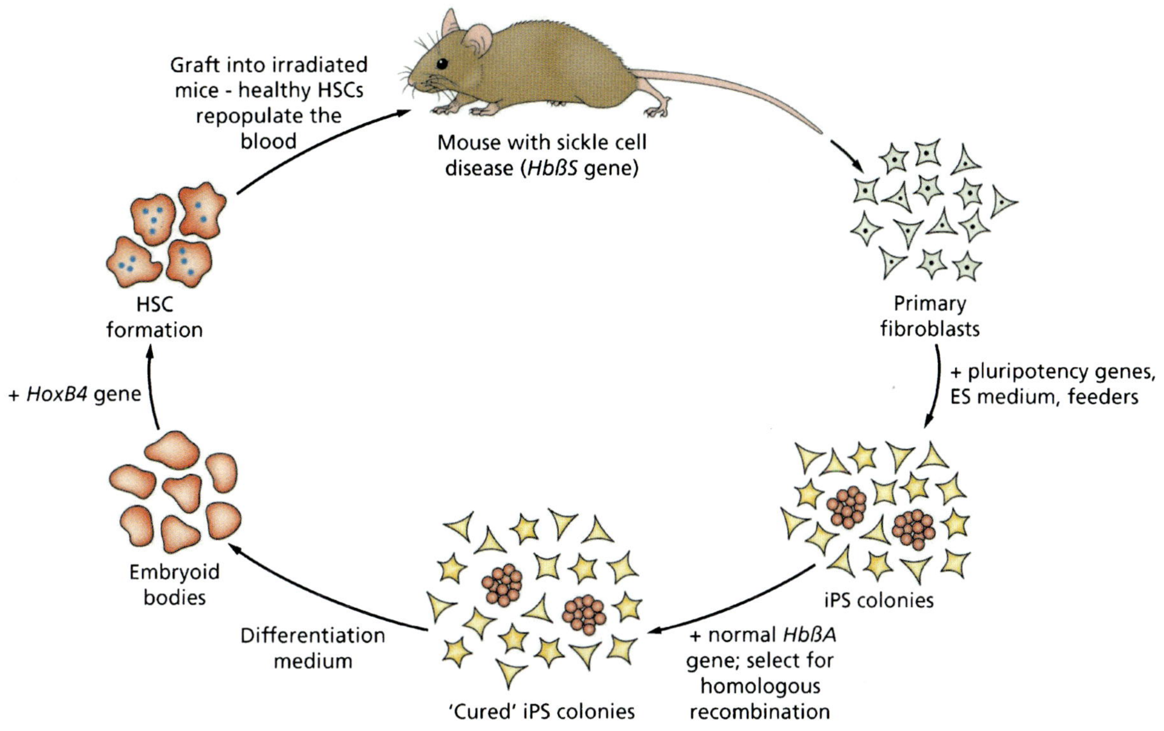

Fig. 13.5 Scenario from the laboratories of Jaenisch and Townes showing a cure of a mouse model of human sickle cell disease using a combination of gene therapy and cell therapy. The method is described in Hanna et al. [84]

2. Second, stem cell biology provides the potential for achieving immunological tolerance of grafted cardiac cell types. With iPS cells, it has been shown possible to create lines from individual patients. These will be a perfect genetic match for the patient, but unlike the autologous bone marrow grafts currently used, they can be differentiated to produce cardiac progenitor cells or the mature cardiac cell types. An alternative method of imparting tolerance to grafts does not require the preparation of patient-specific iPS lines. It involves creating hematopoietic stem cells (HSCs) from ES or iPS cells and making a graft of these to partially repopulate the immune system of the host. This procedure modifies the mechanisms of central and peripheral tolerance that inactivate reactive T cells, and enables a subsequent graft from the same donor to be tolerated [81, 82]. This means that the same cell line could be used first to make HSCs to induce tolerance, and then to make cardiac cells for a subsequent therapeutic graft.

   Which of the two potential strategies for achieving tolerance is ultimately used in clinical practice likely depends on economics as well as technical feasibility. Many consider that bespoke iPS cell production from individual patients will prove much too costly for widespread use, and that economics will force the alternative approach of a panel of standard cell lines that can provide a reasonable HLA match for the majority of individuals. Estimates of the necessary size of such a panel depend on how good a match is required [83]. A panel with at least hundreds of lines is likely, especially in the United States, with its genetically very diverse population.
3. A further dimension of the use of patient-specific iPS lines is the possibility for correcting genetic defects. Because the cells can be expanded without limit in culture, it is possible to introduce targeted genetic changes by homologous recombination [40]. In a remarkable tour de force early in the development of iPS technology, the labs of Townes and Jaenisch achieved a cure for a mouse model of sickle cell anemia, which serves as proof of principle experiment applicable to a wide range of genetic diseases [84] (Fig. 13.5). iPS cells were prepared from tail tip fibroblasts of mice homozygous for the *human beta-S* sickle cell hemoglobin allele. The genetic defect was repaired by introducing a good allele of *Hb beta* and selecting for cells with homologous gene replacement. These cells were then used to generate HSCs, in this case by introducing the *HoxB4* gene, which drives their formation [85]. Then the sickle cell mice were lethally irradiated to destroy their own HSCs and engrafted with the iPS-derived HSCs. The modified iPS cells were able to recolonize the bone marrow and reestablish a donor-derived hematopoietic system with a resulting cure of the sickle cell disease.

In reality, the technologies envisaged are too far off to make reliable estimates of feasibility or cost at the present time. It is true today that patient-specific cell culture is exceedingly expensive, but the history of all technology shows that once large companies compete to bring inventions to the mass market, they can achieve remarkable savings and produce complex and sophisticated products cheap enough for a broad base of consumers to buy and use.

References

1. Evans MJ, Kaufman MH. Establishment in culture of pluripotential cells from mouse embryos. Nature. 1981;292:154–6.
2. Martin GR. Isolation of a pluripotent cell-line from early mouse embryos cultured in medium conditioned by teratocarcinoma stem-cells. Proc Natl Acad Sci USA. 1981;78:7634–8.
3. Thomson JA, Itskovitz-Eldor J, Shapiro SS, et al. Embryonic stem cell lines derived from human blastocysts. Science. 1998;282:1145–7.
4. Nichols J, Silva J, Roode M, Smith A. Suppression of Erk signalling promotes ground state pluripotency in the mouse embryo. Development. 2009;136:3215–22.
5. Brons IGM, Smithers LE, Trotter MWB, et al. Derivation of pluripotent epiblast stem cells from mammalian embryos. Nature. 2007;448:191–5.
6. Tesar PJ, Chenoweth JG, Brook FA, et al. New cell lines from mouse epiblast share defining features with human embryonic stem cells. Nature. 2007;448:196–9.
7. Sato N, Sanjuan IM, Heke M, Uchida M, Naef F, Brivanlou AH. Molecular signature of human embryonic stem cells and its comparison with the mouse. Dev Biol. 2003;260:404–13.
8. Ying Q-L, Wray J, Nichols J, et al. The ground state of embryonic stem cell self-renewal. Nature. 2008;453:519–23.
9. Bradley A, Evans M, Kaufman MH, Robertson E. Formation of germ-line chimeras from embryo-derived teratocarcinoma cell-lines. Nature. 1984;309:255–6.
10. Müller U. Ten years of gene targeting: targeted mouse mutants from vector design to phenotype analysis. Mech Dev. 1999;82:3–21.
11. Daley GQ, Scadden DT. Prospects for stem cell-based therapy. Cell. 2008;132:544–8.
12. Martin GR, Wiley LM, Damjanov I. The development of cystic embryoid bodies in vitro from clonal teratocarcinoma stem cells. Dev Biol. 1977;61:230–44.
13. Beddington RS, Robertson EJ. An assessment of the developmental potential of embryonic stem cells in the midgestation mouse embryo. Development. 1989;105:733–7.
14. ten Berge D, Koole W, Fuerer C, Fish M, Eroglu E, Nusse R. Wnt signaling mediates self-organization and axis formation in embryoid bodies. Cell Stem Cell. 2008;3:508–18.
15. Bauwens CL, Peerani R, Niebruegge S, et al. Control of human embryonic stem cell colony and aggregate size heterogeneity influences differentiation trajectories. Stem Cells. 2008;26:2300–10.
16. Itskovitz-Eldor J, Schuldiner M, Karsenti D, et al. Differentiation of human embryonic stem cells into embryoid bodies comprising the three embryonic germ layers. Mol Med. 2000;6:88–95.
17. Damjanov I, Solter D. Experimental teratoma. Curr Top Pathol. 1974;59:69–130.
18. Silva J, Nichols J, Theunissen TW, et al. Nanog is the gateway to the pluripotent ground state. Cell. 2009;138:722–37.
19. Vallier L, Mendjan S, Brown S, et al. Activin/Nodal signalling maintains pluripotency by controlling Nanog expression. Development. 2009;136:1339–49.
20. Bernstein BE, Mikkelsen TS, Xie XH, et al. A bivalent chromatin structure marks key developmental genes in embryonic stem cells. Cell. 2006;125:315–26.
21. Takahashi K, Yamanaka S. Induction of pluripotent stem cells from mouse embryonic and adult fibroblast cultures by defined factors. Cell. 2006;126:663–76.
22. Lowry WE, Richter L, Yachechko R, et al. Generation of human induced pluripotent stem cells from dermal fibroblasts. Proc Natl Acad Sci. 2008;105:2883–8.
23. Park I-H, Zhao R, West JA, et al. Reprogramming of human somatic cells to pluripotency with defined factors. Nature. 2008;451:141–6.
24. Takahashi K, Tanabe K, Ohnuki M, et al. Induction of pluripotent stem cells from adult human fibroblasts by defined factors. Cell. 2007;131:861–72.
25. Yu JY, Vodyanik MA, Smuga-Otto K, et al. Induced pluripotent stem cell lines derived from human somatic cells. Science. 2007;318:1917–20.
26. Maherali N, Sridharan R, Xie W, et al. Directly reprogrammed fibroblasts show global epigenetic remodeling and widespread tissue contribution. Cell Stem Cell. 2007;1:55–70.
27. Okita K, Ichisaka T, Yamanaka S. Generation of germline-competent induced pluripotent stem cells. Nature. 2007;448:313–7.
28. Aoi T, Yae K, Nakagawa M, et al. Generation of pluripotent stem cells from adult mouse liver and stomach cells. Science. 2008;321:699–702.
29. Eminli S, Utikal J, Arnold K, Jaenisch R, Hochedlinger K. Reprogramming of neural progenitor cells into induced pluripotent stem cells in the absence of exogenous Sox2 expression. Stem Cells. 2008;26:2467–74.
30. Stadtfeld M, Brennand K, Hochedlinger K. Reprogramming of pancreatic beta cells into induced pluripotent stem cells. Curr Biol. 2008;18:890–4.
31. Nagy A, Gocza E, Diaz EM, et al. Embryonic stem cells alone are able to support fetal development in the mouse. Development. 1990;110:815–21.
32. Boland MJ, Hazen JL, Nazor KL, et al. Adult mice generated from induced pluripotent stem cells. Nature. 2009;461:91–4.
33. Zhao XY, Li W, Lv Z, et al. iPS cells produce viable mice through tetraploid complementation. Nature. 2009;461:86–90.
34. Hall VJ, Stojkovic P, Stojkovic M. Using therapeutic cloning to fight human disease: a conundrum or reality? Stem Cells. 2006;24:1628–37.
35. Byrne JA, Pedersen DA, Clepper LL, et al. Producing primate embryonic stem cells by somatic cell nuclear transfer. Nature. 2007;450:497–502.
36. Dimos JT, Rodolfa KT, Niakan KK, et al. Induced pluripotent stem cells generated from patients with ALS can be differentiated into motor neurons. Science. 2008;321:1218–21.
37. Ebert AD, Yu J, Rose FF, et al. Induced pluripotent stem cells from a spinal muscular atrophy patient. Nature. 2009;457:277–80.
38. Maehr R, Chen S, Snitow M, et al. Generation of pluripotent stem cells from patients with type 1 diabetes. Proc Natl Acad Sci. 2009;106:15768–73.
39. Park IH, Arora N, Huo H, et al. Disease-specific induced pluripotent stem cells. Cell. 2008;134:877–86.

40. Raya A, Rodriguez-Piza I, Guenechea G, et al. Disease-corrected haematopoietic progenitors from Fanconi anaemia induced pluripotent stem cells. Nature. 2009;460:53–9.
41. Soldner F, Hockemeyer D, Beard C, et al. Parkinson's disease patient-derived induced pluripotent stem cells free of viral reprogramming factors. Cell. 2009;136:964–77.
42. Yamanaka S. Elite and stochastic models for induced pluripotent stem cell generation. Nature. 2009;460:49–52.
43. Hanna J, Saha K, Pando B, et al. Direct cell reprogramming is a stochastic process amenable to acceleration. Nature. 2009;462:595–601.
44. Brambrink T, Foreman R, Welstead GG, et al. Sequential expression of pluripotency markers during direct reprogramming of mouse somatic cells. Cell Stem Cell. 2008;2:151–9.
45. Huangfu DW, Maehr R, Guo WJ, et al. Induction of pluripotent stem cells by defined factors is greatly improved by small-molecule compounds. Nature Biotechnol. 2008;26:795–7.
46. Kaji K, Norrby K, Paca A, Mileikovsky M, Mohseni P, Woltjen K. Virus-free induction of pluripotency and subsequent excision of reprogramming factors. Nature. 2009;458:771–5.
47. Woltjen K, Michael IP, Mohseni P, et al. piggyBac transposition reprograms fibroblasts to induced pluripotent stem cells. Nature. 2009;458:766–70.
48. Okita K, Nakagawa M, Hong HJ, Ichisaka T, Yamanaka S. Generation of mouse induced pluripotent stem cells without viral vectors. Science. 2008;322:949–53.
49. Stadtfeld M, Nagaya M, Utikal J, Weir G, Hochedlinger K. Induced pluripotent stem cells generated without viral integration. Science. 2008;322:945–9.
50. Kim D, Kim C-H, Moon J-I, et al. Generation of human induced pluripotent stem cells by direct delivery of reprogramming proteins. Cell Stem Cell. 2009;4:472–6.
51. Zhou H, Wu S, Joo JY, et al. Generation of induced pluripotent stem cells using recombinant proteins. Cell Stem Cell. 2009;4(5):381–4.
52. Fusaki N, Ban H, Nishiyama A, Saeki K, Hasegawa M. Efficient induction of transgene-free human pluripotent stem cells using a vector based on Sendai virus, an RNA virus that does not integrate into the host genome. Proc Jpn Acad Ser B. 2009;85:348–62.
53. Darabi R, Gehlbach K, Bachoo RM, et al. Functional skeletal muscle regeneration from differentiating embryonic stem cells. Nat Med. 2009;14:134–43.
54. Buckingham M, Meilhac S, Zaffran S. Building the mammalian heart from two sources of myocardial cells. Nat Rev Genet. 2005;6:826–37.
55. Garry DJ, Olson EN. A common progenitor at the heart of development. Cell. 2006;127:1101–4.
56. Harvey RP. Patterning the vertebrate heart. Nat Rev Genet. 2002;3:544–56.
57. Moretti A, Caron L, Nakano A, et al. Multipotent embryonic Isl1(+) progenitor cells lead to cardiac, smooth muscle, and endothelial cell diversification. Cell. 2006;127:1151–65.
58. Ferdous A, Caprioli A, Iacovino M, et al. Nkx2-5 transactivates the Ets-related protein 71 gene and specifies an endothelial/endocardial fate in the developing embryo. Proc Natl Acad Sci USA. 2009;106:814–9.
59. Nussbaum J, Minami E, Laflamme MA, et al. Transplantation of undifferentiated murine embryonic stem cells in the heart: teratoma formation and immune response. FASEB J. 2007;21:1345–57.
60. He JQ, Ma Y, Lee Y, Thomson JA, Kamp TJ. Human embryonic stem cells develop into multiple types of cardiac myocytes – action potential characterization. Circulation Res. 2003;93:32–9.
61. Kehat I, Kenyagin-Karsenti D, Snir M, et al. Human embryonic stem cells can differentiate into myocytes with structural and functional properties of cardiomyocytes. J Clin Invest. 2001;108:407–14.
62. Passier R, Oostwaard DWV, Snapper J, et al. Increased cardiomyocyte differentiation from human embryonic stem cells in serum-free cultures. Stem Cells. 2005;23:772–80.
63. Behfar A, Perez-Terzic C, Faustino RS, et al. Cardiopoietic programming of embryonic stem cells for tumor-free heart repair. J Exp Med. 2007;204:405–20.
64. Graichen R, Xu XQ, Braam SR, et al. Enhanced cardiomyogenesis of human embryonic stem cells by a small molecular inhibitor of p38 MAPK. Differentiation. 2008;76:357–70.
65. Huber I, Itzhaki I, Caspi O, et al. Identification and selection of cardiomyocytes during human embryonic stem cell differentiation. Faseb J. 2007;21:2551–63.
66. Laflamme MA, Chen KY, Naumova AV, et al. Cardiomyocytes derived from human embryonic stem cells in pro-survival factors enhance function of infarcted rat hearts. Nat Biotechnol. 2007;25:1015–24.
67. Mauritz C, Schwanke K, Reppel M, et al. Generation of functional murine cardiac myocytes from induced pluripotent stem cells. Circulation. 2008;118:507–17.
68. Narazaki G, Uosaki H, Teranishi M, et al. Directed and systematic differentiation of cardiovascular cells from mouse induced pluripotent stem cells. Circulation. 2008;118:498–506.
69. Tanaka T, Tohyama S, Murata M, et al. In vitro pharmacologic testing using human induced pluripotent stem cell-derived cardiomyocytes. Biochem Biophys Res Commun. 2009;385:497–502.
70. Zhang JH, Wilson GF, Soerens AG, et al. Functional cardiomyocytes derived from human induced pluripotent stem cells. Circ Res. 2009;104:E30–41.
71. Zwi L, Caspi O, Arbel G, et al. Cardiomyocyte differentiation of human induced pluripotent stem cells. Circulation. 2009;120:1513–23.
72. Bittner RE, Schofer C, Weipoltshammer K, et al. Recruitment of bone-marrow-derived cells by skeletal and cardiac muscle in adult dystrophic mdx mice. Anat Embryol (Berl). 1999;199:391–6.
73. Jackson KA, Majka SM, Wang HG, et al. Regeneration of ischemic cardiac muscle and vascular endothelium by adult stem cells. J Clin Invest. 2001;107:1395–402.
74. Orlic D, Kajstura J, Chimenti S, et al. Bone marrow cells regenerate infarcted myocardium. Nature. 2001;410:701–5.
75. Wagers AJ, Weissman IL. Plasticity of adult stem cells. Cell. 2004;116:639–48.
76. Passier R, van Laake LW, Mummery CL. Stem-cell-based therapy and lessons from the heart. Nature. 2008;453:322–9.
77. Rosenzweig A. Cardiac cell therapy – mixed results from mixed cells. New Engl J Med. 2006;355:1274–7.
78. Segers VFM, Lee RT. Stem-cell therapy for cardiac disease. Nature. 2008;451:937–42.

79. Zhang G, Wang XH, Wang ZL, Zhang JY, Suggs LA. PEGylated fibrin patch for mesenchymal stem cell delivery. Tissue Eng. 2006;12:9–19.
80. Ott HC, Matthiesen TS, Goh S-K, et al. Perfusion-decellularized matrix: using nature's platform to engineer a bioartificial heart. Nature Med. 2008;14:213–21.
81. Chidgey AP, Layton D, Trounson A, Boyd RL. Tolerance strategies for stem-cell-based therapies. Nature. 2008;453:330–7.
82. Kaufman DS, Thomson JA. Human ES cells – haematopoiesis and transplantation strategies. J Anat. 2002;200:243–8.
83. Taylor CJ, Bolton EM, Pocock S, Sharples LD, Pedersen RA, Bradley JA. Banking on human embryonic stem cells: estimating the number of donor cell lines needed for HLA matching. Lancet. 2005;366:2019–25.
84. Hanna J, Wernig M, Markoulaki S, et al. Treatment of sickle cell anemia mouse model with iPS cells generated from autologous skin. Science. 2007;318:1920–3.
85. Kyba M, Perlingeiro RCR, Daley GQ. HoxB4 confers definitive lymphoid-myeloid engraftment potential on embryonic stem cell and yolk sac hematopoietic progenitors. Cell. 2002;109:29–37.
86. Slack JMW. Essential developmental biology. Oxford: Blackwell Science; 2005. p. 125.

Chapter 14
Regulation of Vasculogenesis and Angiogenesis

Rita C.R. Perlingeiro

Vascular Cell Development and Differentiation

Vasculogenesis vs. Angiogenesis

The earliest functional organ to form during development in the vertebrate embryo is the complex branched network of endothelial cells. This network is crucial for transporting oxygen and nutrients to the developing embryo as well as removing waste products from the tissues. The first blood vessels of the mouse embryo, presumptive blood islands, arise in the extraembryonic yolk sac from the in situ differentiation of mesodermal precursors at approximately embryonic day (E) 7.0–E7.5. Between E8.0 and E9.0, endothelial progenitors or angioblasts, the cells comprising the outer layer of the blood island, differentiate into endothelial cells, while the inner cells differentiate into blood progenitors, in particular, primitive erythroblasts [1].

Endothelial cells then assemble into cord-like vascular structures, with further formation of vascular lumens and organized vascular networks. This process is known as vasculogenesis [2–4]. Slightly later in embryogenesis, angioblasts arise in the proximal lateral mesoderm and migrate to arrange themselves symmetrically at the lateral sides of the embryo. This arrangement establishes the two preendocardial tubes, which then fuse to form the primordial heart [5].

Angiogenesis represents a distinct process that contributes to the vasculature. It involves the proliferation and migration of endothelial cells present in the primary vascular structures, which leads to sprouting and remodeling of the initially homogenous capillary network to form small and large vessels, such as the intersomitic arteries [6] and the organs' vessels. While vasculogenesis occurs primarily during early embryogenesis, angiogenesis is required for the normal growth of both embryonic and postnatal tissues and is also associated with pathological conditions, including tumor growth and wound healing [7–9].

Sites of Vasculogenesis and Origin of Endothelial Cells

Yolk Sac

In the early yolk sac, vasculogenesis begins with the formation of blood islands, which after extensive growth and fusion give rise to the capillary network structure. After the onset of blood circulation, this network differentiates into an arteriovenous vascular system [4]. Angioblasts or endothelial progenitor cells (EPCs) are located at the periphery, while the hematopoietic progenitor cells are located in the center of the blood islands (Fig. 14.1).

The close spatial association between primitive hematopoietic progenitors and angioblasts prompted anatomists, more than a century ago, to hypothesize that these progenitor cells may derive from a common precursor, the so-called heman-

R.C.R. Perlingeiro, PhD, MSc, BSc (✉)
Lillehei Heart Institute, Department of Medicine, University of Minnesota, Minneapolis, MN, USA
e-mail: perli032@umn.edu

Z. Vlodaver et al. (eds.), *Coronary Heart Disease: Clinical, Pathological, Imaging, and Molecular Profiles*,
DOI 10.1007/978-1-4614-1475-9_14, © Springer Science+Business Media, LLC 2012

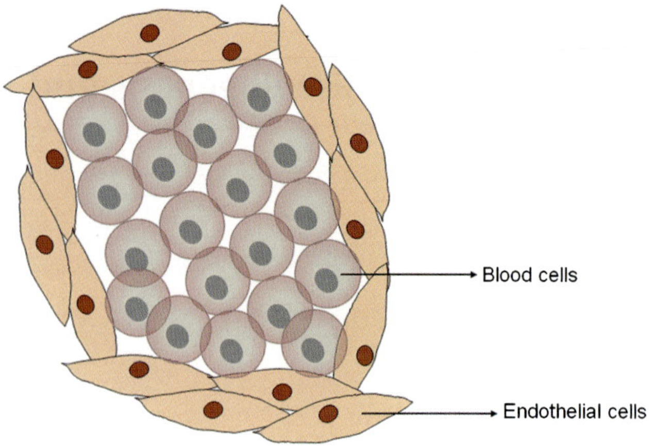

Fig. 14.1 Schematic representation of a blood island

gioblast [10–13]. In addition to their proximity, these two lineages share common expression of crucial regulatory genes and antigenic determinants such as SCL [14], Flk-1 [15–17], endoglin [18], PECAM [19], and CD34 [20].

A cell with properties of the hemangioblast has been identified during in vitro differentiation of embryonic stem (ES) cells into embryoid bodies (EBs) [21] and more recently in the primitive streak of the mouse embryo [22]. These authors have shown that hemangioblast formation within the mouse embryo is restricted to a narrow developmental window (approximately 12–18 h of mouse gestation) – initiated at the midstreak stage, peaking at the late streak/early neural plate and neural plate stages, and severely declining at the head-fold stage. The average number of hemangioblasts detected per embryo varied between 1 and 5.

These results indicate that bipotent progenitors exist in low frequency during embryogenesis, and that the initial stages of hematopoietic and endothelial commitment occur before, and not during, blood island development in the yolk sac, as previously thought [23–27]. This supports the hypothesis that differentiated hemangioblasts, restricted hematopoietic, and vascular progenitor cells migrate from the primitive streak to the yolk sac, where these lineages become morphologically identifiable. Furthermore, clonal analysis experiments of early yolk sac reveal that blood islands have a polyclonal origin, deriving from multiple progenitors [28]. Therefore, it is likely that only a small population of hemangioblasts gives rise to the blood and endothelial lineages of the blood island, and that individual blood islands do not arise from individual hemangioblasts.

It is important to note that in addition to the blood islands, the yolk sac also contains vascular plexuses, located adjacent to the chorion (VPC) and the embryo (VPE), which are formed independently of hematopoietic cells [29]. These distinct types of vasculature, associated or not with the hematopoietic system, may be the result of distinct mesoderm origins. It has been suggested that splanchnopleural mesoderm gives rise to vasculature associated with hematopoiesis, while paraxial mesoderm generates vessels independent of the hematopoietic system [30, 31].

Embryo Proper

The first intraembryonic endothelial structures observed during development are the endocardium and great vessels [23], which are formed in the absence of hematopoiesis, suggesting that they arise solely from angioblasts [31]. Angioblasts that migrate from presomitic cranial mesoderm give rise to a vascular plexus next to the developing myocardium which, following remodeling, forms the endocardial tube.

In parallel to heart development, vasculogenesis is also initiated within the aortic primordia, with the formation of the cardinal veins and dorsal aorta. After bidirectional remodeling, these vessels generate the bilateral embryonic aorta. Throughout development, the region in which this occurs is called the para-aortic splanchnopleural (PAS) and later, the aorta-gonad-mesonephros (AGM) region.

As the heart enlarges, passive diffusion of nutrients and waste becomes limiting, and a coronary vasculature is formed to supply the metabolically active heart tissue. At this point, proepicardium, consisting of angioblasts and smooth muscle cell progenitors, interacts with the developing heart tube and quickly spreads over the entire heart. Following epithelial-to-mesenchymal transformation, these cells invade the underlying mesoderm, giving rise to the capillaries, veins, and arteries of the coronary vasculature [32].

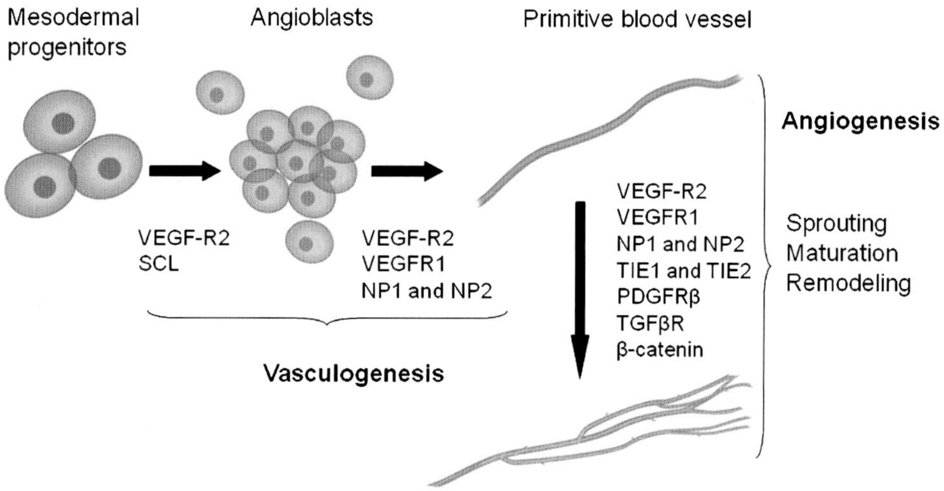

Fig. 14.2 Schematic representation of the molecular mechanisms controlling vasculogenesis and angiogenesis

Molecular Regulation of Vasculogenesis and Angiogenesis

Tremendous knowledge has been gained since the 1990s about the molecular mechanisms that control vasculogenesis and angiogenesis. Figure 14.2 summarizes some of the major signaling pathways involved in these processes. Some pathways are specific to the endothelial lineage, while others have a broader effect on several cell types, including the endothelial lineage.

Vasculogenesis and Its Induction

The initial signals leading to specification of the endothelial lineage in the mammalian embryo primarily include members of the fibroblast growth factor (FGF) [33] and bone morphogenetic protein (BMP) [34] growth factor families. Indian hedgehog signaling from primitive endoderm has also been indicated to play a role in the activation of early vasculogenesis [35].

Regardless of the upstream signals, vascular endothelial growth factor (VEGF) is one of the key cytokines involved in the process of vasculogenesis and angiogenesis. Accordingly, mice lacking the VEGF gene die early in development due to several defects in vasculogenesis [36, 37].

VEGF signals through two tyrosine kinase receptors – Flk-1 and Flt-1 (VEGFR2 and VEGFR1, respectively) – which play a role in vasculogenesis, as embryos deficient in these receptors show impaired vessel formation [16, 38]. Lack of Flk-1 leads to inappropriate endothelial cell differentiation; absence of Flt-1 results in thin-walled vessels of larger-than-normal diameter [16, 38]. This signaling pathway is also critical for angiogenesis, given that VEGF stimulates the migration, proliferation, and tube formation of endothelial cells. High affinity binding of VEGF to the semaphorin receptor neuropilin-1 (NP1) reportedly augments VEGF binding to Flk-1 [39, 40]. Both of the neuropilin coreceptors, NP1 and NP2, are required for proper yolk sac vasculogenesis and embryonic angiogenesis [40].

The bHLH transcription factor SCL, originally thought to be required solely for embryonic hematopoiesis [41–43], is also critical for vasculogenesis and proper vascular remodeling [44, 45].

Angiogenesis

Another family of endothelial-specific tyrosine kinase receptors includes TIE1 and TIE2 (also called Tek). The TIE2 knockout mutation is embryonic lethal. Mice die around E9.5 and E10.5, while mice lacking TIE1 survive a little longer, dying between E13.5 and "birth (need to define "birth, as with "E?") [46–48]. Although both receptors are expressed early during development, they are not required for proper vasculogenesis.

Distinct from Flk-1 and Flt-1 [16, 38], the absence of TIE1/TIE2 leads exclusively to later defects in angiogenic processes, including vascular remodeling and vascular integrity [46–48]. Angiopoietin-1 (ANG1) was the first ligand to be identified for the TIE2 receptor [49] and, as expected, plays a critical role in angiogenesis. ANG1-null embryos display clear defects in endocardial and myocardial development as well as defects in vascular branching and remodeling. This leads to a less complex vascular network in these mice, which usually die by E12.5 [49]. Angiopoietin-2 (ANG2) has been identified as a natural antagonist for the TIE2 receptor, and its absence also leads to impaired angiogenesis [50].

EphrinB2 and its cognate receptor EphB4 are expressed during early vasculogenesis, specifically in developing arterial and venous endothelial cells, respectively [51]. Gene disruption of ephrinB2 [51] or EphB4 [52] results in defective vascular remodeling of the yolk sac and embryo proper, with knockout mice dying by E10.5. Studies indicate that the Notch signaling pathway may act upstream to the ephrin signaling and thus play a critical role in establishing artery vs. vein fate [53].

Platelet-derived growth factor (PDGF) BB and its receptor PDGFRβ [54], as well as signals from the transforming growth factor-β (TGFβ) pathway [55–57], are involved in vessel maturation, which is dependent on the proliferation and migration of vascular smooth muscle cells and pericytes.

β-catenin, which mediates canonical Wnt signals, is important for appropriate vascular patterning and for maintaining vessel integrity. Mice deficient in β-catenin show defective vascular patterning and enhanced vascular fragility, which are restricted to specific areas, including the head's vascular network, large vitelline and umbilical vessels, and the placenta [58].

Sources of Vascular Cells in the Adult

Circulating Endothelial Progenitors

Although reports pointing to the presence of endothelial cells and their progenitors in the blood date from the 1930s [59, 60], it was only in 1997 that this area of research really bloomed with the identification of circulating EPCs in adult human peripheral blood. This seminal study [61] prompted the hypothesis that vasculogenesis and angiogenesis may occur simultaneously in adulthood. It is currently accepted that EPCs reside in adult bone marrow (BM) and are mobilized into peripheral circulation in response to tissue ischemia or cytokine treatment [62, 63].

Transplantation of either culture-expanded EPCs or freshly isolated cells from adult hematopoietic sources (bone marrow, peripheral blood, and umbilical cord blood) results in enhanced blood flow [64, 65] and improved function of ischemic tissues [61, 66–71]. However, engraftment levels vary significantly among these studies. This variability is probably due to the heterogeneity of vascular precursor populations identified in hematopoietic tissues.

To date, a number of cell types obtained using different strategies have been referred to as EPCs, including differentiated endothelial cells [72–74] with more limited proliferation ability and cells associated with the myelomonocytic lineage [74–77]. EPCs were first isolated from peripheral blood on the basis of their expression of VEGFR2 (KDR) or CD34 antigen [61]. The latter has been used by the majority of investigators as a marker for isolating EPCs [64, 68, 70, 78]. Although it is clear that CD34 purification enriches for EPCs, CD34 by itself is not a particularly good marker since it is also expressed in HSCs [79], multiple hematopoietic progenitor cells [80], and mature circulating endothelial cells (ECs) derived from the vessel wall endothelium [81]. This led investigators to raise the possibility that EPCs could be merely differentiated ECs, which also possess some proliferative potential [82].

An elegant study [83] has addressed this issue by analyzing blood samples from BM transplant patients who received gender-mismatched stem cells. These investigators found a significant, proliferative difference between vessel wall and BM-derived endothelial cells. It was shown that in vitro–derived endothelial cells from early phases (9 days in culture) undergo only sixfold expansion and are derived predominantly from the recipient vessel wall, whereas endothelial cells derived from late-outgrowth cells (27 days in culture) undergo 98-fold expansion and mostly originate from transplanted donor BM cells. This corroborates the premise of circulating angioblasts. In any case, CD34 does not distinguish these precursors from hematopoietic or mature ECs. The same applies for KDR (VEGFR2), the receptor for VEGF, which is also present in mature circulating endothelial cells [84].

The hematopoietic stem cell marker CD133 [85] has been suggested as a useful antigen to provide better enrichment for endothelial progenitors since it is expressed in EPCs but downregulated in mature endothelial cells [86]. Consistently, a number of studies support the premise that the $CD133^{+}$ cell fraction is enriched for EPCs and provide evidence for superior perfusion following their transplantation in animal models of ischemia [87–91]. However, given that CD133 is also present in early hematopoietic progenitors [85], phenotypic distinction between hematopoietic and endothelial progenitors has been challenging. To date, it remains controversial whether the source of EPCs in hematopoietic tissues resides within the hematopoietic hierarchy or whether it represents an independent identity.

Recent studies comparing different culture methods suggest that true endothelial progenitors emerge from adherent mononuclear cell cultures after 1–3 weeks [92–94]. These endothelial progenitors, also referred to as endothelial colony-forming cells (ECFCs), differ from other cell types identified as such [73, 74, 76, 77] in their proliferative capacity as well as the kinetics of their colony formation. Conflicting with the reports on $CD133^{+}$ cells described above, some investigators claim that these endothelial outgrowth cells are not derived from $CD133^{+}$ cells or $CD45^{+}$ hematopoietic precursors, but originate independently from the hematopoietic lineage [94–96]. However, the in vivo vascularization potential of these ECFCs has yet to be determined in animal models of ischemia.

Mouse-to-mouse transplantation experiments involving the analyses of mice that had been subjected to unilateral femoral artery occlusion following the engraftment of BM cells isolated from transgenic mice expressing enhanced green fluorescent protein (GFP) revealed that donor GFP^+ cells fail to incorporate into the adult growing vasculature, but were detectable around growing collateral arteries [97]. A similar outcome was obtained following the transplantation of hematopoietic stem cells isolated from GFP transgenic mice directly into the ischemic myocardium of wild-type mice [98]. Although hematopoietic stem cells maintained their hematopoietic cell fate in vivo, stem cell transplantation provided long-term benefit to a certain extent, as evidenced by less severe ventricular dilation and heart dysfunction following infarction [98].

Thus, the mechanism behind these therapeutic effects might be associated with the secretion of growth factors by transplanted cells, which in turn stimulate endogenous angiogenesis [97]. This hypothesis is corroborated by recent studies involving the transplantation of human $CD133^+$ cells [99, 100] or EPCs [101, 102]. The studies indicate that although donor cells tend to disappear of engrafted areas shortly after transplantation [101], these cell types secrete angiogenic factors, including VEGF-A, ANG1, fibroblast growth factor-2 (FGF-2), placenta growth factor (PIGF), hepatocyte growth factor (HGF), and insulin-like growth factor-1 (IGF-1), among others [97, 101].

Bone Marrow and Adipose Stromal Cells

In addition to hematopoietic cells, BM also contains a stromal cell population, known as mesenchymal stem cells or marrow stromal cells (MSCs), that is endowed with the ability to self-renew and differentiate into multiple mesenchymal lineages, including bone, fat, cartilage, and connective tissue [103–106]. Some recent studies have suggested that these cells are also endowed with endothelial potential [107, 108]. Similar endothelial potential has been attributed to the stromal vascular fraction (SVF) within the adipose tissue [109–111].

The SVF is well known as a heterogeneous cell population containing preadipocytes and mature microvascular endothelial cells [112, 113]. Studies by Zuk et al. provide evidence for the presence of a multipotent progenitor able to differentiate into bone, cartilage, and muscle [114]. In this context, another study suggested that adipocytes and endothelial cells may share a common progenitor, and accordingly, cells within the SVF were capable of differentiating into endothelial cells in vitro as well as participating in the process of neovascularization upon injection into ischemic tissues [110].

Since none of these experiments were performed at the clonal level, to date, there is no definitive proof for the existence of an early progenitor in the BM or adipose stroma that is able to differentiate toward the endothelial lineage. Yet there is increasing evidence for a positive effect on perfusion and vascularization following the transplantation of BM or adipose stromal cells in several models of ischemia. This has been attributed to the secretion of angiogenic factors by these cells [111, 115–118].

Angiogenesis/Vasculogenesis and Ischemic Tissue Repair

Several of the studies using animal models of ischemia involved the transplantation of ex vivo expanded EPCs [70, 119, 120]. However, based on data from human EPC transplantation into nude mice, in order to obtain satisfactory reperfusion of the hind limb, $0.5–2 \times 10^4$ EPCs/g of body weight were required. Therefore, about 12 L of human blood would be needed to collect an equivalent dose of EPCs for a human patient [121]. This amount is not viable and suggests that expanded EPCs are not an ideal therapeutic cell population.

Although the identity of EPCs needs additional clarification, the evidence for bone marrow as a reservoir of EPCs prompted several groups of researchers to test the therapeutic effect of autologous cells of medullary origin in human ischemic disease [122–130]. As summarized in Table 14.1, these clinical trials were quite heterogeneous regarding protocol, including distinct sample size, duration of follow-up analyses, cell population and cell number transplanted, and timing of transplantation. Therefore, the extreme difficulty in reconciling diverse outcomes is not surprising. Preliminary data from these early clinical trials suggest that mononuclear cells injected locally in patients with lower limb or cardiac ischemia contribute to the regeneration of vasculature. A recent, systematic meta-analysis of 18 clinical trials including a total of 999 patients suggested that bone marrow cell transplantation is safe. Although, overall, the improvements in terms of physiologic and anatomic parameters are modest in patients with both acute myocardial infarction and chronic ischemic heart disease, they are superior to conventional therapy [131]. Thus, these findings provide scientific rationale for the elaboration of larger randomized clinical trials to assess the long-term therapeutic effects of bone marrow cell transplantation.

Table 14.1 Compilation of recent clinical trial studies

Donor cell population	Number of transplanted cells (×10^6)	Route of injection	Clinical condition	Sample size	Average follow-up duration (months)	Timing from episode (days)	References
BM MNCs	205±110	IC	ICM	28	3	2,470±2,196	[133]
BM MNCs	40	IC	AMI	20	6	1	[134]
BM MNCs	60.25±31	IM	ICM	20	4	217±162	[125]
BM MNCs	172±72	IC	AMI	67	4	1–2	[135]
BM CD133$^+$ cells	12.6±2.2	IC	AMI	35	4	11.6±1.4	[122]
BM MSCs	48,000–60,000	IC	AMI	69	6	18.4±0.5	[123]
PB EPCs	69±14	IC	ICM	26	3	225±87	[124]
PB EPCs	22±11	IC	ICM	24	3	2,348±2,318	[133]
BM MNCs	25.5±6.3	IM	ICM	20	12	NR	[136]
BM MSCs and PB EPCs	2–4	IC	AMI/ICM	22	4	224±470	[137]
BM MNCs	236±174	IC	AMI	204	4	4.3±1.3	[138]
BM MNCs	28±22	IC	AMI	20	3	8±2	[128]
BM MNCs	87±47.7	IC	AMI	100	6	6±1.3	[139]
PB EPCs	72.5±73.3	IC	AMI	70	6	7±5	[140]
BM MNCs	2,460±940	IC	AMI	60	18	4.8±1.3	[141]

Since most of the therapeutic effects associated with stem cell transplantation rely on the secretion of angiogenic factors by engrafted cells, one promising future approach is delivering stem cells genetically engineered to produce angiogenic factors. This approach should provide better enhancement in angiogenesis [132].

References

1. Haar JL, Ackerman GA. A phase and electron microscopic study of vasculogenesis and erythropoiesis in the yolk sac of the mouse. Anat Rec. 1971;170:199–223.
2. Risau W. Embryonic angiogenesis factors. Pharmacol Ther. 1991;51(3):371–6.
3. Risau W. Differentiation of endothelium. FASEB J. 1995;J9:926–33.
4. Risau W, Flamme I. Vasculogenesis. Annu Rev Cell Dev Biol. 1995;11:73–91.
5. Coffin JD, Poole TJ. Endothelial cell origin and migration in embryonic heart and cranial vessel development. Anat Rec. 1991;231:383–95.
6. Coffin JD, Poole TJ. Embryonic vascular development: immunohistochemical identification of the origin and subsequent morphogenesis of the major vessel primordia in quail embryos. Development. 1988;102:735–48.
7. Ferrara N. Leukocyte adhesion. Missing link in angiogenesis. Nature. 1995;376:517–9.
8. Folkman J, Shing Y. Angiogenesis. J Biol Chem. 1992;267:10931–4.
9. Hanahan D, Folkman J. Patterns and emerging mechanisms of the angiogenic switch during tumorigenesis. Cell. 1996;86:353–64.
10. His W. Untersuchungen über die erste Anlage des Wirberthierleibes. Die erste Entwickelung des Hühnchens im Ei. Leipzig: FCW Vogel; 1868.
11. His W. Lecithoblast und Angioblast der Wirbelthiere. Abhandl KS Ges Wiss Math Phys. 1900;22:171–328.
12. Murray PDF. The development "in vitro" of blood of the early chick embryo. Proc Roy Soc London B. 1932;111(773):497–521.
13. Sabin FR. Studies on the origin of blood vessels and of red blood corpuscles as seen in the living blastoderm of chicks during the second day of incubation. Contr Embryol. 1920;9:213–62.
14. Kallianpur AR, Jordan JE, Brandt SJ. The SCL/TAL-1 gene is expressed in progenitors of both the hematopoietic and vascular systems during embryogenesis. Blood. 1994;83:1200–8.
15. Kabrun N, Buhring HJ, Choi K, Ullrich A, Risau W, Keller G. Flk-1 expression defines a population of early embryonic hematopoietic precursors. Development. 1997;124:2039–48.
16. Shalaby F, Rossant J, Yamaguchi TP, et al. Failure of blood-island formation and vasculogenesis in Flk-1 deficient mice. Nature. 1995;376:62–6.
17. Yamaguchi TP, Dumont DJ, Conlon RA, Breitman ML, Rossant J. flk-1, an flt-related receptor tyrosine kinase is an early marker for endothelial cell precursors. Development. 1993;118:489–98.
18. Perlingeiro RC. Endoglin is required for hemangioblast and early hematopoietic development. Development. 2007;134:3041–8.
19. Watt SM, Gschmeissner SE, Bates PA. PECAM-1: its expression and function as a cell adhesion molecule on hemopoietic and endothelial cells. Leuk Lymphoma. 1995;17:229–44.
20. Young PE, Baumhueter S, Lasky LA. The sialomucin CD34 is expressed on hematopoietic cells and blood vessels during murine development. Blood. 1995;85:96–105.
21. Kennedy M, Firpo M, Choi K, et al. A common precursor for primitive erythropoiesis and definitive haematopoiesis. Nature. 1997;386:488–93.
22. Huber TL, Kouskoff V, Fehling HJ, Palis J, Keller G. Haemangioblast commitment is initiated in the primitive streak of the mouse embryo. Nature. 2004;432:625–30.

23. Drake CJ, Fleming PA. Vasculogenesis in the day 6.5 to 9.5 mouse embryo. Blood. 2000;95:1671–9.
24. Moore MA, Owen JJ. Chromosome marker studies in the irradiated chick embryo. Nature. 1967;215:1081–2.
25. Moore MAS, Metcalf D. Ontogeny of the haematopoietic system: yolk sac origin of in vivo and in vitro colony forming cells in the developing mouse embryo. Br J Haematol. 1970;18:279–96.
26. Moore MAS, Owen JJT. Stem-cell migration in developing myeloid and lymphoid systems. Lancet. 1967;II:658–9.
27. Wong PM, Chung SW, Chui DH, Eaves CJ. Properties of the earliest clonogenic hemopoietic precursors to appear in the developing murine yolk sac. Proc Natl Acad Sci USA. 1986;83:3851–4.
28. Ueno H, Weissman IL. Clonal analysis of mouse development reveals a polyclonal origin for yolk sac blood islands. Dev Cell. 2006; 11:519–33.
29. Ema M, Rossant J. Cell fate decisions in early blood vessel formation. Trends Cardiovasc Med. 2003;13:254–9.
30. Hatzopoulos AK, Folkman J, Vasile E, Eiselen GK, Rosenberg RD. Isolation and characterization of endothelial progenitor cells from mouse embryos. Development. 1998;125:1457–68.
31. Pardanaud L, Luton D, Prigent M, Bourcheix LM, Catala M, Dieterlen-Lievre F. Two distinct endothelial lineages in ontogeny, one of them related to hemopoiesis. Development. 1996;122:1363–71.
32. Pérez-Pomares JM, Carmona R, González-Iriarte M, Atencia G, Wessels A, Muñoz-Chápuli R. Origin of coronary endothelial cells from epicardial mesothelium in avian embryos. Int J Dev Biol. 2002;46:1005–13.
33. Cox CM, Poole TJ. Angioblast differentiation is influenced by the local environment: FGF-2 induces angioblasts and patterns vessel formation in the quail embryo. Dev Dyn. 2000;218:371–82.
34. Winnier G, Blessing M, Labosky PA, Hogan BL. Bone morphogenetic protein-4 is required for mesoderm formation and patterning in the mouse. Genes Dev. 1995;9:2105–16.
35. Dyer MA, Farrington SM, Mohn D, Munday JR, Baron MH. Indian hedgehog activates hematopoiesis and vasculogenesis and can respecify prospective neuroectodermal cell fate in the mouse embryo. Development. 2001;128:1717–30.
36. Carmeliet P, Ferreira V, Breier G, et al. Abnormal blood vessel development and lethality in embryos lacking a single VEGF allele. Nature. 1996;380:435–9.
37. Ferrara N, Carver-Moore K, Chen H, et al. Heterozygous embryonic lethality induced by targeted inactivation of the VEGF gene. Nature. 1996;380:439–42.
38. Fong GH, Rossant J, Gertsenstein M, Breitman ML. Role of the Flt-1 receptor tyrosine kinase in regulating the assembly of vascular endothelium. Nature. 1995;376:66–70.
39. He Z, Tessier-Lavigne M. Neuropilin is a receptor for the axonal chemorepellent Semaphorin III. Cell. 1997;90:739–51.
40. Takashima S, Kitakaze M, Asakura M, et al. Targeting of both mouse neuropilin-1 and neuropilin-2 genes severely impairs developmental yolk sac and embryonic angiogenesis. Proc Natl Acad Sci USA. 2002;99:3657–62.
41. Porcher C, Swat W, Rockwell K, Fujiwara Y, Alt FW, Orkin SH. The T cell leukemia oncoprotein SCL/tal-1 is essential for development of all hematopoietic lineages. Cell. 1996;86:47–57.
42. Robb L, Elwood NJ, Elefanty AG, et al. The scl gene product is required for the generation of all hematopoietic lineages in the adult mouse. EMBO J. 1996;15:4123–9.
43. Shivdasani RA, Mayer EL, Orkin SH. Absence of blood formation in mice lacking the T-cell leukaemia oncoprotein tal-1/SCL. Nature. 1995;373:432–4.
44. Elefanty AG, Begley CG, Hartley L, Papaevangeliou B, Robb L. SCL expression in the mouse embryo detected with a targeted lacZ reporter gene demonstrates its localization to hematopoietic, vascular, and neural tissues. Blood. 1999;94:3754–63.
45. Visvader JE, Fujiwara Y, Orkin SH. Unsuspected role for the T-cell leukemia protein SCL/tal-1 in vascular development. Genes Dev. 1998;12:473–9.
46. Dumont DJ, Gradwohl G, Fong GH, et al. Dominant-negative and targeted null mutations in the endothelial receptor tyrosine kinase, tek, reveal a critical role in vasculogenesis of the embryo. Genes Dev. 1994;8:1897–909.
47. Puri MC, Rossant J, Alitalo K, Bernstein A, Partanen J. The receptor tyrosine kinase TIE is required for integrity and survival of vascular endothelial cells. EMBO J. 1995;14:5884–91.
48. Sato TN, Tozawa Y, Deutsch U, et al. Distinct roles of the receptor tyrosine kinases Tie-1 and Tie-2 in blood vessel formation. Nature. 1995;376:70–4.
49. Suri C, Jones PF, Patan S, et al. Requisite role of angiopoietin-1, a ligand for the TIE2 receptor, during embryonic angiogenesis. Cell. 1996; 87:1171–80.
50. Maisonpierre PC, Suri C, Jones PF, et al. Angiopoietin-2, a natural antagonist for Tie2 that disrupts in vivo angiogenesis. Science. 1997;277: 55–60.
51. Wang HU, Chen ZF, Anderson DJ. Molecular distinction and angiogenic interaction between embryonic arteries and veins revealed by ephrin-B2 and its receptor Eph-B4. Cell. 1998;93:741–53.
52. Gerety SS, Wang HU, Chen ZF, Anderson DJ. Symmetrical mutant phenotypes of the receptor EphB4 and its specific transmembrane ligand ephrin-B2 in cardiovascular development. Mol Cell. 1999;4:403–14.
53. Artavanis-Tsakonas S, Rand MD, Lake RJ. Notch signaling: cell fate control and signal integration in development. Science. 1999;284:770–6.
54. Hellström M, Kalén M, Lindahl P, Abramsson A, Betsholtz C. Role of PDGF-B and PDGFR-beta in recruitment of vascular smooth muscle cells and pericytes during embryonic blood vessel formation in the mouse. Development. 1999;126:3047–55.
55. Hirschi KK, Rohovsky SA, D'Amore PA. PDGF, TGF-beta, and heterotypic cell-cell interactions mediate endothelial cell-induced recruitment of 10T1/2 cells and their differentiation to a smooth muscle fate. J Cell Biol. 1998;141:805–14.
56. Li DY, Sorensen LK, Brooke BS, et al. Defective angiogenesis in mice lacking endoglin. Science. 1999;284:1534–7.
57. Yang X, Castilla LH, Xu X, et al. Angiogenesis defects and mesenchymal apoptosis in mice lacking SMAD5. Development. 1999;126: 1571–80.
58. Cattelino A, Liebner S, Gallini R, et al. The conditional inactivation of the beta-catenin gene in endothelial cells causes a defective vascular pattern and increased vascular fragility. J Cell Biol. 2003;162:1111–22.
59. Parker RC. The development of organized vessels in cultures of blood cells. Science. 1933;77:544–6.

60. White JF, Parshley MS. Growth in vitro of blood vessels from bone marrow of adult chickens. Am J Anat. 1950;89:321–45.
61. Asahara T, Murohara T, Sullivan A, et al. Isolation of putative progenitor endothelial cells for angiogenesis. Science. 1997;275:964–7.
62. Asahara T, Masuda H, Takahashi T, et al. Bone marrow origin of endothelial progenitor cells responsible for postnatal vasculogenesis in physiological and pathological neovascularization. Circ Res. 1999;85:221–8.
63. Takahashi T, Kalka C, Masuda H, et al. Ischemia- and cytokine-induced mobilization of bone marrow-derived endothelial progenitor cells for revascularization. Nat Med. 1999;5:434–8.
64. Schatteman GC, Hanlon HD, Jiao C, Dodds SG, Christy BA. Blood-derived angioblasts accelerate blood-flow restoration in diabetic mice. J Clin Invest. 2000;106:571–8.
65. Shintani S, Murohara T, Ikeda H, et al. Augmentation of postnatal neovascularization with autologous bone marrow transplantation. Circulation. 2001;103:897–903.
66. Crosby JR, Kaminski WE, Schatteman G, et al. Endothelial cells of hematopoietic origin make a significant contribution to adult blood vessel formation. Circ Res. 2000;87:728–30.
67. Jackson KA, Majka SM, Wang H, et al. Regeneration of ischemic cardiac muscle and vascular endothelium by adult stem cells. J Clin Invest. 2001;107:1395–402.
68. Kocher AA, Schuster MD, Szabolcs MJ, et al. Neovascularization of ischemic myocardium by human bone-marrow-derived angioblasts prevents cardiomyocyte apoptosis, reduces remodeling and improves cardiac function. Nat Med. 2001;7:430–6.
69. Murayama T, Tepper OM, Silver M, et al. Determination of bone marrow-derived endothelial progenitor cell significance in angiogenic growth factor-induced neovascularization in vivo. Exp Hematol. 2002;30:967–72.
70. Murohara T, Ikeda H, Duan J, et al. Transplanted cord blood-derived endothelial precursor cells augment postnatal neovascularization. J Clin Invest. 2000;105:1527–36.
71. Nagano M, Yamashita T, Hamada H, et al. Identification of functional endothelial progenitor cells suitable for the treatment of ischemic tissue using human umbilical cord blood. Blood. 2007;110:151–60.
72. He T, Smith LA, Harrington S, Nath KA, Caplice NM, Katusic ZS. Transplantation of circulating endothelial progenitor cells restores endothelial function of denuded rabbit carotid arteries. Stroke. 2004;35(10):2378–84.
73. Hill JM, Zalos G, Halcox JP, et al. Circulating endothelial progenitor cells, vascular function, and cardiovascular risk. N Engl J Med. 2003; 348:593–600.
74. Yoon CH, Hur J, Park KW, et al. Synergistic neovascularization by mixed transplantation of early endothelial progenitor cells and late outgrowth endothelial cells: the role of angiogenic cytokines and matrix metalloproteinases. Circulation. 2005;112:1618–27.
75. Elsheikh E, Uzunel M, He Z, Holgersson J, Nowak G, Sumitran-Holgersson S. Only a specific subset of human peripheral-blood monocytes has endothelial-like functional capacity. Blood. 2005;106:2347–55.
76. Rehman J, Jingling L, Orschell CM, March KL. Peripheral blood "endothelial progenitor cells" are derived from monocyte/macrophages and secrete angiogenic growth factors. Circulation. 2003;107:1164–9.
77. Urbich C, Heeschen C, Aicher A, Dernbach E, Zeiher AM, Dimmeler S. Relevance of monocytic features for neovascularization capacity of circulating endothelial progenitor cells. Circulation. 2003;108:2511–6.
78. Pesce M, Orlandi A, Iachininoto MG, et al. Myoendothelial differentiation of human umbilical cord blood-derived stem cells in ischemic limb tissues. Circ Res. 2003;93:1–12.
79. Berenson RJ, Andrews RG, Bensinger WI, et al. Antigen CD34+ marrow cells engraft lethally irradiated baboons. J Clin Invest. 1988;81: 951–5.
80. Manz MG, Miyamoto T, Akashi K, Weissman IL. Prospective isolation of human clonogenic common myeloid progenitors. Proc Natl Acad Sci U S A. 2002;99:11872–7.
81. Fina L, Molgaard HV, Robertson D, et al. Expression of the CD34 gene in vascular endothelial cells. Blood. 1990;75:2417–26.
82. Gupta K, Ramakrishnan S, Browne PV, Solovey A, Hebbel RP. A novel technique for culture of human dermal microvascular endothelial cells under either serum-free or serum-supplemented conditions: isolation by panning and stimulation with vascular endothelial growth factor. Exp Cell Res. 1997;230:244–51.
83. Lin Y, Weisdorf DJ, Solovey A, Hebbel RP. Origins of circulating endothelial cells and endothelial outgrowth from blood. J Clin Invest. 2000;105:71–7.
84. Rafii S. Circulating endothelial precursors: mystery, reality, and promise. J Clin Invest. 2000;105:17 9.
85. Yin AH, Miraglia S, Zanjani ED, et al. A novel five-transmembrane hematopoietic stem cell antigen: isolation, characterization, and molecular cloning. Blood. 1997;90:5013–21.
86. Peichev M, Naiyer AJ, Pereira D, et al. Expression of VEGFR-2 and AC133 by circulating human CD34(+) cells identifies a population of functional endothelial precursors. Blood. 2000;95:952–8.
87. Bonanno G, Mariotti A, Procoli A, et al. Human cord blood CD133+ cells immunoselected by a clinical-grade apparatus differentiate in vitro into endothelial- and cardiomyocyte-like cells. Transfusion. 2007;47:280–9.
88. Gehling UM, Ergun S, Schumacher U, et al. In vitro differentiation of endothelial cells from AC133-positive progenitor cells. Blood. 2000;95:3106–12.
89. Larrivée B, Niessen K, Pollet I, et al. Minimal contribution of marrow-derived endothelial precursors to tumor vasculature. J Immunol. 2005;175:2890–9.
90. Leor J, Guetta E, Feinberg MS, et al. Human umbilical cord blood-derived CD133+ cells enhance function and repair of the infarcted myocardium. Stem Cells. 2006;24:772–80.
91. Wu X, Lensch MW, Wylie-Sears J, Daley GQ, Bischoff J. Hemogenic endothelial progenitor cells isolated from human umbilical cord blood. Stem Cells. 2007;25:2770–6.
92. Ingram DA, Mead LE, Tanaka H, et al. Identification of a novel hierarchy of endothelial progenitor cells using human peripheral and umbilical cord blood. Blood. 2004;104:2752–60.
93. Prater DN, Case J, Ingram DA, Yoder MC. Working hypothesis to redefine endothelial progenitor cells. Leukemia. 2007;21:1141–9.
94. Yoder MC, Mead LE, Prater D, et al. Redefining endothelial progenitor cells via clonal analysis and hematopoietic stem/progenitor cell principals. Blood. 2007;109:1801–9.

95. Case J, Mead LE, Bessler WK, et al. Human CD34(+)AC133(+)VEGFR-2(+) cells are not endothelial progenitor cells but distinct, primitive hematopoietic progenitors. Exp Hematol. 2007;35:1109–18.
96. Timmermans F, Van Hauwermeiren F, De Smedt M, et al. Endothelial outgrowth cells are not derived from CD133+ cells or CD45+ hematopoietic precursors. Arterioscler Thromb Vasc Biol. 2007;27:1572–9.
97. Ziegelhoeffer T, Fernandez B, Kostin S, et al. Bone marrow-derived cells do not incorporate into the adult growing vasculature. Circ Res. 2004;94:230–8.
98. Balsam LB, Wagers AJ, Christensen JL, Kofidis T, Weissman IL, Robbins RC. Haematopoietic stem cells adopt mature haematopoietic fates in ischaemic myocardium. Nature. 2004;428:668–73.
99. Barcelos LS, Duplaa C, Kränkel N, et al. Human CD133+ progenitor cells promote the healing of diabetic ischemic ulcers by paracrine stimulation of angiogenesis and activation of Wnt signaling. Circ Res. 2009;104:1095–102.
100. Invernici G, Emanueli C, Madeddu P, et al. Human fetal aorta contains vascular progenitor cells capable of inducing vasculogenesis, angiogenesis, and myogenesis in vitro and in a murine model of peripheral ischemia. Am J Pathol. 2007;170:1879–92.
101. Cho HJ, Lee N, Lee JY, et al. Role of host tissues for sustained humoral effects after endothelial progenitor cell transplantation into the ischemic heart. J Exp Med. 2007;204:3257–69.
102. Ziebart T, Yoon CH, Trepels T, et al. Sustained persistence of transplanted proangiogenic cells contributes to neovascularization and cardiac function after ischemia. Circ Res. 2008;103:1327–34.
103. Gang EJ, Bosnakovski D, Figueiredo CA, Visser JW, Perlingeiro RC. SSEA-4 identifies mesenchymal stem cells from bone marrow. Blood. 2007;109:1743–51.
104. Pereira RF, Halford KW, O'Hara MD, et al. Cultured adherent cells from marrow can serve as long-lasting precursor cells for bone, cartilage, and lung in irradiated mice. Proc Natl Acad Sci USA. 1995;92:4857–61.
105. Pittenger MF, Mackay AM, Beck SC, et al. Multilineage potential of adult human mesenchymal stem cells. Science. 1999;284:143–7.
106. Prockop DJ. Marrow stromal cells as stem cells for nonhematopoietic tissues. Science. 1997;276:71–4.
107. Nagaya N, Fujii T, Iwase T, et al. Intravenous administration of mesenchymal stem cells improves cardiac function in rats with acute myocardial infarction through angiogenesis and myogenesis. Am J Physiol Heart Circ Physiol. 2004;287:H2670–6.
108. Silva GV, Litovsky S, Assad JA, et al. Mesenchymal stem cells differentiate into an endothelial phenotype, enhance vascular density, and improve heart function in a canine chronic ischemia model. Circulation. 2005;111:150–6.
109. Miyahara Y, Nagaya N, Kataoka M, et al. Monolayered mesenchymal stem cells repair scarred myocardium after myocardial infarction. Nat Med. 2006;12:459–65.
110. Planat-Benard V, Silvestre JS, Cousin B, et al. Plasticity of human adipose lineage cells toward endothelial cells: physiological and therapeutic perspectives. Circulation. 2004;109:656–63.
111. Rehman J, Traktuev D, Li J, et al. Secretion of angiogenic and antiapoptotic factors by human adipose stromal cells. Circulation. 2004;109: 1292–8.
112. Frye CA, Patrick CWJ. Isolation and culture of rat microvascular endothelial cells. In Vitro Cell Dev Biol Anim. 2002;38:208–12.
113. Hutley LJ, Herington AC, Shurety W, Cheung C, Vesey DA, Cameron DP, et al. Human adipose tissue endothelial cells promote preadipocyte proliferation. Am J Physiol Endocrinol Metab. 2001;281:E1037–44.
114. Zuk PA, Zhu M, Ashjian P, et al. Human adipose tissue is a source of multipotent stem cells. Mol Biol Cell. 2002;13:4279–95.
115. Iso Y, Soda T, Sato T, et al. Impact of implanted bone marrow progenitor cell composition on limb salvage after cell implantation in patients with critical limb ischemia. Atherosclerosis. 2010;209(1):167–72. doi:10.1016/j.atherosclerosis.2009.08.028.
116. Wang X, Jameel MN, Li Q, et al. Stem cells for myocardial repair with use of a transarterial catheter. Circulation. 2009;120:S238–46.
117. Zeng L, Hu Q, Wang X, et al. Bioenergetic and functional consequences of bone marrow-derived multipotent progenitor cell transplantation in hearts with postinfarction left ventricular remodeling. Circulation. 2007;115:1866–75.
118. Zhang G, Nakamura Y, Wang X, Hu Q, Suggs LJ, Zhang J. Controlled release of stromal cell-derived factor-1 alpha in situ increases c-kit+cell homing to the infarcted heart. Tissue Eng. 2007;13:2063–71.
119. Kalka C, Masuda H, Takahashi T, et al. Transplantation of ex vivo expanded endothelial progenitor cells for therapeutic neovascularization. Proc Natl Acad Sci USA. 2000;97:3422–7.
120. Kawamoto A, Gwon HC, Iwaguro H, et al. Therapeutic potential of ex vivo expanded endothelial progenitor cells for myocardial ischemia. Circulation. 2001;10:3634–7.
121. Iwaguro H, Yamaguchi JI, Kalka C, et al. Endothelial progenitor cell vascular endothelial growth factor gene transfer for vascular regeneration. Circulation. 2002;105:732–8.
122. Bartunek J, Vanderheyden M, Vandekerckhove B, et al. Intracoronary injection of CD133-positive enriched bone marrow progenitor cells promotes cardiac recovery after recent myocardial infarction: feasibility and safety. Circulation. 2005;112:I178–83.
123. Chen SL, Fang WW, Ye F, et al. Effect on left ventricular function of intracoronary transplantation of autologous bone marrow mesenchymal stem cell in patients with acute myocardial infarction. Am J Cardiol. 2004;94:92–5.
124. Erbs S, Linke A, Adams V, et al. Transplantation of blood-derived progenitor cells after recanalization of chronic coronary artery occlusion: first randomized and placebo-controlled study. Circ Res. 2005;97:756–62.
125. Hendrikx M, Hensen K, Clijsters C, et al. Recovery of regional but not global contractile function by the direct intramyocardial autologous bone marrow transplantation: results from a randomized controlled clinical trial. Circulation. 2006;114:I101–7.
126. Perin EC, Dohmann HF, Borojevic R, et al. Transendocardial, autologous bone marrow cell transplantation for severe, chronic ischemic heart failure. Circulation. 2003;107:2294–302.
127. Stamm C, Westphal B, Kleine HD, et al. Autologous bone-marrow stem-cell transplantation for myocardial regeneration. Lancet. 2003;361:45–6.
128. Strauer BE, Brehm M, Zeus T, et al. Repair of infarcted myocardium by autologous intracoronary mononuclear bone marrow cell transplantation in humans. Circulation. 2002;106:1913–8.
129. Tateishi-Yuyama E, Matsubara H, Murohara T, et al. Therapeutic angiogenesis for patients with limb ischaemia by autologous transplantation of bone-marrow cells: a pilot study and a randomised controlled trial. Lancet. 2002;360:427–35.
130. Tse HF, Kwong YL, Chan JK, Lo G, Ho CL, Lau CP. Angiogenesis in ischaemic myocardium by intramyocardial autologous bone marrow mononuclear cell implantation. Lancet. 2003;361:47–9.

131. Abdel-Latif A, Bolli R, Tleyjeh IM, et al. Adult bone marrow-derived cells for cardiac repair: a systematic review and meta-analysis. Arch Intern Med. 2007;167:989–97.
132. Yang F, Cho SW, Son SM, et al. Genetic engineering of human stem cells for enhanced angiogenesis using biodegradable polymeric nanoparticles. Proc Natl Acad Sci USA. 2010;107(8):3317–22. doi:10.1073/pnas.0905432106.
133. Assmus B, Honold J, Schächinger V, et al. Transcoronary transplantation of progenitor cells after myocardial infarction. N Engl J Med. 2006;355:1222–32.
134. Ge J, Li Y, Qian J, et al. Efficacy of emergent transcatheter transplantation of stem cells for treatment of acute myocardial infarction (TCT-STAMI). Heart. 2006;92:1764–7.
135. Janssens S, Dubois C, Bogaert J, et al. Autologous bone marrow-derived stem-cell transfer in patients with ST-segment elevation myocardial infarction: double-blind, randomised controlled trial. Lancet. 2006;367:113–21.
136. Perin EC, Dohmann HF, Borojevic R, et al. Improved exercise capacity and ischemia 6 and 12 months after transendocardial injection of autologous bone marrow mononuclear cells for ischemic cardiomyopathy. Circulation. 2004;110:II213–8.
137. Katritsis DG, Sotiropoulou PA, Karvouni E, et al. Transcoronary transplantation of autologous mesenchymal stem cells and endothelial progenitors into infarcted human myocardium. Catheter Cardiovasc Interv. 2005;65:321–9.
138. Schächinger V, Erbs S, Elsässer A, et al. Intracoronary bone marrow-derived progenitor cells in acute myocardial infarction. N Engl J Med. 2006;355:1210–21.
139. Lunde K, Solheim S, Aakhus S, et al. Intracoronary injection of mononuclear bone marrow cells in acute myocardial infarction. N Engl J Med. 2006;355:1199–209.
140. Li ZQ, Zhang M, Jing YZ, et al. The clinical study of autologous peripheral blood stem cell transplantation by intracoronary infusion in patients with acute myocardial infarction (AMI). Int J Cardiol. 2007;115:52–6.
141. Meyer GP, Wollert KC, Lotz J, et al. Intracoronary bone marrow cell transfer after myocardial infarction: eighteen months' follow-up data from the randomized, controlled BOOST (BOne marrOw transfer to enhance ST-elevation infarct regeneration) trial. Circulation. 2006;113:1287–94.

Chapter 15
Chronic Stable Angina

Santiago Garcia and Edward O. McFalls

Introduction

More than 16,500,000 Americans live with stable angina (SA), a chronic condition that represents the first clinical manifestation of ischemic heart disease (IHD) in 50% of the patients [1, 2]. In the Framingham Heart Study, the annual incidence of SA was 216 cases/100,000 persons [3].

The direct and indirect costs of treating SA are measured in billions of dollars, and despite our best efforts, many patients remain severely disabled. In the BARI trial, 30% of patients never returned to work after "successful" revascularization [4].

Diagnosis

The diagnosis of stable angina can be established on clinical grounds in the vast majority of patients. When there is diagnostic uncertainty, after a complete anamnesis and physical examination, judicious use of complementary studies can aid the clinician in detecting coronary artery disease while providing important prognostic information.

Typical angina is characterized by left-sided substernal chest discomfort that is precipitated by physical or emotional stress, and relieved by rest or nitroglycerin. *Atypical angina* refers to any chest discomfort that has two of the three characteristics described for typical angina (location, triggers, or alleviating factors). *Noncardiac chest pain* denotes a syndrome where the typical features of angina are lacking and there are features to suggest an alternative diagnosis (e.g., pleuritic chest pain).

Diamond and Forrester [5, 6] used angiographic data to determine the pretest probability of coronary artery disease on the basis of pain characteristics, age, and gender (Table 15.1). According to the "threshold theory of decision-making," also known as Bayesian analysis, patients with pretest probability at the low extreme of the spectrum need no additional testing, whereas patients with intermediate probability of having obstructive coronary disease should undergo noninvasive evaluation (see section "Risk Stratification").

Exercise electrocardiography is the preferred modality for patients who can perform exercise in the absence of specific contraindications that diminish the specificity of abnormal EKG findings. Examples include preexcitation, left ventricular hypertrophy, digitalis use, and paced rhythm or left bundle branch block [1, 7–9]. The reported sensitivity and specificity of pharmacological and exercise stress testing coupled with various imaging techniques is presented in Table 15.2 [1, 7].

Pathophysiology

Angina results from an imbalance between myocardial oxygen supply and myocardial oxygen demand. The major determinants of myocardial oxygen consumption are heart rate, loading condition of the left ventricle (afterload, preload), and contractility. Myocardial oxygen supply is determined by arterial content of oxygen and coronary flow. Unlike other

S. Garcia, MD (✉) • E.O. McFalls, MD, PhD
Department of Cardiology, University of Minnesota, Minneapolis VA Medical Center,
One Veterans Drive (111-C), Minneapolis, MN 55417, USA
e-mail: garci205@umn.edu

Z. Vlodaver et al. (eds.), *Coronary Heart Disease: Clinical, Pathological, Imaging, and Molecular Profiles*,
DOI 10.1007/978-1-4614-1475-9_15, © Springer Science+Business Media, LLC 2012

Table 15.1 Pretest probability of angiography-proven coronary artery disease according to gender, age and pain characteristic

	Nonanginal chest pain		Atypical angina		Typical angina	
Age (years)	Men	Women	Men	Women	Men	Women
30–39	4	2	34	12	76	26
40–49	13	3	51	22	87	55
50–59	20	7	65	31	93	73
60–69	27	14	72	51	94	86

Data from [5, 6]

Table 15.2 Sensitivity and specificity of noninvasive stress test modalities before and after correction for referral bias

	Sensitivity		Specificity	
	Biased	Adjusted	Biased	Adjusted
Exercise SPECT	0.98	0.82	0.14	0.59
Dypiridamole SPECT	0.93	0.88	0.89	0.96
Exercise echo	0.78	0.42	0.37	0.83

Referral bias refers to those studies in which patients with "negative scans" did not undergo routine coronary angiography to confirm the findings of noninvasive stress test. After adjusting for referral bias a significant drop in sensitivity with a concomitant increase in specificity is observed for both nuclear imaging and stress echocardiography

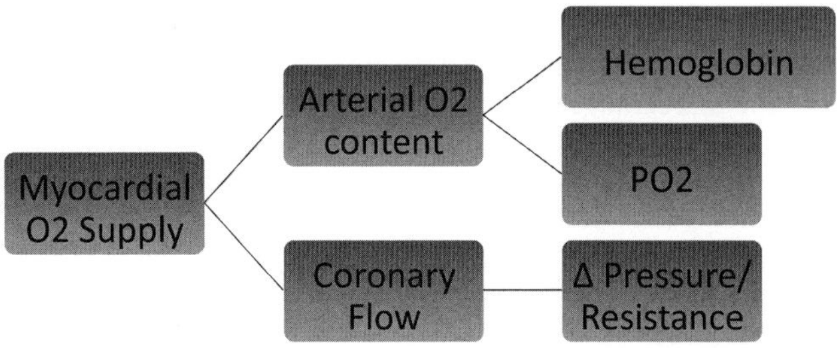

Fig. 15.1 Determinants of myocardial oxygen supply

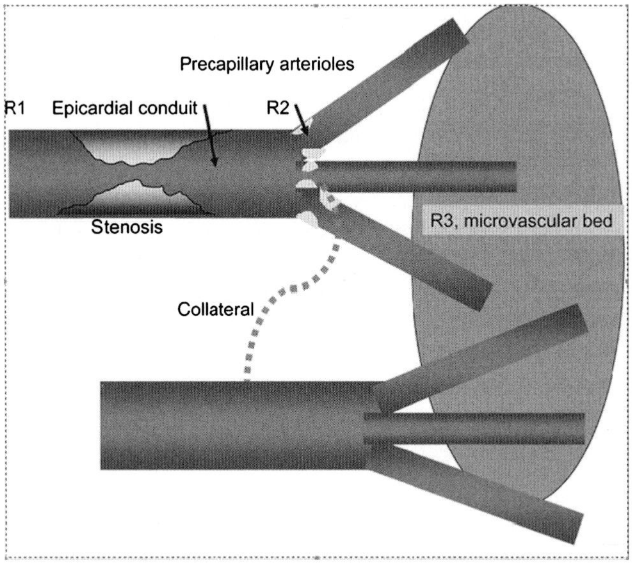

Fig. 15.2 Distribution of coronary resistance (adapted from "Myocardial blood flow and metabolism" in [11], p. 337)

peripheral organs, the heart extracts about 70% of the oxygen it receives; therefore, every increase in myocardial oxygen demand should be matched with a similar increase in myocardial oxygen supply if ischemia is to be avoided.

Under normal circumstances, the *arterial content of oxygen* remains fairly constant and is determined by the concentration of hemoglobin and the partial pressure of O_2 in the artery (PO_2a). *Coronary flow* is directly proportional to the pressure gradient between the aortic root and the right atrium, and inversely proportional to coronary resistance (Fig. 15.1). In a normal heart, perfusion remains fairly constant between ranges of physiologic arterial pressure, a phenomenon known as autoregulation. Therefore, regulation of coronary flow occurs by modulation of coronary resistance [10].

Three serial resistances are in play in coronary physiology (Fig. 15.2) [11]. Epicardial vessels (R1) offer little resistance under normal circumstances. The coronary microvasculature (vessel size <400 μm) is the site where coronary flow is regulated (R2) by paracrine release of adenosine in response to tissue hypoxia [12]. Adenosine leads to vasodilation of the coronary microcirculation, which in turn decreases coronary resistance and increases coronary flow. Finally, systolic compression of coronary vessels traveling through the myocardium, from epicardium into subendocardium, offers a considerable source of "extravascular" resistance (R3), particularly in the left ventricle, which has increased mass and thickness when compared to the right ventricle.

In the presence of significant (>70%) epicardial vessel atherosclerotic disease, R1 becomes the limiting factor for increasing coronary flow in response to increased myocardial oxygen demand. This leads to "effort angina," which is the cardinal feature of stable coronary artery disease. A solid grasp of the pathophysiology of stable angina is crucial to understanding how various medical therapies and revascularization make an impact.

Risk Stratification

Despite the disabling nature of angina pectoris, the majority of patients with stable angina have a good prognosis, with predicted annual mortality rates of approximately 1–2%. Therefore, the role of risk stratification is to identify the minority of patients with high-risk features who benefit from more aggressive interventions such as coronary revascularization. Patients with expected annual mortality rates in excess of 3% generally represent a high-risk group, and those with expected annual mortality rates between 1 and 3% represent an intermediate-risk group.

The two most powerful predictors of long-term survival among patients with stable coronary artery disease are left ventricular function and extent of coronary artery disease (Fig. 15.3). In the landmark Coronary Artery Surgery Study (CASS), patients with severe left ventricular dysfunction (EF<35%) and severe triple-vessel coronary artery disease had survival rates at 12 years of less than 30%. Conversely, patients with single-vessel disease and preserved systolic performance had survival rates in excess of 70% at 12 years [13]. Other important, although less-powerful identifiers of poor prognosis include noncardiac comorbidities such as renal failure and diabetes, demographic factors such as advanced age and male gender, and advanced functional class (CCS III–IV) [14–17].

Noninvasive exercise testing, with or without an imaging modality, remains the most widely used tool to assess prognosis in patients with SA. Invasive angiography is usually reserved for patients with high-risk features on noninvasive imaging tests, or disabling angina, are sudden death survivors, or have heart failure with left ventricular dysfunction [1].

Noninvasive angiography with multisliced CT has recently emerged as a powerful tool able to define the coronary anatomy, cardiac function, and noncardiac structures with acceptable levels of radiation and contrast exposure (Fig. 15.4) [18]. Strengths of exercise testing include relatively high diagnostic accuracy, noninvasiveness, and that it is physiology-based, has a lower cost relative to invasive angiography, and a large body of evidence supporting its role in risk prediction. Limitations include false negatives, inability to localize ischemic territories when imaging is not applied, radiation exposure from nuclear imaging tests, and a lower technical success rate than invasive angiography for stress echocardiography [7, 19, 20]. The relative merits of stress echocardiography vs. myocardial perfusion imaging are summarized in Table 15.3.

High-risk features of noninvasive imaging tests include angina and/or electrocardiographic ischemic changes (horizontal or downsloping ST depressions) at a low functional class, S3 or rales with exercise, multiple perfusion defects, or wall

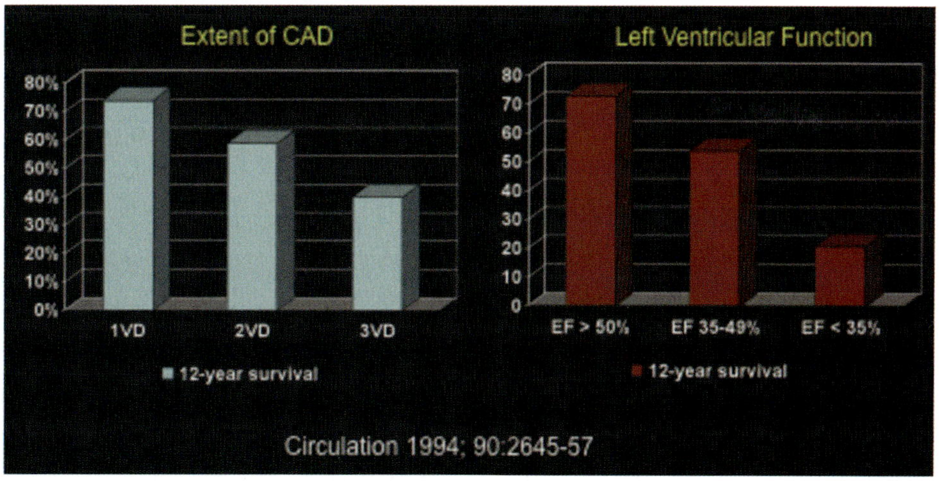

Fig. 15.3 Predictors of long-term survival in the Coronary Artery Surgery Study (CASS) registry (adapted from [120])

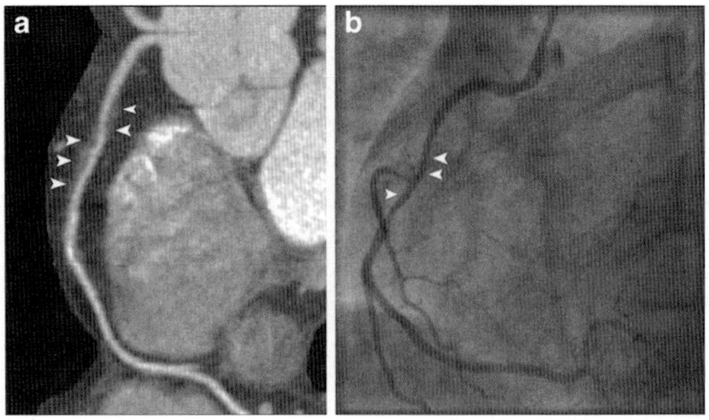

Fig. 15.4 Multislice computed tomography (**a**) and invasive coronary angiography (**b**) in a patient with nonobstructive coronary artery disease of the mid-right coronary artery. Note that soft plaque and positive remodeling (*arrowheads*) can be appreciated in multislice CT images, but not in invasive arteriography (images courtesy of John Lesser, MD)

Table 15.3 Relative merits of different exercise-based imaging modalities to risk-stratify patients with stable coronary artery disease

Stress-echocardiography	Myocardial perfusion imaging
Higher specificity	Higher sensitivity
Versatility	Higher technical success rate
Lower cost, no radiation	Longer follow-up prognostic data

Table 15.4 Survival according to risk groups based on Duke treadmill scores

Risk group (score)	% of Total	4-Year survival	Annual mortality (%)
Low (≥5)	62	0.99	0.25
Moderate (−10 to 4)	34	0.95	1.25
High (<−10)	4	0.79	5

The Duke treadmill score can be calculated using the following formula: Exercise duration (min) − ST-segment deviation (mm) × 5 − angina index × 4. Angina index "0" no angina, "1" angina occurs, "2" angina reason for stopping the test

motion abnormalities in two or more vascular territories suggestive of multivessel or left main disease, low ejection fraction, ischemic transient dilatation of the left ventricular cavity, and thallium uptake in the lungs suggestive of exercise-induced pulmonary edema [1, 19–21]. For patients undergoing an exercise stress test with electrocardiography monitoring and no imaging modality, the Duke treadmill score can be used to estimate disease severity and guide management (Table 15.4) [22]. For patients in the high-risk category (Duke score ≤−11), consideration should be given to coronary angiography and revascularization in addition to optimal medical therapy (OMT). Conversely, patients falling in the low-risk group (Duke score ≥5) should be managed medically and revascularization reserved only to control refractory or disabling symptoms. Patients in the intermediate-risk category (−10 to 4) may benefit from the addition of an imaging modality or coronary angiography to further risk-stratify and help make decisions regarding appropriateness of revascularization.

A summary of noninvasive criteria to assess risk in patients with chronic stable coronary artery disease is presented in Table 15.5, and indications for coronary angiography in Table 15.6 [1, 21].

Therapy

The objectives of therapy in patients with chronic coronary artery disease are to prolong life and improve symptoms. Strategies to achieve these goals include risk factor modification, medical management of anginal symptoms, coronary artery revascularization, and experimental therapies (stem cell transplantation, angiogenesis, transmyocardial revascularization with laser). Risk factor modification is described in detail in other chapters of this book. A brief summary of current recommendations regarding diabetes control, blood pressure management, diet, and exercise can be found in Table 15.7 [23–43].

Table 15.5 Criteria for noninvasive risk stratification

High risk (>3% annual mortality)
Treadmill score ≤11
Severe resting or exercise-induced LV dysfunction (EF<35%)
Stress-induced large perfusion defect (particularly if anterior)
Stress-induced multiple perfusion defects of moderate size
Stress-induced moderate perfusion defect with LV dilatation or increased lung-uptake (thallium-201)
Echocardiographic wall motion abnormality involving two segments developing with low dose dobutamine (≤10 mcg/kg/min) or at a low heart rate (<120 bpm)
Stress echocardiographic evidence of extensive ischemia
Moderate risk (1–3% annual mortality rate)
Treadmill score −10 to 4
Mild/moderate resting LV dysfunction (LVEF: 35–49%)
Stress-induced moderate perfusion defect without LV dilatation or increased lung uptake (thallium-201)
Limited stress echocardiographic ischemia with a wall motion abnormality only with higher doses of dobutamine involving ≤2 segments
Low risk (<1% annual mortality rate)
Treadmill score ≥5
Normal or small perfusion defect at rest or with stress
Normal stress echocardiographic wall motion or no change of limited resting wall motion abnormality during stress

Table 15.6 Indications for invasive coronary angiography in patients with stable coronary artery disease

Disabling angina (CCS III or IV)
High-risk criteria on noninvasive testing
Sudden death survivors
Angina and heart failure
High-likelihood of multivessel disease
LV dysfunction
Inadequate noninvasive testing

Table 15.7 Cardiovascular risk reduction for patients with coronary artery disease

Risk factor	Recommendation	Benefit of treatment
Sedentary lifestyle	30–45 min of Physical activity 7 days a week (minimum 5 day/week)	Decreases mortality after MI Decreases hospitalizations and revascularization Improves exercise tolerance and helps control other risk factors
Overweight	BMI of 18.5–24.9 kg/m^2 Waist circumference of <89 cm in women and <102 cm in men	Mortality reduction
Smoking	Smoking cessation and avoidance to secondhand smoking	Mortality reduction Reduction in nonfatal MI Slow progression of atherosclerosis
Diabetes	Aim for Hb A1c level of <7% with lifestyle and pharmacotherapy	Reduction in nonfatal MI, stroke and CV death
Hypertension	Treat with beta-blockers and/or ACEI initially to target BP of <140/90 mmHg or <130/80 for patients with diabetes or kidney disease	Mortality reduction Reduction in nonfatal CV events (stroke, MI, heart failure) Regression of LV hypertrophy

Medical Therapy

The armamentarium to treat chronic stable angina has increased significantly over the last 4 decades. A look at the medical arm in clinical trials conducted in the 1970s reveals that coronary vasodilators, beta-blockers, diuretics, and digoxin were considered standards of care at that time [44–47]. By contrast, the medical arm of the COURAGE trial (Clinical Outcomes Utilizing Revascularization and Aggressive Drug Evaluation) included aspirin, angiotensin-converting enzyme inhibitors (ACEI) or angiotensin-receptor blockers (ARBs), beta-blockers, calcium antagonists, nitrates, and statins [48].

Medical therapy has become the mainstay of therapy for stable coronary artery disease and has resulted in significant reduction in morbidity and mortality. Conceptually, drugs used to treat patients with stable coronary disease can be divided into antiischemic drugs, antiplatelet and anticoagulant agents, and vasoprotective agents.

Antiischemic Drugs

This group of drugs' mechanism of action is reducing myocardial oxygen demand, primarily by reducing heart rate, but also by modifying the loading conditions of the ventricle (nitrates) and contractile state (beta-blockers, nondihydropyridine calcium antagonists). With few exceptions (beta-blockers post-MI with LV dysfunction, heart failure), this group of drugs does not lead to a mortality reduction.

Beta-blockers: Multiple clinical trials have assessed the role of beta-blockers in the treatment of stable coronary artery disease [49–57]. Beta-blockers have been found to increase time to ST depression during treadmill ergometry, decrease the frequency and duration of angina, and reduce the incidence of cardiovascular events. In addition, among patients with left ventricular dysfunction postmyocardial infarction, beta-blockers have been shown to reduce mortality [58–60]. All beta-blockers appear to be equally effective as antianginal agents provided that they are titrated to reduce heart rate to 55–60 bpm and exercise heart rate to 75% of the heart rate response associated with angina.

Calcium antagonists: Both dihydropyridine and nondihydropyridine calcium antagonists are as effective as beta-blockers in relieving angina and improving exercise time to onset of angina or ischemia [61–66]. Current recommendations stipulate that calcium antagonists be used in conjunction with beta-blockers or as an alternative to beta-blockers when contraindications exist [1]. In patients with vasospastic angina, calcium antagonists completely abolish or control angina in 90% of the patients and are the treatment of choice. Short-acting nifedipine in patients with recent, unstable presentation of coronary artery disease should be avoided as its use has been linked to excess mortality [67].

Nitrates: Nitrates are endothelium-independent venodilators that reduce preload and also improve epicardial and collateral flow. Among patients with chronic stable angina, nitrates improve exercise tolerance and reduce the frequency and duration of ischemic episodes with a neutral effect on mortality [68–75]. Tolerance to the effect of nitrates over time limits the usefulness of these drugs in the long term.

Antiplatelet and Anticoagulants

This group of drugs effectively reduces the risk of myocardial infarction and death by achieving platelet inhibition. Anticoagulants have not shown to be beneficial in the presence of antiplatelet therapy while significantly increasing the risk of stroke.

Aspirin: Aspirin (ASA) is an irreversible inhibitor of platelet thromboxane A2 production. In clinical trials, aspirin use has been associated with a 33% reduction in cardiovascular events, a 34% reduction in MI/sudden death rates, and a 32% reduction in secondary vascular events [76–80]. Current guidelines recommend daily aspirin 75–162 mg in patients with stable coronary artery disease [1].

Clopidogrel: Clopidogrel interferes with the $P2Y_{12}$ receptor on the surface of platelets and leads to potent platelet inhibition. Although clopidogrel is usually recommended for patients with unstable coronary artery disease [81] or after stent implantation [82], its routine use in patients with chronic stable angina is not recommended unless there is a contraindication to aspirin.

In the CHARISMA study (Clopidogrel for High Atherothrombotic Risk and Ischemic Stabilization, Management, and Avoidance), 15,603 patients at risk of atherothrombotic events were randomized to aspirin, 75–162 mg/day monotherapy, or ASA plus clopidogrel 75 mg/daily [83]. Fifty percent of patients in CHARISMA had stable coronary artery disease. The incidence of the primary end point (composite of death from CV causes, myocardial infarction, or stroke) was no different between the two groups (6.8% vs. 7.3%, $p=0.22$). It should be mentioned, however, that in a prespecified subgroup analysis of patients with symptomatic atherothrombosis, many of whom had stable angina, clopidogrel use was associated with a 12% relative risk reduction in the primary end point.

Warfarin: Warfarin interferes with the production of vitamin K-dependent coagulation factors (II, VII, IX, and X) as well as proteins C and S. Although warfarin effectively reduces nonfatal cardiovascular events when compared to placebo in patients with stable coronary disease, it is not superior to ASA monotherapy [84]. Additionally, its use is associated with a

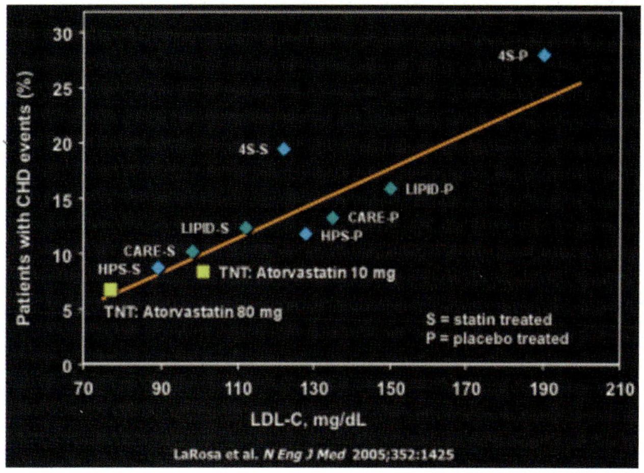

Fig. 15.5 Secondary prevention trials of statins in coronary heart disease. Coronary heart disease events are plotted against LDL levels (adapted from [40], p. 1425. Copyright 2005 by Massachusetts Medical Society)

1.4% absolute increase in the risk of stroke. In the absence of specific indications (e.g., atrial fibrillation, LV clot), the use of warfarin is not recommended [1].

Vasculoprotective Drugs

This group of drugs is believed to have effects beyond lowering blood pressure and reducing cholesterol levels. In effect, ACEI and statins have antiproliferative, antiaggregatory, and antithrombotic effects on the vasculature (i.e., pleiotropic effect). In at-risk populations, these drugs have led to significant reduction in mortality and morbidity and, along with ASA and beta-blockers, constitute the mainstay of therapy for patients with stable coronary disease.

ACEIs: By blocking the production of angiotensin II, ACEI therapy leads to blood pressure reduction and antiproliferative effects on the heart and vasculature. Three trials have evaluated the use of ACEI in patients with stable coronary artery disease [84–86].

In the HOPE (Heart Outcomes Prevention Evaluation) trial, 9,300 patients at risk for vascular events (80% had CAD) were randomized to either 10 mg of ramipril or placebo. The composite outcome of myocardial infarction, stroke, or death from vascular causes was reduced by 22% with ramipril.

In EUROPA (European Trial on Reduction of Cardiac Events with Perindopril in Stable Coronary Artery Disease), 12,218 patients were randomized to either perindopril 8 mg/day or placebo. At 4 years, perindopril use was associated with a 22% reduction in the primary end point of cardiovascular death, MI, or cardiac arrest.

By contrast, trandolapril was not superior to placebo in the PEACE (Prevention of Events with Angiotensin-Converting Enzyme inhibition) trial in preventing deaths or vascular events. A post hoc analysis of PEACE showed a 27% relative risk reduction with trandolapril among patients with chronic kidney disease and creatinine clearance less than 60 mL/min.

Current guidelines recommend the use of ACEI (or ARBs) in patients with stable coronary artery disease and diabetes, LV dysfunction, or kidney disease. The use of ACEI in low-risk patients is "reasonable." [1]

Statins: This group of drugs blocks HMG Co-A reductase, a critical step in the biosynthesis of cholesterol. Although in clinical trials, the degree of CV event reduction parallels the fall in LDL cholesterol (Fig. 15.5), similar reductions in LDL cholesterol by other lipid-lowering agents have not translated into similar positive results, which suggests LDL-independent properties of statins [87–89]. Current guidelines advocate for LDL less than 100 mg/dL for patients with stable coronary disease, with an "optional" goal of LDL <70 mg/dL [40].

Coronary Revascularization

The clinical indication to perform a revascularization procedure in patients with chronic stable angina, either with percutaneous coronary intervention (PCI) or coronary artery bypass graft (CABG), remains one of the most debated topics in clinical cardiology [90, 91]. Two elements are key in understanding the nuances and the two sides in this debate.

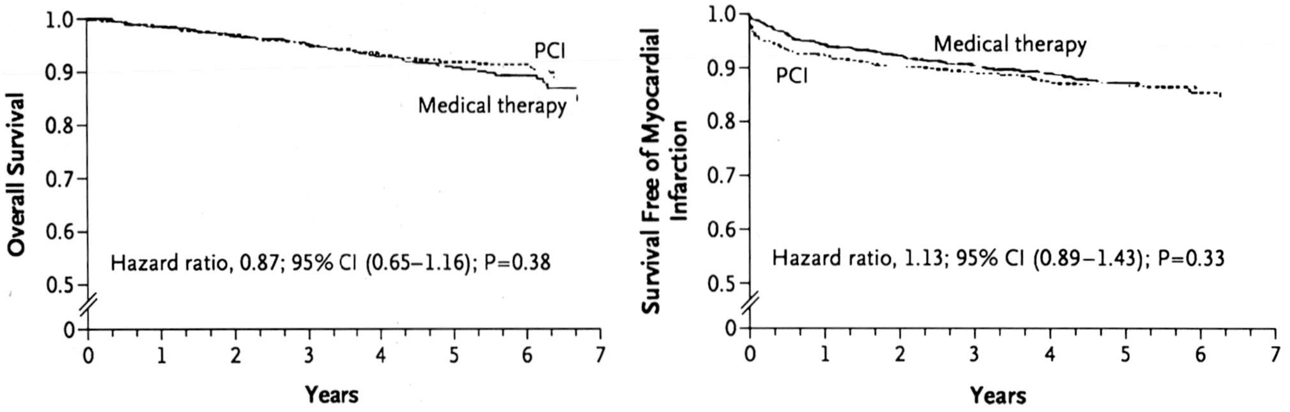

Fig. 15.6 In the Clinical Outcomes Utilizing Revascularization and Aggressive Drug Evaluation (COURAGE) trial, no significant difference was found between patients treated with optimal medical therapy (OMT) and those with percutaneous coronary intervention (PCI) and OMT regarding the primary outcome of death or myocardial infarction (adapted from [48], p. 1512. Copyright 2007 by Massachusetts Medical Society)

Initial Optimal Medical Therapy

First, the results of two large and multicenter, strategy-based, clinical trials have recently been published [48, 92]. Both the COURAGE trial and BARI 2D (Bypass Angioplasty Revascularization Investigation 2 Diabetes) trial unequivocally have shown that a strategy of initial OMT is safe, and as effective, in reducing major cardiovascular events among low- to moderate-risk patients with chronic stable coronary artery disease (annual morality <3%).

Benefits of Coronary Revascularization

On the contrary, coronary revascularization has been shown to be superior to medical therapy in relieving angina and has provided a mortality reduction in patients at high risk of events based on noninvasive testing (moderate or large areas of reversible ischemia with or without LV dysfunction) or coronary angiography (left main or proximal left anterior descending artery disease) [44–47]. It is, therefore, prudent to treat all patients with OMT and reserve invasive revascularization therapies for those patients who remain symptomatic or have high-risk imaging or angiographic features.

Contemporary Trials of Optimal Medical Therapy vs. Revascularization

COURAGE

In COURAGE, 2,287 patients with stable coronary artery disease and evidence of myocardial ischemia were randomized to a strategy of OMT or PCI with OMT. The primary outcome was a composite of death or nonfatal myocardial infarction during a follow-up period of 2.5–7 years. After a median follow-up of 4.6 years, 211 events occurred in the PCI group and 202 in the OMT group (19% vs. 18.5%; hazard ratio, 1.05; 95% confidence interval, 0.87–1.25; $p=0.62$). There were no differences between the groups in rates of admission for acute coronary syndromes or the individual components of the primary end point (Fig. 15.6). COURAGE, therefore, confirms what other small clinical trials have previously shown (Table 15.8) – that a strategy of initial PCI is *not* associated with significant reductions in the rates of "hard" end points such as MI or death.

On the contrary, COURAGE has also shown that PCI is superior to medical therapy in providing angina relief and improving quality of life, although most of these differences attenuate over time, likely a reflection of disease progression in other vascular beds or restenosis of bare-metal stents, which were used in COURAGE.

In a subgroup that focused on a cost-effectiveness analysis of COURAGE, the authors found PCI not to be cost-effective [93]. The cost per patient for a significant improvement in angina frequency, physical limitation, and quality of life were $154,580, $112,876, and $124,333, respectively.

Table 15.8 Summaries of clinical trial comparing PCI and medical therapy for stable CAD ($n>5,000$)

Trial	Mortality and MI	Angina relief	QOL	Repeat revascularization
RITA-2	No difference	PCI	PCI	PCI
ACME	No difference	PCI	PCI	PCI
ACME-2	No difference	PCI	PCI	NA
MASS	No difference	PCI	NA	No difference
MASS-II	No difference	PCI	PCI	No difference
AVERT	No difference	PCI	PCI	No difference
TIME	No difference	PCI	PCI	PCI
COURAGE	No difference	No difference	PCI	PCI

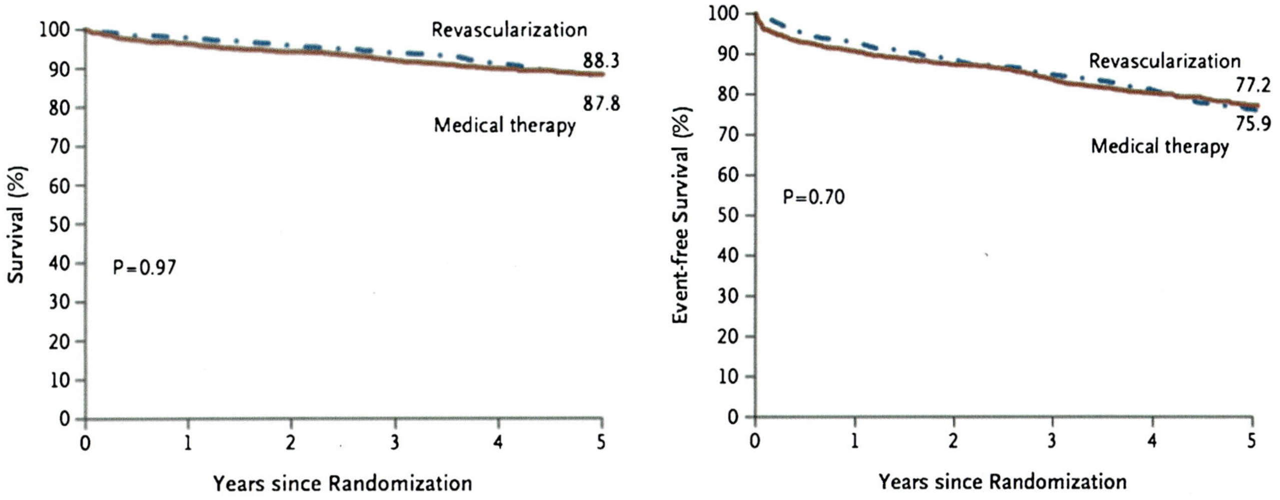

Fig. 15.7 In Bypass Angioplasty Revascularization Investigation 2 Diabetes (BARI 2D), a strategy of prompt revascularization did not reduce overall mortality (*left*), nor the composite of death, MI, or stroke (*right*) (adapted from [92], p. 2510. Copyright 2009 by Massachusetts Medical Society)

BARI 2D

BARI 2D assigned 2,368 patients with type II diabetes mellitus and coronary artery disease to medical therapy or prompt revascularization in addition to medical therapy. The trial had a 2×2 factorial design to allow for a comparison of insulin-sensitization vs. insulin provision. The primary end point of the study was a composite of death and major cardiovascular events (myocardial infarction or stroke) at 5 years. A strategy of prompt revascularization, either with PCI or CABG, did not reduce mortality (88.3% vs. 87.8%, $p=0.97$) or have a beneficial effect on major cardiovascular events (77.2% vs. 75.9%, $p=0.70$) (Fig. 15.7).

Controversies

Misplaced Financial Incentives

Convincing evidence indicates that coronary angioplasty is overutilized in the United States [94, 95]. Revascularization rates also show wide fluctuations according to different geographic regions. For example, Florida has revascularization rates that are 83% higher than Oregon; the number of revascularization procedures correlates in part to the number of surgeons and interventional cardiologists in that particular region. Financial incentives may play a role in the overutilization of PCI [96].

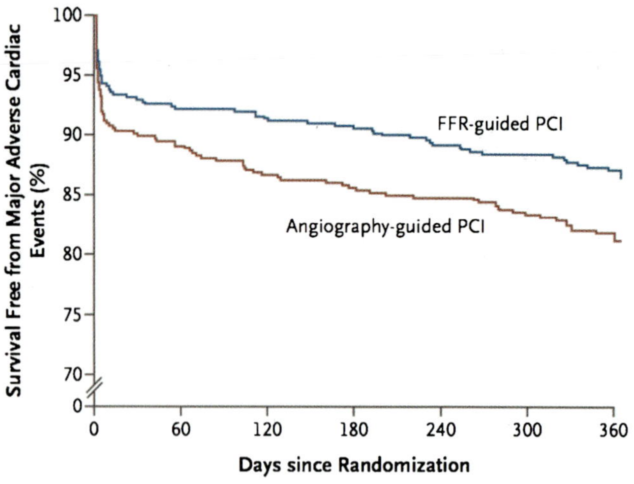

Fig. 15.8 Fractional flow reserve vs. coronary angiography for guiding PCI, based on results from the FAME trial (adapted from [101], p. 222. Copyright 2009 by Massachusetts Medical Society)

Oculostenotic Reflex

Only 44.5% of patients have noninvasive stress testing before PCI in the United States [97], with a marked variation according to geography (22–71%). Although coronary angiography remains the gold standard to risk-stratify symptomatic patients with an abnormal imaging test or severe disabling symptoms, visual estimation of stenosis severity correlates poorly with functional assessment [98–100]. It should not be used to decide on the need for PCI in lesions of intermediate severity (30–70%). Studies have shown that a fractional flow reserve (FFR) strategy is superior to an angiography-based strategy at selecting patients for PCI (Fig. 15.8) [101]. Only patients with hemodynamically significant stenosis (FFR <0.80) stand to benefit from PCI, whereas the prognosis of intermediate lesion with normal FFR is excellent [102].

Ischemic Burden

The benefits of coronary revascularization relative to medical therapy should be considered in the context of the amount of viable myocardium at risk of ischemia. The greater the amount of inducible ischemia, the more likely that coronary revascularization will result in improved clinical outcomes. Hachamovitch et al [103]. analyzed the outcomes of 10,627 patients with myocardial ischemia on SPECT and who had no prior history of myocardial infarction or coronary revascularization according to the therapy received within 60 days. They found that coronary revascularization compared with OMT had greater absolute and relative reductions in cardiac death among patients with moderate or large ischemic burden (>12.5% of the LV mass) (Fig. 15.9a, b).

Ischemia Reduction

A substudy of the COURAGE trial compared reductions in ischemic burden with PCI vs. OMT among 313 patients undergoing nuclear myocardial perfusion imaging studies before and 6–18 months after the intervention [104]. The proportion of patients with ≥5% reductions in ischemic burden was greater with PCI as compared with OMT (33% vs. 19%, $p=0.004$). When outcomes were plotted against reductions in ischemic burden, the authors found that patients with ≥5% reductions had a 50% reduction in composite death and MI when compared to patients with no ischemic reduction (Fig. 15.10). Other studies have shown better outcomes with complete coronary revascularization when compared to partial revascularization or no change in revascularization status [105, 106].

Taken together, these observations suggest that perhaps a high-risk subset of chronic coronary disease patients with a large ischemic burden and suitable coronary anatomy may derive benefit from a strategy of coronary revascularization. A similar observation was made within the Coronary Artery Revascularization Trial (CARP) for patients with anterior wall ischemia undergoing abdominal aortic operations [107]. These observations highlight the importance of using clinical judgment when applying strategy-based studies such as COURAGE into clinical practice.

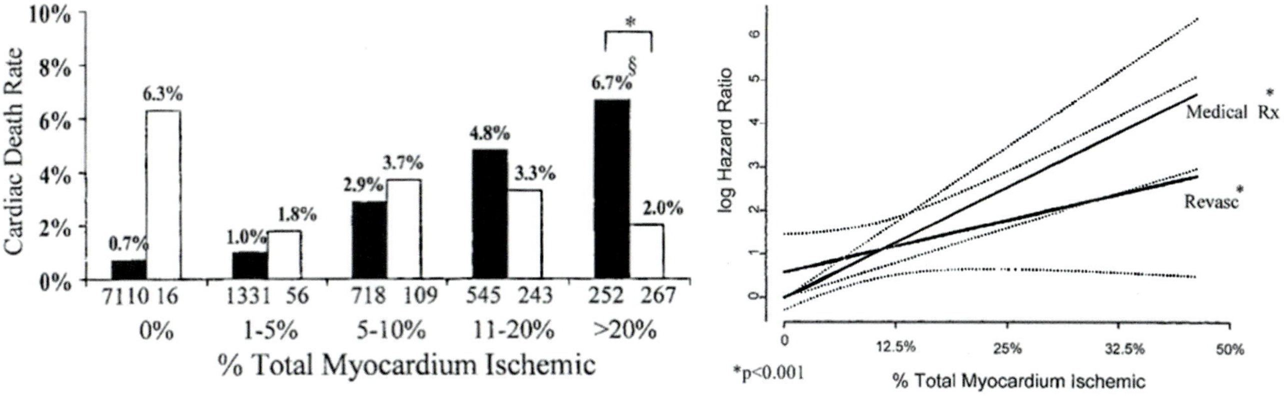

Fig. 15.9 Revascularization vs. medical therapy as a function of ischemic burden. (**a**) Cardiac death rates are lower for revascularization (*white bars*) than for medical therapy (*black bars*) when ischemic burden is moderate or large. (**b**) Hazard ratio for CV death becomes favorable for coronary revascularization above the ischemic threshold of 12.5% of LV mass (adapted from [103], p. 2903. Copyright 2003 by American Heart Association)

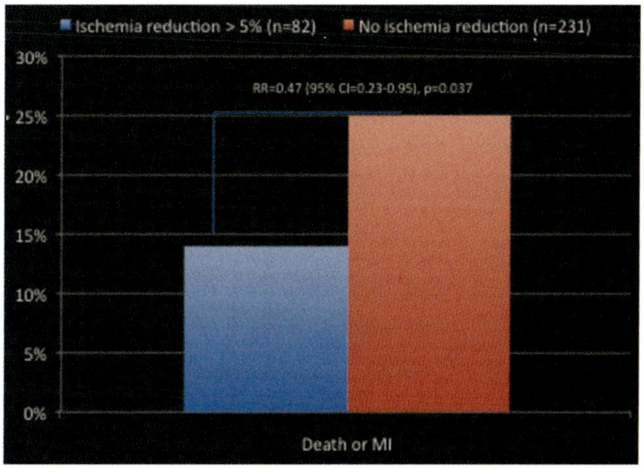

Fig. 15.10 COURAGE Nuclear Substudy: Patients with >5% ischemic reduction had a 53% reduction in the composite of MI or death (adapted from [104]. Copyright 2008 by American Heart Association)

Early Trials of CABG vs. Medical Therapy

Soon after its inception by Favaloro [108], the efficacy and safety of CABG surgery was studied in three large, pivotal, randomized clinical trials conducted in the 1970s [44–47].

VA Cooperative Study

The Veterans Administration Cooperative Study of Surgery for Coronary Arterial Occlusive Disease was conducted in 13 Veterans Administration centers in the United States [44–47]. Entry criteria included presence of stable angina for <6 months, no contraindications to CABG, electrocardiographic evidence of myocardial infarction or ischemia, or a positive exercise test. A total of 1,015 patients were randomized to medical therapy ($n=508$) or CABG ($n=507$). Of these 1,015 patients, 683 had abnormal left ventricular function. Randomization was stratified according to age (< or ≥50 years) and coronary angiography findings.

The first report of the VA cooperative study dealt with 113 patients with significant (>50%) left main disease. Despite a high surgical mortality rate in the first 2 years of the study (25%), a significant reduction in mortality was found with CABG (CABG, 20%, vs. medical treatment, 36%). For patients randomized in the latter 3 years of the study (surgical mortality, 7%), the mortality difference in favor of CABG was even greater (CABG, 7%, vs. medical treatment, 29%). A preliminary report of the VA Cooperative Study of patients without left main disease showed no difference in mortality between the two

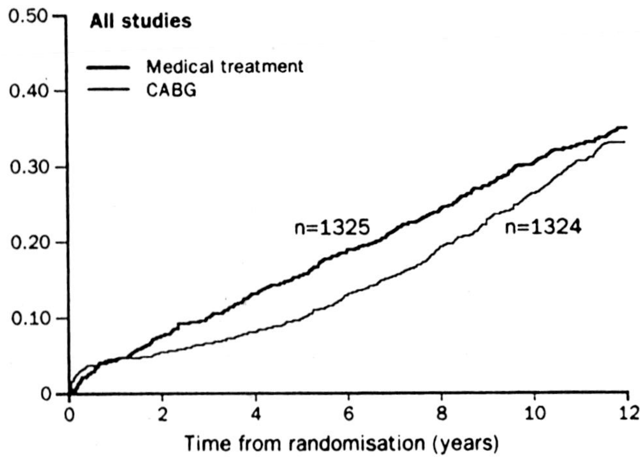

Fig. 15.11 Meta-analysis of seven clinical trials comparing bypass surgery with medical therapy. Surgery was associated with a mortality reduction that persisted at 10 years (adapted from [109]. Copyright 1994 by The Lancet Publishing Group)

treatment arms, with better angina relief among surgically treated patients. A subsequent report showed improved mortality for patients with three-vessel disease when the three centers with the highest operative mortality were excluded.

ECSS Group

The European Coronary Surgery Study (ECSS) Group performed a randomized clinical trial in 12 centers to assess the effect of CABG on the incidence of death and myocardial infarction in patients with angina pectoris (42% with angina class III) [45, 47]. The study included 768 males with preserved systolic function who were randomized to medical therapy ($n=373$) or surgery ($n=395$). Survival was improved by surgery in the entire cohort, including patients with three-vessel disease and those with proximal left anterior descending disease as part of two- or three-vessel disease.

CASS

The CASS consisted of a patient registry (24,959 patients) and a randomized trial (780 patients) [46, 47]. Within the randomized component of the trial, patients were assigned to one of three possible clinical groups: (1) group A ($n=514$): mild angina with normal left ventricular function, (2) group B ($n=106$): mild angina with moderate left ventricular dysfunction, and (3) group C ($n=160$): asymptomatic after myocardial infarction. The 5-year probability of remaining free of death or myocardial infarction was 82% in the group assigned to medical therapy, and 83% in the group assigned to surgery. There was a trend toward better survival in patients with triple-vessel disease and moderate left ventricular dysfunction (group B).

Meta-Analysis of Seven Trials

Yusuf et al. [109] conducted a meta-analysis of seven clinical trials that compared CABG with medical therapy to assess whether surgery conferred a survival advantage over medical therapy. In addition to the three pivotal trials, four smaller trials were also included. Collectively, these trials included 1,649 patients randomized to medical therapy ($n=1{,}325$) or surgery ($n=1{,}324$). Overall, CABG was associated with a significant reduction in mortality at 5 years (OR: 0.61, 95% CI: 0.48–0.77, $p<0.001$) and at 10 years (OR: 0.83, 95% CI: 0.70–0.98, $p=0.03$) (Fig. 15.11).

Percutaneous Coronary Intervention vs. Surgical Revascularization

Since the introduction of coronary angioplasty by Andreas Gruentzig in 1977, the number of PCIs has continued to grow in the USA and worldwide. In 2006, 1,314,000 angioplasty procedures were performed in the USA compared with 448,000 CABG procedures [110].

Many clinical trials have compared the efficacy and safety of both techniques in patients with stable and unstable multivessel coronary artery disease (Table 15.9) [111–117]. The evolution of these trials reflects dramatic changes in the practice

Table 15.9 Summary of trials comparing PCI with CBAG in patients with multivessel CAD

	Overall (*N*=7,812)	ARTS [1] (*N*=1,205)	BARP [2] (*N*=1,829)	CABRI [3] (*N*=1,054)	EAST [4] (*N*=392)	ERAC-II [5] (*N*=450)	GABI [6] (*N*=323)	MASS-II [7] (*N*=1,011)	RITA-1 [8] (*N*=1,011)	SoS [9] (*N*=988)	Toulouse [10] (*N*=152)
Age											
<55 Years	2,185 (28%)	332 (28%)	442 (24%)	286 (27%)	94 (24%)	124 (28%)	107 (33%)	131 (32%)	403 (40%)	253 (26%)	13 (9%)
55–64 Years	2,933 (38%)	420 (35%)	678 (37%)	443 (42%)	143 (36%)	163 (36%)	130 (40%)	135 (33%)	442 (44%)	340 (34%)	39 (26%)
≥65 Years	2,688 (34%)	453 (38%)	709 (39%)	320 (31%)	155 (40%)	162 (36%)	86 (27%)	142 (35%)	166 (16%)	395 (40%)	100 (66%)
Female	1,831 (23%)	283 (23%)	489 (27%)	234 (22%)	103 (26%)	93 (21%)	67 (21%)	125 (31%)	196 (19%)	206 (21%)	35 (23%)
Diabetes	1,233 (16%)	208 (17%)	353 (19%)	124 (12%)	90 (23%)	78 (17%)	41 (13%)	115 (28%)	62 (6%)	142 (14%)	20 (13%)
Current smoker	1,665 (25%)	323 (27%)	463 (25%)	NA	79 (20%)	233 (52%)	36 (11%)	134 (33%)	169 (17%)	149 (15%)	79 (52%)
Hypertension	3,503 (45%)	540 (45%)	896 (49%)	378 (36%)	206 (53%)	318 (71%)	136 (42%)	253 (62%)	265 (26%)	447 (45%)	64 (42%)
Hypercholesterolemia	3,386 (52%)	694 (58%)	725 (44%)	460 (44%)	146 (40%)	275 (61%)	201 (63%)	322 (79%)	NA	509 (52%)	54 (36%)
Peripheral vascular disease	665 (10%)	64 (5%)	303 (17%)	72 (7%)	NA	103 (23%)	26 (8%)	0 (0%)	NA	66 (7%)	31 (20%)
Unstable symptoms	2,653 (41%)	451 (37%)	1,250 (68%)	166 (16%)	NA	412 (92%)	41 (13%)	0 (0%)	NA	202 (20%)	131 (86%)
Previous myocardial infarction	3,506 (45%)	520 (43%)	987 (55%)	439 (43%)	160 (41%)	126 (28%)	150 (47%)	191 (47%)	428 (43%)	448 (45%)	57 (38%)
Heart failure	245 (3%)	0 (0%)	161 (9%)	0 (0%)	13 (3%)	0 (0%)	0 (0%)	0 (0%)	0 (0%)	62 (6%)	9 (6%)
Abnormal left ventricular function	1,166 (17%)	189 (17%)	341 (19%)	138 (15%)	63 (16%)	88 (20%)	25 (13%)	13 (3%)	142 (26%)	153 (20%)	14 (9%)
Three-vessel disease	2,853 (37%)	338 (29%)	754 (41%)	449 (43%)	156 (40%)	219 (49%)	119 (38%)	230 (56%)	125 (12%)	419 (42%)	44 (29%)
Proximal LAD disease	3,391 (51%)	NA	668 (37%)	638 (61%)	283 (72%)	230 (51%)	92 (28%)	389 (95%)	567 (56%)	457 (46%)	67 (44%)
Follow-up (years)	5.9 (5.0–10.0)	5.1 (5.0–5.3)	10.4 (10.0–11.0)	3.0 (2.4–3.7)	8.2 (8.2–8.2)	5.0 (5.0–5.0)	13.0 (12.1–14.5)	5.1 (5.1–5.2)	10.0 (10.0–10.0)	6.0 (5.5–6.7)	4.9 (40–5.7)
Stent use in PCI[a]	1,432 (37%)	580 (98%)	9 (1%)	0 (0%)	0 (0%)	221 (100%)	0 (0%)	157 (82%)	0 (0%)	465 (97%)	0 (0%)
IMA use in CABG[b]	2,573 (83%)	539 (93%)	729 (82%)	NA	NA	198 (96%)	62 (39%)	188 (95%)	364 (74%)	451 (93%)	42 (55%)

ARTS Arterial Revascularization Therapies Study; *BARI* Bypass Angioplasty Revascularization Investigation; *CABRI* Coronary Angioplasty vs. Bypass Revascularisation Investigation; *CABG* coronary artery bypass graft; *EAST* Emory Angioplasty vs. Surgery Trial; *ERACI* Argentine Randomized Trial of Coronary Angioplasty vs. Bypass Surgery in Multivessel Disease; *GABI* German Angioplasty Bypass Surgery Investigation; *IMA* internal mammary artery; *LAD* left anterior descending artery; *MASS* Medicine, Angioplasty, or Surgery Study; *NA* not available; *RITA* Randomized Intervention Treatment of Angina trial; *SoS* Stent of Surgery trial

Data are in (%) or median (IQR). The number of randomized patients in each trial (*N*) is shown. Patients with missing data were omitted from the calculation of percentages for baseline characteristics. For trials from which data were available, between 0 and 51 (0–7%) patients had missing values on baseline characteristics, apart from hypercholesterolemia (228 missing values) and left ventricular function (1,066 missing values). Definitions for hypertension and hypercholesterolemia differed among the trials

[a] Stent use in 3,841 patients assigned to PCI who received this treatment

[b] Eight trials provided individual patient data on IMA use, in which 3,087 patients assigned to GABG received this treatment. The CABRI trial [3] previously reported 81% use of IMA grafts

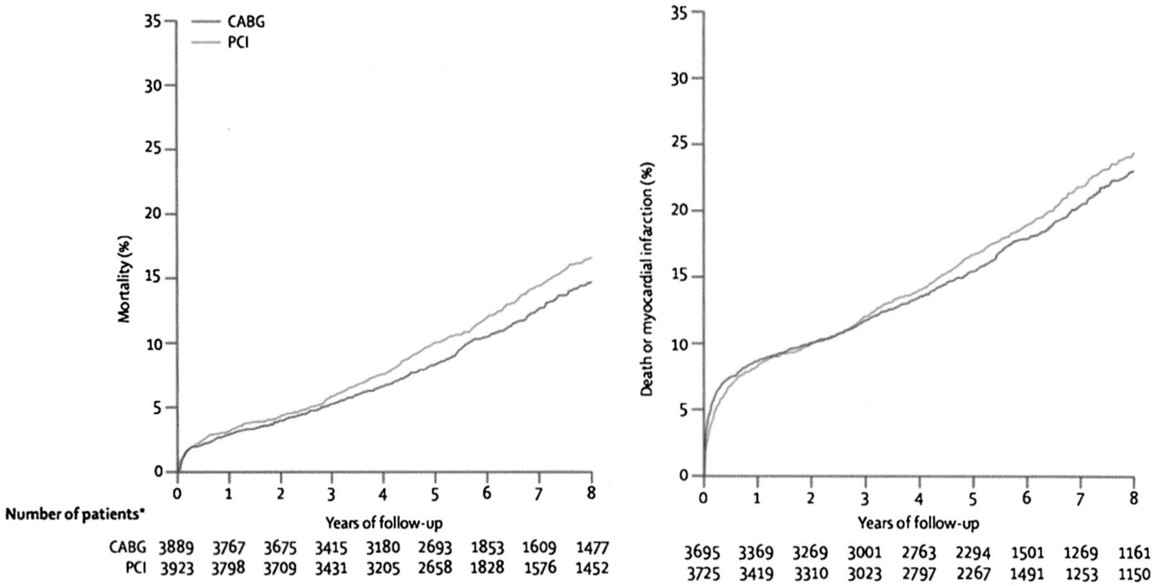

Fig. 15.12 Kaplan–Meier curves for mortality (*left*) and the composite of death and MI (*right*). Individual patient data was obtained from ten randomized clinical trials. No differences between coronary artery bypass graft (CABG) and PCI were detected (adapted from [117]. Copyright 2009 by The Lancet Publishing Group)

Table 15.10 Comparison of CABG and PCI in patients with multivessel disease in a collaborative meta-analysis of ten randomized clinical trials

	5-year event rate (% (95% CI))			
	CABG	PCI	Hazard ratio (95% CI)[a]	*p* Value
Death	8.4% (7.4–9.2)	10.0% (9.0–10.9)	0.91 (0.82–1.02)	0.12
Death or myocardial infarction[b]	15.4% (14.2–16.6)	16.7% (15.4–17.9)	0.97 (0.88–1.06)	0.47
Death or repeat revascularization[c]	9.9% (8.9–10.9)	24.5% (23.0–26.0)	0.41 (0.37–0.45)	<0.0001
Death, myocardial infarction, or repeat revascularization[d]	20.1% (18.7–21.4)	36.4% (34.8–38.0)	0.52 (0.49–0.57)	<0.0001

Event rates are unadjusted, 5-year Kaplan–Meier estimates

[a] Hazard ratios for coronary artery bypass graft (CARG) vs. percutaneous coronary intervention (PCI) are based on the full duration of follow-up from all trials

[b] No data were available on myocardial infarction from the Emory Angioplasty vs. Surgery Trial (EAST) [4]

[c] No data were available on repeat revascularization from the Toulouse trial [10]

[d] No data were available from the EAST [4] and Toulouse [10] trials

of interventional cardiology as well as cardiac surgery in the last 2 decades. Although it is useful to consider these clinical trials in the context of major technological or procedural breakthroughs (i.e., stents, internal mammary artery grafts), most of these strategy-based trials have yielded similar results, establishing equipoise for mortality and MI reductions with superiority of CABG vs. PCI regarding repeat revascularization procedures.

Hlatky et al. [117] conducted a collaborative meta-analysis of individual patient data ($n=7,812$) from ten randomized clinical trials comparing CABG with either balloon angioplasty or bare metal stents. Mortality and myocardial infarction rates at 5 years were similar in the two groups (Fig. 15.12 and Table 15.10), whereas CABG was associated with a significant reduction in repeat revascularization procedures.

In certain angiographic and clinical subgroups (i.e., left main coronary artery disease, diabetics with multivessel coronary disease, multivessel disease with reduced systolic performance, multivessel disease with proximal LAD disease), the superiority of CABG over medical therapy has clouded a direct comparison with PCI. Some clinical trials, registry data, and a meta-analysis [117] have suggested a reduction in death and MI rates with CABG over PCI among patients with diabetes and patients aged 65 years or older (Fig. 15.13).

Theoretical advantages of CABG in these angiographic subsets are more complete revascularization and superior long-term patency for the internal mammary artery graft anastomosed to the left anterior descending artery [118]. Therefore, in

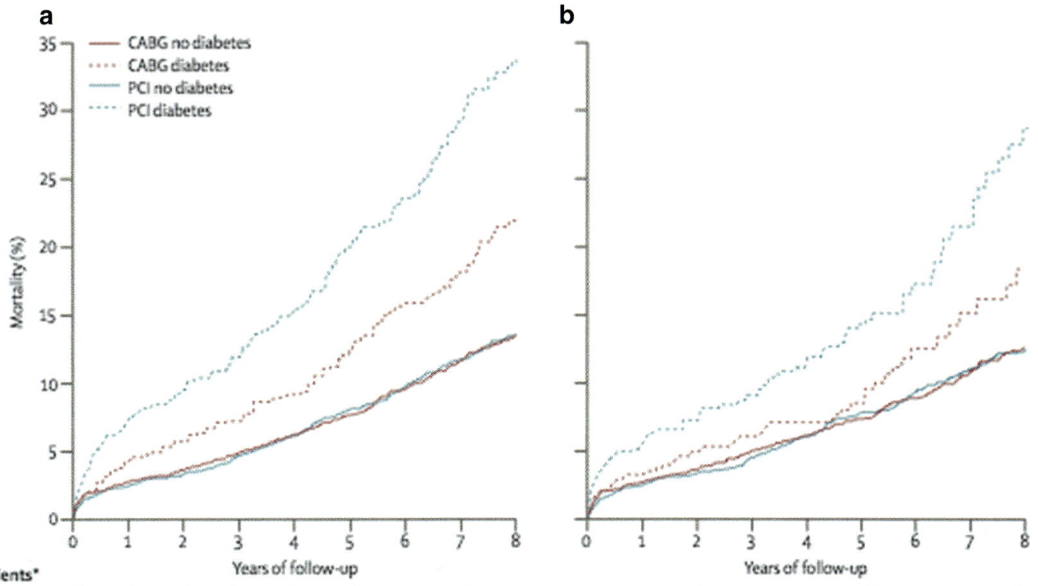

Number of patients*

	a: 0	1	2	3	4	5	6	7	8	b: 0	1	2	3	4	5	6	7	8
CABG no diabetes	3263	3169	3089	2877	2677	2267	1592	1380	1274	2529	2457	2382	2179	1992	1598	940	747	655
CABG diabetes	615	587	575	532	498	421	257	225	200	435	420	410	371	344	278	120	91	73
PCI no diabetes	3298	3217	3148	2918	2725	2281	1608	1393	1288	2556	2493	2432	2215	2031	1606	946	750	655
PCI diabetes	618	574	555	508	475	373	218	179	160	445	421	408	369	344	258	110	81	66

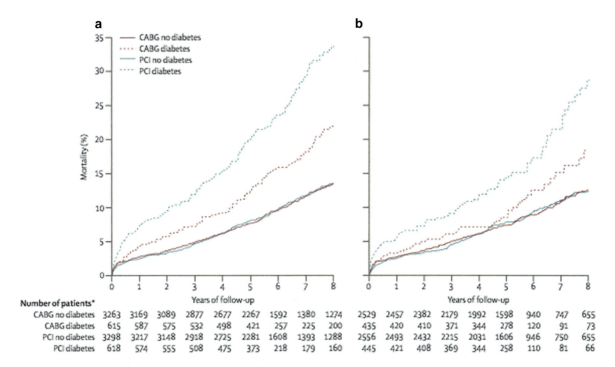

Fig. 15.13 CABG vs. PCI among patients with multivessel disease and diabetes. (**a**) All patients from ten randomized controlled trials are included. (**b**) Patients from the BARI trial have been excluded. The differences in survival between PCI and CABG, however, persisted after exclusion of BARI patients (adapted from [117]. Copyright 2009 by The Lancet Publishing Group)

the above-mentioned subsets, current guidelines recommend CABG as the preferred revascularization modality, whereas PCI remains an option for patients with prohibitive surgical risks [1]. The ongoing debate as to how to best treat these patients underscores the need for adequately powered randomized clinical trials.

Contemporary Trials of CABG vs. Stenting

The SYNergy between PCI with TAXus and Cardiac Surgery (SYNTAX) Trial randomly assigned 1,800 patients with three-vessel or left main disease to undergo CABG or PCI [119]. All patients were considered to have suitable anatomy for either revascularization modality. At 12 months, the composite of death, myocardial infarction, or repeat revascularization was higher for the PCI group compared to the CABG group (17.8% vs. 12.4%, $p=0.002$). The difference between the two groups was driven by higher repeat revascularization rates in the PCI group compared to the CABG group (13.5% vs. 5.9%, $p<0.001$) with similar death (4.4% vs. 3.5%, $p=0.37$) and MI rates (4.8% vs. 3.3%, $p=0.11$) at 12 months (Fig. 15.14). Patients treated with PCI were less likely to have a stroke (2.2% vs. 0.6%, $p=0.003$). The SYNTAX trial once again has confirmed that PCI and CABG are associated with similar rates of death and myocardial infarction in patients with multivessel coronary artery disease.

The superiority of CABG over PCI regarding repeat revascularization procedures remains in the drug-eluting stent era. Interestingly, this benefit is partially offset by an increased risk of stroke. The ongoing FREEDOM, CARDIA, and VA Cards trials are enrolling patients with diabetes and mutivessel coronary artery disease and randomizing them to drug-eluting stents vs. CABG.

Conclusions and Future Directions

The prognosis of the millions of patients who live with chronic stable angina has improved dramatically over the last 4 decades. Annual mortality rates for medically treated patients with stable angina in the VA Cooperative Study and ECSS were 4.25 and 3.2%, respectively. By contrast, the COURAGE trial reported an annual mortality of 0.8% for the medical

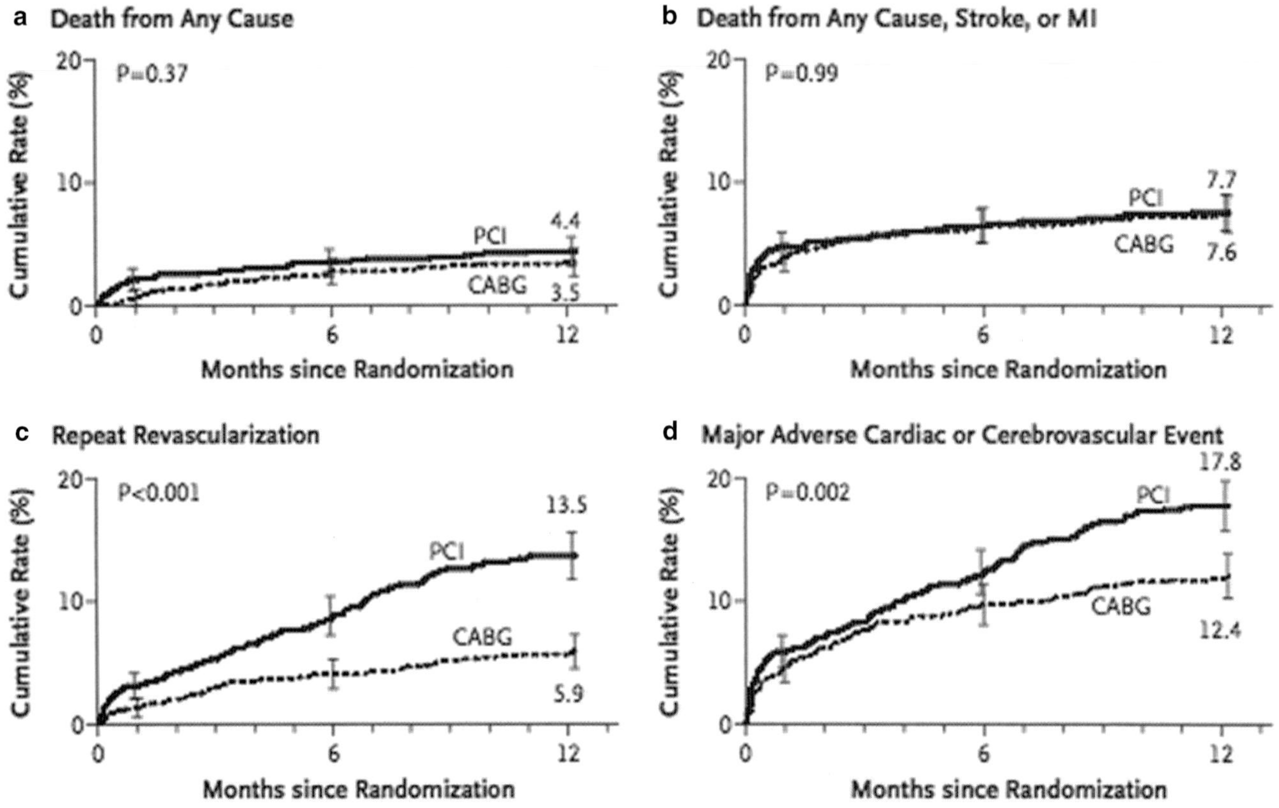

Fig. 15.14 In the The SYNergy between PCI with TAXus and Cardiac Surgery (SYNTAX) trial, PCI with paclitaxel-eluting stents was associated with increased rates of repeat revascularization procedures and similar rates of death and MI when compared to CABG (adapted from [119], p. 968. Copyright 2009 by Massachusetts Medical Society)

arm. Likewise, improvements in surgical and interventional techniques have dramatically reduced the upfront risk of these interventions while improving the long-term patency of the conduits or stented vessels. For example, operative mortality in the VA Cooperative Study was 5.8% compared to 1.4% [44, 92] in the recently reported BARI 2D trial.

Despite our best efforts, the incidence of chronic stable angina, as well as angina refractory to medical and revascularization therapy, is likely to grow in the future as the population ages and risk factors for coronary heart disease increase in prevalence. A new wave of clinical trials is needed to assess the role of experimental therapies such as stem cells and hybrid revascularization procedures.

References

1. Gibbons RJ, Abrams J, Chatterjee K, et al. ACC/AHA 2002 guideline update for the management of patients with chronic stable angina: a report of the American College of Cardiology/American Heart Association Task Force on Practice Guidelines (committee to update the 1999 guidelines for the management of patients with chronic stable angina). 17 Nov 2002. http://www.americanheart.org/downloadable/heart/1044991838085StableAnginaNewFigs.pdf. Accessed 21 May 2010.
2. The American Heart Association. Heart and stroke. Statistical update. Dallas: American Heart Association; 1999.
3. Kannel WB, Feinleib M. Natural history of angina pectoris in the Framingham study. Prognosis and survival. Am J Cardiol. 1972;29:154–63.
4. Writing Group for the Bypass Angioplasty Revascularization Investigation (BARI) Investigators. Five-year clinical and functional outcome comparing bypass surgery and angioplasty in patients with multivessel coronary disease: a multicenter randomized trial. JAMA. 1997;277: 715–21.
5. Diamond GA, Forester JS. Analysis of probability as an aid in the clinical diagnosis of coronary-artery disease. N Engl J Med. 1979;300: 1350–8.
6. Chaitman BR, Bourassa MG, Davis K, et al. Angiographic prevalence of high-risk coronary artery disease in patient subsets (CASS). Circulation. 1981;64:360–7.

7. Gibbons RJ, Balady GJ, Bricker JT, et al. ACC/AHA 2002 guideline update for exercise testing: a report of the American College of Cardiology/American Heart Association Task Force on Practice Guidelines (Committee on Exercise Testing). Circulation. 2002;106(14):1883–92.
8. Morise AP, Diamond GA. Comparison of the sensitivity and specificity of exercise electrocardiography in biased and unbiased populations of men and women. Am Heart J. 1995;130:741–7.
9. Froelicher VF, Lehmann KG, Thomas R, et al. The electrocardiographic exercise test in a population with reduced workup bias: diagnostic performance, computerized interpretation, and multi-variable prediction. Veterans Affairs Cooperative Study in Health Services #016 (QUEXTA) Study Group. Quantitative exercise testing and angiography. Ann Intern Med. 1998;128:965–74.
10. Marcus ML, Chilian WM, Kanatsuka H, Dellsperger KC, Eastham CL, Lamping KG. Understanding the coronary circulation through studies at the microvascular level. Circulation. 1990;82:1–7.
11. Kern M, Lim M. Grossman's cardiac catheterization, angiography and intervention. 7th ed. Philadelphia: Lippincott Williams & Wilkins; 2005.
12. Wilson RF. Assessing the severity of coronary-artery stenoses [editorial]. N Engl J Med. 1996;334:1735–7.
13. Mock MB, Ringqvist I, Fisher LD, et al. Survival of medically treated patients in the Coronary Artery Surgery Study (CASS) registry. Circulation. 1982;66:562–8.
14. Weiner DA, Ryan TJ, McCabe CH, et al. Prognostic importance of a clinical profile and exercise test in medically treated patients with coronary artery disease. J Am Coll Cardiol. 1984;3:772–9.
15. Hammermeister KE, DeRouen TA, Dodge HT. Variables predictive of survival in patients with coronary disease. Selection by univariate and multivariate analyses from the clinical, electrocardiographic, exercise, arteriographic, and quantitative angiographic evaluations. Circulation. 1979;59:421–30.
16. Block Jr WJ, Crumpacker EL, Dry TJ, Gage RP. Prognosis of angina pectoris: observations in 6,882 cases. JAMA. 1952;150:259–64.
17. Califf RM, Armstrong PW, Carver JR, et al. Task Force 5. Stratification of patients into high-, medium-, and low-risk subgroups for purposes of risk factor management. J Am Coll Cardiol. 1996;27:964–1047.
18. Pontone G, Andreini D, Bartorelli AL, et al. Diagnostic accuracy of coronary computed tomography angiography: a comparison between prospective and retrospective electrocardiogram triggering. J Am Coll Cardiol. 2009;54:346–55.
19. Ritchie JL, Bateman TM, Bonow RO, et al. Guidelines for clinical use of cardiac radionuclide imaging. Report of the American College of Cardiology/American Heart Association Task Force on Assessment of Diagnostic and Therapeutic Cardiovascular Procedures (Committee on Radionuclide Imaging), developed in collaboration with the American Society of Nuclear Cardiology. J Am Coll Cardiol. 1995;25:521–47.
20. Cheitlin MD, Alpert JS, Armstrong WF, et al. ACC/AHA Guidelines for the Clinical Application of Echocardiography. A report of the American College of Cardiology/American Heart Association Task Force on Practice Guidelines (Committee on Clinical Application of Echocardiography). Developed in collaboration with the American Society of Echocardiography. Circulation. 1997;95:1686–744.
21. Cassar A, Holmes D, Rihal C, Gersh B. Chronic coronary artery disease: diagnosis and management. Mayo Clin Proc. 2009;84(12):1130–46.
22. Mark DB, Hlatky MA, Harrell Jr FE, Lee KL, Califf RM, Pryor DB. Exercise treadmill score for predicting prognosis in coronary artery disease. Ann Intern Med. 1987;106(6):793–800.
23. Pyorala K, De Backer G, Graham I, Poole-Wilson P, Wood D. Prevention of coronary heart disease in clinical practice: recommendations of the Task Force of the European Society of Cardiology, European Atherosclerosis Society and European Society of Hypertension. Atherosclerosis. 1994;110:121–61.
24. US Department of Health and Human Services. The health benefits of smoking cessation. A report of the surgeon general. Washington, DC: US Department of Health and Human Services; 1990.
25. Multiple Risk Factor Intervention Trial Research Group. Multiple Risk Factor Intervention Trial. Risk factor changes and mortality results. JAMA. 1982;248:1465–77.
26. Hjermann I, Velve Byre K, Holme I, Leren P. Effect of diet and smoking intervention on the incidence of coronary heart disease. Report from the Oslo Study Group of a randomised trial in healthy men. Lancet. 1981;2:1303–10.
27. Singh RB, Rastogi SS, Verma R, et al. Randomised controlled trial of cardioprotective diet in patients with recent acute myocardial infarction: results of one year follow up. BMJ. 1992;304:1015–9.
28. Schuler G, Hambrecht R, Schlierf G, et al. Regular physical exercise and low-fat diet. Effects on progression of coronary artery disease. Circulation. 1992;86:1–11.
29. Smith Jr SC, Blair SN, Criqui MH, et al. AHA consensus panel statement: preventing heart attack and death in patients with coronary disease. The Secondary Prevention Panel. J Am Coll Cardiol. 1995;26:292–4.
30. Superko HR, Krauss RM. Coronary artery disease regression: convincing evidence for the benefit of aggressive lipoprotein management. Circulation. 1994;90:1056–69.
31. Rossouw JE. Lipid-lowering interventions in angiographic trials. Am J Cardiol. 1995;76:86C–92.
32. The fifth report of the Joint National Committee on detection, evaluation, and treatment of high blood pressure (JNC V). Arch Intern Med. 1993;153:154–83
33. Stamler J, Neaton J, Wentworth D. Blood pressure (systolic and diastolic) and risk of fatal coronary heart disease. Hypertension. 1993;13:2–12.
34. MacMahon S, Peto R, Cutler J, et al. Blood pressure, stroke, and coronary heart disease. Part 1, prolonged differences in blood pressure: prospective observational studies corrected for the regression dilution bias. Lancet. 1990;335:765–74.
35. Effects of treatment on morbidity in hypertension: results in patients with diastolic blood pressures averaging 115 through 129 mm Hg. JAMA. 1967;202:1028–34.
36. Effects of treatment on morbidity in hypertension, II: results in patients with diastolic blood pressure averaging 90 through 114 mm Hg. JAMA. 1970;213:1143–52.
37. Collins R, Peto R, MacMahon S, et al. Blood pressure, stroke, and coronary heart disease. Part 2, short-term reductions in blood pressure: overview of randomised drug trials in their epidemiological context. Lancet. 1990;335:827–38.

38. Cutler JA, Psaty BM, McMahon S, Furberg CD. Public health issues in hypertension control: what has been learned from clinical trials. In: Laragh JH, Brenner BM, editors. Hypertension: pathophysiology, diagnosis, and management. 2nd ed. New York: Raven; 1995. p. 253–70.
39. Neaton JD, Grimm RH, Prineas RJ, et al. Treatment of Mild Hypertension Study. Final results. Treatment of Mild Hypertension Study Research Group. JAMA. 1993;270:713–24.
40. LaRosa JC, Grundy SM, Waters DD, et al. Intensive lipid lowering with atorvastatin in patients with stable coronary disease. N Engl J Med. 2005;352:1425–35.
41. UK Prospective Diabetes Study (UKPDS) Group. Intensive blood-glucose control with sulphonylureas or insulin compared with conventional treatment and risk of complications in patients with type 2 diabetes (UKPDS 33). Lancet. 1998;352:837–53.
42. UK Prospective Diabetes Study (UKPDS) Group. Effect of intensive blood-glucose control with metformin on complications in overweight patients with type 2 diabetes (UKPDS 34). Lancet. 1998;352:854–65.
43. Reichard P, Nilsson BY, Rosenqvist U. The effect of long-term intensified insulin treatment on the development of microvascular complications of diabetes mellitus. N Engl J Med. 1993;329:304–9.
44. Takaro T, Hultgren H, Lipton M, Detre K. The Veterans Administration randomized study of surgery for coronary arterial occlusive disease II. Subgroup with significant left main lesions. Circulation. 1976;54(6 Suppl):III107–17.
45. European Coronary Surgery Study Group. Coronary artery bypass surgery in stable angina pectoris: survival at two years. Lancet. 1979;1: 889–93.
46. CASS Principal Investigators and Their Associates. Myocardial infarction and mortality in the Coronary Artery Surgery Study (CASS) randomized trial. N Engl J Med. 1984;310:750–8.
47. Frye R, Fisher L, Schaff H, Gersh B, Vlietstra R, Mock M. Randomized trials in coronary artery bypass surgery. Prog Cardiovasc Dis. 1987; 30:1–22.
48. Boden WE, O'Rourke RA, Teo KK, et al; for the COURAGE Trial Research Group. Optimal medical therapy with or without PCI for stable coronary disease. N Engl J Med. 2007;356:1503–16.
49. Frishman WH, Heiman M, Soberman J, Greenberg S, Eff J. Comparison of celiprolol and propranolol in stable angina pectoris. Celiprolol International Angina Study Group. Am J Cardiol. 1991;67:665–70.
50. Narahara KA. Double-blind comparison of once daily betaxolol versus propranolol four times daily in stable angina pectoris. Betaxolol Investigators Group. Am J Cardiol. 1990;65:577–82.
51. Hauf-Zachariou U, Blackwood RA, Gunawardena KA, O'Donnell JG, Garnham S, Pfarr E. Carvedilol versus verapamil in chronic stable angina: a multicentre trial. Eur J Clin Pharmacol. 1997;52:95–100.
52. Raftery EB. The preventative effects of vasodilating beta-blockers in cardiovascular disease. Eur Heart J. 1996;17(Suppl B):30–8.
53. McLenachan JM, Findlay IN, Wilson JT, Dargie HJ. Twenty-four-hour beta-blockade in stable angina pectoris: a study of atenolol and betaxolol. J Cardiovasc Pharmacol. 1992;20:311–5.
54. Prida XE, Hill JA, Feldman RL. Systemic and coronary hemodynamic effects of combined alpha- and beta-adrenergic blockade (labetalol) in normotensive patients with stable angina pectoris and positive exercise stress test responses. Am J Cardiol. 1987;59:1084–8.
55. Capone P, Mayol R. Celiprolol in the treatment of exercise induced angina pectoris. J Cardiovasc Pharmacol. 1986;8 Suppl 4:S135–7.
56. Ryden L. Efficacy of epanolol versus metoprolol in angina pectoris: report from a Swedish multicentre study of exercise tolerance. J Intern Med. 1992;231:7–11.
57. Boberg J, Larsen FF, Pehrsson SK. The effects of beta blockade with (epanolol) and without (atenolol) intrinsic sympathomimetic activity in stable angina pectoris. The Visacor Study Group. Clin Cardiol. 1992;15:591–5.
58. CAPRICORN Investigators. Effect of carvedilol on outcome after myocardial infarction in patients with left-ventricular dysfunction: the CAPRICORN randomised trial. Lancet. 2001;357:1385–90.
59. Beta-Blocker Heart Attack Trial Research Group. A randomized trial of propranolol in patients with acute myocardial infarction. Mortality results. JAMA. 1982;247:1707–14.
60. Norwegian Multicenter Study Group. Timolol-induced reduction in mortality and reinfarction in patients surviving acute myocardial infarction. N Engl J Med. 1981;304:801–7.
61. Wallace WA, Wellington KL, Chess MA, Liang CS. Comparison of nifedipine gastrointestinal therapeutic system and atenolol on antianginal efficacies and exercise hemodynamic responses in stable angina pectoris. Am J Cardiol. 1994;73:23–8.
62. de Vries RJ, van den Heuvel AF, Lok DJ, et al. Nifedipine gastrointestinal therapeutic system versus atenolol in stable angina pectoris. The Netherlands Working Group on Cardiovascular Research (WCN). Int J Cardiol. 1996;57:143–50.
63. Fox KM, Mulcahy D, Findlay I, Ford I, Dargie HJ. The Total Ischaemic Burden European Trial (TIBET). Effects of atenolol, nifedipine SR and their combination on the exercise test and the total ischaemic burden in 608 patients with stable angina. The TIBET Study Group. Eur Heart J. 1996;17:96–103.
64. Parmley WW, Nesto RW, Singh BN, Deanfield J, Gottlieb SO. Attenuation of the circadian patterns of myocardial ischemia with nifedipine GITS in patients with chronic stable angina. N-CAP Study Group. J Am Coll Cardiol. 1992;19:1380–9.
65. Tatti P, Pahor M, Byington RP, et al. Outcome results of the Fosinopril Versus Amlodipine Cardiovascular Events Randomized Trial (FACET) in patients with hypertension and non-insulin dependent diabetes mellitus. Diabetes Care. 1998;21:597–603.
66. Singh BN. Comparative efficacy and safety of bepridil and diltiazem in chronic stable angina pectoris refractory to diltiazem. The Bepridil Collaborative Study Group. Am J Cardiol. 1991;68:306–12.
67. Furberg CD, Psaty BM, Meyer JV. Nifedipine: dose-related increase in mortality in patients with coronary heart disease. Circulation. 1995;92:1326–31.
68. Kaski JC, Plaza LR, Meran DO, Araujo L, Chierchia S, Maseri A. Improved coronary supply: prevailing mechanism of action of nitrates in chronic stable angina. Am Heart J. 1985;110:238–45.
69. Lacoste LL, Theroux P, Lidon RM, Colucci R, Lam JY. Anti-thrombotic properties of transdermal nitroglycerin in stable angina pectoris. Am J Cardiol. 1994;73:1058–62.
70. Tirlapur VG, Mir MA. Cardiorespiratory effects of isosorbide dinitrate and nifedipine in combination with nadolol: a double-blind comparative study of beneficial and adverse antianginal drug interactions. Am J Cardiol. 1984;53:487–92.

71. Schneider W, Maul FD, Bussmann WD, Lang E, Hor G, Kaltenbach M. Comparison of the antianginal efficacy of isosorbide dinitrate (ISDN) 40 mg and verapamil 120 mg three times daily in the acute trial and following two-week treatment. Eur Heart J. 1988;9:149–58.
72. Ankier SI, Fay L, Warrington SJ, Woodings DF. A multicentre open comparison of isosorbide-5-mononitrate and nifedipine given prophylactically to general practice patients with chronic stable angina pectoris. J Int Med Res. 1989;17:172–8.
73. Emanuelsson H, Ake H, Kristi M, Arina R. Effects of diltiazem and isosorbide-5-mononitrate, alone and in combination, on patients with stable angina pectoris. Eur J Clin Pharmacol. 1989;36:561–5.
74. Akhras F, Chambers J, Jefferies S, Jackson G. A randomised double-blind crossover study of isosorbide mononitrate and nifedipine retard in chronic stable angina. Int J Cardiol. 1989;24:191–6.
75. Akhras F, Jackson G. Efficacy of nifedipine and isosorbide mononitrate in combination with atenolol in stable angina. Lancet. 1991;338: 1036–9.
76. Ridker PM, Manson JE, Gaziano JM, Buring JE, Hennekens CH. Low-dose aspirin therapy for chronic stable angina. A randomized, placebo-controlled clinical trial. Ann Intern Med. 1991;114:835–9.
77. Antiplatelet Trialists Collaboration. Collaborative overview of randomised trials of antiplatelet therapy, I: prevention of death, myocardial infarction and stroke by prolonged antiplatelet therapy in various categories of patients. BMJ. 1995;308:81–106.
78. Lewis HD, Davis JW, Archibald DG, et al. Protective effects of aspirin against acute myocardial infarction and death in men with unstable angina: results of a Veterans Administration cooperative study. N Engl J Med. 1983;309:396–403.
79. Cairns JA, Gent M, Singer J, et al. Aspirin, sulfinpyrazone, or both in unstable angina. Results of a Canadian multicenter trial. N Engl J Med. 1985;313:1369–75.
80. Juul-Moller S, Edvardsson N, Jahnmatz B, Rosen A, Sorensen S, Omblus R. Double-blind trial of aspirin in primary prevention of myocardial infarction in patients with stable chronic angina pectoris. The Swedish Angina Pectoris Aspirin Trial (SAPAT) Group. Lancet. 1992;340: 1421–5.
81. The Clopidogrel in Unstable Angina to Prevent Recurrent Events Trial Investigators. Effects of clopidogrel in addition to aspirin in patients with acute coronary syndromes without ST-segment elevation. N Engl J Med. 2001;3457:494–502.
82. Mehta SR, Yusuf S, Peters RJG, et al. Effects of pretreatment with clopidogrel and aspirin followed by long-term therapy in patients undergoing percutaneous coronary intervention: the PCI-CURE study. Lancet. 2001;358:527–33.
83. Bhatt D, Fox KA, Hacke W, et al; for the CHARISMA Investigators. Clopidogrel and aspirin versus aspirin alone for the prevention of atherothrombotic events. N Engl J Med. 2006;354(16):1706–17.
84. The Medical Research Council's General Practice Research Framework. Thrombosis prevention trial: randomised trial of low-intensity oral anticoagulation with warfarin and low-dose aspirin in the primary prevention of ischaemic heart disease in men at increased risk. Lancet. 1998;351:233–41.
85. The Heart Outcomes Prevention Evaluation Study Investigators. Effects of an angiotensin-converting-enzyme inhibitor, ramipril, on cardiovascular events in high-risk patients. N Engl J Med. 2000;342:145–53.
86. The EURopean trial On reduction of cardiac events with Perindopril in stable coronary Artery disease Investigators. Efficacy of perindopril in reduction of cardiovascular events among patients with stable coronary artery disease: randomised, double-blind, placebo-controlled, multicentre trial (the EUROPA study). Lancet. 2003;362(9399):1935.
87. Larosa JC, Hunninghake D, Bush D, et al. The cholesterol facts: a summary of the evidence relating dietary fats, serum cholesterol, and coronary heart disease. A joint statement by the American Heart Association and the National Heart, Lung, and Blood Institute. The Task Force on Cholesterol Issues, American Heart Association. Circulation. 1990;81:1721–33.
88. Gould AL, Rossouw JE, Santanello NC, Heyse JF, Furberg CD. Cholesterol reduction yields clinical benefit: impact of statin trials. Circulation. 1998;97:946–52.
89. Sacks FM, Pfeffer MA, Moye LA, et al. The effect of pravastatin on coronary events after myocardial infarction in patients with average cholesterol levels. Cholesterol and Recurrent Events Trial investigators. N Engl J Med. 1996;335:1001–9.
90. Diamond GA, Kaul S. COURAGE under fire. On the management of stable coronary disease. J Am Coll Cardiol. 2007;50:1604–9.
91. Kereikaes DJ, Teirstein PS, Sarembock IJ, et al. The truth and consequences of the COURAGE trial. J Am Coll Cardiol. 2007;50:1598–603.
92. BARI 2D Study Group. A randomized trial of therapies for type 2 diabetes and coronary artery disease. N Engl J Med. 2009;360(24):2503–15.
93. Weintraub WS, Boden WE, Zhang Z, et al. Cost-effectiveness of percutaneous coronary intervention in optimally treated stable coronary patients. Circ Cardiovasc Qual Outcomes. 2008;1:12–20.
94. Krone RJ, Shaw RE, Klein LW, et al. Ad hoc percutaneous coronary interventions in patients with stable coronary artery disease – a study of prevalence, safety, and variation in use from the America College of Cardiology National Cardiovascular Data Registry (ACC-NCDR). Catheter Cardiovasc Interv. 2006;68:696–703.
95. Hannan E, Racz MJ, Gold J, et al. Adherence of catheterization laboratory cardiologists to American College of Cardiology/American Heart Association guidelines for percutaneous coronary interventions and coronary artery bypass graft surgery. What happens in actual practice? Circulation. 2010;121:267–75.
96. Gawande A. The cost conondrum. New Yorker, 1 June 2009.
97. Lin GA, Dudley RA, Lucas FL, et al. Frequency of stress testing to document ischemia prior to elective percutaneous coronary intervention. JAMA. 2008;300(15):1765–73.
98. Gould KL, Lipscomb K, Hamilton GW. Physiologic basis for assessing critical coronary stenosis: instantaneous flow response and regional distribution during coronary hyperemia as measures of coronary flow reserve. Am J Cardiol. 1974;33:87–94.
99. Wilson RF, Marcus ML, White CW. Prediction of the physiologic significance of coronary arterial lesions by quantitative lesion geometry in patients with limited coronary artery disease. Circulation. 1987;75:723–32.
100. White CW, Wright CB, Doty DB, et al. Does visual interpretation of the coronary arteriogram predict the physiologic importance of a coronary stenosis? N Engl J Med. 1984;310:819–24.
101. Tonino PA, De Bruyne B, Pijls NHJ, et al. Fractional flow reserve versus angiography for guiding percutaneous coronary intervention. N Engl J Med. 2009;360:213–24.

102. Pijls NH, van Schaardenburgh P, Manoharan G, et al. Percutaneous coronary intervention of functionally nonsignificant stenosis: 5-year follow-up of the DEFER Study. J Am Coll Cardiol. 2007;49:2105–11.
103. Hachamovitch R, Hayes SW, Friedman JD, et al. Comparison of short-term survival benefit associated with revascularization compared with medical therapy in patients with no prior coronary artery disease undergoing stress myocardial perfusion single photon emission computed tomography. Circulation. 2003;107(23):2900–7.
104. Shaw L, Berman D, Baron DJ, et al. Optimal medical therapy with or without percutaneous coronary intervention to reduce ischemic burden. Results from the Clinical Outcomes Utilizing Revascularization and Aggressive Drug Evaluation (COURAGE) Trial Nuclear Substudy. Circulation. 2008;117:1283–91.
105. Hannan EL, Racz M, Holmes DR, et al. Impact of completeness of percutaneous coronary intervention revascularization on long-term outcomes in the stent era. Circulation. 2006;113:2406–12.
106. Van den Brand MJ, Rensing BJ, Morel MA, et al. The effect of completeness of revascularization on event-free survival at one year in the ARTS trial. J Am Coll Cardiol. 2002;39:559–64.
107. Rider J, Ward H, Moritz T, et al. Preoperative coronary artery revascularization and long-term outcome in patients with abdominal aortic operations and myocardial ischemia on SPECT: a post-hoc analysis of the CARP Trial [abstract 3346]. Circulation. 2006;114:II 711.
108. Favaloro RG. Saphenous vein graft in the surgical treatment of coronary artery disease. J Thorac Cardiovasc Surg. 1969;58:178.
109. Yusuf S, Zucker D, Peduzzi P, et al. Coronary artery bypass grafting (CABG): randomized studies comparing survival with CABG vs medical treatment. Lancet. 1994;334:563–70.
110. Lloyd-Jones D, Adams R, Carnethon M, et al. AHA Statistics Committee and Stroke Statistics Subcommittee – 2009 update: a report from the AHA Statistics Committee and Stroke Statistics Subcommittee. Circulation. 2009;119(3):480–6.
111. Bravaia DM, Glenger AL, McDonald KM, et al. Systematic review: the comparative effectiveness of percutaneous coronary interventions and coronary artery bypass graft surgery. Ann Intern Med. 2007;147(10):703–16.
112. BARI Investigators. The final 10-year follow-up results from the BARI randomized trial. J Am Coll Cardiol. 2007;49(15):1600–6.
113. Rodriguez A, Rodriguez Alemparte M, Baldi J, et al. Coronary stenting versus coronary bypass surgery in patients with multiple vessel disease and significant proximal LAD stenosis: results from the ERACl II study. Heart. 2003;89(2):184–8.
114. Investigators SoS. Coronary artery bypass surgery versus percutaneous coronary intervention with stent implantation in patients with multivessel coronary artery disease (the Stent or Surgery trial): a randomised controlled trial. Lancet. 2002;360(9338):965–70.
115. Serruys PW, Ong AT, van Herwerden LA, et al. Five-year outcomes after coronary stenting versus bypass surgery for the treatment of multivessel disease: the final analysis of the Arterial Revascularization Therapies Study (ARTS) randomized trial. J Am Coll Cardiol. 2005; 46(4):575–81.
116. Hannan EL, Racz MJ, Walford G, et al. Long-term outcomes of coronary artery bypass grafting versus stent implantation. N Engl J Med. 2005;352(21):2174–83.
117. Hlatky MA, Boothrnyd DB, Bravata DM, et al. Coronary artery bypass surgery compared with percutaneous coronary interventions for multivessel disease: a collaborative analysis of individual patient data from ten randomised trials. Lancet. 2009;373(9670):1190–7.
118. Taggart DP, D'Amico R, Altman DG. Effect of arterial revascularisation on survival: a systematic review of studies comparing bilateral and single internal mammary arteries. Lancet. 2001;358(9285):870–5.
119. Serruys PW, Morice MC, Kappetein AP, et al. Percutaneous coronary intervention versus coronary-artery bypass grafting for severe coronary artery disease. N Engl J Med. 2009;360(10):961–72.
120. Emond M, Mock MB, David KB, et al. Long-term survival of medically treated patients in the Coronary Artery Surgery Study (CASS) registry. Circulation. 1994;90:2645–57.

Chapter 16
Pathology of Sudden Death in Coronary Arterial Diseases

Shannon M. Mackey-Bojack, Emily R. Duncanson, and Susan J. Roe

Definition and Epidemiology

Sudden death can be defined as unexpected natural death occurring in an apparently healthy individual or in an individual whose illness is not so severe that death is not an expected outcome [1]. In the literature, the time from the onset of symptoms to death is a variable part of the definition [1, 2]. A few minutes up to 24 h have been suggested [1]. The extreme of a few minutes leaves out many deaths that should probably be classified as sudden, and the opposite extreme of 24 h is probably too inclusive. The interval of 6 h from onset of symptoms to a witnessed death, and less than 24 h from being seen in a stable condition to being found dead, has been suggested as a compromise [3].

Sudden cardiac death is one of the causes of sudden death [4]. Most cases of sudden death fall under the jurisdiction of a medical examiner/coroner. The interval of symptoms to death is less relevant to the medical examiner/coroner [5]. An unexpected, natural death of a person not recently seen by a physician and without a medical diagnosis should be investigated by the medical examiner/coroner. These investigations often include patients who collapse and are resuscitated, and later die in a hospital before a diagnosis is made.

Sudden death is estimated to comprise 15–20% of all natural deaths in industrialized countries [1]. Gillum indicated that more than 350,000 people die suddenly each year from cardiovascular disease (sudden cardiac death) in the United States [6]. In people between the ages of 35 and 74, the annual incidence of sudden death is estimated to be 191/100,000 for men and 57/100,000 for women [1]. In the pediatric age group – from ages 1–20 years – 1.3–8.5/100,000 persons die suddenly each year [1, 7], with many of these deaths attributed to a cardiac cause [7, 8]. One study of sudden death in subjects between the ages of 18 and 35 years cited 25% of the deaths were from coronary artery disease [9].

The final, common pathway for most sudden cardiac deaths is an ischemic-induced arrhythmia [1, 3]. The exact cause of the arrhythmia is often unclear [5]. The majority of fatal arrhythmias are ventricular fibrillation, ventricular tachycardia, and asystole [1]. These fatal arrhythmias are most often preceded by recent or prior ischemic myocardial damage.

Less commonly, mechanical arrest from cardiac rupture can lead to sudden death [1]. Fifty percent of sudden cardiac deaths in adults older than 35 years are due to coronary disease. This percentage declines with age, with older patients dying more frequently from complications of heart failure rather than of sudden ventricular arrhythmias [3]. In the pediatric age group, nonatherosclerotic coronary artery disease is more common. The etiology is often decreased regional blood flow leading to myocardial ischemia, causing a fatal arrhythmia [3].

Atherosclerotic Coronary Artery Disease

Atherosclerotic coronary artery disease is the most common cause of sudden, natural death of adults in the United States. Coronary artery disease accounts for the vast majority of sudden unexpected cardiac death in adults autopsied in medical examiners' offices. Sudden cardiac death may be the first indication of coronary artery atherosclerosis [10]. Approximately 25–50% of people dying suddenly from atherosclerotic coronary artery disease had no previous symptoms or diagnoses [11].

S.M. Mackey-Bojack, MD (✉) • E.R. Duncanson, MD • S.J. Roe, MD
Department of Jesse E. Edwards Registry of Cardiovascular Disease, United Hospital, St. Paul, MN, USA
e-mail: Shannon.Mackey-Bojack@allina.com

Z. Vlodaver et al. (eds.), *Coronary Heart Disease: Clinical, Pathological, Imaging, and Molecular Profiles*,
DOI 10.1007/978-1-4614-1475-9_16, © Springer Science+Business Media, LLC 2012

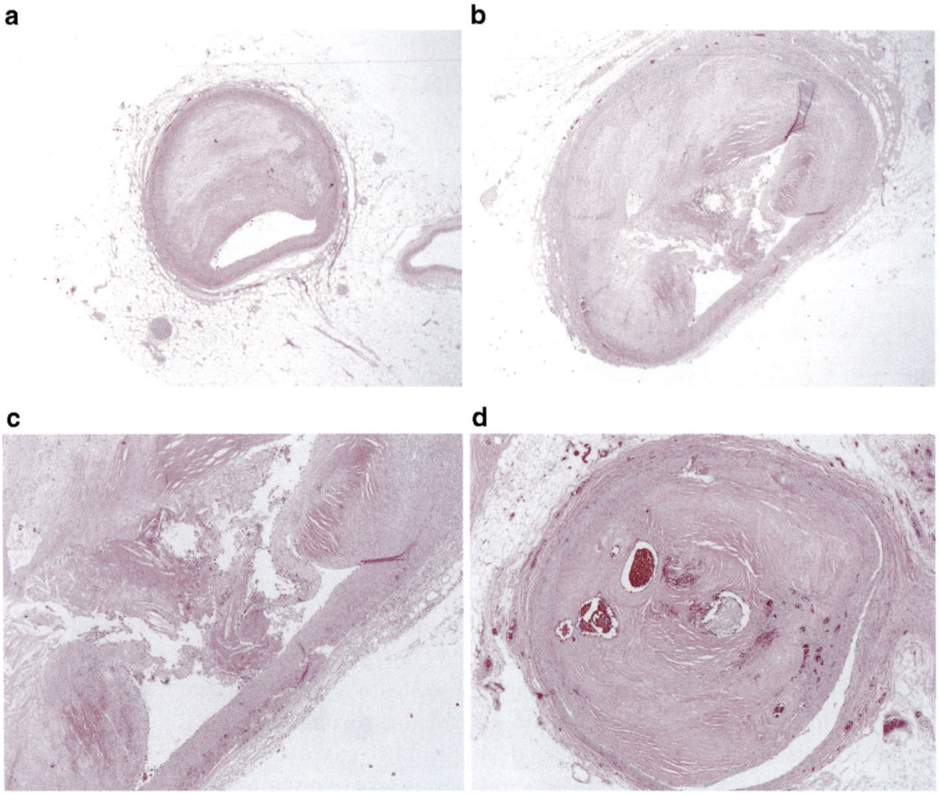

Fig. 16.1 (**a**) Photomicrograph showing 70–75% narrowing of left circumflex coronary artery by minimally calcified atherosclerotic plaque (H&E 2×). (**b**) Photomicrograph showing 80–85% narrowing of left circumflex coronary artery by atherosclerotic plaque, with acute plaque rupture into lumen (H&E 2×). (**c**) Higher magnification of (**b**) showing rupture into the lumen (H&E 4×). (**d**) Photomicrograph showing 95–99% narrowing by calcified, complicated atherosclerotic plaque (H&E 2×)

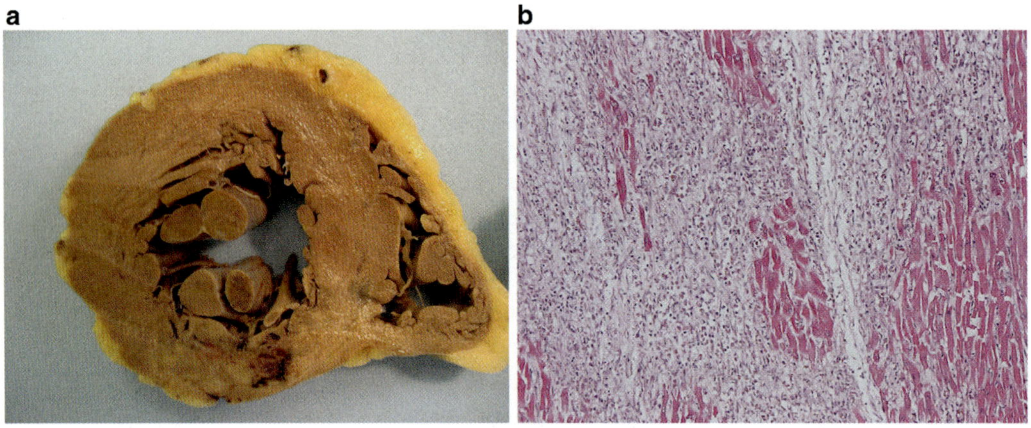

Fig. 16.2 (**a**) Posterior wall infarct in a 76-year-old man who died suddenly the day after angioplasty. (**b**) Photomicrograph of 5–7-day-old infarct, with removal of myocytes, a cellular interstitial inflammatory cell infiltrate, and no collagen deposition (H&E 10×)

Acute Myocardial Infarct

Sudden death due to acute myocardial infarct (MI) is almost always due to critical narrowing of one or more coronary arteries by atherosclerotic plaque. Invariably, the mechanism of death is myocardial ischemia leading to fatal arrhythmia. At least 75% luminal narrowing by atherosclerotic plaque is required to account for sudden cardiac death due to atherosclerotic disease (Fig. 16.1) [11, 12]. Acute plaque hemorrhage with or without rupture is identified in a reported 3–20% of cases [11]. In acute out-of-hospital deaths or in cases of sudden death with no symptoms or symptoms lasting less than 1 h, an acute infarction is seen in less than 25% of cases. Of those, 50% will have grossly visible, transmural infarcts (Fig. 16.2), and 50% will have subendocardial acute infarcts seen only histologically [11].

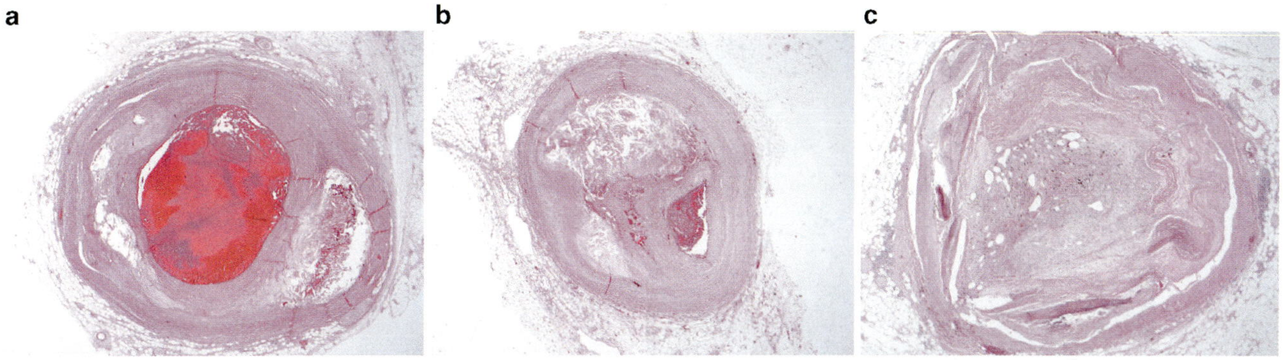

Fig. 16.3 (**a**) Photomicrograph of acute thrombus of right coronary artery (RCA) with intact and degenerating erythrocytes and leukocytes in an 86-year-old man who died of sudden cardiac arrest (H&E 2×). (**b**) Organizing thrombus of left anterior descending (LAD) coronary artery consisting of fibrin with early infiltration by fibroblasts (H&E 2×). (**c**) Organized thrombus of RCA containing multiple, recanalized vascular channels and numerous pigment-laden macrophages (H&E 4×)

The earliest histologic change seen in myocardial infarction (MI) is hypereosinophilia of myocytes. Survival of at least 4 h is required to see these changes; if death occurs rapidly after the ischemic insult, the myocardium will appear normal by light microscopy [12]. In cases of sudden collapse, the survival interval is much too brief to see these histologic changes, and the diagnosis rests on the finding of critical narrowing of coronary arteries, diffuse or focal, in the absence of a competing cause of death. In some cases of sudden death, there may be a history of recent vague or nonspecific symptoms such as fatigue, heartburn, or flu-like symptoms.

A second population of sudden death patients may reportedly have classic symptoms of acute MI such as chest pain or shortness of breath in the days or hours leading up to their sudden collapse. Some may even progress to signs of congestive heart failure, including peripheral edema, increasing abdominal girth, and hemoptysis. In such cases, it is more common to find gross or histologic evidence of acute MI at autopsy, sometimes with associated ascites, hepatosplenomegaly, and pulmonary edema.

These two different presentations suggest that the mechanism of death due to atherosclerotic coronary artery disease may be either from a sudden arrhythmia or a myocardial infarct with subsequent heart failure. Often, patients in the second population will have sought medical attention for their symptoms before dying of coronary artery disease, so their deaths do not fit the definition of "sudden death" and do not fall under the jurisdiction of the medical examiner.

Coronary Arterial Thrombi

The finding of coronary arterial thrombus is the exception rather than the rule in cases of sudden death, with a reported incidence of 8–19% among adults who collapse suddenly, are dead on arrival to an emergency department, or are found dead (Fig. 16.3). This contrasts with findings in hospitalized patients, where 87% of patients admitted with transmural acute myocardial infarcts demonstrate occlusive coronary thrombi on angiography [13, 14].

Healed Myocardial Infarction

A frequent autopsy finding in sudden cardiac death is critical luminal narrowing of one or more coronary arteries associated with a healed infarct, or fibrous scar, in the myocardium (Fig. 16.4). A healed infarct is found in approximately 41% of sudden out-of-hospital deaths from coronary disease [11]. The previous infarction may have been clinically silent, or there may be a history of documented MI. On histologic examination, there is often no evidence of more recent infarction. Within the scar, there often are remaining islands of viable or chronically ischemic myocytes. These myocytes are potentially arrhythmogenic foci, as they retain conductive activity but are isolated from other myocytes by the fibrous scar (Fig. 16.4).

Complications Following MI

A number of complications can follow acute MI; however, sudden death due to these complications in the absence of previous symptoms of myocardial ischemia is unusual. Ventricular free-wall rupture with hemopericardium and tamponade is the most common complication of acute MI in cases of sudden death (Fig. 16.5). It is an unusual finding in patients without

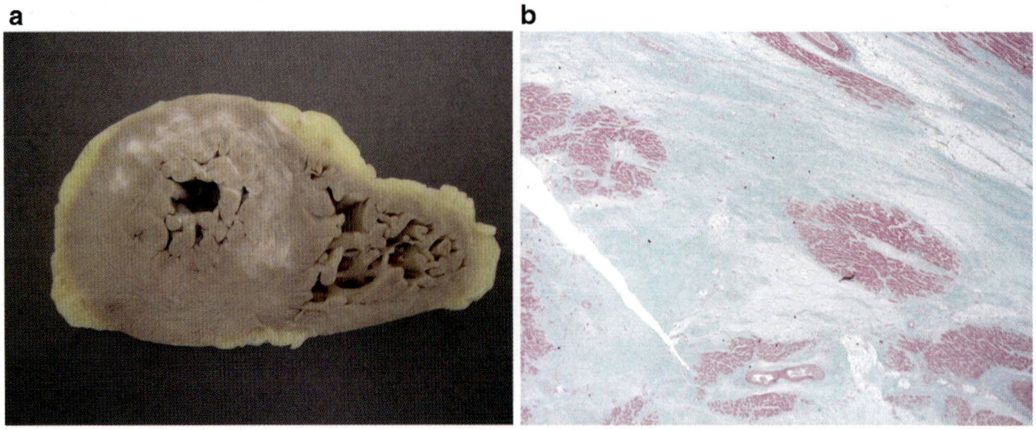

Fig. 16.4 (**a**) Healed fibrous scar in the anterior wall of the left ventricle in a 31-year-old man who collapsed suddenly the day after angioplasty. (**b**) Photomicrograph of the healed infarct, demonstrating remaining islands of viable myocytes completely surrounded by the fibrous scar (Trichrome 2×)

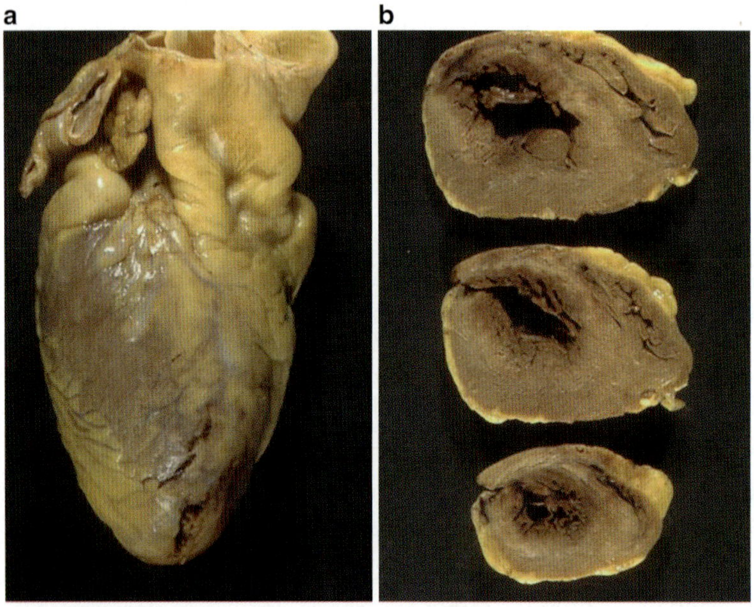

Fig. 16.5 (**a**, **b**) Recent myocardial infarct (histologically, 3–5 days) with rupture of ventricular free wall in a 79-year-old man with sudden cardiac arrest

apparent previous symptoms [15, 16]. The greatest risk of rupture is within 3–7 days postinfarct, with a subpopulation experiencing ruptures in the first 24 h post-MI. Risk factors for ventricular rupture following MI include female sex, greater than 70 years of age, first infarct, sustained hypertension following infarct, anterior wall infarct, and transmural infarct [12, 16].

Septal rupture (Fig. 16.6), papillary muscle rupture (Fig. 16.6), or ventricular aneurysm with mural thrombus (Fig. 16.7) is less commonly found in those presenting with sudden collapse. Such complications may be seen in sudden death cases in patients without previously diagnosed MI, due to lack of medical care or "silent" MI.

Nonatherosclerotic Coronary Disease

Anomalies of Coronary Artery Ostia

Anomalies related to the origins of the coronary arteries are a known cause of sudden death, especially in the young. In a study of young athletes from the United States and Italy, coronary artery anomalies (CAAs) were the third most common abnormality associated with sudden death, after hypertrophic cardiomyopathy and arrhythmogenic right ventricular cardiomyopathy [17].

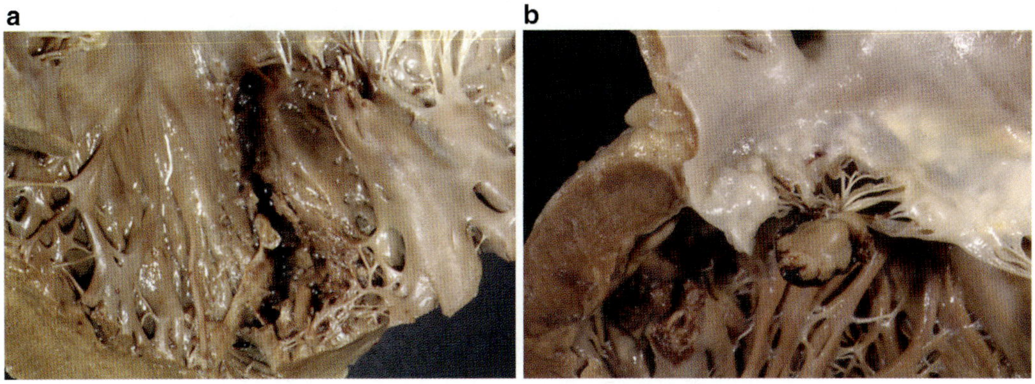

Fig. 16.6 (**a**) Left ventricular view of septal rupture of 7–10-day myocardial infarct creating an acquired ventricular septal defect in a 43-year-old male. (**b**) Recent myocardial infarction (histologically, 5–7 days) with complete rupture of posteromedial papillary muscle in a 60-year-old man

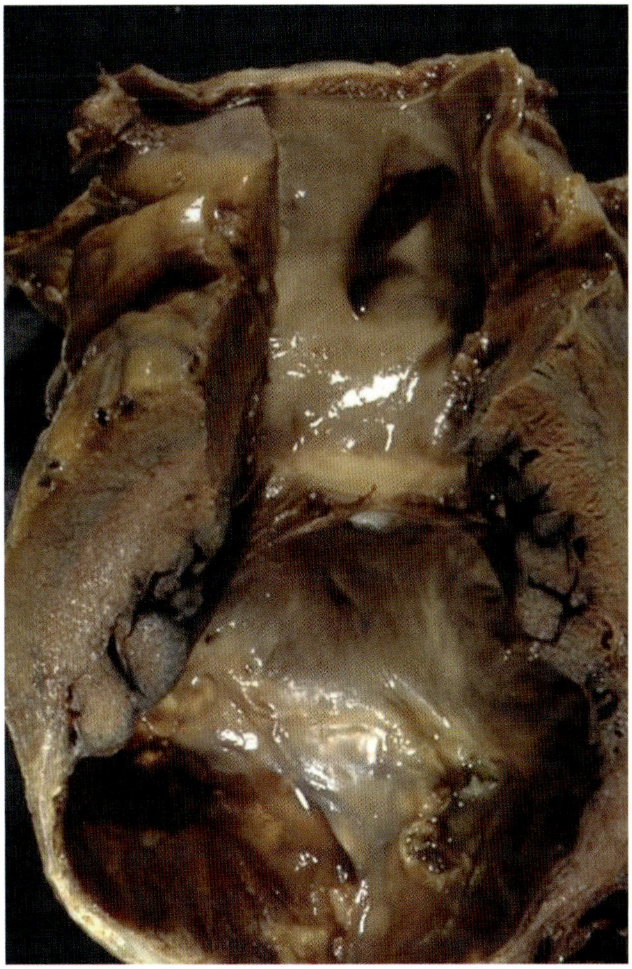

Fig. 16.7 Large aneurysm of the left ventricle with mural thrombus in an asymptomatic 62-year-old man who collapsed suddenly at work. Past medical history of myocardial infarction 12 years prior

The mechanism of sudden death and CAAs is most likely related to myocardial ischemia due to decreased blood flow. Although sudden death may occur while at rest, it is more commonly seen during or immediately after a period of intense exertion, even in someone who exercises regularly [9–18].

Postulated mechanisms of myocardial ischemia with CAAs include ostial obstruction by aortic wall flap, compression of an intramural segment of the coronary artery, and coronary arterial spasm; however, the exact mechanism is unknown [9, 19, 20].

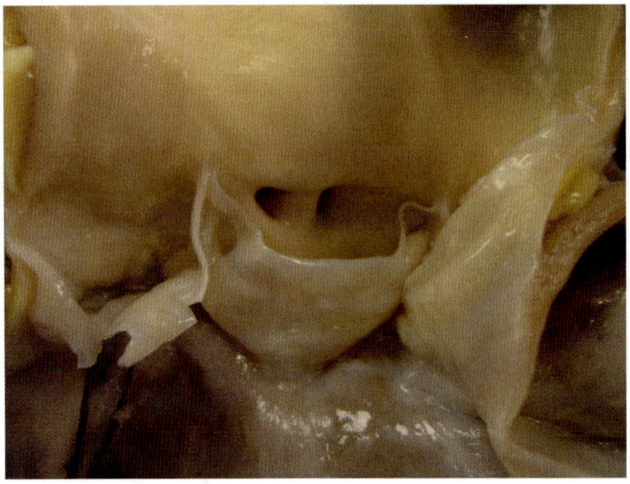

Fig. 16.8 Left coronary artery (LCA) arising from the right sinus of Valsalva in 35-year-old female with sudden death. LCA ostium has a lateral angle of origin and proximal intramural course within the aorta

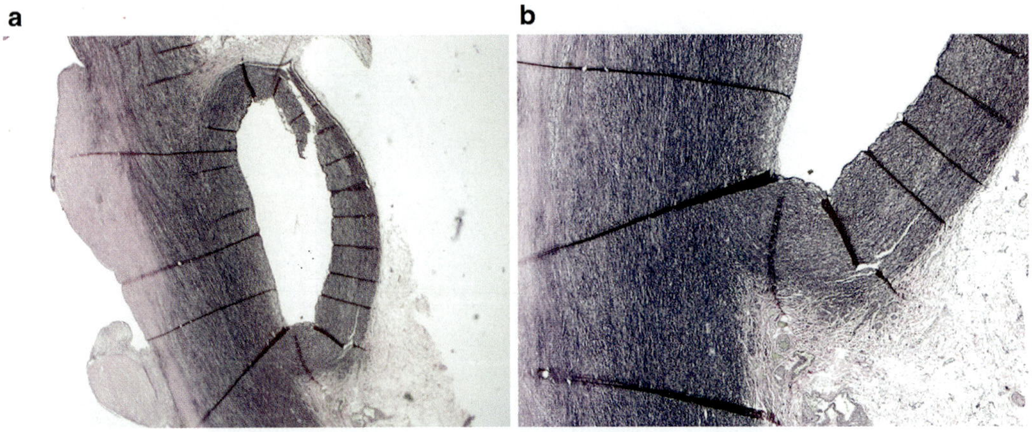

Fig. 16.9 (**a**) Photomicrograph demonstrating intramural aortic segment of proximal LCA (ELVG 2×). (**b**) Higher magnification of (**a**). Coronary artery courses within the aortic media; LCA and aorta share the adventitia (ELVG 10×)

On histologic examination in cases of sudden death associated with CAAs, the myocardium in the distribution supplied by the anomalous artery may show acute ischemic changes such as hypereosinophilic myocytes, wavy myocyte fibers and contraction bands, or chronic ischemic changes consisting of patchy areas of replacement fibrosis. Most commonly, however, no histologic changes of either acute or chronic ischemia are present.

Normally, coronary arteries arise from the central aspect of their respective aortic sinuses at or below the sinotubular ridge and with an angle of origin between 45° and 90°, although there is a spectrum of "normal angles."

Some of the more common anomalies of coronary artery origins associated with sudden death include origin from the wrong sinus [21], high angle of origin with ostial flap, and abnormal course of a coronary artery. Having a single coronary artery originate from outside the sinuses of Valsalva is uncommon, but may also cause sudden death [9, 17–20, 22–25].

Origin from incorrect sinus – Either the right coronary artery (RCA) or left coronary artery (LCA) may originate from the incorrect sinus. Often, the artery arises at a lateral angle from the incorrect sinus with the ostium more oval in shape (Fig. 16.8). There may be an obstructive flap over the ostium. Often, the proximal course of the coronary artery will be intramural within the aortic wall, and the coronary artery and aorta will share the media without an intervening adventitia (Fig. 16.9) [17]. Although this pattern has been the most commonly reported one with sudden death in athletes [20], the artery may also course anterior to the pulmonary artery, posterior to the aorta, or between the aorta and pulmonary artery but without an intramural segment (Fig. 16.10) [17, 19, 24].

One branch arises from incorrect sinus – Cases in which only one of the branches of the LCA – either left anterior descending (LAD) or left circumflex (LCX) – arises from the incorrect sinus and the other branch arises normally from the left sinus

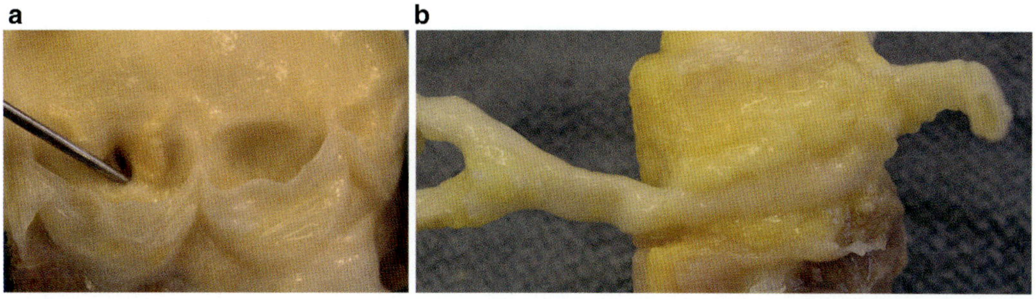

Fig. 16.10 (**a**) Single coronary artery ostium from the right sinus of Valsalva. Probe is in LCA. (**b**) LCA courses posterior to aorta above the anterior leaflet of the mitral valve

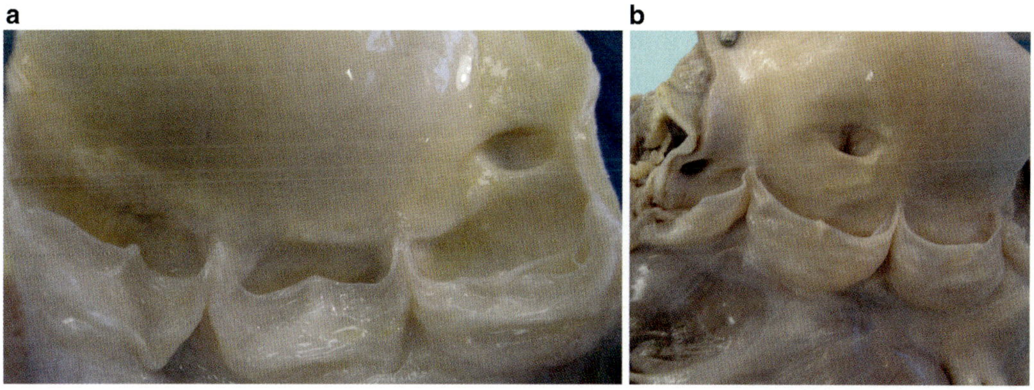

Fig. 16.11 (**a**) LCA ostium with acute angle of origin. LCA arises above the left sinotubular ridge. Possible obstructive aortic wall ostial flap over the inferior aspect of the ostium. (**b**) RCA ostium with acute angle of origin. RCA arises above right sinotubular ridge with aortic wall ostial flap over inferior aspect of ostium

of Valsalva do occur. Variants seen in association with sudden death include LAD from the right sinus of Valsalva with intramural course between the aorta and pulmonary artery, and left circumflex coronary artery arising from the RCA and coursing posterior to the aorta [17, 24, 25].

Ostia with acute angles of origin – Coronary artery ostia arising high above the sinotubular ridge often have an acute angle of origin between 15 and 45°. Angles between 15 and 35° are the most severe and more often related to sudden death. Often, there is a flap of the aortic wall over the inferior aspect of the ostium, resulting in a partial obstruction (Fig. 16.11) [17, 23, 25].

Arteries not arising from aortic sinuses – Coronary arteries arising from locations other than the aortic sinuses are uncommon, with origin from the pulmonary artery the most common variant (Fig. 16.12) [3]. Variants may be isolated or combined with other congenital abnormalities [17, 19, 23–25].

Spontaneous Coronary Artery Dissection

Coronary artery dissections may be spontaneous, trauma-induced, or iatrogenic. Spontaneous coronary artery dissection (SCAD) is a rare condition that was first described by Pretty [26]. Patients with SCAD may present with acute myocardial infarction or heart failure, although sudden death is often the initial presentation [27–31].

SCAD occurs in both men and women; however, it is more common in women. It is most often seen in young peripartum/postpartum women with no prior cardiac history [27–34]. SCAD can occur in pregnancy or in the postpartum period. Although the exact mechanism is unknown, hormonal factors are thought to play a role by creating changes in the arterial wall and extracellular matrix proteins [27–30, 33].

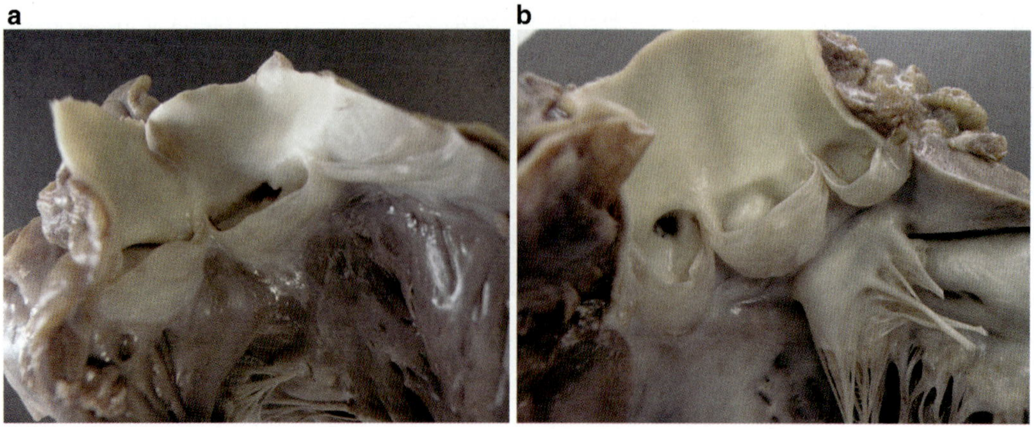

Fig. 16.12 (**a**) Right ventricular outflow tract with LCA arising from posterior left sinus of pulmonary artery in previously healthy 16-year-old male found dead in bed. (**b**) Left ventricular outflow tract with RCA arising from right sinus of Valsalva and absent LCA ostium

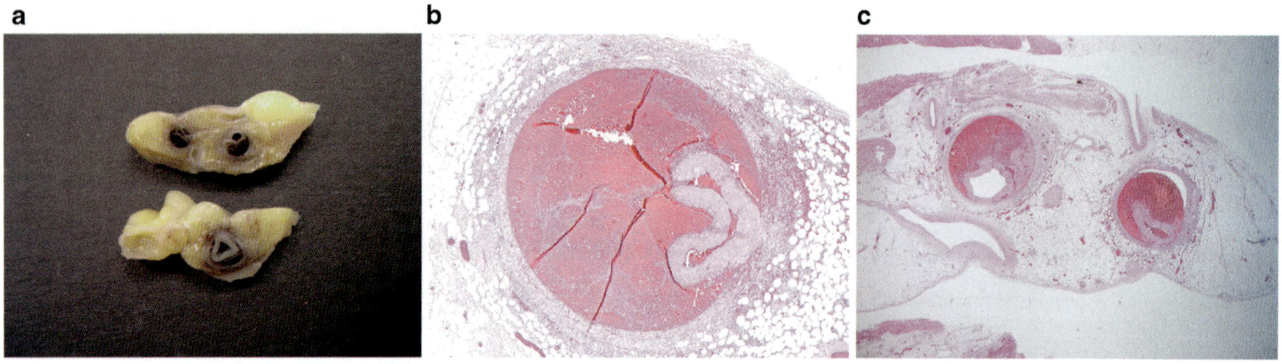

Fig. 16.13 (**a**) Spontaneous coronary artery dissection (SCAD) of left main coronary artery with extension into LAD and first diagonal coronary arteries in previously healthy 38-year-old female with no recent history of pregnancy. (**b**) Photomicrograph of coronary artery dissection of left main coronary artery. Blood accumulates within the media resulting in compression of the true lumen (H&E 2×). (**c**) Extension of the dissection into the LAD and first diagonal coronary arteries (H&E 1.25×)

SCAD may occur in otherwise healthy individuals with no medical history of or risk factors for cardiovascular disease. SCAD has been seen in patients with atherosclerotic coronary artery disease, oral contraceptive use, connective tissue disorders (Ehlers–Danlos syndrome, Marfan syndrome, and systemic lupus erythematosus), systemic hypertension [27, 28, 30, 33], and with cocaine use [34].

SCAD most typically involves a single artery, but multiple arteries may be involved. The LAD is the most commonly involved artery reported in the literature, especially in women, with the RCA reportedly more common in men [30–33]. In our experience with 34 patients, SCAD was diagnosed in 30 females and 4 males.

- Twenty-six cases involved the left main coronary artery or LAD coronary artery.
- Four involved the RCA only.
- Two involved the posterior descending coronary artery only.
- One case each involved only the left circumflex or obtuse marginal coronary artery.
- Eleven cases involved multiple arteries.
- Ten cases occurred in the peripartum/postpartum period.
- In the four men, the artery involved was the RCA (1), obtuse marginal coronary artery (1), LAD coronary artery (1), and LAD *and* first diagonal coronary arteries (1).

The dissection plane occurs between the outer one-fourth/one-third and the inner three-fourths/two-thirds of the media. Blood accumulates within the dissection plane or false channel and compresses the true lumen, leading to decreased myocardial perfusion with subsequent myocardial ischemia (Figs. 16.13 and 16.14).

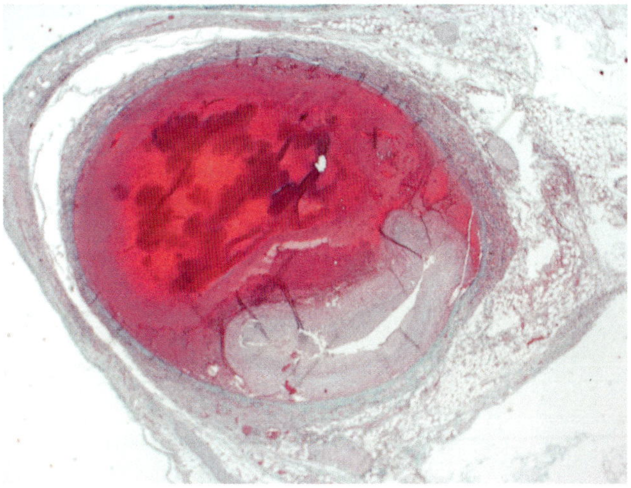

Fig. 16.14 SCAD of left main coronary artery in a 34-year-old postpartum female. Dissection plane is within the media, resulting in accumulation of blood in the false channel and compression of the true lumen (Trichrome 2×)

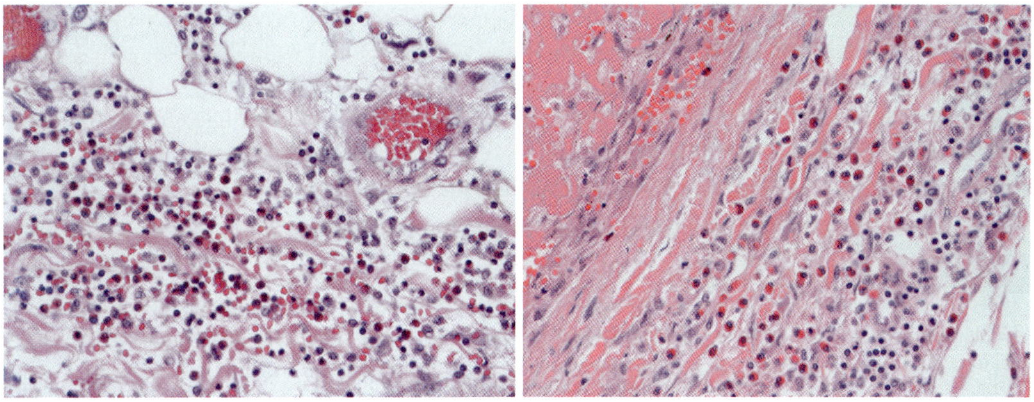

Fig. 16.15 (**a**) Adventitial eosinophils in LAD coronary artery from same case as Fig. 16.6 (H&E 40×). (**b**) Adventitial eosinophils in left main coronary artery from same case as Fig. 16.7 (H&E 40×)

Histologic examination often demonstrates a large number of eosinophils in the adventitia (Fig. 16.15). Although vasculitis has been suggested by some, the inflammation may be a response to the dissection rather than an actual cause [31, 32]. Histologic examination of uninvolved coronary arteries with SCAD may show increased extracellular matrix proteins within the media (Fig. 16.16), but often are unremarkable [31]. Adventitial eosinophils are not seen in arteries uninvolved by the dissection.

Coronary Arteritis

Coronary arteritis is an uncommon condition and a rare cause of sudden death, especially in previously undiagnosed cases. The most commonly encountered coronary arteritis is Kawasaki disease, also called mucocutaneous lymph node syndrome. Kawasaki disease is seen most commonly in infants and children, and clinically is accompanied by fever, rash, cervical lymphadenopathy, and oral and cutaneous lesions. The etiology is unknown, although an immune-mediated reaction to an as-yet-unidentified antigen in genetically susceptible persons is speculated [35].

The acute phase of the illness often involves a necrotizing panvasculitis with involvement of the epicardial coronary arteries, often with aneurysm formation, although aneurysms do not occur in all cases [36]. The healed phase is usually

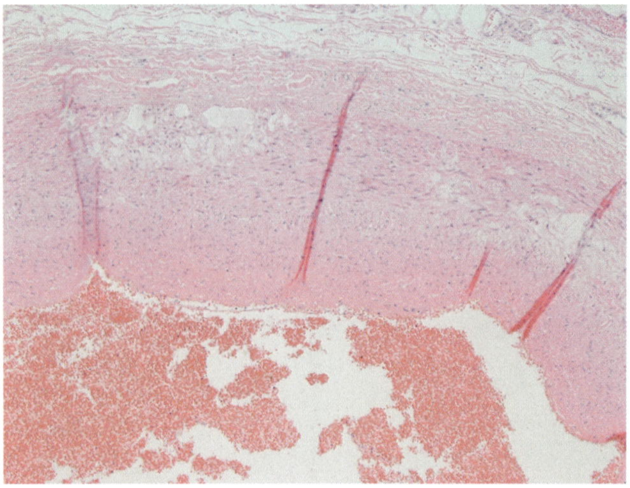

Fig. 16.16 Photomicrograph of RCA from same case as Fig. 16.7. Media has pools of proteoglycans in artery not involved by the dissection. Adventitia is free of eosinophils (H&E 10×)

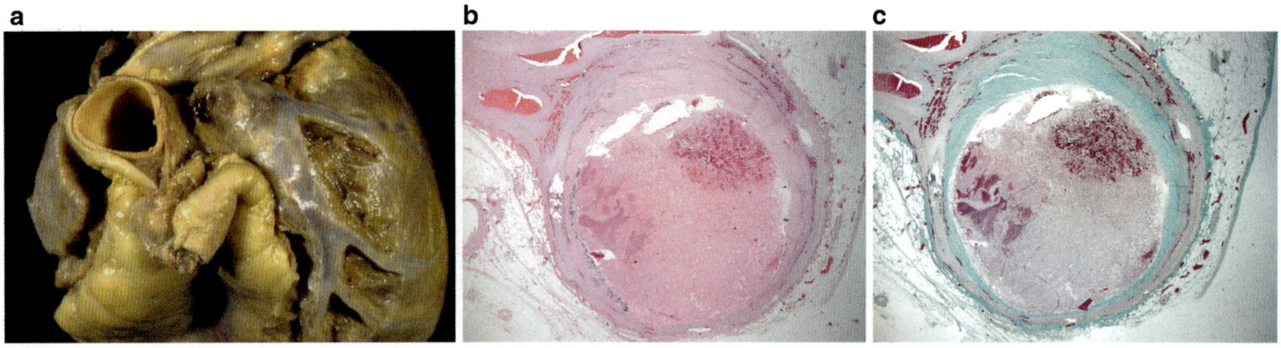

Fig. 16.17 (**a**) Giant coronary artery aneurysm of LCA in a 15-year-old male with sudden death while playing basketball, and no previous diagnosis of Kawasaki disease. (**b**) Photomicrograph of LCA aneurysm with occlusion by organizing thrombus (H&E 2×). (**c**) Trichrome stain of (**b**), demonstrating fibrous replacement of the artery wall (*green*) and thinning of the media (Trichrome 2×)

characterized by fibrointimal proliferation with coronary artery stenosis. Myocardial ischemia, coronary artery aneurysm thrombosis, and aneurysm rupture are potential causes of sudden death (Fig. 16.17) [36, 37].

Takayasu arteritis and giant cell arteritis more commonly involve the aorta and larger-caliber branches; however, coronary artery involvement is known to occur in up to 30% of cases of Takayasu arteritis (Fig. 16.18) [38]. In the healed phase, fibrointimal proliferation without aneurysm formation is the most common histologic finding. Residual inflammation and giant cells may be present. The histologic features of other arteries, especially the thoracic aorta, in correlation with clinical history and age are important features in distinguishing the underlying disease process in coronary arteritis.

Coronary arteritis has been reported with other vasculidities (see Fig. 16.19) such as polyarteritis nodosa and thromboangitis obliterans [39, 40].

Dysplastic Coronary Arteries/Fibromuscular Dysplasia

Fibromuscular dysplasia is a noninflammatory, nonatherosclerotic disease of medium- to small-caliber arteries. It is seen more commonly in women of childbearing age, but can be present in either sex and at any age. The renal artery is most commonly involved, followed by cerebral arteries; however, femoral, iliac, splenic, mesenteric, and the aorta can be involved [41]. Coronary artery involvement has been reported, although it is rare [42–45].

Gross examination of the heart in cases with epicardial coronary arterial involvement by fibromuscular dysplasia shows the arteries are focally severely narrowed, often with only a pinpoint lumen. On cross-section, the artery wall is firm and white.

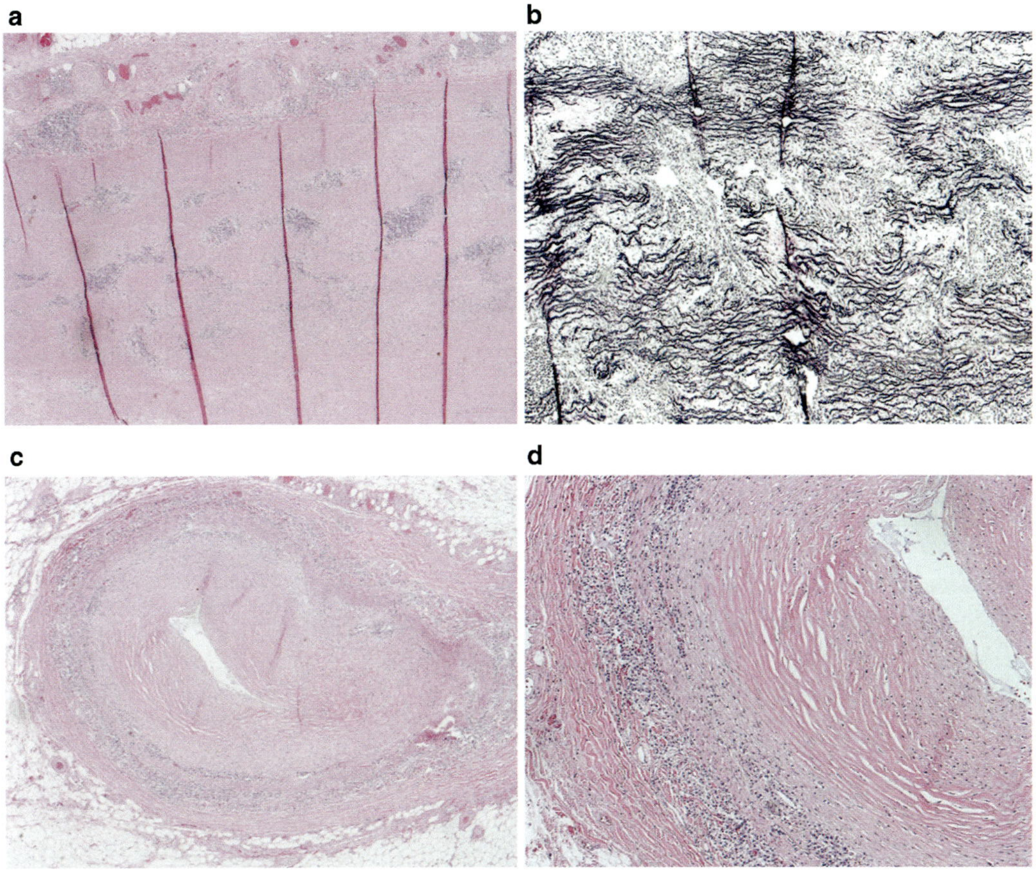

Fig. 16.18 (**a**) Takayasu arteritis in a previously healthy 24-year-old male with witnessed collapse and sudden death. Photomicrograph of ascending aorta, demonstrating healed aortitis with medial fibrosis, inflammatory cell infiltrate, and endarteritis obliterans of vasa vasorum (H&E 10×). (**b**) ELVG stain of ascending aorta, demonstrating the marked loss and fragmentation of elastic fibers (ELVG 10×). (**c**) Takayasu arteritis involvement of RCA with destruction of the media, intimal fibrous thickening, and a residual inflammatory cell infiltrate (H&E 4×). (**d**) Higher magnification of RCA, showing residual inflammation within the media and adventitia (H&E 10×)

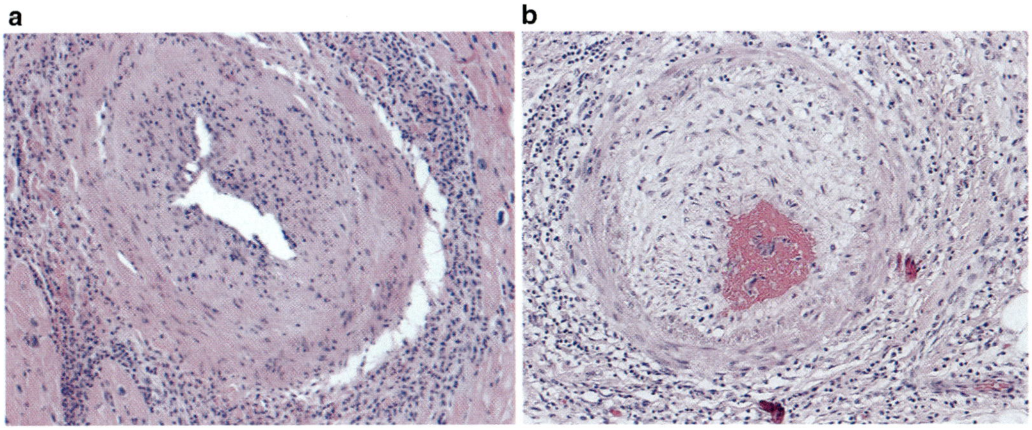

Fig. 16.19 (**a**) Active arteritis involving intramyocardial artery with intimal thickening and an acute inflammatory cell infiltrate within the artery wall (H&E 20×). (**b**) Arteritis involving intramyocardial artery with intimal proliferative-type fibrous thickening, luminal thrombus, and inflammatory cell infiltrate (H&E 20×)

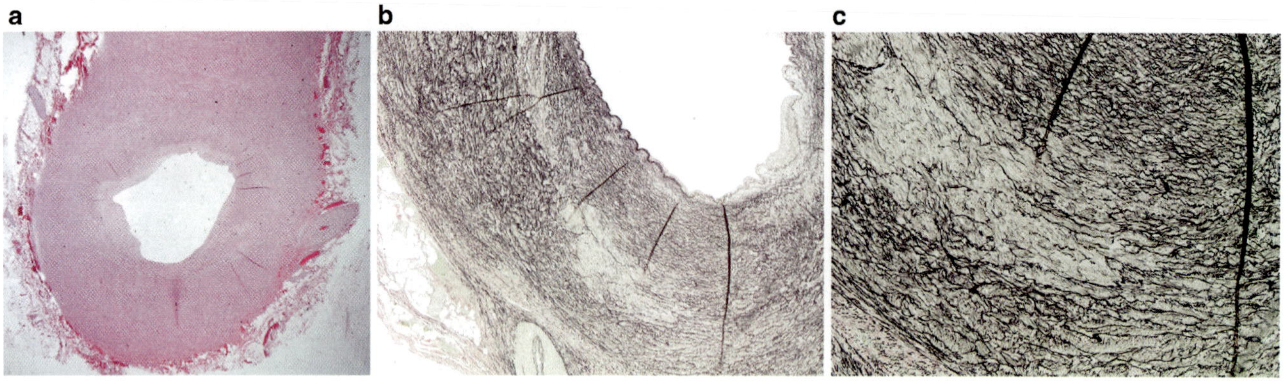

Fig. 16.20 (**a**) Photomicrograph of proximal RCA with 80% luminal narrowing by abnormal media in a 21-year-old previously healthy female found dead at home (H&E 2×). (**b**) ELVG stain of RCA, demonstrating medial disorganization and abnormal elastic fibers (ELVG 10×). (**c**) Higher magnification of (**b**) (ELVG 20×)

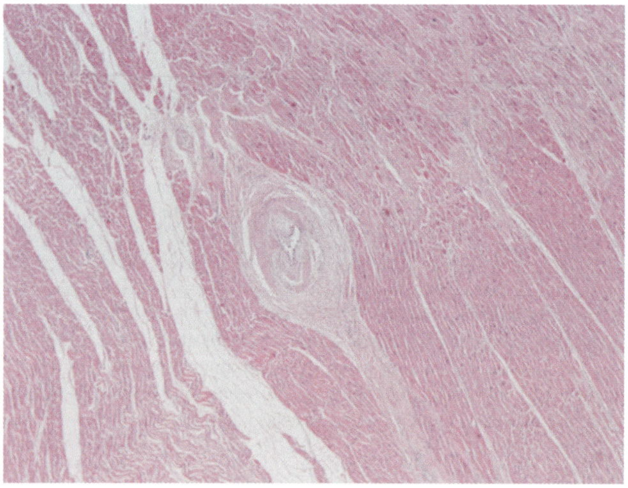

Fig. 16.21 Dysplastic intramyocardial arteries with intimal and medial thickening with associated myocardial fibrosis (*upper right*) in a 29-year-old female with sudden death (H&E 4×)

Histologically, the media is more commonly involved. The media is thickened, with disorganization of the wall and increased proteoglycan deposition (Fig. 16.20). Blunting of the layers may occur, with thickening of both the media and intima, and adventitial fibrosis may be present. Rare cases have predominant or isolated intimal involvement. Concentric or eccentric intimal fibrous thickening is visible, along with numerous myofibroblasts [42, 43].

Intramyocardial arteries may be involved and are best appreciated histologically [46]. Intramyocardial arterial involvement has been reported in cases of hypertrophic cardiomyopathy and mitral valve prolapse [47–49], but can occur independently. Dysplastic intramyocardial arteries are most commonly seen in left ventricular papillary muscles and the ventricular septal base. Isolated case reports of sudden death have been attributed to dysplastic intramyocardial arteries [46], although this diagnosis is controversial. If dysplastic intramyocardial arteries are an isolated finding, it is insufficient as a sole cause of sudden death. Dysplastic intramyocardial arteries associated with significant myocardial fibrosis (Fig. 16.21) or dysplastic atrioventricular nodal or sinoatrial nodal arteries (Fig. 16.22) may be a cause of sudden death [41, 50, 51].

Myocardial Bridge

Myocardial bridge is a segment of coronary artery that is completely within the myocardium, creating a tunneled segment. Any of the myocardial arteries may be involved; however, the mid-LAD is the most common. The incidence of myocardial

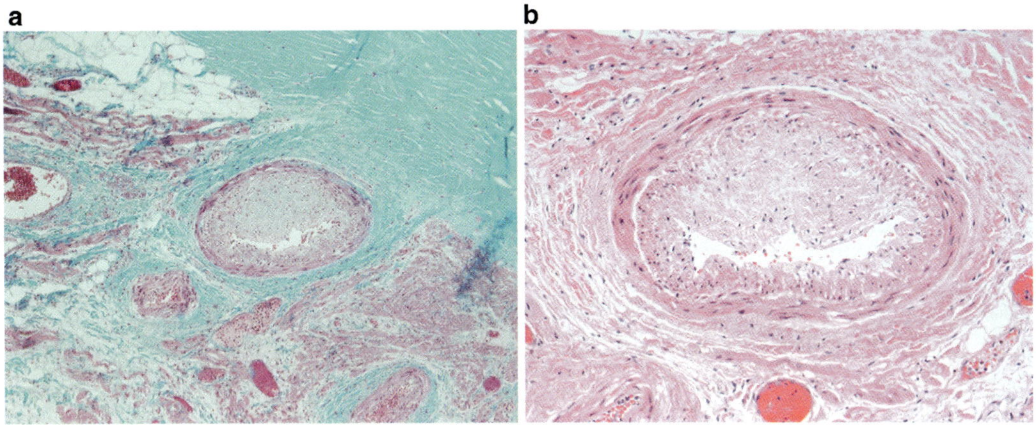

Fig. 16.22 (**a**) Dysplastic AV nodal artery with predominant intimal thickening in a 19-year-old male with witnessed collapse and sudden death (Trichrome 4×). (**b**) Higher magnification of (**a**) (H&E 10×)

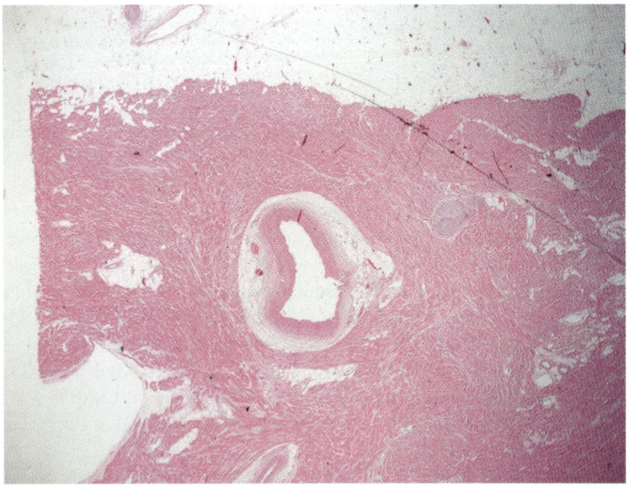

Fig. 16.23 Myocardial bridge of LAD coronary artery in a 33-year-old male with sudden death. Myocardial bridge extended for 2.5 cm with a maximum depth of 6 mm within the myocardium. The bridged coronary artery is patent and there is myocyte disarray surrounding the artery (H&E 4×)

bridge in autopsy studies has been reported from 15 to 85% with an average of 33%, and 0.5–2.5% in angiographic studies [52]. This variation suggests that not all cases with a myocardial bridge are at risk for symptoms [52–54]. In most instances, the myocardial bridge extends for a short distance (5–2 cm) and has a maximum depth within the myocardium of 1–2 mm.

In rare instances, myocardial bridge may be clinically significant and even result in sudden death [9, 55]. In these cases, the diagnosis is reserved for cases with a myocardial bridge in the absence of all other findings, including toxicology. In sudden death cases due to myocardial bridge, the myocardial bridge is often long (>2 cm) and/or deep within the myocardium (>3 mm) (Fig. 16.23) [17]. The intramyocardial segment of the artery is often free of atherosclerotic disease, although there may be significant disease proximally [56]. The mechanism of sudden death is believed to be ischemia or ischemic-induced arrhythmia caused by compression of the tunneled segment by the overlying myocardium [52, 54].

Coronary Artery Emboli

Coronary artery emboli occur from a variety of sources and are a rare cause of sudden death. Coronary emboli should be considered in cases of acute or healed myocardial infarction with normal coronary arteries. Potential sources of emboli include vegetations in infective endocarditis or nonbacterial endocarditis; calcific emboli from aortic or mitral valve stenosis (Fig. 16.24), or mitral valve annular calcification; emboli from a mural thrombus; or paradoxical thromboembolus and tumor emboli from cardiac tumors such as myxoma and papillary fibroelastoma [57].

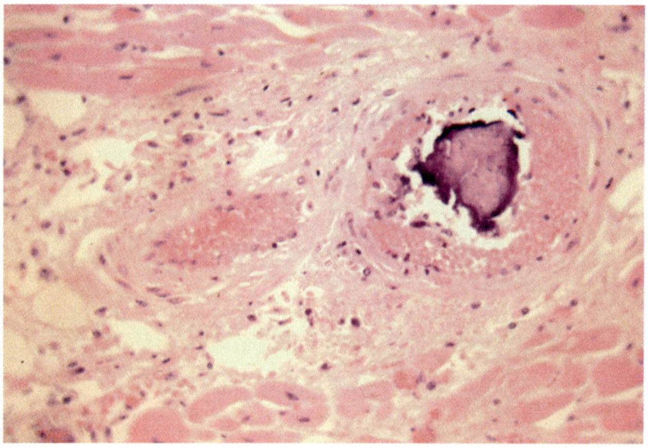

Fig. 16.24 Calcific embolus to left circumflex coronary artery causing an acute myocardial infarct 5 days after aortic valve replacement for aortic valve stenosis (H&E 4×)

References

1. Thiene G, Basso C, Corrado D. Cardiovascular causes of sudden death. In: Silver M, Gotlieb A, Schoen F, editors. Cardiovascular pathology. 3rd ed. Philadelphia: Churchill Livingstone; 2001. p. 326–74.
2. Langlois N. Sudden adult death. Forensic Sci Med Pathol. 2009;5:210–32.
3. Virmani R, Burke A, Farb A. Sudden cardiac death. Cardiovasc Pathol. 2001;10:211–8.
4. Myerburg R, Castellanos A. Cardiac arrest and sudden cardiac death. In: Braunwald E, editor. Braunwald heart disease. 5th ed. Philadelphia: W.B. Saunders Company; 1997. p. 742–56.
5. Virmani R, Burke A, Farb A, et al. Problems in forensic cardiovascular pathology. In: Schoen F, editor. Cardiovascular pathology: clinicopathologic correlations and pathogenetic mechanisms. Philadelphia: Williams & Wilkins; 1995. p. 173–93.
6. Gillum R. Sudden coronary death in the United States, 1980–1985. Circulation. 1989;79:756–65.
7. Liberthson R. Sudden death from cardiac causes in children and young adults. N Engl J Med. 1996;334:1039–44.
8. Driscoll D, Edwards W. Sudden unexpected death in children and adolescents. J Am Coll Cardiol. 1985;5:118B–21.
9. Corrado D, Thiene G, Cocco P, et al. Non-atherosclerotic coronary artery disease and sudden death in the young. Br Heart J. 1992; 68:601–7.
10. Edwards BS, Edwards JE. Atherosclerotic coronary disease. Pathology of sudden death. Malden: Blackwell Futura; 2006. p. 1–25.
11. Virmani R, Burke AP, Farb A. Sudden cardiac death. Cardiovasc Pathol. 2001;10:275–82.
12. Kumar V, Abbas AK, Fausto N, editors. The heart. In: Robbins and Cotran pathologic basis of disease. 7th ed. Philadelphia: Elsevier Saunders; 2005. p. 571–86.
13. DiMaio V, DiMaio D. Incidence of coronary thrombosis in sudden death due to coronary artery disease. Am J Forensic Med Pathol. 1993;14:273–5.
14. Warnes CA, Roberts WC. Sudden coronary death: comparison of patients with to those without coronary thrombus at necropsy. Am J Cardiol. 1984;54:1206–11.
15. Shirani J, Berezowski K, Roberts WC. Out of hospital sudden death from left ventricular free wall rupture during acute myocardial infarction as the first and only manifestation of atherosclerotic coronary artery disease. Am J Cardiol. 1994;73:88–92.
16. Wilansky S, Moreno CA, Lester SJ. Complications of myocardial infarction. Crit Care Med. 2007;35:S348–54.
17. Basso C, Corrado D, Thiene G. Congenital coronary artery anomalies as an important cause of sudden death in the young. Cardiol Rev. 2001;9:312–7.
18. Taylor A, Rogan K, Virmani R. Sudden cardiac death associated with isolated congenital coronary artery anomalies. J Am Coll Cardiol. 1992;20:640–7.
19. Angelini P. Coronary artery anomalies: an entity in search of an identity. Circulation. 2007;115:1296–305.
20. Basso C, Maron B, Corrado D, et al. Clinical profile of congenital coronary artery anomalies with origin from the wrong aortic sinus leading to sudden death in young competitive athletes. J Am Coll Cardiol. 2000;35:493–501.
21. Taylor A, Byers J, Cheitlin M, et al. Anomalous right or left coronary artery from the contralateral coronary sinus: "high-risk" abnormalities in the initial coronary artery course and heterogeneous clinical outcomes. Am Heart J. 1997;133:428–35.
22. Davis J, Cecchin F, Jones T, et al. Major coronary artery anomalies in a pediatric population: incidence and clinical importance. J Am Coll Cardiol. 2001;37:593–7.
23. Frescura C, Basso C, Thiene G, et al. Anomalous origin of coronary arteries and risk of sudden death: a study based on an autopsy population of congenital heart disease. Hum Pathol. 1998;29:689–95.
24. Roberts W. Major anomalies of coronary arterial origin seen in adulthood. Am Heart J. 1985;111:941–63.
25. Vlodaver Z, Neufeld H, Edwards J. Coronary arterial variations in the normal heart and in congenital heart disease. New York: Academic; 1975. p. 23–35.
26. Pretty HC. Dissecting aneurysm of coronary artery in a woman aged 42: rupture. Br Med J. 1931;1:667.

27. Dhawan R, Singh G, Fesniak H. Spontaneous coronary artery dissection: the clinical spectrum. Angiology. 2002;53:89–93.
28. Lodha A, Mirsakov N, Malik B, et al. Spontaneous coronary artery dissection: case report and review of literature. South Med J. 2009;102:315–7.
29. Terrovitis J, Kanakakis J, Nanas J. Spontaneous coronary artery dissection as a cause of acute myocardial infarction in the postpartum period. Cardiol Rev. 2005;13(4):211–3.
30. DeMaio S, Kinsella S, Silverman M. Clinical course and long-term prognosis of spontaneous coronary artery dissection. Am J Cardiol. 1989;64:471–4.
31. Claudon DG, Claudon DB, Edwards J. Primary dissecting aneurysm of coronary artery a cause of acute myocardial ischemia. Circulation. 1972;45:259–66.
32. Koul A, Hollander G, Moskovits N, et al. Coronary artery dissection during pregnancy and the postpartum period: two case reports and review of literature. Catheter Cardiovasc Interv. 2001;52:88–94.
33. Jorgensen M, Aharonian V, Mansukhani P, et al. Spontaneous coronary dissection: a cluster of cases with this rare finding. Am Heart J. 1994;127:1382–7.
34. Steinhauer J, Caulfield J. Spontaneous coronary artery dissection associated with cocaine use: a case report and brief review. Cardiovasc Pathol. 2001;10:141–5.
35. Freeman AF, Shulman ST. Recent developments in Kawasaki disease. Curr Opin Infect Dis. 2001;14:357.
36. Burke A, Virmani R, Lowell P, et al. Fatal Kawasaki disease with coronary arteritis and no coronary aneurysms. Am Acad Pediatr. 1998;101:108–12.
37. Maresi E, Passantino R, Midulla R, et al. Sudden infant death caused by ruptured coronary aneurysm during acute phase of atypical Kawasaki disease. Hum Pathol. 2001;32:1407–9.
38. Rav-Acha M, Plot L, Peled N, et al. Coronary involvement in Takayasu's arteritis. Autoimmun Rev. 2007;6:566–71.
39. Ohno H, Matsuda Y, Takashiba K, et al. Acute myocardial infarction in Buerger's disease. Am J Cardiol. 1986;57:690.
40. Donatelli F, Triggiani M, Nascimbene S, et al. Thromboangiitis obliterans of coronary and internal thoracic arteries in a young woman. J Thorac Cardiovasc Surg. 1997;113:800.
41. James T. Morphologic characteristics and functional significance of focal fibromuscular dysplasia of small coronary arteries. Am J Cardiol. 1990;65:12G–22.
42. Maresi E, Becchina G, Ottoveggio G, et al. Arrhythmic sudden cardiac death in a 3-year-old child with intimal fibroplasia of coronary arteries, aorta, and its branches. Cardiovasc Pathol. 2001;9:43–8.
43. Imamura M, Yokoyama S, Kikuchi K. Coronary fibromuscular dysplasia presenting as sudden infant death. Arch Pathol Lab Med. 1997;121:159–61.
44. Kaneko K, Someya T, Ohtaki R, et al. Congenital fibromuscular dysplasia involving multivessels in an infant with fatal outcome. Eur J Pediatr. 2004;163:241–4.
45. Lee A, Gray P, Gallagher P. Sudden death and regional left ventricular fibrosis with fibromuscular dysplasia of small intramyocardial coronary arteries. Heart. 2000;83:101–2.
46. Burke A, Virmani R. Intramural coronary artery dysplasia of the ventricular septum and sudden death. Hum Pathol. 1998;29:1124–7.
47. Morales A, Romanelli R, Boucek R, et al. Myxoid heart disease: an assessment of extravalvular cardiac pathology in severe mitral valve prolapse. Hum Pathol. 1992;23:129–37.
48. Burke A, Farb A, Tang A, et al. Fibromuscular dysplasia of small coronary arteries and fibrosis in the basilar ventricular septum in mitral valve prolapse. Am Heart J. 1997;134:282–91.
49. Maron B, Wolfson J, Epstein S, et al. Intramural (small vessel) coronary artery disease in hypertrophic cardiomyopathy. J Am Coll Cardiol. 1986;8:545–57.
50. Zack F, Terpe H, Hammer U, et al. Fibromuscular dysplasia of coronary arteries as a rare cause of death. Int J Legal Med. 1996;108:215–8.
51. Burke A, Subramanian R, Smialek J, et al. Nonatherosclerotic narrowing of the atrioventricular node artery and sudden death. J Am Coll Cardiol. 1993;21:117–22.
52. Kim P, Hur G, Kim S, et al. Frequency of myocardial bridges and dynamic compression of epicardial coronary arteries: a comparison between computed tomography and invasive coronary angiography. Circulation. 2009;119:1408–16.
53. Möhlenkamp S, Hort W, Ge J, et al. Update on myocardial bridging. Circulation. 2002;106:2616–22.
54. Boktor M, Mansi I, Troxclair S, et al. Association of myocardial bridge and Takotsubo cardiomyopathy: a case report and literature review. South Med J. 2009;102:957–60.
55. Morales AR, Romanelli R, Boucek RJ. The mural left anterior descending coronary artery, strenuous exercise and sudden death. Circulation. 1980;62:230–7.
56. Ishikawa Y, Akasaka Y, Suzuki K, et al. Anatomic properties of myocardial bridge predisposing to myocardial infarction. Circulation. 2009; 120:376–83.
57. Edwards B, Edwards J. Nonatherosclerotic coronary artery disease. In: Malden MA, editor. Sudden cardiac death. Malden: Blackwell Futura; 2006. p. 27.

Chapter 17
Acute Coronary Syndromes

Robert F. Wilson

The Etiology of ACS

Based on postmortem studies in the 1950s and 1960s, the cause of acute coronary syndrome (ACS) was believed to be intracoronary thrombosis related to an atherosclerotic plaque within the coronary lumen [1]. In the 1970s, investigators postulated that an intraluminal coronary clot was a postmortem event and proposed that the actual cause was an imbalance of myocardial oxygen supply and demand, whereby the supply was restricted by a worsening coronary stenosis. In the 1980s and 1990s, definitive angiographic and pathology studies demonstrated conclusively that the *primary* cause of ACS is the rupture of an atherosclerotic, lipoprotein-laden plaque into the arterial lumen with subsequent thrombosis over the newly exposed, inflammatory plaque contents [2].

Relatively fresh atherosclerotic plaque is highly inflammatory and its contents are soft (Fig. 17.1). The plaque is often eccentrically positioned within the intimal layer of the artery, covering only a portion of the arterial cross-section. Plaque often develops at arterial bifurcation points.

In the initial steps of fresh plaque development, lipoprotein particles in the blood infiltrate the intima through "leaky" endothelium covering the artery [3]. Most risk factors for coronary heart disease – such as diabetes, smoking, elevated low-density lipoprotein (LDL) cholesterol, and hypertension – are associated with increased endothelial permeability to these lipoprotein molecules. Macrophages engulf the lipoprotein particles but cannot digest them, leading the giant macrophages with lipid-laden vesicles. Macrophages rupture, releasing their contents. The plaque becomes rich in metalloproteinases and inflammatory cytokines which attract additional inflammatory cells. This creates an "atherosclerotic abscess."

This fresh, inflammatory atherosclerotic plaque is often termed "vulnerable" plaque because it is prone to rupture into the arterial lumen [4, 5]. In addition to the inflammatory erosion of the intimal plaque, the plaque is subjected to the pulsatile stress of arterial blood pressure [6]. Since the junction between the intimal cap over the abscess and the adjacent artery concentrates the fatigue-related stress of arterial pulsation, rupture is most likely to occur in this area. It has been postulated that this pulsatile stress is one factor leading to plaque rupture; that might explain the cluster of acute coronary events associated with sudden hypertension and tachycardia (which markedly increase the mechanical stress) seen after natural disasters.

When atherosclerotic plaque ruptures, the contact of its inflammatory constituents initiates platelet activation, and to a lesser extent, clotting factor coagulation (Figs. 17.2 and 17.3). This can be a fairly prolonged process whereby an initial layer or clump of platelets forms over the rupture site and then the surface of the clot becomes inactive [7]. This may end the process or the surface can reactivate, creating a new round of thrombosis. Urinary thromboxane B2 (the metabolite of thromboxane A2 liberated from platelets during activation) is elevated on days that patients with ACS have a flare of symptoms, suggesting that the waxing and waning of symptoms is driven by recurrent episodes of thrombosis [8].

Eventually, the clot either completely occludes the artery, the clot dissolves through endogenous thrombolysis, or the clot organizes and heals into a fibrotic lesion. At autopsy, the thrombotic lesion leading to death can often be seen to have multiple layers, suggesting successive activations that eventually lead to lumen closure [9]. The etiology of the activations is not clear, but enhanced coagulation due to smoking, sympathetic nervous system activation, and systemic factors (e.g., surgery or injury-induced procoagulation, infection, or other inflammatory disorders) have been implicated.

R.F. Wilson, MD (✉)
Division of Cardiovascular Medicine, University of Minnesota, Minneapolis, MN, USA
e-mail: wilso008@umn.edu

Z. Vlodaver et al. (eds.), *Coronary Heart Disease: Clinical, Pathological, Imaging, and Molecular Profiles*,
DOI 10.1007/978-1-4614-1475-9_17,

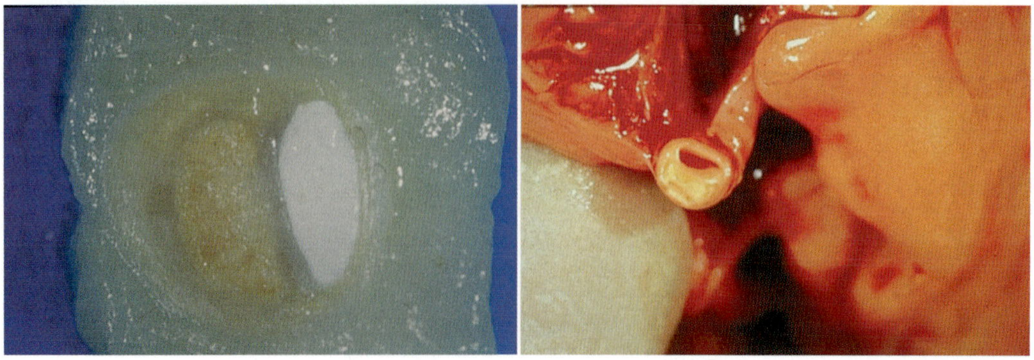

Fig. 17.1 *Left*: Cross-section of coronary artery showing an eccentric fresh atherosclerotic plaque with a fibrous cap. *Right*: Cross-section of another coronary artery showing an eccentric fresh atherosclerotic plaque. The majority of the arterial cross-section has no plaque and is capable of vasoconstriction

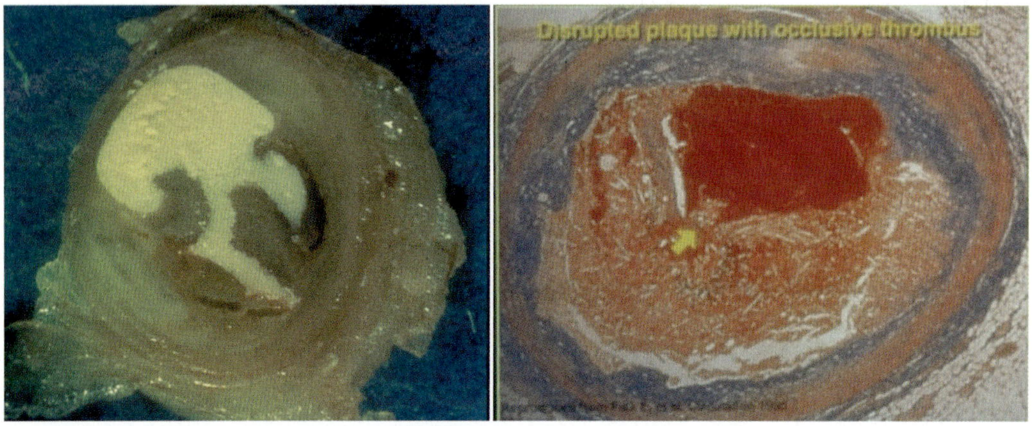

Fig. 17.2 *Left*: A ruptured atherosclerotic plaque in a coronary artery of a patient with ACS (courtesy of Ehrling Falk, MD). *Right*: A ruptured and thrombosed atherosclerotic coronary lesion with a clot adherent to the ulcerated rupture site

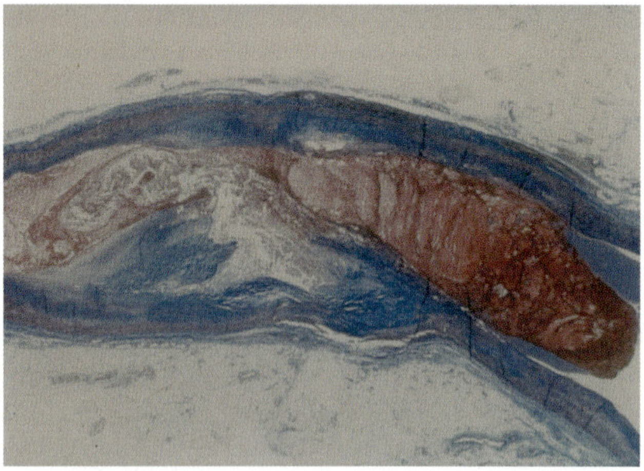

Fig. 17.3 A longitudinal section of ruptured and thrombosed atherosclerotic coronary lesion with a clot adherent to the ulcerated rupture site (courtesy of Ehrling Falk, MD)

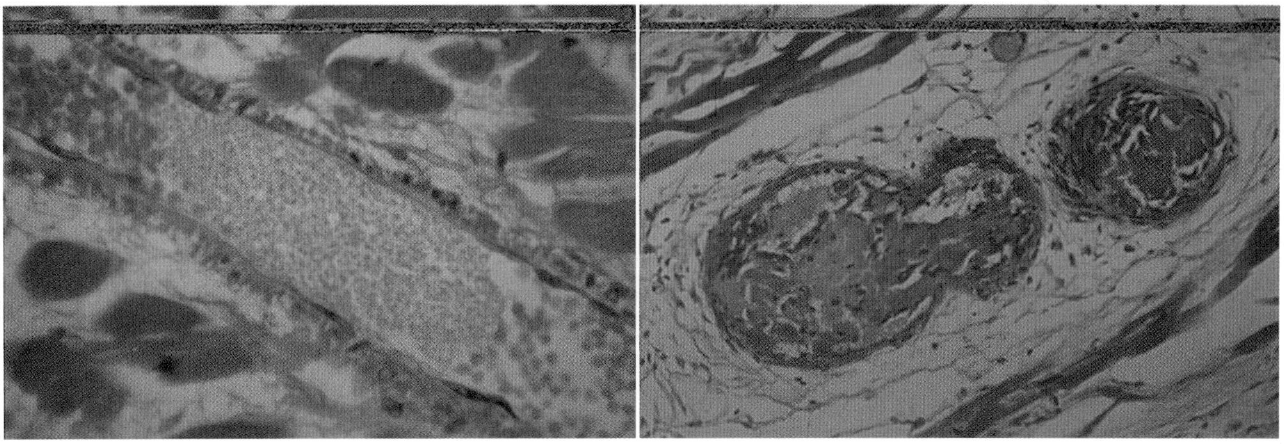

Fig. 17.4 *Left*: A photomicrograph of a platelet embolus in the myocardium distal to a thrombotic coronary lesion associated with ACS. *Right*: A microinfarction in the myocardium distal to a thrombotic coronary lesion associated with ACS

Associated Effects of Intracoronary Thrombosis

Thrombotic, inflammatory lesions also release vasoactive and procoagulant factors (thrombin, serotonin, and thromboxane A2) that lead to vasospasm at the site of the lesion and in the downstream microcirculation [10]. In a seminal study, Bertrand et al. found that 14–38% of lesions related to a thrombotic syndrome had vasospasm inducible with ergonovine at the site of the unstable lesion, as opposed to only 1% of patients with atypical chest pain [11].

In addition to release of vasoactive material, most thrombotic coronary lesions have some degree of downstream clot embolization (Fig. 17.4). The size of these platelet-rich emboli is highly variable, but typically they are small. In some patients, the contents of the liquid-filled plaque also embolize. Occlusion of small branch vessels – often too small to be detected on angiography – with resultant microinfarction is the rule in patients with ACS.

Alternative Causes for ACS

In a smaller group of patients, symptoms may abruptly worsen due to changes in myocardial oxygen consumption or supply (e.g., acute anemia, marked tachycardia, or hypertension) or sudden sympathetic nervous system discharge in response to sudden emotional or physical stress, or pain. Acute or severe anemia can lead to angina in the presence of a coronary stenosis when the hemoglobin concentration falls below 10 g/dL, but typically much more severe levels of anemia are required, particularly if the anemia is chronic. This is because blood viscosity falls as the red blood cell concentration is reduced. The reduced oxygen-carrying capacity of the anemic blood is compensated in part by the lower viscous resistance of flow through the stenotic lesion. Typically, the anemia-related reduction in viscosity compensates for the reduced O_2-carrying capacity to a hemoglobin concentration of 10 g/dL. Below that level, the reduction in oxygen delivery exceeds the improvement in viscosity.

Other conditions can lead to an increase in myocardial oxygen demand which, in the presence of a flow-limiting coronary stenosis, can lead to accelerated angina symptoms. These conditions include hyperthyroidism, infection, sudden beta blocker withdrawal, and postoperative state.

Finally, coronary constriction, primarily at the microcirculatory level, can be induced by sympathetic discharge or exogenous catecholamine-like vasoconstrictors such as cocaine [12]. Systemic sympathetic discharge can be caused by extreme stress or fright, subarachnoid hemorrhage, or extreme pain. The myocardium is very densely innervated and release of large amounts of catecholamines can lead to marked microvascular constriction [13]. This leads to chest discomfort and loss of ventricular contraction, particularly involving the anterior and apical left ventricle. Although markers of necrosis are often elevated (e.g., troponin) and myocardial biopsy shows contraction band necrosis typical of catecholamine-induced myocardial necrosis, recovery of left ventricular function after withdrawal of the stress is the rule.

Clinical Diagnosis and Natural History

Clinical Symptoms

As noted, the hallmark of ACS is the relatively sudden onset of ischemic symptoms such as angina or dyspnea. Since the thrombotic event plays out over time with cycles of clot activation and passivation, symptoms also wax and wane from day to day. The clinical presentation of ACS can be classified using the Braunwald criteria (Table 17.1) [14]. The symptoms, however, can be nonspecific, leading to reliance on coronary risk-factors and laboratory data to make the diagnosis.

The likelihood that a patient's symptoms of ischemia are due to a thrombotic coronary lesion must be interpreted in the context of other risk factors for atherosclerosis and thrombosis. Elevated serum LDL, low serum high-density lipoprotein (HDL), a family history of premature coronary disease, diabetes, smoking, and hypertension suggest that the individual is at increased risk of having the substrate for ACS – an unstable, ruptured atherosclerotic plaque. Smoking or working in a smoke-filled environment, having diabetes or one of several collagen-related vascular diseases places patients at higher risk of thrombosing a ruptured plaque (Fig. 17.5).

Laboratory Tests

The electrocardiogram (ECG) is an important but low-specificity tool for diagnosing ACS. In many patients, localized ST-segment depression or T wave inversion reflects recurrent ischemia or microinfarction in the affected perfusion field. The size of the perfusion field and the risk of a cardiac event is proportional to the number of leads showing ST-depression or T wave inversion, and the magnitude of ST-depression. ST-depression of $\geq$0.1 mV is associated with an 11% rate of death and myocardial infarction (MI) at 1 year. ST-depression of $\geq$0.2 mV carries about a sixfold increased mortality risk.

Two additional ECG findings have significance [15]. Transient ST-elevation is an ominous sign of impending ST-segment elevation MI (STEMI) [16]. Similarly, deep, symmetrical inversion of the T waves in the anterior chest leads is often related

Table 17.1 Braunwald classification system for unstable angina

Severity	Clinical precipitating factor	Therapy during symptoms
Symptoms with exertion	Secondary	No treatment
Subacute symptoms at rest (onset 2–30 days prior)	Primary	Usual angina therapy
Acute symptoms at rest (<48 h)	Post-myocardial infarction	Maximal therapy

Adapted from Braunwald [14]. Copyright 1989 by the American Heart Association

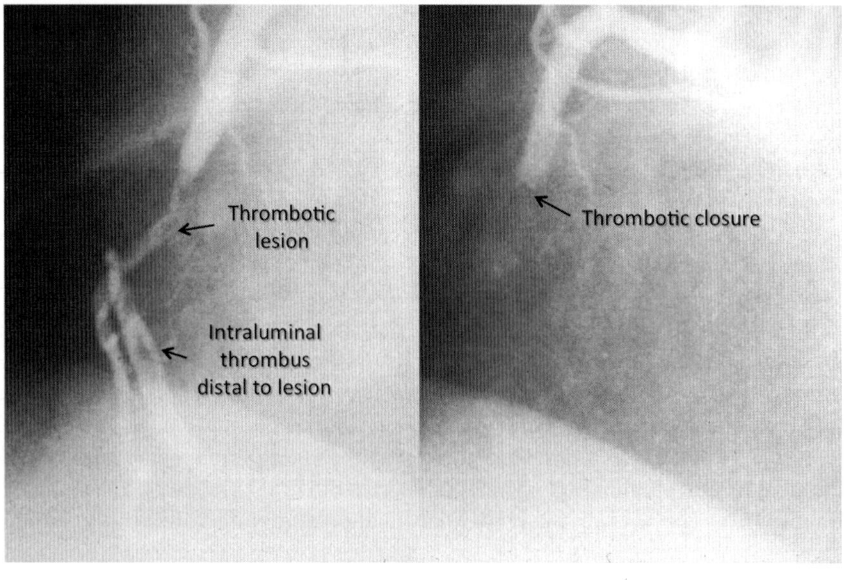

Fig. 17.5 *Left*: A 54-year-old male smoker presented with a recent onset of episodic chest pain and nausea. ECG showed transient ST-elevation that normalized after nitroglycerin. The angiogram showed a large thrombus adherent to the mid-right coronary artery. *Right*: After completion of the angiogram, the patient developed chest discomfort with inferior ST-elevation. The angiogram showed occlusion of the RCA at the site of thrombosis

Table 17.2 TIMI ACS risk score calculation

Add one point for each of the following (score range = 0–7)
Age ≥ 65 years
≥3 risk factors for coronary disease
Coronary stenosis ≥50%
ST-segment deviation on ECG
Severe angina symptoms (≥2 episodes within 24 h)
Use of aspirin in the prior 7 days
Elevated cardiac biomarkers (CK MB, troponin)

Modified from Antman et al. [21]. Copyright by the American Medical Association

to a significant thrombotic lesion in the proximal left anterior descending coronary artery or left main lesion. This finding also predicts a poor prognosis without revascularization therapy [17].

Serum biomarkers of myocardial infarction are commonly elevated in ACS and have a high level of sensitivity for making the diagnosis [18]. Thrombotic lesions are usually associated with some degree of downstream embolization and microinfarction. This *microinfarction* can now be detected with a high level of sensitivity using ultrasensitive measurements of serum troponin. Because troponin is very cardioselective and, under normal conditions, is present in vanishingly small concentrations, even small elevations in serum level are indicative of cardiac myocyte necrosis. The weakness of troponin measurements is that a number of other factors, such as hypotension or sepsis, can lead to a very small, but measureable, rise. Due to this lack of specificity of small troponin elevations, it is necessary to evaluate its prognostic significance in the clinical setting.

Incidence and prognosis of ACS: ACS is common. In the United States alone, ACS accounts for more than 733,000 hospital admissions in 1 year [19]. In addition, approximately 57% of patients suffering out-of-hospital cardiac arrest are found at angiography to have a thrombotic coronary lesion as the culprit [20].

ACS is associated with a significant risk of myocardial infarction and death in the 6 months after development of symptoms. Unlike STEMI, where the risk of death occurs soon after presentation, ACS-related death occurs cumulatively over the ensuing 6–9 months, likely reflecting the indolent nature of the thrombotic lesion.

Without revascularization, the aggregate risk of ACS appears to mimic or exceed the risk of STEMI, but the risk is spread out over a much longer time period. The in-hospital mortality risk of about 5% grows to about 13% during the 6 months after presentation. In addition, patients with ACS tend to be older and have more comorbidities than patients presenting with STEMI. This might account for the several-fold greater risk of cardiac death in the first 2–4 years after presentation.

ACS Risk Classification Methods

The risk of death or acute MI can be estimated from several "risk scores" that combine risk factors to determine the risk that an individual patient will suffer an adverse event (Tables 17.2–17.4) [21–23]. These risk scores can be useful in determining which patients likely have a thrombotic coronary lesion and would benefit from coronary angiography and revascularization. In general, the risk is proportional to the number of risk factors for coronary atherosclerosis, and evidence of acute ischemia or infarction on the ECG, or elevated biomarkers.

Although counterintuitive, patients with a new onset of ischemic symptoms (Braunwald class III) have a higher risk of an adverse event or death than do patients with an abrupt worsening of preexisting ischemic symptoms [24, 25]. Two potential reasons for this difference are the development of collateral blood supply to the ischemic myocardium and myocardial preconditioning.

Collateral blood vessels develop or enlarge very rapidly after profound ischemic events. In one study, collateral blood flow could be detected in 46% of patients with an occluded coronary artery at presentation, and that rose to 92% within 1–14 days. Of note, within 45 days, all patients had some degree of collateral blood flow to an occluded artery; 83% has Rentrop grade 2–3 collateral blood flow [26].

Another potential explanation for the better prognosis associated with a longer duration of symptoms is a condition known as ischemic preconditioning [27]. Preconditioning is a process in which repetitive ischemic episodes cause a change in the cardiac myocyte physiology whereby the myocyte tolerates and survives longer periods of ischemia than it could prior to preconditioning. This process is quite rapid and can even be seen with progressive episodes of ischemia during balloon angioplasty. In that setting, the time required for ischemic ST-depression after balloon inflation progressively lengthens with each balloon inflation. Patients with repetitive ischemic episodes due to preexisting stable coronary atherosclerosis appear to develop a degree of preconditioning that protects the myocardium from the adverse events of repetitive ischemia associated with ACS.

Table 17.3 Calculation of the GRACE score to predict 6-month mortality risk in patients with ACS[a]

Parameter		Points
Age (years)	≤40	0
	40–49	18
	50–59	36
	60–69	55
	70–79	73
	80–89	91
	≥90	100
Heart failure		24
Prior myocardial infarction		12
Resting heart rate		12
Resting heart rate	50–69	3
	70–89	9
	90–109	14
	110–149	23
	150–199	35
	≥200	43
Systolic blood pressure	≤80	24
	80–99	22
	100–119	18
	120–139	14
	140–159	10
	160–199	4
	≥200	0
ST-segment depression on ECG		11
Initial serum creatinine	0–0.39	1
	0.4–0.79	3
	0.8–1.19	5
	1.2–1.59	7
	1.6–1.99	9
	2.0–3.99	15
	≥4	20
Elevated cardiac biomarkers		15
No PCI during hospitalization		14

Modified from Eagle et al. [23]. Copyright by the American Medical Association
[a] Select the appropriate point score in each category and add them together to obtain the GRACE risk score

Table 17.4 Risk of a cardiac event based on different risk scores

Risk category	Score name	Score	Death in hospital to 30 days (%)	Death within 6 months (%)
Low	GRACE [23]	≤108	<1	<3
	TIMI [21]	0/1	1.2 (14 day)	
	Troponin [18]	Normal	<2	<5
Moderate	GRACE [23]	109–140	1–3	3–8
	TIMI [21]	2–4	1–2.5	
High	GRACE [23]	>140	>3	>8
	TIMI [21]	5–7	5.6–6.5	
	Troponin [18]	Elevated	15–20	25

Angiographic Findings in ACS

McMahon et al. described the angiographic appearance of coronary lesions responsible for ACS [28]. They found that ACS lesions caused a severe obstruction of the coronary lumen (>85% stenosis, minimal cross-sectional area: <0.4 mm^2). Subsequent studies showed that not only do these “culprit” lesions usually cause severe coronary obstruction, they also have a morphology similar to that associated with acute myocardial infarction [29]. In such patients, the angiogram can have a high predictive value in determining the culprit lesion responsible for the abrupt change in symptoms.

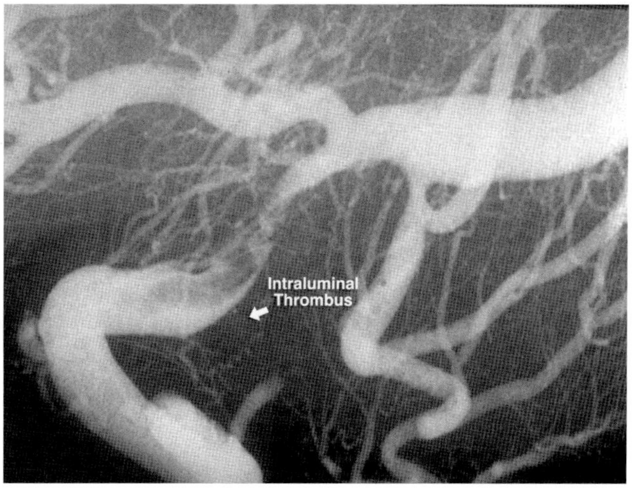

Fig. 17.6 An angiogram demonstrating an intraluminal filling defect (*arrow*) in the circumflex coronary artery. The clot is adherent to the coronary wall and projects down the lumen

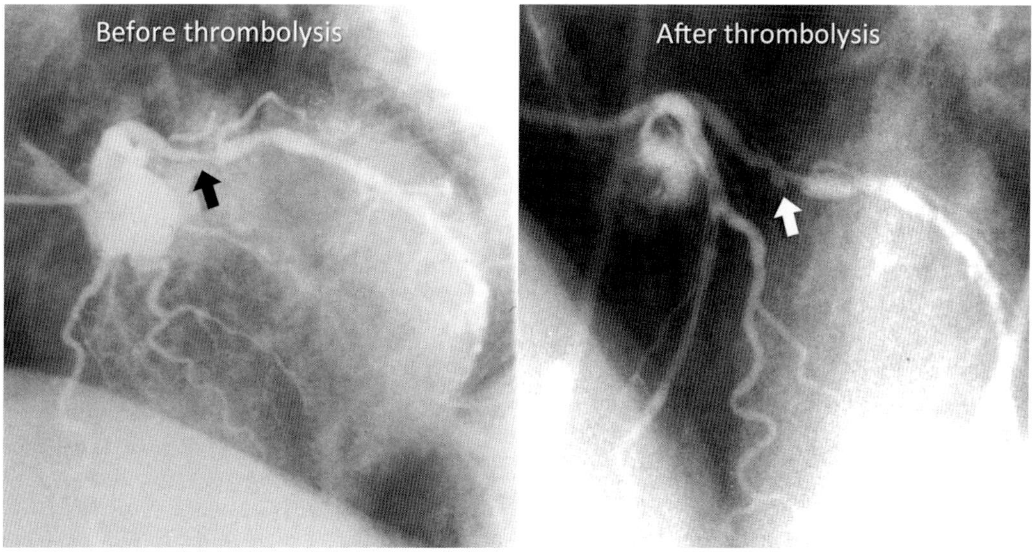

Fig. 17.7 *Left*: An angiogram obtained from a patient 1 day after a non-ST-elevation myocardial infarction of the posterior wall. A hazy stenosis of the proximal circumflex (*black arrow*) is visible. *Right*: An angiogram from the same patient 1 week after treatment with heparin anticoagulation shows an ulcerated lesion (*white arrow*) at the site of the prior smooth stenosis. Endogenous thrombolysis led to a reduction in stenosis and revelation of the ulcer crater

The angiographic appearance of thrombotic coronary lesions is characterized by:

1. Intraluminal filling defects (the tail of the clot projects into the lumen) (Fig. 17.6)
2. Indistinct or hazy outline of the vessel's lumen
3. The presence of an "ulcer crater" in the vessel wall, indicating a ruptured atherosclerotic plaque (Figs. 17.7 and 17.8)
4. Downstream abrupt occlusion of smaller branches due to clot embolization; these occlusions usually have an abrupt "soft" edge which distinguishes it from a chronic occlusion
5. In some cases, complete occlusion of the parent artery at the site of plaque rupture, with the typical, abrupt "soft" edge which distinguishes it from a chronic occlusion

The risk of progression to acute infarction or death can be predicted from several factors, most of which relate to:

1. The likelihood that the symptoms are due to a thrombotic lesion
2. The extent of myocardium served by the thrombotic coronary
3. The vulnerability of the myocardium to ischemia

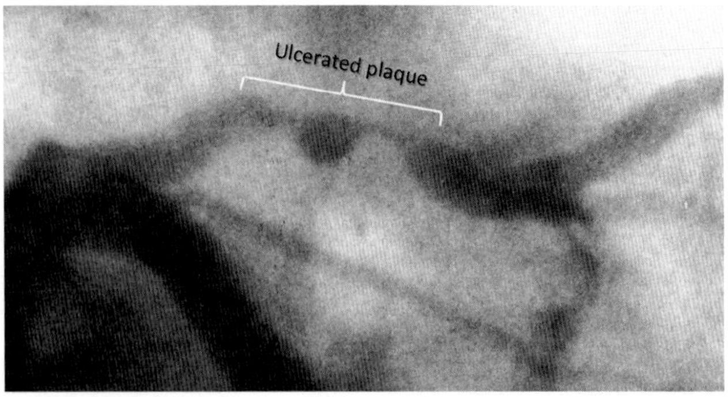

Fig. 17.8 An angiogram obtained from a 62-year-old man presenting with abrupt onset of angina and deep symmetrical T wave inversion in the anterior precordial leads. The proximal left anterior descending artery has a severe ulcerated stenosis characteristic of ACS

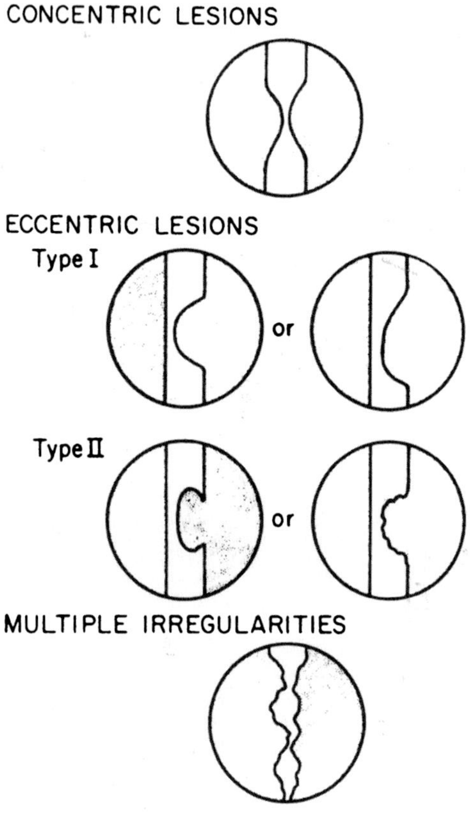

Fig. 17.9 The Ambrose classification of coronary lesion morphology. Type IIB is associated with the eccentric, thrombotic lesions characteristic of ACS

Ambrose et al. developed a system for classifying coronary stenosis morphology based on its angiographic appearance (Fig. 17.9) [30]. Lesions associated with acute thrombotic syndromes (unstable angina and infarction) were usually of Type II eccentric morphology, and in most thrombotic lesions, the edges were irregular and scalloped.

Visual interpretation of stenosis morphology is fraught with marked intraobserver and interobserver variability. For these reasons, quantitative indices of lesion irregularity applicable for use with computer-assisted quantitative angiography have been developed (Fig. 17.10). One such quantitative measure, the "Ulceration Index," is defined as the diameter of the least-severe narrowing within the lesion (the downward lip of the ulcer) divided by the maximum intralesional diameter. This index decreases as the irregularity increases, and is independent of stenosis severity (in terms of lumen obstruction). In one study of patients with stable angina, unstable angina, or recent myocardial infarction, the severity of the coronary lesion measured either as percent stenosis, or in absolute terms as minimal cross-sectional area was similar in all groups, although lesions causing unstable angina tended to be more severe (Fig. 17.11) [31]. The Ulceration Index, however, was significantly lower in lesions causing unstable angina (0.62 ± 0.05) or infarction (0.61 ± 0.03), than in lesions causing stable angina (0.90 ± 0.01) ($N = 351$).

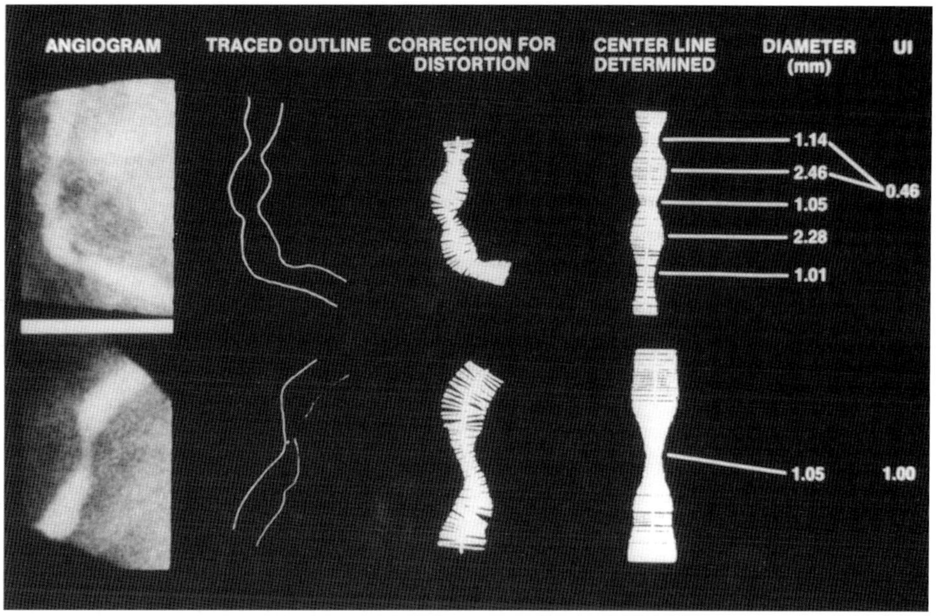

Fig. 17.10 A quantitative angiographic diagram (Brown-Dodge method) of the angiographic characteristics of ulcerated coronary lesions and calculation of the Ulceration Index

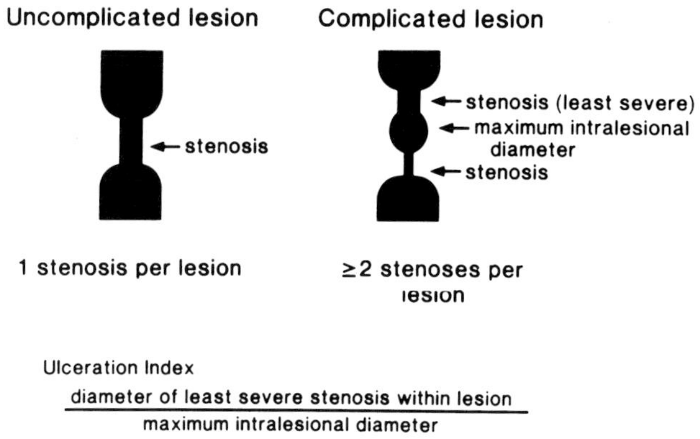

Fig. 17.11 A diagram of the angiographic characteristics of uncomplicated and complicated (ulcerated) coronary lesions and calculation of the Ulceration Index

Coronary Imaging in ACS

Intravascular ultrasound (IVUS) of unstable plaque shows a relatively echolucent area inside the plaque and a thin intimal covering that separates the inflammatory "abscess" from the vessel lumen [32]. The thickness of the intimal cap over the plaque varies significantly [33]. The thinner the intimal covering, the more likely is the plaque to rupture. With time, the intimal thickness increases, reducing the likelihood of rupture (see Fig. 21.12).

Optical coherence tomography (OCT) imaging, using near-infrared (NIR) reflectance, provides images of the coronary wall similar to IVUS, but with much greater spatial resolution [34]. This enables more accurate measurement of the thickness of the cap on atherosclerotic plaque [35]. In addition, the structure of the contents of the plaque can be better visualized and the constituents of the plaque contents can be better predicted from the high-resolution images. The disadvantages, however, are its shallow depth of imaging penetration of the arterial wall and the need for a saline flush into the coronary artery during imaging to remove the blood. (The infrared light is absorbed by the red cells). Like IVUS, OCT shows that plaque lesions associated with ACS have semiliquid contents and a thin tissue cap.

Intracoronary temperature measurements made using thermistors mounted on a catheter show that these inflammatory plaques have elevated temperatures typical of inflamed tissue [36]. In one study, temperature heterogeneity in the arterial wall indicated a higher risk of a subsequent cardiac event.

NIR spectroscopy obtained using a catheter inside the coronary lumen can provide an automated, detailed image of the location and chemical characteristics of lipid core plaque [37]. NIR light is absorbed or scattered by certain chemical groups. Measurement of this absorption or scatter can provide a "chemical signature" of the constituents of atherosclerotic plaque.

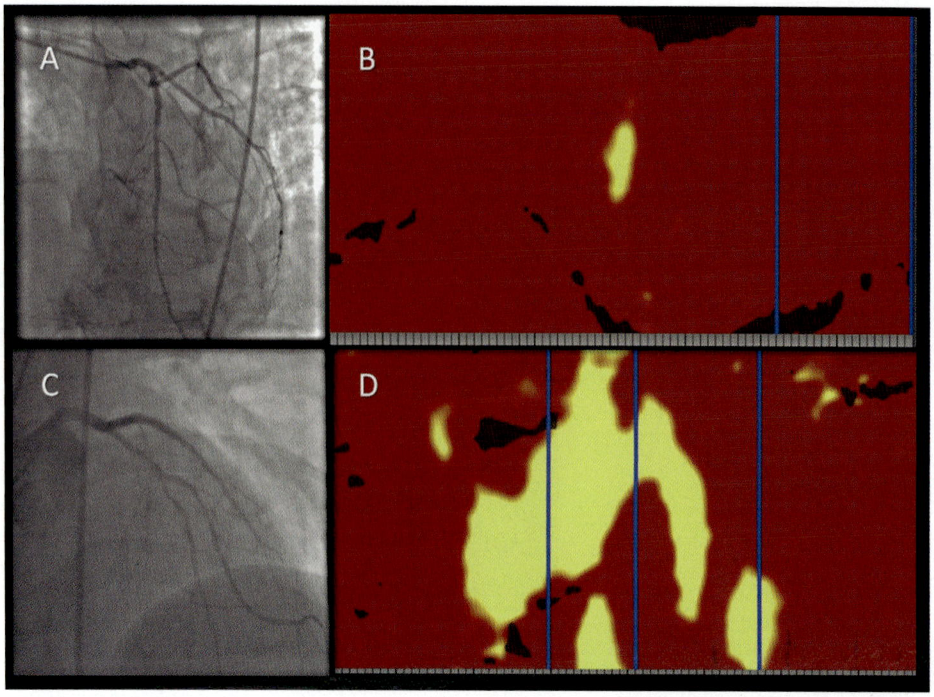

Fig. 17.12 Near-infrared chemograms taken from the LAD of two patients. (**a**) An angiogram showing moderate diffuse disease in the mid-LAD. (**b**) The associated chemogram shows minimal lipid content of the LAD plaque, suggesting low risk (courtesy of Emmanouil S. Brilakis, MD, Dallas TX). (**c**) An angiogram from another patient showing similar, moderate diffuse disease in the mid-LAD. (**d**) The associated chemogram showing marked lipid accumulation in the plaque, suggesting that the plaque is vulnerable to rupture and poses a higher risk of ACS (courtesy of David Rizik, MD, Scottsdale, AZ)

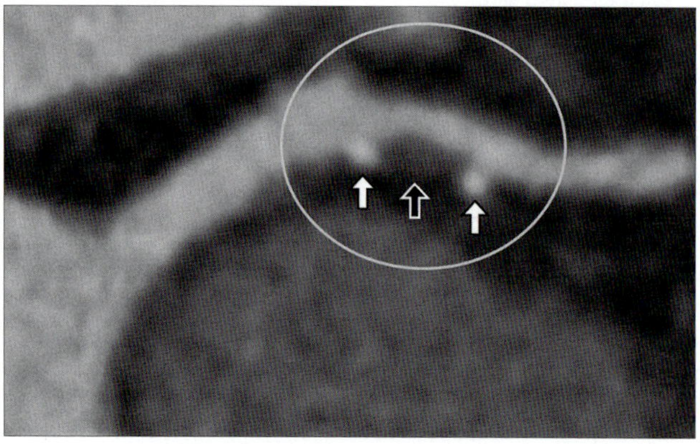

Fig. 17.13 A CT coronary angiogram demonstrating a "soft" plaque in the proximal LAD (hypodense area, *black arrow*) with calcific plaque on both sides (*white arrows*) (courtesy of Uma Valeti, MD, University of Minnesota)

Fresh inflammatory plaque has a different infrared signature from established, fibrotic plaque. Image maps called "chemograms" of the artery generated by the InfraReDx catheter system show the localization of fresh plaque within the lumen (Fig. 17.12).

Coronary plaque can also be imaged less invasively using computed tomography (CT) coronary angiography. CT angiography, unlike invasive, catheter-based angiography, displays images of the coronary wall in addition to the lumen (Fig. 17.13) "Soft plaque" is relatively radiolucent compared to fibrotic or calcific plaque. Thrombi can be difficult to delineate with certainty, but the marked luminal obstruction associated with ACS can be defined with a high level of accuracy using CT angiography [38, 39].

Treatment of ACS

Antithrombotic Treatment

Treatment of ACSs centers on passivation of the thrombotic lesion and relief of the coronary obstruction. Anticoagulants, particularly antiplatelet agents, are the cornerstone of therapy [40]. Theroux et al. showed definitively in 1988 that aspirin, intravenous unfractionated heparin, or both are effective in reducing the subsequent incidence of acute infarction [41].

Compared to either agent alone, however, the combination of heparin and aspirin increased the risk of bleeding without a reduction in the risk of adverse event. Low-molecular weight heparin (LMWH) appears to be as effective as unfractionated heparin, but has a lower risk of bleeding [42]. Concerns about its long therapeutic half-life and use in patients subsequently undergoing angiography or percutaneous coronary intervention (PCI) have limited its use.

More recently, the CURE trial demonstrated that the addition of clopidogrel, an ADP platelet receptor-mediated antiplatelet agent, to aspirin significantly reduced the likelihood of an adverse event for as long as 9 months after the initial presentation [43]. In contrast, the powerful intravenous 2B3A antiplatelet agents (e.g., abciximab, tirofiban, and integrilin) and their oral counterparts appear to have no beneficial effect in patients with ACSs, and one (abciximab) may be harmful, due to increased risk of infarction after cessation [44].

Additional Medical Therapy

Additional medical therapy usually consists of drugs to reduce myocardial oxygen consumption (beta adrenergic receptor antagonists and antihypertensive drugs) and drugs that limit arterial spasm (nitrates and calcium channel antagonists) [45]. Beta receptor antagonists reduce heart rate and blood pressure. Use of these drugs may reduce progression to STEMI, but there is no clear evidence that they reduce mortality. Similarly, nitrates can reduce ischemic symptoms, but there is no definitive evidence that they alter outcomes of ACS [46].

In distinction to vasoactive drugs, emerging evidence indicates that statin-type medications do reduce the risk of ACS [47]. These drugs have anti-inflammatory properties (e.g., inhibition of matrix metalloproteinases) that may lead to more rapid resolution of inflammatory plaque. Administration at hospital admission and use in high doses appears to reduce the risk of a cardiac event.

Revascularization

The first significant trial of revascularization for patients with ACS was the VA Cooperative Trial on Unstable Angina. Patients presenting with ACS were randomized to treatment with bypass surgery or medical therapy (at the time, consisting of aspirin, beta blockers, and nitrates). Patients with reduced left ventricular ejection fraction had a clear survival advantage if they were revascularized with surgery. Patients with normal LV function, however, had similar mortality regardless of therapy. Of note, 43% of patients failed medical treatment and crossed over to surgery.

Subsequently, numerous clinical trials have compared PCI to medical therapy alone for patients with ACS [48–50]. Taken as a whole, these trials show a reduction in mortality and recurrent ischemia in the groups treated with PCI compared to medical therapy (Fig. 17.14) [51]. In addition, the cost of revascularization appears to be less than the cost of therapy needed for recurrent infarction and hospitalization associated with medical therapy alone.

PCI of these lesions can be complicated by embolization of thrombus and plaque material, vasospasm, and enhanced rethrombosis of the PCI site. Balloon inflation in the thrombotic lesion causes platelet barotrauma, causing the platelets to release their alpha granules filled with thromboxane A2 and serotonin. These cause local and downstream vasospasm and slow, transient blood flow in the artery, often leading to immediate ischemia (with symptoms and ST-segment changes on the ECG). In addition, the release of procoagulant agents from the plaque (such as tissue factor) and further tissue trauma exposing collagen can lead to marked thrombosis at the site of dilation.

The incidence of balloon dilation-induced embolization, thrombosis, and vasospasm has been reduced by the use of intravenous or intracoronary-administered 2B3A platelet receptor antagonists and by pretreatment with clopidogrel antiplatelet therapy. Trials of embolic protection devices have not proven effective in treatment of native coronary-related ACS [52].

Coronary Bypass Surgery

About 10% of patients presenting with ACS subsequently undergo coronary bypass surgery [53, 54]. Compared to patients undergoing PCI, patients revascularized with bypass surgery have a higher incidence of more widespread coronary atherosclerosis and a higher incidence of diabetes.

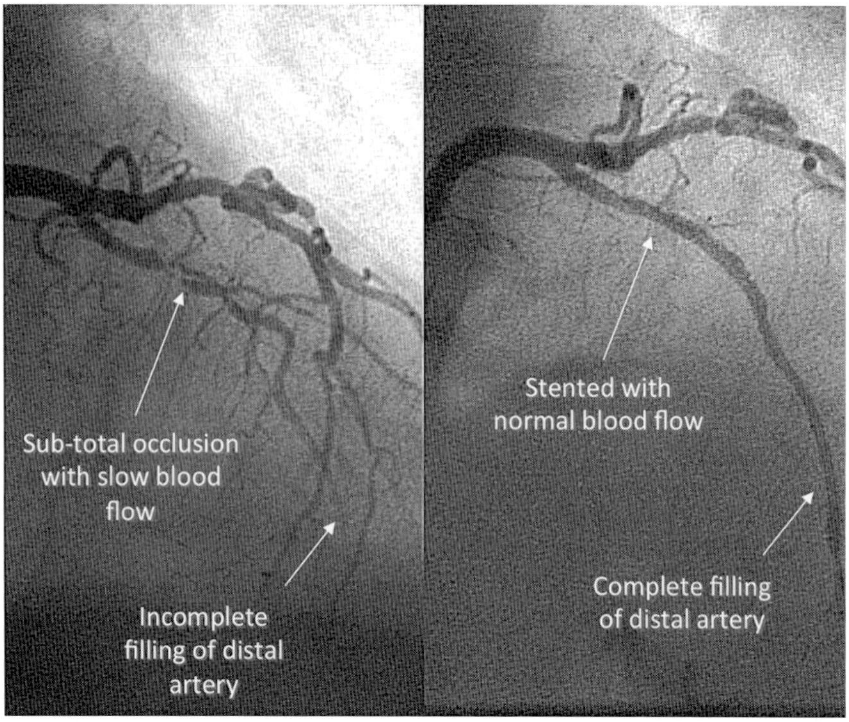

Fig. 17.14 *Left*: Angiogram from a 65-year-old diabetic woman who presented with a 4-day history of exertional dyspnea and vague episodic left jaw pain. The ECG showed ST-depression in the anterior leads. Troponin I was slightly elevated. The angiogram showed subtotal occlusion of the proximal LAD and incomplete filling (TIMI 1 blood flow) of the distal vessel. *Right*: After treatment with the 2B3A platelet inhibitor abciximab, the LAD was stented, with restoration of blood flow to the distal vessel

Performing bypass surgery soon after presentation with myocardial infarction has been associated with a higher mortality risk [55]. The risk of bypass surgery and the timing relative to symptom onset of ACS (without ST-elevation MI) have been controversial. In the VA Cooperative Trial, bypass surgery was delayed by a mean of 9 or more days from presentation, and the overall operative mortality was 3% [56]. In the more recent VANQWISH trial, patients revascularized with surgery (performed an average of 8 days after presentation) had a 7.7% risk of mortality, compared to no mortality in the patients treated with PCI [57]. The mechanism for this early risk is unclear but may involve microcirculatory injury related to the upstream lesion, and the pro-inflammatory and procoagulant effects of bypass surgery. No such time-dependency of risk occurs for patients treated with PCI [58].

References

1. Fulton M, Lutz W, Donald KW, et al. Natural history of unstable angina. Lancet. 1972;1:860.
2. Tanaka A, Imanishi T, Kitabata H, et al. Morphology of exertion-triggered plaque rupture in patients with acute coronary syndrome: an optical coherence tomography study. Circulation. 2008;118(23):2368–73.
3. Shah PK. Pathophysiology of coronary thrombosis: role of plaque rupture and plaque erosion. Prog Cardiovasc Dis. 2002;44:357–68.
4. Davignon J, Ganz P. Role of endothelial dysfunction in atherosclerosis. Circulation. 2004;109(23 Suppl 1):III27–32.
5. Kolodgie FD, Burke AP, Farb A, et al. The thin-cap fibroatheroma: a type of vulnerable plaque: the major precursor lesion to acute coronary syndromes. Curr Opin Cardiol. 2001;16:285–92.
6. Takano M, Mizuno K, Okamatsu K, Yokoyama S, Ohba T, Sakai S. Mechanical and structural characteristics of vulnerable plaques: analysis by coronary angioscopy and intravascular ultrasound. J Am Coll Cardiol. 2001;38:99–104.
7. Falk E. Unstable angina with fatal outcome: dynamic coronary thrombosis leading to infarction and/or sudden death. Autopsy evidence of recurrent mural thrombosis with peripheral embolization culminating in total vascular occlusion. Circulation. 1985;71:699–708.
8. Fitzgerald DJ, Roy L, Catella F, et al. Platelet activation in unstable coronary disease. N Engl J Med. 1986;315:983–9.
9. Falk E, Shah PK, Fuster V. Coronary plaque disruption. Circulation. 1995;92:657–71.
10. Willerson JT, Golino P, Eidt J, et al. Specific platelet mediators and unstable coronary artery lesions. Experimental evidence and potential clinical implications. Circulation. 1989;80:198–205.
11. Bertrand ME, LaBlanche JM, Tilmant PY, et al. Frequency of provoked coronary arterial spasm in 1089 consecutive patients undergoing coronary arteriography. Circulation. 1982;65:1299–308.
12. Isner JM, Estes III NA, Thompson PD, et al. Acute cardiac events temporally related to cocaine abuse. N Engl J Med. 1986;315:1438–43.
13. Cangella F, Medolla A, De Fazio G, et al. Stress-induced cardiomyopathy presenting as acute coronary syndrome: Tako-tsubo in Mercogliano, southern Italy. Cardiovasc Ultrasound. 2007;5:36.
14. Braunwald E. Unstable angina: a classification. Circulation. 1989;80:410–4.

15. Savonitto S, Ardissino D, Granger CB, et al. Prognostic value of the admission electrocardiogram in acute coronary syndromes. JAMA. 1999;281:707–13.
16. Bassand J, Hamm CW, Ardissino D, et al. Guidelines for the diagnosis and treatment of non-ST-segment elevation acute coronary syndromes. Eur Heart J. 2007;13:1598–660.
17. Cannon CP, McCabe CH, Stone PH, et al. The electrocardiogram predicts one-year outcome of patients with unstable angina and non-Q-wave myocardial infarction: results of the TIMI III Registry ECG Ancillary Study. Thrombolysis in myocardial ischemia. J Am Coll Cardiol. 1997;30:133–40.
18. Hamm CW, Braunwald E. A classification of unstable angina revisited. Circulation. 2000;102:118–22.
19. American Heart Association Statistics Committee and Stroke Statistics Subcommittee. Heart disease and stroke statistics – 2010 update: a report from the American Heart Association. Circulation. 2010;121:e46–215.
20. Farb A, Tang AL, Burke AP, Sessums L, Liang Y, Virmani R. Sudden coronary death. Frequency of active coronary lesions, inactive coronary lesions, and myocardial infarction. Circulation. 1995;92:1701–9.
21. Antman EM, Cohen M, Bernink PJ, et al. The TIMI risk score for unstable angina/non-ST elevation MI: a method for prognostication and therapeutic decision making. JAMA. 2000;284:835–42.
22. Goldman L, Cook EF, Johnson PA, Brand DA, Rouan GW, Lee TH. Prediction of the need for intensive care in patients who come to the emergency departments with acute chest pain. N Engl J Med. 1996;334:1498–504.
23. Eagle KA, Lim MJ, Dabbous OH, et al. GRACE Investigators. A validated prediction model for all forms of acute coronary syndrome: estimating the risk of 6-month postdischarge death in an international registry. JAMA. 2004;291:2727–33.
24. Ottani F, Galvani M, Ferrini D, et al. Prodromal angina limits infarct size. A role for ischemic preconditioning. Circulation. 1995;91:291–7.
25. Mladenovic ZT, Angelkov-Ristic A, Tavciovski D, Mijailovic Z, Gligic B, Cosic Z. The cardioprotective role of preinfarction angina as shown in outcomes of patients after first myocardial infarction. Tex Heart Inst J. 2008;35:413–8.
26. Schwartz H, Leiboff RH, Bren GB, et al. Temporal evolution of the human coronary collateral circulation after myocardial infarction. J Am Coll Cardiol. 1984;4:1088–93.
27. Liu GS, Thornton J, Van Winkle DM, Stanley AW, Olsson RA, Downey JM. Protection against infarction afforded by preconditioning is mediated by A1 adenosine receptors in rabbit heart. Circulation. 1991;84:350–6.
28. McMahon MM, Brown BG, Cukingnan R, et al. Quantitative coronary angiography: measurement of the "critical" stenosis in patients with unstable angina and single-vessel disease without collaterals. Circulation. 1979;60(1):106–13.
29. Levin DC, Fallon JT. Significance of the angiographic morphology of localized coronary stenoses: histopathologic correlations. Circulation. 1982;66:316–20.
30. Ambrose JA, Tannenbaum MA, Alexopoulos D, et al. Angiographic progression of coronary artery disease and the development of myocardial infarction. J Am Coll Cardiol. 1988;12:56–62.
31. Wilson RF, Holida MD, White CW. Quantitative angiographic morphology of coronary stenoses leading to myocardial infarction or unstable angina. Circulation. 1986;73:286–93.
32. Hamdan A, Assali A, Fuchs S, Battler A, Kornowski R. Imaging of vulnerable coronary artery plaques. Catheter Cardiovasc Interv. 2007; 70:65–74.
33. Rodriguez-Granillo GA, Garcia-Garcia HM, Mc Fadden EP, et al. In vivo intravascular ultrasound-derived thin-cap fibroatheroma detection using ultrasound radiofrequency data analysis. J Am Coll Cardiol. 2005;46:2038–42.
34. Jang IK, Tearney GJ, MacNeil B, et al. In vivo characterization of coronary atherosclerotic plaque by use of optical coherence tomography. Circulation. 2005;111:1551–5.
35. Mizukoshi M, Imanishi T, Tanaka A, et al. Clinical classification and plaque morphology determined by optical coherence tomography in unstable angina pectoris. Am J Cardiol. 2010;106:323–8.
36. Stefanadis C, Diamantopoulos L, Vlachopoulos C, et al. Thermal heterogeneity within human atherosclerotic coronary arteries detected in vivo: a new method of detection by application of a special thermography catheter. Circulation. 1999;99:1965–71.
37. Caplan JD, Waxman S, Nesto RW, Muller JE. Near-infrared spectroscopy for the detection of vulnerable coronary artery plaques. J Am Coll Cardiol. 2006;47:C92–6.
38. Manini AF, Dannemann N, Brown DF, et al. Rule Out Myocardial Infarction using Coronary Artery Tomography (ROMICAT) study investigators. Limitations of risk score models in patients with acute chest pain. Am J Emerg Med. 2009;27:43–8.
39. Henneman MM, Schuijf JD, Pudziute G, et al. Noninvasive evaluation with multislice computed tomography in suspected acute coronary syndrome: plaque morphology on multislice computed tomography versus coronary calcium score. J Am Coll Cardiol. 2008;52:216–22.
40. Telford AM, Wilson C. Trial of heparin versus atenolol in prevention of myocardial infarction in intermediate coronary syndrome. Lancet. 1981;1:1225–8.
41. Theroux P, Ouimet H, McCans J, et al. Aspirin, heparin, or both to treat acute unstable angina. N Engl J Med. 1988;319:1105–11.
42. Ferguson JJ, Califf RM, Antman EM, et al. SYNERGY Trial Investigators: enoxaparin vs unfractionated heparin in high-risk patients with non-ST-segment elevation acute coronary syndromes managed with an intended early invasive strategy: primary results of the SYNERGY randomized trial. JAMA. 2004;292(1):45–54.
43. Peters RJ, Mehta SR, Fox KA, et al. Effects of aspirin dose when used alone or in combination with clopidogrel in patients with acute coronary syndromes: observations from the Clopidogrel in Unstable angina to prevent Recurrent Events (CURE) study. Circulation. 2003;108:1682–7.
44. Simoons ML. GUSTO IV-ACS Investigators: effect of glycoprotein IIb/IIIa receptor blocker abciximab on outcome in patients with acute coronary syndromes without early coronary revascularisation: the GUSTO IV-ACS randomised trial. Lancet. 2001;357(9272):1915–24.
45. Yusuf S, Wittes J, Friedman L. Overview of results of randomized clinical trials in heart disease. II. Unstable angina, heart failure, primary prevention with aspirin, and risk factor modification. JAMA. 1988;260:2259–63.
46. Curfman GD, Heinsimer JA, Lozner EC, Fung HL. Intravenous nitroglycerin in the treatment of spontaneous angina pectoris: a prospective, randomized trial. Circulation. 1983;67:276–82.
47. Murphy SA, Cannon CP, Wiviott SD, et al. Effect of intensive lipid-lowering therapy on mortality after acute coronary syndrome (a patient-level analysis of the Aggrastat to Zocor and Pravastatin or Atorvastatin Evaluation and Infection Therapy-Thrombolysis in Myocardial Infarction 22 trials). Am J Cardiol. 2007;100:1047–51.

48. de Winter RJ, Windhausen F, Cornel JH, et al. Early invasive versus selectively invasive management for acute coronary syndromes. N Engl J Med. 2005;353:1095–104.
49. Lagerqvist B, Husted S, Kontny F, et al. A long-term perspective on the protective effects of an early invasive strategy in unstable coronary artery disease: two-year follow-up of the FRISC-II invasive study. J Am Coll Cardiol. 2002;40:1902–14.
50. Mehta SR, Cannon CP, Fox KA, et al. Routine vs. selective invasive strategies in patients with acute coronary syndromes: a collaborative meta-analysis of randomized trials. JAMA. 2005;293:2908–17.
51. Montalescot G, Cayla G, Collet JP, et al. Intervention timing and acute coronary syndromes. JAMA. 2010;303:131–2.
52. Mauri L, Rogers C, Baim DS. Devices for distal protection during percutaneous coronary revascularization. Circulation. 2006;113:2651–6.
53. Eagle KA, Lim MJ, Dabbous OH, et al. GRACE Investigators. A validated prediction model for all forms of acute coronary syndrome: estimating the risk of 6-month postdischarge death in an international registry. JAMA. 2004;291:2727–33.
54. McCormick JR, Schick Jr EC, McCabe CH, Kronmal RA, Ryan TJ. Determinants of operative mortality and long-term survival in patients with unstable angina – the CASS experience. J Thorac Cardiovasc Surg. 1985;89:683–8.
55. Tu JV, Sykora K, Naylor CD. Assessing the outcomes of coronary artery bypass graft surgery: how many risk factors are enough? J Am Coll Cardiol. 1997;30:1317–23.
56. Rahimtoola SH, Nunley D, Grunkemeier G, Tepley J, Lambert L, Starr A. Ten-year survival after coronary bypass surgery for unstable angina. N Engl J Med. 1983;308:676–81.
57. Boden WE, O'Rourke RA, Crawford MH, et al. Outcomes in patients with acute non-Q-wave myocardial infarction randomly assigned to an invasive as compared with a conservative management strategy. Veterans Affairs Non-Q-Wave Infarction Strategies in Hospital (VANQWISH) Trial Investigators. N Engl J Med. 1998;338:1785–92.
58. Neumann FJ, Kastrati A, Pogatsa-Murray G, et al. Evaluation of prolonged antithrombotic pretreatment ("cooling-off" strategy) before intervention in patients with unstable coronary syndromes: a randomized controlled trial. JAMA. 2003;290:1593–9.

Chapter 18
Complications of Acute Myocardial Infarction

Zeev Vlodaver and Robert F. Wilson

Definition

Complications of acute myocardial infarction include mechanical failure, arrhythmia, thromboembolism from the heart, and pericarditis. Circulatory failure from severe left ventricle (LV) dysfunction or one of the other mechanical complications of acute myocardial infarction accounts for most fatalities.

Mechanical Complications

Mechanical complication of acute myocardial infarction (MI) include left ventricular failure and cardiogenic shock, cardiac rupture, and mitral insufficiency.

Left Ventricular Failure

The degree of LV pump failure is generally related to the size of the perfusion field distal to the thrombotic coronary occlusion. Infarction of more than 40% of the LV muscle mass usually results in cardiogenic shock and death. Prior infarction, mitral insufficiency, an acquired left-to-right shunt (usually from an infarct-related rupture of the ventricular septum [VSD]), or large aneurysm potentiate the effects of acute infarction on overall pump function, dramatically increasing the risk of death.

Other conditions not immediately related to the myocardial infarction, such as chronic pulmonary disease, non-infarct related valvular heart disease, left ventricular hypertrophy, and hypertension further increase the risk of heart failure and shock. Before reperfusion therapy was available large infarcts often resulted in death due to low cardiac output or intractable arrhythmia. While these patients are still very ill, prompt reperfusion and temporary circulatory support can sometimes allow the muscle time to recover function and sustain life.

In instances where extensive myocardial infarction is responsible for LV failure, the infarction may be both acute and healed, in part. When the infarction is only acute, LV failure usually means that the infarction is transmural, and involves an extensive portion of the LV. Less commonly, the LV failure results from extensive, acute subendocardial infarction (circumferential infarction). When lesser amounts of acute myocardial infarction are present, LV failure may result from the acute infarction damage plus extensive damage from an old myocardial infarction. Preexisting diastolic noncompliance, much more common in women and patients with hypertension, doubles the risk of heart failure after MI. Conversely,

Z. Vlodaver, MD (✉) • R.F. Wilson, MD
Division of Cardiovascular Medicine, University of Minnesota, Minneapolis, MN, USA
e-mail: zeev.vlodaver@gmail.com

Z. Vlodaver et al. (eds.), *Coronary Heart Disease: Clinical, Pathological, Imaging, and Molecular Profiles*,
DOI 10.1007/978-1-4614-1475-9_18,

Table 18.1 Killip classification of degree of CHF severity

Class	Characteristics
I	No evidence of CHF
II	Rales, jugular venous distension, or S3
III	Pulmonary edema
IV	Cardiogenic shock

Adapted from Killip and Kimball [1]. Copyright 1967 by Elsevier Ltd.

patients with small, more distal infarctions may have discrete regional wall motion abnormalities with preserved overall LV function because of compensatory hyperkinesis of unaffected segments.

In their landmark research published in 1967, Killip and Kimball demonstrated increased mortality among hospitalized patients who had acute myocardial infarction with greater degree of congestive heart failure (CHF) severity [1]. The authors developed a classification scheme to categorize patients' prognosis based on their hemodynamics profile. Patients were classified into four subgroups, from "no evidence of congestive heart failure (CHF)" to "cardiogenic shock" (Table 18.1).

CHF occurs in approximately 15–25% of patients who experience MI and is associated with an in-hospital mortality rate of 15–40%. In their 2002 report based on the Second National Registry of Myocardial Infarction (NRMI-2), Wu et al. analyzed the outcomes for patients with ST-elevation MI with CHF (Killip classes II and III), and they found that 19% had CHF on admission [2]. Patients presenting with CHF were older, more often female, had longer time to hospital presentation, and higher prevalence of anterior/septal AMI, diabetes, and hypertension. They also had longer lengths of stay and greater risk for in-hospital death. Patients with CHF were less likely to receive aspirin, heparin, oral beta-blockers, fibrinolytics, or primary angioplasty, and more likely to receive angiotensin-converting enzyme inhibitors. CHF on admission was one of the strongest predictors of in-hospital death.

Left Ventricular Failure and Cardiogenic Shock

Cardiogenic shock is defined as a state of inadequate tissue perfusion resulting from severe impairment of ventricular pump function in the presence of adequate intravascular volume. It is the leading cause of death for patients with acute myocardial infarction.

Despite advances in the treatment of myocardial infarction, the incidence of cardiogenic shock has remained at 7–10% during the last 25 years. In a prospective study of 293,633 patients with ST-elevation myocardial infarction (STEMI), Babaev et al. found that 8.6% had cardiogenic shock [3]. Hospital mortality was about 90% in the 1970s. It has improved over the years, but in-hospital mortality is still estimated to be about 50% [3]. For persons older than 75 years, the mortality rate is higher. The short-term survival rate has increased in recent years – at the same time that use of coronary reperfusion and temporary circulatory support strategies have increased.

The vast majority of patients with cardiogenic shock have LV failure; in about 12% of cases, cardiogenic shock is related to other infarct-related mechanical causes, including acute mitral insufficiency, ventricular septal rupture, and ventricular free wall rupture.

Risk factors for developing cardiogenic shock include older age, anterior myocardial infarction location, hypertension, diabetes mellitus, multivessel coronary artery disease, prior MI, prior CHF, ST-elevation MI, or left bundle branch block (LBBB). All of these risk factors are correlated with either a large perfusion field distal to the thrombosed coronary lesion or to reduced diastolic compliance of the ventricle.

Most patients develop cardiogenic shock because of extensive myocardial ischemia or necrosis, which directly impairs myocardial contractility and results in diminished stroke volume and arterial pressure. On a mechanical level, a marked decrease in contractility, reduced ejection fraction and cardiac output, and ultimately ventricular failure, result in systemic hypotension and/or pulmonary edema.

Varying pathological stages of infarction confirm the stuttering and progressive nature of the myocardial necrosis. A combination of new and old infarctions consistently involves at least 40% of the myocardium.

A systemic inflammatory response syndrome-type mechanism has been implicated in the pathophysiology of cardiogenic shock. Elevated levels of white blood cells, interleukins, and C-reactive proteins are often seen in large infarcts. Inflammatory nitric oxide synthetase (iNOS) is also released in high levels and induces nitric oxide (NO) production, which may uncouple calcium metabolism in the myocardium, resulting in stunned myocardium. Additionally, iNOS leads to the expression of interleukins, which may themselves cause hypotension.

Elevated sympathetic neural tone and elevated circulating catecholamines increase systemic vascular resistance, cause pulmonary vein constriction, and may reduce blood flow to non-infarct related coronary perfusion fields. The result can be a limitation of hyperemic blood flow to the remaining muscle, exhibiting compensatory hyperkinesis to make up for the loss of function in the infarct zone. All of these factors and the diminished coronary artery perfusion from hypotension trigger a vicious cycle of further myocardial ischemia and necrosis, resulting in even lower blood pressure, lactic acidosis, multiple organ failure, and ultimately, death.

Patients in cardiogenic shock generally will have a sustained blood pressure less than 90 mmHg (or 30 mmHg below baseline mean arterial pressure) for at least 30 min, or the need for vasopressors or intra-aortic balloon pump (IABP) counter pulsation to maintain the systolic blood pressure above 90 mmHg [4]. These patients may have a cardiac index less than 2.2 L/min/m^2 not related to hypovolemia (pulmonary artery wedge pressure less than 12 mmHg), arrhythmia, hypoxemia, acidosis, or atrio-ventricular block. Outcomes significantly improve only when rapid revascularization can be achieved. The Shock Trial Registry demonstrated that overall mortality when rapid revascularization occurs is 38%. When rapid revascularization is not attempted, mortality rate approaches 70% [5].

Patients in cardiogenic shock generally have severe orthopnea, dyspnea, and oliguria, and may have altered mental status, as well multisystem organ failure from hypoperfusion. Additionally, an S3 gallop, pulmonary rales, and elevated jugular venous pressure are common findings on physical examination.

Patients with cardiogenic shock caused by acute myocardial infarction generally have extensive electrocardiographic changes demonstrating a large infarct, diffuse ischemia, or multiple prior infarcts. Chest radiography likely reveals pulmonary edema. Laboratory tests may demonstrate lactic acidosis, renal failure, and arterial hypoxemia.

Two-dimensional echocardiography and pulsed-wave and color Doppler imaging provide a comprehensive assessment of the anatomic and hemodynamic status at the bedside. They also help identify other mechanical complications of myocardial infarction that may contribute to cardiogenic shock.

In a small fraction of patients, hypovolemia (e.g., from vomiting or lack of oral intake) in the setting of acute MI can cause hypotension. When the intravascular volume status is unclear, patients in cardiogenic shock pulmonary artery wedge pressure should be assessed. This may help distinguish between primary LV failure and other mechanical causes of cardiogenic shock.

Illustrative Case: Left Ventricular Failure and Cardiogenic Shock Resulting from Healed Anterior and Acute Inferior Infarction

The case portrayed in Figs. 18.1–18.7 is one of extensive loss of muscle incidental to an acute myocardial infarction complicating a healed infarction and a dilated LV. The combination resulted in death attributed to the ventricle's grossly inadequate pump function.

The patient was a 49-year-old man with a history of episodes of acute myocardial infarctions 1, 3, and 7 years previously. Angina pectoris persisted and he was admitted to the hospital for surgery. A recent ECG showed evidence of an old anteroseptal myocardial infarction (Fig. 18.1). A coronary arteriogram revealed occlusion of the left anterior descending (LAD) artery (Fig. 18.2). On the third day in the hospital, the patient developed new episodes of chest pain, and enzyme and ECG changes that indicated an acute posteroinferior myocardial infarction. During the next few days, he experienced recurrent thoracic pain, supraventricular tachycardia (rate, 150), followed by hypotension (BP, 80–90, systolic), and signs of LV failure, including shortness of breath and pulmonary edema. During further study, hypotension continued and oliguria developed. His extremities were pale and cold, and a gallop rhythm with a third sound developed. The patient died in a state of cardiogenic shock on the seventh day of illness.

On pathologic examination, the heart was hypertrophied (700 g). Atherosclerosis was widely distributed in the three main coronary arteries. The LAD was occluded proximally by organized thrombi (Fig. 18.3) and a recent thrombus was present in the intermediate segment of the RCA (Fig. 18.4a). The CX showed moderate disease (Fig. 18.4b).

The anteroseptal region of the LV showed extensive scarring related to a healed myocardial infarction, and the posteromedial papillary muscle was scarred as part of another healed myocardial infarction (Fig. 18.5a). The inferior wall of the LV and juxtaposed ventricular septum were the sites of acute transmural myocardial infarction consistent histologically with 7 days' duration (Fig. 18.5b).

The lungs showed extensive pulmonary edema (right lung, 1,000 g; left lung, 800 g) (Fig. 18.6). The liver showed central hemorrhagic necrosis (Fig. 18.7). Hydrothorax of about 1 L was present in each pleural cavity.

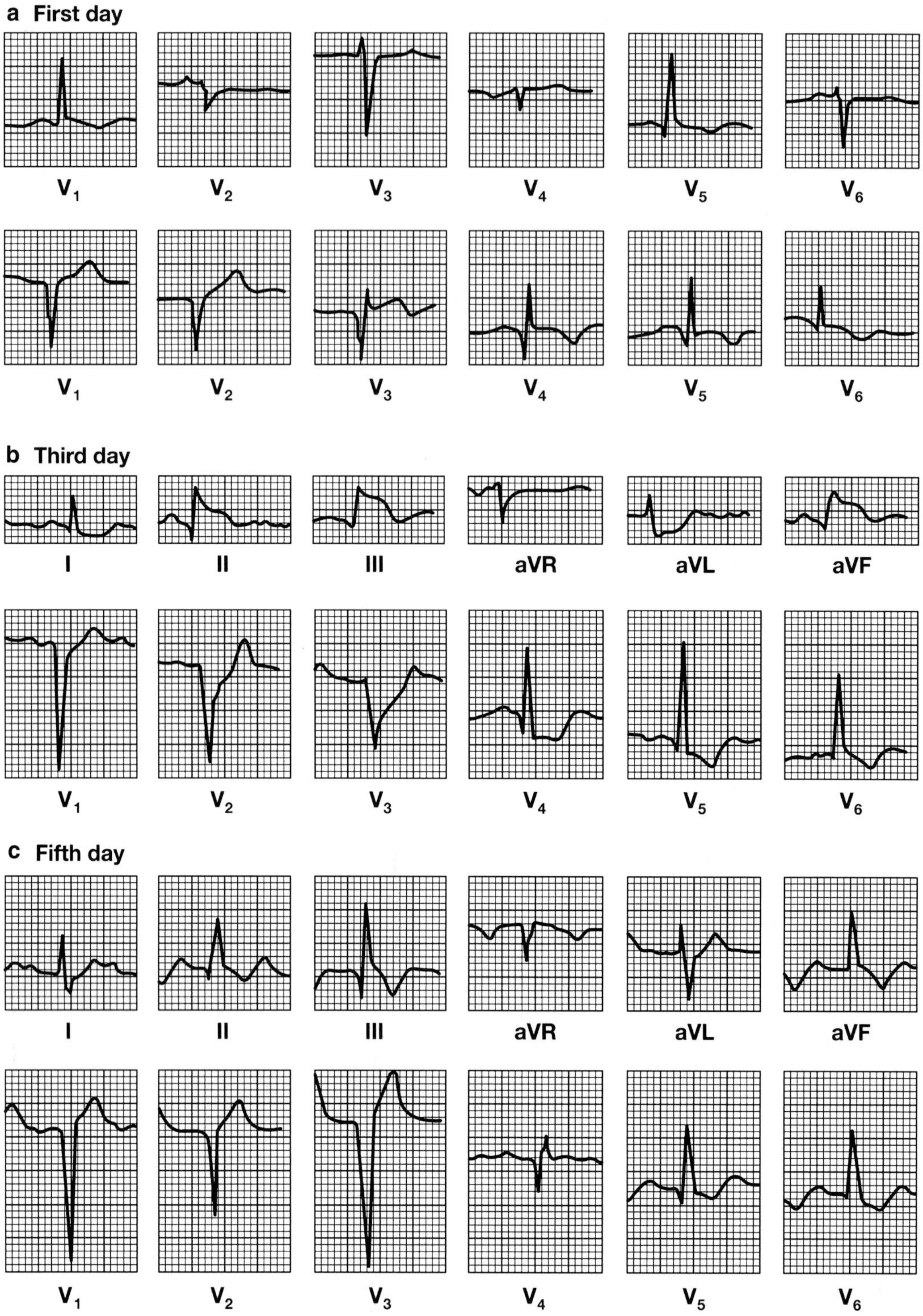

Fig. 18.1 (**a**) ECG on day 1 shows changes typical of an old, anteroseptal myocardial infarction: left axis deviation and nonspecific T-wave changes in the left precordial leads. (**b**) Day 3: ECG shows additional changes, typical of acute inferior wall myocardial infarction and disappearance of the left axis deviation. (**c**) Day 5: Evolutionary changes of the inferior myocardial infarction are apparent with a slight increase in the intraventricular conduction defect, in which the fault in the posterior fasciculus predominates, giving rise to a definite right axis shift

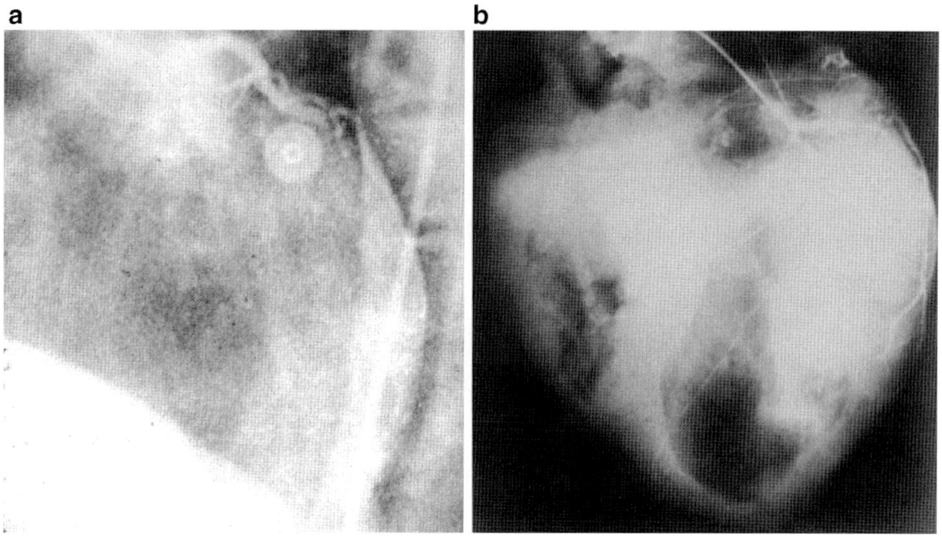

Fig. 18.2 (**a**) LC arteriogram in RAO view 4 months before death shows occlusion of the LAD. (**b**) Postmorten LC arteriogram shows the LAD occluded shortly after its origin

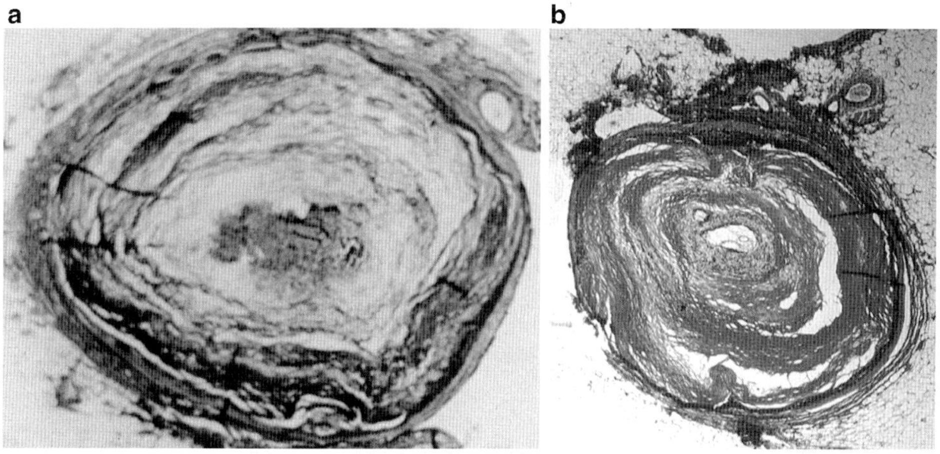

Fig. 18.3 Photomicrographs of LAD. (**a**) Proximal segment with the arterial lumen occluded by dense fibrous tissue considered to represent an old, organized thrombus. Elastic tissue stain: 15×. (**b**) Artery distal to site of organized thrombus shows extensive atherosclerosis. Elastic tissue stain: 18×

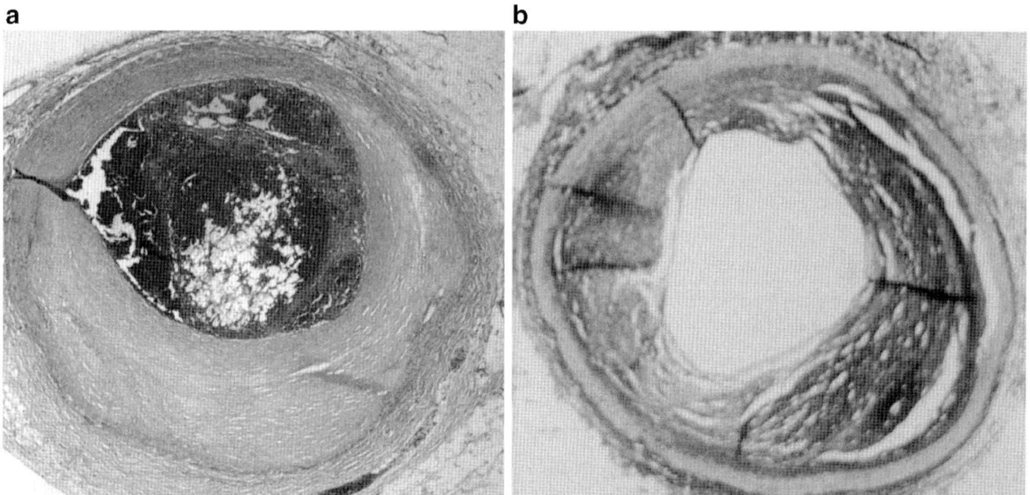

Fig. 18.4 (**a**) RC approximately 7 cm from origin showing atherosclerosis and occlusion by a recent thrombus. Hematoxylin and eosin stain: 18×. (**b**) CX 3.5 cm from origin shows moderate narrowing. Elastic tissue stain: 55×

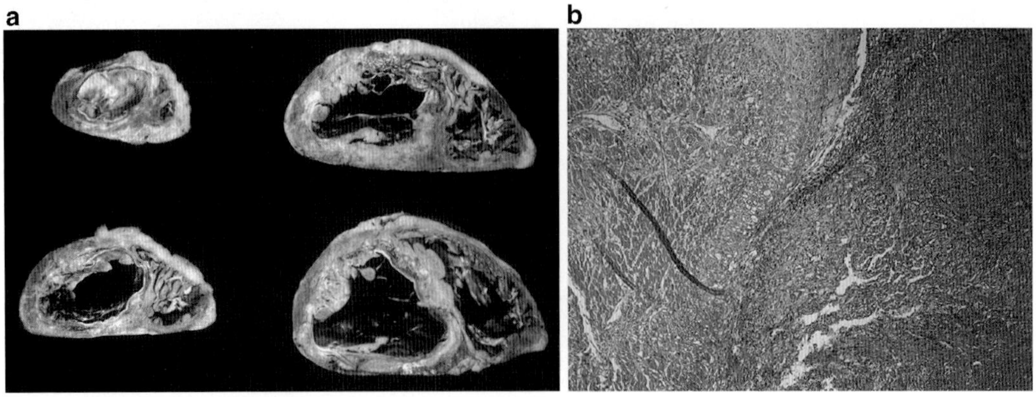

Fig. 18.5 (**a**) Cross sections of ventricular portion of heart show evidence of healed anteroseptal and acute inferior myocardial infarction. (**b**) Photomicrograph of inferior wall of LV. At periphery of myocardial infarction there is removal of tissue, a picture consistent with an infarction of 7 days duration. Hematoxylin and eosin stain: 69×

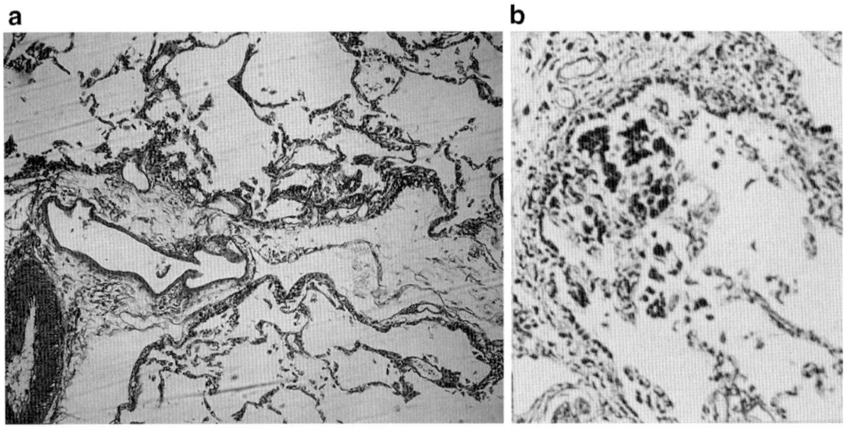

Fig. 18.6 Photomicrographs of lung. (**a**) Congestion and edema. Hematoxylin and eosin stain: 45×. (**b**) Dilatation of lymphatics. Hemosiderosis as sign of LV failure. Hematoxylin and eosin stain: 98×

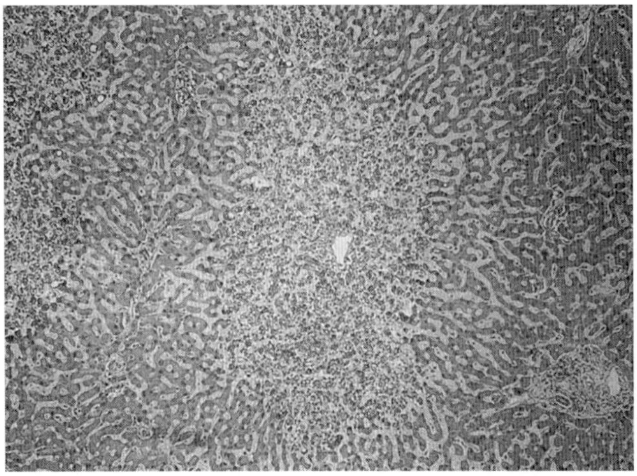

Fig. 18.7 Photomicrograph of liver, showing central hemorrhagic necrosis. Hematoxylin and eosin stain: 67×

Cardiac Rupture

Rupture of the Free Wall of the LV

Rupture of the free wall of the left ventricle is found in less than 1% of living patients with an acute myocardial infarction [6], but myocardial rupture was a frequent cause of death in those patients dying in the acute or early phases after their first myocardial infarction [7].

The profile of rupture of the heart following infarction has certain characteristics:

1. Age 70 or older
2. Female gender
3. Preexistent hypertension with little or no ventricular hypertrophy
4. Transmural MI
5. Myocardial rupture that may occur from 1 day to 3 weeks after infarction (vs. most ruptures, which occur 3–5 days after infarction)
6. The rupture site is devoid of scars, although scars from previous infarctions may be present in other areas
7. The rupture occurs in the periphery of the infarction near the non-infarcted muscle
8. Poor collateral vessels

An additional potential risk – and one that is controversial – is thrombolytic therapy. Honan et al. [8] studied the relationship between the risk of cardiac rupture and the timing of thrombolytic therapy for acute MI. Thrombolytic therapy early after MI improves survival and decreases the risk of cardiac rupture. Late administration of thrombolytic therapy also appears to improve survival, but may increase the risk of cardiac rupture. The risk of myocardial rupture was significantly decreased by successful angioplasty in all age groups studied. In a retrospective study review of 2,209 patients with acute MI treated with percutaneous coronary intervention (PCI), the risk of cardiac rupture was 0.7% when successful reperfusion was achieved within 12 h, 0.9% when reperfusion occurred within 12–24 h, and 3.8% after failed reperfusion [9]. Prompt reperfusion with PCI appears to have reduced the incidence of rupture.

Specific types of rupture of the heart include rupture of the ventricular septum, of a papillary muscle, and of the free wall of the LV.

When the free wall of the LV ruptures, the lesion represents laceration of the wall's endocardium with secondary extravasation of blood through the free wall and into the pericardial sac. Typically, rupture of the free wall of the LV is associated with hemopericardium, pericardial tamponade, and cardiogenic shock, but cases of incomplete rupture or rupture without hemopericardium have been reported. Many autopsy specimens show abundant epicardial fat, which has been postulated to contain the tear and prevent hemopericardium. As to sites of infarction which underlie rupture of the free wall, Van Tassel and Edwards [10] found equal distribution of cardiac rupture of the anterior, lateral, and posterior wall of the LV. The high incidence of rupture through the lateral wall of the LV compared to relatively low incidence of isolated transmural infarction in this area is of interest. It suggests that the zone of the LV between the papillary muscles, when infarcted, is more susceptible to the forces leading to rupture than is the case with other sites of myocardial infarction.

Early diagnosis of myocardial rupture is crucial if life saving therapy is to be applied. Recent chest pain with further ST-segment elevation, hypotension, and cardiogenic shock in the setting of an acute or recent myocardial infarction should alert clinicians to the possibility of this complication, particularly in patients with an extensive transmural (Q-wave) infarction. Transthoracic or transesophageal echocardiography (TEE) affords a rapid, potentially definitive diagnostic tool. Pericardial fluid can be visualized, overall LV function assessed, the area of infarction localized, and the presence of psudoaneurysm or true aneurysm revealed.

Definitive treatment is surgical, with infarctectomy, if possible, to repair the rupture. Coronary bypass may or may not be necessary. Before surgery, hemodynamic monitoring and stabilization with appropriate fluids, vasopressors, and inotropic agents should be promptly initiated. Pericardiocentesis can provide temporary relief of hemodynamic compromise. Intra-aortic balloon counterpulsation has been used for emergency stabilization, but its role is controversial.

Illustrative Case: Rupture of the Free Wall of the LV 1 Day Following Onset of Infarction

The case shown in Figs. 18.8–18.10 illustrates an uncommon event: rupture of the free wall occurring approximately 24 h after the onset of myocardial infarction. The patient was an 83-year-old woman with mild diabetes known for 40 years. On admission, she felt weak and appeared anorexic, and substernal pain had been present for some hours. Physical examination revealed BP of 148/72; pulse, 100 and irregular. No murmurs were detected. Blood sugar was 285 mg/dL.

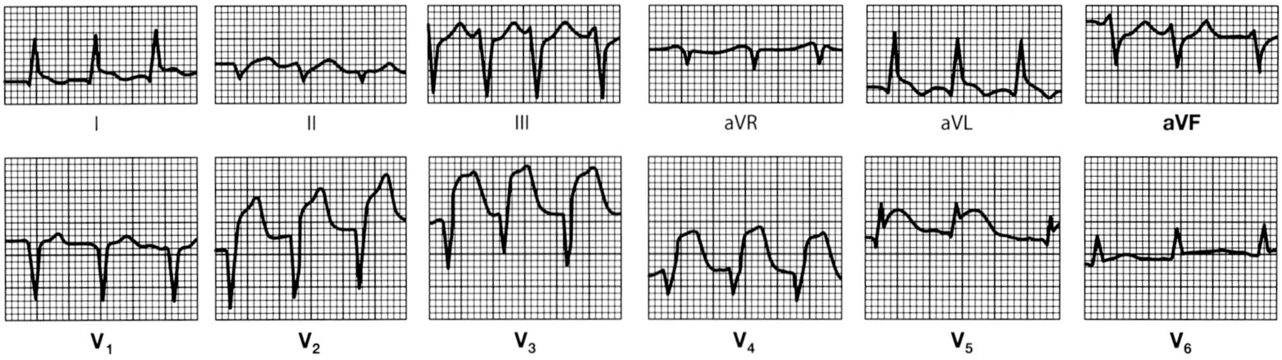

Fig. 18.8 ECG on admission. Taken approximately 20 h after the onset of symptoms, shows tachycardia, presumably atrial fibrillation, left axis deviation, and Q and ST abnormalities characteristic of anterolateral acute myocardial infarction

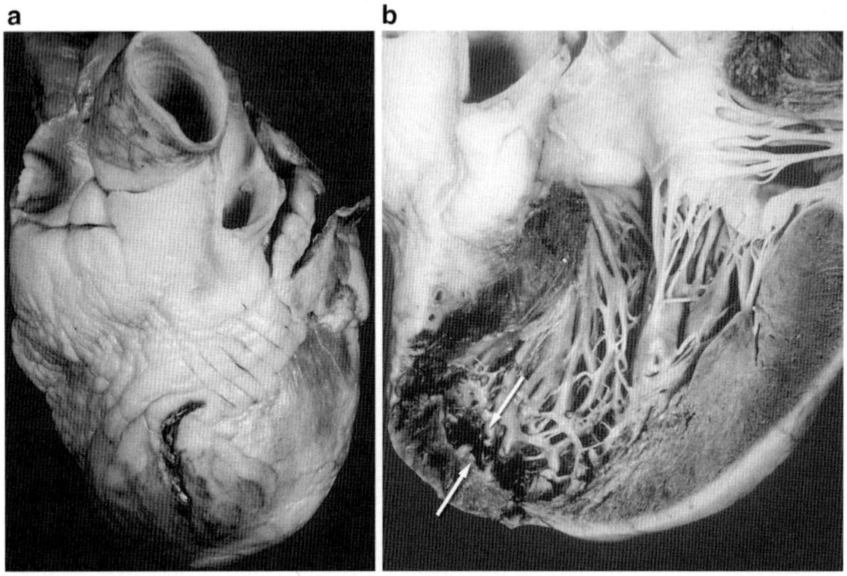

Fig. 18.9 (**a**) External view of heart showing laceration to the left of the anterior interventricular sulcus. (**b**) Interior of LV. A zone of discoloration in the anterior wall represents acute transmural myocardial infarction. The site of internal tear of the LV lies between the *arrows*

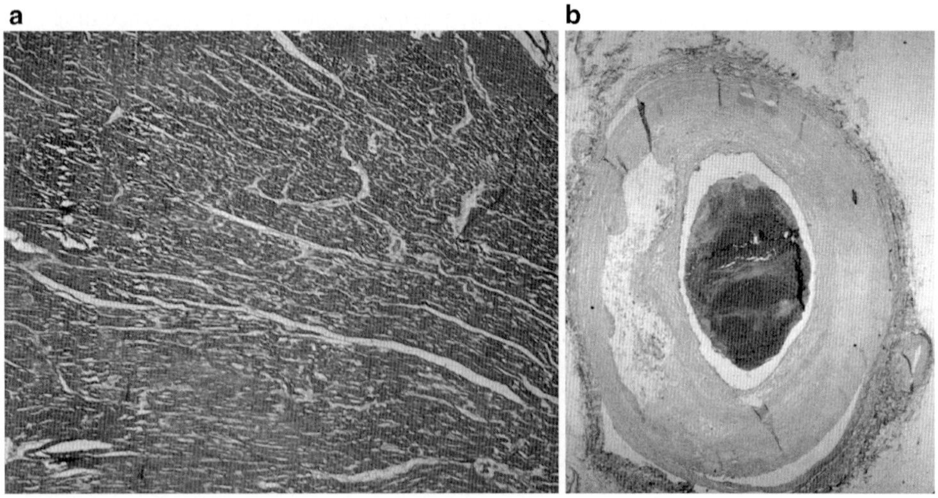

Fig. 18.10 (**a**) Photomicrograph of the LV's anterior wall shows signs of early acute myocardial infarction; the mobilized leukocytes have not yet penetrated the individual muscle fibers. In the original section, the involved muscle fibers showed a high degree of eosinophilia. Hematoxylin and eosin stain: 73×. (**b**) Photomicrograph of LAD 2.5 cm from its origin. Lumen narrowed by atherosclerosis has been occluded by a recent thrombus. Hematoxylin and eosin stain: 15×

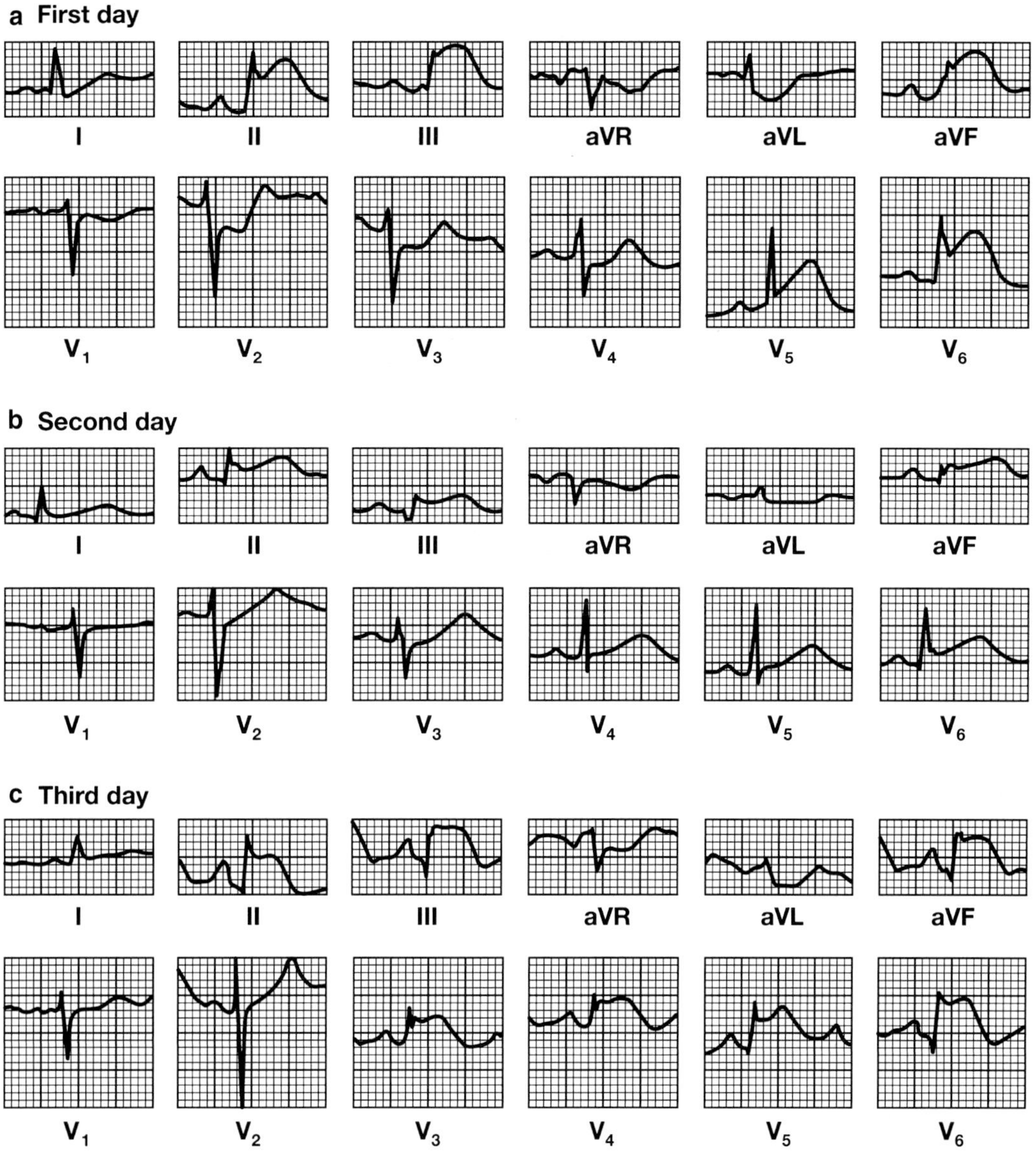

Fig. 18.11 (**a**) The ECG first day post-resuscitation shows segmental changes characteristics of injury to the posteroinferior wall and apex of the LV. (**b**) On the second hospital day, a moderate decrease in ST-segmental changes is visible. (**c**) The tracings on the third hospital day (day of death) show further increase in the injury effect (ST shift and Q waves in leads II, III, and aVF), with a nearly monophasic-appearing potential in leads aVF and V6. The prominent P waves in leads II and III are also noteworthy and may reflect pulmonary hypertension consequent to LV failure

Several hours after admission, she complained of further pain in the neck, throat, upper chest, and back. The ECG was interpreted as indicating acute myocardial infarction (Fig. 18.8). About 7 h after admission, the patient's cardiovascular status rapidly deteriorated and death occurred.

Pathological examination revealed hemopericardium. The cardiac weight was normal (250 g). An acute infarction involved the anterolateral region of the LV associated with laceration leading to the hemopericardium (Fig. 18.9). Each of the three coronary arteries showed zones of severe narrowing and a recent thrombus was present in the LAD approximately 2.5 cm beyond its origin (Fig. 18.10b).

Illustrative Case: Rupture of the Free Wall of the LV 3 Days Following Onset of Infarction

The case shown in Figs. 18.11–18.13 is more typical, in that rupture of the free wall of the LV occurred about 3 days after the onset of myocardial infarction.

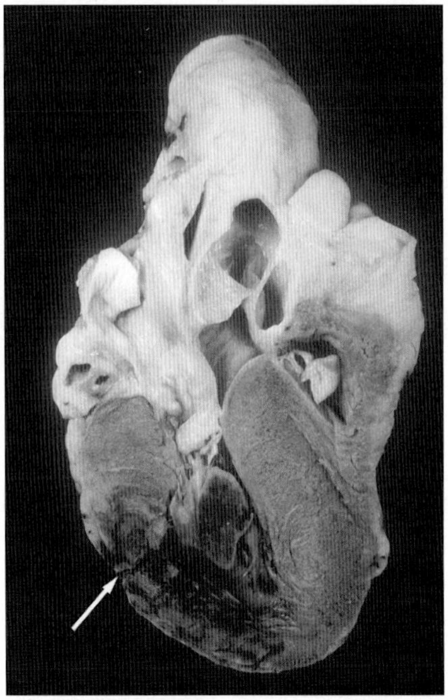

Fig. 18.12 Gross photograph of sagittal section of heart viewed from behind. The discolored area involves the lateral wall of the LV and represents the site of acute infarction. The rupture tract begins (*arrow*) near the upper portion of the periphery of the infarction

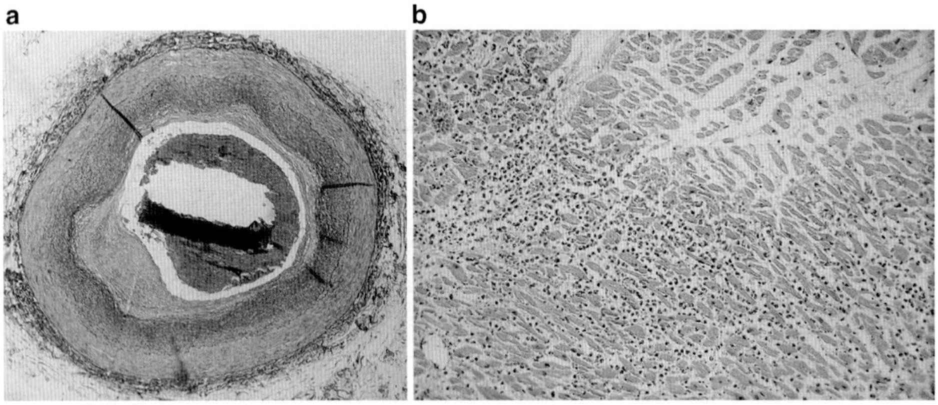

Fig. 18.13 (**a**) CX 1.5 cm from its origin shows relatively mild atherosclerosis with occlusion of the lumen by a thrombus. Elastic tissue stain: 16×. (**b**) Photomicrograph of lateral wall of the LV. Leukocytic infiltration is prominent, while evidence of removal is absent. The picture is compatible with an infarction of 3-day duration. Hematoxylin and eosin stain: 122×

The patient was a 65-year-old woman admitted after a few hours of unrelenting thoracic pain, nausea, and dyspnea. The previous day, while walking in the snow, she experienced severe chest distress from which she recovered after going indoors, warming, and resting. On the day of admission, an ECG performed in the emergency room (showed) ST-segmental depression. Initially, the patient's condition was satisfactory, but after a few hours, an episode of ventricular fibrillation occurred. Following defibrillation, ECG features of classical acute posteroinferior and lateral myocardial infarction were present (Fig. 18.11). Cardiac enzymes were elevated. The patient's condition was relatively stable until the third day, at which time she become comatose and BP was undetectable.

Pathologic examination showed distention of the pericardium with blood. The heart weighed 240 g. The lateral wall of the LV had a small perforation (Fig. 18.12). The coronary arteries showed marked narrowing by atherosclerosis. The CX was occluded by a thrombus about 1.5 cm from its origin (Fig. 18.13a). The myocardium was discolored near the LV rupture. The myocardial infarction was concentrated in the lateral and apical region.

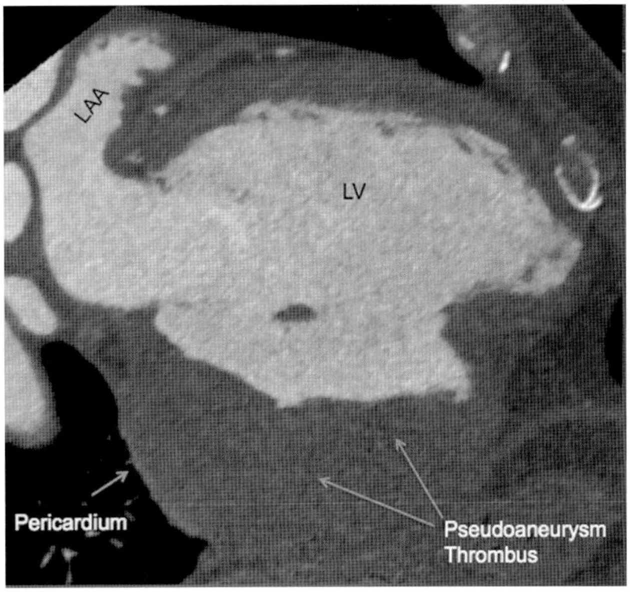

Fig. 18.14 Multidetector computed tomographic angiography (MCTA) long axis view illustrates a case with inferobasal pseudoaneurysm of the LV, complicating myocardial infarction. Image courtesy of Dr. John R. Lesser, Minneapolis Heart Institute

Histologic examination of the myocardium showed increased eosinophilia with heavy leukocytic infiltration in the periphery of the infarcted zone. No removal of muscle fibers was evident. The histologic age was compatible with an infarction of 3 days duration (Fig. 18.13b).

Rupture of the Free Wall of the Left Ventricle Formation of False or Pseudoaneurysm

In exceptional instances of rupture of the free wall of the LV complicating acute myocardial infarction, the leak is restricted. The pericardial hematoma is contained and the patient survives. With time, the periphery of the hematoma becomes organized to form the wall of a false aneurysm. The latter maintains communication with the cavity of the LV. A false aneurysm may mimic classical LV aneurysm clinically, and usually shows a relatively narrow communication with the cavity of the LV. This feature contrasts with that of a true aneurysm, in which, characteristically, a wide communication is present between the aneurysm and the LV cavity. The tendency for false aneurysm to rupture contrasts with the very low tendency for a true ventricular aneurysm to rupture [11].

False aneurysm may be associated with pericardial effusion. Some patients may have recurrent tachyarrythmia, systemic embolization, and heart failure. Patients may have systolic, diastolic, or to-and-fro murmurs related to the blood flow across the narrow neck of the false aneurysm [12]. A chest radiograph may show cardiomegaly, with an abnormal bulge on the cardiac border. There may be persistent ST-segment elevation on the ECG. The diagnosis of false aneurysm can be confirmed by echocardiography, MRI, or CT angio. See Fig. 3.14 – an echocardiogram showing rupture of the free wall of the LV contained by a hematoma and formation of a pseudoaneurysm.

Features of rupture of the free wall of the LV and formation of pseudoaneurysm can be clearly defined with multidetector computed tomography angiography (MCTA), as shown in Figs. 18.14 and 18.15.

Spontaneous rupture can occur without warning in approximately 45% of patients with false LV aneurysms, even when small [11]. Therefore, surgical intervention is recommended for all patients, regardless of symptoms or the size of the aneurysm, to prevent sudden death [13].

Angiographic Demonstration

Angiographic features in a case of false left ventricular aneurysm are shown in Fig. 18.16.

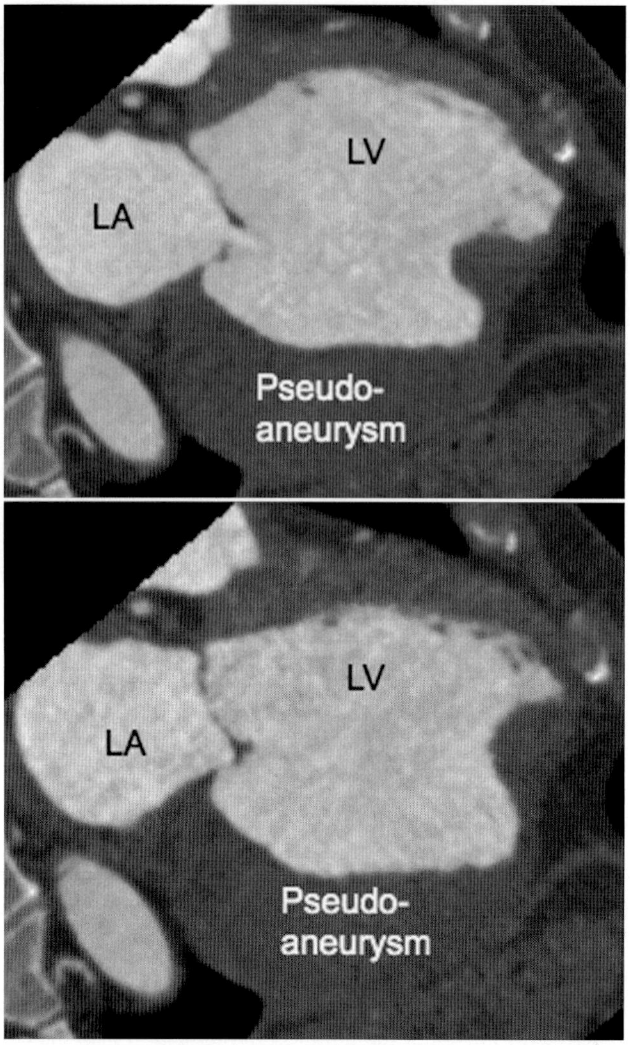

Fig. 18.15 From the case shown in Fig. 18.14, MCTA long axis view at end-diastole and systole. Image courtesy of Dr. John R. Lesser, Minneapolis Heart Institute

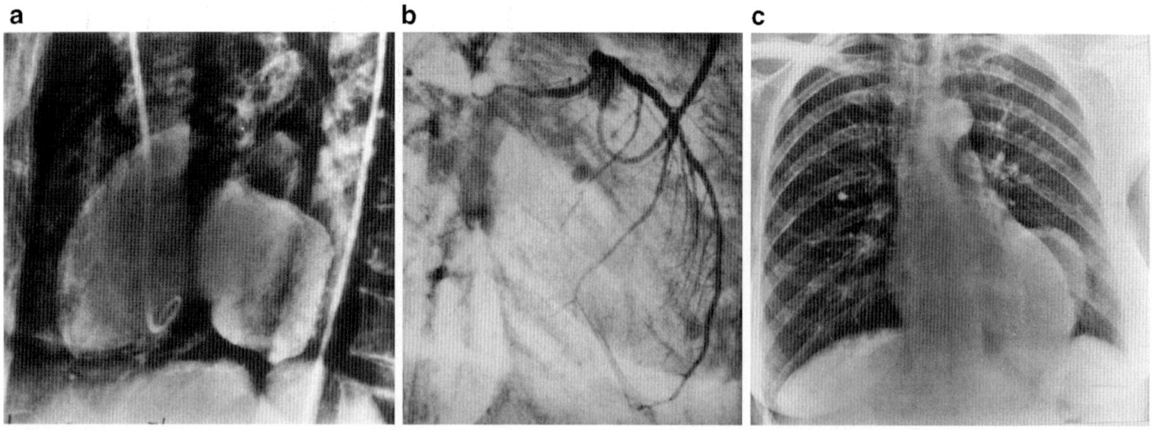

Fig. 18.16 (**a**) Lateral view of LV shows a distinct "neck" between the LV and the aneurysm. Note the unusually thick wall of the false aneurysm. (**b**) LC arteriogram in lateral view shows severe disease in the proximal segment of the LAD and occlusion in the proximal portion of the CX. (**c**) Thoracic roentgenogram in frontal view shows a large protrusion from the anterolateral aspect of the LV

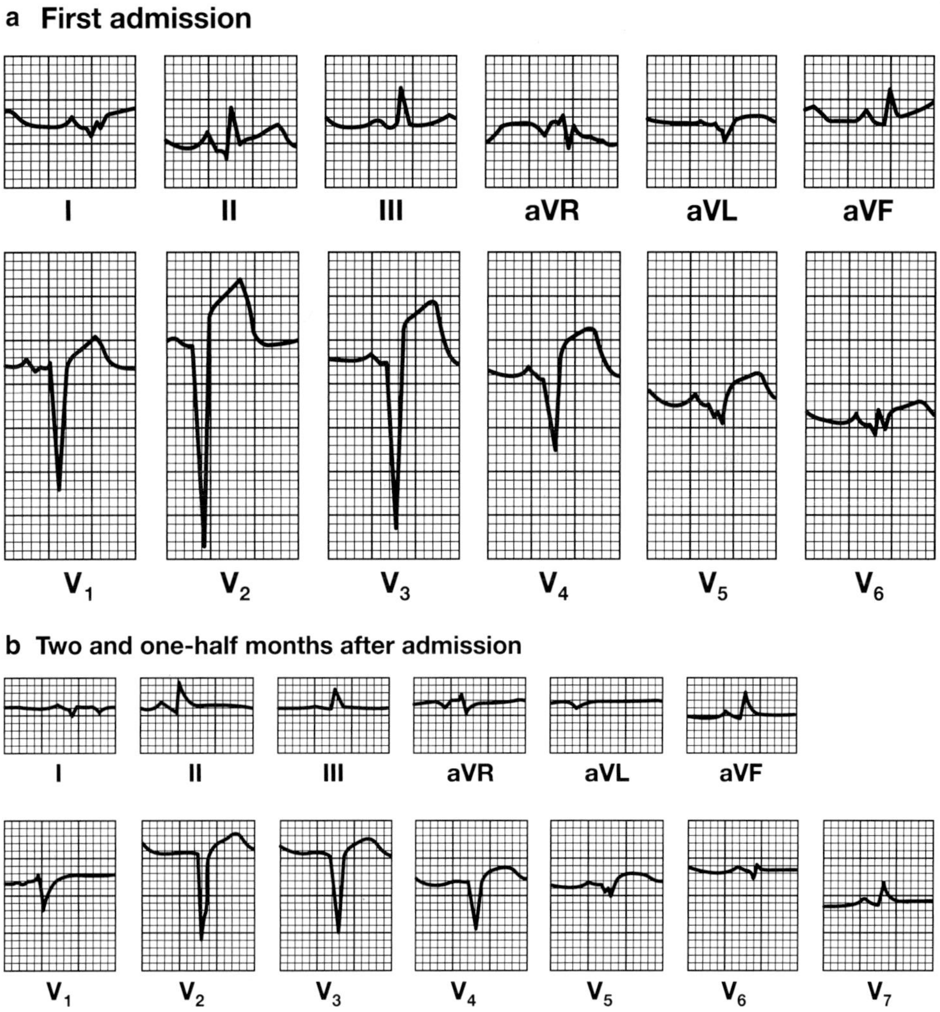

Fig. 18.17 From a 65-year-old man hospitalized for acute myocardial infarction. (**a**) ECG on first admission shows signs of acute anteroseptal myocardial infarction, probably extensive, with involvement of the apex and lateral wall. (**b**) ECG 2-½ months after the onset of acute myocardial infarction shows signs of old, anterior myocardial infarction with persistent ST elevation. The QRS voltage is low, consistent with pericardial effusion, but the nature of the ST segments primarily in leads V4 and V5 suggests LV aneurysm

Illustrative Case with Postmortem Study

Rupture of a Large False Aneurysm of the Left Ventricle

Figures 18.17–18.20 show images from a patient hospitalized for acute myocardial infarction [14]. Two and one-half months later, the patient was readmitted because of increasing dyspnea and findings of pericardial effusion and cardiac tamponade. Pericardiocentesis removed 200 mL of bloody fluid. Clinical improvement occurred following the procedure. Two weeks after the second admission, the patient suddenly become hypotensive, dyspneic, and cyanotic, and died.

At autopsy, the pericardium was distended with blood. A large aneurysmal deformity of the LV (11 × 5 cm) was discovered (Fig. 18.20). A narrow neck connected the aneurysm with the LV wall. The site of the narrow neck is interpreted as that of rupture of the free wall, which communicated with a false aneurysm.

Rupture of a Small False Aneurysm of the Left Ventricle

The case shown in Fig. 18.21 illustrates that false aneurysm may rupture, even when small. A 70-year-old man was found dead. The autopsy revealed hemopericardium resulting from rupture of one or two small aneurysms of the LV. Each was considered a complication of myocardial infarction.

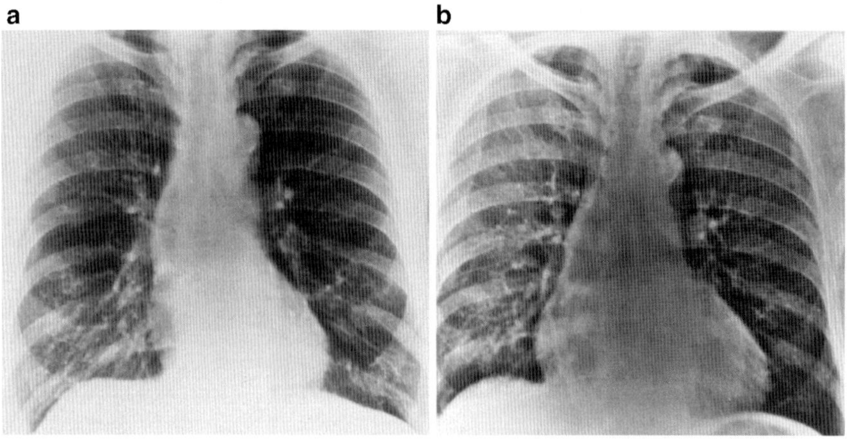

Fig. 18.18 (**a**) Roentgenogram of thorax from patient illustrated in Figs. 18.14 and 18.15, taken 2 months before first admission. It shows normal features. (**b**) Roentgenogram taken during first admission shows mild cardiac enlargement. Adapted from Gobel et al. [14]. Copyright 1971 by American College of Chest Physicians

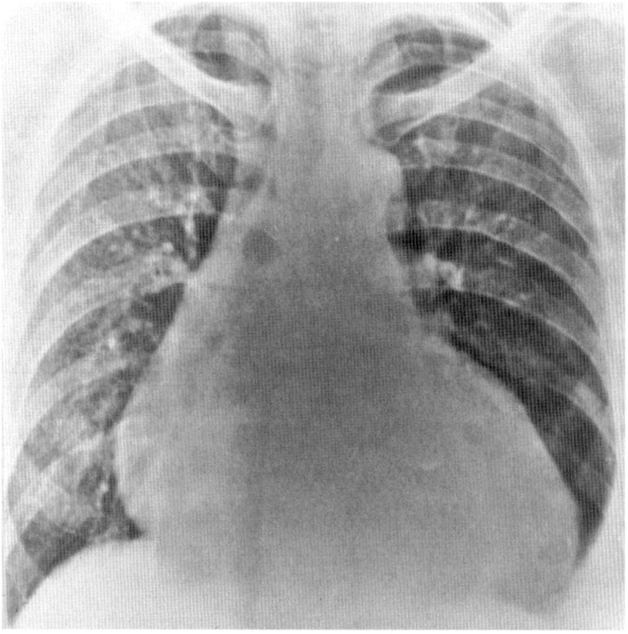

Fig. 18.19 Thoracic roentgenogram taken during the patient's second admission, before pericardiocentesis, shows enlargement of the cardiac silhouette – in part, the result of hemorrhagic pericardial effusion

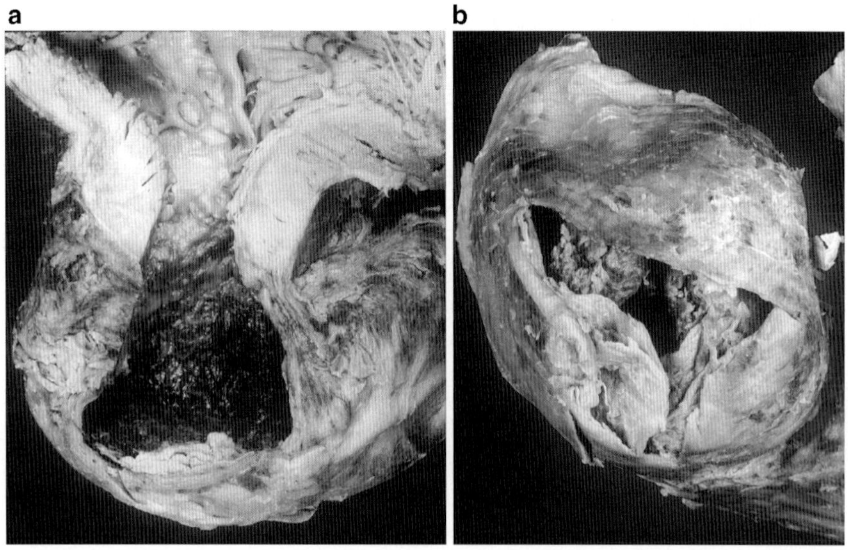

Fig. 18.20 (**a**) Interior of the LV and false aneurysm. The characteristic narrow neck connecting the false aneurysm with the LV cavity. *AA* ascending aorta. (**b**) Close-up view of the pericardial surface of the false aneurysm shows the extensive laceration which led to fatal hemopericardium. Adapted from Gobelet al. [14]. Copyright 1971 by American College of Chest Physicians

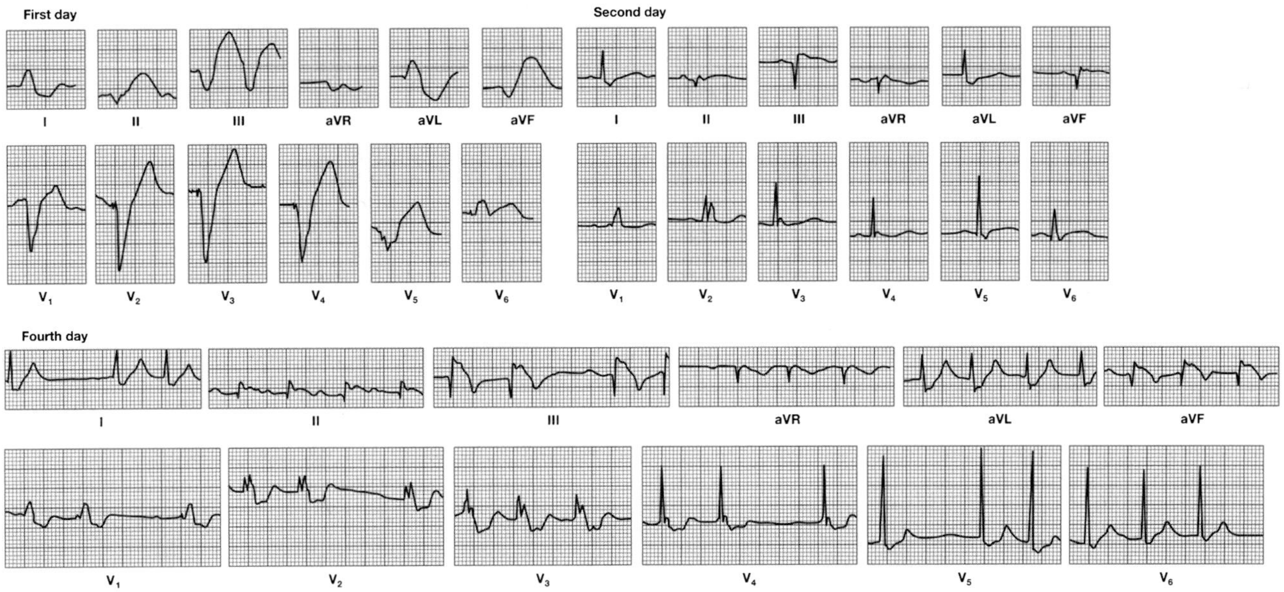

Fig. 18.23 Images from a 64-year-old man with rupture of the interventricular septum, complicating acute myocardial infarction. ECG day 1: The demand type-R innervated pacemaker is in position. The QRS complexes simulate left bundle branch block with prolonged QRS duration (0.20). The marked segmental change in leads III and aVF is noteworthy. Day 2: Sinus rhythm. The ST-segmental elevation in leads II, III, and aVF indicates an acute inferior myocardial infarction. Right bundle branch block is also present. Day 4: The signs of right bundle branch block and acute inferior infarction persist, with ST depression in leads V1 through V5 supporting true posterior infarction. Evidence of incomplete heart block and sequences of junctional rhythm with retrograde conduction to the atria are present.

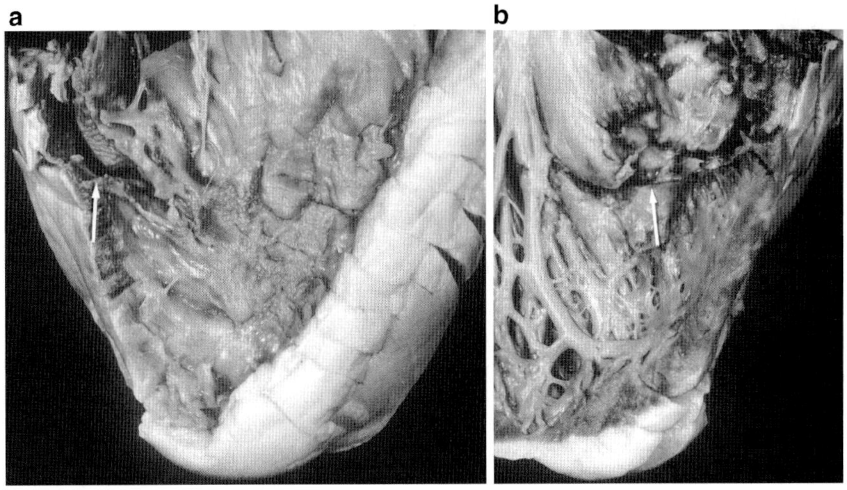

Fig. 18.24 (**a**) RV view. The *arrow* points to the rupture tract within the ventricular septum. (**b**) Inferior wall of LV, with zone of discoloration and the beginning of a tract (*arrow*), representing the LV aspect of ventricular septum rupture

Transthoracic echocardiography (TTE) confirms wall motion abnormalities, assesses the degree of mitral regurgitation, and often demonstrates flail mitral leaflets. TEE is the diagnostic imaging tool of choice, and is more definitive for evaluating the degree of mitral regurgitation and the status of the posterior papillary muscle. Color flow velocity mapping documents the presence of mitral regurgitation and (semiquantitative evaluation of its severity) (see Figs. 3.6a, b). Prompt surgery is the best choice for survival for most patients with acute severe mitral regurgitation postinfarction [19]. A few highly screened patients without papillary muscle rupture early in their presentation have been treated by emergency percutaneous transluminal coronary angioplasty (PTCA) in an attempt to reduce the size of the infarct and, thereby, reduce mitral regurgitation.

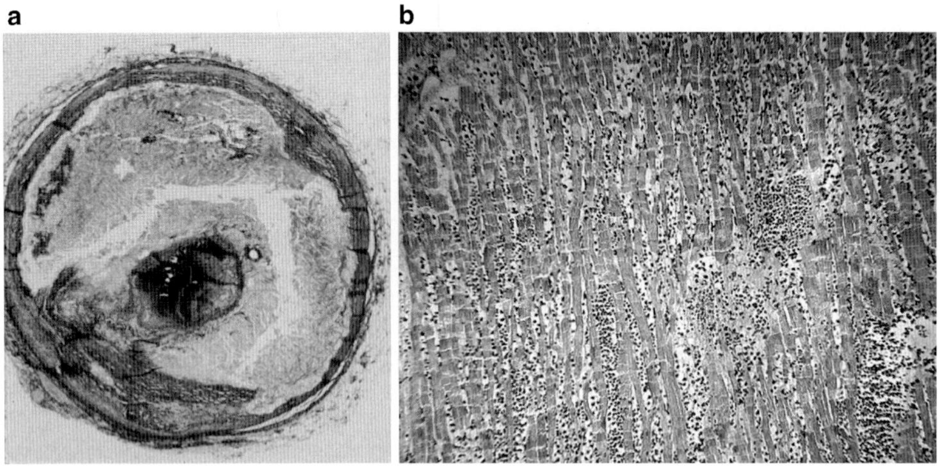

Fig. 18.25 (**a**) Photomicrograph of RCA shows extensive atherosclerosis with numerous cholesterol crystals. The narrowed lumen is occluded by a recent thrombus. Elastic tissue stain: 9×. (**b**) Photomicrograph shows lining of tract leading through ventricular septum. The tract is lined with infarcted myocardial tissue in which interstitial leukocytes have infiltrated. Hematoxylin and eosin stain: 80×

Pathological Demonstration

Rupture of a Papillary Muscle

(a) The classical situation involves rupture of the entire posteromedial papillary muscle.
(b) An unusual situation is rupture of the anterolateral papillary muscle.

In each case, the flail papillary muscle has looped through the interchordal space.

Rupture of a Papillary Muscle and of the Left ventricle's Free Wall

Figures 18.26 and 18.27 pertain to a patient admitted from a nursing home because of sternal pain of 3-day duration and diagnosis of acute inferior myocardial infarction. On the day after admission, the patient developed hypotension, tachycardia (120), and signs of LV failure, and a systolic murmur was noted for the first time. The patient was treated with digitalis and diuretics, but she remained in a state of cardiac failure. On the tenth day of the initial symptoms, cardiac arrest occurred and resuscitation was unsuccessful.

Pathologically, the pericardial sac was distended. The heart weighed 425 g. The epicardium showed a fibrinous reaction and rupture of the posterolateral wall of the LV was identified. The myocardium was discolored, indicative of acute myocardial infarction. The posteromedial papillary muscle of the LV was ruptured. The coronary arteries showed obstructive lesions and there was a recent thrombus in the CX. Pulmonary edema was also present.

Rupture of a Papillary Muscle: Chronic Mitral Insufficiency

The case in Figs. 18.28–18.30 illustrates the uncommon phenomenon of chronic mitral insufficiency from rupture of a papillary muscle [20].

A 70-year-old man was admitted because of shortness of breath. Two months before admission, he had noticed a feeling of sudden tightness in his chest associated with shortness of breath. He was treated for CHF; improvement resulted.

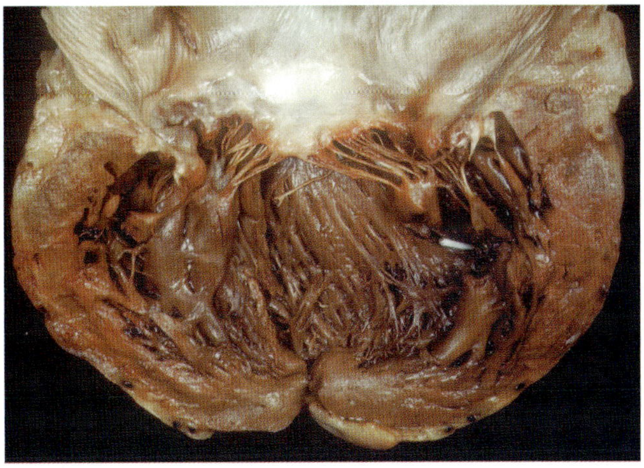

Fig. 18.26 Image from an 86-year-old woman with a ruptured papillary muscle of the mitral valve complicating acute myocardial infarction. Interior of the LV shows the posteromedial papillary muscle rupture (near probe).

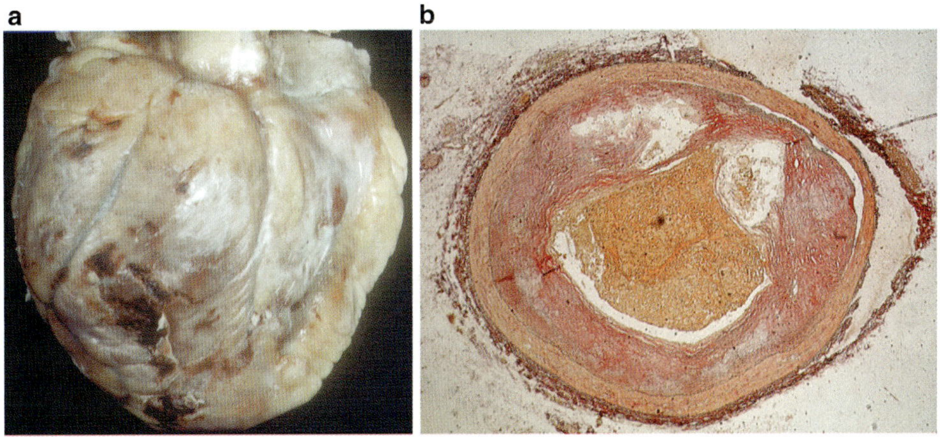

Fig. 18.27 (**a**) Exterior of inferior aspect of LV. The laceration of the posterolateral wall of the LV represents rupture of the free wall. (**b**) Photomicrograph of the CX 4 cm from its origin. In addition to atherosclerotic thickening of the intima, the lumen is occluded by a thrombus. Elastic tissue stain: 16×

Physical examination revealed a systolic thrill at the cardiac apex associated with a loud grade 3+ holosystolic murmur, which was transmitted to the axilla. An ECG showed ST changes suggestive of subendocardial ischemic injury plus possible digitalis effect. A thoracic roentgenogram revealed LV and LA enlargement, and pulmonary congestion.

Cardiac catheterization showed the pulmonary arterial pressure to be elevated (75/23). The pulmonary arterial wedge pressure was characterized by a huge cv wave (70 mm). The cardiac index was 2.1 and systemic arterial saturation was 96%. A cardiac shunt was excluded. Left ventriculography showed gross mitral regurgitation with systolic expansion of the LA. Both left-sided chambers were moderately enlarged; ventricular contractions were vigorous.

The patient was referred for surgery. The surgeon reported a rupture on the head of the posteromedial papillary muscle. The mitral valve was resected and replaced with a prosthetic valve. Histological examination of the ruptured segment of the papillary muscle showed signs of myocardial infarction with phagocytes and fibroblastic reaction.

The patient died suddenly about 7 months after replacement of the mitral valve. No specific cause for the sudden death was found at autopsy other than existing coronary disease. The heart was moderately enlarged, weighing 415 g. The posterior wall showed extensive scarring. Sections of the coronary arteries showed severe atherosclerotic lesions compromising all three main vessels.

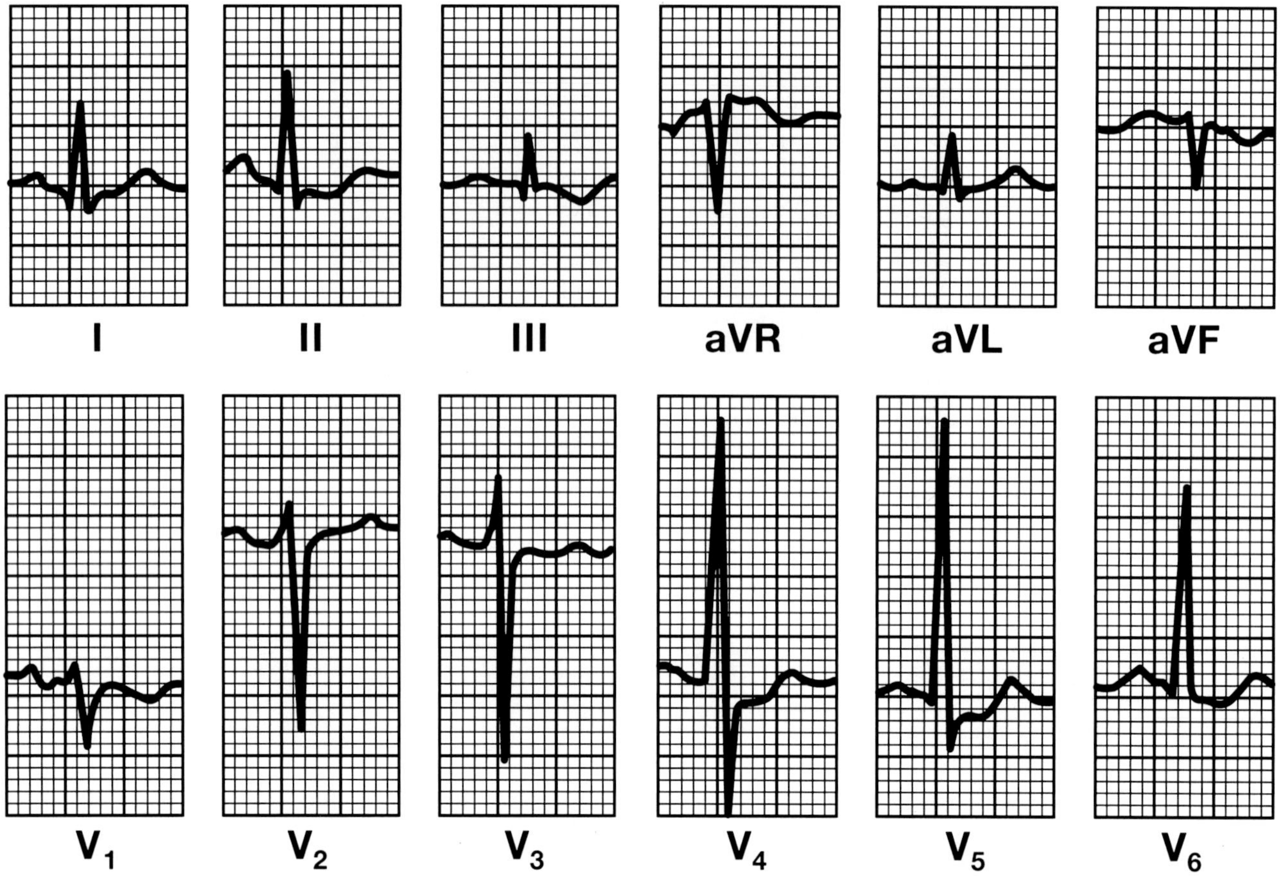

Fig. 18.28 From a case with chronic mitral regurgitation following rupture of a papillary muscle. ECG taken 2 months after the onset of chest pain and when mitral insufficiency was apparent shows ST changes suggestive of subendocardial injury and possibly associated digitalis effect. Adapted from Lee et al. [20]. Copyright 1970 by Elsevier

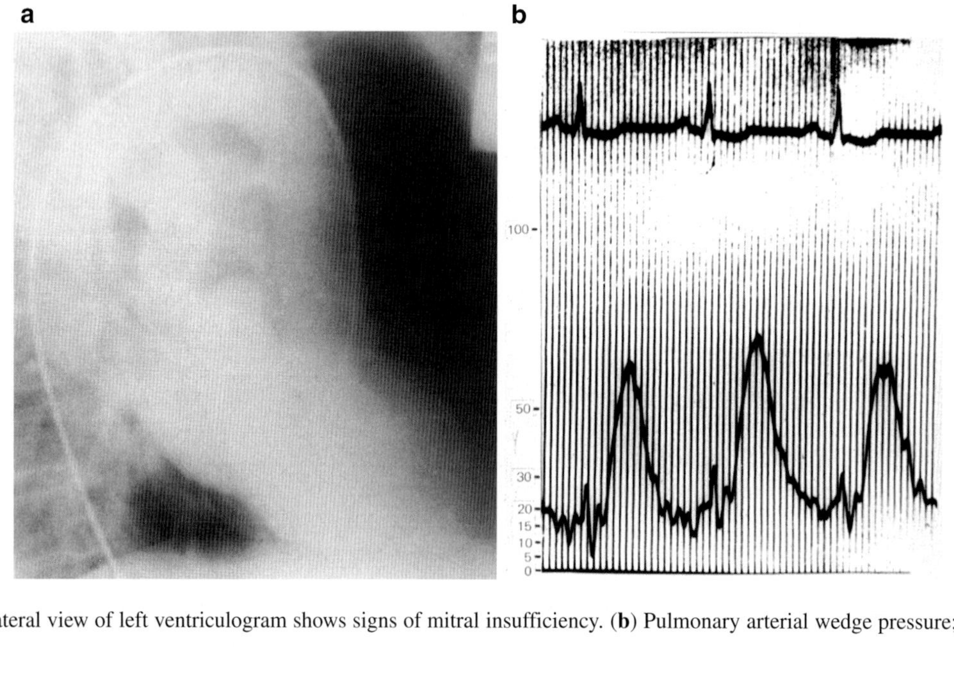

Fig. 18.29 (**a**) Lateral view of left ventriculogram shows signs of mitral insufficiency. (**b**) Pulmonary arterial wedge pressure; huge cv wave

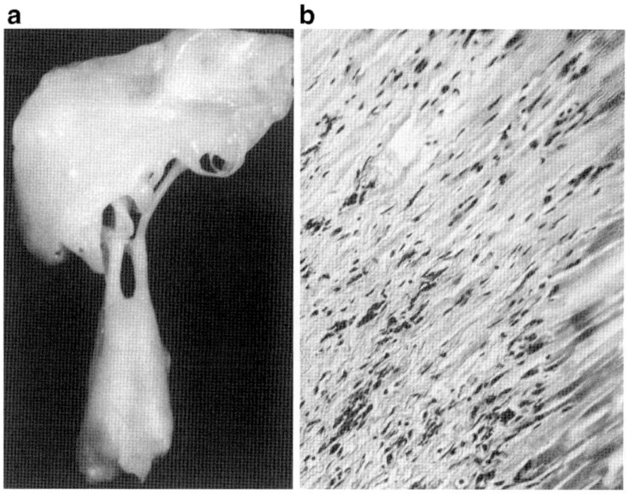

Fig. 18.30 (**a**) The surgical specimen of resected mitral valve shows the ruptured head of the posteromedial papillary muscle. (**b**) Photomicrograph of the excised flail head of the papillary muscle at the junction of infarcted muscle and phagocytic and fibroblastic reaction in which removal of muscle has occurred and fibrosis has developed. Hematoxylin and eosin stain: 73×

Arrythmias

Ventricular arrhythmia is a common complication of acute myocardial infarction, occurring in most patients experiencing an MI. It is related to formation of reentry circuits at the confluence of the necrotic and viable myocardium. Premature ventricular contractions (PVCs) occur in about 90% of patients. The incidence of ventricular fibrillation is approximately 2–4%.

The significance of ventricular fibrillation in myocardial infarction has been reevaluated in the context of the interaction between severe systolic dysfunction and the potential for sudden cardiac death. Although implantable defibrillators have been shown to reduce mortality in patients with an ejection fraction less than 30%, regardless of the presence of ventricular dysrhythmia, their placement in the first month after MI has not proven beneficial, in part because many patients given prompt reperfusion have a significant recovery of LV function in that time period [21]. These patients also have a lower risk of serious dysrhythmias later on.

Supraventricular arrythmias (mainly atrial fibrillation) occur in fewer than 10% of patients with acute myocardial infarction. These patients tend to have more severe ventricular dysfunction, and potentially, a worse outcome.

Bradyarrythmias, including AV block and sinus bradycardia, occur most frequently with inferior myocardial infarction. Complete AV block occurs in about 20% of patients with right ventricular infarction. These episodes of heart block are usually associated with a narrow QRS complex; the site of conduction block is in the AV node. Infranodal conduction disturbances with wide, complex ventricular escape rhythms occur most often in large anterior myocardial infarction and portend a very poor prognosis.

Illustrative Case: Subendocardial Infarction

The case portrayed in Figs. 18.31–18.33 is an example of acute myocardial infarction in a 69-year-old man that was complicated early by ventricular arrythmias which, in turn, led to the patient's death.

Following the episode of bradycardia that was not responsive to atropine and isoproterenol, a pacemaker was inserted. Fourteen hours after the initial event, the patient experienced cardiac arrest from which he could not be resuscitated.

Pathological findings:

- The heart weighed 550 g.
- Each of the three main coronary arteries showed multiple, severe atherosclerotic lesions. The LAD, additionally, showed a focus of intimal hemorrhage beyond which the lumen was occluded by a blood clot containing cholesterol crystals, a process suggesting embolism from an atheroma at a proximal level.
- The anteroseptal segment region of the LV showed healed subendocardial infarction, and in a circumferential manner there was eosinophilia involving the subendocardial region of the anterior, lateral, and inferior walls of the LV.

The overall picture was that of an acute myocardial infarction consistent with the history of about 14-h duration.

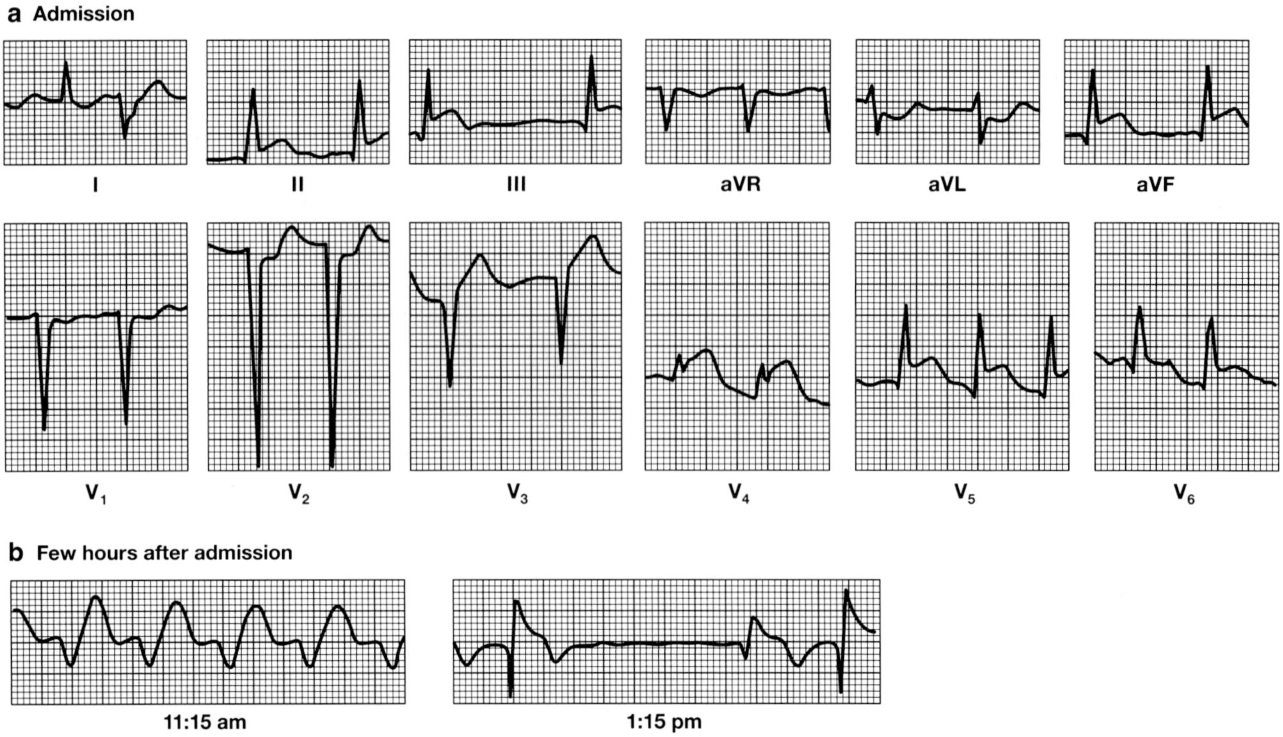

Fig. 18.31 Images from a 60-year-old man with early arrythmias complicating acute myocardial infarction. (**a**) Admission ECG shows atrial fibrillation, signs of an anteroseptal myocardial scar, and classical ST-segmental shift of ischemic injury involving the inferior and anterolateral walls. (**b**) ECG taken a few hours after admission (11:15 A.M.) with ventricular tachycardia present at the time of circulatory collapse. At 1:15 P.M., after resuscitation from previous episode, bradycardia developed, presumably atrial fibrillation and bigeminy

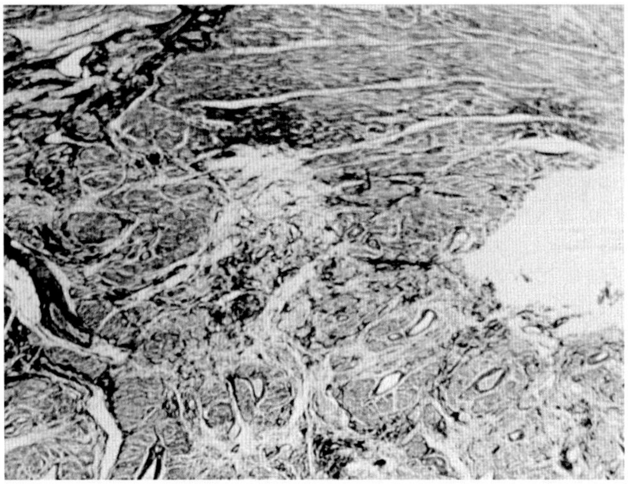

Fig. 18.32 Low-power photomicrograph of anterior wall of the LV. The *dark areas* represent scarring of the healed myocardial infarction. Some retained muscle among the scar tissue showed eosinophilia without leukocytic infiltration, a picture interpreted as that of early acute myocardial infarction. Elastic tissue stain: 12×

Thromboembolism

Thromboembolic complications may be either systemic or pulmonary.

Systemic Thromboembolism

Systemic thromboembolic complications occur in fewer than 2% of acute myocardial infarctions [22]. The overall incidence of mural thrombus complicating myocardial infarction is approximately 20%. Mural thrombus with embolism occurs in the setting of a large, especially anterior ST-segment elevation acute MI and heart failure, associated with extensive wall motion

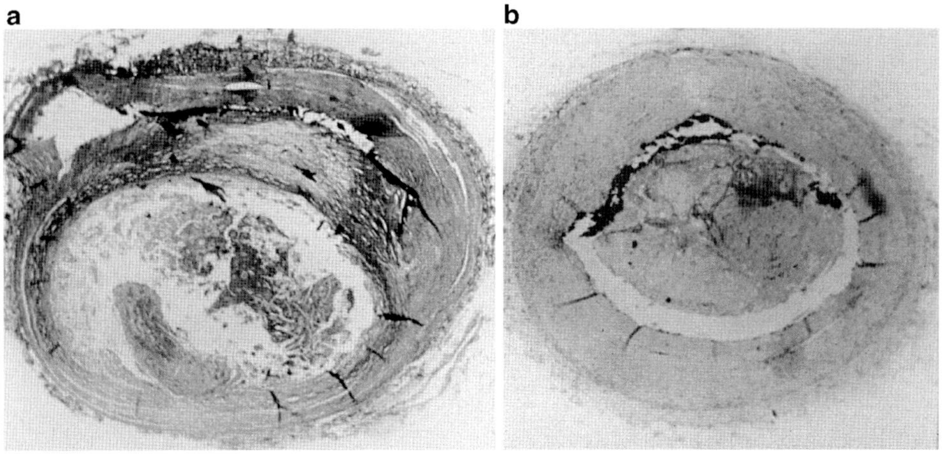

Fig. 18.33 (**a**) Photomicrograph of proximal segment of LC. Rupture of an atheroma is visible with extrusion of atheromatous material into the lumen. Elastic tissue stain: 18×. (**b**) Photomicrograph shows LAD distal to the lesion in (**a**). The lumen is occluded by thrombotic material in which foam cells and cholesterol crystals are present. The lesion is considered to be embolic from the site of atheroma rupture shown in (**a**). Hematoxylin and eosin: 18×

abnormalities or aneurysm. Atrial fibrillation in the setting of ischemia may also contribute to systemic embolism. The widespread use of anticoagulation during the first treatment of acute infarction with reperfusion therapy may have diminished the incidence of intracardiac thrombosis and embolism.

The most common clinical manifestation of embolism is stroke, although patients may have limb ischemia, renal infarction, or intestinal ischemia. Most episodes of systemic embolism occur in the first 10 days after acute myocardial infarction. Arterial embolism can cause dramatic clinical events such as hemiparesis, loss of pulse, ischemic bowel, or sudden hypertension, depending on the regional circulation involved.

TTE remains the imaging modality of choice and is 92% sensitive and 89% specific for detecting LV thrombus (see Fig. 3.15 showing LV protruding thrombus in a case with acute myocardial infarction). Sensitivity and specificity increase with transesophageal echo or MRI with contrast. Their use is indicated when diagnosis with routine transthoracic echo is not definitive.

Pulmonary Embolism

Pulmonary embolism, most often resulting from thrombus in the leg veins, previously was the cause of death in about 4% of fatal cases of acute myocardial infarction. Current management with anticoagulants for patients with acute myocardial infarction have resulted in marked reduction of the incidence of pulmonary embolism as a complication of acute MI.

Illustrative Case: Thromboembolism Complicating Myocardial Infarction

Figures 18.34–18.37 portray thromboembolic complications of myocardial infarction in a 75-year-old man who was admitted because of vague discomfort in the upper abdomen for 1 week. He had no pain or dyspnea.

Physical examination revealed BP of 130/80, atrial fibrillation (rate, 110), and rales over the pulmonary bases. An ECG showed evidence of anteroseptal infarction of uncertain age consistent with either recent infarction or an older lesion with aneurysm formation. On day 2, signs of CHF became apparent, and on day 3, pain appeared in the lower right extremity. Examination showed a cold, pulseless lower right extremity. Femoral thrombectomy was performed. Postoperatively, ventricular tachycardia occurred followed by the appearance of pulmonary edema and, finally, ventricular fibrillation.

Pathologic examination revealed cardiac hypertrophy (550 g). Focal scars were apparent in the inferior wall of the LV and acute transmural anteroseptal myocardial infarction. Mural thrombi were present at the apex of the LV and in the LA appendage. The LC showed moderate narrowing of its lumen by grade II atherosclerosis, while the RC and LAD showed marked narrowing by grade III + atherosclerosis.

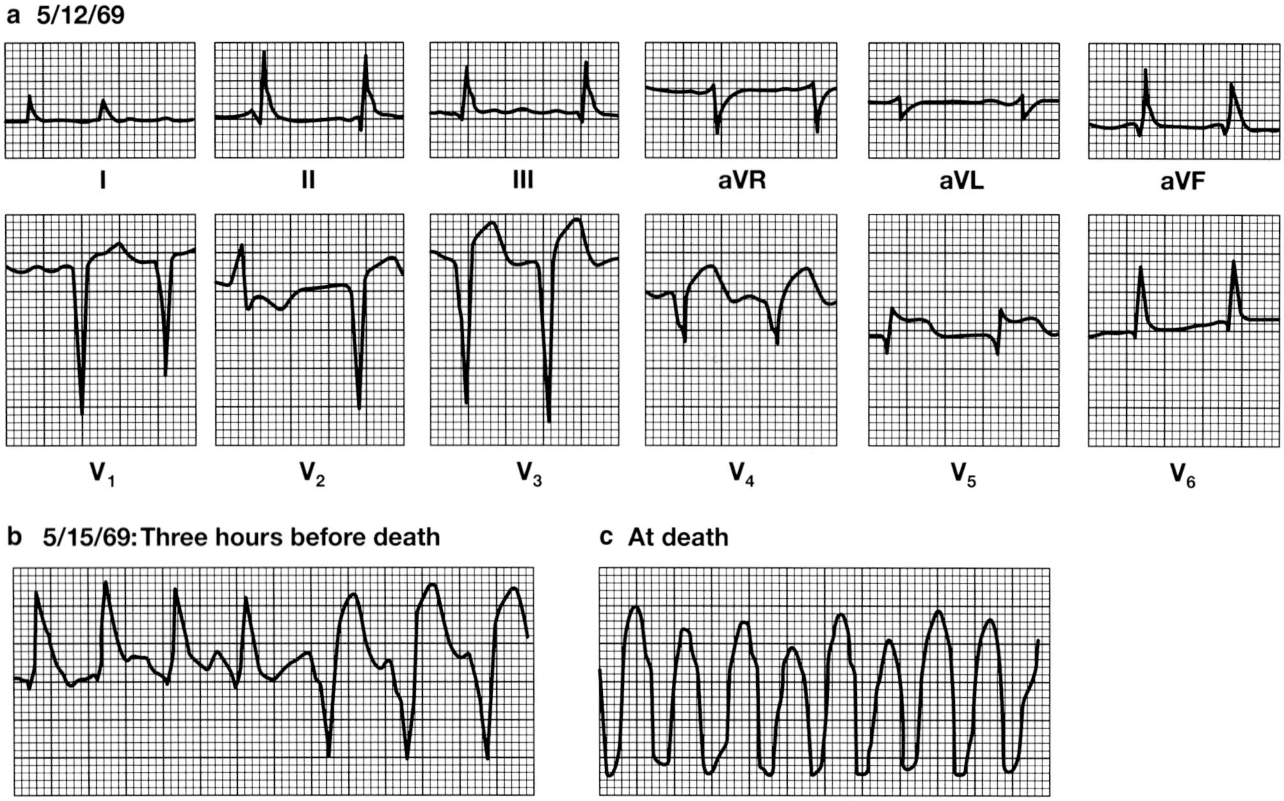

Fig. 18.34 From case with thromboembolism complicating acute myocardial infarction. (**a**) ECG day of admission shows atrial fibrillation and changes typical of anteroseptal myocardial infarction, the age of which is not clear. The *bottom panel* shows (**b**) ventricular tachycardia (3 h before death) followed by (**c**) ventricular fibrillation (at death)

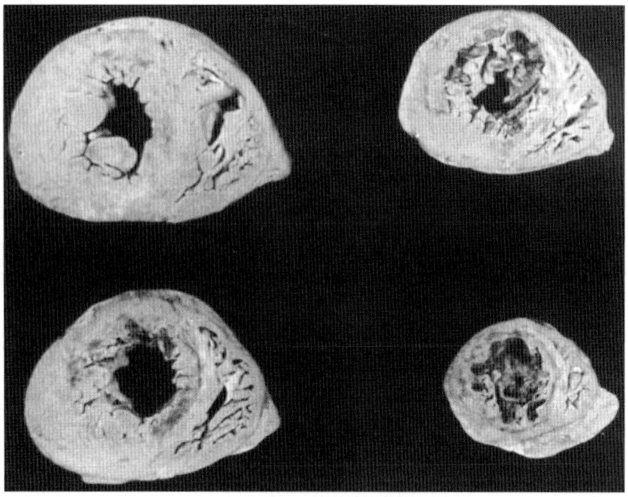

Fig. 18.35 Cross sections of ventricular portion of the heart. The anteroseptal region shows discoloration of acute myocardial infarction. Mural thrombosis is present in the LV apex. Focal scars are present in the inferior wall of the LV at its base

Histologic examination of the infarcted anteroseptal region showed necrotic muscle associated with early removal. The LV thrombus was undergoing organization. A recent infarction was apparent in the lower lobe of the left kidney.

It is believed that an embolism from thrombi either in the LV or LA had occurred to the left kidney and to the left femoral artery. In addition, extensive ulcerative atherosclerosis with thrombosis of the aorta was visible. This case indicates that myocardial infarction and thromboembolic complications may, at times, be the result of coincident atherosclerotic disease of other organs. In this instance, however, the femoral artery occlusion and renal infarction were believed to have resulted from emboli originating in the heart.

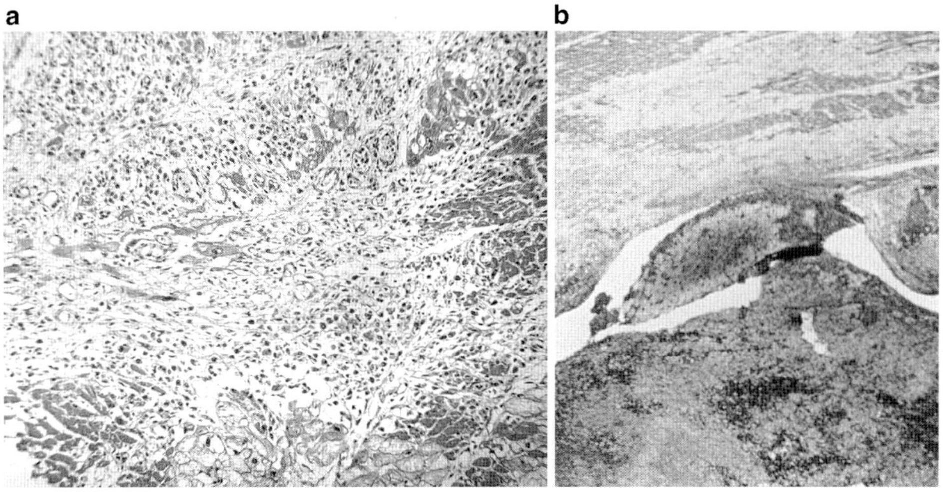

Fig. 18.36 (**a**) Photomicrograph of anterior wall of the LV. At the periphery of the infarcted myocardium is a zone of removal of tissue. Hematoxylin and eosin stain: 40×. (**b**) Junction of LV wall and mural thrombus (*below*). The process of organization of the thombus is faily extensive and suggests an older age than the related myocardial infarction. This, in turn, suggests that the patient may have been suffering from ventricular failure before the onset of myocardial infarction. Hematoxylin and eosin stain: 23×

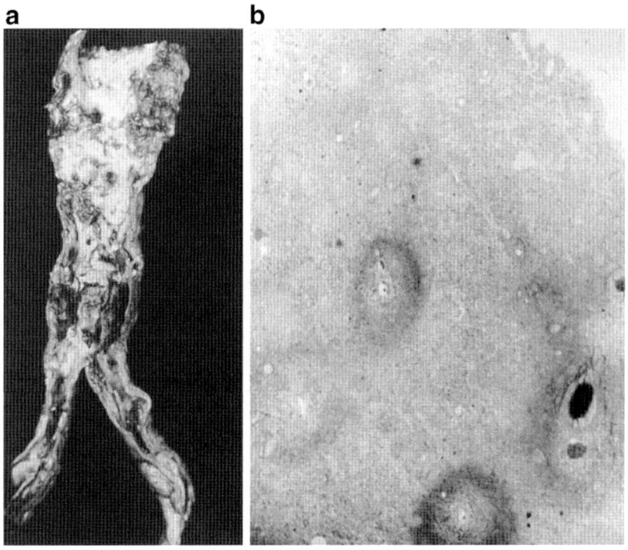

Fig. 18.37 (**a**) Abdominal aorta and terminal branches. Extensive thrombotic atherosclerosis is present. (**b**) Photomicrograph of left kidney shows acute infarction. Hematoxylin and eosin stain: 8×

Right Ventricular Failure

Right ventricular infarction is almost invariably caused by thrombotic occlusion of the right coronary artery proximal to the RV branches in the setting of inferior wall infarction. Hemodynamically significant RV dysfunction occurs in only 10% of patients with inferior or inferoposterior wall infarction. Despite the younger age, lower rate of anterior myocardial infarction, and higher prevalence of single-vessel disease of the RV compared with LV shock patients, mortality is unexpectedly high and similar to patients with LV shock [23].

Most acute "RV infarctions" are initially diagnosed by right-sided ST-elevations (typically, lead V4R). Interestingly, they generally do not progress to myocardial necrosis and subsequent scar formation. This accounts for the far lower percentage of autopsy-reported RV infarcts than clinically suspected infarcts. The latter group includes many patients with a stunned or hibernating RV free wall, which recovers more readily than a similarly injured LV wall. This more rapid recovery occurs in part because of the rich collateral perfusion of the RV free wall and septum from the LC, and the relatively greater penetration from the blood cavity by the thebesian veins [24].

Approximately one-third to one-half of patients with acute inferior LV infarction and accompanying RV infarction will show the effects of LV volume underload [25]. The hemodynamic effect may include elevated jugular venous pressure and a noncompliant pattern of the right atrial pulse wave form similar to that of constrictive pericarditis. Reduced RV contractility may lead to a serious deficit in LV preload with a resultant drop in cardiac output and consequent hypotension that will require vigorous fluid administration. Cases with occlusion of the proximal segment of the RC can compromise the blood supply of the sinus node and AV node, producing sinus bradycardia, atrial infarction, AV block, or atrial fibrillation. The triad of hypotension, jugular venous distension with clear lungs, and absence of dyspnea has high specificity but low sensitivity for RV infarction.

A rare but clinically important complication is right to left shunting secondary to increased pressures in the RA and RV, and opening of the foramen ovale, resulting in systemic hypoxemia unresponsive to supplemental oxygen.

Echocardiography is the diagnostic study of choice for RV infarction. It demonstrates inferior wall motion abnormalities in conjunction with dilated RV and hypokinetic RV walls.

Hemodynamic monitoring with a pulmonary artery catheter reveals high right atrial pressure with low pulmonary capillary wedge pressure (PCWP), unless severe LV dysfunction is also present. Cardiac output is often depressed.

References

1. Killip T, Kimball JT. Treatment of myocardial infarction in a coronary care unit: a two-year experience with 250 patients. Am J Cardiol. 1967;20:457–64.
2. Wu AH, Parsons L, Every NR, Bates ER. Hospital outcomes in patients with congestive heart failure complicating acute myocardial infarction: a report from the Second National Registry of Myocardial infarction (NRMI-2). J Am Coll Cardiol. 2002;40:1389–94.
3. Babaev A, Frederick PD, Pasta DJ, et al. Trends in management and outcomes of patients with acute myocardial infarction complicated by cardiogenic shock. JAMA. 2005;294:448–54.
4. Sanborn TA, Sleeper LA, Bates ER, et al. Impact of thrombolysis, intraaortic balloon pump counterpulsation in cardiogenic shock complicating acute myocardial infarction: a report from the Shock Trial Registry. J Am Coll Cardiol. 2000;36:1123–9.
5. Hochman JS, Buller CE, Sleeper LA, et al. Cardiogenic shock complicating acute myocardial infarction — etiologies, management and outcome: a report from the Shock Trial Registry. J Am Coll Cardiol. 2003;36:1063–70.
6. Becker RC, Gore JM, Lambrew C, et al. A composite view of cardiac rupture in the United States National Registry of myocardial infarction. J Am Coll Cardiol. 1996;27:1321–6.
7. Stevenson WG, Linssen GC, Havenith MG, et al. The spectrum of death after myocardial infarction: a necropsy study. Am Heart J. 1989;118:1182–8.
8. Honan MB, Harrel Jr FE, Reimer KA, et al. Cardiac rupture, mortality and the timing of thrombosis therapy: a meta-analysis. J Am Coll Cardiol. 1990;16:359–67.
9. Nakatani D, Sato H, Kinjo K, et al. Effect of successful late reperfusion by primary angioplasty on mechanical complications of acute myocardial infarction. Am J Cardiol. 2003;92:785–8.
10. Van Tassel RA, Edwards JE. Rupture of heart complicating myocardial infarction. Analysis of 40 cases including nine examples of left ventricular false aneurysm. Chest. 1972;61:104.
11. Vlodaver Z, Coe JI, Edwards JE. True and false left ventricular aneurysms. Propensity for the latter to rupture. Circulation. 1975;51:567–72.
12. Yeo TC, Malouf JF, Reeder GS, Oh JK. Clinical characteristics and outcome in post infarction pseudoaneurysm. Am J Cardiol. 1999;84:592–5.
13. Giltner A, Marelli D, Halpern E, Savage M. Subepicardial aneurysm with impending cardiac rupture: a case of antemortem diagnosis and review of the literature. Clin Cardiol. 2007;30:44–7.
14. Gobel FL, Visudh-Arom K, Edwards JE. Pseudoaneurysm of the left ventricle leading to recurrent pericardial hemorrhage. Chest. 1971;59:23.
15. Crenshaw BS, Granger CB, Birmbaum Y, et al. Risk factors, angiographic patterns and outcomes in patients with ventricular septal defect complicating acute myocardial infarction. Circulation. 2000;101:27–32.
16. Edwards BS, Edwards WD, Edwards JE. Ventricular septal rupture complicating acute myocardial infarction: identification of simple and complex types in 53 autopsied hearts. Am J Cardiol. 1984;54:1201–5.
17. Poulsen SH, Praestholm M, Munk K, Wierup P, Egeblad H, Nielsen-Kudsk JE. Ventricular septal rupture complicating acute myocardial infarction. Clinical characteristics and contemporary outcome. Ann Thorac Surg. 2008;85:1591–6.
18. Wei JY, Hutchins GM, Bulkely BH. Papillary muscle rupture complicating acute myocardial infarction. Ann Intern Med. 1979;90:149–56.
19. Chevalier P, Burri H, Fahrat F, et al. Perioperative outcome and long-term survival of surgery for acute post-myocardial mitral regurgitation. Eur J Cardiothorac Surg. 2004;26:330–5.
20. Lee KS, Johnson T, Karnegis JN, et al. Acute myocardial infarction with long-term survival following papillary muscle rupture. Am Heart J. 1970;79:258.
21. Moss AJ, Zareba W, Hall WJ, et al. Prophylactic implantation of a defibrillator in patients with myocardial infarction and reduced LV ejection fraction. N Engl J Med. 2002;346:877–83.

22. Puletti M, Cusmano E, Testa MG, et al. Incidence of systemic thromboembolic lesions in acute myocardial infarction. Clin Cardiol. 1986;9(7):331–3.
23. Jacobs AK, Leopold JA, Bates E, et al. Cardiogenic shock caused by right ventricular infarction. A report from the SHOCK registry. J Am Coll Cardiol. 2003;41:1273–9.
24. Kinch JW, Ryan JJ. Right ventricular infarction. N Engl J Med. 1994;330:1211–7.
25. Cohen A, Guyon P, Johnson N, et al. Hemodynamic criteria for diagnosis of right ventricular ischemia associated with inferior wall left ventricular acute myocardial infarction. Am J Cardiol. 1995;76:220–5.

Chapter 19
Healed Myocardial Infarction

Gary S. Francis and Daniel J. Garry

Ischemic Heart Failure

Among the most important clinical determinants of prognosis in HF is the etiology of LV dysfunction. Hypertension and valvular heart disease have been replaced by coronary artery disease (CAD) as the most common cause of HF in the Western world. The term "ischemic cardiomyopathy" is now commonly used to describe patients with HF and concomitant CAD or a history of myocardial infarction, although this can lead to an incorrect assignment. The coronary angiogram as the sole arbiter can be wrong, possibly because of coronary recanalization after infarction [1]. Gadolinium-enhanced magnetic resonance imaging (MRI) indicating epicardial scar formation may be a better arbiter than coronary angiography, but the two imaging tests are quite complimentary.

Heart failure due to an ischemic etiology is known to be independently associated with a poorer long-term outlook than for patients with HF from other causes [2, 3]. Moreover, HF due to myocardial ischemia may impact the decision to pursue coronary revascularization or use certain therapies. The mode of death in patients with so-called ischemic HF may also be quite different than in patients with nonischemic dilated cardiomyopathy, as acute coronary events may more often trigger sudden death in patients with ischemic cardiomyopathy [4].

Despite lingering uncertainty about the definition of ischemic cardiomyopathy or ischemic HF, the diagnosis is important because substantial prognostic and therapeutic implications are attached. The presence of CAD and HF is not the equivalent of ischemic HF. True ischemic HF is associated with a worse prognosis and a shortened survival relative to nonischemic HF [5]. It is important to remember that a patient with single-vessel coronary disease not involving the proximal left anterior descending or left main coronary artery who manifests no history of myocardial infarction or coronary revascularization despite a poorly functioning, dilated LV probably does not have ischemic HF [4].

CAD and dilated cardiomyopathy are both common disorders, and may sometimes simply coexist in patients by random chance, with no clear causal relation. In an estimated 15% of patients with HF and CAD, the CAD plays no etiologic role in the development of HF. The patient with true ischemic HF typically has severe CAD involving a single large area of the LV or substantial scar involving several distributions of blood flow. In most cases, one or more acute myocardial infarctions (AMIs) is documented, an epicardial scar is visible by MRI, and Q waves are present on the electrocardiogram (EKG). Such patients manifest a dilated LV chamber with impaired systolic performance with signs and symptoms of HF. An estimated 50% of incident HF in the general population is due to CAD [6], and CAD is the underlying etiology of HF in nearly 70% of patients [7], at least in the Western world.

The case illustrating HF and CAD shown in Figs. 19.1–19.6 is of a 55-year-old man who had experienced acute anteroseptal myocardial infarction 3 months before death. While in the hospital convalescing from the acute event, he was diagnosed with a large pulmonary embolus and prescribed anticoagulants. One month after discharge, the patient was readmitted because of HF and for consideration of special studies. Selective coronary arteriography revealed occlusion of the proximal portion of the proximal LAD (Fig. 19.2). LV ventriculography showed akinesis of the apex of the LV and

G.S. Francis, MD (✉)
Division of Cardiovascular Medicine, University of Minnesota, 420 Delaware Ave S.E, Minneapolis, MN 55455, USA
e-mail: franc354@umn.edu

D.J. Garry, MD, PhD
Division of Cardiovascular Medicine, University of Minnesota, Minneapolis, MN, USA

Z. Vlodaver et al. (eds.), *Coronary Heart Disease: Clinical, Pathological, Imaging, and Molecular Profiles*,
DOI 10.1007/978-1-4614-1475-9_19, © Springer Science+Business Media, LLC 2012

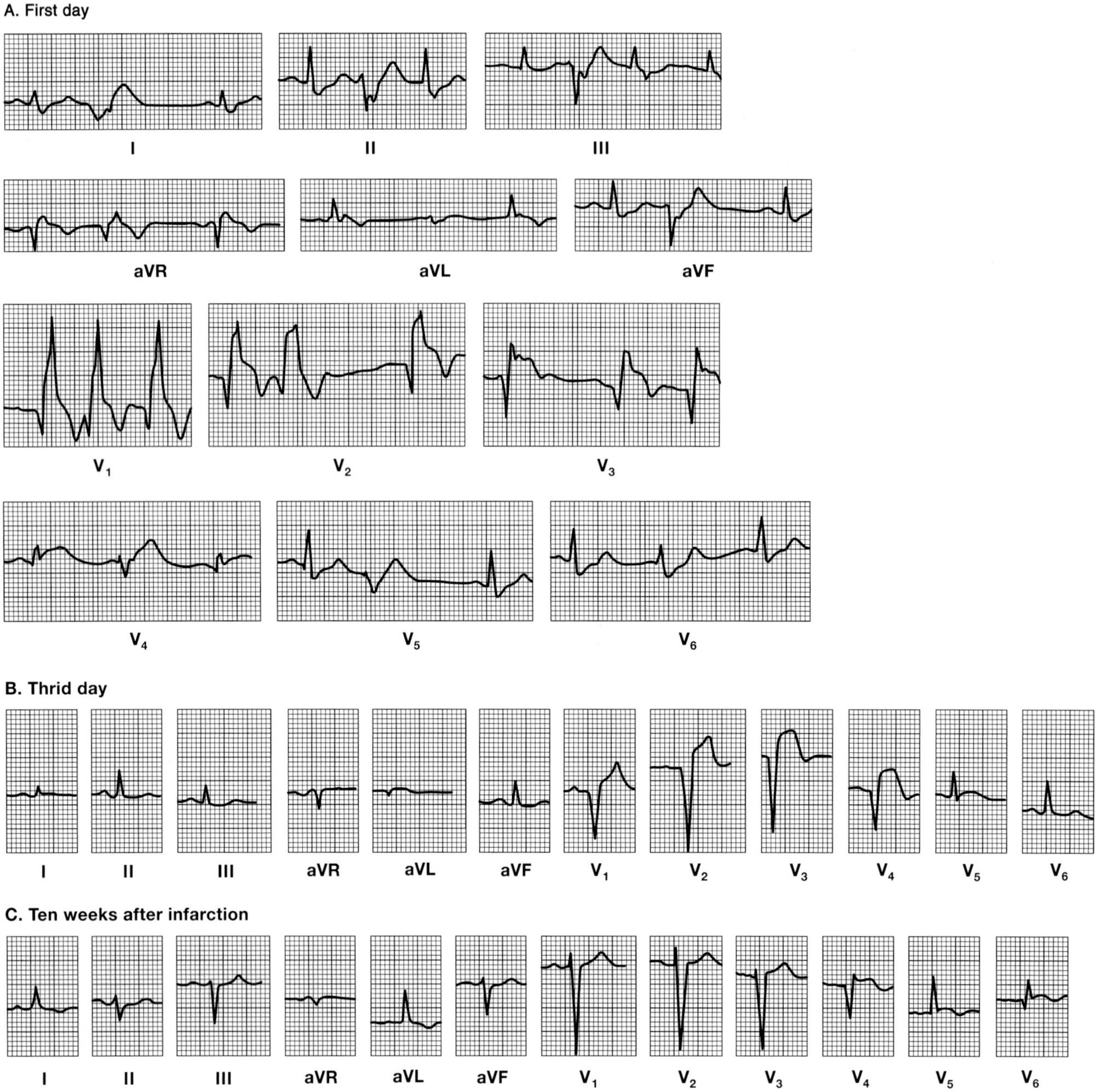

Fig. 19.1 ECGs. (**a**) First day after onset of myocardial infarction. There are right bundle branch block, junctional, and ventricular ectopic beats (retrograde conduction to atrium), and evidence of acute anteroseptal myocardial infarction. (**b**) On the third day after the onset of acute myocardial infarction, classic changes of acute anterior infarction are visible (Q wave in leads V1 through V4, and ST-segment elevation). (**c**) Ten weeks after the onset of myocardial infarction, a left axis deviation (anterior fascicular block) and return of R waves in the right precordial leads are visible. A prominent Q wave and ST-segment elevation persist in left precordial leads

mitral insufficiency. The left ventricular end-diastolic pressure (LVEDP) was elevated to 26 mmHg and the ejection fraction was 20%. The patient's HF progressed. Pulmonary edema and distended neck veins appeared, and he died suddenly, about 3 months after the onset of AMI.

The autopsy revealed coronary arterial lesions consistent with those demonstrated angiographically. The heart showed hypertrophy (650 g) and a greatly enlarged LV (Fig. 19.3). The anteroseptal region revealed a large, transmural scar with moderate bulging of the ventricular septum toward the RV. The papillary muscles were neither infarcted nor scarred. Mural thrombi were found in both ventricles and in the right atrial appendage (Figs. 19.3 and 19.4). Other signs of HF were supported by chronic passive congestion of the liver (Fig. 19.5), and spleen and bilateral pleural effusion. There were no signs

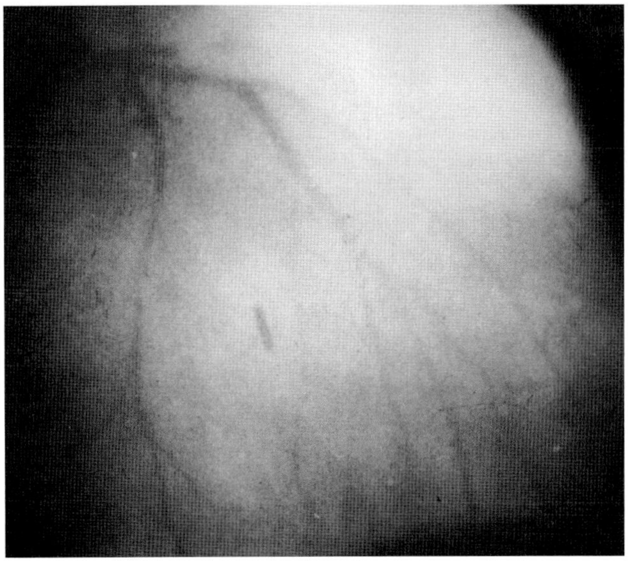

Fig. 19.2 LC arteriogram in RAO view. Occlusion of the proximal LAD

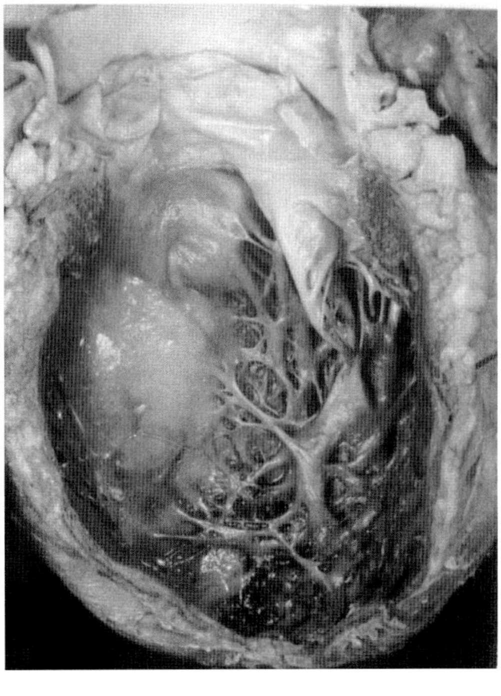

Fig. 19.3 Interior of LV. Scarring of the thinned anterior wall and bulging of the interventricular septum toward the RV. Mural thrombus in the apex. The papillary muscles are not infarcted

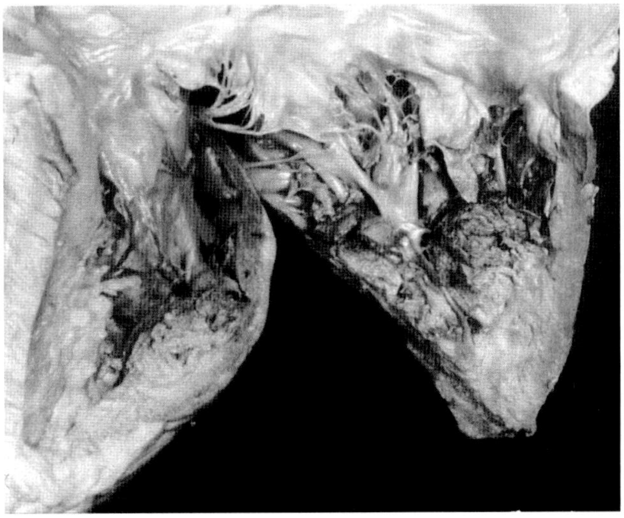

Fig. 19.4 RV. Mural thrombus at apex – an important anatomic signs of congestive heart failure

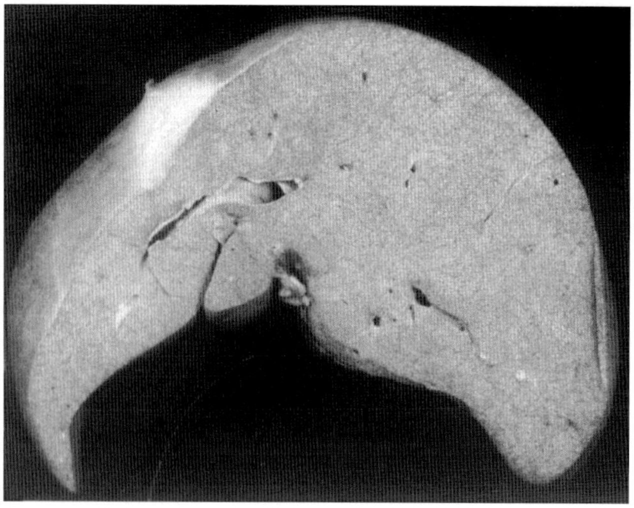

Fig. 19.5 Liver. Prominent central zones characteristic of chronic passive congestion of the organ (so-called "nutmeg appearance")

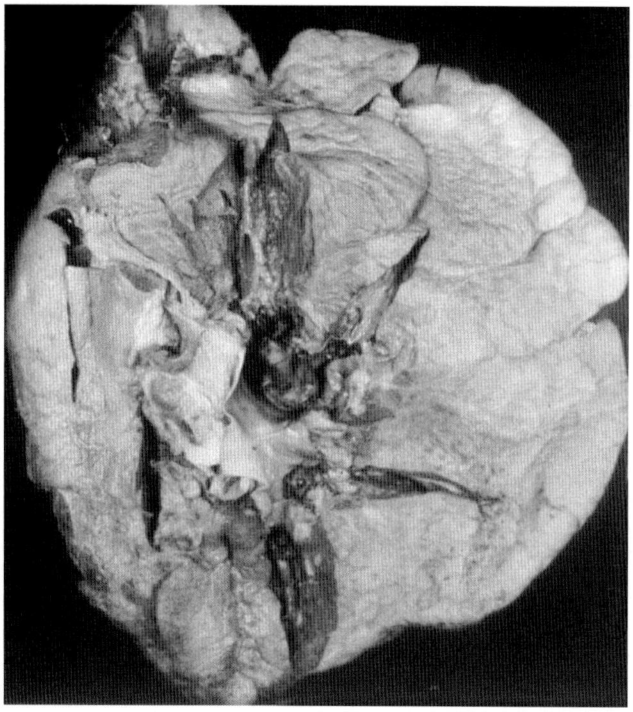

Fig. 19.6 Right lung. The main pulmonary artery of this lung is occluded by organizing thrombus

of AMI grossly or microscopically. The myocardium beyond the gross scar showed no scarring histologically. Pulmonary emboli of varying ages were present (Fig. 19.6). The degree of pulmonary arterial obstruction seemed of such magnitude as to have been a significant factor contributing to the right heart failure.

Trends in HF have changed in recent decades [8]. CAD has clearly increased as a cause of HF in the Framingham cohort [8], whereas valvular heart disease has markedly declined as a causal factor. The data on hypertension and HF are less clear. More recently, hypertension has appeared to play a diminished causal role in the Framingham population [8]. The reduced prevalence of left ventricular hypertrophy with more effective treatment of hypertension has paralleled the declining incidence of HF in various treatment trials, and may underlie the declining causal role of hypertension as a cause of heart failure. This is in contrast to the prevalence of diabetes mellitus, which is clearly rising in the HF population. In the Framingham cohort, the rate of increase in diabetes is 20% per decade [8]. Reduced glucose tolerance and insulin resistance favor the development of HF. Diabetes mellitus is associated with the development of atherosclerosis, and atherosclerosis accounts for up to 60% of deaths from diabetes. Overall, CAD, hypertension, and diabetes mellitus account for most of the HF in the western world.

Systolic Heart Failure: Heart Failure with Reduced Left Ventricular Ejection Fraction

For years, systolic heart failure was the main type of HF familiar to cardiologists. It is classic HF characterized by a reduction in systolic performance from a myriad of causes, leading to increased filling pressures, shortness of breath, and, in the later stages, is accompanied by a low cardiac output, fatigue, and edema. The primary feature is progressive remodeling of the heart so that it assumes a more spherical, globular shape. The LV internal dimension increases in size, and the LV ejection fraction is reduced. Essentially, the heart does not empty its contents with sufficient force and power. The afterload increases commensurate with the increase in LV radius and wall tension, and the preload rises commensurate with the increase in filling pressures. For any given increase in sarcomere length, there is little or no further development of contractile force (reduced Starling effect).

The combination of perverse loading conditions and reduced contractile strength are responsible for impaired systolic function [9]. In chronic ischemic HF or ischemic cardiomyopathy, contractile tissue is partially replaced by noncontractile, dense scar tissue. Acute myocardial ischemia may be superimposed on chronic ischemic HF, and can lead to further reductions in contractile muscle strength.

Chronic myocardial under-perfusion of the heart can lead to a condition known as "hibernating myocardium." In this state, the metabolism of the myocardium is reduced to a lower level of activity, presumably in an adaptive attempt to conserve energy, resulting in a less forceful contraction [10]. This is a potentially reversible condition, and serves as part of the basis for revascularization therapy. Hibernating myocardium can be diagnosed by a combination of coronary arteriography and positron emission tomography, which has emerged as an important step in the identification of chronically ischemic but viable myocardium [11].

In some patients with chronic ischemic HF and extensive hibernating myocardium, revascularization can occasionally lead to spectacular improvement in LV function. For some, the combination of an angiotensin-converting enzyme inhibitor (ACEi), angiotensin receptor blocker (ARB), β-adrenergic blocker, aldosterone receptor blocker, or diuretic and coronary revascularization can relieve at least some of the signs and symptoms of chronic ischemic HF [12]. The development of HF leads to activation of the renin-angiotensin-aldosterone axis and the sympathetic nervous system, and these contribute importantly to the remodeling process [13]. Blocking these systems pharmacologically with ACE inhibitors or ARBs, β-blockers, and aldosterone inhibitors slows progressive remodeling and improves survival in patients with HF [14]. When LV scarring is extensive, however, and little myocardium is viable, there may be a poor response to either medical, device, or revascularization therapy [15].

Patients who develop systolic HF in the setting of a healed myocardial infarction have an annual mortality of 8–20% per year, depending on NYHA class, duration of symptoms, age, severity of LV dysfunction, and comorbidities. Sudden unexpected death occurs in 30–50% of these patients, depending on how one defines sudden death. The sudden death rate has probably been reduced by the widespread use of implantable cardioverter-defibrillators (ICDs), cardiac resynchronization therapy (CRT), and improved medical therapy over the past few decades. Still, the relative importance of an acute coronary event as a trigger for sudden death in patients with ischemic cardiomyopathy is high, as acute coronary findings are frequent in these patients at autopsy, even though they are not usually clinically diagnosed [16].

Recurrent myocardial infarction is likely a frequent cause of terminal HF in patient with chronic CAD. Therefore, improved strategies to prevent or treat acute myocardial ischemia are still very important in this patient group.

Acute systolic HF syndromes occur in patients with CAD and healed myocardial infarction, and may take many forms. These syndromes are defined as a rapid or gradual change in signs and symptoms in patients with chronic HF or new-onset HF that requires urgent therapy [17]. Such episodes may present as acute coronary syndromes, often with some element of mitral regurgitation, and usually require investigation that includes coronary arteriography.

The in-hospital mortality rate varies from 4 to 7%, and the rehospitalization rate is quite high – 30% in the first 90 days after discharge [18]. Treatment usually consists of optimal medical HF therapy, optimal medical therapy for CAD, control of cardiac risk factors, and myocardial revascularization. Treatment, of course, must be tailored to the individual patient, and must take into account multiple variables such as the patient's age, expectations, and desires, and is influenced greatly by concomitant comorbid conditions. Previous heart surgery, the presence or absence of mitral regurgitation, the size and the performance of the LV, and the extent of myocardial viability are of major importance when considering revascularization strategies.

Diastolic Heart Failure: Heart Failure with Preserved Ejection Fraction

About 40% of patients with HF have a normal or near-normal ejection fraction, but estimates vary widely. Of course, the two conditions of systolic and diastolic HF may coexist to some extent in some patients. Predominant systolic HF results in impaired ventricular pump performance, whereas predominant diastolic heart failure results in impaired ventricular filling [19, 20]. Patients with diastolic HF often have underlying CAD, hypertension, and diabetes mellitus. It is more common in elderly women.

The two conditions cannot be easily distinguished by history and bedside examination, so echocardiography is usually performed to help diagnose diastolic HF. Other cardiac imaging techniques and cardiac catheterization can also be used to distinguish these two basic types of HF. Typically, the LV ejection fraction is 40% or more in patients with diastolic HF. The LV in these patients may be stiffer than normal, and less compliant. This can be caused by fibrosis from a previous but now healed myocardial infarction, or from a restrictive or infiltrative form of cardiomyopathy. Wall thickness may be increased, and the internal LV chamber size may be normal or even smaller than normal. Left ventricular hypertrophy is not infrequently present, usually from long-standing, poorly controlled hypertension, or in response to previous myocardial infarction. Therefore, any given LV end-diastolic volume may be higher than normal, thus, in some cases pushing the filling pressures above normal, and creating the sensation of dyspnea for the patient. Although cardiac output may be intact, the full-blown syndrome of HF can ensue, with all its typical signs and symptoms. Biomarkers such as brain natriuretic peptide (BNP) rise in the serum in response to increased LV wall tension, similar to but less robustly than with systolic HF. Neurohumoral systems are activated, very similar to that which occurs with systolic HF.

The prognosis for patients with early diastolic HF in its pre-hospitalization stage may be somewhat better than that of systolic HF, but once patients with diastolic HF are hospitalized for decompensated heart failure, that early advantage is lost in a few months [21]. Moreover, treatment with ACE inhibitors, ARBs, or β-blockers does not improve post-discharge outcomes for patients with diastolic HF over the short term. Clinical trials indicate that treatment with an ARB [22] or an ACE inhibitor [23] also failed to provide long-term survival benefit. Spironolactone, an aldosterone receptor inhibitor, is presently being studied as possible therapy for diastolic HF. For now, treatment includes control of hypertension, optimal medical therapy for comorbidities, revascularization for CAD, and diuretics to control fluid overload.

Cardiac Resynchronization Therapy

CRT has emerged as an important form of device therapy for patients with NYHA class III or ambulatory class IV systolic HF who manifest cardiac dyssynchrony despite standard pharmacologic therapy [24]. CRT improves symptoms and quality of life, and reduces complications and the risk of death. In the United States, CRT is often implanted with an ICD [25]; in Europe, CRT is often used as a single device [24]. Guidelines require that its use be restricted to patients with an LV ejection fraction £35%, a QRS duration ^{3}120 ms, and sinus rhythm [26].

Mechanical dyssynchrony can lead to marked disparities in regional LV loading. Regions activated earlier are under less load because their shortening reciprocally stretches the still-inactive opposing wall. In contrast, late-stimulated regions must operate at higher loads because of pre-stretch and late contraction against an already stiffened muscle. Such unequal loading can affect localized expression of genes that control myocyte size and function.

The rationale behind CRT is that reversal of LV dyssynchrony leads to reversal of disparate regional loading conditions, reverse remodeling with improvement in LV ejection fraction, less mitral regurgitation, and a smaller LV cavity [27, 28]. However, selection of patient responders to CRT is not always possible despite careful preimplantation echocardiography [29]. Moreover, not all patients with left bundle branch block (LBBB) have mechanical dyssynchrony [30]. Additionally, viable muscle and location of the pacing lead in the appropriate position in the coronary sinus seems necessary. This can be an obvious problem in patients with HF due to a healed myocardial infarction or ischemic cardiomyopathy, where large amounts of fibrous tissue or a strategically placed scar may preclude the benefit of CRT.

Very dilated ventricles are unlikely to respond to either revascularization or CRT. Patients with a narrow QRS, right bundle branch block (RBBB), diastolic HF, or atrial fibrillation may not respond to CRT. Current iterations of echocardiographic and tissue Doppler-based indices of mechanical synchrony are unsuited to everyday clinical use in CRT selection.

The QRS width is probably the single most important factor in predicting which patient with systolic HF is going to respond to CRT. More recently, NYHA class II patients appear to gain a survival benefit from CRT [31, 32], as well as demonstrate reversal of LV remodeling [33–35], thus expanding the potential utility of this evolving form of device therapy.

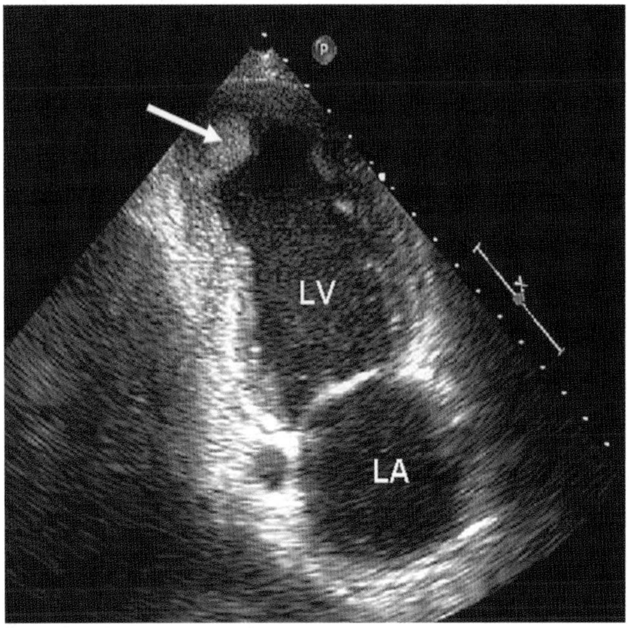

Fig. 19.7 Two-dimensional echocardiogram, apical two-chamber view. Mural thrombus in the LV apex (*arrow*)

Thrombus in the Chambers

The incidence of left ventricular thrombus formation after ST-elevation myocardial infarction (STEMI) appears to have dropped from about 20 to 5% with more aggressive use of antithrombotic strategies. When a mural thrombus does develop within 48–72 h of a STEMI, the prognosis is poor because of complications of a large infarction such as shock, reinfarction, rupture, and ventricular arrhythmia rather than emboli from the LV thrombus. Factors that predispose to thromboembolic events in patients with HF include low cardiac output, relative stasis of blood in the cardiac chambers, very impaired myocardial performance, regional wall motion abnormalities, and concomitant atrial fibrillation. Myocardial thrombi are most commonly seen in the LV apex.

Figure 19.7 shows an echocardiogram from a patient with a history of extensive anteroseptal infarction and LV apical thrombus. Figure 19.8 illustrates a large thrombus in the LV apex.

An estimated 10% of mural thrombi result in systemic embolization. Heart failure is believed to be a hypercoagulable state, with impaired endothelial function in the heart's chambers and peripheral vasculature. It is clear that patients with HF and atrial fibrillation benefit from therapy with warfarin, but the role of anticoagulation with antiplatelet drugs and/or warfarin for patients with HF and normal sinus rhythm (NSR) remains understudied.

Although left ventricular thrombus is well-known to form acutely on the endocardial surface of the heart in patients with AMI, approximately 20–40% undergo spontaneous resolution without anticoagulant therapy in the first year, and another 42–88% resolve with anticoagulant therapy. Persistence of LV thrombus is more common when anticoagulant therapy is not used [36].

Thromboembolic events occurred at a rate of about 1.7% per year in patients entering the relatively recent Sudden Cardiac Death in Heart Failure Trial (SCD-HeFT) [37]. Older retrospective natural history studies reported an annual incidence of thromboembolic events in patients with HF at 2.7–3.5% per year. To this day, it is not certain that patients with HF who are in NSR clearly benefit from anticoagulation with aspirin, warfarin, or clopidogrel [38]. Randomized clinical trials such as the Warfarin and Antiplatelet Therapy in Chronic Heart Failure (WATCH) Trial demonstrated relatively few thromboembolic events, were slow to enroll patients, and have generally not provided clear and convincing evidence to justify warfarin, aspirin, or clopidogrel use on a routine basis for patients with HF and impaired LV function who are in NSR.

The use of aspirin for these patients remains controversial. Current clinical practice guidelines recommend antiplatelet therapy for patients with HF and CAD. However, patients randomized to aspirin in WATCH had a higher hospitalization rate for HF. Nevertheless, the study does not have the power to refute or recommend its routine use. Aspirin may be beneficial in patients who have HF with recent myocardial infarction or multiple vascular risk-factors.

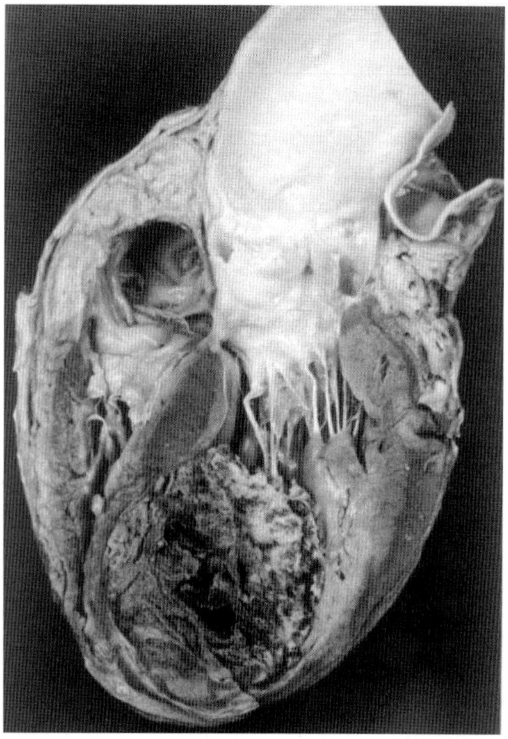

Fig. 19.8 True aneurysm of anteroseptal region. Frontal section of the heart. The apical and septal walls of the LV are thin and show an aneurysm bulge. The cavity of the aneurysm is filled with thrombus. Characteristically, this example of a true ventricular aneurysm shows a wide neck leading into the fundus

Left Ventricular Aneurysm

The term "LV aneurysm" or "true aneurysm" implies a discrete, dyskinetic area of the LV wall with a wide "neck" that is observed months or years after a STEMI. It should be differentiated from the far more common dyskinetic or akinetic areas of the left ventricle that occur early after STEMI and that may resolve or improve over time. Poorly contracting areas of the LV that are frequently seen early after STEMI are referred to as regional wall motion abnormalities and not LV aneurysms. In fact, true LV aneurysms develop in only about 5% of patients with STEMI, and are most commonly seen after large anterior myocardial infarction [39].

The wall of a true aneurysm is "old," thinned out, and composed of a combination of fibrous tissue, necrotic muscle, and, occasionally, some viable myocardium. True LV aneurysms vary in size, but can be up to 8 cm in diameter. After many years, they may become somewhat calcified. Unlike false aneurysms, they rarely rupture. This is especially the case when they are quite old. One feature of true LV aneurysms is that they are usually subserved by a totally occluded coronary artery and have no collaterals, or are very poorly collateralized.

Although true LV aneurysms are relatively inert, they can be a source of lethal ventricular arrhythmias [40]. When death occurs, it can be sudden. Such aneurysms can also be a source of mural thrombus and systemic embolization.

The cases shown in Fig. 19.9a, b portrays anatomic features of LV aneurysm. From a pathologist's point of view, a true aneurysm is characterized by extreme thinning of the cardiac wall with a convex distortion of the external contour, corresponding to the zone of previous infarction.

Figure 19.10 illustrates the echocardiographic features of LV apical aneurysm. The echocardiographic finding is a thin wall that fails to thicken during systolic contraction, producing a "bulge" during systole and diastole.

The case shown in Figs. 19.11 and 19.12 portrays several features of an LV aneurysm. These are the suggestive ECG, the finding of mural thrombus in the aneurysm, and calcification. The terminal complication was gangrene of a lower extremity associated with heart failure.

The patient was a 65-year-old man with a "heart attack" 16 years prior. He was admitted with signs of early gangrene of the right leg. Physical examination revealed signs of congestive HF and tachycardia. BP was 140/100, roentgenogram showed enlargement of the LV with calcification, and central pulmonary venous congestion. Arteriogram revealed occlusion of the right superficial femoral artery and occlusion of the popiteal, tibial, and peroneal trunk. Sudden death occurred on the fifth hospital day.

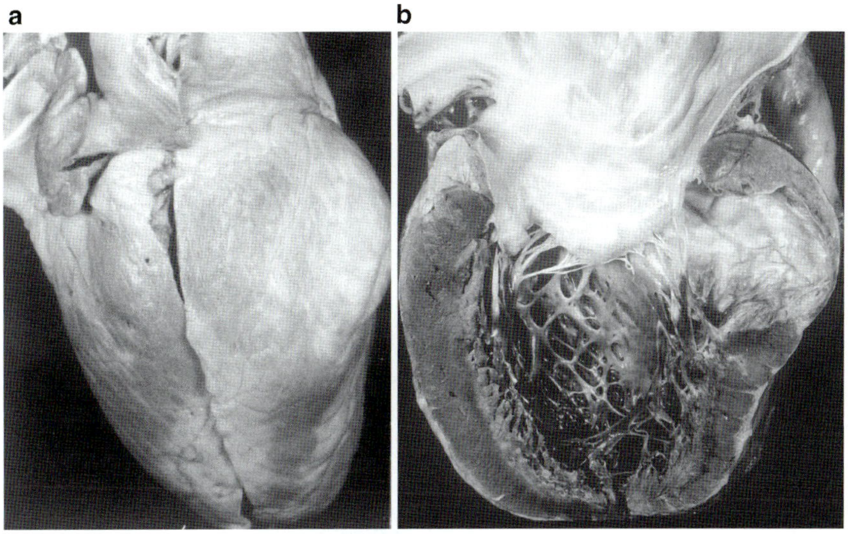

Fig. 19.9 LV aneurysm of the inferior type. (**a**) View of the heart from left, showing a bulge in the posterobasal region of the LV. (**b**) Interior of the LA and LV, showing the aneurysm bulge externally. Aneurysms in this location are frequently associated with infarction of papillary muscles, as is present here

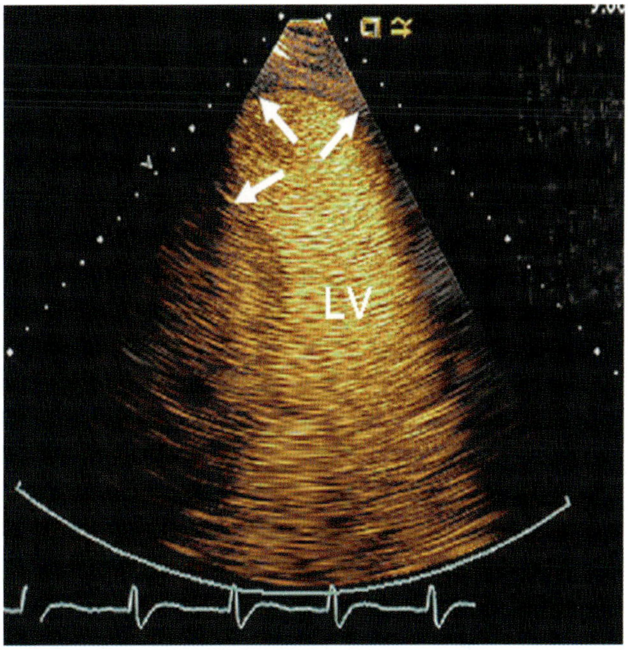

Fig. 19.10 Two-dimensional imaging in the four chambers apical view, demonstrates a thin distal septum and dilatation of apical LV segment (*arrows*). A hinge point demarcates the transition from contractile area to the aneurysmal segment

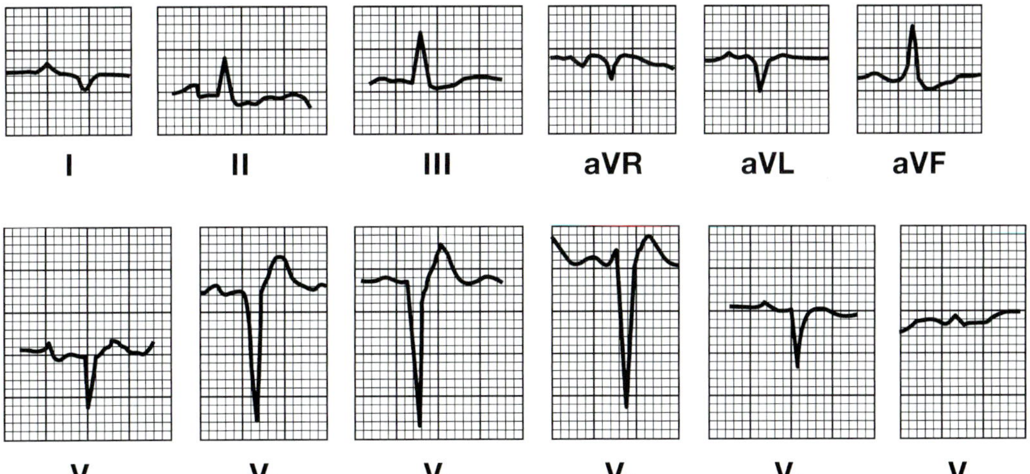

Fig. 19.11 ECG. QS deflection is shown in leads I and AVL, minimal R waves in lead V5 with negative T wave, slanting ST-segment elevation in leads V2 through V4 indicative of healed lateral apical transmural myocardial infarction

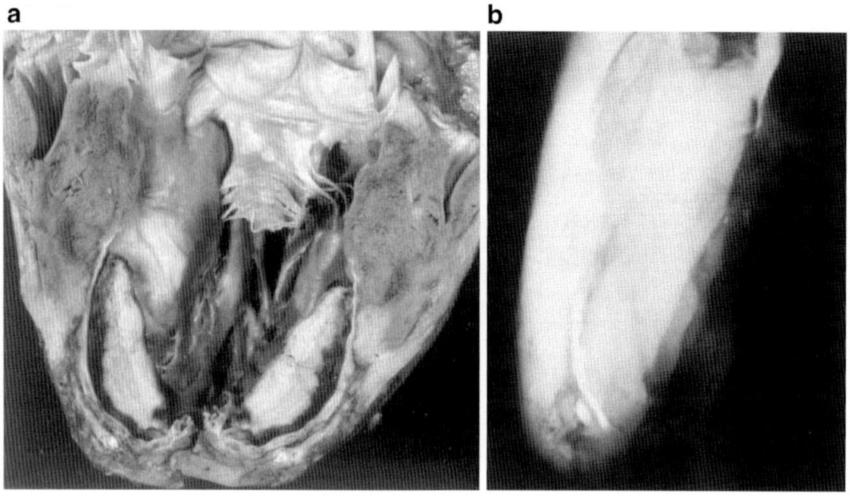

Fig. 19.12 (**a**) LV. At the apex of the LV is an aneurysm containing a thrombus. (**b**) Roentgenogram of specimen of heart showing calcification at the base of the LV thrombus

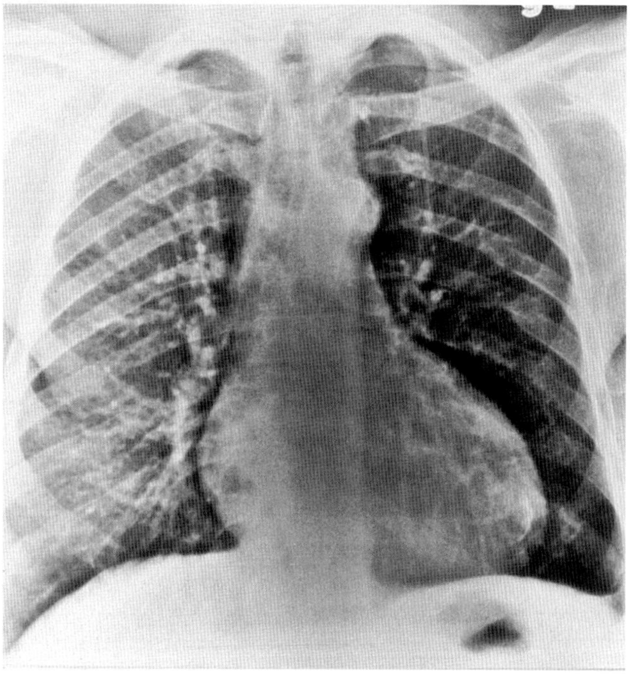

Fig. 19.13 Frontal view of thoracic roentgenogram shows slight distortion of the LV contour, associated with calcification

Some physicians favor long-term anticoagulation with warfarin in these patients. Surgical aneurysmectomy is rarely performed today, unless contractile performance in the remaining ventricle is relatively preserved, and the patient has refractory angina, heart failure, arrhythmias, or systemic embolization.

Figure 19.13 portrays calcification in the wall of an LV aneurysm observed in a plain X-ray film and correlated with coronary arteriography (Fig. 19.14).

Another case of LV aneurysm shown in Figs. 19.15 and 19.16 illustrates not only distortion of the LV shape, as seen in left ventriculograms, but also the lack of visualization of small vessels over the zone of aneurysm, as shown in the coronary arteriogram.

A pseudoaneurysm or false aneurysm is much different than a true aneurysm. It is basically a contained, incomplete myocardial rupture, and typically has a narrow neck. Pseudoaneurysm occurs when an organizing hematoma and thrombus, along with the pericardium, essentially seal off a myocardial rupture of the LV and prevent the development of a hemopericardium. Over time, a pseudoaneurysm forms a narrow "neck" that maintains communication with the LV cavity.

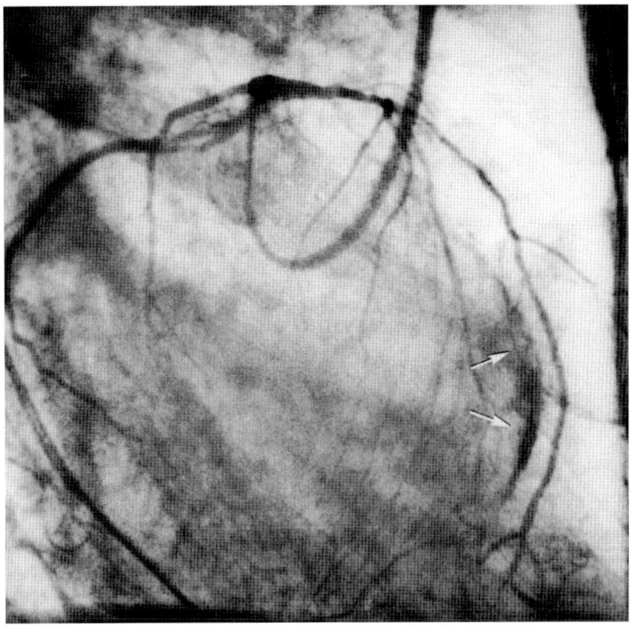

Fig. 19.14 Lateral view of LC arteriogram shows occlusion in the midportion of the Cx and severe stenosis of the LAD. Dense calcification in aneurysmal wall (*arrows*)

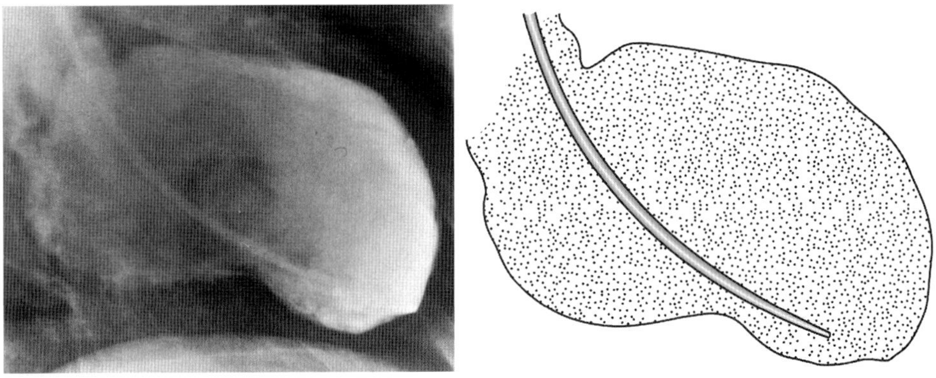

Fig. 19.15 Left ventriculogram in RAO view during systole. A distorted enlargement of an akinetic apical portion of the LV is visible – the characteristic appearance of an LV aneurysm

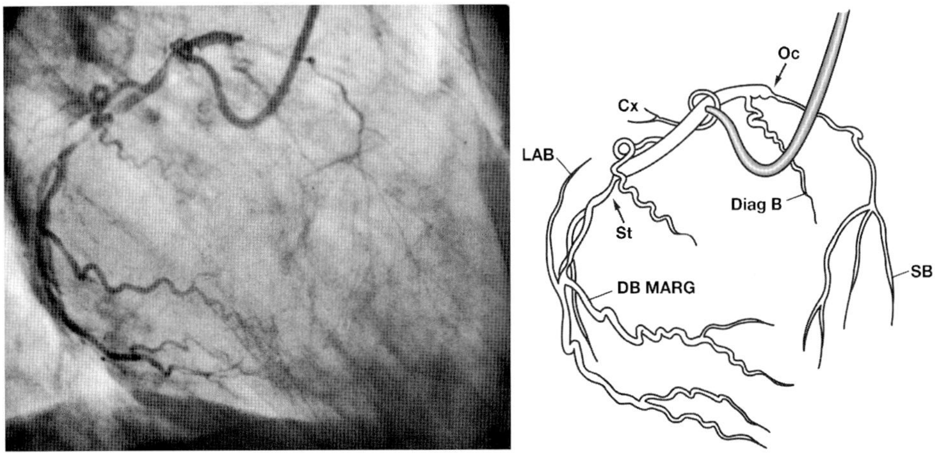

Fig. 19.16 LC arteriogram in lateral view. The LAD is occluded. There is paucity of small vessels over the entire anterolateral aspect of the LV, the latter being an indirect sign of the presence of extensive scarring. Severe disease in the Cx is also present

A pseudoaneurysm can become quite large. It may contain a thrombus, which can be a source of systemic emboli. The diagnosis of a pseudoaneurysm or false aneurysm can be made by contrast ventriculography or echocardiography, but differentiation from a true LV aneurysm can be difficult. Because rupture of a pseudoaneurysm can occur at any time and is not infrequent, prompt elective surgery is usually indicated.

Mitral Insufficiency

Mitral insufficiency stems from a structural problem involving the "mitral valve"; this can include the subvalvular apparatus, the annulus, the valve leaflets' chordae tendineae, papillary muscles, and left ventricular wall [41]. While there are many causes of mitral insufficiency, it is a well-known complication of AMI.

Mitral regurgitation as a consequence of AMI can be acute, where it can be associated with acute pulmonary edema and cardiogenic shock, or it can be chronic and lead to progressive LV remodeling and chronic congestive HF. Acute mitral regurgitation can result from ischemic or infarcted papillary muscle, ruptured chordae tendineae, or even ruptured (infarcted) papillary muscle. Ruptured papillary muscle is usually a catastrophic event, not infrequently leading to torrential mitral insufficiency, shock, and death, unless surgically repaired on an urgent basis. What happens more commonly, especially following a large STEMI, is that LV remodeling occurs as a response to the acute myocardial injury [42], the LV changes shape (becomes more spheroid) and dilates, the papillary muscles are displaced to some extent, and mitral regurgitation more gradually ensues. Such cases are referred to as "functional" mitral insufficiency to distinguish them from mitral insufficiency as a consequence of structural abnormality of the mitral leaflets themselves, as might occur in mitral valve prolapse. So-called functional mitral insufficiency can become quite severe and can cause signs and symptoms of HF, requiring coronary artery bypass grafting (CABG) and repair or replacement of the mitral valve.

Preoperative echocardiography often indicates papillary muscle dyssynchrony, widened vena contracta, mitral valve tenting, alteration of the mitral regurgitation color flow jet area to the left atrial area ratio, displacement of mitral leaflet coaptation, and often an eccentric mitral regurgitant jet. Echocardiographic features of "functional" mitral regurgitation from a patient with a history of previous inferior myocardial infarction and chronic heart failure is illustrated in Fig. 19.17.

With mitral insufficiency, the LV internal chamber dimension is usually increased and the LV ejection fraction may be diminished. The left atrium may be enlarged if the mitral insufficiency has been chronic. Preoperative LV viability studies are needed to plan surgical intervention, as the surgery can be high risk and some patients do not derive obvious benefit.

The case selected to show mitral insufficiency as a complication of healed myocardial infarction is that of a 55-year-old man who exhibited progressive dyspnea on exertion and angina following AMI 2 years previously. Physical examination revealed a systolic murmur of mitral insufficiency. An ECG at this time suggested a healed posterior myocardial infarction and the voltage features of LVH (Fig. 19.18). A left ventriculogram showed gross mitral insufficiency with moderate enlargement of the LA and the LV (Fig. 19.19).

The patient's symptoms deteriorated and the mitral valve was replaced the following year with a prosthetic mitral valve. After surgery, the patient developed LV failure, hypotension, and tachycardia, and ECG signs suggesting acute infarction of the posterior wall. Five days after surgery, the patient developed signs of acute cholecystitis and pyelonephritis. Despite antibiotic therapy, he died 3 days later.

Autopsy showed the heart to be enlarged (600 g). Its posterior wall showed transmural healed infarction (Fig. 19.20a, b). Both papillary muscles were scarred and atrophic. Scarring and a recent myocardial infarction were found in the lateral wall of the LV. A myocardial infarction had occurred in the early postoperative period. Severe obstructive disease was noted in the RC, LAD, and CX (Fig. 19.20c). Acute cholecystitis (nonruptured) and acute pyelonephritis were present.

Whether mitral insufficiency is due to a dilated mitral annulus or distortion of LV geometry is a matter of some controversy, as is the architecture of the subvalvular apparatus. Although both mechanisms may be operative, it is likely that LV geometric distortion and ischemia/infarction of the LV wall and the subvalvular apparatus are primarily responsible for the functional mitral insufficiency that occurs in patients with healed myocardial infarction and ischemic cardiomyopathy. Some element of mitral annular dilation may be present in patients with extremely dilated left ventricles, but for the most part, this probably plays a minor role in the genesis of functional ischemic mitral insufficiency.

Another myth is that surgically correcting the mitral insufficiency will mitigate the low pressure circuit into the left atrium, thus causing an acute afterload stress on the heart and acute left HF following surgery. Although this can probably occur when there is little or no contractile reserve, more often than not, the wall stress (afterload) is actually *reduced* following correction of severe mitral insufficiency. As progressive LV remodeling is abrogated, the LV actually becomes smaller, and the wall stress diminishes gradually over time.

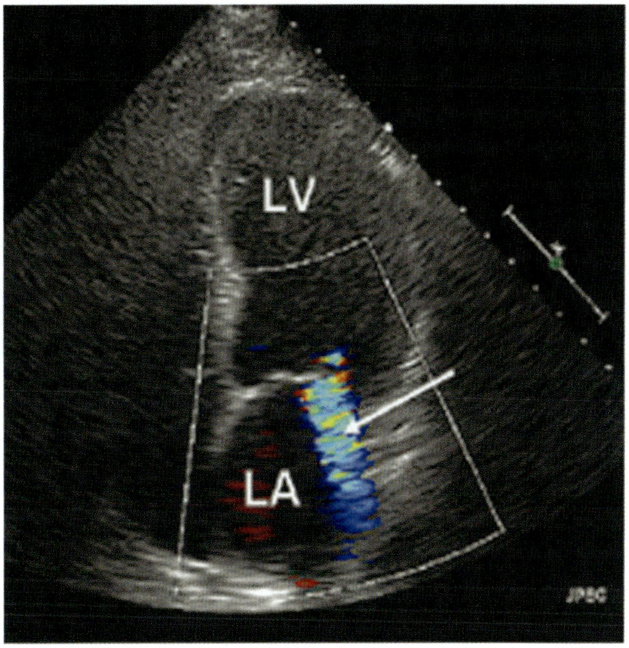

Fig. 19.17 Two-dimensional imaging in the apical two-chamber view, demonstrating an eccentric jet of mitral regurgitation (arrow) caused by the incomplete mitral leaflet closure from a patient with a history of previous inferior myocardial infarction and chronic heart failure

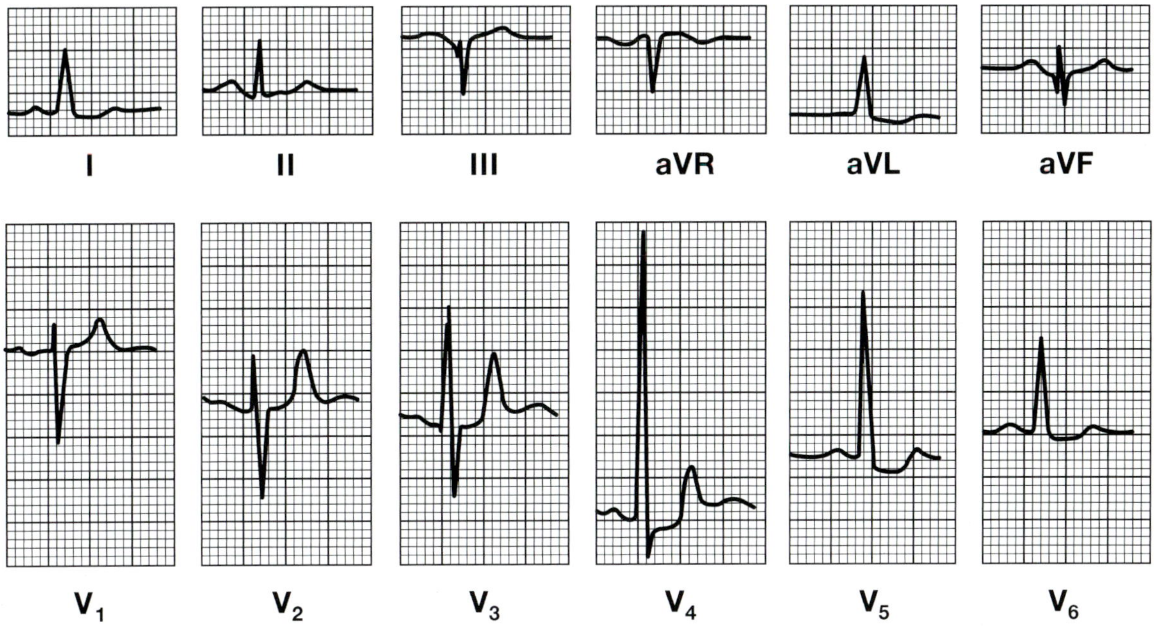

Fig. 19.18 ECG taken approximately 1 year before death and 2 years after the initial myocardial infarction. This shows features of healed inferior-posterior myocardial infarction, as well as signs of LV and LA enlargement

Evidence from observational studies suggests that surgical intervention is beneficial [43]. Depressed LV function is an independent predictor of poor outcomes but is not a contraindication to mitral valve repair. In fact, earlier surgery seems to be creeping into our consideration of surgical treatment for this condition. It is unclear if asymptomatic patients with severe mitral insufficiency who demonstrate no LV dysfunction or dilatation, atrial fibrillation, or pulmonary hypertension should undergo early surgery. Improved preoperative viability testing, better anesthesia, intraoperative transesophageal echocardiography, better control of rapid perioperative atrial fibrillation, and the ability to repair the mitral valve in most cases has, in recent years, led to improved survival for patients undergoing mitral valve surgery for functional ischemic mitral insufficiency.

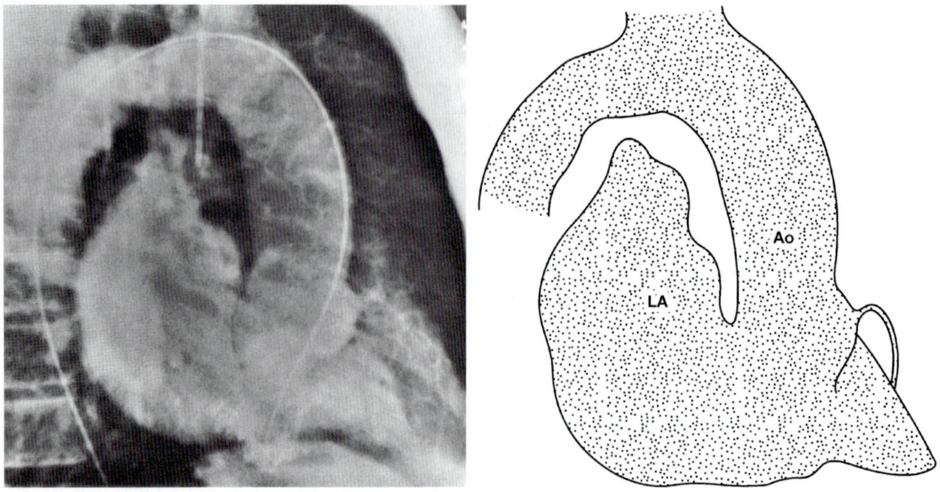

Fig. 19.19 Left ventriculogram showing marked opacification of an enlarged LA related to gross mitral regurgitation

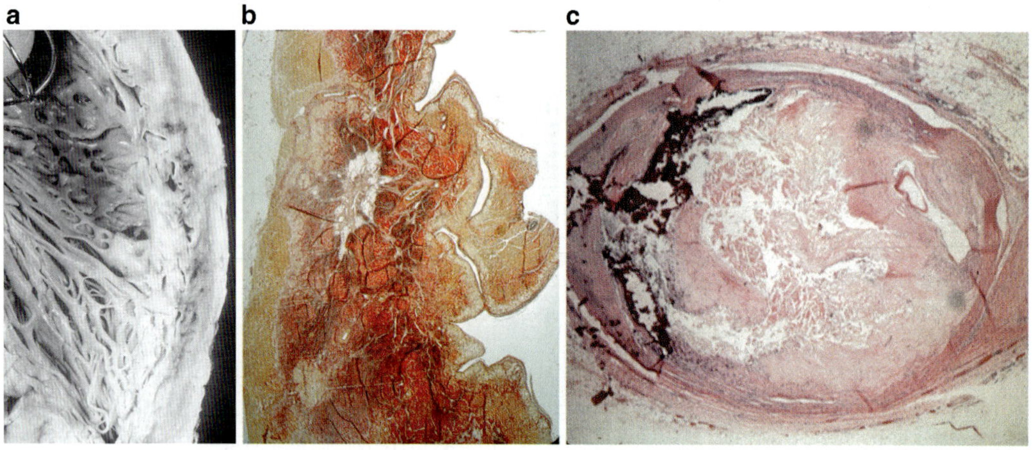

Fig. 19.20 (**a**) Interior of LV showing the prosthesis that has replaced the mitral valve. The subjacent posteromedial papillary muscle is atrophic. Scarring and discoloration of acute infarction are present in the cut surface representing the lateral wall. The inferior wall, lying immediately below the prosthesis, has thinned and was scarred histologically. (**b**) Low-power photomicrograph of the lateral wall of the LV shows extensive scarring. Residual muscle shows signs of acute infarction. Elastic tissue stain: 7×. (**c**) Photomicrograph. (**a**) LAD. The lumen is almost totally occluded by extensive atherosclerosis with focal calcification. Hematoxylin and eosin stain: 12×

References

1. Felker GM, Shaw LK, O'Conner CM. A standardized definition of ischemic cardiomyopathy for use in clinical research. J Am Coll Cardiol. 2002;39:210–8.
2. Bart BA, Shaw LK, McCants CB, et al. Clinical determinants of mortality in patients with angiographically diagnosed ischemic or nonischemic cardiomyopathy. J Am Coll Cardiol. 1997;30:1002–8.
3. Likoff MJ, Chandler SL, Kay HR. Clinical determinants of mortality in chronic congestive heart failure secondary to idiopathic dilated or to ischemic cardiomyopathy. Am J Cardiol. 1987;59:634–8.
4. Farb A, Tang AL, Burke AP, et al. Sudden coronary death: frequency of active coronary lesions, inactive coronary lesions, and myocardial infarction. Circulation. 1995;92:1701–9.
5. Adams KF, Dunlap SH, Sueta CA, et al. Relation between gender, etiology and survival in patients with symptomatic heart failure. J Am Coll Cardiol. 1996;28:1781–8.
6. Tavazzi L. Towards a more precise definition of heart failure aetiology. Eur J Cardiol. 2002;22:192–5.

7. Kannel WB, Ho K, Thom K. Changing epidemiological features of cardiac failure. Eur Heart J. 1994;72(Suppl):S3–9.
8. Levy D, Larson MG, Vasan RS, et al. The progression from hypertension to congestive heart failure. JAMA. 1996;275:1557–62.
9. Fox C, Coady S, Sorlie PD, et al. Increasing cardiovascular disease burden due to diabetes mellitus. The Framingham heart study. Circulation. 2007;115:1544–50.
10. Braunwald E, Rutherford J. Reversible ischemic left ventricular dysfunction: evidence of the "hibernating myocardium". J Am Coll Cardiol. 1986;8:1467–70.
11. Underwood SR, Bax JJ, vom Dahl J, et al. Imaging techniques for the assessment of myocardial hibernation. Eur Heart J. 2004;25:815–36.
12. Gheoghiade M, Sopko G, DeLuca L, et al. Navigating the crossroads of coronary artery disease and heart failure. Circulation. 2006;114:1202–13.
13. Cohn J, Ferrari R, Sharpe N. Cardiac remodeling-concepts and clinical implications: a consensus paper from an international forum on cardiac remodeling. J Am Coll Cardiol. 2000;35:569–82.
14. Solomon SD, Skali H, Anavekar NS, et al. Changes in ventricular size and function in patients treated with valsartan, captopril or both after myocardial infarction. Circulation. 2005;111:3411–9.
15. Cheong BYC, Muthupillai R, Wilson JM, et al. Prognostic significance of delayed-enhancement magnetic resonance imaging. Survival of 857 patients with and without left ventricular dysfunction. Circulation. 2009;120:2069–76.
16. Uretsky BF, Thygesen K, Armstrong P, et al. Acute coronary findings at autopsy in heart failure patients with sudden death. Results from the assessment of treatment with lisinopril and survival (ATLAS) trial. Circulation. 2000;102:611–6.
17. Flaherty JD, Bax JJ, De Luca L, et al. Acute heart failure syndromes in patients with coronary artery disease. Early assessment and treatment. J Am Coll Cardiol. 2009;53:254–63.
18. Goldberg RJ, Ciampa J, Lessard D, et al. Long-term survival after heart failure: a contemporary population based perspective. Arch Intern Med. 2007;167:490–6.
19. Zile M, Brutsaert D. New concepts in diastolic dysfunction and diastolic heart failure: Part 1. Diagnosis, prognosis, and measurement of diastolic function. Circulation. 2002;105:1387–93.
20. Chatterjee K, Massie B. Systolic and diastolic heart failure: differences and similarities. J Card Fail. 2007;13:569–76.
21. Dauterman KW, Go AS, Rowell R, et al. Congestive heart failure with preserved systolic function in a statewide sample of community hospitals. J Card Fail. 2001;7:221–8.
22. Yusuf S, Pfeffer MA, Swedberg K, et al. Effects of candesartan in patients with chronic heart failure and preserved left-ventricular ejection fraction: the CHARM-Preserved trial. Lancet. 2003;362:777–81.
23. Cleland JG, Tendera M, Freemantle N, Polonski L, Taylor J. The perindopril in elderly people with chronic heart failure (PEP-CHF) study. Eur Heart J. 2006;27:2338–45.
24. Cleland JGF, Daubert J-C, Erdmann E, et al., on behalf of the CARE-CHF Investigators. The effect of cardiac resynchronization on morbidity and mortality in heart failure. N Engl J Med. 2005;352:1539–49.
25. Bristow MR, Saxon LA, Boehmer J, et al. Comparison of Medical Therapy, Pacing, and Defibrillation in Heart Failure (COMPANION) Investigators. Cardiac-resynchronization therapy with or without an implantable defibrillator in advanced chronic heart failure. N Engl J Med. 2004;350:2140–50.
26. Epstein AE, DiMarco JP, Ellebogen KA, et al. ACC/AHA/HRS 2008 Guidelines for Device-Based Therapy of Cardiac Rhythm Abnormalities: a report of the American College of Cardiology/American Heart Association Task Force on Practice Guidelines (Writing Committee to Revise the ACC/AHA/NASPE 2002 Guideline Update for Implantation of Cardiac Pacemakers and Antiarrhythmia Devices). J Am Coll Cardiol. 2008;51:e1–62.
27. Yu CM, Chau E, Sanderson JE, et al. Tissue Doppler echocardiographic evidence of reverse remodeling and improved synchronicity by simultaneously delaying regional contraction after biventricular pacing therapy in heart failure. Circulation. 2002;105:438–45.
28. St. John Sutton MG, Plappert T, Abraham WT, et al. Effect of cardiac resynchronization therapy on left ventricular size and function in chronic heart failure. Circulation. 2003;107:1985–90.
29. Cleland J, Freemantle N, Ghio S, et al. Predicting the long-term effects of cardiac resynchronization therapy on mortality from baseline variables and the early response. A report from the CARE-CHF (Cardiac Resynchronization in Heart Failure) Trial. J Am Coll Cardiol. 2008;52:438–45.
30. Marwick TH. Hype and hope in the use of echocardiography for selection for cardiac resynchronization therapy. The Tower of Babel revisited. Circulation. 2008;117:2573–6.
31. Moss AJ, Hall WJ, Cannom DS, et al., for the MADIT-CRT Trial Investigators. Cardiac-resynchronization therapy for the prevention of heart-failure events. N Engl J Med. 2009;361:1329–38.
32. Linde C, Abraham WT, Gold MR, St. John Sutton M, Ghio S, Daybert C, on behalf of the REVERSE Study Group. Randomized trial of cardiac resynchronization in mildly symptomatic heart failure patients and in asymptomatic patients with left ventricular dysfunction and previous heart failure symptoms. J Coll Cardiol. 2008;52:1834–43.
33. St. John Sutton M, Ghio S, Plappert T, et al., on behalf of the REVERSE Study Group. Cardiac resynchronization induces major structural and functional reverse remodeling in patients with New York Heart Association class I/II heart failure. Circulation. 2009;120:1858–65.
34. Francis GS, Tang WHW. Early cardiac resynchronization therapy and reverse remodeling in patients with mild heart failure. Is it time? Circulation. 2009;120:1845–6.
35. Daubert C, Gold MR, Abraham WT, et al., on behalf of the REVERSE Study Group. Prevention of disease progression by cardiac resynchronization therapy in patients with asymptomatic or mildly symptomatic left ventricular dysfunction. J Am Coll Cardiol. 2009;54:1837–46.
36. Stratton JR, Nemanich JW, Johannessem K-A, Resnick AD. Fate of left ventricular thrombi in patients with remote myocardial infarction or idiopathic cardiomyopathy. Circulation. 1998;78:1388–93.
37. Freudenberger RS, Hellkamp AS, Halpern JL, et al., for the SCD-HeFT Investigators. Risk of thromboembolism in heart failure. An analysis from Sudden Cardiac Death in Heart Failure Trial (SCD-HeFT). Circulation. 2008;115:2637–41.
38. Massie B, Cillins JF, Ammon SE, et al., for the WATCH Trial Investigators. Randomized trial of warfarin, aspirin, and clopidogrel in patients with chronic heart failure. The Warfarin and Antiplatelet Therapy in Chronic Heart Failure (WATCH) trial. Circulation. 2009;119:1616–24.

39. Vargas SO, Sampson BA, Schoen FJ. Pathological detection of early myocardial infarction: a critical review of the evolution and usefulness of modern techniques. Mod Pathol. 1999;12:635–45.
40. Abildstrom SZ, Ottesen MM, Rask-Madsen C, et al. Sudden cardiovascular death following myocardial infarction: the importance of left ventricular systolic dysfunction and congestive heart failure. Int J Cardiol. 2005;104:184–9.
41. Verma S, Mesana TG. Mitral valve repair for mitral-valve prolapse. N Engl J Med. 2009;361:2261–9.
42. Pfeffer MA, Braunwald E. Ventricular remodeling after myocardial infarction. Experimental observations and clinical implications. Circulation. 1990;81:1161–72.
43. Enriquez-Sarano M, Avierinos JF, Messika-Zeitoun D, et al. Quantitative determinants of the outcome of asymptomatic mitral regurgitation. N Engl J Med. 2005;352:875–83.

Chapter 20
Nonatherosclerotic Ischemic Heart Disease

Uma S. Valeti, Robert F. Wilson, and Zeev Vlodaver

Coronary Vasospasm

Spontaneous coronary vasospasm leads to an anginal syndrome (often referred to as Printzmetal angina), occurring at rest or with exertion. Coronary spasm occurs in two broad settings – spasm associated with atherosclerosis or other arterial diseases, and spasm that occurs in the absence of identifiable arteriopathy [1–5]. The former is common, but the latter is not [1]. Bertrand administered ergonovine, a compound that precipitates spasm in predisposed individuals, to 1,089 patients undergoing coronary arteriography and found that spasm was relatively common in patients with recent coronary thrombosis (Fig. 20.1) [3]. Vasospasm could be induced in 20% of patients with a recent infarction and 38% of patients with unstable or rest angina, but in only 4.3% of patients with stable, exertional angina. Equally important, only 1.2% of patients with chest pain atypical for angina had inducible spasm, emphasizing that spasm is not a common cause of atypical chest pain.

Patients with inducible vasospasm and a significant (>75%) stenotic lesion have a higher incidence of death, infarction, and atherosclerosis progression than patients with isolated stenotic lesions without inducible vasospasm or vasospasm alone [6–8]. Harding et al. [9] retrospectively analyzed ergonovine provocative studies and found that smoking (odds ratio 4.7–7.7:1 compared to nonsmokers) and atherosclerosis were significant risk factors for inducible spasm [9, 10]. More recently, vascular inflammation, polymorphism of eNOS genes, and enhanced phospholipase C activity have been linked to coronary spasm [11, 12]. The diagnosis of coronary vasospasm can be made at the time of angiography by giving drugs that provoke spasm or occasionally by observing spontaneous spasm [1, 2, 13–18]. The most commonly administered agent is an ergot derivative, usually ergonovine maleate or ergometrine, although methacholine was used to induce vasospasm in pioneering studies in the catheterization laboratory. Ergot derivatives are potent constrictors of vascular smooth muscle. Muscarinic receptor agonists (acetylcholine and methacholine) appear to cause vasospasm in a large fraction of patients with ergonovine-induced spasm [19]. Other agents have also been reported to induce spasm (cold pressor test, histamine, hyperventilation), but not enough information is known to assess the potency and specificity of these agents [20, 21].

Prior to a provocative test for vasospasm, an electrocardiogram should be obtained and a coronary arteriogram should show the absence of severe coronary obstruction. When vasospasm is suspected, acetylcholine or ergonovine generally is given in incremental intravenous doses – starting at 50 mg and increasing doses until a total dose of 350–400 mg intravenously is reached for ergonovine. Although ergonovine appears safe in doses up to 800 mg, the vast majority of patients

U.S. Valeti, MD, FACC (✉)
Cardiovascular Division, Department of Medicine, University of Minnesota, Minneapolis, MN, USA
e-mail: uvaleti@umn.edu

R.F. Wilson, MD • Z. Vlodaver, MD
Division of Cardiovascular Medicine, University of Minnesota, Minneapolis, MN, USA

Z. Vlodaver et al. (eds.), *Coronary Heart Disease: Clinical, Pathological, Imaging, and Molecular Profiles*,
DOI 10.1007/978-1-4614-1475-9_20, © Springer Science+Business Media, LLC 2012

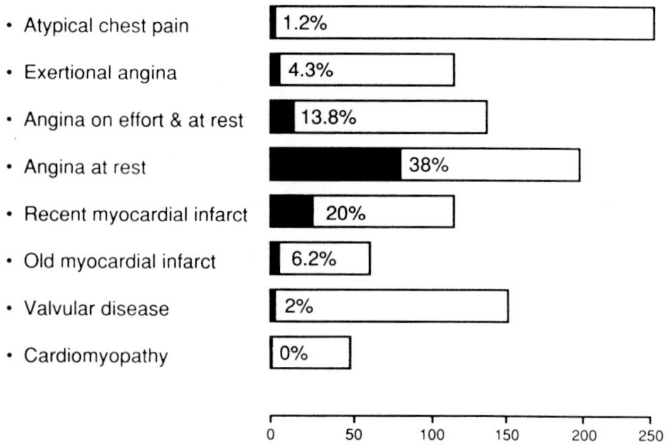

Fig. 20.1 The frequency of coronary vasospasm induced by ergonovine in 1,089 patients undergoing cardiac catheterization. The incidence of provokable spasm was high in patients with angina at rest and recent myocardial infarction, but uncommon in patients with chest pain, which is atypical for myocardial ischemia

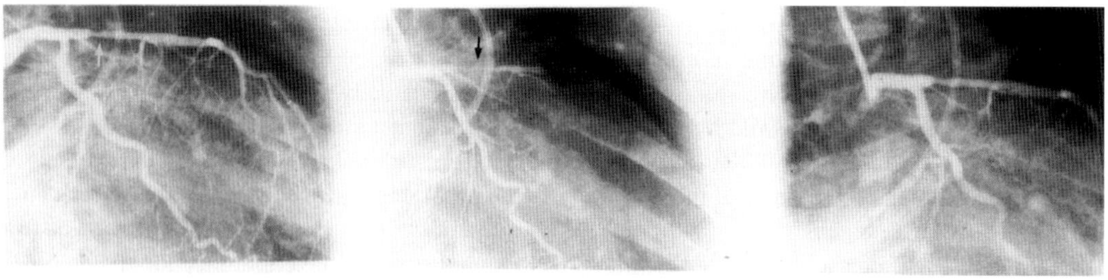

Fig. 20.2 An angiogram from a patient with vasospasm induced by ergonovine. *Left*: Before ergonovine, there is a 50% diameter stenosis in the proximal LAD. *Center*: After ergonovine (100 mg intravenously), the LAD develops spasm at the site of the lesion (*arrow*), with minimal antegrade blood flow. *Right*: After nitroglycerin (200 mg intracoronary), the spasm is relieved and blood flow is restored

with vasospastic angina develop spasm at doses of <200 mg [1, 2, 15–17, 22]. More recently, intracoronary acetylcholine (25–50 mg and an intracoronary bolus) has been used to provoke spasm [23].

In normal patients, ergonovine causes mild, diffuse coronary constriction in the epicardial arteries (10–20% decrease in diameter) [16]. The response is more pronounced in the distal vessels. In patients with vasospastic angina, ergonovine or acetylcholine causes focal, usually severe, large-vessel coronary constriction – frequently leading to transient, total coronary occlusion (Fig. 20.2). The peak response occurs 2–5 min after administration, although onset of spasm 15–20 min later has been reported. In its classical description, coronary spasm leads to chest pain, ST-segment elevation on the electrocardiogram, increased left ventricular end-diastolic pressure, and myocardial lactate release [18]. In as many as half of patients with vasospastic angina, the response to ergonovine is less intense. ST-segment depression (rather than elevation) is often observed in patients with incomplete coronary occlusion with spasm, in patients with collateral arteries to the ischemic bed, and if spasm occurs in a small vessel [23–28]. Most would consider the test positive if the patient's symptoms are reproduced, if focal spasm >75% is demonstrated, and if there are electrocardiographic changes (ST-segment elevation or depression) [1].

Coronary spasm may be slightly more likely in the right coronary artery (RCA), followed by the left anterior descending (LAD) and circumflex arteries (CX). Vein bypass grafts also can exhibit spasm, but rarely do [29]. Patients with vasospastic angina appear to have more constriction in nonspastic coronary segments, suggesting a generalized coronary abnormality, and also may have enhanced resting tone, as evidenced by a greater degree of relaxation after nitroglycerin [30–33].

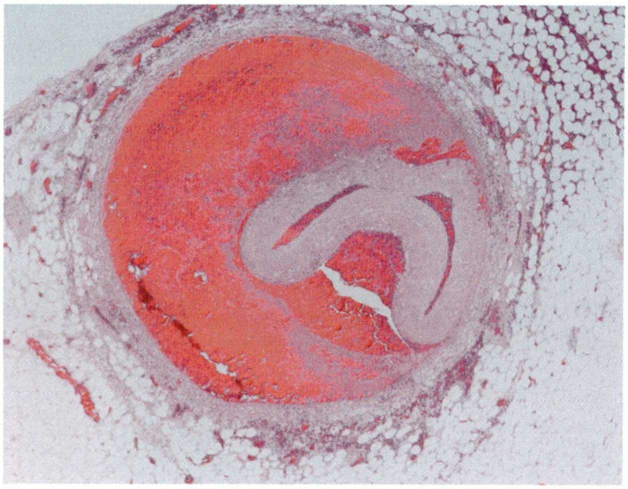

Fig. 20.3 Photomicrograph is from a 48-year-old female with sudden death and spontaneous dissection of the LAD, with acute thrombus within a false channel compressing the true lumen. Hematoxylin and eosin stain: 2×

Catheter- and Device-Induced Vasospasm

Coronary cannulation can cause vasospasm at the catheter tip, usually thought to result from mechanical traction on the artery. Catheter-induced spasm is much more common in the right compared to the left coronary artery, and rarely, may occur distal to the catheter tip or in vein grafts [34, 35]. It may occur more frequently in patients with vasospastic disease in other coronary segments, but an association with clinical vasospasm is very uncommon. Implanted devices such as coronary stents can also cause diffuse coronary spasm resulting in symptoms [36].

Spontaneous Coronary Artery Dissection

Isolated spontaneous coronary artery dissection is a rare event that occurs in all coronary arteries with approximately equal incidence [37–42]. It occurs most frequently in young women, particularly in the peripartum period, but may be associated with blunt chest trauma, atherosclerosis (possibly related to plaque rupture), obstruction immediately above the aortic valve (e.g., an obstructed prosthetic ball valve), and from iatrogenic complications of coronary artery cannulation [38, 43–47]. Coronary dissection also occurs in conjunction with aortic dissection and involves the RCA more often than the left. Histological examinations have shown a variety of abnormalities [38, 40, 42, 45]. The most common observation is a hematoma within the arterial media and luminal compression (Fig. 20.3) [38, 42]. A rent in the intima leading to the medial hematoma is observed inconsistently, as are changes of cystic medial necrosis [40]. Atherosclerosis with aneurysm or plaque rupture has been reported [40]. Perivascular eosinophilia has also been found late after dissection, but it is not clear whether eosinophils were related to the cause or occur as a response to the dissection [48].

At angiography, spontaneous dissection appears as a radiolucent linear filling defect that spirals down the coronary artery [37, 39, 42, 49–51]. After intracoronary contrast injection, contrast material frequently persists in the false lumen. The dissection may be complicated by total thrombotic coronary occlusion (Figs. 20.4 and 20.5). Distal emboli with abrupt vessel cut-offs are common [42]. Unless complicated by lumen thrombosis or death, most spontaneous dissections heal, but permanent true and false channel lumens may persist [44, 49–51]. A similar dual-lumen vessel can be seen late after angioplasty complicated by a spiral dissection. In one series of patients with spontaneous dissection, the mortality rate was 18% [37]. Thrombolytic therapy has been used successfully to treat acute coronary occlusion related to spontaneous dissection [52], but stenting is now the therapy of choice if the operator can negotiate through the true lumen to place the stent [53]. Recurrent dissection in another artery is uncommon, but may occur more frequently in women.

Figures 20.6 and 20.7 illustrate two cases with iatrogenic coronary dissection following cannulation (Fig. 20.6) and postcoronary arteriography (Fig. 20.7).

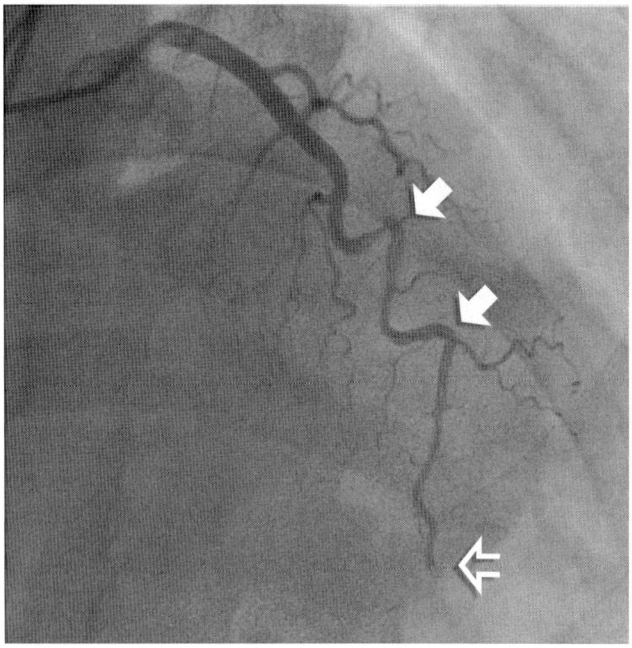

Fig. 20.4 A 67-year-old male with spontaneous LAD dissection shown in this RAO cranial projection. The dissection originates in the mid-LAD (*arrows*) and extends all the way into the apical LAD with distal occlusion (*white arrow*). The circumflex artery had an anomalous origin from the right coronary cusp (courtesy Dr. Abhiram Prasad. Mayo Clinic)

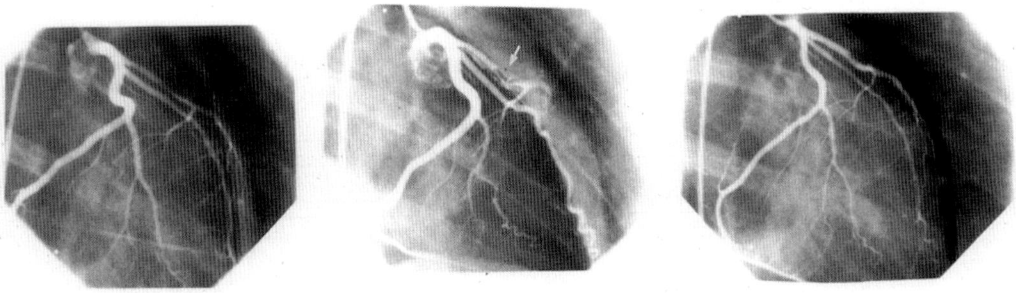

Fig. 20.5 Serial angiograms obtained from a patient with spontaneous dissection of the LAD. *Left*: An angiogram obtained before presentation revealed mild, diffuse narrowing of the LAD. *Center*: After developing signs of acute myocardial infarction, the angiogram revealed subtotal occlusion of the LAD and a linear intraluminal filling defect along the occlusion (*arrow*). *Right*: Angiography months after presentation and treatment with streptokinase showed healing of the dissection and minimal stenosis

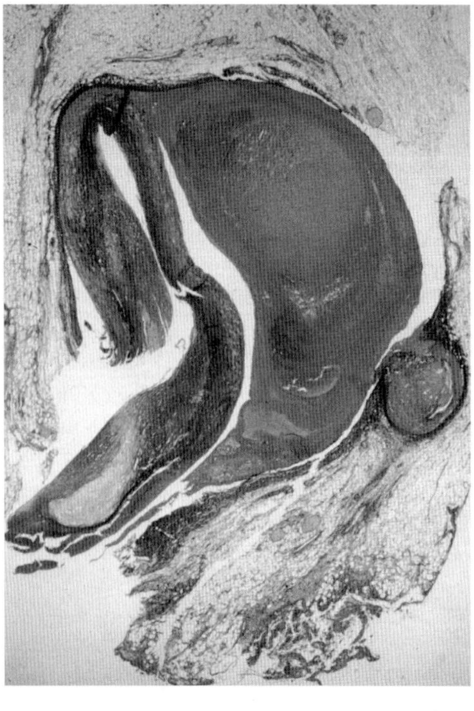

Fig. 20.6 An example of intramural hematoma of the ML following aortic valve replacement with cannulation of the ML. Elastic tissue stain: 11×

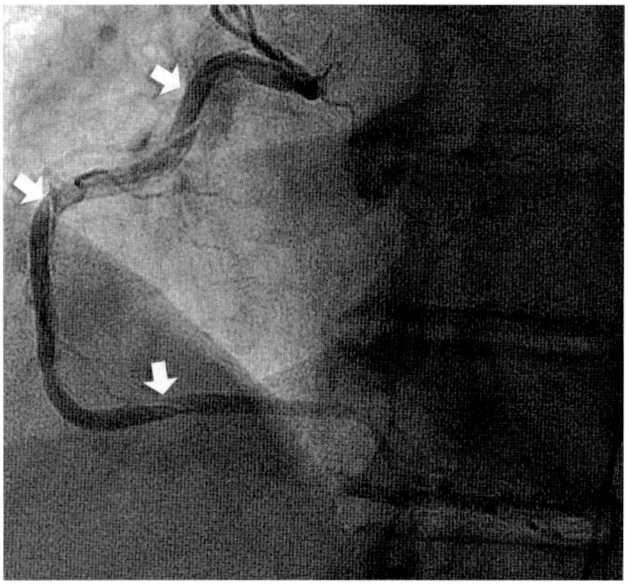

Fig. 20.7 A 46-year-old woman with fibromyalgia and atypical anginal symptoms underwent a coronary CT angiogram that was normal. She presented to another hospital 2 weeks later with atypical symptoms and underwent a coronary angiogram that revealed no coronary disease, but resulted in a large, spiral coronary dissection extending into the distal RCA, requiring stenting (*arrows*)

Myocardial Infarction in Patients with Angiographically Normal

Coronary Arteries

One percent to 16% of patients with documented acute myocardial infarction are found at angiography to have normal or nearly normal coronary arteries [54–57]. Coronary embolism, in situ coronary thrombosis with spontaneous lysis, stress-induced cardiomyopathy (takotsubo syndrome), and vasospasm have been proposed as possible mechanisms [58–61].

Compared to patients with infarction associated with coronary atherosclerosis, those with a normal coronary angiogram after infarction tend to be younger (16–22% of patients are under 35 years of age) and have fewer antecedent symptoms of angina and fewer risk factors for atherosclerosis [62, 63]. In contrast to the male predominance of atherosclerosis-associated infarction, men and women are approximately equally affected [60, 63]. Associations with tobacco smoking, a prior history of migraine headaches, Raynaud phenomenon, mitral valve prolapse, cocaine abuse, and birth control pill use have been reported [63–65]. Cocaine, sumatriptan, nifedipine, or excessive alcohol use also may precipitate infarction, presumably by causing vasospasm or transient thrombosis. . Coronary spasm induced by ergonovine can be demonstrated in a minority of patients, but no definitive underlying mechanism can be found in most [60].

Sudden sympathetic discharge (e.g., with emotional stress, shock, or postoperative pain) has also been associated with transient anterior wall dysfunction, chest pain, and deep T-wave inversion across the precordial leads on the ECG in the presence of normal coronary angiography (Fig. 20.8). Although blood markers of infarction are elevated, nearly all patients have recovery of ventricular function. Myocardial biopsies have shown contraction band necrosis, which is pathognomonic of catecholamine excess-mediated infarction. This syndrome associated with sudden sympathetic discharge has been underappreciated and may actually account for the majority of cases of infarction with normal angiography [66, 67].

Infarctions associated with a normal coronary angiogram tend to be smaller than those associated with atherosclerosis, and their mortality rate may be lower [63]. The long-term prognosis is generally good in terms of mortality, but recurrent infarction and stroke may be more common than in patients with atherosclerosis [56, 63].

Patients with stress cardiomyopathy who underwent myocardial biopsy have shown interstitial infiltrates primary of mononuclear lymphocytes, leukocytes, macrophages, myocardial fibrosis, and contraction bands (Fig. 20.9). The inflammatory changes and contraction bands in stress cardiomyopathy distinguish it from myocardial infarction showing coagulation necrosis resulting from coronary artery occlusion.

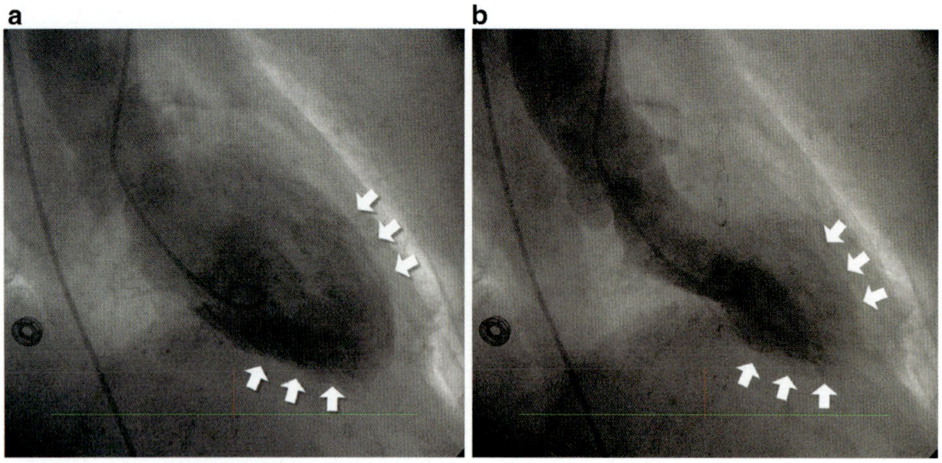

Fig. 20.8 A 67-year-old woman experienced stress cardiomyopathy after the unexpected death of her son. Panel (**a**) shows the left ventricular end-diastolic image on LV angiogram and (**b**) shows the left ventricular end-systolic image. The anterolateral wall, apex, and mid inferior wall in (**b**) do not contract, resulting in appearance of an apical balloon (or Takosubo, a Japanese narrow-necked pot-like device used to capture an octopus). Patient had normal coronary arteries

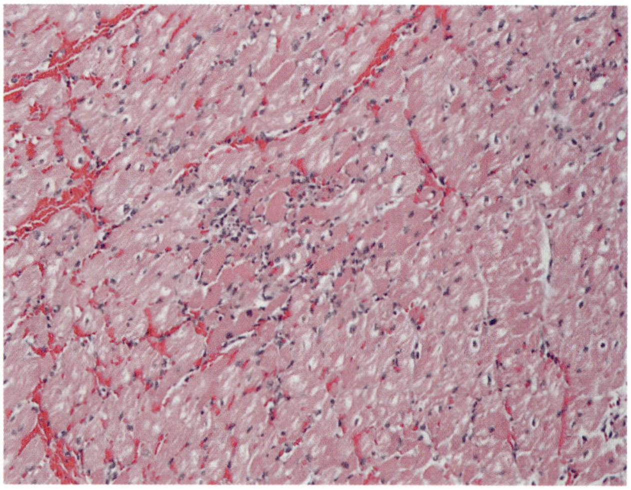

Fig. 20.9 Photomicrograph from a 28-year-old female with features of contraction band necrosis with focal area of hypereosinophilic myocytes and mixed inflammatory cell infiltrate. Hematoxylin and eosin stain: 20×

Microcirculatory Coronary Disease

Studies in highly selected patient populations suggest that microvascular coronary dysfunction may be a frequent cause of symptoms in the 10–25% of patients undergoing coronary angiography for chest pain, but in whom no significant obstruction to blood flow is found in the epicardial vessels [68–71]. Of patients with angiographically normal coronary arteries, Cannon reported that 71% had abnormal microvascular function [72] and Geltman found reduced coronary flow reserve in 50% [73]. It is now accepted that microvascular dysfunction can cause clinically important myocardial ischemia, including anginal syndromes, exertional dyspnea, and left ventricular dysfunction, but the mechanism(s) and incidence are unclear [70, 71, 74].

A number of diseases are associated with or cause microvascular dysfunction. These include prolonged hypertension, cardiac hypertrophy, cardiomyopathies, collagen vascular diseases, and atherosclerosis [74–78] – diseases associated with endothelial dysfunction. Although common entities, these specific disease entities are present in less than half of patients found at catheterization to have microvascular disease. Hence, it is likely that other, still uncharacterized syndromes alter microvascular function in these patients.

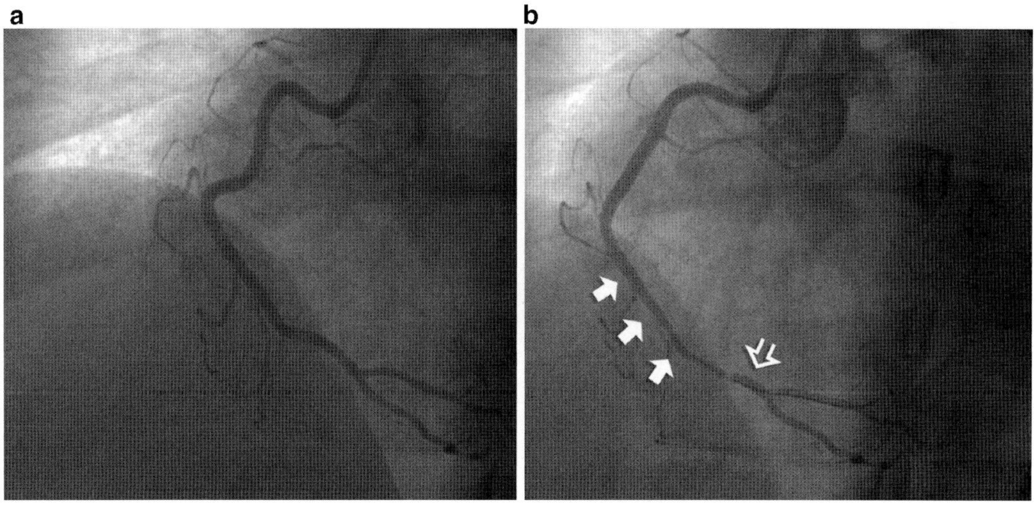

Fig. 20.10 A 45-year-old woman with persistent anginal symptoms with normal coronary arteries noted on coronary CT angiography. Evaluation with invasive angiography before (**a**) and after infusion of intracoronary acetylcholine (**b**) revealed obvious endothelial dysfunction with diffuse epicardial coronary vasoconstriction (*arrows*, **b**) with infusion of acetylcholine and focal spasm (*white arrow*, **b**)

The functioning of the microcirculation can be tested in several ways at the time of angiography, although the clinical significance of any abnormalities found in the absence of symptoms is not yet certain. Maximal coronary conductance can be assessed by measurements of coronary flow reserve, the ratio of peak hyperemic blood flow to resting flow [79–82]. In patients with a severe epicardial coronary stenosis (e.g., atherosclerotic stenosis), treadmill exercise performance is reduced proportionately to coronary reserve [83]. Patients with fixed microvascular disease may have similarly reduced coronary reserve, suggesting a fixed reduction in maximal coronary conductance.

Endothelial dysfunction may play an important, etiologic role in microvascular disease syndromes [84]. The functional integrity of the endothelium can be tested at the time of angiography by measuring the amount of large-vessel dilation and change in blood flow (i.e., microvascular dilation) during intracoronary infusion of pharmacologic agents that normally elicit the release of endothelial dilating factor(s). When normal endothelium is present, acetylcholine causes a dose-dependent, epicardial, coronary, and microvascular dilation [85]. In the absence of endothelium, acetylcholine causes short-acting constriction. Hence, the response to intracoronary acetylcholine infusion (dilation or no change/constriction) is one marker of endothelial function that can be tested in humans (Fig. 20.10).

The acetylcholine response is abnormal in several diseases with known endothelial dysfunction (atherosclerosis, transplantation) [86, 87]. The endothelial response to acetylcholine also was abnormal in both the large conduit coronary arteries and the coronary microcirculation (i.e., constriction or subnormal dilation) in a series of nine patients with anginal symptoms and normal coronary angiography, even though the response to nonendothelial-dependent pharmacological vasodilators was preserved [88]. These suggest that functional as well as fixed abnormalities in the coronary microcirculation may be causes of ischemia in the absence of epicardial atherosclerosis.

Radiation-Induced Coronary Artery Disease

Chest irradiation can lead to narrowing or occlusion of the epicardial and intramural coronary arteries, typically presenting several months to 12 years after the exposure [89–99]. Radiation-induced injury usually leads to adventitial fibrosis, smooth muscle cell loss in the media, and intimal proliferation [89, 92]. Atherosclerotic changes have also been observed, although lipid deposition is less marked than in patients with typical atherosclerosis. The angiographic findings are similar to atherosclerosis [94]. The coronary lumen can be diffusely narrowed or occluded entirely from radiation-induced fibrosis (Fig. 20.11). Acute myocardial infarction following radiation is reported [97]. The proximal vessels are more commonly affected.

Generally, a dose over 3,000R is associated with increased risk of radiation-induced coronary disease. In one series of 16 patients <33 years of age who had received >3,500R to the heart, six had severe, focal, epicardial coronary stenoses [94, 95]. In another series, patients treated for Hodgkin disease with mantle radiation had a 2.7-fold increase in risk for coronary disease [91].

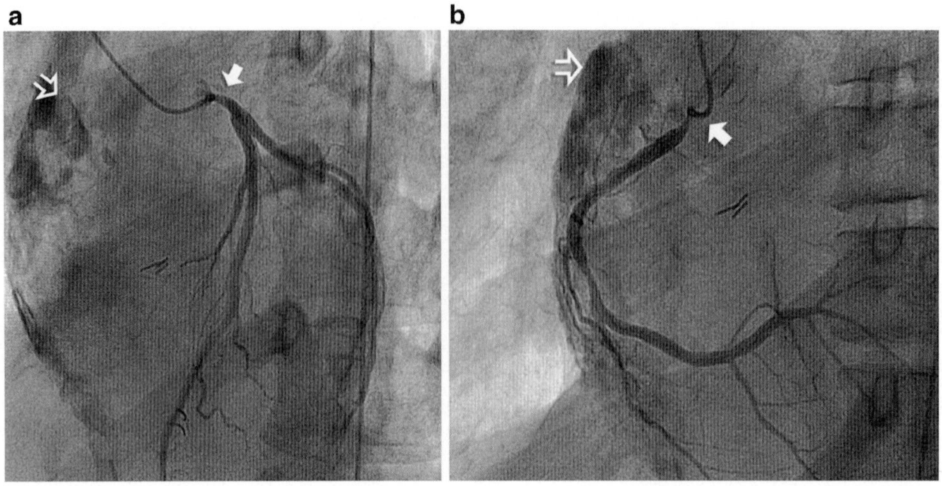

Fig. 20.11 A 60-year-old woman underwent chest radiation for breast carcinoma presented with severe angina and biventricular heart failure and ascites. Coronary angiography revealed severe ostial stenosis of the left main coronary artery (**a**) and the right coronary artery (**b**, *arrows*). Also visible is severe anterior pericardial calcification (*white arrow*) that correlated with hemodynamics consistent with constrictive physiology

Transplant-Related Arteriopathy

The most persistent problem in patients surviving more than 1 year after heart transplantation has been the development of coronary arteriopathy characterized by diffuse intimal thickening of the transplanted arterial wall [100–104]. The process extends from the large conduit arteries into smaller branch vessels >400 mm in diameter. In its classical angiographic description, transplant vasculopathy is characterized by diffuse luminal obliteration, which is most marked in the smaller branch vessels seen during angiography (Fig. 20.12).

The intimal thickening process affects the entire conduit artery. Focal stenoses in the large epicardial arteries – similar in angiographic morphology to atherosclerotic lesions – are not infrequent (Fig. 20.13). The typical angiographic patterns of transplant vasculopathy were described by Gao et al. [105] (Fig. 20.14). Of note, the angiographic hallmarks of beaded vasculitis are absent.

Serial angiographic studies demonstrate the development of luminal irregularities or frank stenosis within 3 years of transplantation in 25–45% of patients [106–113]. Serial angiographic measurements of coronary luminal cross-sectional areas using quantitative angiography show that the large conduit arteries decrease in diameter by 6–10% in the first year after transplantation, but thereafter, the lumen diameter remains fairly stable until more advanced vasculopathy occurs [109].

Angiographic studies underestimate the frequency of arteriopathy because they detect only narrowing of the coronary lumen, and not increased coronary wall thickening [104]. Intravascular ultrasound (IVUS) imaging of transplanted coronary arteries generally demonstrates a substantially greater degree of intimal thickening than is observed using angiography [114, 115]. Many angiographers routinely image the coronary arteries using IVUS at the time of angiography. Development of angiographically detectable vasculopathy is associated with shortened survival [113]. Endothelial function is frequently abnormal in transplanted coronary arteries [116]. In many patients, intracoronary acetylcholine administration fails to elicit the expected coronary dilation and increase in blood flow, suggesting a failure of the endothelium to normally release endothelium-derived relaxing factor (nitric oxide) [117]. Some transplant recipients have frank vasoconstriction in response to acetylcholine [27]. Epicardial coronary tone is also reduced in the first several months after transplantation [118], but returns to normal by 1 year after transplantation. Diffuse coronary constriction due to elevated vascular tone can be misinterpreted as diffuse intimal thickening. Nitroglycerin should be administered immediately prior to angiography to enable a true assessment of the lumen caliber.

Histological features of transplant arteriopathy are marked intimal thickening in the coronary arteries with epicardial inflammatory changes (Fig. 20.15).

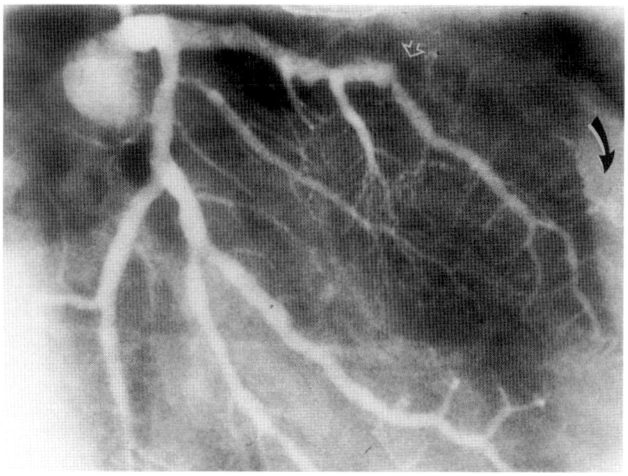

Fig. 20.12 An angiogram of the left coronary artery of a patient with transplant-related vasculopathy. The left anterior descending (LAD) artery is occluded (*open arrow*) and fills distally by faint collaterals (*solid arrow*). The remainder of the coronary tree has diffuse irregularities and pruning of the distal brunches

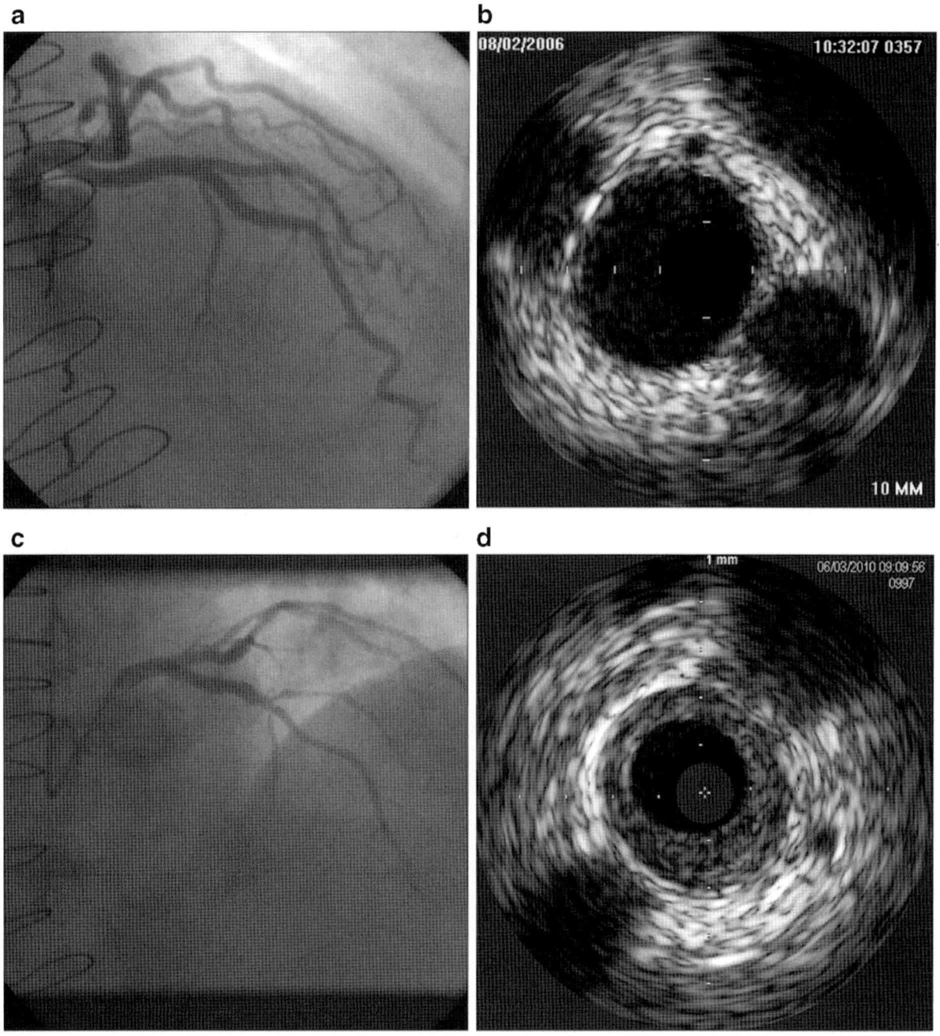

Fig. 20.13 A 52-year-old male, s/p postheart transplant, had idiopathic, dilated cardiomyopathy with normal coronary arteries on angiography (*top left*) and IVUS (*top right*) 3 months after transplant. He subsequently developed moderate posttransplant coronary arteriopathy 4 years post-transplant as shown on angiography of the LAD artery (*bottom left*) and IVUS (*bottom right*) (courtesy Dr. Abhiram Prasad. Mayo Clinic)

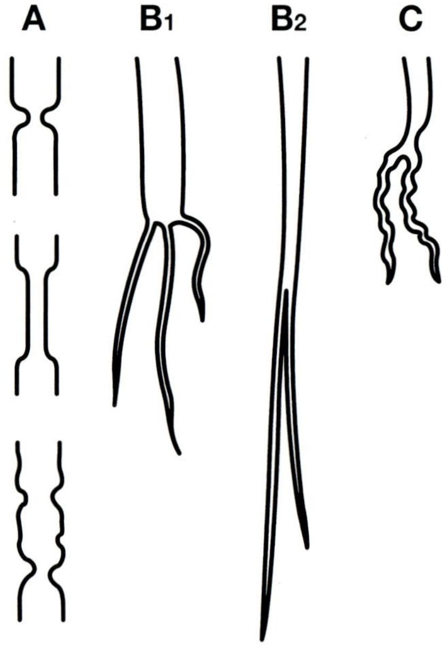

Fig. 20.14 Angiographic morphologies of coronary lesions associated with transplant vasculopathy. Lesion type A: discrete tubular or multiple stenoses. Lesion type B1: distal concentric narrowing and obliterated vessels with sparing of the proximal vessel. Lesion type B2: Diffuse concentric narrowing. Lesion type C: Narrow irregular distal branches with abrupt terminations. Adapted from Gao et al. [105]. Elsevier Inc.

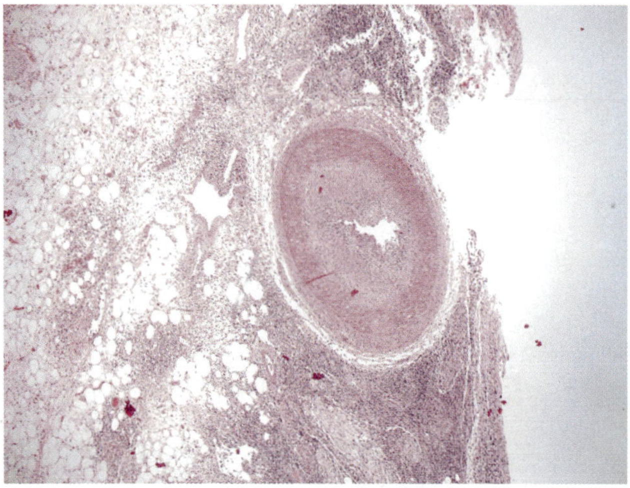

Fig. 20.15 Photomicrograph of epicardium of a 3-year-old male, 2 months following transplantation and acute cellular rejection, showing LAD coronary artery with marked intimal thickening and epicardial inflammation. Hematoxylin and eosin stain: 2×

Coronary Abnormalities Associated with Vasculitis

Coronary vasculitis can result from vascular infection or collagen-related vascular diseases. It causes four angiographically detectable coronary abnormalcies: focal stenotic lesions, diffuse narrowing, thrombosis, and late aneurysmal dilation [40, 41]. Lesions may be located from the aortic origin of the coronary arteries to the microcirculation. Aortitis associated with syphilis, Takayasu arteritis, and more rarely, tuberculosis can cause stenosis of the coronary ostia [42]. Involvement of the larger epicardial coronary arteries is reported, but is rare [40, 43].

Of the collagen-related vascular diseases, systemic lupus erythematosus most commonly involves the angiographically visible epicardial coronary vessels, although large coronary involvement can be seen in polyarteritis nodosa, progressive systemic sclerosis, and more rarely, giant cell arteritis and rheumatoid arthritis [44–48]. The epicardial lesions associated with vasculitis typically resemble atherosclerotic lesions [41]. Diffuse luminal narrowing is less common and the typical beaded appearance of beaded vasculitis seen in other vascular beds is notably absent, although one case of a huge coronary aneurysm associated with systemic lupus erythematosus is reported [44, 46, 49]. Thrombosis of vasculitic segments can occur, leading to total arterial occlusion or the typical angiographic appearance of a thrombotic lesion.

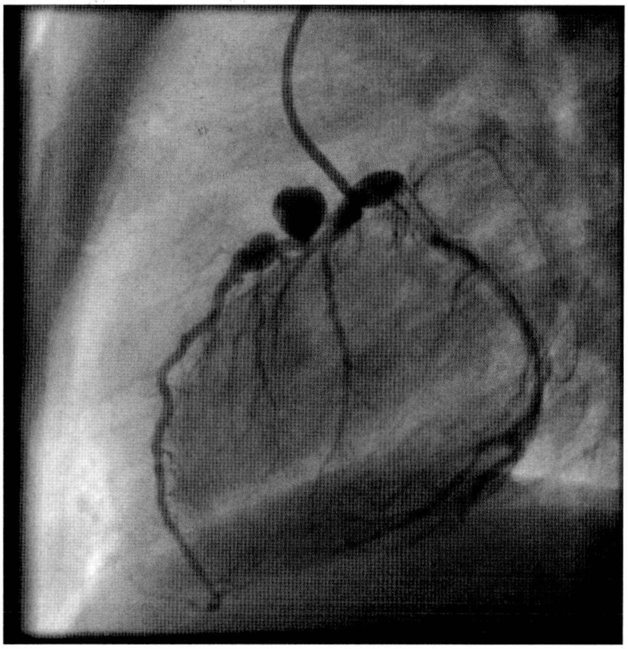

Fig. 20.16 Patient with Kawaski vasculitis and giant coronary artery aneurysms in the LAD artery shown in this RAO projection (courtesy Dr. Abhiram Prasad. Mayo Clinic)

The incidence of coronary vasculitis is probably underestimated by angiography because the findings are so similar to atherosclerosis [44]. In young patients with systemic lupus erythematosus and no important risk factors for atherosclerosis, coronary lesions and myocardial infarction should be assumed to be due to vasculitic involvement of the coronary arteries until shown otherwise, although accelerated atherosclerosis due to corticosteroid therapy may also account for angiographically detected lesions. Late aneurysmal dilation of the large coronary arteries, especially in periarteritis nodosa, has been reported to occur in nearly all of the vasculitic syndromes, and rupture of the aneurysm has been reported as a rare consequence [44, 46, 50].

Microcirculatory vasculitis occurs frequently in patients with systemic lupus erythematosus, scleroderma, and rheumatoid arthritis. In these patients, coronary flow reserve is typically reduced and ischemia due to microvascular obstruction or dysfunction has been proposed as the cause [51, 52].

The most common infectious agent to involve the angiographically visible coronary vessels is Kawasaki disease (mucocutaneous lymph node syndrome). It is characterized by coronary aneurysmal dilation, stenosis, and thrombosis occurring primarily in the proximal coronary arteries [53]. The aneurysms can be huge (Figs. 20.16 and 20.17). Late after the acute illness, about one-half of the aneurysms present during the initial febrile episode resolve [54, 55]. In angiographic studies of 1,100 patients at an average of 25 months after disease onset, Suzuki et al. found that 36% had frank aneurysms, 28% had coronary dilation, 24% had localized coronary stenosis, and 8% had an occluded coronary artery [56]. Aneurysmal calcification can occur [57].

Most of the Kawasaki disease-associated aneurysms appear in the proximal coronary arteries, but about 1 in 5 are in the more distal vessels. Large aneurysms (>9 mm in diameter) are particularly prone to occlude or develop stenotic lesions [58]. Rarely, aneurysms can rupture. Basal coronary blood flow is usually normal, but coronary flow reserve is usually reduced in the microvascular bed of arteries affected by Kawasaki disease. Kawasaki disease should be considered in the differential diagnosis of young adults presenting with aneurysmal coronary artery disease or myocardial infarction.

The most prominent histopathological feature of late coronary artery lesions in Kawasaki disease is intimal thickening, which consists of extracellular matrix and smooth muscle cells that probably migrated through the disrupted internal elastic lamina. Destruction of the arterial wall leads to aneurysm formation and thrombosis occluding the lumen of the vessel (Figs. 20.18 and 20.19).

In polyarteritis nodosum, widespread necrotizing vasculitis occurs, most commonly involving medium-sized arteries, usually in a patchy segmental pattern. Small aneurysms may develop and may either rupture or become thrombosed. Myocardial infarction may be the presenting manifestation of polyarteritis nodosa. Figure 20.20 shows the histological features of acute and healed coronary arteritis.

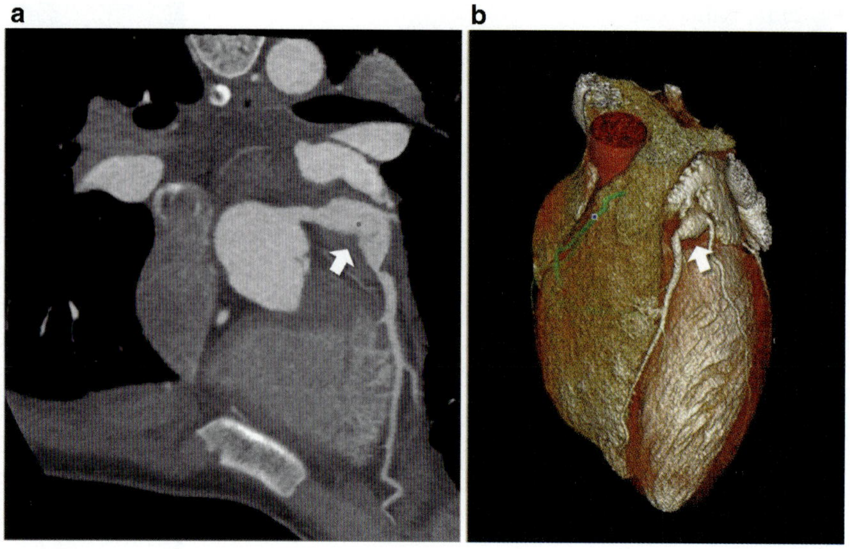

Fig. 20.17 Patient with Kawasaki vasculitis and giant coronary artery aneurysms in the LAD artery shown in this coronary CT angiogram. (**a**) and (**b**) (*arrows*) (courtesy Dr. Szilard Voros. Piedmont Heart Institute)

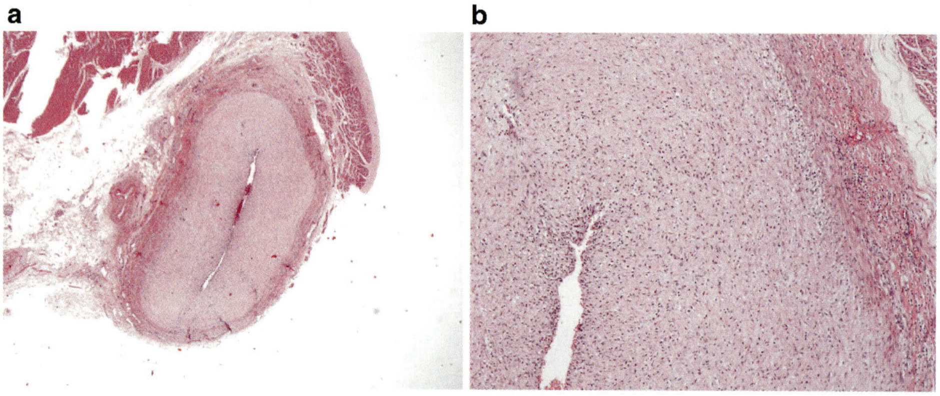

Fig. 20.18 Coronary arteritis involvement in healing phase of Kawasaki disease. From a 15-month-old male with sudden death. (**a**) Cross-section of epicardial coronary artery showing marked intimal thickening. Hematoxylin and eosin stain: 4×. (**b**) Higher magnification of (**a**), showing proliferative fibrous intimal thickening. Residual inflammation is within the media. Hematoxylin and eosin stain: 10×

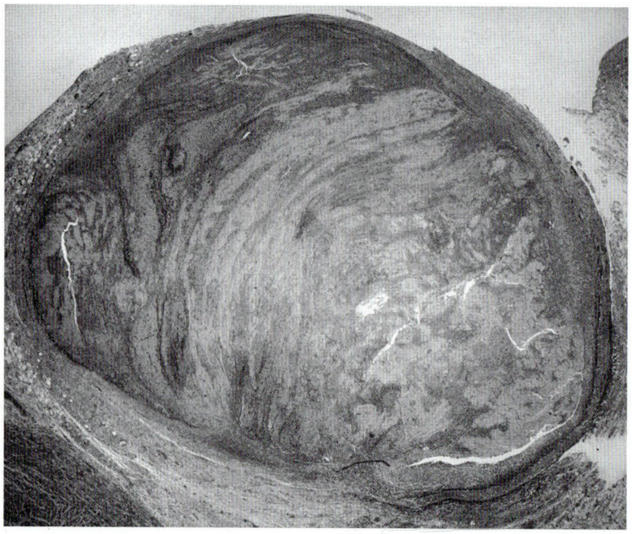

Fig. 20.19 Acute coronary arteritis involvement in Kawasaki disease from a 6-month-old child. An epicardial artery with aneurismal dilatation and lumen occluded by organized thrombi. Elastic tissue stain: 10.6×

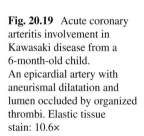

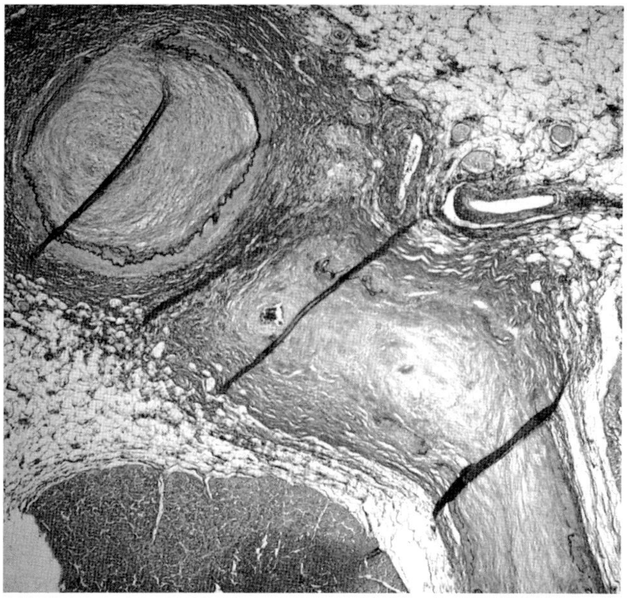

Fig. 20.20 An epicardial artery and a major branch are each occluded by fibrous tissue considered to be organized thrombi from a 60-year-old woman with polyarteritis nodosa. Elastic tissue stain: 14×

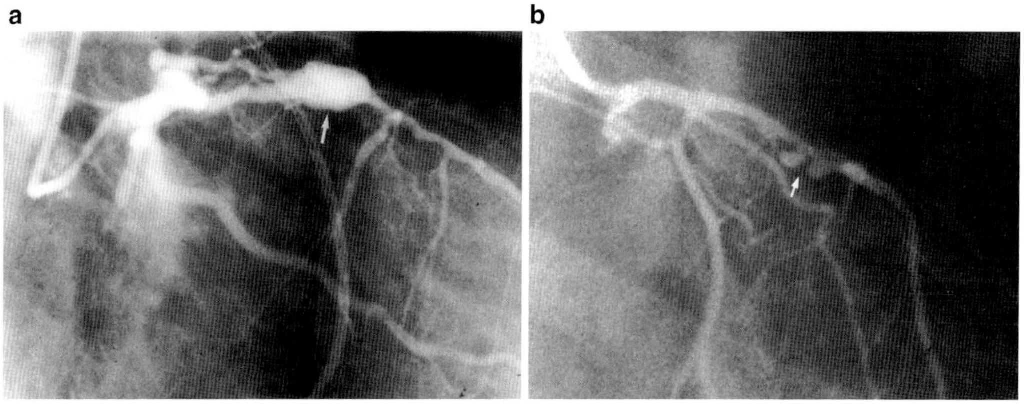

Fig. 20.21 (**a**) A large fusiforme aneurysm of the LAD considered to be a true or congenital aneurysm (*arrow*). (**b**) Left coronary arteriogram of a patient who underwent angioplasty 6 months previously and developed an irregular, saccular pseudoaneurysm at the site of dilation (*arrow*)

Coronary Artery Aneurysms

The angiographic morphology of coronary aneurysms can be saccular or fusiform (Fig. 20.21a). They frequently contain thrombotic material laminated against the borders of an aneurysm that may not be identifiable on the angiogram. Occasionally, most of the aneurysmal cavity can be filled with thrombus, leaving the angiographic appearance of a relatively normal artery. After angioplasty or thrombolytic drug treatment, a portion of the aneurysm cavity can be revealed and at first may resemble a coronary perforation. Pseudoaneurysms can occur after coronary rupture from balloon dilation (Fig. 20.21b) [68].

True aneurysms of the coronary arteries are associated with thinning of the tunica media and are very uncommon, but when present, can reach more than 2 cm in diameter [59–61, 119] (Fig. 20.22).

Aneurysms can be congenital in origin, or result from atherosclerosis, inherited diseases of connective tissue (e.g., periarteritis nodosa, systemic lupus erythematosis), inflammatory arteritis (e.g., Kawasaki disease), mycotic-embolic events [61], or coronary trauma, usually iatrogenic. True atherosclerotic coronary aneurysms are very uncommon, occurring in only 0.2% of coronary arteriographic studies [59, 61]. The overall incidence from all causes ranges from 0.5 to 1.1% of coronary angiographic studies [62]. When associated with atherosclerosis, coexistent stenotic lesions are usually present in

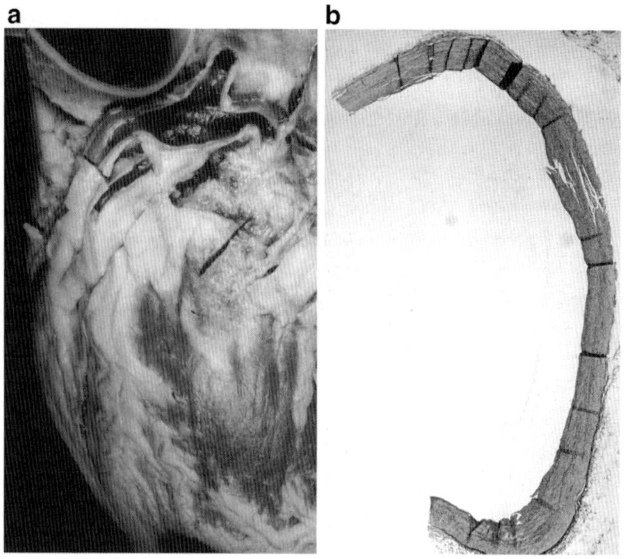

Fig. 20.22 A 59-year-old man with pulmonary emphysema and in whom an aneurysm of the bifurcation of the LC was an incidental finding. (**a**) Left lateral aspect of the heart and ascending aorta. At the bifurcation of the LC is an aneurysm considered to be a true or congenital aneurysm. (**b**) Photomicrograph of the aneurysm with atrophy of the media. Elastic tissue stain: 5×

multiple vessels. Atherosclerotic aneurysms almost never rupture, but they may contain thrombotic material and can cause myocardial infarction by in situ thrombosis or embolization. Dissection of atherosclerotic aneurysms has been reported, but also is uncommon [120].

Congenital disorders of connective tissue are associated with multiple aneurysms, particularly of the proximal arteries. Ehlers-Danlos syndrome type IV is characterized by dilation of the proximal and midcoronary arteries [63]. One case of rupture and another of thrombosis have been reported. Both angiography-related dissection of the coronary ostium and peripheral vascular pseudoaneurysm have been linked to the syndrome.

Interventional coronary artery procedures also can result in true coronary aneurysms, including laser angioplasty, atherectomy, stent placement, and balloon dilation [64, 65, 121]. One report suggests that use of corticosteroids around the time of stent placement may promote aneurysm formation [121]. Aneurysms have also developed at the site of coronary anastomosis of vein bypass grafts [122]. Paclitaxel-coated stents have rarely caused aneurysms [68].

Cocaine and Other Drug-Induced Ischemic Heart Disease

Many studies reported the link of cocaine use to myocardial ischemia and myocardial infarction. Various studies revealed a 6% rate of myocardial infarction in patients who presented to the Emergency Department with chest pain after cocaine ingestion [123]. Cocaine has multiple cardiovascular and hematologic effects that contribute to the development of ischemia and/or myocardial infarction Potential factors include:

- Increasing myocardial oxygen demand caused by increased heart rate, blood pressure, and contractility
- Decreasing oxygen supply caused by vasoconstriction
- Inducing a prothrombotic state by stimulating platelet activation and altering the balance between procoagulant and anticoagulant factors
- Accelerating atherosclerosis [124]

The majority of patients with cocaine-associated myocardial infarction are young (mean age, 38 years), nonwhite (72%), and smokers (91%) and had a history of cocaine use in the preceding 24 h (88%) [125].

Frequent symptoms among cocaine users are chest pain perceived as pressure-like in quality, dyspnea, and diaphoresis. Cocaine-associated myocardial infarction shows equal distribution between anterior and inferior wall, and most are a non-Q-wave infarction.

An acute pulmonary syndrome called "crack lung" involves hypoxemia, hemoptysis, respiratory failure, and diffuse pulmonary infiltrates and occurs after inhalation of freebase cocaine [126].

Cocaine-associated myocardial infarction appears to occur most often within 3 h of cocaine ingestion; however, the onset of ischemic symptoms could still occur several hours after cocaine ingestion, when blood concentration is low or undetectable. These findings are attributed to cocaine metabolites which rise in concentrations several hours after cocaine ingestion, persist in the circulation for up to 24 h, and may cause delayed or recurrent coronary vasoconstriction [127].

About one third of patients admitted for cocaine-associated myocardial infarction had cardiac complications including heart failure and arrhythmias.

The use of cocaine can be diagnosed by self-report or by urine analysis. Qualitative immunoassay detection of the cocaine metabolite benzoylecgonine in the urine is the most commonly used laboratory method. Cocaine use is reported as positive when the level of benzoylecgonine is above 300 ng/mL.

Abnormal ECG results have been reported in about 75% of patients with cocaine-associated chest pain, but the sensitivity of an ECG revealing ischemia or myocardial infarction to predict a true myocardial infarction in the COCHPA study was only 36%. Many of these patients are young and may have the normal variant of early repolarization, which may be interpreted as an abnormal ECG finding.

Cardiac troponins are the most sensitive and specific markers for diagnosing cocaine-associated myocardial infarction.

Long-term cocaine use appears to be associated with concentric LV hypertrophy. Echocardiography will reveal information regarding LV systolic and diastolic function, and the presence of wall motion abnormalities.

Of patients with cocaine-associated myocardial infarction, 77% had significant coronary artery disease on coronary angiography. Of patients without myocardial infarction, only 35% had significant coronary disease [128]. Patients with cocaine-associated chest pain, unstable angina, or myocardial infarction should be treated similarly to those with traditional acute coronary syndrome or possible acute coronary syndrome. In addition, cocaine users should be treated with benzodiazepines as early management for relieving chest pain and for its beneficial cardiac hemodynamics effects. Benzodiazepines decrease the central stimulatory effects of cocaine and often lead to resolution of anxiety, hypertension, and tachycardia [127].

Few reports indicate the safety and efficacy of phentolamine, an alpha-antagonist, for treating cocaine-associated acute coronary syndrome [129]. Instead, routine administration of aspirin is recommended, as is unfractioned heparin or low-molecular-weight heparin for patients with cocaine-associated MI, unless there is a contraindication [125].

Cessation of cocaine use should be the primary goal of secondary prevention. Recurrent chest pain is less common, and myocardial infarction and death are rare among patients who discontinue cocaine.

Coronary Embolism

A variety of conditions may be sources of embolism, including bacterial endocarditis, left-sided bland mural thrombi or vegetations, left-sided intracavitary tumors, and particles from calcified valves. Emboli may involve either the epicardial trunks or the intramyocardial arteries. The former tend to be solitary, while the latter frequently are multiple. In some settings where myocardial infarction occurs, the underlying basis seems reasonable on the basis of embolism, even though the latter process may not be proved. Angiography soon after embolization of the coronary circulation can reveal abrupt occlusion of a coronary artery with persistence of contrast media proximal to the occlusion (usually to the nearest proximal branch) or a filling defect with the coronary lumen (Fig. 20.23).

Coronary Embolism from Bacterial Endocarditis

Figure 20.24 pertains to a 70-year-old man with calcification of the aortic valve and staphylococcal bacterial endocarditis. The myocardium showed numerous emboli of vegetations containing bacteria. With this high degree of virulence of organisms, the embolic lesions became abscessed.

Coronary Embolism from Marantic Valvular Vegetations

A second valvular condition that may be responsible for coronary embolism is marantic vegetation. This process tends to occur in individuals with wasting disease, commonly malignant tumors. The vegetative process is composed of fibrin and platelets, but no bacteria are present. The vegetations of marantic nature usually involve the left-side valves, occasionally occurring on the right-side valves (Fig. 20.25).

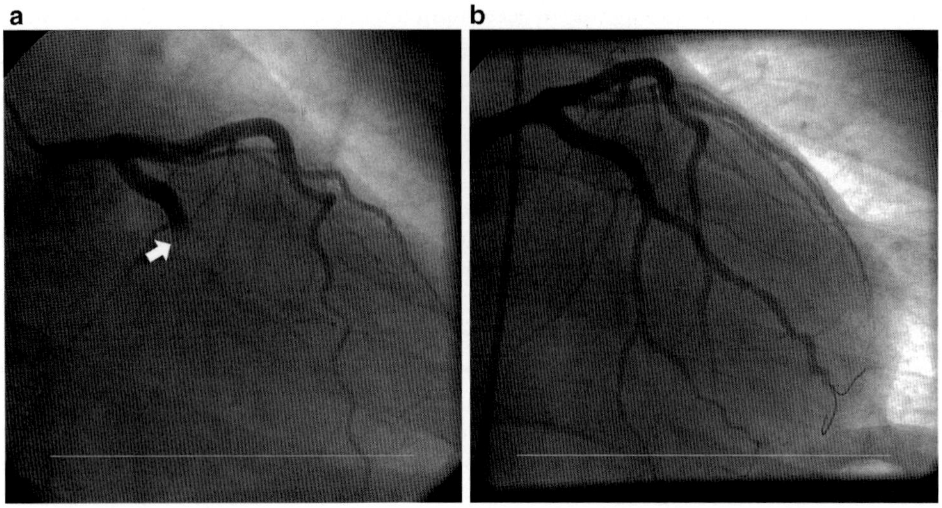

Fig. 20.23 From a 26-year-old male with lateral ST elevation myocardial infarction. Coronary angiography revealed an abrupt occlusion of the proximal circumflex with large thrombus burden (arrow) (**a**). After aspiration with a thrombectomy catheter, the underlying coronary artery was noted to be widely patent (**b**) without any atherosclerotic plaque on intravascular ultrasound. Patient was noted to have a patent foramen ovale with a prominent right to left shunt and a DVT. He underwent successful closure of the PFO

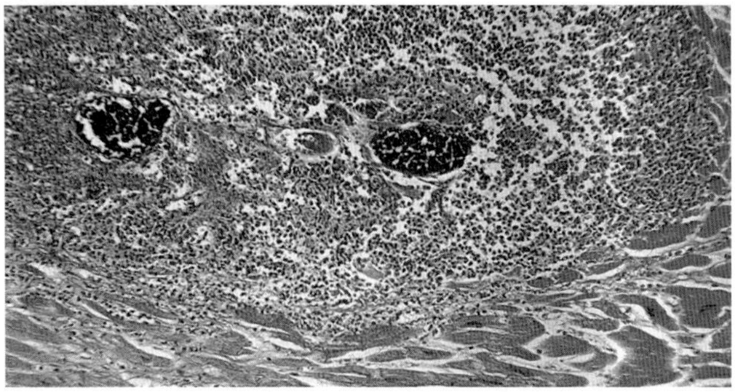

Fig. 20.24 Photomicrograph of the myocardium. Two arterioles contain obstructive emboli composed of bacteria. An abscess surrounds this process. Hematoxylin and eosin stain: 92×

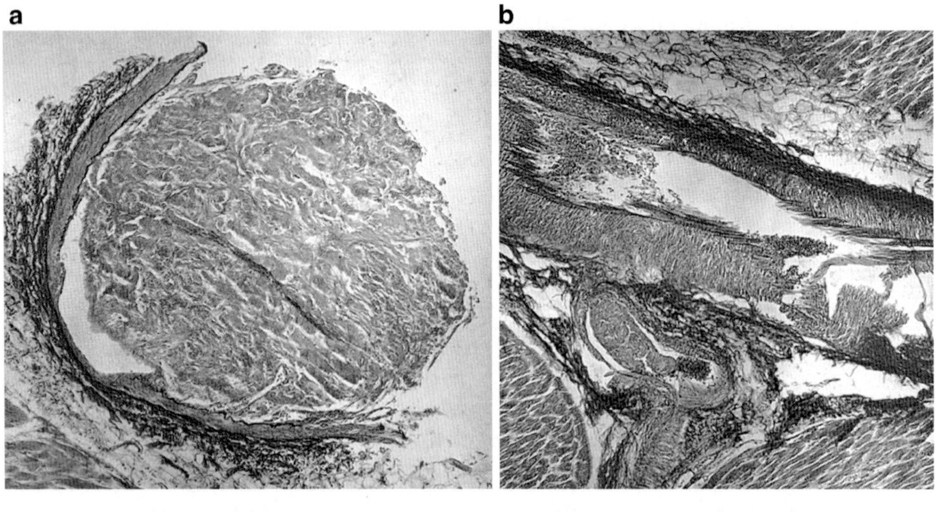

Fig. 20.25 A 32-year-old woman with carcinoma of the breast and marantic vegetations involving the aortic and mitral valves and vegetative material occluding the posterior descending coronary artery and intramyocardial branches. Acute myocardial infarction was present in the distribution of the PDA. (**a**) PDA. The lumen is occluded by vegetative material. Hematoxylin and eosin stain: 61×. (**b**) A branch of the PDA shows occlusion by a process similar to that shown in (**a**)

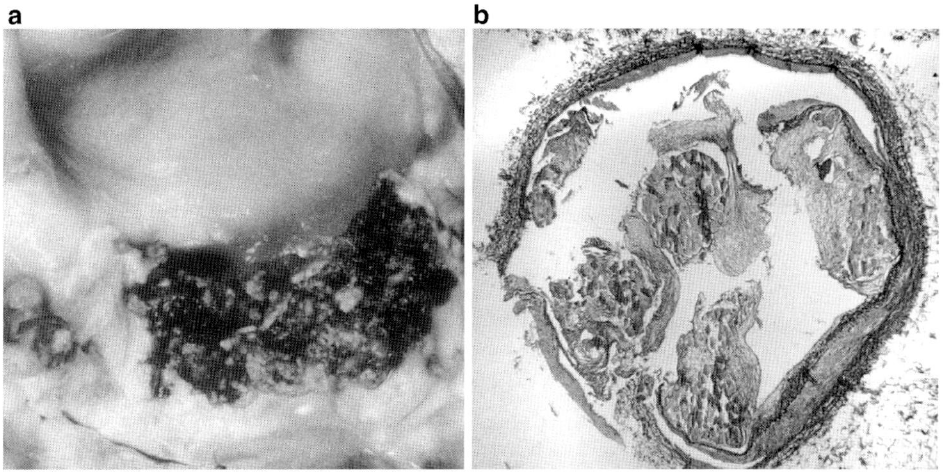

Fig. 20.26 A 50-year-old man with calcific aortic stenosis who died suddenly. An embolus of calcific aortic material was found in the PDA adherent to the wall. (**a**) Calcified and ulcerated aortic valve. (**b**) Photomicrograph of PDA. Fragments of calcific material are adherent to the wall of the artery. Elastic tissue stain: 16×

Figure 20.25 is from a 32-year-old woman with carcinoma of the breast and marantic vegetations involving the aortic and mitral valves, and vegetative material occluding the posterior descending coronary artery (PDA) and intramyocardial branches. Acute myocardial infarction was present in the distribution of the PDA.

Coronary Embolism from Calcified Valves

Calcification of valves, particularly the aortic valve, is a source of coronary embolism. This may occur spontaneously or be a complication of surgical replacement of the diseased valves (Fig. 20.26).

Figure 20.26 is from a 50-year-old man with calcific aortic stenosis who died suddenly. An embolus of calcific aortic material was found in the PDA adherent to the wall.

In association with aortic valve replacement, coronary embolism of fragments of calcific material may occur at the time of operation. In other circumstances, late thrombosis in relation to the prosthesis may serve as a basis for coronary embolism.

Coronary Embolism from Calcification of the Aortic Wall

The section in this book dealing with coronary ostial stenosis described a condition of Ao calcification at the junction of its tubular and sinus portion. The calcific material may occlude a coronary ostium, particularly the right, and may also serve as a basis for embolism to a coronary artery. The latter situation is interpreted as having occurred in the case illustrated in Figs. 20.27 and 20.28.

Coronary Embolism from Left Atrial Myxoma

Figure 20.29 illustrates left atria myxoma in a 42-year-old woman who died suddenly.

Coronary Embolism Complicating Cardiac Catheterization

Coronary embolism may follow right-sided cardiac catheterization in individuals with septal defects. Figures 20.30 and 20.31 are from a 16-year-old girl with persistent truncus arteriosus who experienced an episode of hypotension 8 h after cardiac catheterization. Death occurred 8 days later. The autopsy showed persistent truncus arteriosus, as well as an acute

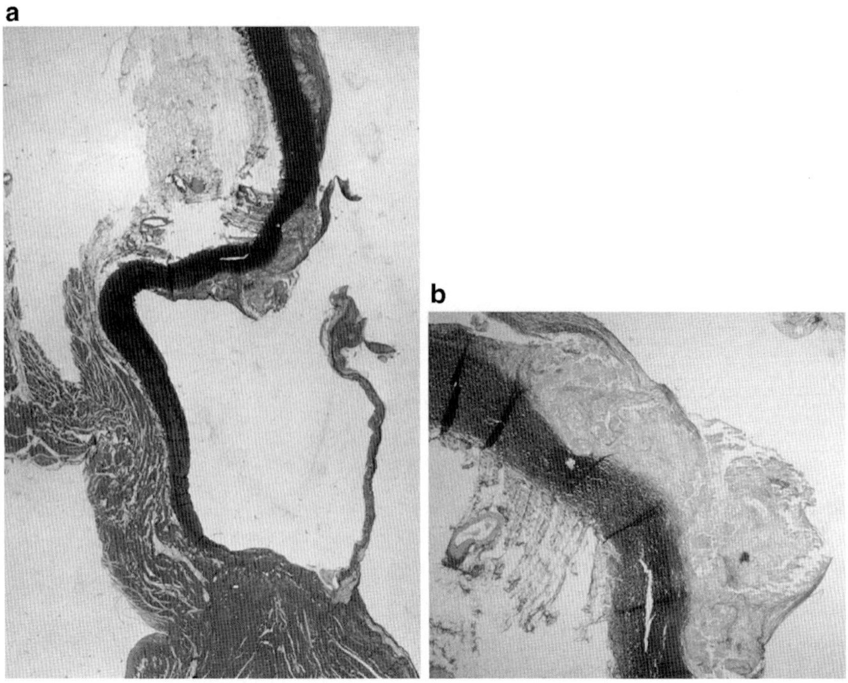

Fig. 20.27 The patient was a 53-year-old man in whom extensive coronary atherosclerosis was associated with healed myocardial infarction. The origin of the RC was occluded by a calcific embolus, which was considered to have originated in the calcific process involving the aortic wall. Acute myocardial infarction was present in the distribution of the RC. (**a**) Photomicrograph of the right aortic cusp and related aortic wall. A residual calcific lesion is present at the junction of the sinus and tubular portions of the aorta. (**b**) Higher magnification of the calcific area in the aortic wall shown in Fig. 19.27a. Elastic tissue stain: 32×

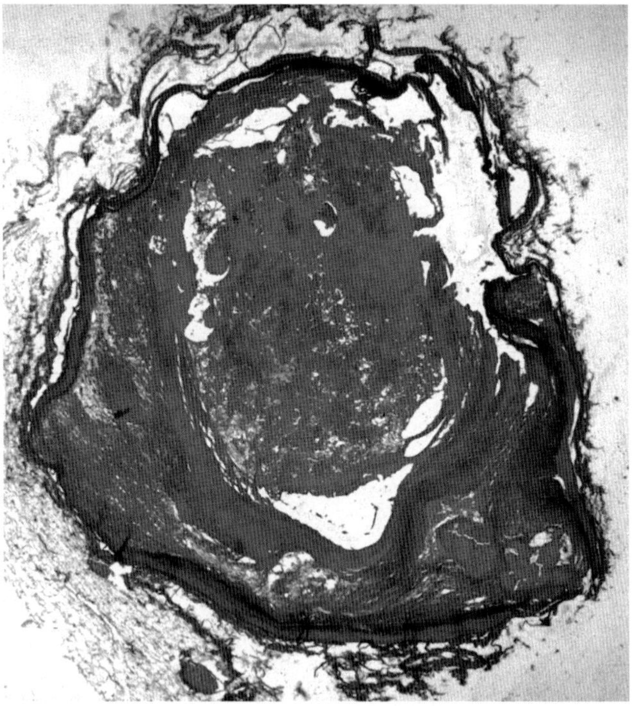

Fig. 20.28 From patient illustrated in Fig. 19.27. Slightly atherosclerotic segment of RCA shows occlusion by a calcific mass considered to be an embolus from the aortic lesion. Elastic tissue stain: 24×

Fig. 20.29 From a patient with left atrial myxoma. (a) LA and LV. A large polyploid left atrial myxoma partially obscures the mitral valve. (b) Photomicrograph of an intramyocardial coronary artery. An embolus of myxomatous tumor is present. Numerous microinfarcts were present in the LV myocardium. Hematoxylin and eosin stain: 54×

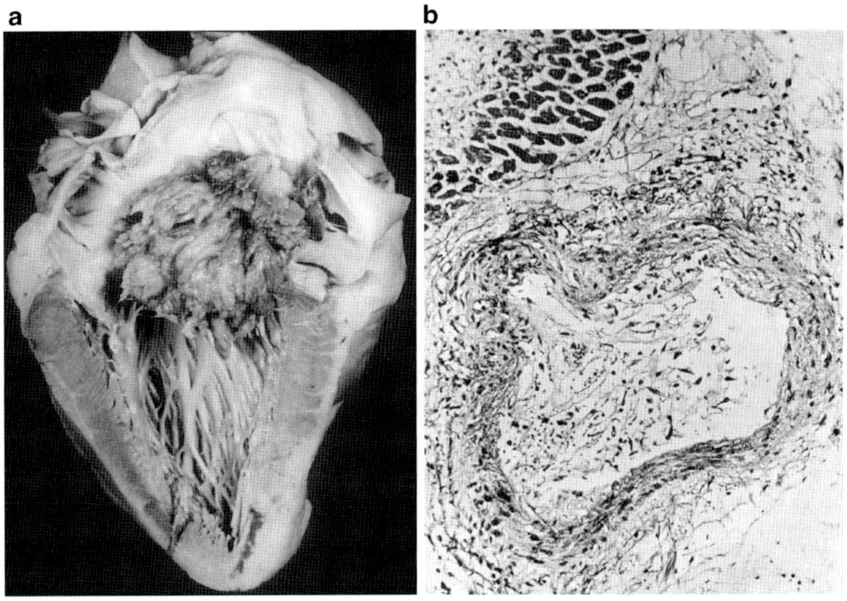

Fig. 20.30 A 16-year-old girl with persistent truncus arteriosus who experienced an episode of hypotension 8 h after cardiac catheterization. Death occurred 8 days later. (a) Base of the RV. A persistent truncus arteriosus arises above a VSD (D). (b) LV. Discoloration in apical portion is that of acute myocardial infarction

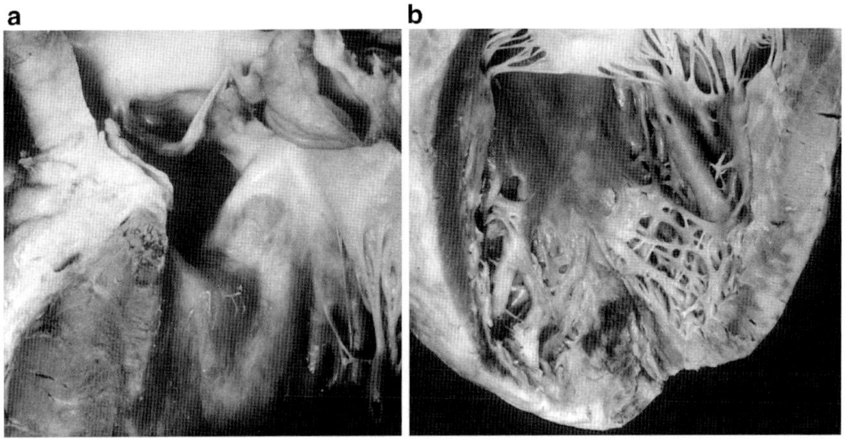

Fig. 20.31 From case illustrated in Fig. 20.30. LAD. The lumen is occluded by thrombotic material considered to be an embolus. Elastic tissue stain: 32×

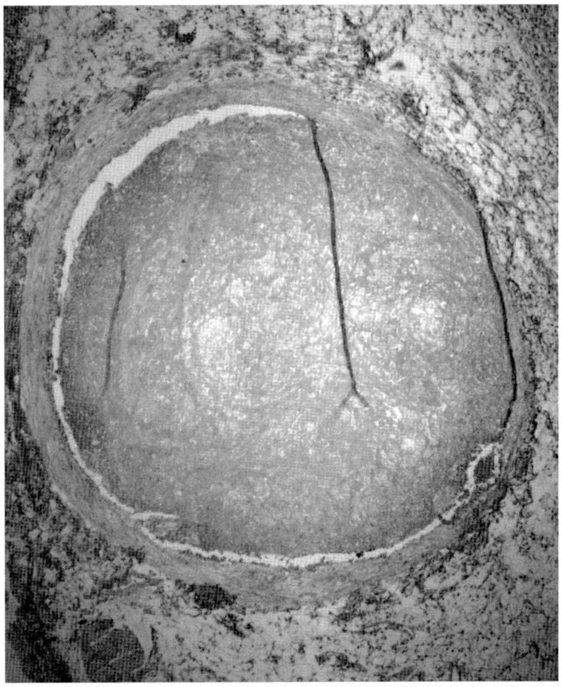

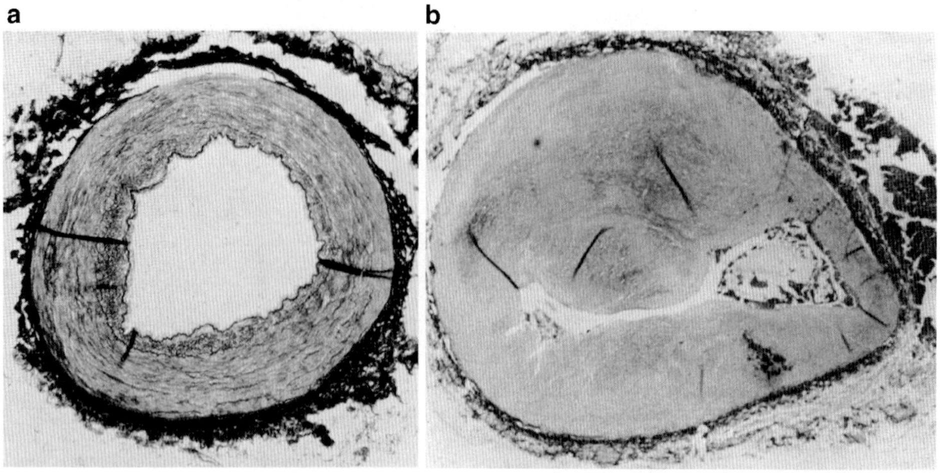

Fig. 20.32 (**a**) In a case of supravalvular aortic stenosis, the media of the LC shows major hypertrophy with numerous elastic tissue fibers present in the thickened layer. Elastic tissue stain: 28×. (**b**) In a case of Marfan syndrome showing an epicardial coronary artery, the intima is greatly thickened with mucoid connective tissue causing luminal narrowing. Elastic tissue stain: 15×

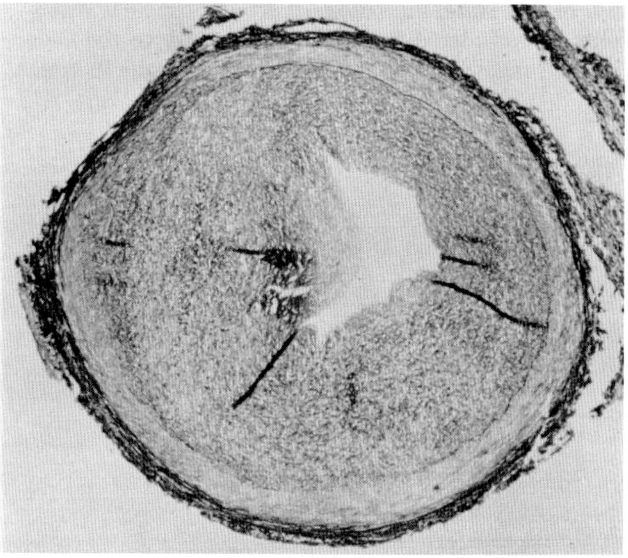

Fig. 20.33 In a case with Hurler syndrome, the lumen is markedly narrowed by loose connective tissue that thickened the intima. Elastic tissue stain: 20×

myocardial infarct at the LV apex. Histologically, the infarct was estimated to be between 7 and 10 days old. A mass of thrombotic material occluded the lumen of the LAD. No intracardiac or venous thrombi were found. The thrombotic lesion in the LAD was believed to result from embolism of material which had formed on the surface of the catheter during the procedure.

Embolism from an infected mitral or aortic valve can lead to mycotic aneurysm formation and rupture. Embolism should be suspected in patients with an acute ischemic syndrome, otherwise normal coronary arteries with a smooth luminal surface, and a source of emboli (e.g., abnormal native or prosthetic valves with thrombus or infectious vegetation, and left atrial or ventricular thrombus, or atrial fibrillation) [130–133]. Additionally, embolism should be considered in patients with multiple acute coronary occlusions and in patients with acute vascular occlusions in other beds (e.g., stroke).

Coronary Changes in Congenital Conditions

Among certain congenital diseases, the coronary arterial wall may be altered in some conditions, including supravalvular aortic stenosis (Fig. 20.32a), Marfan syndrome (Fig. 20.32b), and Hurler syndrome (Fig. 20.33).

References

1. Maseri A, Chierchia S. Coronary artery spasm: demonstration, definition, diagnosis, and consequences. Prog Cardiovasc Dis. 1982; 25:169–92.
2. Heupler FA, Proudfit WL, Razavi M, et al. Ergonavine maleate provocative test for coronary artery spasm. Am J Cardiol. 1978;41:631–40.
3. Bertrand ME, LaBlance JM, Tilmant PY, et al. Frequency of provoked coronary arterial spasm in 1089 consecutive patients undergoing coronary arteriography. Circulation. 1982;65:1299–308.
4. Bentivoglio LG, Leo LR, Wolf NM, et al. Frequency and importance of unprovoked coronary spasm in patients with angina pectoris undergoing percutaneous transluminal coronary angioplasty. Am J Cardiol. 1983;51:1067–71.
5. Bott-Silverman C, Heupler FA, Yiannikas J. Variant angina: comparison of patients with and without fixed severe coronary artery disease. Am J Cardiol. 1984;54:1173–5.
6. Mark DB, Califf RM, Morris KG, et al. Clinical characteristics and long-term survival of patients with variant angina. Circulation. 1984;69:880–8.
7. Egashira K, Kikuchi Y, Sagara T, et al. Long-term prognosis of vasospastic angina without significant atherosclerotic coronary artery disease. Jpn Heart J. 1987;28:841–9.
8. Nobuyoshi M, Tanaka M, Nosaka H, et al. Progression of atherosclerotis: is coronary spasm related to progression? J Am Coll Cardiol. 1991;18:904–10.
9. Harding MB, Leithe ME, Mark DB, et al. Ergonavine maleate testing during cardiac catheterization: a 10-year perspective in 3,447 patients without significant coronary artery disease or Prinzmetal's variant angina. J Am Coll Cardiol. 1992;20:107–11.
10. Carlis DG, Deligonul U, Kern MJ, et al. Smoking is a risk factor for coronary spasm in young women. Circulation. 1992;85:905–9.
11. Nakano T, Osanai T, Yomita H, et al. Enhanced activity of variant phospholipase C-1 protein (R257H) detected in patients with coronary artery spasm. Circulation. 2002;105:2024–9.
12. Suzuki S, Yoshimura M, Nakayama M, et al. A novel genetic marker for coronary spasm in women from a genome-wide single nucleotide polymorphism analysis. Pharmacogenet Genomics. 2007;17:919–30.
13. Ginsburg R, Schroeder JS. Coronary spasm producing coronary thrombosis. N Engl J Med. 1983;309:648.
14. Oliva PB, Potts DE, Plus RG. Coronary arterial spasm in Prinzmetal angina. N Engl J Med. 1973;288:745–51.
15. Schroeder JS, Bolen JL, Quint RA, et al. Provocation of coronary spasm with ergonovine maleate. Am J Cardiol. 1977;40:487–91.
16. Curry RC, Pepine CJ, Sabom MB, et al. Effects of ergonavine in patients with and without coronary artery disease. Circulation. 1977;56:804–9.
17. Chahine RA, Raizner AE, Ishimori T, et al. The incidence and clinical implications of coronary artery spasm. Circulation. 1975;52:972–8.
18. Curry RC, Pepine CJ, Sabom MB, et al. Hemodynamic and myocardial metabolic effects of ergonavine in patients with chest pain. Circulation. 1978;58:648–54.
19. Suzuki Y, Tokunaga S, Ikeguchi S, et al. Induction of coronary artery spasm by intracoronary acetylcholine: comparison with intracoronary ergonovine. Am Heart J. 1992;124:39–47.
20. Wright CM, Engler R, Maisel A. Coronary thrombosis precipitated by hyperventilation-induced vasospasm. Am Heart J. 1988;116:867–9.
21. Ginsburg R, Bristow MR, Kantrowitz N, et al. Histamine provocation of clinical coronary artery spasm: implications concerning pathogenesis of variant angina pectoris. Am Heart J. 1981;102:819–22.
22. Feldman RL, Curry RC, Pepine CJ, et al. Regional coronary hemodynamic effects of ergonovine in patients with and without variant angina. Circulation. 1980;62:149–59.
23. Kugiyama K, Ohgushi M, Motoyama T, et al. Enhancement of constrictor response of spastic coronary arteries to acetylcholine but not to phenylephrine in patients with coronary spastic angina. J Cardiovasc Pharmacol. 1999;33:414–9.
24. Magder SA, Johnstone DE, Huckell VF, et al. Experience with ergonovine provocative testing for coronary arterial spasm. Chest. 1981;79:638–46.
25. Kodma K, Yamagishi M, Nanto S, et al. Comparison of coronary hemodynamic and cardiac metabolic alterations during coronary spasm associated with ST segment elevation or depression. Jpn Circ J. 1985;49:422–31.
26. Whittle JL, Feldman RL, Pepine CJ, et al. Variability of electrocardiographic responses to repeated ergonovine provocation in variant angina patients with coronary artery spasm. Am Heart J. 1982;103:161–7.
27. Matsuda Y, Ogawa H, Moritani K, et al. Transient appearance of collaterals during vasospastic occlusion in patients without obstructive coronary atherosclerosis. Am Heart J. 1985;109:759–63.
28. Takeshita A, Koiwaya Y, Nakamura M, et al. Immediate appearance of collaterals during ergonovine-induced arterial spasm. Chest. 1982;82:319–22.
29. Maleki M, Manley JC. Venospastic phenomena in saphenous vein grafts: possible causes for unexplained postoperative recurrence of angina or early or late occlusion of vein bypass grafts. Br Heart J. 1989;62:57–60.
30. Hosio A, Kotake H, Mashiba H. Significance of coronary artery tone in patients with vasospastic angina. J Am Coll Cardiol. 1989;14:604–9.
31. Hill JA, Feldman RL, Pepine CJ, et al. Regional coronary artery dilation response in variant angina. Am Heart J. 1982;104:226–33.
32. Kaski JC, Maseri A, Vejar M, et al. Spontaneous coronary artery spasm in variant angina is caused by a local hyperactivity to a generalized constrictor stimulus. J Am Coll Cardiol. 1989;14:1456–63.
33. Feldman RL, Pepine CJ, Whittle JL, et al. Coronary hemodynamic findings during spontaneous angina in patients with variant angina. Circulation. 1981;64:76–83.
34. Deckelbaum LI, Isner JM, Konstam MA, et al. Catheter-induced versus spontaneous spasm – do these coronary bedfellows deserved to be estranged? Am J Med. 1985;79:1–4.
35. Schwartz RE, Butman S. Catheter-induced nonproximal coronary artery spasm. Am J Cardiol. 1984;53:352–4.
36. Rabih R, Azar I. Diffuse coronary spasm in a patient with a recent stent. JACC Cardiovasc Interv. 2010;3:459–60.

37. DeMaio S, Kinsella SH, Silverman ME. Clinical course and long-term prognosis of spontaneous coronary artery dissection. Am J Cardiol. 1989;64:471–4.
38. Bulkley BH, Roberts WC. Dissecting aneurysm (hematoma) limited to coronary artery. Am J Med. 1973;55:747–56.
39. Mathieu D, Larde D, Vasile N. Primary dissecting aneurysms of the coronary arteries: case report and literature review. Cardiovasc Intervent Radiol. 1984;7:71–4.
40. Claudon DG, Claudon DB, Edwards JE. Primary dissecting aneurysm of coronary artery. Circulation. 1972;45:259–66.
41. Brody GL, Burton JF, Zawadzki ES, et al. Dissecting aneurysm of the coronary artery. N Engl J Med. 1965;273:10–5.
42. Yeoh J, Choo H, Soo C, et al. Spontaneous coronary artery dissection in a young man with anterior myocardial infarction. Cathet Cardiovasc Diagn. 1991;24:186–8.
43. Heilbrunn A, Zimmerman JM. Coronary artery dissection: a complication of cannulation. J Thorac Cardiovasc Surg. 1965;49:767.
44. Roy P, Finci L, Boop P, et al. Emergency balloon angioplasty and digital subtraction angiography in the management of an acute iatrogenic occlusive dissection of a saphenous vein graft. Cathet Cardiovasc Diagn. 1989;16:176–9.
45. Thayer JO, Healy RW, Maggs PR. Spontaneous coronary artery dissection. Ann Thorac Surg. 1987;44:97–102.
46. Orbe LC, Gallego FG, Sobrino N, et al. Acute myocardial infarction after blunt chest trauma in young people. Cathet Cardiovasc Diagn. 1991;24:182–5.
47. Lee FH, Yeung AC, Fowler MB, et al. Spontaneous postpartum dissection. Circulation. 1999;99:271.
48. Rabinowitz M, Virmani R, McAllister H. Spontaneous coronary artery dissection and eosinophilic inflammation: a cause and effect relationship? Am J Med. 1982;72:923–7.
49. Nishikawa H, Nakanishi S, Nishiyama S, et al. Primary coronary dissection observed at coronary angiography. Am J Cardiol. 1988;61:645–8.
50. Alvarez J, Deal CW. Spontaneous dissection of the left main coronary artery: case report and review of the literature. Aust N Z J Med. 1991;21:891–2.
51. Himbert D, Makowski S, Laperche T, et al. Left main coronary spontaneous dissection: progressive angiographic healing without coronary surgery. Am Heart J. 1991;22:747–56.
52. Behnan R, Tillinghast S. Thrombolytic therapy in spontaneous coronary dissection. Clin Cardiol. 1991;14:611–4.
53. Vale PR, Baron DW. Coronary stenting for spontaneous coronary dissection: a case report and review of the literature. Cathet Cardiovasc Diagn. 1998;45:280–6.
54. Betriu A, Pare JC, Sanz GA, et al. Myocardial infarction in normal coronary arteries: a prospective clinical-angiographic study. Am J Cardiol. 1981;48:28–38.
55. Rigatelli G, Rossi P, Docali G. Normal angiogram in acute coronary syndromes: the underestimated role of alternative substrates of myocardial ischemia. Int J Cardiovasc Imaging. 2004;20:471–5.
56. Thompson SI, Vieweg WVR, Alpert JS, et al. Incidence and age distribution of patients with myocardial infarction and normal coronary arteriograms. Cathet Cardiovasc Diagn. 1977;3:1–9.
57. Thompson EA, Ferraris S, Gress T, et al. Gender differences and predictors of mortality in spontaneous coronary artery dissection: a review of reported cases. J Invasive Cardiol. 2005;17:59–61.
58. Cipriano PR, Koch FH, Rosenthal SJ, et al. Myocardial infarction in patients with coronary spasm demonstrated by angiography. Am Heart J. 1983;105:542–7.
59. Gersh BJ, Chesebro JH, Bove AA. Myocardial infarction with angiographically "normal:" coronary arteries: is this rapid progression of early coronary artery disease? Chest. 1984;84:654–6.
60. Legrand V, Deliege M, Henrard L, et al. Patients with myocardial infarction and normal coronary arteries. Chest. 1982;82:678–85.
61. Lindsay J, Pichard AD. Acute myocardial infarction with normal coronary arteries. Am J Cardiol. 1984;54:902–4.
62. Rosenblatt A, Selzer A. The nature and clinical features of myocardial infarction with normal coronary arteriogram. Circulation. 1977;55:578–80.
63. Ciraulo DA, Bresnahan GF, Frankel PS, et al. Transmural myocardial infarction with normal coronary arteriograms and with single vessel coronary obstruction. Chest. 1983;83:196–202.
64. Glover MU, Kuber MT, Warren SE, et al. Myocardial infarction before age 36: risk factor and arteriographic analysis. Am J Cardiol. 1982;49:1600–3.
65. Smith HWB, Liberman HA, Brody SL, et al. Acute myocardial infarction temporally related to cocaine use: clinical, angiographic and pathophysiologic observations. Ann Intern Med. 1987;107:13–8.
66. Sharkey SW, Windenburg DC, Lesser JR, et al. Natural history and expansive clinical profile of stress (tako-tsubo) cardiomyopathy. J Am Coll Cardiol. 2010;55:333–41.
67. Sharkey SW, Lesser JR, Zenovich AG, et al. Acute and reversible cardiomyopathy provoked by stress in women from the United States. Circulation. 2005;111:472–9.
68. Likoff W, Segal BL, Kasparian H. Paradox of normal selective coronary arteriograms in patients considered to have unmistakable coronary heart disease. N Engl J Med. 1967;276:1063.
69. Kemp HG. Left ventricular function in patients with the anginal syndrome and normal coronary arteriograms. Am J Cardiol. 1973;32:375.
70. Cannon RO, Schenke WH, Leon MB, et al. Limited coronary flow reserve after dipyridamole in patients with ergonovine-induced coronary vasoconstriction. Circulation. 1987;75:163.
71. Cannon RO, Schenke WH, Leon MB, et al. Limited coronary flow reserve in patients with angina pectoris, normal epicardial coronary arteries, and abnormal vasodilator reserve. Circulation. 1985;7:218.
72. Cannon RO. Microvascular angina. In: Braunwald E, editor. Heart disease: a textbook of cardiovascular medicine. 3rd ed. New York: WB Saunders; 1991. p. 343–50.
73. Geltman EM, Henes CG, Senneff MJ, et al. Increased myocardial perfusion at rest and diminished perfusion reserved in patient with angina and angiographically normal coronary arteries. J Am Coll Cardiol. 1990;16:586–95.
74. Lanza G, Crea F. Primary coronary microvascular dysfunction: clinical presentation, pathophysiology, and management. Circulation. 2010;121:2317–25.

75. Opherk D, Schwartz F, Mall G, et al. Coronary dilatory capacity in idiopathic dilated cardiomyopathy: analysis of 16 patients. Am J Cardiol. 1983;51:1657–62.
76. Brush JE, Cannon RO, Schenke WH, et al. Angina due to microvascular disease, in hypertensive patients without left ventricular hypertrophy. N Engl J Med. 1988;319:1302–7.
77. Ryan TJ, Treasure CB, Yeung AC, et al. Impaired endothelium-dependent dilation of the coronary microvasculature in patients with atherosclerosis [abstract]. Circulation. 1991;84:II624.
78. Selke FW, Armstrong ML, Harrison DC. Endothelium-dependent vascular relaxation is abnormal in the coronary microcirculation of atherosclerotic primates. Circulation. 1990;81:586.
79. Wilson RF, Marcus ML, White CW. Prediction of the significance of coronary arterial lesions by quantitative coronary angiography in patients with limited coronary artery disease. Circulation. 1987;75:723–32.
80. Wilson RF, Laughlin DE, Ackell PH, et al. Transluminal, subselective measurement of coronary artery blood flow velocity and vasodilator reserve in man. Circulation. 1985;72:82.
81. McGinn AL, White CW, Wilson RF. Interstudy variability of coronary flow reserve: influence of heart rate, arterial pressure, and ventricular preload. Circulation. 1990;81:1319–28.
82. Wilson RF, Christensen BV, Zimmer S, et al. The effects of adenosine on human coronary circulation. Circulation. 1990;82:1595–606.
83. Wilson RF, Marcus ML, Christensen BV, et al. The accuracy of exercise electrocardiography in predicting the physiologic significance of coronary arterial stenosis. Circulation. 1991;83:412–21.
84. Egashira K, Inou T, Hirooka Y, et al. Evidence of impaired endothelium dependent coronary vasodilation in patients with angina pectoris and normal coronary angiograms. N Engl J Med. 1993;328:1659–64.
85. Zir LM, Miller SW, Dinsmore RE, et al. Interobserver variability in coronary arteriography. Circulation. 1976;53:627–32.
86. Ludmer PL, Selwyn AP, Shook TL, et al. Paradoxical vasoconstriction induced by acetylcholine in atherosclerotic coronary arteries. N Engl J Med. 1986;315:1046–51.
87. Fish RP, Nabel EG, Selwyn AP, et al. Responses of coronary arteries of cardiac transplant patients to acetylcholine. J Clin Invest. 1988;81:21–31.
88. Vogt M, Rabenau O, Motz W, et al. Evidence of endothelial dysfunction in patients with angina pectoris and angiographically normal coronary arteries [abstract]. Circulation. 1989;80:II436.
89. McReynolds RA, Gold GL, Roberts WC. Coronary heart disease after mediastinal irradiation for Hodgkin disease. Am J Med. 1976;60:39–45.
90. Hancock SL, Tucker MA, Hoppe RT. Factors affecting late mortality from heart disease after treatment of Hodgkin disease. JAMA. 1993;270:1949–55.
91. Reinders JG, Heijmen BJ, Olofsen-van-Acht MJ, et al. Ischemic heart disease after mantle field irradiation for Hodgkin disease in long-term follow-up. Radiother Oncol. 1999;51:35–42.
92. Steward JR, Cohn KE, Fajardo LF, Hancock EW, et al. Radiation-induced heart disease. Radiology. 1967;89:302–10.
93. Pohjola-Sintonen S, Totterman KJ, Almo M, et al. Late cardiac effects of mediastinal radiotherapy in patients with Hodgkin disease. Cancer. 1987;60:31–7.
94. Brosius FC, Waller BF, Roberts WC. Radiation heart disease: analysis of 16 young (aged 15–33 years) necropsy patients who received over 3,500 rads to the heart. Am J Med. 1981;70:519–30.
95. Theodoulou M, Seiman AD. Cardiac effects of adjuvant therapy for early breast cancer. Semin Oncol. 2003;30:730–9.
96. Tracy GP, Brown DE, Johnson LW, et al. Radiation-induced coronary artery disease. JAMA. 1974;228:1660–2.
97. Prentice RTW. Myocardial infarction following radiation. Lancet. 1965;2:388.
98. Rademaker J, Schoder H, Ariaratnam NS, et al. Coronary artery disease after radiation therapy for Hodgkin lymphoma: coronary CT angiography findings and calcium scores in nine asymptomatic patients. Am J Radiol. 2008;191:32–7.
99. Carmel RJ, Kaplan HS. Mantle irradiation in Hodgkin disease: an analysis of technique, tumor eradication and complications. Cancer. 1976;37:2813–25.
100. Ogum S, Okazaki H, Jimbo M, et al. Vascular rejection and arteriosclerosis. Transplant Proc. 1987;19:63–70.
101. Schmauss D, Weis M. Cardiac allograft vasculopathy. Recent developments. Circulation. 2008;117:2131–41.
102. Pucci AM, Forbes RDC, Billingham ME. Pathologic features in long-term cardiac allografts. J Heart Transplant. 1990;9:339–45.
103. Johnson DE, Gao SZ, Schroeder JS, et al. The spectrum of coronary artery pathologic findings in heart cardiac allografts. J Heart Transplant. 1989;8:349–59.
104. Libby P, Salomon RN, Payne DD, et al. Functions of vascular wall cell related to development of transplantation-associated coronary atherosclerosis. Transplant Proc. 1989;21:3677–84.
105. Gao SZ, Alderman EL, Schroeder JS, Silverman JF, Hunt SA. Accelerated coronary vascular disease in the heart transplant patient: coronary arteriographic findings. J Am Coll Cardiol. 1988;12:334–40.
106. Uretsky BF, Murali S, Reddy PS, et al. Development of coronary artery disease in cardiac transplant patients. Circulation. 1987;76: 827–34.
107. Gao SZ, Alderman EL, Schroeder JS, et al. Prevalence of accelerated coronary artery disease in heart transplant survivors. Circulation. 1989;80(Suppl III):100–5.
108. Olivari MT, Homans DC, Wilson RF, et al. Coronary artery disease in cardiac transplant patients receiving triple-drug immunosuppressive therapy. Circulation. 1989;80(Suppl III):111–5.
109. Gao SZ, Alderman EL, Schroeder JS, et al. Progressive coronary luminal narrowing after cardiac transplantation. Circulation. 1990;82 (Suppl IV):269–75.
110. Nitkin RS, Hunt SA, Schroeder JS. Accelerated atherosclerosis in a cardiac transplant patient. J Am Coll Cardiol. 1985;6:243–5.
111. Mulvagh SL, Thornton B, Frazier OH, et al. The older cardiac transplant donor: relation to graft function and recipient survival longer than 6 years. Circulation. 1989;80(Suppl III):126–32.
112. O'Neill B, Pflugfelder PW, Singh NR, et al. Frequency of angiographic detection and quantitative assessment of coronary arterial disease one and three years after cardiac transplantation. Am J Cardiol. 1989;63:1221–3.

113. Sharples LD, Mullin PA, Cary NRB, et al. A method of analyzing the onset and progression of coronary occlusive disease after transplantation and its effect on patient survival. Transplantation. 1993;12:381–7.
114. Kapadia SR, Nissen SE, Ziada KM, et al. Impact of intravascular ultrasound in understanding transplant coronary artery disease. Curr Opin Cardiol. 1999;14(2):140–50.
115. Kapadia SR, Nissen SE, Ziada KM, et al. Development of transplantation vasculopathy and progression of donor-transmitted atherosclerosis: comparison by serial intravascular ultrasound imaging. Circulation. 1998;98(24):2672–8.
116. Gao HZ, Hunt SA, Alderman EL, et al. Relation of donor age and preexisting coronary artery disease on angiography and intracoronary ultrasound to later development of accelerated allograft coronary artery disease. J Am Coll Cardiol. 1997;29(3):623–9.
117. Davis SF, Yeung AC, Meredith IT, et al. Early endothelial dysfunction predicts the development of transplant coronary artery disease at 1 year post-transplant. Circulation. 1996;93(3):457–62.
118. McGinn AL, Christensen BV, Meyer S, et al. Early impairment of nitroglycerin-induced coronary dilation after human cardiac transplantation [abstract]. J Am Coll Cardiol. 1991;17(2):309A.
119. Vlodaver Z, Neufeld HN, Edwards JE. Coronary arterial variations in the normal heart and in congenital heart disease. New York: Academic; 1975.
120. Fulton WF. The coronary arteries. Springfield: Charles C. Thomas; 1965.
121. Ottervanger JP, Wilson JH, Stricker BH. Drug-induced chest pain and myocardial infarction. Report to a national center and review of the literature. Eur J Clin Pharmacol. 1997;53(2):105–10.
122. Sharkey SW, Lesser JR, Zenovich AG, et al. Acute and reversible cardiomyopathy provoked by stress in women of the United States. Circulation. 2005;111:472–9.
123. Hollander JE, Hoffman RS, Gennis P, et al. Prospective multicenter evaluation of cocaine-associated chest pain. Cocaine Associated Chest Pain (COCHPA) study group. Acad Emerg Med. 1994;1:330–9.
124. Weber EJ, Chudnofsky CR, Boczar M, Boyer EW, Wilkerson MD, Hollander JE. Cocaine associated chest pain, how common is myocardial infarction? Acad Emerg Med. 2000;7:873–7.
125. McCord J, Jneid H, Hollander JE, et al. Management of cocaine-associated chest pain and myocardial infarction. Circulation. 2008;117:1897–907.
126. Forrester JM, Steele AW, Waldron JA, Parsons PE. Crack lung: an acute pulmonary syndrome with a spectrum of clinical and histopathologic findings. Am Rev Respir Dis. 1990;42:462–7.
127. Brogan III WC, Lange RA, Kim AS, et al. Alleviation of cocaine-induced coronary vasoconstriction by nitroglycerin. J Am Coll Cardiol. 1991;18:581–6.
128. Kontos MC, Jesse RJ, Tatum JL, Ornato JP. Coronary artery findings in patients with cocaine-associated chest pain. J Emerg Med. 2003;24:9–13.
129. Lange RA, Hillis LD. Cardiovascular complications of cocaine use. N Engl J Med. 2001;345:351–67.
130. Walley VM, Giannoccaro P, Beanlands DS, et al. Dead at cardiac catheterization: coronary artery embolization of calcium debris from Ionescu-Shiley bioprosthesis. Cathet Cardiovasc Diagn. 1990;21:92–4.
131. Johnson D, Gonsalez-Lavin L. Myocardial infarction secondary to calcific embolization: an unusual complication of bioprosthetic valve degeneration. Ann Thorac Surg. 1986;42:102–3.
132. Tannike M, Nishino M, Egami Y, et al. Acute myocardial infarction caused by septic coronary embolism diagnosed and treated with thrombectomy catheter. Heart. 2005;91(5):e34.
133. Vlodaver Z, Neufeld HN, Edwards JE. Pathology of angina pectoris. Circulation. 1972;46:1048–64.

Chapter 21
Transcatheter Treatment of Coronary Artery Disease

Robert F. Wilson

Balloon Angioplasty

Balloon angioplasty, also referred to as POBA ("plain old balloon angioplasty"), is a method of enlarging the lumen of coronary arteries by stretching the narrowed segment of the artery with a balloon. Typically, a guiding catheter is advanced from the femoral, brachial, or radial arteries to the ostium of the left or right coronary artery (Fig. 21.1). Once the ostium is engaged, a 0.014-in diameter, radiopaque guidewire is advanced through the guide catheter into the narrowed artery. The wire is steered through the stenotic lesion and the wire tip is "parked" in the distal vessel. Next, a balloon catheter is slid over the guidewire and positioned across the narrowed portion of the artery. The balloon is then inflated with a radiopaque fluid for 20–60 s, stretching the artery and enlarging the narrowed lumen. The arterial lumen at the stenotic site increases in diameter immediately, although there usually is some degree of elastic recoil that can be seen minutes to hours after the procedure.

Balloon angioplasty causes a semicontrolled dissection of the artery (Fig. 21.2) [2]. Typically, the atherosclerotic plaque is fractured and split. The internal elastic lamina of the artery is also torn and often is accompanied with a small hematoma in the media of the artery. The increase in lumen caliber is the result of three factors: enlargement of the outer diameter of the artery (accounting for 57% on average), compression of the plaque material (some of which probably embolizes downstream), and eventual reabsorption of plaque by the healing process that ensues after dilation of the artery [3].

The improvement in arterial caliber varies, but averages 250% (minimum stenosis diameter 0.8–2.0 mm, percent stenosis 90–36%). With that increase in arterial cross-sectional area, the translesional pressure gradient falls from an average of 56–13 mmHg, and coronary flow reserve improves from 1.6 to 4.3 [4]. Of interest, coronary flow reserve continues to improve for several weeks after the procedure, possibly due to continued remodeling of the arterial lumen and improvement of the downstream microcirculation [5]. Nuclear perfusion studies often normalize late after the procedure as well [6]. Symptoms of angina improve almost immediately after the procedure, although the artery can be prone to spasm at the site of the dilation for several weeks [7].

Complications of POBA

The most important immediate complications of POBA are related to vascular trauma from the guiding catheter, balloon catheter, or guidewire; inadvertent injection of air into the coronaries; and embolization of a clot or atheromatous material.

Balloon dilation initiates a disruption of the arterial intima that extends into the media. A large dissection can cause a blind pocket or flap that leads to arterial closure. Untreated, and in the absence of significant collateral blood flow, closure usually causes a myocardial infarction of the downstream perfusion field. Large dissections often cause immediate arterial close, but in some cases, the closure can occur 1–2 days after the procedure. The likelihood of closure is related to the size

R.F. Wilson, MD (✉)
Division of Cardiovascular Medicine, University of Minnesota, Minneapolis, MN, USA
e-mail: wilso008@umn.edu

Z. Vlodaver et al. (eds.), *Coronary Heart Disease: Clinical, Pathological, Imaging, and Molecular Profiles*,
DOI 10.1007/978-1-4614-1475-9_21, © Springer Science+Business Media, LLC 2012

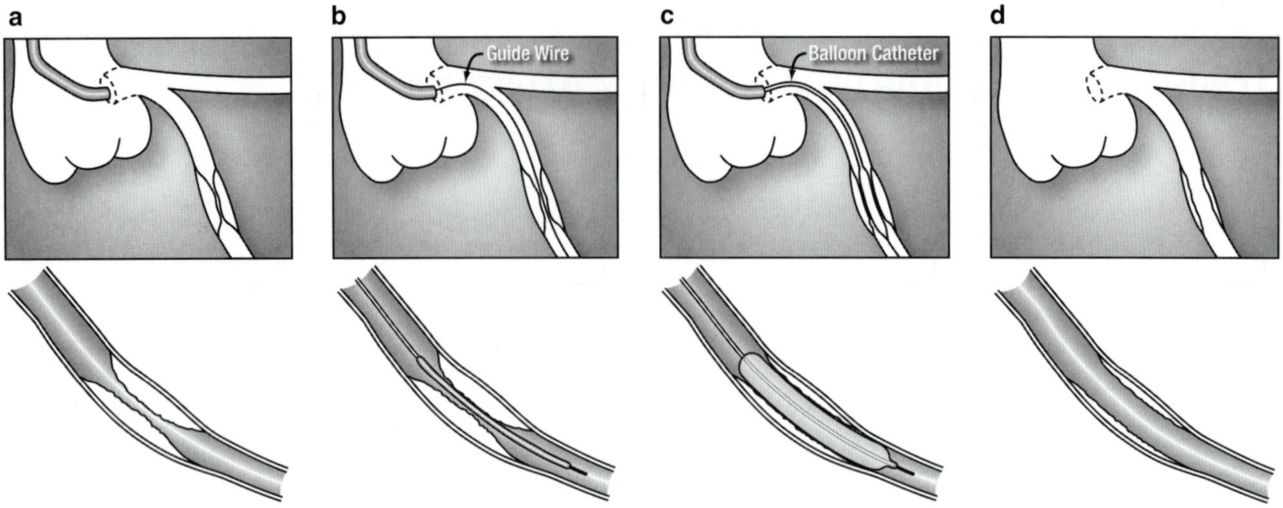

Fig. 21.1 Typical technique of balloon angioplasty and stenting. (**a**) A guide catheter is advanced to the coronary ostium. (**b**) A small radiopaque guidewire is advanced through the stenotic area of the artery. (**c**) A balloon catheter is advanced over the guidewire to the stenotic portion of the artery and inflated. (**d**) The balloon is withdrawn, leaving the dilated artery

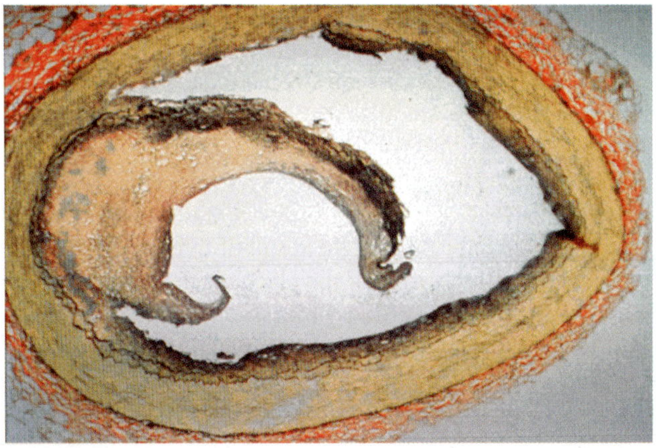

Fig. 21.2 A micrograph of an artery subjected to balloon dilation. The thickened, atherosclerotic, intimal layer has been dissected off of the media by balloon inflation

of the dissection and the presence of a blind pouch identified by persistent contrast staining after an angiographic injection. Dissections are graded using a standard National Heart, Lung, and Blood Institute (NHLBI) dissection scale [8].

Arterial perforation by the balloon or the guidewire can lead to anything from a localized hematoma on the epicardial surface of the heart to frank bleeding into the pericardial sac and cardiac tamponade. Balloon-initiated perforation occurs most commonly when the artery is overdilated (balloon:artery diameter >1.1). It is usually treated by immediate reinflation of the balloon to tamponade the bleeding from inside the arterial lumen, and reversal of the anticoagulants (if possible) (Fig. 21.3). Prolonged balloon inflation – 10–30 min – can often allow the vessel to seal itself. Definitive treatment is either placement of a stent covered with polytetrafluoroethylene (PTFE) or other impermeable material, or open-chest cardiac surgery [9].

The guiding catheters used to deliver intracoronary guidewires and balloons can also cause injury to the ostium of the coronary arteries, usually leading to a dissection flap. During percutaneous coronary intervention (PCI), the guide catheters often need to be manipulated so that they are pushed against the ostium or threaded partially down the artery being treated to provide more "back-up" force to advance the balloon catheter or other device through a narrowed or tortuous segment downstream. Since the guide catheters have a thin wall thickness and a wide mouth, they can dig into the arterial wall as

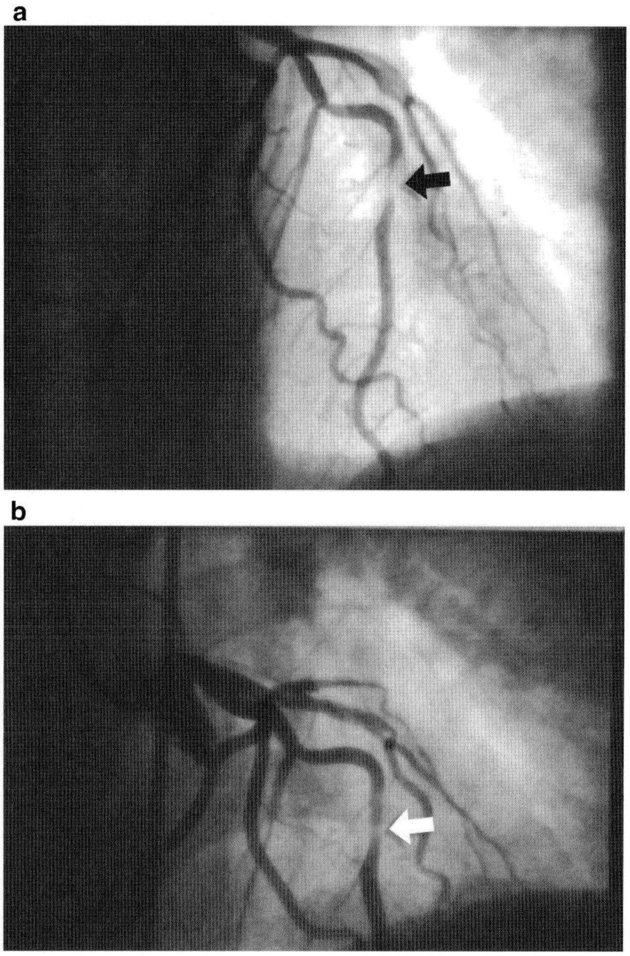

Fig. 21.3 Balloon coronary angioplasty. (**a**) A stenotic lesion is present in the mid-LAD (*arrow*). (**b**) After balloon angioplasty, the stenosis is reduced to 30% (*arrow*)

they are advanced. This can lead to a closure of the ostium or a spiral dissection down the entire length of the artery. In rare cases, the dissection can extend backward into the sinus of Valsalva and up the aorta. Ostial dissection is usually treated with stenting of the dissection. In severe cases, coronary bypass surgery or aortic root replacement can be required [10].

The Achilles' heel of balloon angioplasty is that the violent stretching of the artery results in a fibrotic healing response of variable magnitude (Fig. 21.4) [11]. The initial gain in lumen cross-sectional area is usually reduced by 30%, but the response can vary from a slight, further improvement in the lumen caliber with healing, to severe or complete obliteration of the lumen by the fibrotic response.

Histologically, the response to injury is characterized by smooth muscle cell transformation into fibroblasts, with migration of these cells from the arterial media through the torn internal elastic lamina to the intima, where they lay down collagen-based scar tissue. At the same time, monocytes from the luminal blood and arterial media set up an inflammatory reaction that results in reabsorption of the torn arterial intima and media. These cells also transform into fibroblasts and participate in the fibrotic response [12].

Predictors of restenosis after balloon angioplasty are (1) small vessel size (diameter of the normal portion of the artery), (2) an initial poor result (>50% diameter stenosis after POBA, residual pressure gradient >15 mmHg, or FFR < 0.90), (3) the presence of diabetes, and (4) prior restenosis of the same segment after POBA [13] (Fig. 21.5).

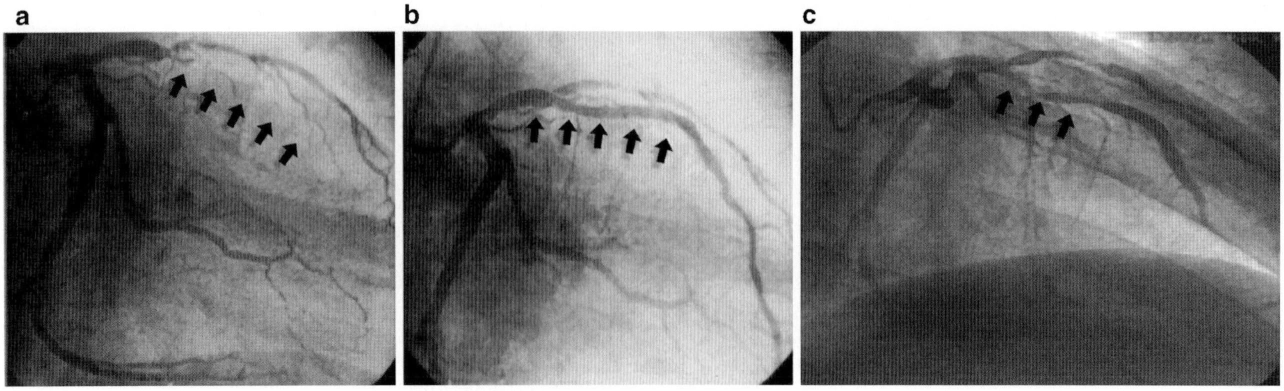

Fig. 21.4 Restenosis after coronary angioplasty. (**a**) The patient presented with recent onset of exertional and rest angina. The proximal LAD was found to be completely occluded (*arrows*). (**b**) After angioplasty and stenting, the LAD is fully patent (*arrows*). The patient's symptoms resolved entirely. (**c**) Seven months after angioplasty, the patient had recurrence of symptoms. Angiography showed severe restenosis (*arrows*)

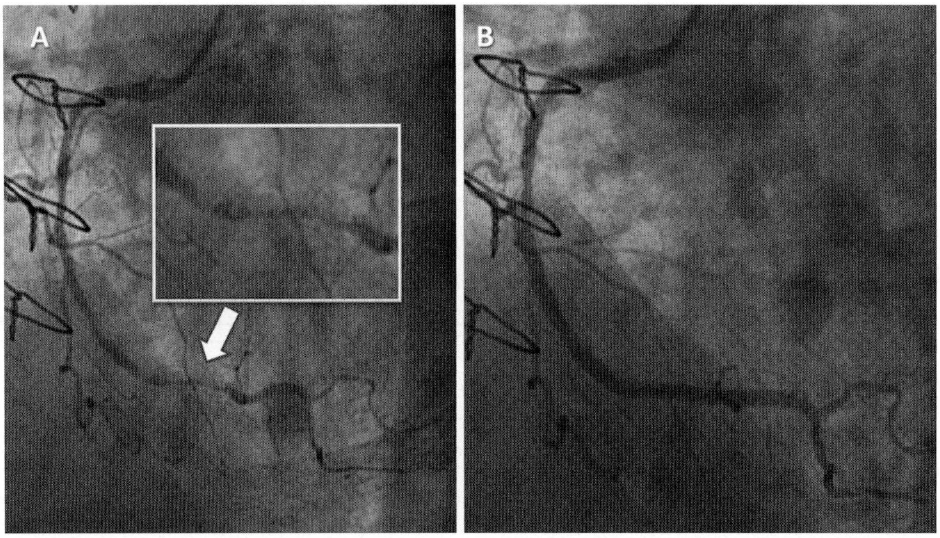

Fig. 21.5 Coronary stent restenosis with restenting. A 65-year-old man had stenting of the distal and mid-RCA with 3.0 and 2.5 mm everolimus drug-eluting stents (DESs). Eight months later, he had reonset of chest discomfort with exertion and a presyncopal spell with bradycardia after exertion. (**a**): Angiography showed in-stent restenosis of the distal RCA, (*arrow*), likely related to the small diameter of the implanted stent (for the size artery) and fibrosis. (**b**) Angiogram of the RCA after implantation of two 3.0 mm stents and high-pressure (19-bar) dilation

Stenting

Bare-Metal Stents

The stents used initially for coronary revascularization were composed of stainless steel fashioned into a tubular structure that could be crimped onto a balloon, passed into the narrowed portion of an artery, and then deployed by inflation and deflation of the balloon, leaving the expanded stent in place to prevent any recoil and seal the disrupted arterial intima [14] (Fig. 21.6). The initial generation of stents had several problems. First, they were bulky and could not always be delivered to the narrowed portion of the artery, even when the lesion had been predilated with a balloon. That problem was reduced by changing the design to a slotted, laser-cut tube with improved longitudinal flexibility and by changing the material to a cobalt

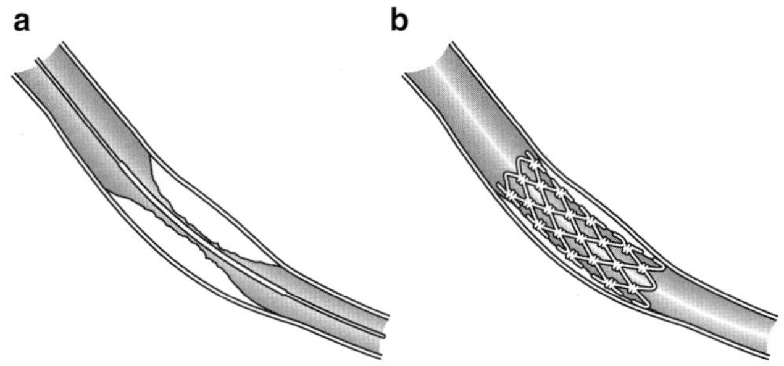

Fig. 21.6 A diagram of coronary stenting. (**a**) A stent crimped onto a balloon is passed through the stenotic area of the artery. The balloon is then inflated, deflated, and withdrawn. (**b**) The stent left in place prevents elastic recoil of the artery

chromium alloy. Its greater radial strength allowed a reduction in stent wall thickness. The second problem with stents is that they often initiated a thrombotic reaction within the artery, leading to acute myocardial infarction from vessel closure.

Although most of these closures occurred within several days of stent placement, a disturbing minority occurred up to several months after placement. The incidence of thrombosis is reduced markedly by combination antiplatelet therapy (a theinopyridine and aspirin) and better dilation of the stents so that they are better apposed to the vessel lumen through correct sizing and high-pressure balloon dilation. Renal failure, hypercoagulable states (e.g., malignancy, very recent surgery) and extensive stenting (e.g., bifurcation lesions) increase the risk of thrombosis.

The third problem with bare-metal stents is that, although the lumen cross-sectional area after stenting was substantially larger than after POBA, the fibrotic response and late lumen loss was more intense [15]. Bare-metal coronary stents usually develop a 400-mm-thick layer of fibrotic tissue within the stent, reducing arterial diameter by 800 mm. Because the initial improvement in lumen caliber was so great, however, the incidence of clinically relevant restenosis was still somewhat less than that after POBA. This problem was solved in large part by drug-eluting stents (DESs).

Drug-Eluting Stents

A number of antiproliferative drugs can reduce the fibro-proliferative response to arterial dilation when applied locally in the correct concentration for a defined time [16]. The challenge of placing these drugs on a stent was identifying the concentration and exposure time needed to reduce scarring, but not so much as to cause drug-induced arterial injury, leading to aneurysm formation or vessel necrosis. To meet this challenge, stents were covered with a drug-embedded polymer that controlled the drug's time-release kinetics. Two families of drugs are used today: the immunosuppressant "limus" family (sirolimus, everolimus, zotarolimus) and the cancer chemotherapy drug paclitaxol. These DES have reduced late-diameter lumen loss from about 800 mm with bare-metal stents to 150–300 mm [17]. The incidence of clinically relevant restenosis has likewise fallen from about 20% with bare-metal stents to about 4–8% with DES. Moreover, when restenosis occurs in a DES, it is usually much more focal and easy to treat with restenting.

The primary concern about DES is that the delay in arterial healing induced by the drug can lead to increased vulnerability to stent thrombosis for at least a year after placement [18–20]. The incidence of thrombosis is markedly reduced by dual antiplatelet therapy, but interruption in antiplatelet agents, and the hypercoagulable states induced by noncardiac surgery and cancer, can lead to thrombosis (Fig. 21.7).

Thrombectomy

Coronary lesions causing the acute coronary syndromes of unstable angina and acute myocardial infarction result from atherosclerotic plaque rupture and subsequent coronary thrombosis. PCI of thrombotic coronary lesions can lead to embolization of a clot to the downstream vessel, sometimes further extending the infarct (Fig. 21.8) [21]. In addition, the PCI activates the existing clot at the site of the lesion, leading to release of platelet products that cause intense microvascular constriction in the downstream bed and accelerated thrombosis within the lesion. Transcatheter removal of the thrombus can reduce the complications and lead to a lower mortality risk. There are two basic methods of thrombectomy (1) using a simple aspiration catheter and (2) using a catheter that mechanically aspirates and disrupts the clot.

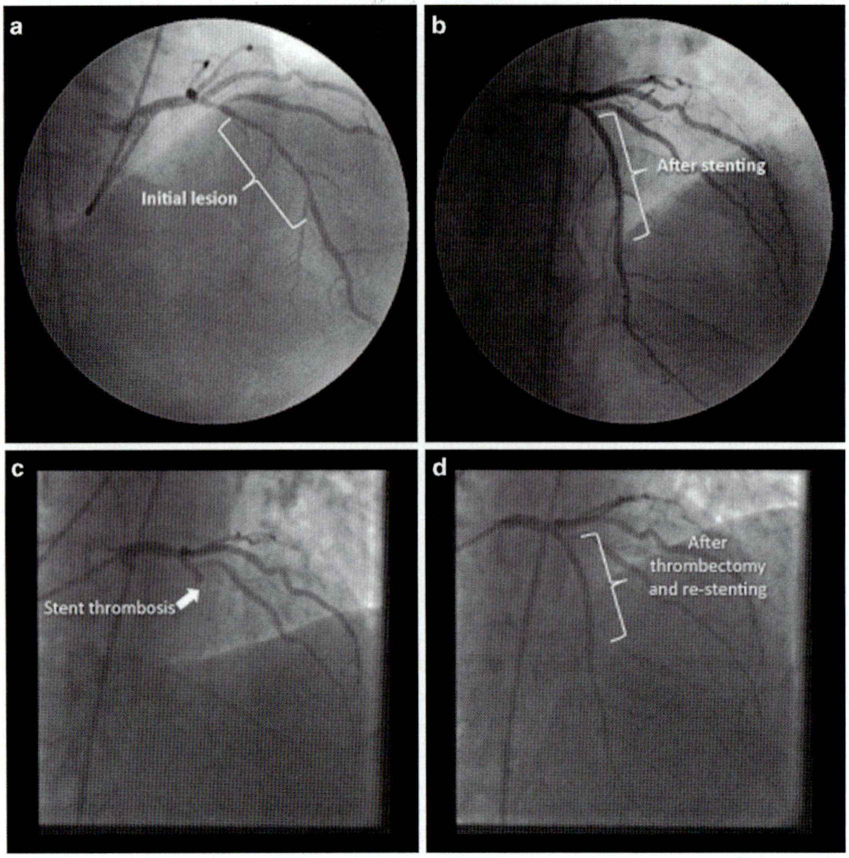

Fig. 21.7 A 42-year-old man with multiple myeloma presented with an abnormal stress myocardial perfusion scan (anterior wall defect). (**a**) Angiography showed a long stenosis of the mid-LAD. (**b**) After stenting with a 3.5 × 28 mm DES, vessel patency was restored. (**c**) One month later, he presented with an anterior STEMI and hypotension. Angiography showed complete proximal stent thrombosis (*arrow*). (**d**) After thrombectomy and restenting, arterial patency was restored

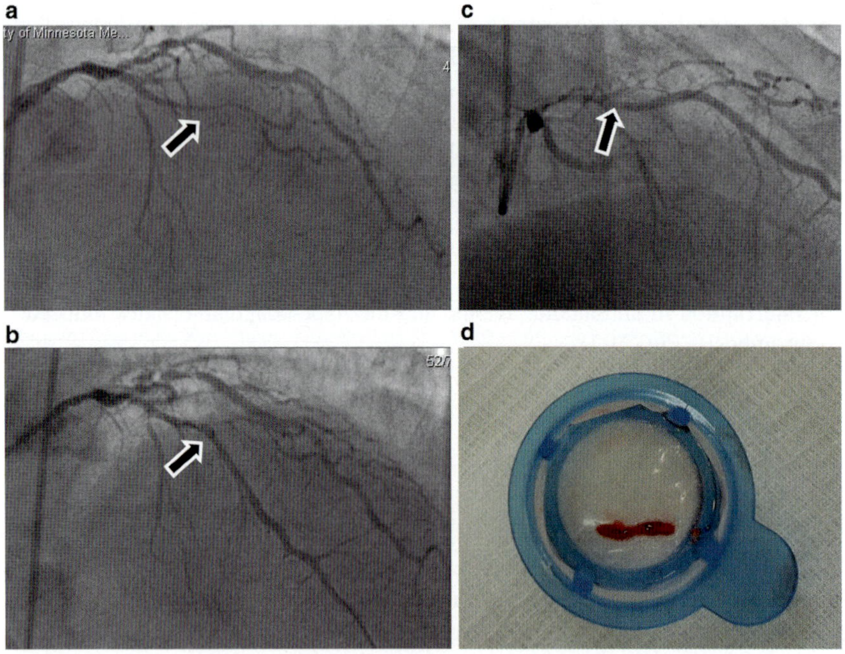

Fig. 21.8 A 56-year-old man presented with an acute anterior STEMI. (**a**) Emergency angiography showed acute occlusion of the proximal LAD (*arrow*). The left main and all three coronary arteries were severely and diffusely narrowed. (**b**) Simple aspiration thrombectomy restored blood flow (*arrow*). (**c**) The LAD was balloon dilated, stabilizing the artery. The patient later had bypass surgery. (**d**) A photograph of the thrombus aspirated from the LAD

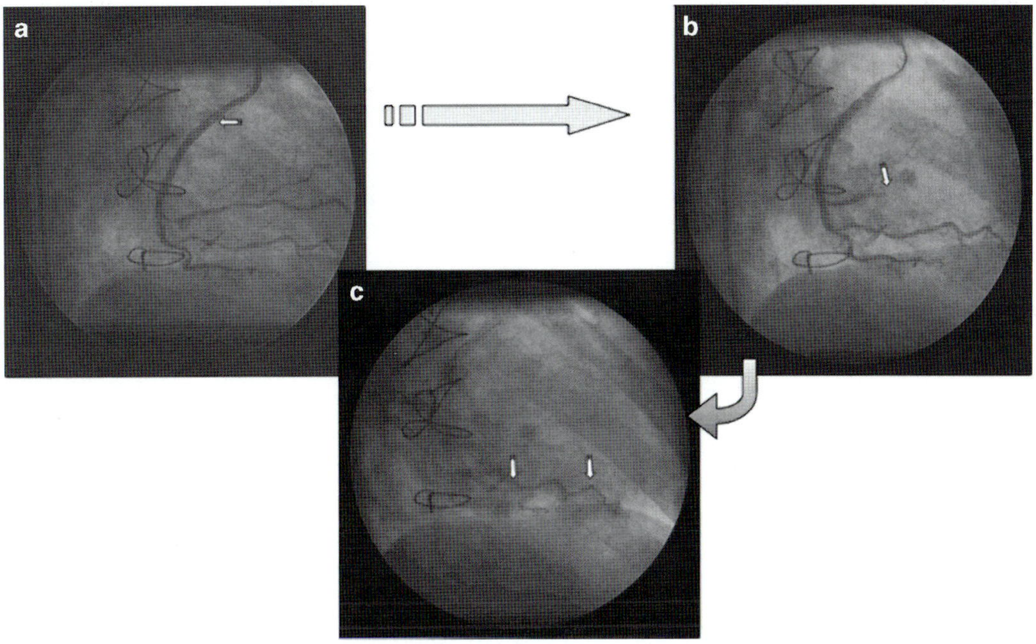

Fig. 21.9 A 58-year-old man presented with recent onset angina and new T-wave inversion in the inferior ECG leads. Creatine-kinase-MB was elevated. (**a**) Angiography showed a clot adherent to the proximal vessel at the site of moderate stenosis (*arrow*). After balloon dilation, the patient developed angina and inferior ST elevation on the ECG. Angiography showed occlusion of an RV marginal branch (**b**) (*arrow*), and very slow blood flow in the distal vessel with persistent hang-up of contrast (**c**) (*arrows*)

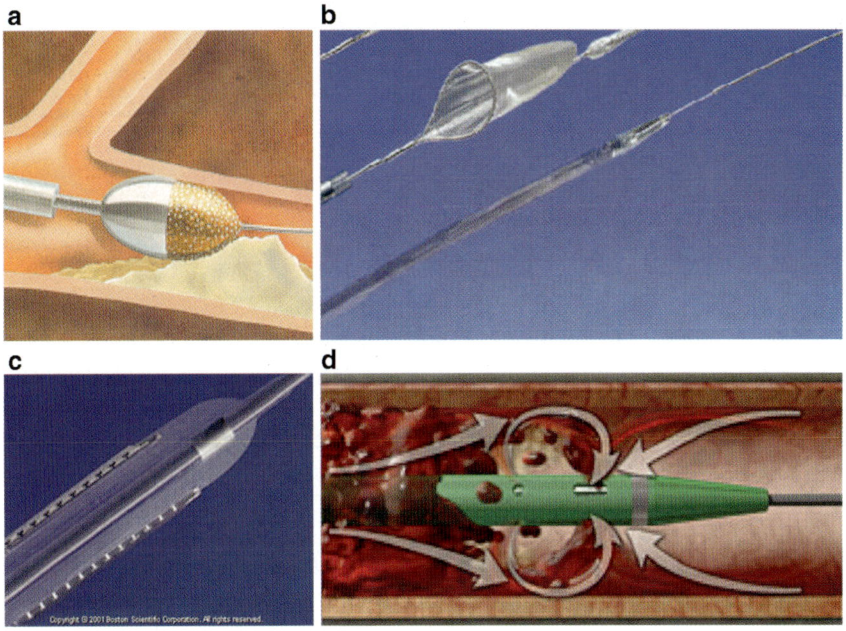

Fig. 21.10 A composite of "ancillary" devices used for percutaneous coronary intervention (PCI). (**a**) A Rotablator® burr (Boston Scientific, Natick MA). (**b**) A FilterWire EZ™ embolic protection device (Boston Scientific, Natick MA). (**c**) A Cutting Balloon™ (Boston Scientific, Natick MA). (**d**) AngioJet® thrombectomy device (Possis/Medrad, Minneapolis, MN)

Simple aspiration thrombectomy is carried out using a thin-wall catheter that rides on a standard coronary guidewire (Fig. 21.9). The catheter has one or more large holes at the distal lumen. When the catheter is positioned just in front of the thrombotic lesion, a syringe aspirates the clot as the catheter is advanced forward.

The other method uses a device (AngioJet®, MEDRAD, Inc.) that consists of a catheter that has a lumen for a high-pressure saline jet released entirely within the distal lumen of the catheter (Fig. 21.10). This jet causes suction within the catheter tip. A clot aspirated into the tip is then macerated by the jet, and the clot and fluid are continuously aspirated by a mechanized console. This device has been generally less effective [22] in improving outcomes, compared to a simple thrombectomy.

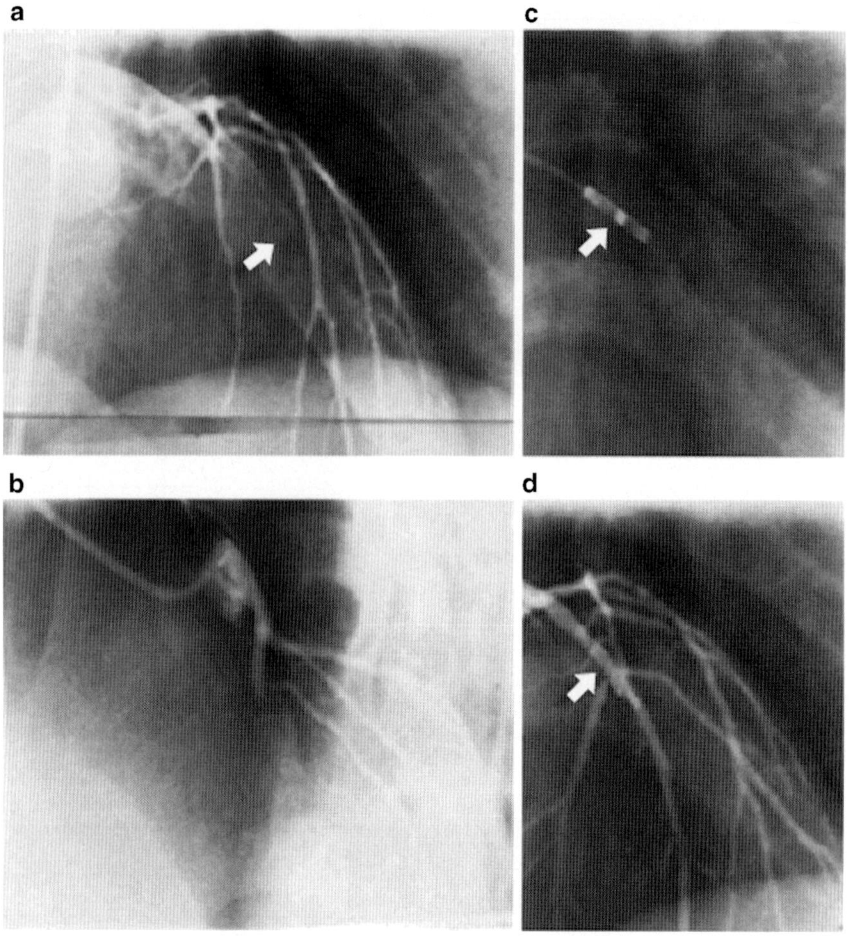

Fig. 21.11 Directional atherectomy of an occluded LAD. (**a**, **b**) A patient with exertional angina was found to have an occluded LAD (*arrow*). (**c**) After crossing the occlusion with a guidewire and predilating with a 2.0 mm balloon, a directional atherectomy cutter was advanced across the stenotic segment. Multiple passes with the cutting device yielded a white, fibrotic material that was packed into the nose cone of the device. (**d**) After atherectomy, the artery was fully patent (*arrow*) and symptoms abated

Atherectomy

Atherectomy catheters remove intraluminal tissue by cutting or abrasion (Fig. 21.11). The most commonly used device is the Rotablator® rotational atherectomy system (Boston Scientific, Natick, MA) [23]. The Rotablator consists of an olive-shaped, diamond-encrusted burr attached to a long, hollow drive shaft. The Rotablator catheter is passed into the coronary artery over a special guidewire. When positioned above the lesion, the burr is rotated by a gas-driven console at 140,000–160,000 rpm and the burr is slowly advanced in and out of the coronary narrowing, "sanding off" the inner layer of intima.

As a standalone device or when used routinely, the Rotablator has not improved outcomes. However, the Rotablator is particularly useful in pretreating calcified, rigid arteries that are difficult to balloon dilate and stent. Outcomes are improved when more than 240° of the arterial cross section is calcified, as assessed by intravascular ultrasound, or when significant intraluminal surface calcium spicules are present. The Rotablator is limited to a 2.25 mm maximum burr diameter. A newer rotational atherectomy device from Cardiovascular Systems, Inc., that rotates in an off-center ellipse may allow removal of more tissue using a small burr size [24].

The cutting atherectomy devices developed in the late 1980s and 1990s – used in "directional atherectomy" – have been abandoned because of a higher complication rate and poor outcomes [25]. Newer devices, however, are under development.

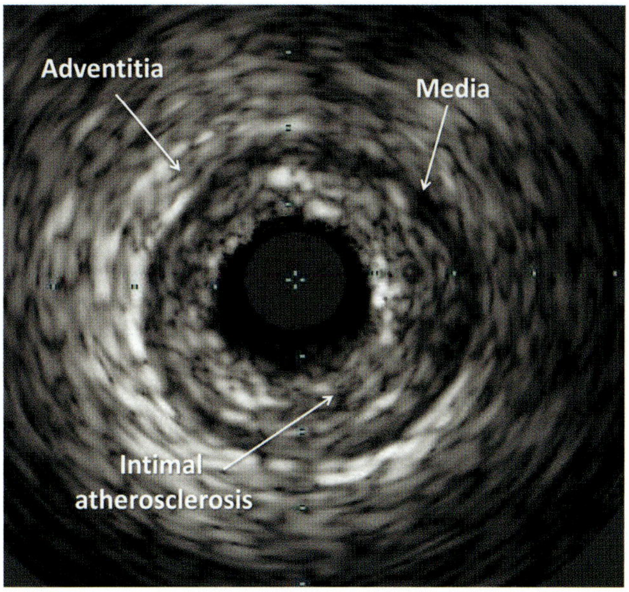

Fig. 21.12 A typical example of an intravascular ultrasound image from a patient with coronary atherosclerosis. The medial layer is echolucent and appears black. Inside the media, the intima is thickened

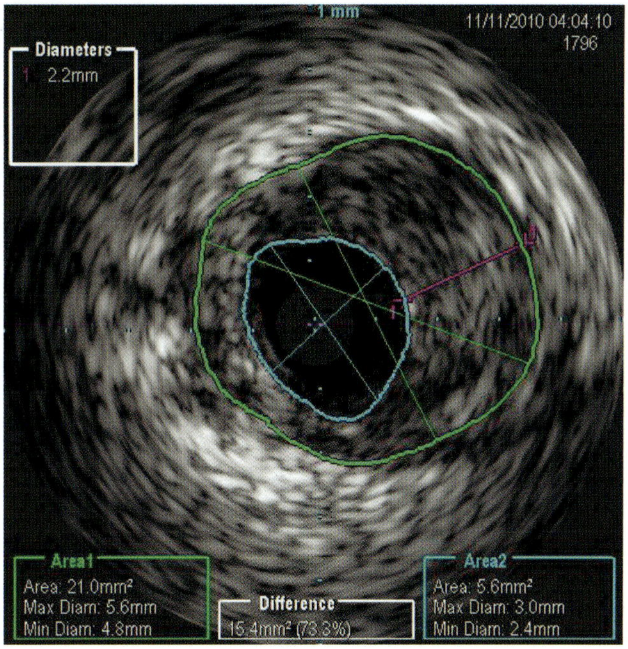

Fig. 21.13 Analysis of IVUS images of the coronary artery. The inner circle of the arterial lumen is used to derive the lumen cross-sectional area and diameters. The other circle is drawn at the intimal medial border to define the area within the internal elastic lamina (the "normal artery cross-sectional area"). The difference between the two areas is the "plaque area." By measuring the plaque area along the length of the artery, plaque volume can be calculated

Intravascular Ultrasound

Intravascular coronary ultrasound (IVUS) is a catheter-based ultrasound system that enables the operator to obtain a cross-sectional ultrasound of a coronary artery. Two types of ultrasound systems are used: mechanical transducers and solid state transducers. Mechanical transducers operate at 20–40 MHz and are located at the end of a monorail-style catheter. The transducer consists of a fixed piezoelectric crystal and an ultrasound "mirror" that rotates within the end of a catheter. Solid state transducers consist of an array of 32–64 piezoelectric crystals near the catheter tip. The resultant image is an ultrasound cross section of the arterial lumen and coronary wall.

Typical measurements are shown in Figs. 21.12 and 21.13, and consist of the arterial lumen diameters and cross-sectional area (CSA), internal elastic lamina CSA, and external elastic lamina CSA. Indicators of the quantity of disease are measures of intima thickness and volume (also known as plaque volume). The difference between the internal elastic lamina CSA and

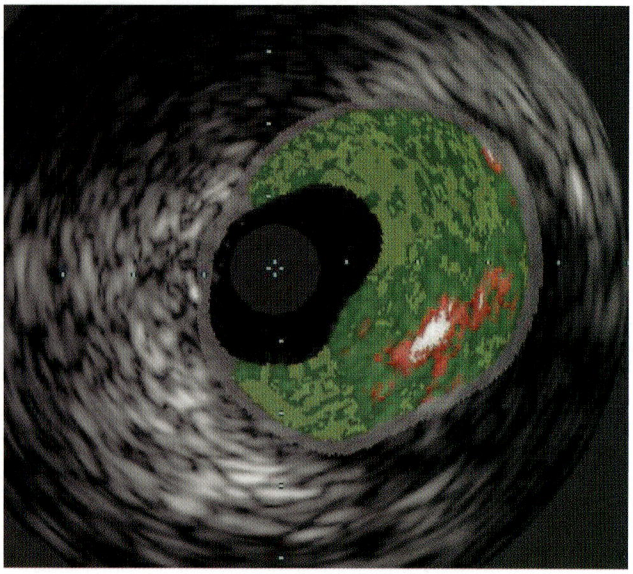

Fig. 21.14 An intravascular ultrasound of a coronary segment with a large atherosclerotic plaque. Using "virtual histology" analysis of the plaque composition, the plaque is composed of fibrofatty tissue (*green*) and necrotic core (*red*). The white areas represent calcification

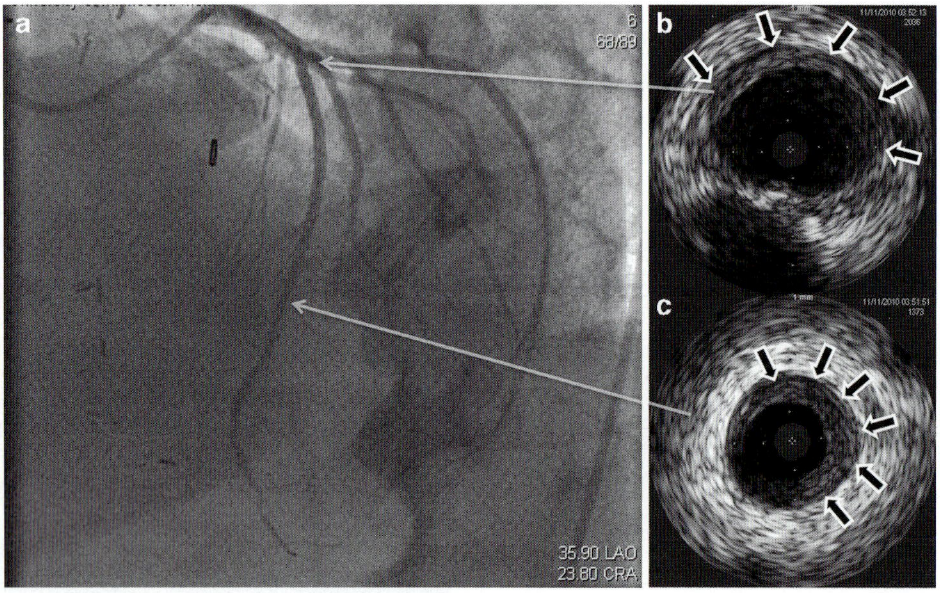

Fig. 21.15 Transplant arteriopathy detected by intravascular ultrasound (IVUS). (**a**) An angiogram of the left coronary artery from a patient 3 years after cardiac transplantation, showing minimal luminal obstruction. (**b**) An IVUS image from the proximal LAD around the area of the diagonal take-off, showing a large atherosclerotic plaque not apparent on the angiogram (*black arrows*). (**c**): IVUS examination of the mid-LAD showing diffuse luminal thickening (*black arrows*)

the lumen CSA defines the cross-sectional area of plaque. Using an automated pullback device to obtain a 3D view of the vessel, plaque volume can be quantified [26]. In addition, the presence of calcium deposits within the plaque or muscular layer can be detected as bright, ultrasound reflectors that cause ultrasound shadowing (Fig. 21.14). The presence of severe calcification increases the risk of PCI. Pretreatment with rotational atherectomy can improve outcomes in such cases. In addition, disease unappreciated on an angiogram can frequently be seen clearly on IVUS (Fig. 21.15).

IVUS measurements can be useful when choosing the size of an interventional device (balloon, Rotablator burr, stent) to match the size of the adjacent "normal artery." [27] In addition, the physiologic significance of a stenosis (its ability to impair myocardial blood flow under physiologic circumstances) can be predicted by measuring the minimal CSA of the artery and matching that to the arterial segment. For example, a minimum CSA <4.0 mm [2] in the proximal LAD is a surrogate for a flow-limiting lesion.

The length of the total occlusion, and the position and caliber of the distal vessel can be assessed by retrograde filling of the distal artery by collateral filling.

In many cases, a stiff, hydrophilic guidewire can be used to work through the occlusion and be positioned in the distal vessel – particularly if the length of the occlusion is short (<10 mm). Simultaneous injection of contrast into the artery, providing collateral flow, can aid in determining if the distal end of the guidewire is intraluminal. Once a guidewire is in place, the artery can be dilated with a small balloon and be treated in the usual fashion.

The likelihood of successful recannulation is dependent on the duration of occlusion, the length of the occlusion, and the presence of a "nipple" at the proximal edge, where the tip of a wire can be engaged [31]. Overall, about 50% of CTOs are not amenable to percutaneous revascularization. The major risk is perforation of the coronary artery and late reocclusion. Owing to limited means of assessing the position of the guidewire in the CTO and distal vessel, entry into the medial and adventitial layers of the artery is frequent, although bleeding into the pericardial space is not. Most perforations result in an epicardial hematoma. Reocclusion after recannulation can be mitigated by stenting, particularly with a DES. Reocclusion remains more frequent than with nonoccluded arteries, possibly due in part to the higher distal collateral pressure, which favors cessation of blood flow with relatively less proximal occlusion.

Several tools have been developed to assist in reopening CTOs. The Bridgewater device helps the user create a tunnel with the guidewire through the wall of the artery and around the CTO, and then reenter the distal lumen. Another approach involves passing a guidewire through a contralateral collateral artery retrograde through the CTO, which is usually easier to pass retrograde. Finally, a new, forward-looking intracoronary ultrasound device from Volcano, Inc., may assist the operator by enabling better negotiation of the occluded lumen.

Severe Calcification

Severe coronary calcification complicates PCI by two mechanisms: making passage of catheters though the lumen difficult and preventing effective luminal expansion [32]. Intracoronary ultrasound can be very helpful by imaging the position and extent of calcification. If catheter passage is difficult, surface calcification should be treated with rotational atherectomy [33]. With extensive calcification of the arterial intima and media (>240° arc), rotational atherectomy can reduce the likelihood of dissection and incomplete dilation.

Aneurysmal Disease

Ectasia and aneurysmal disease can complicate percutaneous treatment. First, stenotic lesions frequently occur at the inflow or outflow of ecstatic segments [34]. Stenting these lesions requires very precise placement so that the stent is not "hanging" into the ecstatic segment, where it will not be apposed to the vessel wall and will be a risk for thrombosis. The second problem with aneurysmal segments is that they are prone to thrombosis due to the low flow and stasis at the edges of the aneurysm. Distal embolization from an in situ clot or catheter and guidewire movement can cause distal occlusion. Stenting with covered stents can seal the aneurysmal segment and prevent thrombotic closure, but presently available covered stents have some risk of occlusion from restenosis. In general, the risk of coronary aneurysm rupture is low – less than 1% of atherosclerotic aneurysms.

Bypass Grafts

PCI of vein bypass grafts is common but can be complicated by distal embolization and slow graft blood flow, leading to myocardial infarction [35]. To prevent embolization, two types of devices have been developed: filters and aspiration devices (Fig. 21.19) [36]. The most commonly used are filter devices, which are usually deployed over a guidewire distal to the target lesion [37, 38]. Once the deployment catheter is in the distal graft, the filters are unsheathed and provide a 100–150-mm-diameter blood filter to catch embolized fragments. After PCI, the devices (with the emboli caught in the filter) are resheathed in a retrieval catheter and pulled out using the guiding catheter. These devices reduce the incidence of infarction after vein graft PCI, but smaller emboli can pass through or around the filter. In addition, the initial passage of the filter delivery catheter through the vein graft can cause embolization.

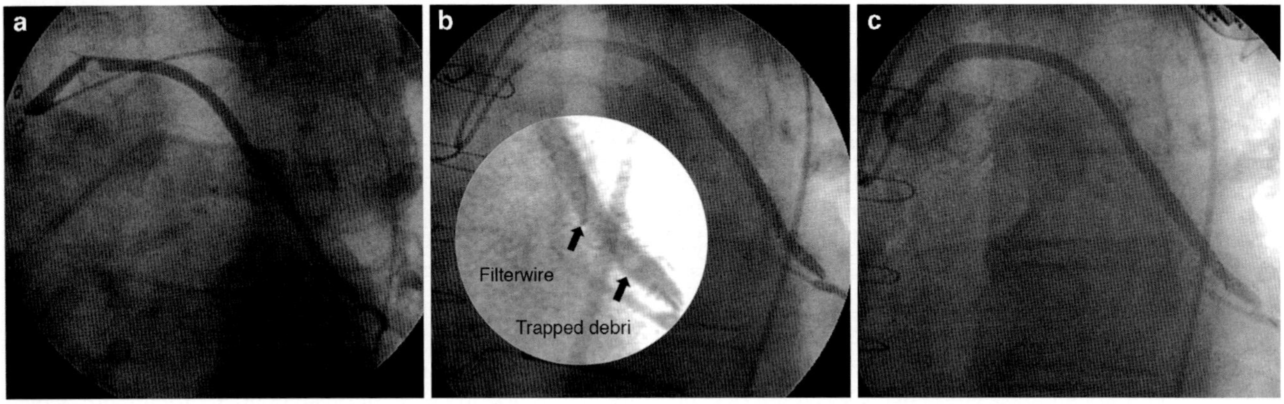

Fig. 21.19 A 76-year-old man presented with angina at rest and with exertion. Three years prior, he underwent coronary bypass surgery (LIMA graft to the mid-LAD; vein graft to the circumflex OM2 and vein graft to the first diagonal branch). (**a**) Angiography showed a severe stenosis of the vein bypass graft to OM2. Prior to stenting, a FilterWire EZ™ embolism protection device was passed to the mid-section of the graft. The proximal stenosis was stented. (**b**) Radiolucent embolized material is seen in the FilterWire after stenting (*inset, round white circle*). (**c**) The FilterWire was recaptured, along with the embolic material. The distal vessel remained patent. Symptoms resolved

The second category of devices occludes the artery during the intervention. Medtronic's GuardWire® uses a small balloon on a 0.014-in. guidewire. It is passed beyond the lesion and inflated at low pressure, stopping blood flow. The intervention is then carried out over the same wire. At the end of the intervention, a catheter is advanced to aspirate the blood and emboli in the work zone.

All of the devices discussed require a certain length of undiseased bypass graft distal to the lesion where the embolism protection device can be "landed." The The Proxis™ catheter (St. Jude Medical, Maple Grove, MN), a proximal embolic protection system, occludes the graft proximally using a low-pressure balloon around a guide catheter [39]. The intervention is performed through the device, while liberated emboli are aspirated retrograde. This obviates the need for a distal landing zone.

References

1. Andreas R, Grüntzig MD, Åke Senning MD, Siegenthaler WE. Nonoperative dilatation of coronary-artery stenosis — percutaneous transluminal coronary angioplasty. N Engl J Med. 1979;301:61–8.
2. Tenaglia AN, Buller CE, Kisslo KB, Stack RS, Davidson CJ. Mechanisms of balloon angioplasty and directional coronary atherectomy as assessed by intracoronary ultrasound. J Am Coll Cardiol. 1992;20:685–91.
3. Jain A, Demer LL, Raizner AE, Hartley CJ, Lewis JM, Roberts R. In vivo assessment of vascular dilatation during percutaneous transluminal coronary angioplasty. Am J Cardiol. 1987;60(13):988–92.
4. Fischman DL, Leon MB, Baim DS, et al., Stent Restenosis Study Investigators. A randomized comparison of coronary-stent placement and balloon angioplasty in the treatment of coronary artery disease. N Engl J Med. 1994;331:496–501.
5. Wilson RF, Marcus ML, Aylward PE, Talman CT, White CW. The effect of coronary angioplasty on coronary flow reserve. Circulation. 1988;77:873–85.
6. Manyari DE, Knudtson M, Kloiber R, Roth D. Sequential thallium-201 myocardial perfusion studies after successful percutaneous transluminal coronary artery angioplasty: delayed resolution of exercise-induced scintigraphic abnormalities. Circulation. 1988;77:86–95.
7. Writing Group for the Bypass Angioplasty Revascularization Investigation (BARI) Investigators. Five-year clinical and functional outcome comparing bypass surgery and angioplasty in patients with multivessel coronary disease. A multicenter randomized trial. JAMA. 1997;277:715–21.
8. Coronary artery angiographic changes after PTCA: manual of operations NHLBI PTCA Registry. 1985;6:9.
9. Ellis SG, Vandormael MG, Cowley MJ, et al. Coronary morphologic and clinical determinants of procedural outcome with angioplasty for multivessel coronary disease. Implications for patient selection. Multivessel Angioplasty Prognosis Study Group. Circulation. 1990;82:1193–202.
10. Goldstein JA, Casserly IP, Katsiyiannis WT, et al. Aortocoronary dissection complicating a percutaneous coronary intervention. J Invasive Cardiol. 2003;15:89–92.
11. Eberli FR, Meier B. Restenosis after angioplasty: an Achilles' heel well covered-up [editorial]. Eur Heart J. 1998;19:976–7.
12. Schwartz RS, Henry TD. Pathophysiology of coronary artery restenosis. Rev Cardiovasc Med. 2002;3 suppl 5:S4–9.
13. Kastrati A, Dibra A, Mehilli J, et al. Predictive factors of restenosis after coronary implantation of sirolimus- or paclitaxel-eluting stents. Circulation. 2006;113(19):2293–300. doi:10.1161/CIRCULATIONAHA.105.601823.

14. Serruys PW, de Jaegere P, Kiemeneij F, et al. A comparison of balloon-expandable-stent implantation with balloon angioplasty in patients with coronary artery disease. Benestent Study Group. N Engl J Med. 1994;331:489–95.
15. Farb A, Weber DK, Kolodgie FD, Burke AP, Virmani R. Morphological predictors of restenosis after coronary stenting in humans. Circulation. 2002;105:2974–80.
16. Park DW, Kim YH, Yun SC, et al. Comparison of zotarolimus-eluting stents with sirolimus- and paclitaxel-eluting stents for coronary revascularization. J Am Coll Cardiol. 2010;56:1187–95.
17. Shishehbor MH, Goel SS, Kapadia SR, et al. Long-term impact of drug-eluting stents versus bare-metal stents on all-cause mortality. J Am Coll Cardiol. 2008;52:1041–8.
18. Iakovou T, Schmidt T, Bonizzoni E, et al. Incidence, predictors, and outcome of thrombosis after successful implantation of drug-eluting stents. JAMA. 2005;293:2126–30.
19. Kuchulakanti PK, Chu WW, Torguson R, et al. Correlates and long-term outcomes of angiographically proven stent thrombosis with sirolimus- and paclitaxel-eluting stents. Circulation. 2006;113:1108–13.
20. Nakazawa G, Finn AV, Joner M, et al. Delayed arterial healing and increased late stent thrombosis at culprit sites after drug-eluting stent placement for acute myocardial infarction patients: an autopsy study. Circulation. 2008;118:1138–45.
21. Porto I, Selvanayagam JB, Van Gaal WJ, et al. Plaque volume and occurrence and location of periprocedural myocardial necrosis after percutaneous coronary intervention: insights from delayed-enhancement magnetic resonance imaging, thrombolysis in myocardial infarction myocardial perfusion grade analysis, and intravascular ultrasound. Circulation. 2006;114(7):662–9.
22. Migliorini A, Stabile A, Rodriguez AE, et al., JETSTENT Trial Investigators.. Comparison of AngioJet rheolytic thrombectomy before direct infarct artery stenting with direct stenting alone in patients with acute myocardial infarction: the JETSTENT Trial. J Am Coll Cardiol. 2010;56:1298–306.
23. Vom Dahl J, Dietz U, Haager PK, et al. Rotational atherectomy does not reduce recurrent in-stent restenosis: results of the angioplasty versus rotational atherectomy for treatment of diffuse in-stent restenosis trial (ARTIST). Circulation. 2002;105:583–8.
24. Casserly IP. Orbital atherectomy – another tool in the art of peripheral arterial intervention. Catheter Cardiovasc Interv. 2009;73(3):413–4.
25. Albiero R, Silber S, Di Mario C, et al. Cutting balloon versus conventional balloon angioplasty for the treatment of in-stent restenosis: results of the restenosis cutting balloon evaluation trial (RESCUT). J Am Coll Cardiol. 2004;43:943–9.
26. Sales FJ, Falcão BA, Falcão JL, et al. Evaluation of plaque composition by intravascular ultrasound "virtual histology:" the impact of dense calcium on the measurement of necrotic tissue. EuroIntervention. 2010;6:394–9.
27. Russo RJ, Silva PD, Teirstein PS, et al. AVID investigators: a randomized controlled trial of angiography versus intravascular ultrasound-directed bare-metal coronary stent placement (the AVID Trial). Circ Cardiovasc Interv. 2009;2:113–23.
28. Finn AV, Nakazawa G, Ladich E, Kolodgie FD, Virmani R. Does underlying plaque morphology play a role in vessel healing after drug-eluting stent implantation? JACC Cardiovasc Imaging. 2008;1:485–8.
29. Vlaar PJ, Svilaas T, Damman K, et al. Impact of pretreatment with clopidogrel on initial patency and outcome in patients treated with primary percutaneous coronary intervention for ST-segment elevation myocardial infarction: a systematic review. Circulation. 2008;118:1828–36.
30. Weisz G, Moses JW. Contemporary principles of coronary chronic total occlusion recanalization. Catheter Cardiovasc Interv. 2010;75 suppl 1:S21–7.
31. Paizis I, Manginas A, Voudris V, Pavlides G, Spargias K, Cokkinos DV. Percutaneous coronary intervention for chronic total occlusions: the role of side-branch obstruction. EuroIntervention. 2009;4:600–6.
32. Hodgson JM. Oh no, even stenting is affected by calcium [editorial]. Cathet Cardiovasc Diagn. 1996;38:236–7.
33. Rathore S, Matsuo H, Terashima M, et al. Rotational atherectomy for fibro-calcific coronary artery disease in drug eluting stent era: procedural outcomes and angiographic follow-up results. Catheter Cardiovasc Interv. 2010;75:919–27.
34. Bajaj S, Parikh R, Hamdan A, Bikkina M. Covered-stent treatment of coronary aneurysm after drug-eluting stent placement: case report and literature review. Tex Heart Inst J. 2010;37:449–54.
35. Baim DS, Wahr D, George B, et al. Saphenous vein graft Angioplasty Free of Emboli Randomized (SAFER) Trial investigators: randomized trial of a distal embolic protection device during percutaneous intervention of saphenous vein aorto-coronary bypass grafts. Circulation. 2002;105(11):1285–90.
36. Kelbaek H, Terkelsen CJ, Helqvist S, et al. Randomized comparison of distal protection versus conventional treatment in primary percutaneous coronary intervention: the drug elution and distal protection in ST-elevation myocardial infarction (DEDICATION) trial. J Am Coll Cardiol. 2008;51:899–905.
37. Roffi M, Mukherjee D. Current role of emboli protection devices in percutaneous coronary and vascular interventions. Am Heart J. 2009;157:263–70.
38. Stone GW, Rogers C, Hermiller J, et al. FilterWire EZ Randomized Evaluation Investigators: randomized comparison of distal protection with a filter-based catheter and a balloon occlusion and aspiration system during percutaneous intervention of diseased saphenous vein aorto-coronary bypass grafts. Circulation. 2003;108:548–53.
39. Mauri L, Cox D, Hermiller J, et al. The PROXIMAL trial: proximal protection during saphenous vein graft intervention using the Proxis embolic protection system: a randomized, prospective, multicenter clinical trial. J Am Coll Cardiol. 2007;50:1442–9.

Chapter 22
Surgical Treatment of Coronary Artery Disease

Kenneth Liao

History

Development of coronary angiogram by Sones at the Cleveland Clinic during the early 1960s made possible precise identification of anatomical coronary artery disease and laid foundation for modern coronary artery surgery [1]. In 1967 Favaloro at the Cleveland Clinic began performing coronary artery bypass grafting (CABG) with reversed vein grafts [2]. In 1968 Green et al. [3] at New York University used a dissecting microscope to perform anastomosis of the internal mammary artery (IMA) to the left anterior descending artery (LAD). Largely overlooked by the western world is the first CABG, in which an IMA was anastomozed to the LAD, was performed by Russian surgeon Kolessov [4] prior to 1967.

Between the 1970s and early 1980s, the CABG technique was made simpler and safer especially with the introduction of potassium cardioplegia for myocardium protection. A few landmark studies of CABG such as the Veterans Administration Study, the European Coronary Cooperative Study, and the Coronary Artery Surgery Study (CASS) have demonstrated the efficacy and safety of CABG to treat CAD [5, 6]. Prior to 1990s most CABG techniques were performed using saphenous veins only and at 10 years after surgery majority of vein grafts were occluded or had significant stenoses. In 1986 Loop et al. [7] reported the long-term result of CABG and found that, at 10 years after surgery the longevity was much better in patients who had the IMA as one of the bypass grafts compared to those who had only vein grafts. This important report has led to widespread use of IMA and the use of IMA in CABG is considered the standard practice worldwide [8].

Indications for CABG

The main goals of treating CAD are to improve the patient's quality of life (i.e., relief of angina and increased exercise tolerance), and prolong the patient's survival. The indications for CABG are established based on the comparative benefits and risks of surgery relative to those of medical treatment or percutaneous coronary intervention (PCI) to achieve the above goals. There is a large body of literature comparing medical management with CABG, medical management with PCI, and CABG with PCI. Although useful, the data must be interpreted critically in the context of the selection and exclusion criteria of patients within the trials. The impact of recent technological advances in both interventional cardiology and cardiac surgery on the selection of treatment modality needs to be factored in as well. However, there is a general consensus among cardiac surgeons that CABG should be the treatment of choice for CAD with the following pathologies: (1) left main stenosis, (2) triple-vessel disease, (3) double vessel disease with proximal LAD stenosis, (4) impaired left ventricular function, and (5) diabetes.

Based on the original American College of Cardiology (ACC)/American Heart Association (AHA) guidelines for Coronary Artery Bypass Graft Surgery published in 1999, a joint ACC/AHA task force on practice guidelines revised the existing guidelines in 2004 [9]. The current common class I indications for CABG are outlined as follows:

For Stable Angina

1. CABG is recommended for patients with stable angina who have significant left main coronary artery stenosis (greater than 50% stenosis); who have left main equivalent: significant (greater than or equal to 70%) stenosis of the proximal

K. Liao, MD, PhD (✉)
University of Minnesota, 420 Delaware Street SE, MMC 207, Minneapolis, MN 55455, USA
e-mail: liaox014@umn.edu

Z. Vlodaver et al. (eds.), *Coronary Heart Disease: Clinical, Pathological, Imaging, and Molecular Profiles*,
DOI 10.1007/978-1-4614-1475-9_22, © Springer Science+Business Media, LLC 2012

LAD and proximal left circumflex artery; who have three-vessel disease (survival benefit is greater when LVEF is less than 0.50); who have two-vessel disease with significant proximal LAD stenosis and either EF less than 0.50 or demonstrable ischemia on noninvasive testing (*Level of Evidence: A*).
2. CABG is beneficial for patients with stable angina who have one- or two-vessel CAD without significant proximal LAD stenosis but with a large area of viable myocardium and high-risk criteria on noninvasive testing (*Level of Evidence: B*).

For Unstable Angina/Non-ST-Segment Elevation MI

1. CABG should be performed for patients with unstable angina/non-ST-segment elevation MI with significant left main coronary artery stenosis; with left main equivalent: significant (greater than or equal to 70%) stenosis of the proximal LAD and proximal left circumflex artery (*Level of Evidence: A*).
2. CABG is recommended for unstable angina/non-ST-segment elevation MI in patients in whom revascularization is not optimal or possible and who have ongoing ischemia not responsive to maximal nonsurgical therapy (*Level of Evidence: B*).

For ST-Segment Elevation MI (STEMI)

Emergency or urgent CABG in patients with STEMI should be undertaken in the following circumstances: (a) Failed angioplasty with persistent pain or hemodynamic instability in patients with coronary anatomy suitable for surgery. (b) Persistent or recurrent ischemia refractory to medical therapy in patients who have coronary anatomy suitable for surgery, who have a significant area of myocardium at risk, and who are not candidates for PCI (Level of Evidence: B).

For Poor LV Function

CABG should be performed in patients with poor LV function who have significant left main coronary artery stenosis; who have left main equivalent: significant (greater than or equal to 70%) stenosis of the proximal LAD and proximal left circumflex artery; who have proximal LAD stenosis with two- or three-vessel disease (Level of Evidence: B).

Life-Threatening Ventricular Arrhythmias

CABG should be performed in patients with life-threatening ventricular arrhythmias caused by left main coronary artery stenosis and by three-vessel coronary disease (*Level of Evidence: B*).

Contraindications to Operation

In the last 30 years the advancement of medical knowledge and technology has made CABG a routine and safe operation. In elective operation the patient is medically optimized prior to surgery. Improvement in cardiopulmonary bypass (CPB) support and myocardium preservation has minimized ischemia-reperfusion injury. Vigorous training and high volume of CABG have made cardiac surgeons technically skilled. The cardiac ICU care and cardiac rehabilitation have reduced the postoperative complications and shortened the postoperative recovery time. Current operative risk for CABG is low, with a national average mortality rate of 2.5% based on STS data [10].

Virtually no absolute contraindications to CABG exist. The following conditions are generally considered high risks for CABG: recent stroke, acute MI within 2 weeks, ongoing sepsis, severe chronic congestive heart failure, pulmonary hypertension, severe chronic obstructive pulmonary disease, coagulopathy due to liver failure. Since the introduction of minimally invasive cardiac surgery technique and the increased use of mechanical circulatory support, advanced age and poor left ventricular function are not considered as serious risks as they were used to.

Preoperative Preparation

Most patients who come for elective CABG are taking B-adrenergic receptor or calcium channel blocking agents, angiotension converting enzyme (ACE) inhibitors, and platelet antiaggregating drugs. The above medications except antiplatelet agents are continued to operative day. Clopidogrel (Plavix) is discontinued for 5 days prior to surgery if feasible while aspirin is typically continued to operative day. For patients with unstable angina, intravenous heparin is continued up to surgery. Intra-aortic balloon pump is indicated for patients who have critical left main disease, unstable angina that fails to respond to medical therapy and who are unstable hemodynamically.

Operative Technique

Operative Strategy

Most patients undergoing CABG have three-vessel disease, many of them with impairment of LV function and diabetes. The primary goal of CABG is to revascularize all coronary artery branches completely with significant stenosis (i.e., more than 50% of luminal narrowing). At least one of the IMAs is used as bypass conduit and left IMA (LIMA) is routinely anastomozed to LAD. At least one or more saphenous vein grafts are bypassed to the remaining left and right coronary arteries. A typical CABG with three-vessel grafting is illustrated in Fig. 22.1.

At present, CABG with the use of CPB through a full sternotomy remains the most widely used surgical technique, comprising 80% of total CABG performed in the US. About 20% of total CABG is performed through a full sternotomy but without CPB (OPCAB). A small portion of CABG is performed without sternotomy, with or without the use of CPB (MIDCAB) [11]. Robot is recently introduced into the field of cardiac surgery and is being increasingly used in MIDCAB [12, 13]. The choices of above approaches are made typically based on the institutional and individual surgeon's experience and preference.

Choices of Bypass Conduits

IMA

Multiple clinical studies have clearly demonstrated that the patency rate of pedicled LIMA bypassed to LAD is over 90% after 10 years and such patency rate is maintained up to 15 years. The early and late patient survival benefits have been observed in patients who had a pedicled LIMA to LAD as compared to only vein grafts. Furthermore, the patient's survival rate is higher and reoperative rate lower if both IMAs are used. Bilateral IMAs are used in patients who are young and have inadequate veins or whose radial arteries are not suitable for use. If the IMA is injured or is not long enough to reach the target vessel, it can be used as a free graft. Diabetes, obesity, severe COPD, and chronic renal insufficiency pose increased risk of sternal infection if both IMAs are harvested. There is some evidence to suggest that harvesting of IMA with skeletonized technique might preserve blood supply to sternum and reduce sternal infection (Fig. 22.2). IMA can be harvested through sternotomy (Fig. 22.3), thoracotomy, and more recently endoscopic Robot.

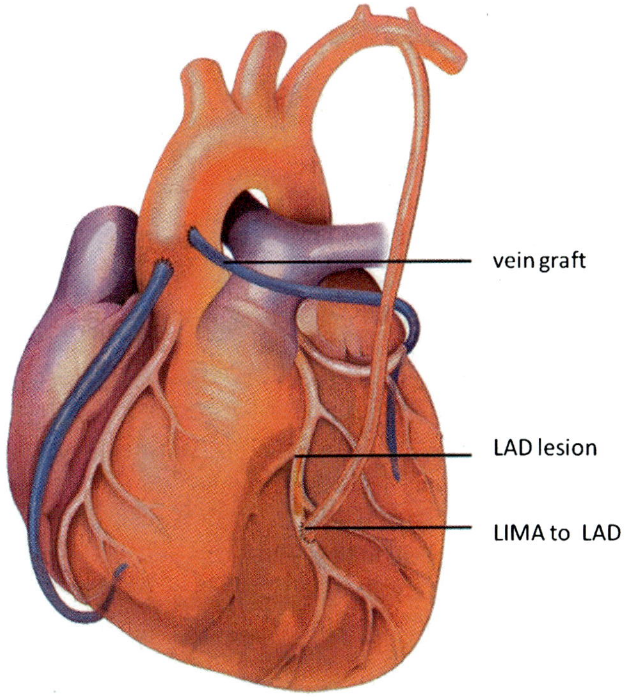

Fig. 22.1 Typical three-vessel coronary artery bypass grafting (CABG) configuration with left internal mammary artery (LIMA) to left anterior descending artery (LAD) and saphenous veins to obtuse marginal artery and right coronary artery

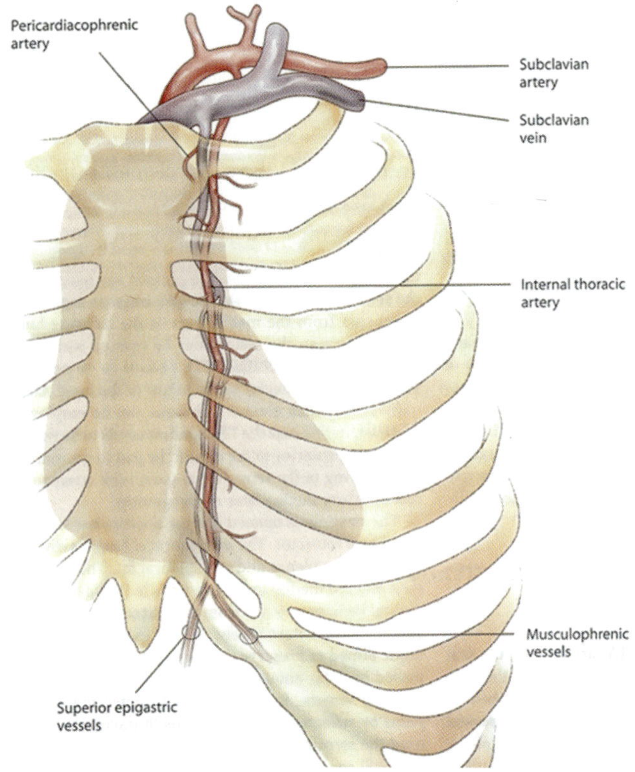

Fig. 22.2 Anatomy of LIMA and its relation with the sternum

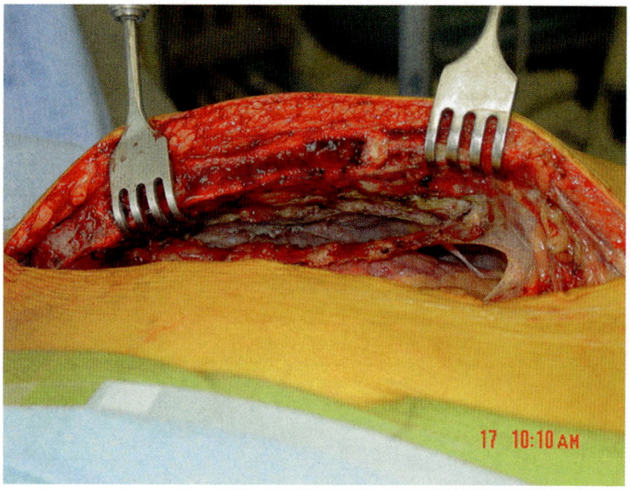

Fig. 22.3 Technique used to harvest LIMA via sternotomy which causes trauma in the sternum

Vein Grafts

The greater saphenous vein remains the primary source of free grafts. If it is absent or inadequate, the lesser saphenous vein can be used. The main advantages of the vein graft include that it provides excellent blood flow to the target arteries and has lower flow resistance and higher flow compared to arterial grafts initially; it is easy to harvest and handle the vein including sewing and it is long enough to reach most target vessels. The disadvantages of vein graft are that its quality varies among individuals and it has a tendency to develop early degenerative change and has poor long-term patency rate. The average patency rate of vein graft is about 50% in 10 years. At 10 years of bypass most vein grafts would develop significant atherosclerotic disease and stenoses (Fig. 22.4). Saphenous vein can be harvested through conventional incision (Fig. 22.5), mini bridge incisions, and endoscope (Fig. 22.6).

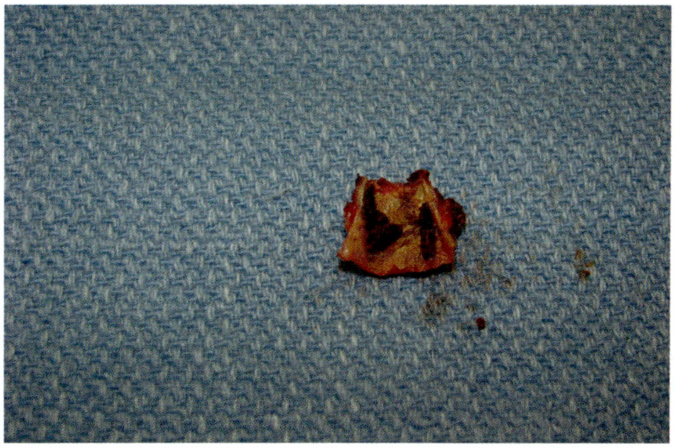

Fig. 22.4 Gross view of a segment of saphenous vein graft 10 years after CABG. Severe degenerative change is noted inside the lumen of vein

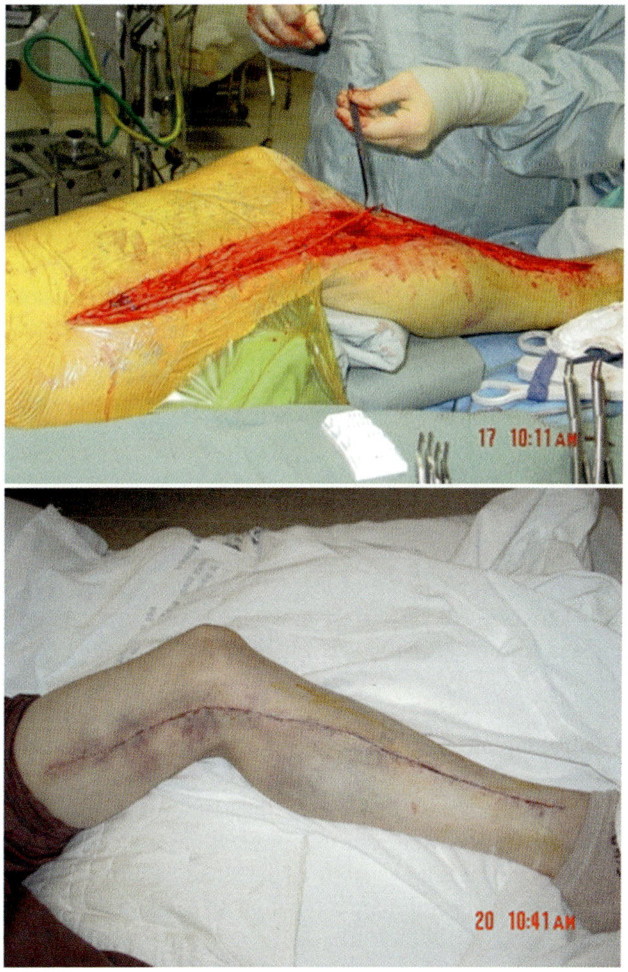

Fig. 22.5 Harvesting of saphenous vein with conventional open technique. A large scar is noted

Radial Artery

Radial artery is typically harvested in the patient whose saphenous vein is inadequate. Though it has a lower rate of graft failure than that of vein graft in the short and intermediate term, it has a tendency to develop spasm in the early postoperative phase and develops "string sign." It works better when it is bypassed to a large target vessel (>1.5 mm) with more than 70% of stenosis. Radial artery however has a lower graft patency rate than that of the IMA. It has different histological

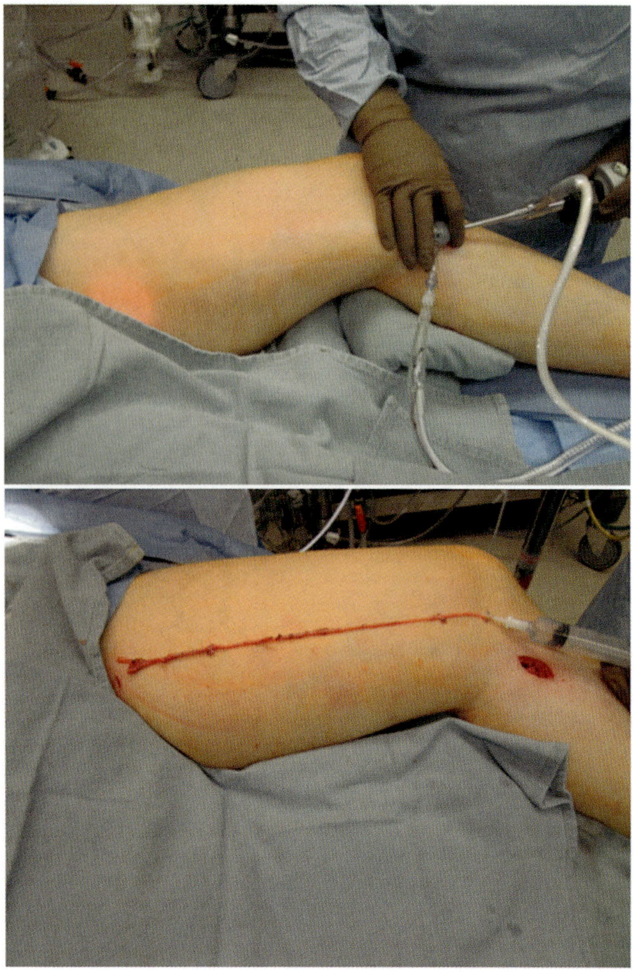

Fig. 22.6 Harvesting of saphenous vein with an endoscope. A small incision in noted

characteristics from that of IMA. Intimal changes and the presence of atheromatous plaque are observed in coronary and radial arteries, but very rarely in the IMA. Like coronary artery, radial artery is muscular artery and aging results in thickening and fibrosis of the intima and media of the wall. IMA has no such changes even after years of bypass.

Gastroepiploic Artery

Its harvesting is achieved through laparatomy and mobilization of the greater curvature of the stomach. It can be used as a pedicled graft as well as a free graft. It has a patency rate of >80% at 5 years. Due to limitations on length, tendency to spasm, inconsistent availability, and small caliber and tedious dissection, this artery is infrequently used. However, it can become very useful for reoperation bypass to the inferior target vessel, which can be performed off pump without sternotomy.

Coronary Artery Bypass Grafting

A median sternotomy is made and at the same time a segment of great saphenous vein or radial artery is harvested. Before the pericardium is opened the LIMA is fully mobilized. The LIMA is dissected out together with its accompanying veins and a 1 cm chest wall muscle pedicle. Heparin (300 units/kg) is administered and the LIMA is divided distally just above the bifurcation. The proximal LIMA is occluded by a bulldog clamp and distal LIMA is cut to the appropriate length and prepared. The pericardium is opened and the heart is inspected for target vessels. The ascending aorta is palpitated to detect

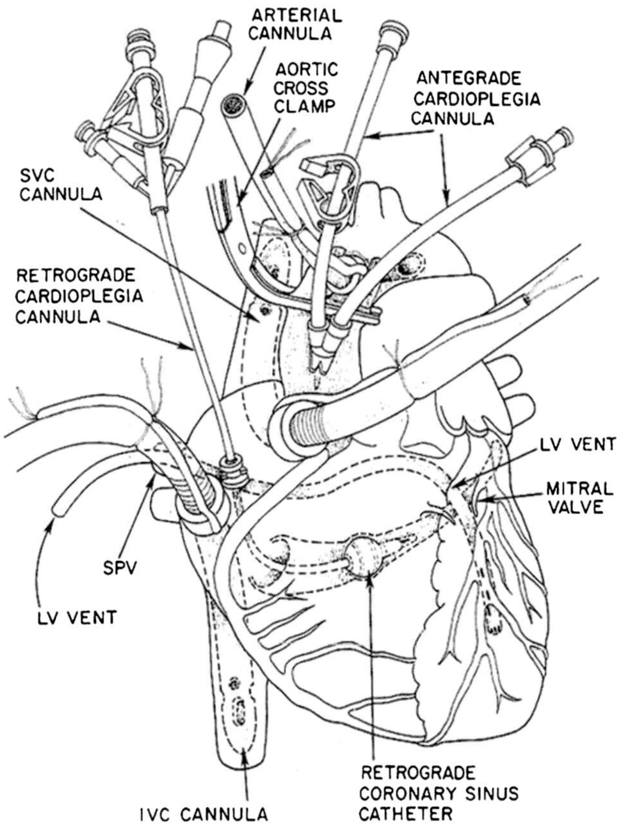

Fig. 22.7 Setup of conventional cardiopulmonary bypass (CPB) and myocardial preservation during CABG

potential plaques and select a cannulation site. We place two 2-0 braided purse-string sutures in distal ascending aorta. A 20–22 Fr Medtronic metal-tip aortic cannula (Medtronic, St Paul, MN) is inserted into the aorta and connected to the arterial limb of the CPB circuit. For isolated CABG we use a single dual-stage cannula (32/34 Fr) for venous drainage and the venous cannula is inserted into the inferior vena cava through a 2-0 braided purse-string suture placed in the right atrial appendage. If other cardiac procedure such as mitral valve repair is anticipated in addition to CABG, two separate single stage venous cannulae are inserted into the superior vena cava and inferior vena cava separately for venous drainage. Two catheters for administering cardioplegia solution are inserted into the ascending aorta and coronary sinus separately. Once the activated clotting time (ACT) of over 500 s is achieved, the CPB is initiated. The CPB flow is maintained from 1.8 to 2.2 L/min/m^2 with a target mean arterial pressure of 50–60 mmHg. The aorta is clamped and cold blood cardioplegia is given via antegtrade and retrograde routes. The heart is covered with cold saline during administration of cardioplegia. The setup of CPB is illustrated in Fig. 22.7.

The heart is lifted toward the head of the patient and rotated toward his left shoulder to expose distal right coronary artery or posterior descending artery (PDA). A vein graft or radial artery is brought over the heart and the distal end of the graft is spatulated. An arteriotomy is made in the target segment of coronary artery and the distal end of the vein graft or radial artery is anastomozed to the arteriotomy in an end-to-side manner with a running 7-0 prolene suture. A dose of cardioplegia is given to the graft to check the flow and bleeding in the anastomosis. High pressure in the graft flow suggests poor distal target vessel run-off, poor graft quality and/or technique error of anastomosis. The bleeding from the anastomosis and graft can be identified and repaired easily. The graft is then distended with cardioplegia, positioned along the right atrium up to the right side of the ascending aorta, and transected at the point where it touches the aorta. The proximal end of the graft is spatulated for proximal anastomosis later.

The heart is then retracted to the patient's right shoulder to expose the obtuse marginal branches of the circumflex artery. A separate vein graft or radial artery is brought to the operative field and its distal end is anastomozed to the targeted marginal branch using similar technique described above. The graft is properly oriented to avoid twisting, and the heart is placed back into the pericardial sac. The graft is distended by infusing cardioplegia and cut to the appropriate length while the heart is distended to its natural size. The graft is positioned along the atrioventricular groove and anterior to pulmonary artery to reach the ascending aorta. The proximal end of the graft is spatulated.

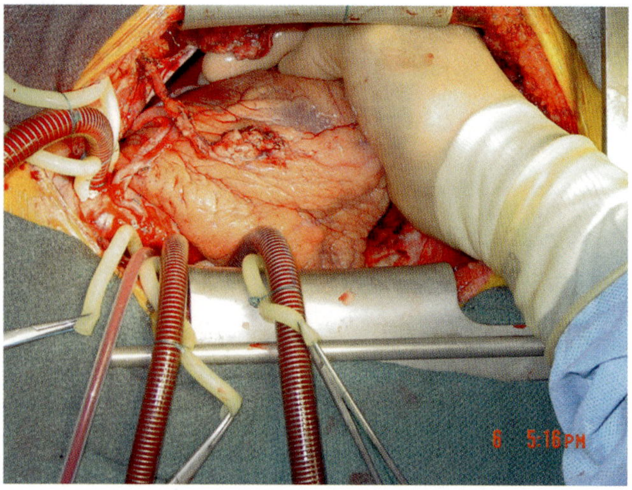

Fig. 22.8 View of heart after a three-vessel CABG. LIMA to LAD and two vein grafts are seen. The arterial and venous cannulae are used during CPB

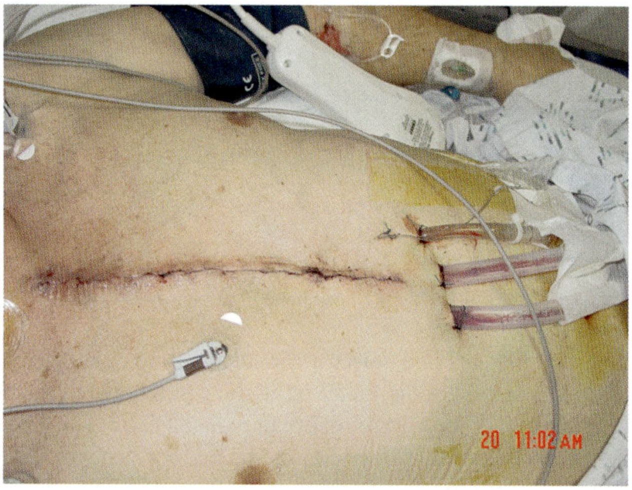

Fig. 22.9 The chest incision after a conventional CABG via full sternotomy. Three mediastinal drainage tubes are noted coming out under the xyphoid

The LIMA is cut to the appropriate length and its distal end is saptulated. The proper orientation of LIMA is ensured. The heart is gently rotated to the right side to bring the LAD to the center of operative field. A 6-mm anterior arteriotomy is made in the targeted segment of LAD and the distal end of LIMA is anastomozed to the LAD in an end-to-side manner with a running 8-0 prolene suture. The bulldog clamp on the LIMA is temporarily released to check the bleeding at the anastomosis. The muscle pedicle of LIMA is sutured to the epicardium near the anastomosis to maintain the proper orientation of the LIMA graft and release the tension on the anastomosis. The pericardium is incised laterally and proximal LIMA is placed laterally outside pericardium to ensure proper alignment of the LIMA with LAD and to prevent possible injury to the LIMA should a redo sternotomy is needed in the future.

The aortic clamp is removed and a partial occluding clamp is placed on the anterior wall of ascending aorta. Two or more 5 mm openings are made in the occluded aortic wall by a punch. The proximal ends of the vein or radial artery grafts are anastomozed to the aortic openings with running 6-0 prolene sutures. The clamp is then removed and the air inside the vein or radial artery grafts is evacuated with a fine tip needle. If the atherosclerotic or calcified ascending aorta is noted or suspected, the partial aortic clamping is avoided and the proximal anastomoses are performed with the heart arrested using the single aortic cross clamp technique (Fig. 22.8). Once the aortic cross clamp is removed, the heart should be perfused on CPB for adequate time until it is beating well. Once the systemic rewarming is completed CPB is terminated and the cannulae are removed. The protamine is given and the hemostasis is achieved. The mediastinal and pleural drainage tubes are placed and the sternum is closed with wires. The rest of incision is closed with Vicryle sutures (Fig. 22.9).

Less Invasive CABG

For years, CABG has been performed routinely with CPB and sternotomy by cardiac surgeons worldwide. Though it is considered somewhat standardized by most cardiac surgeons, continued improvements as well as recognition of the importance of postoperative recovery and quality of life remain significant concerns for patients as well as physicians. In recent years, there has been a major push to develop and provide "less invasive CABG" as an alternative or standard care.

Four major steps used in conventional CABG contribute to the majority of its complications. Any of these steps can impose significant risks or adverse effects.

1. Full Sternotomy: It typically requires over 8 weeks for bone to heal. It can cause deep wound nonhealing or infection especially in diabetic and COPD patients. It can also create a noticeable scar, and occasionally cause chronic pain. For years, the physical and emotional impact of a large incision on the individual patient has been ignored by most cardiac surgeons. Historically, adequate exposure of the target tissues or organs through large skin incisions took priority over concern about incision size; this mindset remained unchallenged until the early 1990s. Since 2000 partial sternotomy or nonsternotomy approaches have been increasingly used by cardiac surgeons and various studies have reported the advantages of such approaches in terms of pain, blood loss, postoperative respiratory function, time to recovery, infection, and cosmesis [14, 15].
2. Cardiopulmonary Bypass: CPB has been associated with a complex systemic inflammatory reaction in the host patient. The hallmarks of this reaction are typically increased microvascular permeability in multiple organs, resulting in an increase in interstitial fluid and the activation of humoral amplification systems. This inflammatory response can affect multiple organs, examples of this systemic response can vary: (1) from transient subtle cognitive impairment to a permanent stroke; (2) from coagulopathy requiring transfusion of blood products to disseminated intravascular coagulation; (3) from pulmonary edema to adult respiratory distress syndrome requiring prolonged ventilation support; (4) from low cardiac output to acute heart failure requiring inotropic or mechanical circulatory support; and/or (5) from transient kidney insult with increased creatinine to permanent kidney failure requiring hemodialysis. Any of these, or a combination thereof, commonly results in prolonged intensive care unit stays requiring intense monitoring and often increased patient mortality [16–21].
3. Arresting the Heart by Administering Cardioplegia: Cardiac arrest is initiated with infusion of cardioplegia to the myocardium during conventional CABG. Unfortunately, subsequent reperfusion of the heart can cause ischemic reperfusion injury to the myocardium and result in depressed cardiac function which can be more detrimental to the hearts with chronic impairment [17].
4. Manipulating the Ascending Aorta: Coronary artery disease is often considered as a component of systemic vascular disease. The same risk factors that contribute to coronary artery disease, such as smoking, diabetes, hypertension, and hyperlipidemia, also contribute to carotid artery disease and atherosclerotic changes in the aorta, especially in the ascending aorta. Atheroma in the aorta can present with calcified plaques or with "cheese like" soft plaques, which can be disrupted (dislodged) during: (1) cannulation of the ascending aorta for CPB, (2) cross-clamping in general; and/or (3) side-clamping of ascending aorta for attachment of proximal anastomoses of bypassed grafts. The mobilized plaques can then cause microembolization or macroembolization of brain vessels, resulting in neurologic deficits [22, 23].

In the last 15 years less invasive CABG has emerged with the goal to minimize or eliminate complications that may occur relative to each or all of the above four steps commonly used in conventional CABG. The initial efforts were made to avoid CPB by performing CABG without CPB, i.e., off-pump CABG (OPCABG). Subsequent efforts were made to avoid full sternotomy by performing OPCABG via left thoracotomy (minimally invasive direct coronary artery bypass, MIDCAB). About 5 years ago endoscopic Robot was subsequently introduced to facilitate MIDCAB. More recently a hybrid approach to treat CAD with Robotic assisted CABG (Rob-CABG) and drug eluting stents (Hybrid Rob CABG) has been started in a few centers in the US.

OPCABG

In contrast to conventional CABG, OPCABG is performed without CPB. Special instruments are employed to stabilize the targeted vessel when the heart is beating. The instruments are composed of a suction cup to hold the heart to a desirable position and a myocardium stabilizer to compress the area of myocardium where the targeted coronary vessel is located. Compared to conventional CABG lower dose of Heparin is administered to achieve a goal ACT of 300–400 s.

A pair of elastic tapes are encircled proximally and distally to the site of arteriotomy of targeted artery. The artery is temporally occluded and a 6 mm arteriotomy is made. An intracoronary shunt can be placed to enhance visualization of the target lumen and to maintain distal myocardium perfusion which can be crucial in performing bypass to a vessel supplying a large territory of myocardium. The anastomotic sewing technique and sutures used in OPCABG are similar to that in conventional CABG. The graft length and positioning and proximal anastomosis of OPCABG are similar to that of conventional CABG. One main challenge of OPCABG is to maintain hemodynamic stability during positioning of the heart to expose the target vessel. Anesthetic management plays an important role in stabilizing the patient's hemodynamics during OPCABG. Close communication between surgeon and anesthesiologist is essential for the success of the surgery.

An increasing number of studies, including prospective randomized studies, have demonstrated that when compared to conventional CABG, OPCABG procedures result in: (1) a lower incidence of postoperative neurologic deficits; (2) fewer blood transfusions; (3) shorter intubation times; (4) less release of cardiac enzyme; (5) less renal insult; (6) shorter ICU stays; (7) less release of cytokines IL8 and IL10; and/or (8) lower mortality [21, 24–26]. It should be noted that the difference in these parameters between OPCABG and CABG procedures mostly ranges from 2 to 10%. In most OPCABG procedures, however, there has been the tendency to bypass fewer vessels; this may result in an incomplete revascularization. Moreover, certain anatomic locations and the nature of target coronary arteries may preclude safe and reliable anastomoses with OPCABG, e.g., arteries located in the posterolateral wall of hypertrophied hearts, intramyocardial arteries, and severely calcified arteries. Furthermore, with today's available methodologies, OPCABG is more challenging technically for most cardiac surgeons. It should also be noted that emergency conversion of OPCABG to conventional CABG because of hemodynamic instability carries a significantly higher morbidity and mortality rate than conventional CABG (about 6 times higher mortality); fortunately the overall conversion is rare, with a rate of only 3.7% [27].

Though OPCABG surgery took off rapidly in the earlier part of the last decade, the initial enthusiasm for OPCABG has cooled down in recent years due to the lack of highly anticipated "drastic" clinical benefits of OPCABG over conventional CABG and the additional technical challenges the surgeons have to face. Currently OPCABG comprises 20–25% of all CABG procedures performed in the US which has not changed much compared to 5 years ago. Yet although isolated centers perform virtually all CABG procedures off pump, in many centers OPCABG is a seldom-used procedure. Such a large discrepancy appears to be from the lack of effective education of practicing surgeons and a steep learning curve to master the tricks of performing OPCABG.

Aortic Nontouch Technique

Several methodologies have been described to avoid disrupting plaques when working in the region of the ascending aorta. For example, topical ultrasound devices have been used to identify hidden plaques, especially the soft types. In addition, a single aortic cross-clamp technique has been shown to reduce the risk of plaque disruption during conventional CABG surgery [28].

Aortic cross-clamping or side-clamping can be avoided by using proximal anastomotic devices during OPCABG. Boston Scientific Inc.'s Heartstring proximal seal system is a facilitator for proximal hand-sewn suture anastomosis. It temporarily occludes aortotomy during direct suture anastomosis of the proximal vein graft to the aortotomy; yet, to date, one of the major drawbacks of its use is that the suture can catch the device, which requires that the anastomosis be redone.

A newer proximal anastomotic device, PAS-Port (Cardica Inc., Redwood City, CA) has obtained FDA approval for use after encouraging success from a multicenter clinical trial. Its impact on the long-term patency rate of the grafts has yet to be determined.

Totally aortic "nontouch" techniques have been described that can be applied during OPCABG by using: (1) bilateral in situ internal mammary arteries; (2) sequential grafts; (3) in situ gastroepiploic arteries; (4) radial artery Y or T grafts from internal mammary arteries; (5) radial artery or vein grafts from innominate, subclavian, axillary arteries; or (6) descending thoracic aorta (Fig. 22.10). Currently, nontouch techniques during OPCABG are gaining popularity, especially in high-risk patients. Nevertheless, given limited patient numbers and short follow-up times, the long-term graft patency rate for the latter procedures remains unknown.

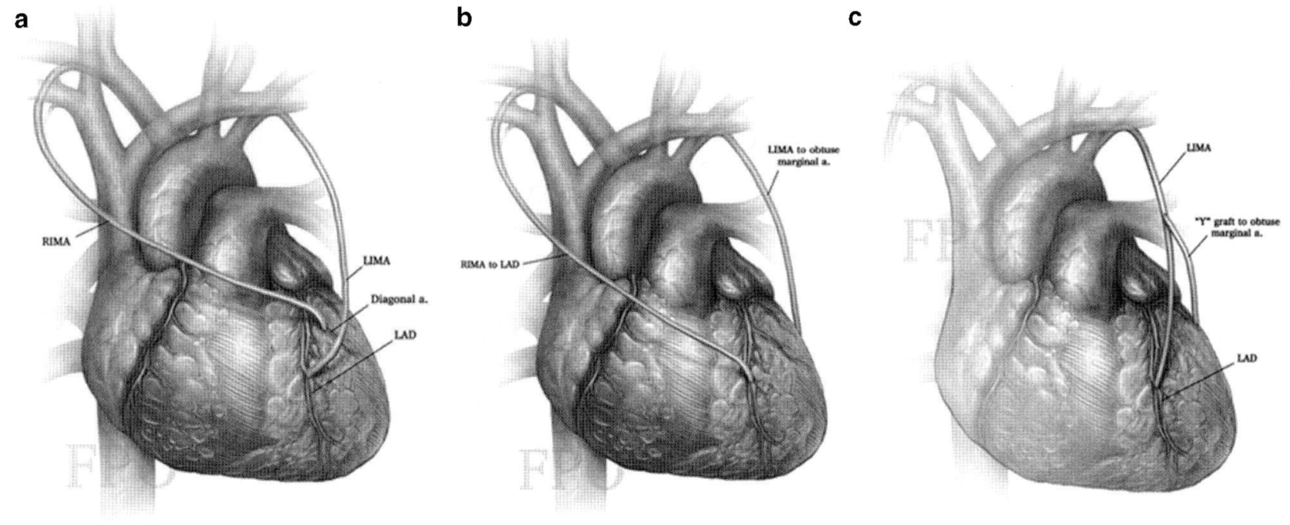

Fig. 22.10 Different configurations of internal mammary artery (IMAs) used in CABG to ensure aortic "nontouch" technique, which can be achieved with Robotic assistance. (**a**) LIMA to LAD and RIMA to Diagonal artery; (**b**) LIMA to Obtuse marginal artery and RIMA to LAD; (**c**) LIMA to LAD and 'Y' grant to Obtuse marginal artery

MIDCABG and Robotic Assisted CABG

For years, the physical and emotional impact of a large incision on the individual patient has been ignored by most cardiac surgeons. Historically, adequate exposure of the target tissues or organs through large incisions took priority over concern about incision size; this mindset remained unchallenged until the early 1990s. Subsequently, with novel specially designed instruments, experience with laparoscopic surgery demonstrated that those surgical procedures traditionally performed through large incisions could actually be accomplished with much smaller incisions. The patient benefits of small incisions have been clearly shown; advantages include: less pain, quicker recovery, lower infection rate, shorter hospital stays, and/or better quality of life. In some studies, less immune function disturbance has also been reported.

Encouraged by positive results from the laparoscopic surgical community, some cardiac surgeons began to adopt less invasive approach to perform CABG. MIDCAB was developed in the mid 1990s with the intent to avoid sternotomy and perform CABG through a limited left anterior thoracotomy [29]. The LIMA is harvested under direct vision and anastomozed to LAD with beating heart. MIDCAB is typically performed off-pump via an 8–10 cm incision and it can be performed with peripherally inserted CPB support as well if needed. If done properly it can minimize surgical trauma by sparing the sternum and avoiding CPB. Medium-term LIMA patency rates were similar to those achieved with CABG [11]. The limited thoracotomy preserves sternal integrity and allows for a more rapid return to daily activities. More important, the avoidance of CPB reduces the immune response, preserves blood components, and improves postoperative neurocognitive function as compared with CABG. However, due to the lack of appropriate instruments to facilitate LIMA harvesting via the limited access, the harvesting of LIMA posed a significant technique challenge upon most cardiac surgeons. Sometimes poor exposure compromised the length of LIMA graft and the thoracotomy incision was too large to cause longer than expected postoperative discomfort. The drawbacks in this technique in early MIDCAB probably hampered the widespread adoption of this approach.

In recent years, Intuitive Surgical's daVinci robotic system (Fig. 22.11) has made significant improvement in cardiothoracic surgery and has made operating inside the chest cavity possible [12, 13, 30–32]. Its second generation Robot is smaller and more user friendly. It has a "third arm" (one more than the first generation) for clinical use. Its 3D visualization, 7° of endo-wrist motion, and capability to eliminate human hand tremors facilitate fine dissecting, cutting, and suturing tasks. The second generation of robotic system has made both IMA takedown and OPCABG surgery via thorocoscopy or minithoracotomy easier. It can precisely locate the target vessel and correlate it to the overlying intercostal space thus making it possible to perform direct anastomosis between LIMA and LAD possible via a tiny incision and achieving true non-rib-spreading mini-thoracotomy (Figs. 22.12–22.19).

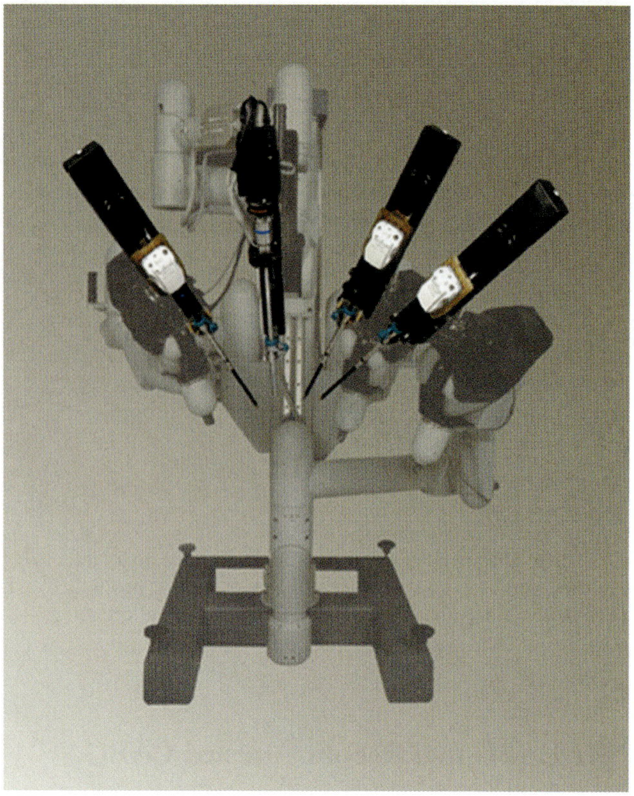

Fig. 22.11 Intuitive Surgical Da Vinci Robot instrument cart with four robotic arms

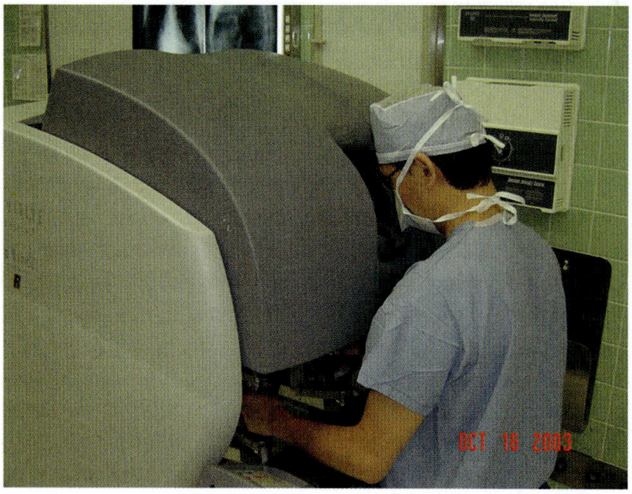

Fig. 22.12 The surgeon operates the Robot instruments at the console

Additional complementary innovations have been required to allow for robotic surgery on the heart. For example, to make OPCABG surgery easier when it is performed via minithoracotomy or total endoscopic robotic approaches, an "endo suction device" and an "endo myocardium stabilizer" (Medtronic, St Paul, MN) have been developed to position the heart and stabilize the target artery through port accesses (Fig. 22.20). Other devices that are currently available for robotic assisted or total endoscopic Robotic graft anastomosis are the distal anastomotic devices such as C-Port Flex A™ (Cardica Inc., Redwood City, CA) and endo "U" clip (Medtronic, St Paul, MN). The employment of such devices will lead the way in moving toward total endoscopic CABG surgery.

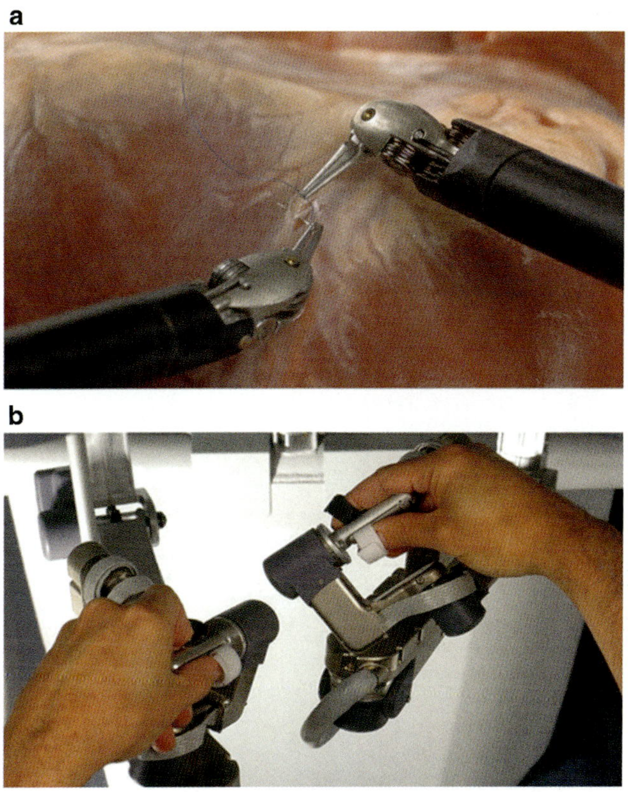

Fig. 22.13 (**a**) Surgeon's view at the top of console and (**b**) surgeon's hands controlling the robotic instruments

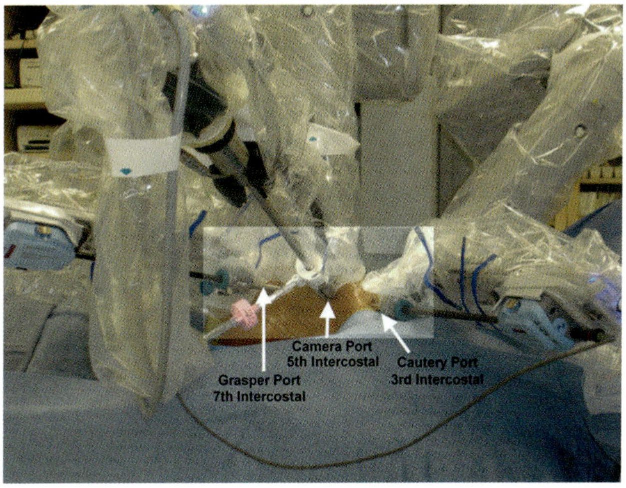

Fig. 22.14 The patient's left chest is exposed and the head is to the *right* of the photo. A camera is inserted in the center port and the robotic cautery spatula and grasper are inserted at the proximal and distal ports respectively. The instruments are connected to the instrument cart which is positioned to the patient's right side. Note that the three ports are placed along the same line slightly medial to the anterior axillary line

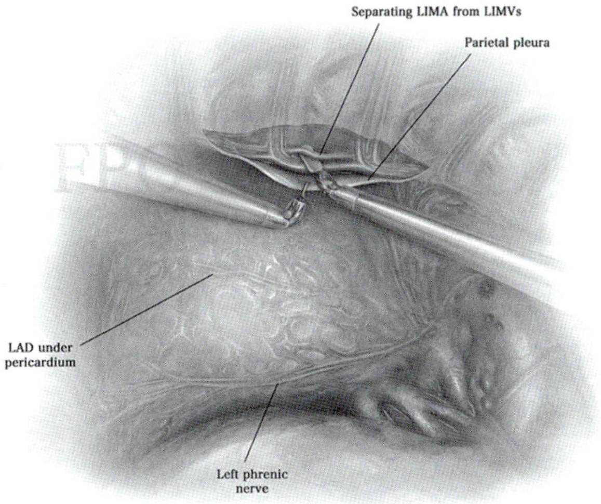

Fig. 22.15 The skeletonized LIMA harvesting technique is shown here. With the microvascular grasper in the left arm and the cautery spatula in the right arm the pleura over the LIMA is opened. The LIMA is separated from its accompanying vein using a spatula with blunt dissection. The vein adjacent to the artery (*below*) is pushed away from the artery

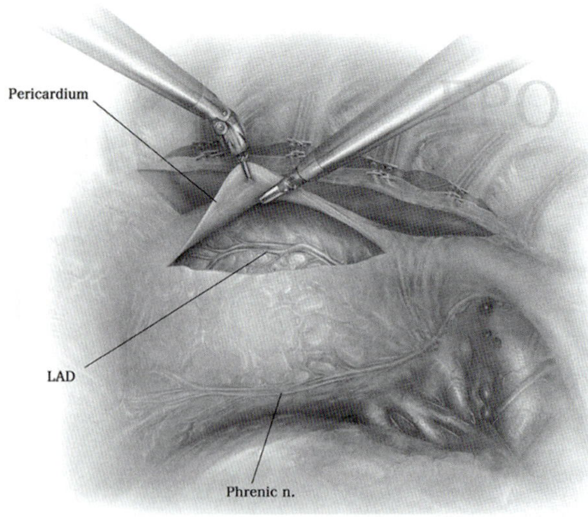

Fig. 22.16 The pericardium is opened longitudinally. The target vessels (LAD and Diagonal) are visualized. The target segment for bypass grafting is located and a spinal needle is inserted into the corresponding intercostal space from the outside chest wall

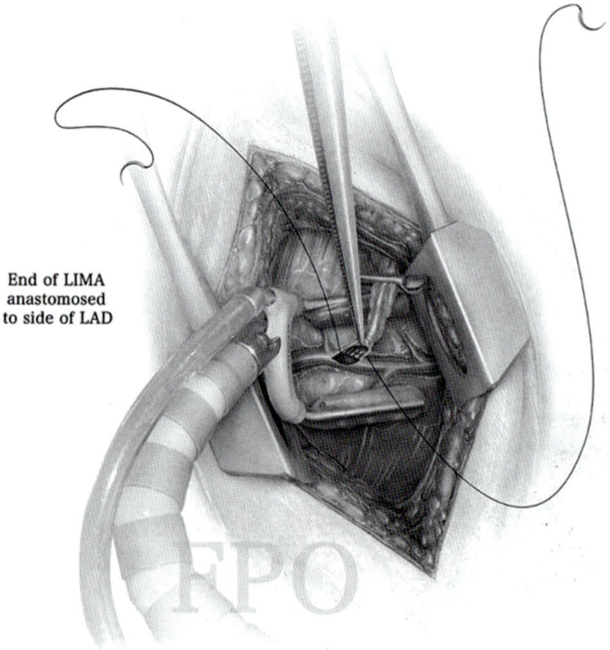

Fig. 22.17 A 5–6 cm left mini thoracotomy is made over the target segment of LAD. A small retractor is placed to gently open the rib space. An epicardial stabilizer is placed over the target LAD segment and the LAD is occluded with elastic vessel loops. LAD is opened and the LIMA is anastomozed to the LAD off pump with an 8-0 prolene suture in a running suture fashion, similar to off pump sternotomy technique

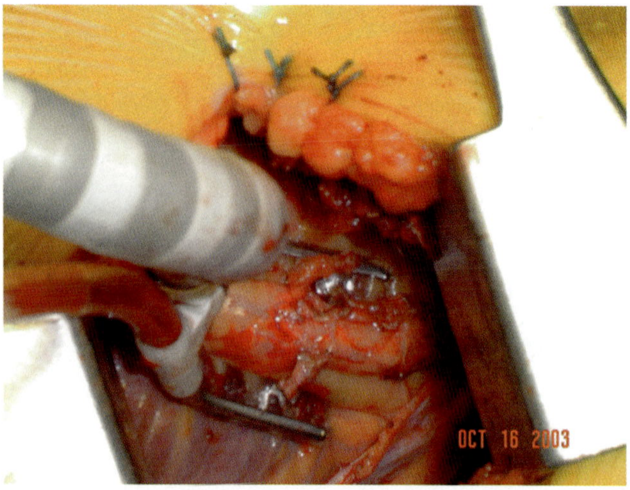

Fig. 22.18 An "octopus" myocardium stabilizing device (Medtronic, St Paul, MN) is used to steady the coronary artery during direct bypass grafting anastomosis

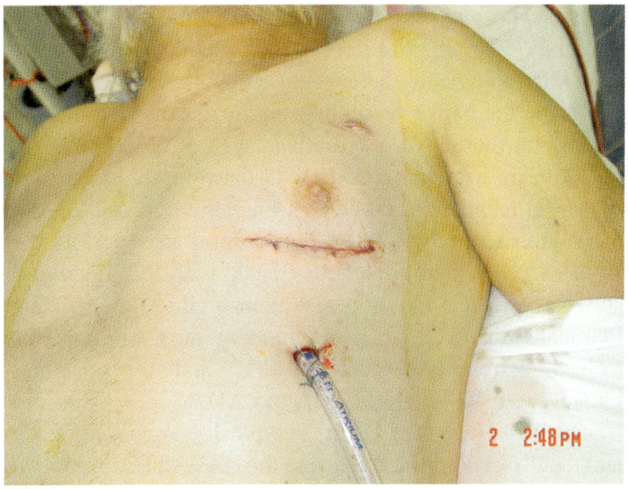

Fig. 22.19 The typical skin incision and chest tube placement after a RCAB with either LIMA to LAD or LIMA and RIMA to LAD and other left CABG

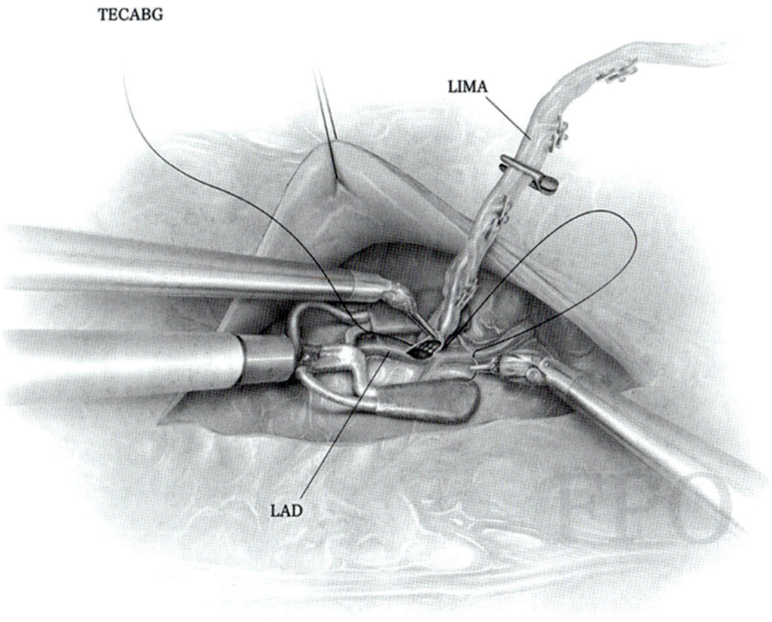

Fig. 22.20 TECAB with robotic anastomosis of LIMA to LAD with a 7-0 prolene suture. A robotic epicardial stabilizer which is held by the fourth arm is placed to stabilize LAD via the subxyphoid port. The robotic grasper holds the tip of LIMA and the needle holder places the suture through the LIMA and LAD. The LAD is temporally occluded with elastic vessel loops

CABG vs. PCI

The two primary interventions for patients with multivessel CAD are CABG and PCI. CABG with the use of LIMA and saphenous veins as bypass conduits is considered the treatment of choice for three-vessel or left main coronary artery disease. Literature has shown, when compared to PCI, CABG has advantages of improved patient event-free survival and less re-intervention rate in patients with three-vessel CAD, diabetes, and decreased left ventricular function [33, 34]. Recently reported landmark randomized multicenter clinical trial (SYNTAX Trial) [35] comparing CABG and PCI with drug-eluting stents in treating "all-comer" CAD has shown that rates of major adverse cardiac or cerebrovascular events at 12 months were significantly lower in the CABG group than in the PCI group. The advantages of CABG over PCI are attributed mainly to the use of in situ LIMA bypass to the LAD. The use of LIMA to LAD grafting is the most remarkable achievement in coronary artery surgery since CABG's introduction in 1968. In the past 3 decades, numerous studies have confirmed that the patency rates of LIMA grafts are excellent with patency rates over 90% even after 15 years of implantation. They result in an improvement in survival of 10–30% and greater freedom from major cardiac events, as compared with the rates in patients whose bypass surgery was performed with vein grafts only. An important feature of this arterial conduit is relative immunity from atherosclerosis, a characteristic not found in either native coronary arteries or saphenous-vein grafts [36]. LIMA is biologically better than either saphenous veins or stents including drug-eluting stents. Only progressive arterial disease in the native vessel beyond the distal anastomosis will compromise the results, and that occurs infrequently.

Despite the above stated advantages of CABG over PCI, including drug-eluting stents, PCI has sharply increased in recent years in treating CAD with three-vessel or left main lesions, mostly because of its minimally invasive nature and improved technology especially since the introduction of drug-eluting stents in 2003. In 2006, a total of 253,000 CABG procedures and 1,131,000 PCI procedures were performed in the US, with drug-eluting stents used in 90% of the PCI [37]. In the SYNTAX trial, patients treated with PCI involving drug-eluting stents had similar rates of death from any cause, stroke, or myocardial infarction compared to the CABG group (7.6% for PCI and 7.7% for CABG). Patients undergoing PCI were more likely than those undergoing CABG to require repeat revascularization (13.5% vs. 5.9%) but were less likely to have a stroke (0.6% vs. 2.2%). The long-term patency rate of drug-eluting stents remains unknown at present, but is unlikely to match that of LIMA to LAD.

The invasiveness of CABG is typically composed of sternotomy, CPB, and manipulation of ascending aorta. Sternotomy and the dissection of LIMA from the chest wall are associated with bleeding, wound infection, most notably in patients with diabetes and delayed recovery. CPB and manipulation of ascending aorta can cause systemic inflammatory reaction and stroke.

Hybrid Rob CABG

Rob-CABG utilizes the state-of-art Robotic technology and harvests the pedicled LIMA and RIMA if needed via three 1 cm trocar ports. The operative field visualization is enhanced by a 10× magnification 3D scope. The coronary target vessel is fully visualized and labeled before direct LIMA to LAD is performed via a 2–3 in. left anterior intercostal incision without sternotomy, CPB, and manipulation of the ascending aorta, thus eliminating the potential complications associated with conventional CABG. LIMA to LAD anastomosis can also be performed with total endoscopic robotic approach with only port accesses [38]. The limitation of Rob-CABG is that non-LAD vessels are difficult to access due to small intercostal incisions.

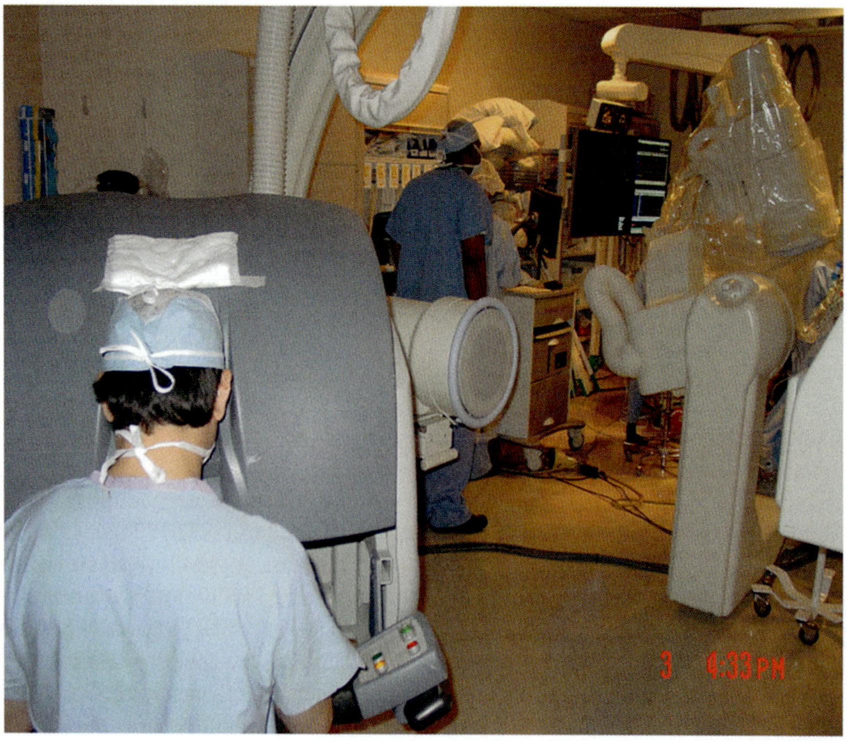

Fig. 22.21 Surgeon is performing Robotic assisted hybrid surgery in the cathlab

The main limitations in treating CAD with three-vessel or left main lesions with the current standard approaches are either being "too" invasive upfront as in CABG or "less" effective in long-term patency as in PCI. Though conventional CABG, OPCABG, MIDCAB, Rob-CABG, and PCI each has its advantages and disadvantages, a hybrid Rob-CABG/PCI approach combining the minimally invasive LIMA to LAD bypass, the best part of CABG and PCI with drug eluting stents which are equivalent or superior to saphenous vein grafts to the non-LAD coronaries might be the best approach to treat CAD with three-vessel or left main lesions.

Hybrid Robotic PCI offers an attractive option of minimally invasive coronary revascularization. At present only a few centers in the US have started such hybrid approach in treating CAD (Fig. 22.21). Initial experience including ours has being encouraging. Hybrid Rob PCI appears to have less major adverse cardio/cerebrovascular events (MACCE), shorter recovery time, and less total cost when compared to OPCABG in treating multivessel CAD [39, 40].

With almost 1.5 million/year coronary revascularization procedures being performed in the US, and the continually increasing use of these procedures due to an aging population, it is imperative that we identify the optimal coronary intervention strategies that reduce the morbidity, risks, and costs of these procedures. Hybrid Robotic PCI approach appears to offer the best service of both cardiology and cardiac surgery.

References

1. Sones Jr FM, Shirey EK. Cine coronary arteriography. Mod Conc Cardiovasc Dis. 1962;31:735.
2. Favaloro RG. Saphenous vein graft in the surgical treatment of coronary artery disease: operative technique. J Thorac Cardiovasc Surg. 1969;58:178.
3. Green GE, Stertzer SH, Reppert EH. Coronary artery bypass grafts. Ann Thorac Surg. 1968;5:443.
4. Kolessov VI. Mammary artery-coronary artery anastomosis as method of treatment for angina pectoris. J Thorac Cardiovasc Surg. 1967;54:535.
5. CASS Principal Investigators and Their Associates. Coronary artery surgery study (CASS): a randomized trial of coronary artery bypass surgery: survival data. Circulation. 1983;68:939.
6. European Coronary Surgery Study Group. Long-term results of prospective randomized study of coronary artery bypass surgery in stable angina pectoris. Lancet. 1982;2:1173.
7. Loop FD, Lytle BW, Cosgrove DM, et al. Influence of internal mammary artery grafts on 10 year survival and other cardiac events. N Engl J Med. 1986;314:1.
8. Cameron A, Davis KB, Green G, Schaff HV. Coronary bypass surgery with internal-thoracic-artery grafts – effects on survival over a 15-year period. N Engl J Med. 1996;334:216–9.
9. Eagle KA, Guyton RA, Davidoff R, et al. ACC/AHA 2004 guideline update for coronary artery bypass graft surgery: summary article, a report of the American College of Cardiology/American Heart Association task force on practice guidelines (committee to update the 1999 guidelines for coronary artery bypass graft surgery). Circulation. 2004;110:1168–76.
10. DiSesa VJ, O'Brien SM, Welke KF, et al. Contemporary impact of state certificate-of-need regulations for cardiac surgery, an analysis using the Society of Thoracic Surgeons' national cardiac surgery database. Circulation. 2006;114:2122–9.
11. Calafiore A, Giammarco GD, Teodori G, et al. Midterm results after minimally invasive coronary surgery (last operation). J Thorac Cardiovasc Surg. 1998;115:763–71.
12. Subramanian V, Patel NU, Patel NC, et al. Robotic assisted multivessel minimally invasive direct coronary artery bypass with port-access stabilization and cardiac positioning: paving the way for outpatient coronary surgery? Ann Thorac Surg. 2005;79:1590–6.
13. Oehlinger A, Bonaros N, Schachner T, et al. Robotic endoscopic left internal mammary artery harvesting: what have we learned after 100 cases? Ann Thorac Surg. 2007;83:1030–4.
14. Cosgrove DM, Sabik JF, Navia JL. Minimally invasive valve operations. Ann Thorac Surg. 1998;65:1535–9.
15. Svensson LG. Minimally invasive surgery with a partial sternotomy "J" approach. Semin Thorac Cardiovasc Surg. 2007;19(4):299–303.
16. Zilla P, Fasol R, Groscurth P, et al. Blood platelets in cardiopulmonary bypass operations. J Thorac Cardiovasc Surg. 1989;97:379.
17. Ko W, Hawes AS, Lazenby WD, et al. Myocardial reperfusion injury. J Thorac Cardiovasc Surg. 1991;102:297.
18. Sladen RN, Berkowity DE. Cardiopulmonary bypass and the lung. In: Gravlee GP, Davis RF, Utley JR, editors. Cardiopulmonary bypass. Baltimore, MD: William & Wilkins; 1993. p. 468.
19. Tuman KJ, McCarthy RJ, Najafi H, et al. Differential effects of advanced age on neurologic and cardiac risks of coronary artery operations. J Thorac Cardiovasc Surg. 1992;104:1510.
20. Abel RM, Buckley MJ, Austen WG, et al. Etiology, incidence and prognosis of renal failure following cardiac operations: results of a prospective analysis of 500 consecutive patients. J Thorac Cardiovasc Surg. 1976;65:32.
21. Ascione R, Lloyd CT, Underwood MJ, et al. Inflammatory response after coronary revascularization with or without cardiopulmonary bypass. Ann Thorac Surg. 2000;69:1198–204.
22. Stump DA, Newman SP. Embolic detection during cardiopulmonary bypass. In: Tegler CH, Babikian VL, Gomez CR, editors. Neurosonology. St. Louis, MO: Mosby; 1996. p. 252–5.
23. Goto T, Baba T, Matsuyama K, et al. Aortic atherosclerosis and postoperative neurological dysfunction in elderly coronary surgical patients. Ann Thorac Surg. 2003;75:1912–8.
24. Cleveland JC, Shroyer AJ, Chen AY, et al. Off-pump coronary artery bypass grafting decrease risk-adjusted mortality and morbidity. Ann Thorac Surg. 2001;72:1282–9.

25. Diegeler A, Doll N, Rauch T, et al. Humoral immune response during coronary artery bypass grafting: a comparison of limited approach, "off-pump" technique, and conventional cardiopulmonary bypass. Circulation. 2000;102:III95–100.
26. Reston JT, Tregear SJ, Turkelson CM. Meta-analysis of short-term and mid-term outcomes following off-pump coronary artery bypass grafting. Ann Thorac Surg. 2003;76:1510–5.
27. Edgerton JR, Dewey TM, Magee MJ, et al. Conversion in off-pump coronary artery bypass grafting: an analysis of predictors and outcomes. Ann Thorac Surg. 2003;76:1138–42.
28. Tsang JC, Morin JF, Tchervenkov CI, et al. Single aortic clamp versus partial occluding clamp technique for cerebral protection during coronary artery bypass: a randomized prospective trial. J Card Surg. 2003;18:158–63.
29. Subramanian V, Stelzer P. Clinical experience with minimally invasive coronary artery bypass grafting (CABG). Eur J Thorac Cardiovasc Surg. 1996;10:1058–63.
30. Loulmet D, Carpentier A, d'Attellis N, et al. Endoscopic coronary artery bypass grafting with the aid of robotic assisted instruments. J Thorac Cardiovasc Surg. 1999;118:4–10.
31. Bonatti J, Schachner T, Bonaros N, et al. Technical challenges in totally endoscopic robotic coronary artery bypass grafting. J Thorac Cardiovasc Surg. 2006;131:146–53.
32. Argenziano M, Katz M, Bonatti J, et al.; TECAB Trial Investigators. Results of the prospective multicenter trial of robotically assisted totally endoscopic coronary artery bypass grafting. Ann Thorac Surg. 2006;81:1666–75.
33. Booth J, Clayton T, Pepper J, et al. Randomized, controlled trial of coronary artery bypass surgery versus percutaneous coronary intervention in patients with multivessel coronary artery disease: six-year follow-up from the Stent or Surgery Trial (SoS). Circulation. 2008;118:381–8.
34. Daemen J, Boersma E, Flather M, et al. Long-term safety and efficacy of percutaneous coronary intervention with stenting and coronary artery bypass surgery for multivessel coronary artery disease: a meta-analysis with 5-year patient-level data from the ARTS, ERACI-II, MASS-II, and SoS trials. Circulation. 2008;118:1146–54.
35. Serruys P, Morice M, Kappetein A, et al. Percutaneous coronary intervention versus coronary-artery bypass grafting for severe coronary artery disease. N Engl J Med. 2009;360:961–72.
36. Loop F. Internal-thoracic-artery grafts – biologically better coronary arteries. N Engl J Med. 1996;334:263–5.
37. Lange RA, Hillis LD. Coronary revascularization in context. N Engl J Med. 2009;360:1024–6.
38. Srivastava S, Gadasalli S, Agusala M, et al. Beating heart totally endoscopic coronary artery bypass. Ann Thorac Surg. 2010;89:1873–80.
39. Vassiliades TA, Douglas JS, Morris DC, et al. Integrated coronary revascularization with drug-eluting stents: immediate and seven-month outcome. J Thorac Cardiovasc Surg. 2006;131:956–62.
40. Poston RS, Tran R, Collins M, et al. Comparison of economic and patient outcome with minimally invasive versus traditional off-pump coronary artery bypass grafting techniques. Ann Surg. 2008;248:638–46.

Chapter 23
Noncoronary Surgical Therapy for Ischemic Heart Disease

Christopher B. Komanapalli, Balaji Krishnan, and Ranjit John

The natural history of coronary artery disease involves progressive atherosclerotic arteriopathy leading to eventual acute coronary syndrome. This may present classically as exertional angina leading to unstable angina, and in some patients, the only symptom is sudden cardiac death. In other patients, more complicated scenarios may present, requiring complex decision-making in order to save these critically ill patients. These presentations involve ischemic ventricular septal defects (VSDs), ventricular dyskinesia/aneurysmal changes, ventricular free wall rupture/pseudo aneurysms, and ischemic mitral regurgitation (MR).

Patients with these complications may present acutely with hemodynamic instability. They are often the most difficult to manage as they present in a moribund state with multi-organ dysfunction. Still others present in a subacute fashion, giving clinicians time to stabilize the patients and manage attendant pulmonary and renal dysfunction in order to facilitate operative management in a delayed manner. Discussion of each of these subacute scenarios follows, along with data on the most recent management strategies for these challenging situations.

Ischemic Ventricular Septal Defects

Ischemic VSDs are a rare but frequently fatal outcome of acute myocardial infarction (AMI). The incidence of these complications has been reported to be about 0.2% of all patients with AMI [1].

Presentation and Pathology of Ruptured Interventricular Septum

The occurrence of a new, pansystolic murmur in the setting of a first transmural anteroseptal or posterior myocardial infarction should create a high degree of suspicion of a ruptured interventricular septum. Sinus tachycardia and signs of right and left heart failure are usually present. Initially, clinical signs of right heart failure may predominate, with raised jugular venous pressure and acute hepatic congestion. Heart sounds become muffled and a third heart sound becomes audible only after cardiac dilatation occurs. Left heart failure can develop rapidly. The murmur is pansystolic, may be accompanied by a systolic thrill in about one-half of cases, and usually does not radiate to the apex; however, the murmur may be indistinguishable from that of acute MR.

C.B. Komanapalli, MD
Division of Cardiovascular and Thoracic Surgery, University of Minnesota Medical Center-Fairview, 420 Delaware Street SE, MMC207, Minneapolis, MN 55455, USA
e-mail: ckomanap@umn.edu

B. Krishnan, MD, MS
Department of Medicine, Division of Cardiovascular Medicine, University of Minnesota Medical Center – Fairview, Minneapolis, MN, USA

R. John, MD (✉)
Division of Cardiothoracic Surgery, University of Minnesota Medical Center-Fairview, Minneapolis, MN, USA

Z. Vlodaver et al. (eds.), *Coronary Heart Disease: Clinical, Pathological, Imaging, and Molecular Profiles*,
DOI 10.1007/978-1-4614-1475-9_23, © Springer Science+Business Media, LLC 2012

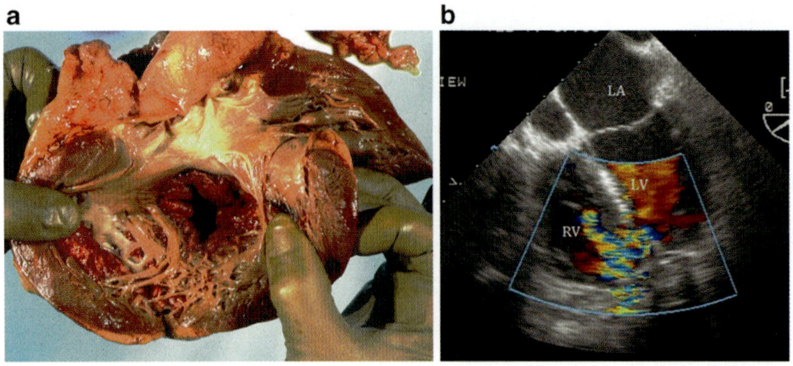

Fig. 23.1 (**a**) Gross photo of a ventricular septal rupture complicating myocardial infarction. (**b**) Gross photo of a left ventricular free wall rupture with patch for repair. (**c**) Transesophageal echocardiogram with color Doppler from the patient with ventricular apical septal rupture shows a turbulent flow jet across the septum

Classically, interventricular septal rupture may develop following a myocardial infarction in its anterior or posterior segments. Anteriorly located septal ruptures are usually associated with an anteroseptal MI and often present in the apical area as a single, transeptal defect of variable size; multiple defects are uncommon. The morphology is that of an endocardial tear with associated transmural hemorrhage leading to perforation. The defect size determines the degree of shunt from left to right ventricle. A typical rupture usually follows a fairly direct course but may zig and zag. Histologically, an anteriorly located septal rupture is usually associated with a transmural infarction.

Ruptures of the posterior septum are often associated with an extensive transmural inferoseptal MI that extends into the right ventricular wall. Involvement of the right ventricular wall makes prognosis in these cases worse than in patients with a ruptured anterior interventricular septum. Lesions may present a direct transeptal passage as described above, or may be associated with a gaping endocardial tear on the left ventricular aspect. This complicates surgical repair.

Complex septal ruptures, sometimes classified as posteroventricular ruptures, are classified separately because of their different gross morphology and different mechanics in the area of the myocardium [1]. Posteroventricular ruptures morphology differs from anterior interventricular and posterior septum ruptures because part of the right ventricle is usually infarcted. Prognosis is worse and surgical treatment may be more difficult. Typically, the pathway of the dissecting hematoma is often very long and serpiginous, passing from the endocardial tear on the inferior left ventricular wall, often at the junction of the septal wall posteriorly, and then in the posterior septal wall, sometimes in the subepicardial fat, before rupturing back into the right ventricle through its inferior wall. This lesion is very often associated with a gaping, chasm-like, left ventricular endocardial tear which extends well into the myocardium. It may have diverticular dilation along its course. Due to the difficulty associated with surgical repair, it is important to distinguish ruptures of the inferior wall with echocardiography prior to surgery.

Figure 23.1a, b shows representative pathological images of rupture of the interventricular septum complicating AMI. See Fig. 3.5 in Chap. 3 – a transthoracic echocardiographic image in a case of AMI and rupture of the interventricular septum. Figure 23.1b shows a representative transesophageal echocardiographic and color Doppler image of rupture of the interventricular septum complicating AMI.

Recently, percutaneous approaches to closure of these VSDs have been used successfully, but traditional, nonoperative management has yielded poor outcomes with as high as 85–90% mortality [2, 3]. Surgical repair, as well, is fraught with risk, with 30-day mortality as high as 21–60% [1, 4].

An operative approach to treating these lesions is similar in most series. It involves institution of cardiopulmonary bypass (CPB) followed by exposure of the VSD through a ventriculotomy. The patch may be closed using either a single- or double-patch technique or interrupted sutures alone. The ventriculotomy is typically closed using felt strips to buttress the repair. Coronary revascularization is then performed using a combination of internal mammary artery pedicled grafts and saphenous vein grafts.

A controversy in the management of these patients is the benefit of coronary revascularization in reducing short- and long-term mortality, and in improving survival. A cogent distillation of the literature on the management of ischemic VSDs with concomitant coronary bypass is presented by Perrotta and Lentini [5]. In their review of the multiple case series from 1950 to 2009, they found that coronary revascularization reduces mortality from 26.3 to 21.2% with an improvement in survival from 29 to 72%. Lundblad et al. [6] described in their series of 102 patients an improved survival in patients undergoing complete revascularization, compared to patients undergoing culprit vessel revascularization alone. Furthermore, they delineated predictors for 30-day mortality, including large AMI (by biochemical markers), large shunt (Qp/Qs > 2.5), intraoperative hemodynamic instability, long CPB time, and no revascularization of the culprit artery. Independent risk factors both at 30-day and at long-term follow-up (5 and 10 years) included incomplete revascularization and no revascularization of the culprit artery.

Ischemic Ventricular Aneurysms

Ischemic cardiomyopathy is the natural outcome of end-stage coronary artery disease. In the advanced stages of ischemic cardiomyopathy, the normal elliptical geometry of the ventricle is lost with subsequent development of a dilated globoid configuration.

Presentation and Pathology of the Ventricular Aneurysm

Clinical recognition alone of a ventricular aneurysm is difficult but clinical suspicion should be aroused in the presence of abnormal, palpable, precordial pulsation. A summation gallop may be present as well as ventricular arrhythmias. Persistent ST-segment elevation in the electrocardiogram may be shown with Q-waves. An echocardiogram must follow these findings in order to verify the diagnosis.

Post-MI aneurysms have been classified as being true, false, or pseudo [7–11]. Classically, a true aneurysm develops when some congenital or acquired process weakens the ventricular wall and allows all of it in the affected area to fall beyond the heart's normal contour. A false aneurysm develops following rupture of the heart with the resultant hemorrhage contained by fibrous pericardial adhesions or the pericardium itself.

True ventricular aneurysms have two pathogenic mechanisms. In one, the entire ventricular wall bulges beyond its usual outline. This is also called an expansion aneurysm. In this circumstance, aneurysm rupture is unlikely. Rather, the aneurysm induces intractable cardiac failure. The second type of true aneurysm forms as a result of an endocardial tear or its complications. One can draw a parallel with aortic aneurysms, mainly thoracic, resulting from a localized dissection following an intimal medial tear. Furthermore, in contrast to expansion aneurysms, the latter often has an ostium with sharply defined edges – as though punched out with a cookie cutter – that, in diameter, is less than that of the resultant aneurysm.

Histologically, an expansion aneurysm demonstrates all components of the ventricle in their wall. Endocardial tear aneurysms, however, demonstrate just myocardium and epicardium or can be confined to epicardial tissues, including epicardial coronary arteries.

Expansion aneurysms occur a few hours to days after an acute transmural MI. The pressure and contraction of the left ventricle acting on the totally or relatively immobile necrotic and structurally weak part of the ventricle may cause it to stretch thin and bulge. This remodeling alters the shape, size, and volume of the left ventricular cavity, but not the size of the MI. The extent of ventricular deformation is governed by the percentage of ventricular wall thickness that is infarcted or subsequently becomes fibrotic.

It is not clear why some transmural infarcts produce expansion aneurysms and others do not. One possibility is that their development may be related to the presence or absence of coronary collaterals. While MIs and consequent left ventricular aneurysms may occur at any site in the ventricular wall, more than 80% occur at the apex and the anteroseptal region.

False aneurysms are complications of endocardial tears that were produced by two different mechanisms. In the first, the heart ruptures, and in the second, a true aneurysm formed following an endocardial tear that subsequently ruptured into the pericardial cavity. However, with the passage of time and adaptive changes in the aneurysm wall, differentiation between the two types of false aneurysm and true and false aneurysms becomes more and more difficult histologically. False aneurysms are uncommon and differentiation may have no clinical relevance.

Right ventricular aneurysms are rare largely because of the ventricle's dual blood supply from left and right coronary arteries. Right coronary artery occlusion proximal to the origin of the acute marginal branches is associated with significant right ventricular infarction.

Figure 23.2a–c shows representative pathological images. Figure 23.2d, e shows representative transthoracic echocardiographic images. Surgical attempts to reverse this pathologic remodeling date to 1944. The first successful correction of an LV aneurysm occurred in 1957 by Dr. Charles Bailey through a left thoracotomy with a clamp placed at the base of the aneurysm, followed by aneurysmectomy and closure with a horizontal mattress suture [12]. One year later, Denton Cooley performed an aneurysmectomy on pump, which has become the gold standard technique [12].

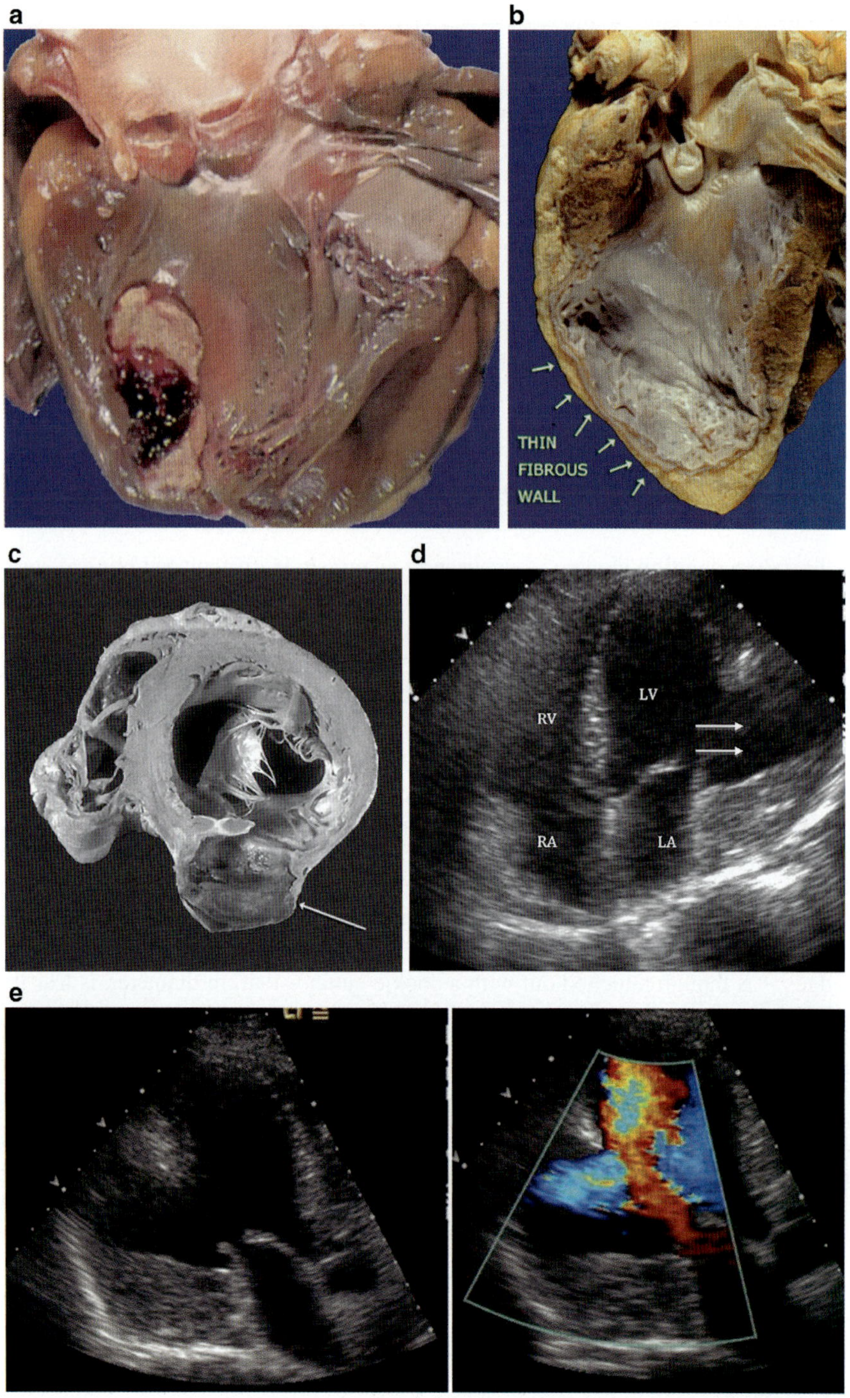

Fig. 23.2 (**a**) Left ventricular aneurysm: mural thrombus formation is often seen after myocardial infarctions, especially when a ventricular aneurysm has formed. Parts of this thrombus may embolize and cause ischemic damage, most commonly going to the brain. (**b**) There has been a previous extensive transmural myocardial infarction involving the free wall of the left ventricle. Note the thickness of the myocardial wall is normal superiorly but inferiorly is only a thin fibrous wall. (**c**) Cross section through the heart reveals a ventricular aneurysm with a very thin wall at the *arrow*. Note how the aneurysm bulges out. The stasis in the aneurysm allows mural thrombus, which is present here, to form within the aneurysm. (**d**) Echocardiogram from a patient with a lateral left ventricular aneurysm. The aneurysm is seen as an outpouching of the lateral wall as a break in the myocardial contour (*white arrows*). (**e**) Echocardiogram apical long axis view with Color Doppler from a patient with a lateral ventricular aneurysm. The *right panel* shows a large jet filling the left ventricular aneurysm

Further advances in left ventricular remodeling have involved attempts with dynamic cardiomyoplasty, with latissimus dorsi muscle wrapped around the heart. The Batista procedure, invented in 1994, involved resection of the left ventricle, but was associated with perioperative mortality and morbidity [13]. The Acorn CorCap™ cardiac support device is a ventricular cap developed to prevent further dilation of the left ventricle [14]. The newest device uses a "mannequin" to facilitate appropriate shaping of the left ventricle.

The Surgical Treatment of Ischemic Heart Failure (STICH) trial in 2001 sought to answer the question of whether patients with revascularizable coronary artery disease and a low ejection fraction (<35%) would benefit from concomitant surgical ventricular reconstruction [15]. Despite a reduction in left ventricular volume by 19%, compared to 6% alone, there was no significant reduction in mortality or freedom from readmission by adding ventricular reconstruction. Furthermore, no improvement in exercise tolerance or symptom relief was shown [15]. Limitations of the study included its lack of blind-

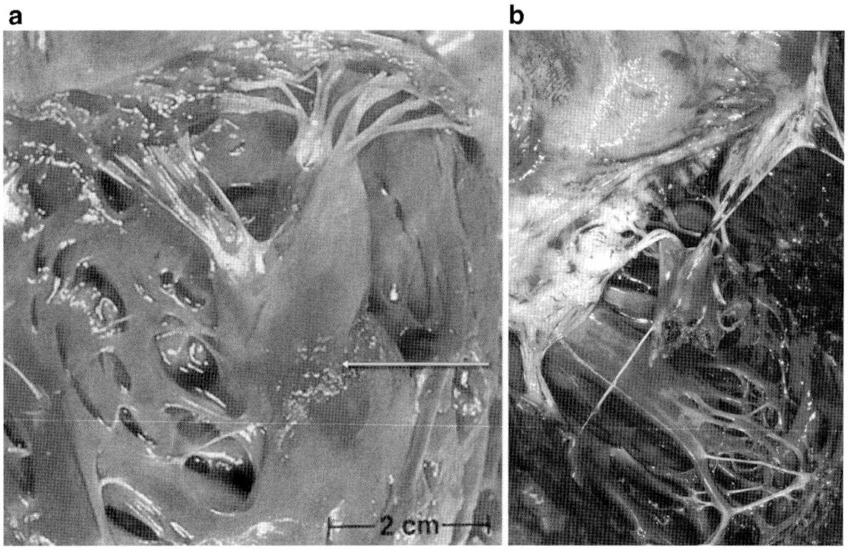

Fig. 23.3 (**a**) Mitral valve with necrotic papillary muscle in a case with acute myocardial infarction (*arrow*). (**b**) Intraoperative view of ruptured of a necrotic papillary muscle

ness procedures regarding the treating physicians' treatment arm, thus the possibility of treatment bias. Another assertion raised was a potential learning curve bias associated with poorer outcomes.

Ischemic Mitral Regurgitation

MR from papillary rupture occurs in 1 to 3% of patients with AMI, which leads to acute pulmonary edema and cardiogenic shock. Medical treatment for ischemic MR can lead to an in-hospital mortality of up to 70–80% [16, 17]. Surgical treatment of ischemic MR has an operative mortality of 19–85%. Sudden death can occur in 0.4–5% of patients following AMI due to acute ischemic MR [16].

Presentation and Pathology of Ischemic Mitral Regurgitation

Many different mechanisms cause pathological MR following an MI; some do so frequently while others are less common. Many result from pathology affecting the papillary muscle in induced papillary muscle dysfunction. They include (1) avulsion of chordae tendineae; (2) rupture of the tip of a papillary muscle; (3) rupture of the belly or base of the papillary muscle; (4), infarction of the tissues; (5) fibrosis and/or atrophy of a papillary muscle. The pathophysiology of papillary muscle rupture may involve subendocardial ischemia leading to infarction, which occurs more prominently in the posteromedial papillary muscle due to its single blood supply (80–90%) [18]. The posteromedial papillary muscle in the left ventricle seems more prone to rupture, and in most cases occurs 3–5 days after the infarct. A papillary muscle can rupture in its upper third, middle third, or at its base. Nine percent of ischemic MR involves the anterolateral papillary muscle bundle, thought to result from its dual blood supply [17, 19].

Sudden mitral insufficiency presents with the abrupt onset of acute pulmonary edema and the advent of a widely propagated apical holosystolic murmur with sinus tachycardia. The first heart sound may become inaudible, the second heart sound increases in intensity, and hypotension quickly follows. Rupture of the entire trunk of a papillary muscle is a sudden, catastrophic event resulting in severe MR followed by fulminant pulmonary edema, cardiogenic shock, and death.

Figure 23.3a, b shows representative pathological images of necrotic and ruptured papillary muscle. See Fig. 3.6a, b in Chap. 3 – echocardiographic features of rupture of a papillary muscle and "flail" mitral valve complicating AMI.

Research on the largest series of patients with ischemic MR was published by Chevalier et al. in 2004 [17]. The authors described 55 patients admitted with AMI necessitating mitral valve surgery – with roughly one-third of them needing concomitant coronary revascularization. They found a 24% operative mortality and a higher incidence of mortality in patients who did *not* undergo revascularization (34 vs. 9%). The 4-year mortality of patients who survived surgery was about 12%. Thus, the authors recommended concomitant coronary revascularization in all patients undergoing valve surgery for ischemic MR.

Ischemic Left Ventricular Free Wall Rupture/Pseudoaneurysm

Myocardial rupture is a frequently fatal and rarely salvageable complication of AMI. The incidence of rupture is between 1 and 3% in patients following AMI, with up to 20% experiencing sudden cardiac death after AMI. Patients present with one of two scenarios: (1) a "blow-out" rupture with sudden cardiovascular collapse, or (2) an oozing-type aneurysm which may present more subacutely with varying symptoms [20].

Presentation and Pathology of Free Wall Rupture/Pseudoaneurysm

With free wall rupture, the patient's condition suddenly deteriorates. Recurrent chest pain may occur. The presentation is variable, with signs of acute cardiac tamponade, sinus tachycardia, hypotension, low pulse pressure, and cyanosis of the upper half of the body, followed rapidly by cardiogenic shock, electromechanical dissociation, and death. The whole sequence of events may happen in less than 3 min.

Characteristic, new electrocardiographic changes are visible, in addition to those showing previous transmural Q-wave myocardial damage. If the condition is recognized and the physician happens to be at the bedside when the rupture occurs, the occasional patient may undergo acute relief of tamponade from a pericardiocentesis. This will lessen cardiac compression and, if time permits, a bedside echocardiogram diagnosis may encourage the cardiac surgeon to intervene immediately.

Most often, lesions cause a rapid accumulation of 150–300 mL of blood in the pericardium, producing cardiac tamponade and leading to sudden death associated with electromechanical dissociation. Rupture of the free wall is most often associated with an extensive full thickness infarct. It often occurs in patients suffering their first infarct. An acute rupture does not occur through scarred tissue. Histologically, the rupture is often associated with a very brisk inflammatory reaction in the infarcted myocardium.

The dissecting hematoma found with an acute rupture in the anterior or lateral free wall is usually not associated with a gaping endocardial tear or a diverticulum. But that is not the case when ruptures occur in the inferior wall of the left ventricle. Possibly, the buttressing of the inferior wall afforded by the diaphragm enables the variation in morphology recorded. Thus, delayed ruptures are more common in this area and ruptures of the wall may be associated with the gaping of the endocardial tear, diverticulum development, or a dissection pathway of long course. Rupture of the left ventricle following an MI is far more common than rupture of the right ventricle. The atria are ruptured most infrequently [21].

Clinically, these events are usually associated with sudden onset of a new holosystolic cardiac murmur; a palpable thrill may be obvious. Figure 23.4a–c shows representative pathological images of left ventricular free wall rupture. See Fig. 3.14 in Chap. 3 – echocardiogram features of rupture of the free wall of the LV and "false" aneurysm. In 2007, Atik et al. reported research findings from the largest series of patients with ventricular pseudoaneurysms [22]. Their group saw patients presenting a median of 50 days following infarct. Twenty-one patients were treated with concomitant coronary revascularization and/or valve surgery. Lower body mass index and greater left ventricle dysfunction were identified as risk factors for death. Mitral valve surgery, reoperation, and operation immediately following AMI were associated with increased risk of mortality.

Surgical techniques involved groin cannulation with hypothermic circulatory arrest [23].

During pericardial opening, sites for cannulation are exposed. Manipulation of the heart should only be performed following aortic cross-clamping and cardioplegia administration. After 4 weeks, fibrous tissue was tough enough to anchor sutures, and primary repair can be attempted. Operative mortality with this approach is between 25 and 35.7% [23].

Surgical repair involves infarctectomy with patch reconstruction. Recently, a sutureless approach has been developed, using a prosthetic patch and glue for "oozing-type" ruptures, and direct mattress sutures and a patch for the more "blow out" type of rupture [24].

Summary

Mechanical complications of coronary artery disease are rare but frequently may lead to poor outcomes. Salvage of these critically ill patients may be afforded by appropriate timing of surgical intervention and often aggressive medical management. While risk stratifying the most appropriate patients for these life-saving therapies is challenging, there are perioperative factors which may aid the clinician in this decision-making.

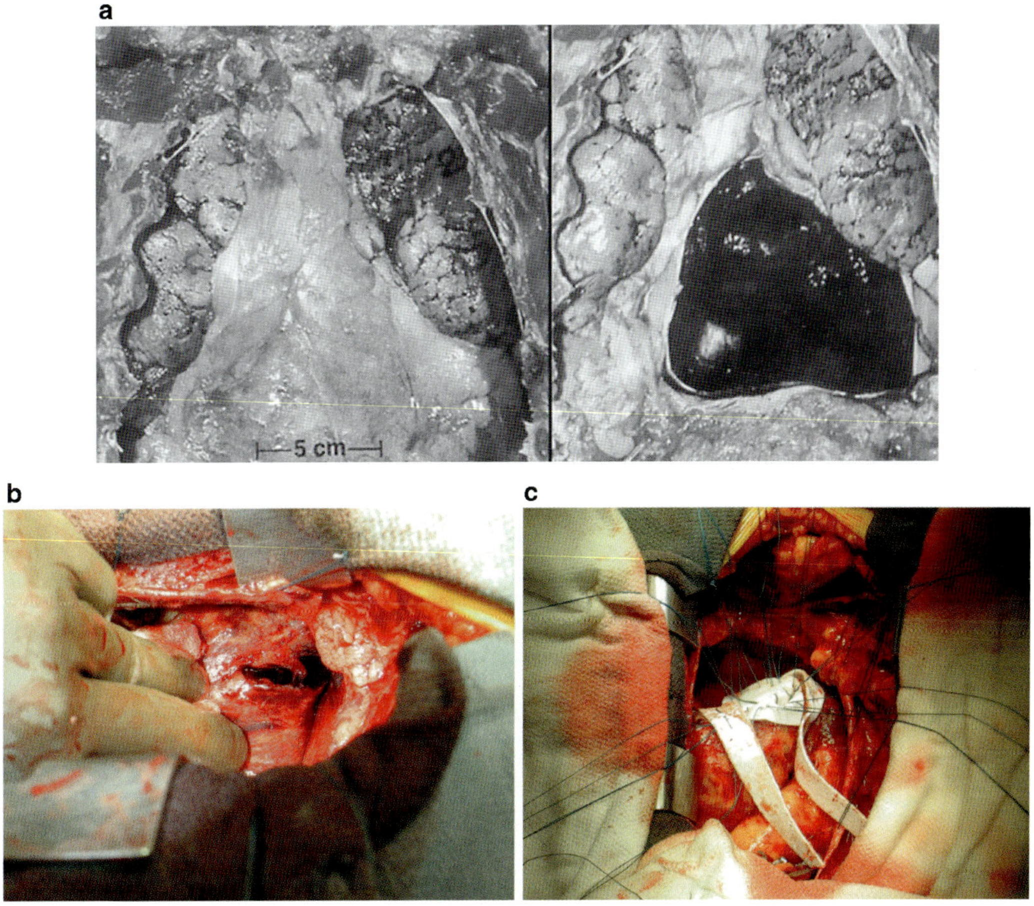

Fig. 23.4 (**a**) Gross photo of a left ventricular free wall rupture and hemopericardium in a case with acute myocardial infarction. (**b**) Intraoperative photo of a left ventricular free wall rupture prior to repair. (**c**) Intraoperative photo of a left ventricular free wall rupture with patch repair

References

1. Jeppsson A, Liden H, Johnsson P, Hartford M, Kjell R. Surgical repair of post-infarction ventricular septal defects: a national experience. Eur J Cardiothorac Surg. 2005;27(2):216–21.
2. Birnbaum Y, Fishbein MC, Blanche C, Siegel RJ. Ventricular septal rupture after acute myocardial infarction. N Engl J Med. 2002;347(18):1426–32.
3. Crenshaw BS, Granger CB, Birnbaum Y, et al. Risk factors, angiographic patterns, and outcomes in patients with ventricular septal defect complicating acute myocardial infarction. GUSTO-I (Global Utilization of Streptokinase and TPA for Occluded Coronary Arteries) Trial Investigators. Circulation. 2000;101(1):27–32.
4. Barker TA, Ramnarine IR, Woo EB, et al. Repair of post-infarct ventricular septal defect with or without coronary artery bypass grafting in the northwest of England: a 5-year multi-institutional experience. Eur J Cardiothorac Surg. 2003;24(6):940–6.
5. Perrotta S, Lentini S. In patients undergoing surgical repair of post-infarction ventricular septal defect, does concomitant revascularization improve prognosis? Interact Cardiovasc Thorac Surg. 2009;9(5):879–87.
6. Lundblad R, Abdelnoor M, Geiran OR, Sennevig E. Surgical repair of postinfarction ventricular septal rupture: risk factors of early and late death. J Thorac Cardiovasc Surg. 2009;137(4):862–8.
7. Braunwald E, Bonow R. Braunwald's heart disease: a textbook of cardiovascular medicine. Philadelphia: Saunders; 2001.
8. Cabin H, Roberts W. True left ventricular aneurysm and healed myocardial infarction. Clinical and necropsy observations including quantification of degrees of coronary arterial narrowing. Am J Cardiol. 1980;46(5):754–63.
9. Lascault G, Reeves F, Drobinski G. Evidence of the inaccuracy of standard echocardiographic and angiographic criteria used for the recognition of true and *"false"* left ventricular inferior aneurysms. Br Heart J. 1988;60(2):125–7.
10. Levin D, Fallon J. Significance of the angiographic morphology of localized coronary stenoses: histopathologic correlations. Circulation. 1982;66(2):316–20.
11. March KL, Sawada SG, Tarver RD, Kesler KA, Armstrong WF. Current concepts of left ventricular pseudoaneurysm: pathophysiology, therapy, and diagnostic imaging methods. Clin Cardiol. 1989;12(9):531–40.

12. Lee R, Hoercher K, McCarthy P. Ventricular reconstruction surgery for congestive heart failure. Cardiology. 2004;101(1–3):61–71.
13. Franco-Cereceda A, McCarthy EH, Blackstone KJ, et al. Partial left ventriculectomy for dilated cardiomyopathy: is this an alternative to transplantation? J Thorac Cardiovasc Surg. 2001;121(5):879–93.
14. Bredin F, Franco-Cereceda F. Midterm results of passive containment surgery using the acorn Cor Cap cardiac support device in dilated cardiomyopathy. J Card Surg. 2010;25(1):107–12.
15. Jones RH, Velazquez EJ, Michler RE, et al. Coronary bypass surgery with or without surgical ventricular reconstruction. N Engl J Med. 2009;360(17):1705–17.
16. Bizzarri F, Consalvo M, Massimo R, et al. Cardiogenic shock as a complication of acute mitral valve regurgitation following posteromedial papillary muscle infarction in the absence of coronary artery disease. J Cardiothorac Surg. 2008;3:61.
17. Chevalier P, Burri H, Fahrat F, et al. Perioperative outcome and long-term survival of surgery for acute post-infarction mitral regurgitation. Eur J Cardiothorac Surg. 2004;26(2):330–5.
18. Estes EH, Dalton FM, Entman ML, et al. The anatomy and blood supply of the papillary muscles of the left ventricle. Am Heart J. 1966;71(3):356–62.
19. Jouan J, Tapia M, Cook RC, Lansac E, Acar C. Ischemic mitral valve prolapse: mechanisms and implications for valve repair. Eur J Cardiothorac Surg. 2004;26(6):1112–7.
20. Kan CB, Chu IT, Chang RY, Chang JP. Postinfarction left ventricular rupture salvaged by resuscitation-induced pericardial tear. Ann Thorac Surg. 2010;89(6):2030–2.
21. Edwards J. An atlas of acquired diseases of the heart and great vessels. Philadelphia: Saunders; 1961.
22. Atik FA, Navia JL, Vega PR, et al. Surgical treatment of postinfarction left ventricular pseudoaneurysm. Ann Thorac Surg. 2007;83(2):526–31.
23. Eren E, Bozbuga N, Keles C, et al. Surgical treatment of post-infarction left ventricular pseudoaneurysm: a two-decade experience. Tex Heart Inst J. 2007;34(1):47–51.
24. Sakaguchi G, Komiya T, Tamura N, Kobayashi T. Surgical treatment for postinfarction left ventricular free wall rupture. Ann Thorac Surg. 2008;85(4):1344–6.

Chapter 24
Refractory Angina

Mohammad Sarraf, Daniel J. Hellrung, and Timothy D. Henry

Definition

The aging population and reduced mortality of patients with coronary artery disease (CAD) has resulted in an increase in patients with severe angina symptoms despite maximal medical therapy [1–3]. When further revascularization is not an option, these patients are described as "no-option" or "nonrevascularizable," but perhaps a better term is refractory angina [1–3].

The European Society of Cardiology (ESC) Joint Study Group on the Treatment of Refractory Angina [3] has defined refractory angina as "a chronic condition (≥3 months) characterized by the presence of angina caused by coronary insufficiency in the presence of CAD, which is not amenable to a combination of medical therapy, angioplasty, or coronary bypass surgery" in patients with objective evidence of ischemia. Reasons for being a poor candidate for further revascularization include diffuse atherosclerosis, unsuitable anatomy, multiple prior procedures – percutaneous coronary intervention (PCI) or coronary artery bypass graft (CABG) – lack of conduits, absence of reasonable targets for bypass surgery, significant comorbidities such as severe left ventricular (LV) dysfunction, chronic kidney disease, carotid artery disease, and advanced age. Unfortunately, despite the increasing prevalence, the American Heart Association/American College of Cardiology guidelines provide limited information regarding the epidemiology, evaluation, or treatment options for patients with refractory angina [4].

Epidemiology

Noting the limited data available from small selected cohorts or observation studies, the ESC Joint Study Group recognized "an urgent need to clarify the epidemiology of this condition" [3]. Based on a number of small trials in northern Europe, the Joint Study Group estimated the incidence of refractory angina as between 5 and 10% of patients undergoing cardiac catheterization [3]. In a retrospective analysis from the Cleveland Clinic, the incidence of patients with no-option coronary anatomy was 11.8% in a cohort of 500 consecutive patients undergoing catheterization [5]. In a more contemporary series from the Minneapolis Heart Institute, 29% of patients had incomplete revascularization, including 16% of patients who were not candidates for revascularization [6].

Considerable controversy exists regarding the prognosis for these patients, as well. In the Cleveland Clinic series, the 1-year mortality was 16.9%, but that was based on only 59 patients [7]. Using data from the Duke cardiac catheter-

M. Sarraf, MD
Cardiovascular Division, University of Minnesota Hospital, Minneapolis, MN, USA

D.J. Hellrung, MD
Mercy Hospital, Coon Rapids, MN, USA

T.D. Henry, MD (✉)
Minneapolis Heart Institute Foundation, Minneapolis, MN, USA
e-mail: henry003@umn.edu

Z. Vlodaver et al. (eds.), *Coronary Heart Disease: Clinical, Pathological, Imaging, and Molecular Profiles*,
DOI 10.1007/978-1-4614-1475-9_24,

ization database, Kandzari et al. reported a mortality rate of 38% at a median follow-up of 2.2 years in patients with severe CAD who did not undergo revascularization, compared with 15% among patients undergoing PCI and 19% for the group undergoing CABG [8]. Recently, several randomized controlled trials designed to evaluate the efficacy of alternative therapies such as transmyocardial revascularization (TMR) [9–12] and therapeutic angiogenesis [13–17] have reported a wide range of mortality from 1 to 22% up to 1 year of follow-up. Data on more than 1,200 patients with confirmed refractory angina from our dedicated refractory angina clinic and who are followed in the Options In Myocardial Ischemic Syndrome Therapy (OPTIMIST) registry demonstrate a mortality rate of 3.9% at 1 year and 28.4% at 9 years [18].

This disparity in outcomes illustrates the importance of national and international registries for systematically recording data about this disease. The registries would help clinicians understand the behavior and natural history of this challenging patient population who are left with minimal options. Nonetheless, these recent results indicate that if these patients are aggressively treated, including risk factor modification, and followed carefully in a systematic approach, long-term survival can be significantly improved.

Clinical Features

Clinical features of patients with refractory angina are similar to patients with chronic stable angina. They may exhibit angina-equivalent symptoms such as dyspnea on exertion or atypical chest discomfort. The diagnosis of ischemia is similar to patients with CAD and chronic stable angina, but can be more challenging since these patients frequently have multivessel disease, previous myocardial infarction, and previous revascularization and diabetes, and therefore, frequently have multiple areas of infarction and/or ischemia.

Understanding the pathophysiology of angina, and thus refractory angina, is essential and helps to understand the rationale for treatment. Angina pectoris results from an imbalance of myocardial oxygen requirements and supply [19]. The myocardial oxygen requirement may be elevated by an increase in one or a number of the following factors: heart rate, LV wall stress, and contractility, while myocardial oxygen supply is mainly determined by coronary blood flow and oxygen content [19]. Therefore, in evaluating these patients, it is important to search for any potential etiology that may increase the myocardial oxygen requirement independent of coronary blood flow, such as aortic stenosis and hyperthyroidism. Additionally, the endothelium of atherosclerotic coronary vessels elaborates a series of vasoconstrictors such as thromboxane A2 and serotonin, while it has an impaired endogenous or pharmacologic response to vasodilators (e.g., nitric oxide). The imbalance between vasoconstrictors and vasodilators at the level of the arterial wall may lead to a dynamic stenosis, hence angina, in the absence of an increased metabolic demand.

While the ESC definition includes only patients with severe CAD and objective evidence of ischemia, another cohort of patients who may present with refractory angina includes those with microvascular disease [20].

Patients in our OPTIMIST refractory angina clinic and the International EECP (Enhanced External Counterpulsation) Patient Registry (IEPR), which includes 7,973 patients with refractory angina, have similar clinical presentations [18, 21]. The majority are male (75–78%) with a high prevalence of cardiac risk factors, including hyperlipidemia (84–95%), hypertension (70–75%), history of smoking (67–69%), and diabetes mellitus (37–47%) [18, 21]. Additionally, previous revascularization either by CABG or PCI (87–93%), peripheral arterial disease (PAD) (23%), myocardial infarction (MI) (69–73%), congestive heart failure (CHF) (31–33%), and LV dysfunction (54%) are common and consistent with long-standing, serious CAD [18, 21].

The etiology of atherosclerosis is extensively discussed in Chap. 10.

Treatment Options

As discussed previously, myocardial ischemia occurs due to a mismatch between myocardial oxygen supply and demand (Fig. 24.1). The main determinants of myocardial oxygen consumption are heart rate, myocardial contractility, wall stress, and fatty acid uptake [19, 22]. The management of chronic stable angina is reviewed in detail in Chap. 15. Patients with refractory angina should have their cardiac risk factors treated aggressively with secondary prevention measures, and should be on an optimal regimen of antiplatelet and antianginal medications.

The following describes novel pharmacologic and nonpharmacologic approaches for patients with refractory angina.

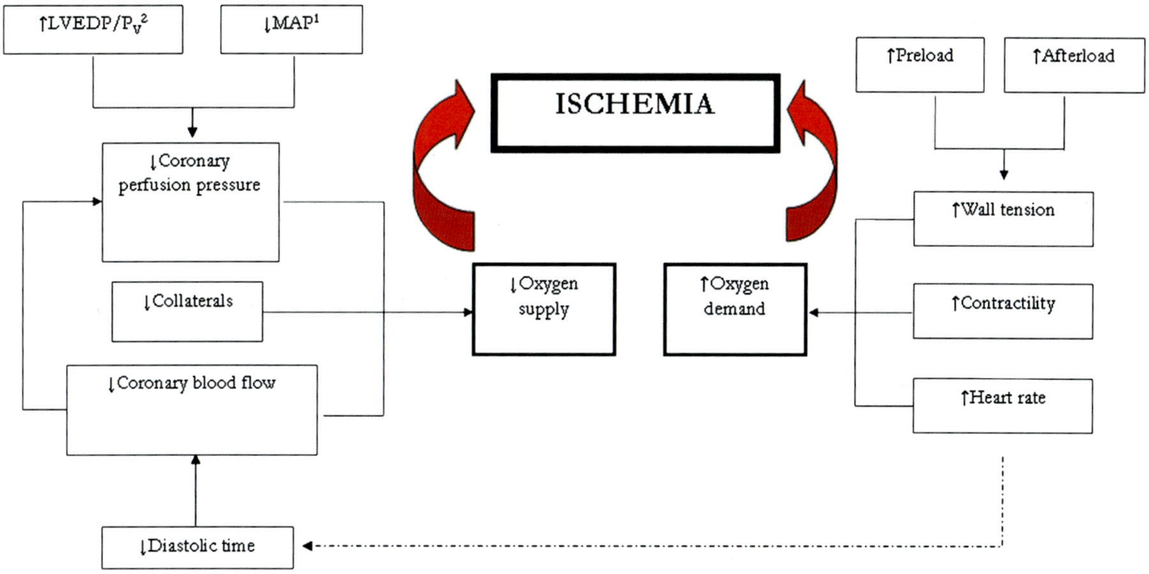

Fig. 24.1 Determinant of angina pectoris and potential therapeutic targets

Novel Pharmacologic Therapies

Conventional pharmacologic therapy of angina focuses on a reduction in heart rate, myocardial contractility, preload, and afterload. The heart uses fatty acids as a primary source of energy in the absence of ischemia, since fatty acids produce more ATP than glucose oxidation, but this occurs at the expense of higher oxygen requirement [22, 23]. During ischemia, however, this preferential source of energy utilization is shifted to glucose oxidation – which is more oxygen-efficient and, potentially, may balance the mismatch between oxygen requirement and demand. Since the heart seems to be an "omnivore" for metabolizing different sources of energy, searching for pharmacologic agents such as trimetazidine and perhexiline that divert oxidation of fatty acids to glucose or other sources of energy in patients with CAD is intriguing. Both nicorandil and ranolazine have a unique mechanism of action as well, as described below.

Trimetazidine

Metabolic-modulating agents can be classified into two broad categories: (1) free fatty acid β-oxidation inhibitors (e.g., trimetazidine) and (2) free fatty acid uptake inhibitors (e.g., perhexiline) [24] (Fig. 24.2). Trimetazidine is widely used in Europe but is not approved in the United States. It has little effect on blood pressure or heart rate. In the Trimetazidine in Angina Combination Therapy (TACT) study [25], the investigators compared the efficacy of trimetazidine to placebo in patients on combination therapy with long-acting nitrates or beta blockers. After 12 weeks of treatment with trimetazidine (20 mg orally 3 times a day), patients in the trimetazidine group had a longer exercise test duration (418 ± 14 to 507 ± 18 s vs. 435 ± 15 to 459 ± 16 s in the placebo group, $p < 0.05$) as well as the time to 1 mm ST depression (389 ± 15 to 480 ± 19 s in the treatment group vs. 412 ± 15 to 429 ± 17 s in the placebo group, $p < 0.05$). Time to onset of anginal pain, mean number of angina attacks per week, and mean consumption of short-acting nitrates per week were all decreased in favor of trimetazidine [25].

Perhexiline

Perhexiline was introduced more than 40 years ago as an antianginal agent, but its widespread use has been limited by hepatotoxicity and peripheral neuropathy [26, 27]. This molecule has a number of diverse biochemical properties (e.g., calcium and beta blocker activities), but it mainly inhibits carnitine palmitoyltransferase-1 (CPT-1) and CPT-2 (Fig. 24.2). CPT transfers the long free fatty acids across the mitochondrial membrane [26].

A "perhexiline resurgence" has occurred recently, especially in Australia and New Zealand. It appears that the liver and neurological toxicity of perhexiline is prevented by keeping the drug concentration in the range of 150–600 μg/L [26, 27]. This drug is not currently approved in Europe or the US.

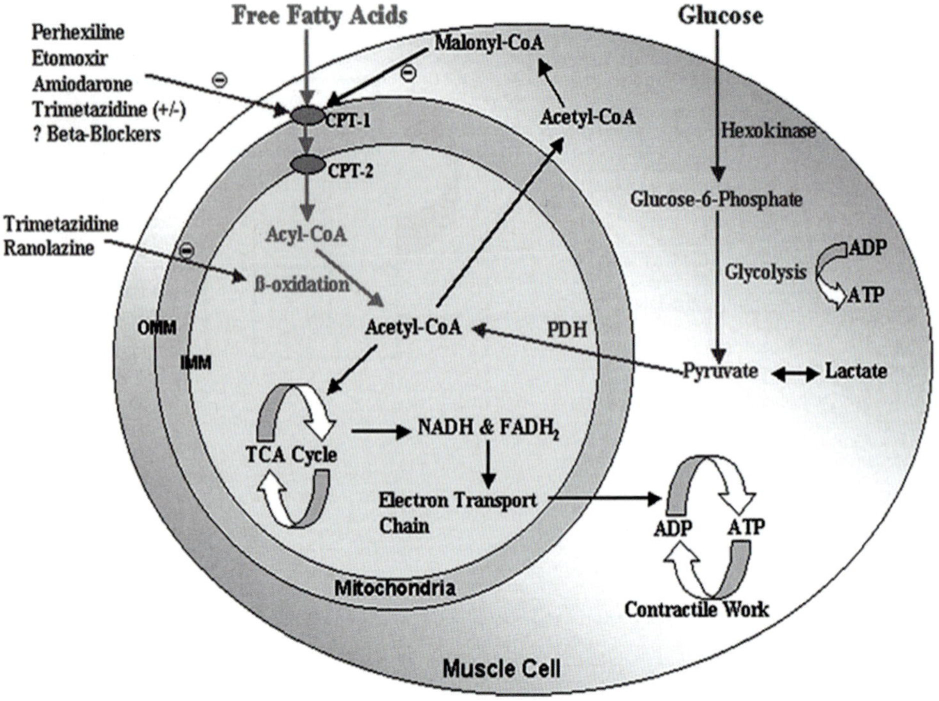

Fig. 24.2 Perhexiline's mechanism of action. By blocking the FFA uptake at the mitochondrial level, the cardiac myocyte will be forced to utilize glucose as the substrate for ATP production. From Baim and Grossman [22]. Copyright 2006

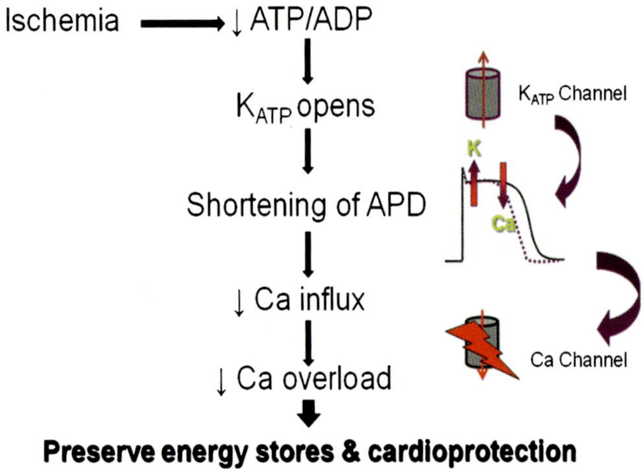

Fig. 24.3 The protective action of K_{ATP} channels during ischemia in cardiac myocytes

Nicorandil

Nicorandil has both a nicotinamide ester and a nitrate moiety, which acts as a nitrate donor that reduces preload and afterload, similar to other nitrate derivatives. In addition, it acts on the ATP – ATP-sensitive potassium (K_{ATP}) channels [28]. K_{ATP} channels couple cell metabolism with electrical activity of the plasma membrane by adjusting membrane potassium flux in response to metabolic deprivation [29]. During ischemia, K_{ATP} channels open and shorten the action potential duration, which decreases the calcium overload in the cytoplasm and conserves energy and the myocardium's ATP pool (Fig. 24.3). Therefore, nicorandil has pharmacological effects by reducing preload and afterload (through nitrate moiety), and it offers cardioprotection through conserving energy by activating K_{ATP} channels.

In the Impact Of Nicorandil in Angina (IONA) trial [30], 5,126 patients with stable angina were randomly assigned to nicorandil (20 mg orally, twice daily) or placebo, in addition to standard antianginal therapy. The primary endpoint was a composite of coronary heart disease death, nonfatal MI, or unplanned hospital admission for cardiac chest pain. The primary composite endpoint in patients treated with nicorandil was reduced by 17% (hazard ratio, HR = 0.83, 95% CI, 0.72–0.97; $p = 0.014$). Furthermore, the rate of acute coronary syndrome (ACS) was significantly lowered – by 21% – in the nicorandil-treated group (HR = 0.79, 95% CI, 0.64–0.98, $p = 0.028$) as well as a 14% reduction in all cardiovascular events (HR = 0.86, 95% CI, 0.75–0.98; $p = 0.027$) [30]. Nicorandil is currently available in Europe but not in the US.

Ranolazine

Ischemia impairs mitochondrial oxidative phosphorylation, which leads to accumulation of ischemia-driven metabolites (through activation of glycolytic pathways or lipophilic amphiphiles) that open late I_{Na} channels [31]. When these channels are activated, the cytosolic Na concentration increases and results in the efflux of Na and influx of Ca through a cell-membrane Na/Ca exchanger that causes calcium overload of the cardiac myocyte. Calcium overload contributes to increased ATP utilization (by actin–myosin filament coupling), decreases LV relaxation, and increases LV wall tension, a very important determinant of MVO2 [31–33]. In addition to the contraction–relaxation dysfunction, calcium overload may stimulate electrophysiological irritability, resulting in ventricular tachycardia or ventricular fibrillation [31, 34]. Ranolazine appears to prevent the pathophysiological consequences of ischemia by inhibiting late I_{Na} channels.

The Monotherapy Assessment of Ranolazine In Stable Angina (MARISA) trial [35], designed to determine the dose–response relationship of ranolazine, enrolled 191 patients with chronic stable angina who were randomized into a double-blind, four-period, crossover study of sustained-release ranolazine 500, 1,000, or 1,500 mg or placebo, twice daily. Duration of exercise increased with ranolazine 500, 1,000, and 1,500 mg twice daily by 94, 103, and 116 s, respectively ($p<0.005$) compared to the 70-s increase on placebo. A dose-related increase in exercise time also occurred, as well as an increase in time to 1 mm ST-segment depression ($p<0.005$) [35].

The Combination Assessment of Ranolazine In Stable Angina (CARISA) trial [36] was a double-blind, placebo-controlled, three-group parallel trial of 823 patients with symptomatic chronic stable angina, who were randomly assigned to receive placebo ($n=269$) or ranolazine 750 mg ($n=279$), or 1,000 mg ($n=275$) orally twice a day. Similar to MARISA, treadmill exercise at peak and trough levels after dosing was assessed after 2, 6, and 12 weeks of treatment. In the combined ranolazine-treated patients (750 and 1,000 mg doses), exercise duration increased by 116 s compared to 92 s in the placebo group ($p=0.01$). Time to angina and time to electrocardiographic ischemia in the ranolazine groups also increased, a finding more evident at peak than at trough. Ranolazine was able to decrease the number of angina attacks and number of sublingual nitroglycerin doses by about 1/week compared to placebo ($p<0.02$) [36].

The Efficacy of Ranolazine in Chronic Angina (ERICA) Trial [37] was a double-blind, placebo-controlled, and parallel-group study designed to assess the antianginal effects of ranolazine in comparison to a maximum dose of amlodipine (10 mg orally, once daily). The study included 565 patients with symptomatic chronic stable angina with at least three angina attacks per week. They were randomly assigned to ranolazine vs. placebo. The primary endpoint was angina frequency, which was decreased by 23% in the ranolazine-treated patients compared to placebo (mean number of angina attacks, 4.3 vs. 3.3; $p=0.028$), and supported by a decrease in nitroglycerine use by 25% ($p=0.014$) [37]. This finding was more prominent in men than women (1.3 for men and 0.3 for women).

In the Metabolic Efficacy with Ranolazine for Less Ischemia in Non-ST-segment elevation ACS – Thrombolysis in Myocardial Infarction 36 (MERLIN-TIMI-36) trial, ranolazine was tested in patients with ACS (unstable angina and non-ST elevation myocardial infarction) [38]. Ranolazine significantly reduced the incidence of recurrent ischemia vs. placebo (13.9 vs. 16.1%; HR=0.87; 95% CI, 0.76–0.99; $p=0.03$), but the primary endpoint of the study (a composite of cardiac death and recurrent ischemia) was not different between the groups. More importantly, the investigators noticed that despite an increase in QT interval, there was no increase in the incidence of malignant ventricular arrhythmias [38].

While ranolazine has not been specifically tested in patients with refractory angina, it appears to be a useful agent based on an ongoing registry of refractory angina patients. Data show that 56% of patients had a ≥2 CCS class improvement in angina symptoms [39]. Overall, ranolazine appears to be an excellent antianginal agent and well-tolerated, with the advantage of no significant effect on hemodynamics.

L-Arginine

Coronary endothelial dysfunction is one of the hallmarks of patients with angina. Thus, retaining the integrity of the vasodilator tone by mechanisms other than nitrate therapy is an important goal. As a precursor of nitric oxide, L-arginine has been proposed to improve the coronary blood flow by improving endothelium-dependent vasodilation [40].

In a study of patients with chest pain without significant CAD, Lerman et al. randomized 26 patients to L-arginine (3 g orally 3 times a day) and placebo. After 6 months of treatment, a marked increase in coronary blood flow was shown in response to acetylcholine in patients who were taking L-arginine compared to the placebo arm, and a significant decrease in plasma concentration of endothelin [41]. In a Polish study, 22 subjects with chronic stable angina were treated with L-arginine (6 g/day for 3 days), resulting in an improvement in exercise capacity. Mean exercise time increased from 501 ± 101 to 555 ± 106 s in placebo vs. 530 ± 195 to 700 ± 173 s in patients treated with L-arginine ($p<0.0002$) [42]. While there is a paucity of well-conducted randomized controlled trials using L-arginine in patients with refractory angina, the available data suggest that the use of 6–9 g of L-arginine may be effective in select patients.

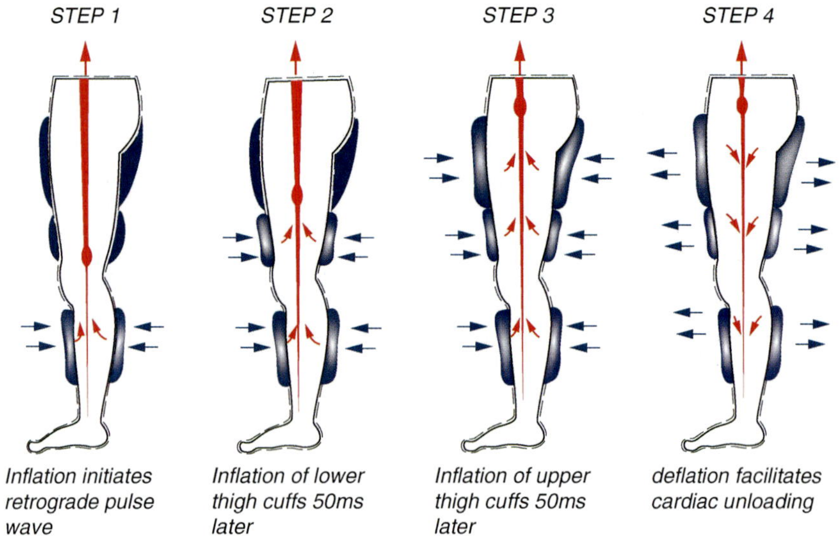
STEP 1
STEP 2
STEP 3
STEP 4
Inflation initiates retrograde pulse wave
Inflation of lower thigh cuffs 50ms later
Inflation of upper thigh cuffs 50ms later
deflation facilitates cardiac unloading

Fig. 24.4 Mechanism of action of enhanced external counterpulsation (EECP). Reprinted with permission from Institute for Progressive Medicine: www.iprogressivemed.com/therapies/eecp.html. Accessed 21 Feb 2011

Nonpharmacologic Therapies

Although effective in many cases, antianginal medications are insufficient or have side effects in a significant number of patients with severe CAD. This has stimulated the investigation of nonpharmacologic approaches for patients with refractory angina, including EECP, TMR, neuromodulation by spinal cord stimulation (SCS), or stellate ganglion blockade, and therapeutic angiogenesis using protein, gene, or cell therapy.

Enhanced External Counterpulsation (EECP)

EECP shares the same principal with intra-aortic balloon counterpulsation, which is a precisely timed diastolic pressure augmentation. Three pairs of pneumatic cuffs are placed around the lower extremities, at the level of the calves, and lower and upper thighs. An electrocardiographic trigger is synchronized to the pneumatic cuffs. With each diastole, the cuffs inflate from distal to proximal (calves to upper thighs), and with the beginning of each systole, all cuffs deflate simultaneously (Fig. 24.4). The diastolic augmentation increases coronary perfusion pressure, which results in an increase in shear stress, while the cuff deflation decreases ventricular afterload, and increases venous return [21, 43].

The randomized, placebo-controlled Multicenter Study of EECP (MUST-EECP) trial studied [44] 139 patients with refractory angina and documented CAD, using a positive exercise treadmill test to assess whether 35 h of active counterpulsation (active CP) compared to inactive counterpulsation (inactive CP) over a 4–7-week period would change the exercise duration and time to ≥1 mm ST-segment depression, and average daily anginal attack count and nitroglycerin usage. No difference in exercise duration existed between the groups ($p<0.3$), but time to ≥1 mm ST-segment depression increased significantly in active CP compared with inactive CP ($p=0.01$). Also, active-CP patients experienced a lower incidence of anginal episodes compared to inactive-CP patients ($p<0.05$). Only 10% of patients were unable to complete the therapy due to side effects [1, 44].

Furthermore, in the randomized, controlled, single-blind, parallel-group, multicenter Prospective Evaluation of Enhanced External Counterpulsation in Congestive Heart Failure (PEECH) study [45], 187 patients with ischemic (70% of cohort) and nonischemic (30% of cohort) CHF patients were randomized to 5 weeks of 1-h EECP sessions. All patients had New York Heart Association (NYHA) Functional Class II or III and a left ventricular ejection fraction <35%. There was a marked improvement in both cohorts in exercise tolerance, quality of life, and NYHA functional class without an accompanying increase in peak VO_2. The subgroup analysis of this study indicated that the benefit of EECP was greater in patients with ischemic HF [45].

A number of mechanisms have been proposed to explain the clinical benefits seen with EECP, including recruitment of myocardial collaterals through activation of vascular endothelial growth factor (VEGF) [46, 47], improvement of endothelial function [48], the release of proangiogenic cytokines, and a peripheral training effect [49]. EECP also increases nitric

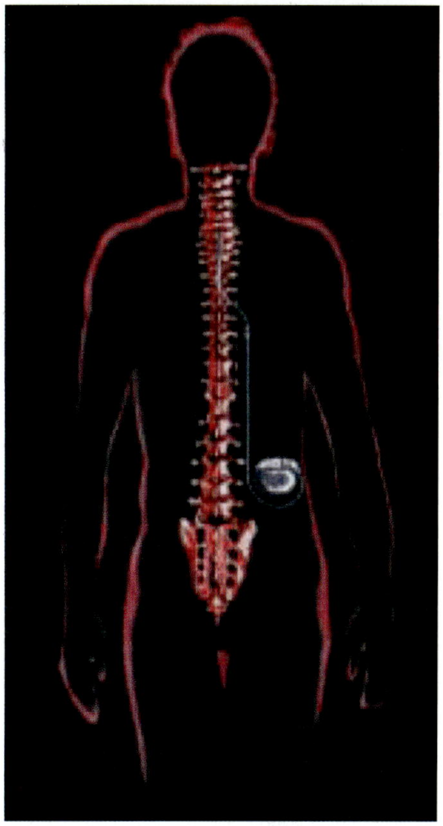

Fig. 24.5 Spinal cord stimulator system, consisting of epidural lead (C7–T1), the extension wire, and a pulse generator. From Yang et al. [75]. Copyright 2004 by Mayo Foundation for Medical Education and Research

oxide, decreases endothelin [50], and is associated with an increase in circulating CD34+ progenitor cells [51]. A number of these potential mechanisms may contribute to the observed improvement in systolic, diastolic, and mean arterial blood pressure [52]. EECP may be contraindicated in select patients with decompensated CHF, severe PAD, and severe aortic insufficiency [1, 21]. Currently, EECP is approved by the FDA and is reimbursed for the management of patients with Canadian Cardiovascular Society (CCS) III and IV refractory angina in the US. The treatment includes 35 1-h sessions over 7 weeks.

Neuromodulation

Spinal Cord Stimulation

A disparity often exists between the presence of ischemia and angina resulting from two independent phenomena: (1) presence of ischemia due to supply–demand imbalance and (2) perception of angina, which is the result of nervous system activity due to presence of ischemia [3]. Thus, it is important to understand the pain pathway and its relationship to myocardial flow.

The potential modulation of angina through the peripheral nervous system and autonomic nervous system, as well as central nervous pathways, may have therapeutic applications. Therefore, investigators have treated refractory angina using neuromodulation over the past 3 decades with transcutaneous electric nerve stimulation, left stellate ganglion blockade, and SCS. With SCS performed under local anesthesia, an electrode is placed in the epidural space, entering the T1–6 spinal cord segments. The lead is connected to a subcutaneously placed generator, which provides intermittent stimulation (Fig. 24.5). SCS decreases angina and improves myocardial ischemia through a number of proposed mechanisms, including a decrease in sympathetic tone [53], increased secretion of endorphins [54], and redistribution of myocardial blood flow from nonischemic to ischemic areas [55, 56].

Mannheimer et al. [57] randomly assigned 104 patients to SCS ($n=53$) or CABG ($n=51$). At 6-month follow-up, no difference in symptom relief was identified between the groups. Patients in the CABG group had a significant increase in exercise capacity ($p=0.02$), less ST-segment depression on maximum workloads ($p=0.005$), and an increase in the rate-pressure product ($p=0.03$) but higher mortality (13 vs. 2%, $p=0.02$) compared to patients in the SCS group. A follow-up study from the same group showed similar results up to 3 years [58].

The only randomized controlled trial stopped early due to slow enrollment. The Stimulation Therapy for Angina Refractory to Standard Treatments, Interventions, and Medications (STARTSTIM) trial randomized 68 patients with CCS III and IV to 1 min vs. 8 h of stimulation and found no difference in angina, although the trial was designed to enroll 310 patients [59]. In the US, SCS is approved for chronic pain management but not for treatment of refractory angina.

The ESC Joint Study Group indicates SCS as the preferred nonpharmacological strategy for patients with refractory angina [3]. In the US, however, SCS is approved for chronic pain management but not for treatment of refractory angina.

Left Stellate Ganglion Blockade

During normal conditions, the coronary vessels have minimal sympathetic tone; therefore, denervation of the sympathetic system has minimal effect on coronary flow in a normal physiologic state. In contrast, when ischemia is present, the interaction of ά1 (vasoconstriction) and β2 (vasodilatation) receptors on the coronary vessels becomes vital to the perfusion of myocardium. In the presence of atherosclerotic disease, the sympathetic nervous drive on the coronary vessels favors vasoconstriction, especially in the presence of dysfunctional endothelium [60, 61]. Before the development of antianginal medications, paravertebral injection of alcohol or lidocaine to block the sympathetic system was used to treat angina [3]. Although left SBG is approved in the UK for treatment of chronic refractory angina, it requires frequent injections and has significant complications, including apnea, unconsciousness, seizures, and locked-in syndrome [62], which has limited its widespread use.

Therapeutic Angiogenesis

Patients with refractory angina have advanced CAD, which is not amenable to revascularization, yet frequently they have preserved LV function due to the development of collateral blood vessels. Therapeutic angiogenesis can be defined as the use of protein growth factors, gene therapy, which encodes these growth factors or stem cell therapy to enhance the natural process of angiogenesis. Preclinical studies have demonstrated successful angiogenesis with protein, gene, and stem cell therapies in animal models [63–65]. These preliminary findings resulted in a number of clinical trials hoping to demonstrate successful therapeutic angiogenesis.

Protein Therapy

The Vascular endothelial growth factor in Ischemia for Vascular Angiogenesis (VIVA) [13] as a double-blind, placebo-controlled trial designed to evaluate the efficacy and safety of recombinant human VEGF using intracoronary and intravenous injection. Patients with stable exertional angina were randomized to receive placebo ($n=63$), low-dose rhVEGF (17 ng/kg/min, $n=56$), or high-dose rhVEGF (50 ng/kg/min, $n=59$) by intracoronary infusion on day 1 followed by intravenous infusions on days 3, 6, and 9. The primary endpoint of the study was the change in exercise tolerance time from baseline to 60 days between groups, and the secondary endpoints included a change in exercise tolerance time from baseline to 120 days, rest and exercise myocardial perfusion imaging on day 60, and an angina class as well as quality-of-life measurements at days 60 and 120 [13]. The primary endpoint was not different between rhVEGF-treated groups (low dose, 30 s; high dose, 30 s) vs. placebo-treated patients (48 s) at day 60. At the end of 120 days, the high-dose rhVEGF-treated group demonstrated significant improvement in angina class ($p=0.05$), with trends in exercise time ($p=0.15$) and improved frequency of anginal episodes ($p=0.09$) as compared with placebo or low-dose rhVEGF-treated patients [13].

The FGF Initiating RevaScularization Trial (FIRST) trial was a randomized, double-blind, placebo-controlled trial of a single intracoronary infusion of rFGF2 at 0.3, 3, or 30 μg/kg or placebo in 337 patients (placebo = 86, 0.3 μg/kg = 82, 3 μg/kg = 84, and 30 μg/kg = 85 patients) [15]. The primary efficacy endpoint was the change in exercise duration at 90 days, and the secondary endpoint included change in exercise duration at 180 days and changes from baseline to 90- and 180-day follow-up in CCS angina class and in quality of life; and ischemic changes on single-photon emission computed tomography (SPECT) imaging from baseline to 90 and 180 days [15]. Although there was no difference between placebo and rFGF2 in the primary efficacy endpoint, there was an improvement in angina at 90 but not 180 days [15].

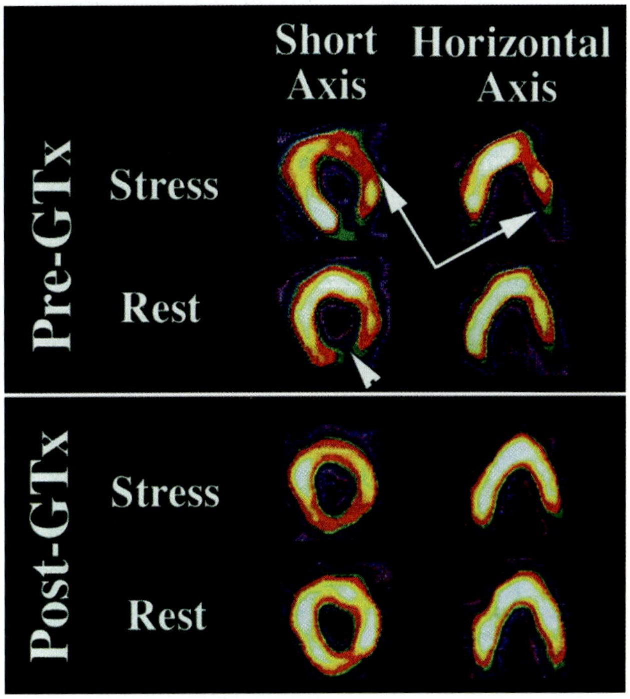

Fig. 24.6 Persantine SPECT-sestamibi scans recorded before and after phVEGF-2 gene therapy in a patient with refractory angina. From Vale et al. [76]. Copyright 2001 by American Heart Association. *Pre-GTx* before gene therapy; *post-GTx* after gene therapy

Gene Therapy

Gene therapy is a novel treatment approach in which target cells are transfected with RNA or DNA. The gene may be delivered using viral vectors (most commonly, adenovirus) or using naked DNA plasmids. When the target gene is incorporated into the genome, the cell will produce the protein of interest. Multiple different angiogenic factors have been identified, but the ones most investigated are VEGF and bFGF. Preclinical models have demonstrated clear evidence for successful angiogenesis [63, 64], but it has been more challenging to demonstrate conclusive evidence of clinical improvement in human gene therapy studies (Fig. 24.6).

A series of clinical trials known as Angiogenic Gene Therapy (AGENT trials) used intracoronary administration of an adenovirus-encoding FGF5 (Ad5FGF) to stimulate angiogenesis. The first trial (AGENT-1) studied 79 patients with refractory angina documented by coronary angiography and objective evidence of ischemia by exercise test [66]. Sixty patients received intracoronary delivery of Ad5FGF and 19 patients received a placebo. At 4 and 12 weeks follow-up, patients in the rFGF-treated group had a significantly improved exercise tolerance time compared to the group who received a placebo.

AGENT-2 randomized 52 patients in a placebo-controlled trial and demonstrated an improvement in adenosine SPECT ischemic defect size at 8 weeks (4.2% absolute reduction, $p<0.001$), while there was no change in placebo-treated patients ($p=0.32$). However, it did not result in a change in reversible perfusion defect size between treatment and placebo arms (4.2 vs. 1.6%, $p=0.14$) [67].

AGENT-3 and AGENT-4 were phase 3 studies designed to enroll more patients (450 patients in each trial) in order to determine the benefits of FGF gene therapy. The primary endpoint was the change in exercise time from baseline and 12 weeks. Both trials were designed as parallel-group, double-blind, placebo-controlled, randomized studies using two different dose groups (low dose of Ad5FGF-4, 1×10^{9} viral particles [vp], a high dose of 1×10^{10} vp, and placebo) in a 1:1:1 randomization ratio with preplanned interim analyses. Both trials were discontinued because the interim analysis showed neither study would reach statistical significance with the current design, but there was a reduction in angina class (a prespecified secondary endpoint) [17]. In a pooled analysis of AGENT-3 and -4, a substantial benefit was shown in high-risk patients – defined as those older than age 55, angina class III/IV, and baseline exercise time less than 300 s. This finding was more prominent in women [17].

The Euroinject One trial investigators randomized 80 no-option patients within CCS III to IV to receive either 0.5 mg of phVEGF-A(165) ($n=40$) or placebo plasmid ($n=40$) using electromechanical mapping and injections with the NOGA-MyoStar system in the region with established myocardial perfusion defects [14]. After a 3-month follow-up, there was no difference in myocardial perfusion defects between the VEGF-treated and placebo-treated groups (primary endpoint). But there was a statistically significant improvement in local wall motion abnormalities, assessed either by NOGA ($p=0.04$) or contrast ventriculography ($p=0.03$). The CCS classification improved in both groups, but there was no difference between the groups. Although there was no difference in the safety between the groups, five patients had complications due to the NOGA procedure [14].

A similar study in Canada, the NOGA angiogenesis Revascularization Therapy: assessment by RadioNuclide imaging (NORTHERN) trial used the NOGA system to deliver plasmid VEGF165 DNA to the LV myocardium in patients with severe ischemia who were not suitable for standard revascularization procedures using a higher dose than Euroinject [68]. The primary endpoint of the study was the change in myocardial perfusion from baseline to 3 or 6 months. The study randomized a total of 93 patients with CCS III or IV. Forty-eight patients received VEGF165. There was no difference between the VEGF-treated and the placebo groups in the primary endpoint of change in myocardial perfusion imaging, although a significant reduction in the ischemic area was demonstrated in both groups [68].

The Randomized Evaluation of VEGF for Angiogenesis (REVASC) study [16] was designed to compare the efficacy and safety of adenovirus containing $VEGF^{121}$ (AdVEGF-121) administered intramyocardially via a thoracotomy [16]. The primary endpoint of the study was exercise time to 1 mm ST-segment depression at 12 weeks. Thirty-five patients continued maximal medical therapy and 32 patients received AdVEGF-121. There was no significant difference between the groups in the primary endpoint, but the AdVEGF-121-treated group demonstrated a statistically significant improvement in time to exercise-induced ischemia at week 26 ($p=0.026$) [16]. Moreover, total exercise duration as well as time to angina improved in the AdVEGF-121-treated group compared to control at weeks 12 ($p=0.008$ and 0.006) and 26 ($p=0.015$ and 0.003) [16].

In another Canadian study, 19 patients with severe three-vessel disease and severely, diffusely diseased left anterior descending arteries received ten 200-μg injections of VEGF-165 plasmid DNA or a placebo along with oral L-arginine (6 g/day for 3 months) in a 2×2 factorial design [69]. The efficacy outcomes included changes in myocardial perfusion and contractility of the anterior myocardium, using (13)N-ammonia positron emission tomography (PET) and echocardiography at 3 months. Patients treated with a combination of VEGF and L-arginine had a significant improvement in anterior wall perfusion on PET ($p=0.02$), but the perfusion defect was not different between the groups ($p=0.10$). An improvement in anterior wall contractility also was shown ($p=0.02$) at 3 months [69]. The protein and gene therapy trials demonstrated excellent safety and some suggestions of efficacy, but definitive proof of successful therapeutic angiogenesis remains inconclusive. This simulated interest in the use of cardiovascular stem cells to provide a more potent angiogenic agent.

Stem Cell Therapy

A significant portion of coronary perfusion involves the microcirculation; evidence suggests microcirculation dysfunction in patients with chronic stable angina [20, 70, 71]. In a double-blind, randomized, placebo-controlled, dose-escalating phase I/IIa study, Losordo et al. provided evidence of safety and feasibility of percutaneous, intramyocardial injection of autologous CD-34+ cells in 24 patients with angina class III/IV [71].

This trial led to a phase II double-blind, randomized, placebo-controlled study to determine the safety and efficacy of intramyocardial injection of G-CSF mobilized auto-CD34+ cells in patients with chronic refractory angina [72]. The phase II study randomized 167 patients to 1×10^5 (low dose), 5×10^5 (high dose), or placebo. The primary outcome of the study, weekly anginal frequency at 6 and 12 months, was significantly lower in the low-dose group compared to placebo (6.8 ± 1.1 vs. 10.9 ± 1.2, $p=0.020$), an effect that was reproduced in the high-dose arm, although it did not reach statistical significance. Furthermore, a marked increase in exercise tolerance occurred in low dose compared to placebo, an effect that was also consistent with high dose [72]. This is the first double-blind, placebo-controlled trial (using any therapy) in patients with refractory angina leading to a significant improvement in exercise time.

A large phase III, multicenter, randomized, placebo-controlled trial will begin in 2011. A large number of trials are underway using a variety of cells and methods of delivery. Still, early results indicate cardiovascular stem cell therapy may well play a key role in the treatment of patients with refractory angina.

Transmyocardial Laser Revascularization (TMLR)

The use of transmyocardial laser revascularization (TMLR) for patients with refractory angina was based on the hypothesis that development of channels in the myocardium can carry blood from the ventricular cavity to the channels and, eventually, to the myocardium [2]. This observation was inspired from the reptilian heart, which has minimal epicardial arteries; a majority of myocardial perfusion occurs through channels formed between the ventricle and myocardium.

There are currently two approaches to TMR: (1) TMLR (performed epicardial during a surgical procedure) and (2) endocardial percutaneous transmyocardial laser revascularization (PTMLR). Based on a number of trials, TMLR – both standalone and in conjunction with CABG – has been approved by the FDA for the treatment of refractory angina.

Horvath et al. reported significant improvement in anginal symptoms as well as myocardial perfusion imaging in more than 75% of patients treated with TMLR up to 12 months after the procedure [73]. Frazier et al. reported a significant improvement in angina class (at least by 2 classes from CCS) and improvement of myocardial perfusion imaging in 91 patients compared to 101 patients with conventional management [11].

The Angina Treatments–Lasers And Normal Therapies In Comparison (ATLANTIC) study compared TMLR + medical therapy vs. medical therapy alone. In a group of 182 patients, those randomized to TMLR performed better according to an exercise tolerance test and they improved their anginal class [10]. In a prospective study, Allen et al. randomized 275 patients with medically treated refractory angina class IV to TMLR (132 patients) and medical therapy alone (143 patients). The primary endpoints were a change in angina symptoms, treatment failure, and a change in myocardial perfusion. After 1-year follow up, patients treated with TMLR had a marked improvement in angina (reduced by 2 classes or more) vs. medical therapy alone (76 vs. 32%, $p<0.001$). TMLR-treated patients also had better survival, free of cardiac events, freedom from treatment failure, and freedom from cardiac-related rehospitalization [9].

The successful TMLR trials led to a series of PTMLR trials using the less-invasive, percutaneous approach. The Potential Angina Class Improvement From Intramyocardial Channels (PACIFIC) trial randomly assigned 221 patients with refractory angina or severe chronic stable angina (CCS III) to PTMLR + medical therapy vs. medical therapy alone [12]. Exercise tolerance significantly improved in PTMLR patients, but there was no difference in mortality by 12 months.

These promising preliminary results were not recapitulated in the DMR In Regeneration of Endomyocardial Channels Trial (DIRECT). In this trial, 298 patients were blindly randomized to placebo PTMLR ($n=98$ patients), low-dose ($n=98$ patients, 10–15 channels), and high-dose ($n=102$ patients, 20–25 channels) PTMLR. The primary endpoint of the study was the change in exercise duration from baseline examination to 6-month follow-up. The 30-day risk of myocardial infarction was higher in the aggregate of low- and high-dose-treated patients vs. placebo (9 vs. 0, $p=0.03$).

All patients in both arms of the study had significant improvement in symptoms compared to baseline, highlighting the importance of the placebo effect [74]. The results of the DIRECT trial led to a decrease in enthusiasm for TMLR, as well, although it should be pointed out that the two approaches are not necessarily equivalent. TMLR is not recommended in patients with ACS or LV dysfunction, since morbidity and mortality is substantially higher in these patients [3].

Selected Issues

Much of the challenge in designing clinical trials in refractory angina patients lies in the blood flow measurement and the marked placebo effect of any advanced nonpharmacologic therapeutic option. Using advanced imaging (MRI or PET) in future clinical trials may enable more accurate assessment of myocardial blood flow. In addition to the pharmacologic and nonpharmacologic approaches outlined above, advances in the treatment of chronic total occlusion and novel approaches such as the coronary sinus occlusion offer hope for clinical improvement.

References

1. Jolicoeur EM, Granger CB, Henry TD, et al. Clinical and research issues regarding chronic advanced coronary artery disease: part I: contemporary and emerging therapies. Am Heart J. 2008;155(3):418–34.
2. Jolicoeur EM, Ohman EM, Temple R, et al. Clinical and research issues regarding chronic advanced coronary artery disease part II: trial design, outcomes, and regulatory issues. Am Heart J. 2008;155(3):435–44.
3. Mannheimer C, Camici P, Chester MR, et al. The problem of chronic refractory angina; report from the ESC joint study group on the treatment of refractory angina. Eur Heart J. 2002;23(5):355–70.
4. Gibbons RJ, Abrams J, Chatterjee K, et al. American College of Cardiology. American Heart Association Task Force on Practice Guidelines (Committee on the Management of Patients with Chronic Stable Angina). ACC/AHA 2002 guideline update for the management of patients with chronic stable angina – summary article: a report of the American College of Cardiology/American Heart Association Task Force on Practice Guidelines (Committee on the Management of Patients with Chronic Stable Angina). J Am Coll Cardiol. 2003;41(1):159–68.
5. Mukherjee D, Bhatt DL, Roe MT, Patel V, Ellis SG. Direct myocardial revascularization and angiogenesis – how many patients might be eligible? Am J Cardiol. 1999;84(5):598–600.
6. Williams B, Menon M, Satran D, et al. Patients with coronary artery disease not amenable to traditional revascularization: prevalence and 3-year mortality. Catheter Cardiovasc Interv. 2010;75(6):886–91.
7. Mukherjee D, Comella K, Bhatt DL, Roe MT, Patel V, Ellis SG. Clinical outcome of a cohort of patients eligible for therapeutic angiogenesis or transmyocardial revascularization. Am Heart J. 2001;142(1):72–4.
8. Kandzari DE, Lam LC, Eisenstein EL, et al. Advanced coronary artery disease: appropriate end points for trials of novel therapies. Am Heart J. 2001;142(5):843–51.

9. Allen KB, Dowling RD, Fudge TL, et al. Comparison of transmyocardial revascularization with medical therapy in patients with refractory angina. N Engl J Med. 1999;341(14):1029–36.
10. Burkhoff D, Schmidt S, Schulman SP, et al. Transmyocardial laser revascularization compared with continued medical therapy for treatment of refractory angina pectoris: a prospective randomized trial. ATLANTIC investigators. Angina treatments – lasers and normal therapies in comparison. Lancet. 1999;354(9182):885–90.
11. Frazier OH, March RJ, Horvath KA. Transmyocardial revascularization with a carbon dioxide laser in patients with end-stage coronary artery disease. N Engl J Med. 1999;341(14):1021–8.
12. Oesterle SN, Sanborn TA, Ali N, et al. Percutaneous transmyocardial laser revascularization for severe angina: the PACIFIC randomised trial. Potential class improvement from intramyocardial channels. Lancet. 2000;356(9243):1705–10.
13. Henry TD, Annex BH, McKendall GR, et al. The VIVA trial: vascular endothelial growth factor in ischemia for vascular angiogenesis. Circulation. 2003;107(10):1359–65.
14. Kastrup J, Jorgensen E, Ruck A, et al. Direct intramyocardial plasmid vascular endothelial growth factor-A165 gene therapy in patients with stable severe angina pectoris. A randomized double-blind placebo-controlled study: the Euroinject One Trial. J Am Coll Cardiol. 2005;45(7):982–8.
15. Simons M, Annex BH, Laham RJ, et al. Pharmacological treatment of coronary artery disease with recombinant fibroblast growth factor-2: double-blind, randomized, controlled clinical trial. Circulation. 2002;105(7):788–93.
16. Stewart DJ, Hilton JD, Arnold JM, et al. Angiogenic gene therapy in patients with nonrevascularizable ischemic heart disease: a phase 2 randomized, controlled trial of (AdVEGF121) versus maximum medical treatment. Gene Ther. 2006;13(21):1503–11.
17. Henry TD, Grines CL, Watkins MW, et al. Effects of Ad5FGF-4 in patients with angina: an analysis of pooled data from the AGENT-3 and AGENT-4 trials. J Am Coll Cardiol. 2007;50(11):1038–46.
18. Henry TD, Satran D, Campbell AR, et al. Long-term mortality in patients with refractory angina. J Am Coll Cardiol. 2008;51:A227.
19. Bache RJ, Dymek DJ. Local and regional regulation of coronary vascular tone. Prog Cardiovasc Dis. 1981;24(3):191–212.
20. Lanza GA, Crea F. Primary coronary microvascular dysfunction: clinical presentation, pathophysiology, and management. Circulation. 2010; 121(21):2317–25.
21. Michaels AD, McCullough PA, Soran OZ, et al. Primer: practical approach to the selection of patients for and application of EECP. Nat Clin Pract Cardiovasc Med. 2006;3(11):623–32.
22. Baim DS, Grossman W. Grossman's cardiac catheterization, angiography, and intervention. 7th ed. Philadelphia: Lippincott, Williams & Wilkins; 2006.
23. Khan SN, Dutka DP. A systematic approach to refractory angina. Curr Opin Support Palliat Care. 2008;2(4):247–51.
24. Cesar LA, Gowdak LH, Mansur AP. The metabolic treatment of patients with coronary artery disease: effects on quality of life and effort angina. Curr Pharm Des. 2009;15(8):841–9.
25. Chazov EI, Lepakchin VK, Zharova EA, et al. Trimetazidine in angina combination therapy – the TACT study: trimetazidine versus conventional treatment in patients with stable angina pectoris in a randomized, placebo-controlled, multicenter study. Am J Ther. 2005;12(1):35–42.
26. Ashrafian H, Horowitz JD, Frenneaux MP. Perhexiline. Cardiovasc Drug Rev. 2007;25(1):76–97.
27. Killalea SM, Krum H. Systematic review of the efficacy and safety of perhexiline in the treatment of ischemic heart disease. Am J Cardiovasc Drugs. 2001;1(3):193–204.
28. Yang EH, Barsness GW. Evolving treatment strategies for chronic refractory angina. Expert Opin Pharmacother. 2006;7(3):259–66.
29. Ashcroft FM. ATP-sensitive potassium channelopathies: focus on insulin secretion. J Clin Invest. 2005;115(8):2047–58.
30. IONA Study Group. Effect of nicorandil on coronary events in patients with stable angina: the impact of nicorandil in angina (IONA) randomised trial. Lancet. 2002;359(9314):1269–75.
31. Hale SL, Shryock JC, Belardinelli L, Sweeney M, Kloner RA. Late sodium current inhibition as a new cardioprotective approach. J Mol Cell Cardiol. 2008;44(6):954–67.
32. Fraser H, Belardinelli L, Wang L, Light PE, McVeigh JJ, Clanachan AS. Ranolazine decreases diastolic calcium accumulation caused by ATX-II or ischemia in rat hearts. J Mol Cell Cardiol. 2006;41(6):1031–8.
33. Takeo S, Tanonaka K, Shimizu K, Hirai K, Miyake K, Minematsu R. Beneficial effects of lidocaine and disopyramide on oxygen-deficiency-induced contractile failure and metabolic disturbance in isolated rabbit hearts. J Pharmacol Exp Ther. 1989;248(1):306–14.
34. Noble D, Noble PJ. Late sodium current in the pathophysiology of cardiovascular disease: consequences of sodium-calcium overload. Heart. 2006;92 Suppl 4:1–5.
35. Chaitman BR, Skettino SL, Parker JO, et al. Anti-ischemic effects and long-term survival during ranolazine monotherapy in patients with chronic severe angina. J Am Coll Cardiol. 2004;43(8):1375–82.
36. Chaitman BR, Pepine CJ, Parker JO, et al. Combination Assessment of Ranolazine In Stable Angina (CARISA) Investigators. Effects of ranolazine with atenolol, amlodipine, or diltiazem on exercise tolerance and angina frequency in patients with severe chronic angina: a randomized controlled trial. JAMA. 2004;291(3):309–16.
37. Stone PH, Gratsiansky NA, Blokhin A, Huang IZ, Meng L. Erica I Antianginal efficacy of ranolazine when added to treatment with amlodipine: the ERICA (efficacy of ranolazine in chronic angina) trial. J Am Coll Cardiol. 2006;48(3):566–75.
38. Morrow DA, Scirica BM, Karwatowska-Prokopczuk E, et al. Effects of ranolazine on recurrent cardiovascular events in patients with non-ST-elevation acute coronary syndromes: the MERLIN-TIMI 36 randomized trial. JAMA. 2007;297(16):1775–83.
39. Bennett NM, Arndt TL, Iyer V, et al. Ranolazine refractory angina registry trial: 1-year results [abstract]. J Am Coll Cardiol. 2011;57:E1050.
40. Egashira K, Hirooka Y, Kuga T, Mohri M, Takeshita A. Effects of L-arginine supplementation on endothelium-dependent coronary vasodilation in patients with angina pectoris and normal coronary arteriograms. Circulation. 1996;94(2):130–4.
41. Lerman A, Burnett Jr JC, Higano ST, McKinley LJ, Holmes Jr DR. Long-term L-arginine supplementation improves small-vessel coronary endothelial function in humans. Circulation. 1998;97(21):2123–8.
42. Ceremuzynski L, Chamiec T, Herbaczynska-Cedro K. Effect of supplemental oral L-arginine on exercise capacity in patients with stable angina pectoris. Am J Cardiol. 1997;80(3):331–3.
43. Sinvhal RM, Gowda RM, Khan IA. Enhanced external counterpulsation for refractory angina pectoris. Heart. 2003;89(8):830–3.
44. Arora RR, Chou TM, Jain D, et al. The multicenter study of enhanced external counterpulsation (MUST-EECP): effect of EECP on exercise-induced myocardial ischemia and anginal episodes. J Am Coll Cardiol. 1999;33(7):1833–40.

45. Feldman AM, Silver MA, Francis GS, et al. Enhanced external counterpulsation improves exercise tolerance in patients with chronic heart failure. J Am Coll Cardiol. 2006;48(6):1198–205.
46. Kersten JR, Pagel PS, Chilian WM, Warltier DC. Multifactorial basis for coronary collateralization: a complex adaptive response to ischemia. Cardiovasc Res. 1999;43(1):44–57.
47. Braith RW, Conti CR, Nichols WW, et al. Enhanced external counterpulsation improves peripheral artery flow-mediated dilation in patients with chronic angina: a randomized sham-controlled study. Circulation. 2010;122(16):1612–20.
48. Bonetti PO, Barsness GW, Keelan PC, et al. Enhanced external counterpulsation improves endothelial function in patients with symptomatic coronary artery disease. J Am Coll Cardiol. 2003;41(10):1761–8.
49. Michaels AD, Raisinghani A, Soran O, et al. The effects of enhanced external counterpulsation on myocardial perfusion in patients with stable angina: a multicenter radionuclide study. Am Heart J. 2005;150(5):1066–73.
50. Akhtar M, Wu GF, Du ZM, Zheng ZS, Michaels AD. Effect of external counterpulsation on plasma nitric oxide and endothelin-1 levels. Am J Cardiol. 2006;98(1):28–30.
51. Kiernan TJ, Boilson BA, Tesmer L, Harbuzariu A, Simari RD, Barsness GW. Effect of enhanced external counterpulsation on circulating CD34+ progenitor cell subsets. Int J Cardiol. 2010 Sep 13.
52. Campbell AR, Satran D, Zenovich AG, et al. Enhanced external counterpulsation improves systolic blood pressure in patients with refractory angina. Am Heart J. 2008;156(6):1217–22.
53. Norrsell H, Eliasson T, Mannheimer C, et al. Effects of pacing-induced myocardial stress and spinal cord stimulation on whole body and cardiac norepinephrine spillover. Eur Heart J. 1997;18(12):1890–6.
54. Eliasson T, Mannheimer C, Waagstein F, et al. Myocardial turnover of endogenous opioids and calcitonin-gene-related peptide in the human heart and the effects of spinal cord simulation on pacing-induced angina pectoris. Cardiology. 1998;89(3):170–7.
55. Hautvast RW, DeJongste MJ, Horst GJ, Blanksma PK, Lie KI. Angina pectoris refractory for conventional therapy – is neurostimulation a possible alternative treatment? Clin Cardiol. 1996;19(7):531–5.
56. Hautvast RW, Blanksma PK, DeJongste MJ, et al. Effect of spinal cord stimulation on myocardial blood flow assessed by positron emission tomography in patients with refractory angina pectoris. Am J Cardiol. 1996;77(7):462–7.
57. Mannheimer C, Eliasson T, Augustinsson LE, et al. Electrical stimulation versus coronary artery bypass surgery in severe angina pectoris: The ESBY study. Circulation. 1998;97(12):1157–63.
58. Ekre O, Eliasson T, Norrsell H, Wahrborg P, Mannheimer C. Electrical stimulation versus coronary artery bypass surgery in severe angina pectoris. Long-term effects of spinal cord stimulation and coronary artery bypass grafting on quality of life and survival in the ESBY study. Eur Heart J. 2002;23(24):1938–45.
59. Zipes DP, Svorkdal N, Breman D, et al. Spinal cord simulation therapy for patients with refractory angina who are not candidates for revascularization. Eur Heart J. 2002;23:355–70.
60. Heusch G, Baumgart D, Camici P, et al. Alpha-adrenergic coronary vasoconstriction and myocardial ischemia in humans. Circulation. 2000; 101(6):689–94.
61. Tune JD, Richmond KN, Gorman MW, Feigl EO. Control of coronary blood flow during exercise. Exp Biol Med (Maywood). 2002;227(4): 238–50.
62. Chaturvedi A, Dash HH. Locked-in syndrome during stellate ganglion block. Indian J Anaesth. 2010;54(4):324–6.
63. Henry TD. Review of preclinical and clinical results with vascular endothelial growth factors for therapeutic angiogenesis. Curr Interv Cardiol Rep. 2000;2(3):228–41.
64. Giordano FJ, Ping P, McKirnan MD, et al. Intracoronary gene transfer of fibroblast growth factor-5 increases blood flow and contractile function in an ischemic region of the heart. Nat Med. 1996;2(5):534–9.
65. Kocher AA, Schuster MD, Szabolcs MJ, et al. Neovascularization of ischemic myocardium by human bone-marrow-derived angioblasts prevents cardiomyocyte apoptosis, reduces remodeling and improves cardiac function. Nat Med. 2001;7(4):430–6.
66. Grines CL, Watkins MW, Helmer G, et al. Angiogenic Gene Therapy (AGENT) trial in patients with stable angina pectoris. Circulation. 2002;105:1291–7.
67. Grines CL, Watkins MW, Mahmarian JJ, et al. Angiogene GENe Therapy (AGENT-2) Study Group. A randomized, double-blind, placebo-controlled trial of Ad5FGF-4 gene therapy and its effect on myocardial perfusion in patients with stable angina. J Am Coll Cardiol. 2003;42(8): 1339–47.
68. Stewart DJ, Kutryk MJ, Fitchett D, et al. NORTHERN Trial I. Mol Ther. 2009;17(6):1109–15.
69. Ruel M, Beanlands RS, Lortie M, et al. Concomitant treatment with oral L-arginine improves the efficacy of surgical angiogenesis in patients with severe diffuse coronary artery disease: the endothelial modulation in angiogenic therapy randomized controlled trial. J Thorac Cardiovasc Surg. 2008;135(4):762.
70. Erbs S, Linke A, Schachinger V, et al. Restoration of microvascular function in the infarct-related artery by intracoronary transplantation of bone marrow progenitor cells in patients with acute myocardial infarction: the doppler substudy of the reinfusion of enriched progenitor cells and infarct remodeling in acute myocardial infarction (REPAIR-AMI) trial. Circulation. 2007;116(4):366–74.
71. Losordo DW, Schatz RA, White CJ, et al. Intramyocardial transplantation of autologous CD34+ stem cells for intractable angina: a phase I/ IIa double-blind, randomized controlled trial. Circulation. 2007;115(25):3165–72.
72. Losordo DW, Henry TD, Davidson C, et al. for the ACT34-CMI Investigators. Intramyocardial, autologous CD34+ cell therapy for refractory angina. Circ Res. 2011;109(4):428-36.
73. Horvath KA, Cohn LH, Cooley DA, et al. Transmyocardial laser revascularization: results of a multicenter trial with transmyocardial laser revascularization used as sole therapy for end-stage coronary artery disease. J Thorac Cardiovasc Surg. 1997;113(4):645–53.
74. Leon MB, Kornowski R, Downey WE, et al. A blinded, randomized, placebo-controlled trial of percutaneous laser myocardial revascularization to improve angina symptoms in patients with severe coronary disease. J Am Coll Cardiol. 2005;46(10):1812–9.
75. Yang EH, Barsness GW, Gersh BJ, Lerman A. Current and future treatment strategies for refractory angina. Mayo Clin Proc. 2004;79(10): 1284–92.
76. Vale PR, Losordo DW, Milliken CE, et al. Randomized, single-blind, placebo-controlled pilot study of catheter-based myocardial gene transfer for therapeutic angiogenesis using left ventricular electromechanical mapping in patients with chronic myocardial ischemia. Circulation. 2001;103:2138–43.

Chapter 25
Acute Catheter-Based Mechanical Circulatory Support

Gladwin S. Das, Ganesh Raveendran, and Jason C. Schultz

Historical Overview

With the advent of percutaneous coronary balloon angioplasty [1–3] and the increasing acceptance of PCI in the 1980s and 1990s, PCI increasingly became an option for patients with high-risk coronary anatomies. The circulatory support technology initially adopted was the intraaortic balloon pump (IABP), which was invented by Adrian Kantrowitz, M.D., and engineer Arthur Kantrowitz, PhD, in the late 1960s [4].

The IABP's initial use was in patients in cardiogenic shock, refractory heart failure, or recurrent ventricular tachycardia [4–8]. With the rapid adoption of coronary balloon angioplasty in several centers, the IABP was used to support patients with cardiogenic shock or a high-risk coronary anatomy undergoing PCIs.

The IABP effectively produces afterload reduction, increases diastolic pressure, and improves coronary blood flow [9]. By can we say markedly reducing the afterload, it decreases cardiac oxygen consumption. The balloon is inflated in diastole, thereby increasing diastolic pressure, increasing coronary blood flow, and coronary-perfusion pressure. Balloon deflation, which occurs at end-diastole, effectively reduces ventricular afterload and increases cardiac output [10].

Following the widespread adoption of the IABP during PCI, percutaneous cardiopulmonary bypass (CPB) was investigated as a technique, particularly for patients who experienced acute decompensation, those at high risk of complications, and subsequently, its prophylactic potential was evaluated in comparison to using it only emergently [11–13].

During the era of balloon angioplasty, PCI was associated with a high incidence of acute closure in intervened arteries [14, 15]. In that era, acute closure required treatment with emergent coronary artery bypass surgery for a significant proportion of patients. With the advent of coronary stents and much higher procedural success rates, the incidence of acute closure has been reduced to less than 1%. The incidence of emergency coronary artery bypass grafting is now less than 0.2% [16]. For this reason, the need for transcatheter-based circulatory support was much higher during the balloon angioplasty-only era than in the contemporary stent-dominant period. With the widespread use of coronary stents and much higher procedural success rates than balloon angioplasty, the need for circulatory support has dwindled.

Standby use of supported PCI increased in the late 1980s and 1990s. The advent of coronary stenting resulted in extremely high procedural success rates, markedly reducing the incidence of acute closure and, consequently, the need for emergent coronary artery bypass surgery. This also lowered the mortality of PCIs. Therefore, the need for percutaneous support has substantially decreased in all but three groups of patients: (1) those who present with cardiogenic shock, (2) those who experience acute hemodynamic collapse in the cardiac catheterization laboratory, and (3) and those who have high-risk coronary anatomies and/or a markedly reduced left ventricular ejection fraction. A patient is considered to have high-risk anatomy when the vessel needing intervention supplies more than half of the viable myocardium, and/or when the patient has an ejection fraction of 15–25%. When a patient has only one patent vessel or an ejection fraction of <15%, the patient is considered *very* high risk.

G.S. Das, MD • G. Raveendran, MD
Cardiovascular Division, University of Minnesota
Minneapolis, MN, USA
e-mail: dasxx007@umn.edu

J.C. Schultz, MD
University of Minnesota Medical Center-Fairview and
Minnesota Cardiovascular Division, Minneapolis, MN, USA

Z. Vlodaver et al. (eds.), *Coronary Heart Disease: Clinical, Pathological, Imaging, and Molecular Profiles*,
DOI 10.1007/978-1-4614-1475-9_25, © Springer Science+Business Media, LLC 2012

With the introduction of newer devices such as the Impella® transcatheter, axially driven impeller (Abiomed Impella®, Abiomed Inc., Danvers, MA) and the TandemHeart™ percutaneous ventricular-assist device (pVAD) (Cardiac Assist, Pittsburg, PA), high-risk patients are increasingly considered as PCI candidates. The current challenge is to develop algorithms and protocols for the appropriate use of these technologies. With increasing experience of newer technologies, we will have a better understanding of the subsets of patients where usage should be routine. The narrative that follows will describe each individual device in clinical use, the data that supports their usage, and finally, suggested protocols for their use.

Percutaneous Circulatory-Assist Devices

Intraaortic Balloon Pump (IABP)

The contemporary indications for IABP support are summarized in Table 25.1. The IABP is the first device to be used in cardiogenic shock that does not respond to pressors. This permits the patient to be stabilized before more definitive measures are adopted. In patients with refractory unstable angina, its use is largely limited to patients who are being considered for emergent bypass surgery. The IABP, which relieves angina and helps stabilize patients, is often used in high-risk angioplasty patients. IABPs can be inserted prophylactically; during procedures when patients are hypotensive and do not respond quickly to pressors, volume loading, and intravenous fluids; and also when patients experience hemodynamic collapse.

Data on the use of IABPs are limited to a number of studies that are not often randomized, evaluate smaller groups of patients, and suggest that while IABP use during PCI may be helpful, mortality reduction is not consistently shown. In a study published by Brigouri et al. in the *American Heart Journal* in 2003, 133 patients with ejection fractions <30% underwent elective PCI [17]. Sixty-one had elective preprocedural IABP support and 72 had conventional PCI. In this study, elective IABP support was found to be useful in reducing procedural complications. However, results also suggest that a high jeopardy score and female sex were determinants of adverse elective cardiac support.

Mishra et al. [18] reported that patients who undergo high-risk PCI and then receive rescue IABP for intraprocedural complications have worse outcomes than patients who receive prophylactic IABP. At 6 months, the mortality and major adverse cardiac event rates were lower in the prophylactic IAPB group (8 vs. 29%, $p<0.01$, and 12 vs. 32%, $p=0.02$, respectively). Multivariate analysis showed that prophylactic insertion of an IABP is the only independent predictor of survival at 6 months. The PAMI II trial showed that a prophylactic IABP strategy after primary PTCA in hemodynamically stable high-risk patients with AMI does not decrease the rates of infarct-related artery reocclusion or reinfarction, promote myocardial recovery, or improve overall clinical outcome [19].

The contraindications to IABP support are few and include severe aortic regurgitation, aortic dissection or aneurysm, and severe aortoiliac disease. In patients with focal, high-grade stenosis in the iliac arteries, it is possible to dilate and stent the stenosis prior to the placement of the IABP.

Use of the IABP is associated with significant complications in a proportion of patients. The incidence of complications has progressively declined over the decades. Early studies [20] reported complication rates as high as 29%. Reports from the decade prior to 2000 quote an incidence of 15% [21, 22]. With the introduction of 8 Fr systems in current practice, the complication rates are lower than historical data. Meisel et al. [23] reported in 2004 on their experience using 8 Fr sheathless IABP catheters in 161 consecutive patients. The overall complication rate was 6.6%. This included mild transient limb ischemia in two patients (1.2%), minor bleeding episodes in four patients (2.4%), one major puncture site bleeding (0.6%), a pseudoaneurysm treated percutaneously in two patients (1.2%), and limb ischemia due to embolization or local thrombosis requiring vascular intervention in two patients (1.2%). Peripheral vascular disease and female sex are important determinants of vascular complications. With the availability of low-profile systems, surgical cutdown is rarely performed for IABP insertion in our practice. The potential complications of IABP are listed in Table 25.2.

Table 25.1 Indications for IABP insertion

Cardiogenic shock
Refractory unstable angina
High-risk PCI
Postoperative hemodynamic compromise
Acute myocardial infarction with mechanical impairment as a result of mitral regurgitation or ventricular septal defect
Intractable ventricular tachycardia as a result of myocardial ischemia
Patients with left main coronary stenosis or severe three-vessel disease undergoing anesthesia for cardiac surgery
Maintenance of vessel patency after PTCA with slow flow

Adapted from Kern [10]. Copyright 2003 by Mosby Publishers, St. Louis, MO

Table 25.2 Complications associated with intraaortic balloon pump use

Vascular complications
Bleeding
Limb ischemia
Compartment syndrome
Arterial dissection
Groin hematoma
Embolic events
Cerebrovascular accident
Bowel infarction
Renal infarction
Emboli to extremities
Infection
Balloon rupture or failure
Aortic rupture
Death

Adapted from Hasdai et al. [60]. Copyright 2002 by Humana Press

Percutaneous Cardiopulmonary Bypass

In the cardiac catheterization laboratory, circulatory support can be established utilizing percutaneous CPB [24]. Percutaneous CPB implies a system of femoral-femoral bypass and requires the placement of a 20 or 21 Fr venous cannula in the right atrium and a 17 Fr arterial cannula though the femoral artery in the aorta. During femoral–femoral bypass, patients are fully heparinized. Long sheaths are passed over stiff guidewires with progressively larger dilators and then are connected to a primed pump oxygenator. Blood is drawn using an external centrifugal pump and passes through a membrane oxygenator before being pumped back into the arterial system. Blood flow rates of 3.5–5 L/min can be achieved.

Because large cannulae are necessary, one significant concern is the need for a patent iliac system without significant tortuosity or stenosis. In order to ensure the absence of significant peripheral vascular disease that may contraindicate cannula placement, pre-CPB diagnostic aortography and arteriography are essential. Initial experience with this technology required surgical cutdowns for the introduction of the large-bore cannulae. However, the procedure soon evolved to percutaneous introduction of these large-bore cannulae, permitting rapid establishment of systemic support. Following prophylactic CPB support in patients with high-risk anatomies and subsequent heparin elimination, cannulae can be pulled with manual support. Alternately, femoral arteries can be surgically repaired. If necessary, patients can be assisted by femoral-femoral bypass for up to 6–12 h.

CPB's advantage is that it is not dependent on a cardiac rhythm: patients with recurrent ventricular fibrillation or even asystole can be adequately supported. Reports show that patients at extremely high risk of adverse hemodynamic complications in the cardiac catheterization laboratory can be safely supported by CPB [24–27]. Patients with severe unstable angina and dilatable lesions, target vessels supplying more than half the residual, viable, left-ventricular myocardium or a left-ventricular ejection fraction <25% were selected for a national registry of supported PCI.

In the era prior to coronary stenting, studies reported that patients with low ejection fractions or single patent arteries tolerate PCI with percutaneous CPB well [24–26]. In a study of 149 patients who underwent high-risk coronary angioplasty [27], 58 underwent cardio pulmonary support (CPS) and 91 underwent IABP support prior to the angioplasty. Patients on CPS had a higher risk profile. Interestingly, the rate of major cardiac events such as myocardial infarction, bypass surgery, stroke, and death did not differ between the groups. Peripheral vascular complications such as hematomas (36 vs. 24%, $p=0.160$), vascular repair (14 vs. 3%, $p=0.03$), and transfusions (60 vs. 27%, $p=0.0001$) were higher in the CPS group. The authors concluded that either method of support may be acceptable during high-risk PTCA.

With the widespread introduction of coronary stenting and the rapid increase in procedural success rates for PCIs, there has been a marked reduction in the use of CPB for even high-risk patients. With the introduction of size 8 Fr IABP balloon catheters, the complication rates of IABP use have reduced substantially, providing a distinct advantage in its use over CPB.

However, CPB continues to have a credible role for the rapid resuscitation of "cath lab crashes" associated with persistent profound hypotension and unstable rhythms, recurrent ventricular fibrillation, or asystole. The delays are primarily related to system set-up and priming. In addition, newer technologies such as the Impella® minimally invasive, catheter-based cardiac assist device and the TandemHeart™ pVAD require no cumbersome "prep" time and are quicker to institute. However, they are dependent on a stable rhythm and some forward flow. The CPB is unique in its ability to support patients who are even in asystole or ventricular fibrillation. Hence the decision to institute CPB is one of logistics. A few cath labs have a CPB unit primed and on standby 24-7, permitting rapid institution of CPB. Newer portable CPB systems that require a set up time of a few minutes may usher in a wider use of this method of support.

Percutaneous Left-Ventricular Assist Devices

In contrast to IABPs, pVADs provide improved hemodynamic support. Comparing pVADs to surgically implanted left-ventricular-assist devices (LVADs), pVADs can be rapidly deployed and used as a bridge to recovery or surgical LVAD implantation. Two pVAD systems are approved in the USA: the AbioMed Impella® and the TandemHeart™.

Impella

Abiomed's Impella (Abiomed Inc., Danvers, MA) is a microaxial-flow, catheter-based left-ventricular-assist system. Impella produces a nonpulsatile flow, unloads the ventricle, increases cardiac output, and decreases wall stress. The Impella 2.5 is a partial support system capable of generating 2.5 L/min of output, whereas the Impella 5.0 is capable of generating 5.0 L/min of output [28]. The Impella 2.5 is inserted percutaneously and placed across the aortic valve. This device is capable of pumping blood from the left ventricle into the aorta using a turbine pump. Inflow, outflow, and the actual pump measure 12 Fr and this system is mounted on a 9 Fr delivery system (Fig. 25.1). The Impella 5.0 has a 21 Fr pump and is mounted on the same 9 Fr delivery system [29].

This system can be placed using a surgical cutdown via the femoral or axillary approach, or femoral percutaneous approach. The average time required for implantation is 10–20 min [30]. The system is FDA-approved for 6 h of use.

Implantation technique: The Impella is inserted through a size 13 Fr femoral sheath over a 0.018 Platinum Plus™ wire across the aortic valve. The patient should have systemic anticoagulation for the duration of the procedure.

Indications for impella:

1. Cardiogenic shock
   (a) Myocardial infarction
   (b) Acute myocarditis
   (c) Decompensated heart failure
2. Refractory ventricular arrhythmia
3. High-risk PCI
4. Complex electrophysiology ablation
5. Patients who fail to wean from CPB following heart surgery
6. Failed transplant patients
7. Bridge to destination therapy
   (a) Transplant
   (b) LVAD placement

The safety and feasibility of Impella 2.5 were evaluated in high-risk PCI patients in the AMC MACHI study [31]. Nineteen high-risk patients deemed poor risk for surgery underwent Impella®-assisted PCI. No device-related complications were noted in this study. Procedural success was achieved in all 19 patients with no procedural deaths. Mean decrease in hemoglobin level was 0.7 mmol/L.

In the PROTECT 1 trial [32], 20 patients underwent high-risk PCI due to poor LV function. PCI was performed in the setting of an unprotected LMCA or last patent coronary conduit. The Impella 2.5 device was implanted successfully in all patients. Mean pump flow during PCI was 2.2±0.3 L/min. None of these patients developed hemodynamic compromise during the procedure. Two patients developed transient hemolysis without clinical sequelae. Free hemoglobin in these patients ranged from 67.8 to 75.8 mg/dL; none required a blood transfusion.

The ISAR Shock trial [33] randomized 25 patients ($n=13$ IABP, $n=12$ LP 2.5) with cardiogenic shock, which revealed an increase in cardiac index (CI) of 0.49±0.46 L/min/m^2 compared to IABP of only 0.11±0.31 L/min/m^2. Overall, 30-day mortality was 46% in both groups. A recent meta-analysis comparing both pVAD to IABP showed that pVADs provide superior hemodynamic support. After device implantation with pVAD, patients had higher CI (weighted mean difference, MD, 0.35 L/min/m^2, 95% CI 0.09–0.61), higher MAP (MD 12.8 mmHg, 95% CI 3.6–22.0), and lower PCWP (MD −5.3 mmHg, 95% CI −9.4 to −1.2). However, the improved hemodynamic support did not translate into early survival for patients with cardiogenic shock, and 30-day mortality (RR 1.06, 95% CI 0.68–1.66) observed using the pVAD was similar to the IABP [34]. Using a random effect model, similar incidence of leg ischemia was noted using pVAD compared to IABP (RR 2.59, 95% CI 0.75–8.97, $p=0.13$). Hemolysis was assessed by measurements of free hemoglobin, which was significantly higher in Impella patients ($p<0.05$) [34]. PROTECT II was a randomized, multicenter trial comparing the Impella

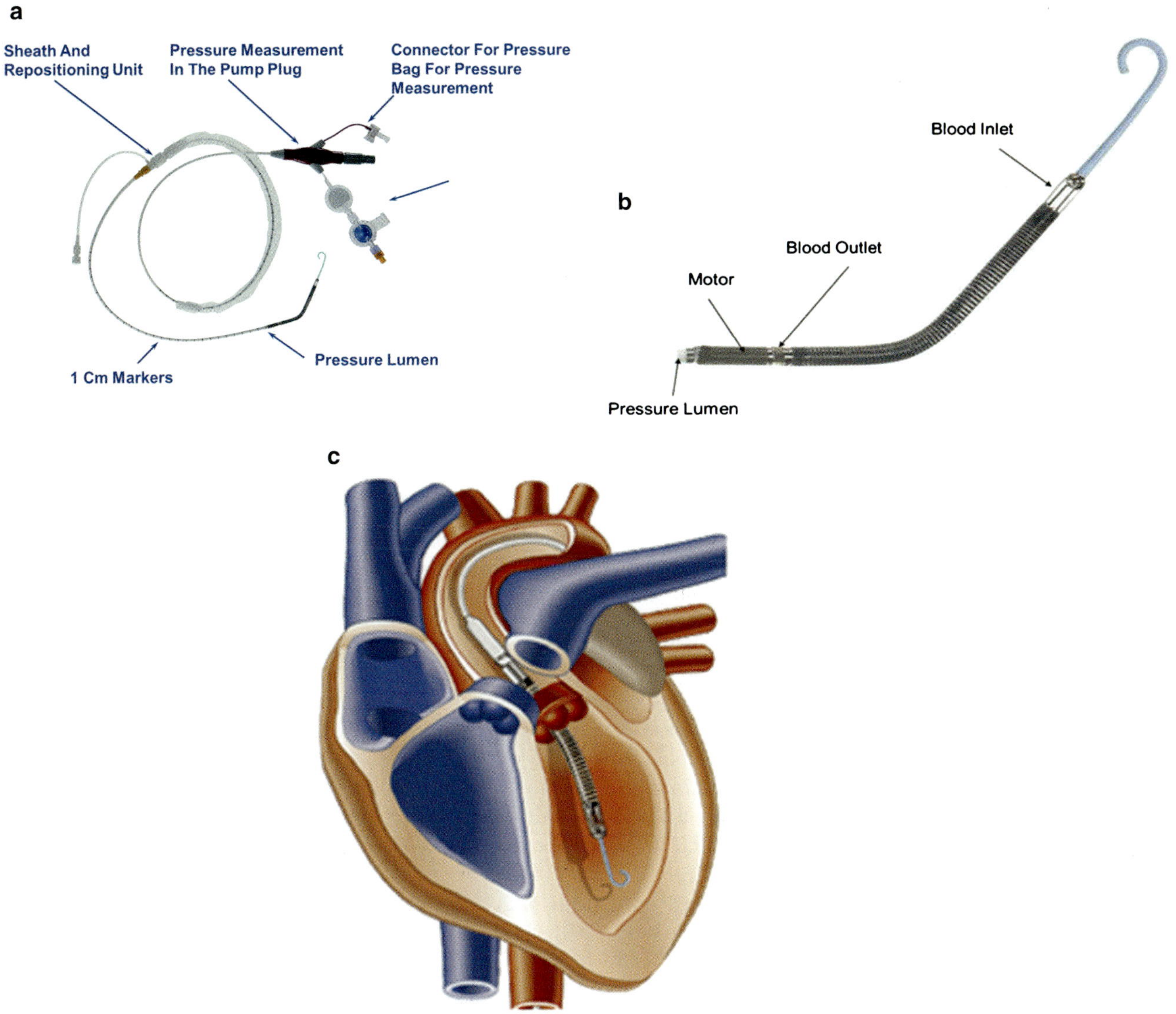

Fig. 25.1 Impella® minimally invasive, catheter-based cardiac assist device. (**a**) Catheter. (**b**) Inlet, outlet, and the pump. (**c**) Showing pump across the aortic valve

system with IABP in patients requiring hemodynamic support during nonemergent high-risk PCI in an unprotected left main coronary or the last patent conduit and an LVEF under 35% or three-vessel disease and an LVEF over 30%.Study was stopped early for futility. 426 met all the criteria to be included in the per-protocol analysis. The per-protocol analysis showed that the Impella patients had 21% fewer major adverse events at 90 days than the IABP patients (40.8% vs 51.4%; p=0.029).

Contraindications for the Impella device:

1. Mechanical aortic valve
2. Aortic valve stenosis moderate to severe
3. Severe peripheral arterial disease (PAD)
4. LV thrombus

Relative contraindications for impella:

1. Hematological disease causing cell fragility or hemolysis
2. Hypertrophic cardiomyopathy

3. Ventricular septal defect (VSD) after myocardial infarction
4. Thoracoabdominal aortic aneurysm
5. Aortic dissection

Potential impella adverse events:

1. Aortic insufficiency
2. Bleeding
3. Hemolysis
4. Perforation
5. Cerebrovascular accident (CVA)
6. Thrombocytopenia
7. Cardiac tamponade
8. Arrhythmia

TandemHeart™

The TandemHeart (Cardiac Assist, Pittsburg, PA) is a percutaneous circulatory-support device designed for short-term circulatory support. It is a centrifugal pump and is capable of generating 5 L/min cardiac output at 7,500 rpm [28, 35]. The TandemHeart is FDA-approved for 6 hours. However, it has been used for a longer duration than 6 hours in clinical practice [3, 36].

TandemHeart device setup: Like the Impella, TandemHeart is placed in the cardiac catheterization laboratory using a transseptal puncture [35–38]. A 21 Fr venous catheter is placed in the femoral vein and advanced into the left atrium (LA) through the transseptal puncture. Blood from the LA is withdrawn through this venous catheter into the pump and propelled via a magnetically driven impeller into the 17 Fr arterial cannula placed in the femoral artery (Fig. 25.2). In case the femoral artery is unfavorable, a two-14 Fr arterial system could be used [35].

A controller console continuously infuses heparinized saline into the pump, eliminating the need for systemic anticoagulation. After removal of the transseptal cannula, the residual atrial septal defect usually closes within 4–6 weeks [36]. TandemHeart also could be used as a right ventricular-assist device to drain blood from the right ventricle and to pump it back in the pulmonary artery [38, 39].

TandemHeart efficacy was compared with IABP in patients with cardiogenic shock after AMI [39, 40]. Forty-one patients were randomized ($n=20$ IABP, $n=21$ pVAD) [40]. Primary outcome measures of cardiac power index ($CPI = CI \times MAP \times 0.0022$), hemodynamic variables, and metabolic variables improved significantly with pVAD. CPI improved in the TandemHeart group from 0.22 (IQR 0.19–0.30) to 0.37 W/m^2 (IQR 0.30–0.47, $p<0.001$) when compared with IABP 0.22 (IQR 0.18–0.30) to 0.28 W m^2 (IQR 0.24–0.36, $p=0.02$; $p=0.0004$ for intergroup comparison).

Burkhoff et al. randomized 42 patients with cardiogenic shock between IABP and TandemHeart™ [41]. Compared with the IABP group, the TandemHeart group had significantly greater CI and greater decrease in PCWP. Complications such as limb ischemia and bleeding were encountered more frequently after pVAD implantation in the earlier studies; however, subsequent studies showed that using a percutaneous closure device to seal the arteriotomy significantly improved bleeding complications [42, 43]. As described above, similar to Impella findings, TandemHeart use showed significant improvement in hemodynamics during the usage; however, it did not reveal any early mortality benefits. However, comparing Impella to TandemHeart, bleeding was more frequently reported as a complication of the TandemHeart (RR 2.59, 95% CI 1.40–3.93, $p<0.01$) [43]. Technical expertise in performing a transseptal puncture and large-size femoral sheaths are factors limiting its utilization.

Contraindications for TandemHeart:

1. Right-ventricular failure is a relative contraindication
2. Severe aortic insufficiency

Potential TandemHeart adverse events:

1. Complications of transseptal puncture
2. Cardiac perforation
3. Femoral access site bleeding/complications
4. Limb ischemia

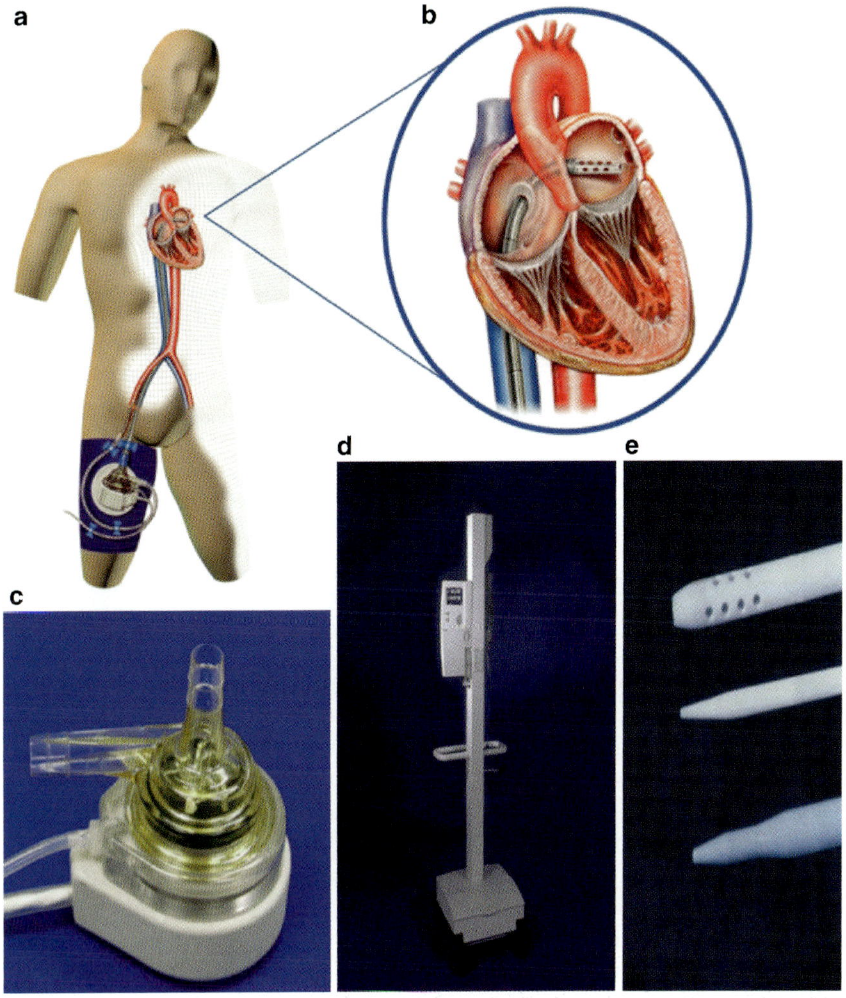

Fig. 25.2 TandemHeart™ percutaneous ventricular assist device. (**a**) Setup through the femoral vein and femoral artery. (**b**) Transseptal puncture showing the venous catheter in the left atrium. (**c**) Pump. (**d**) Console with the backup pump. (**e**) Outflow and inflow catheters

Contemporary Practice of Catheter-Based Circulatory Support

The contemporary practice of circulatory support includes three groups of patients: (1) those needing elective support for high-risk PCI, (2) those who present with cardiogenic shock, and (3) those who experience hemodynamic collapse (acute decompensation) in the cardiac catheterization laboratory. For patients with cardiogenic shock or "cath lab crashes," the four available technologies – the IABP, Impella device, TandemHeart, and percutaneous CPB – are used based on operator experience and institutional experience. Our strategy involves use of the IABP first and if the patient has persistent severe hypotension, use of the Impella device or peripheral CPB.

Elective support for high-risk PCI is planned based on several factors: ejection fraction, amount of myocardium supplied by the artery on which to intervene, presence of heart failure and hemodynamics assessed by right heart cardiac catheterization, single patent artery or bypass graft intervention, and the complexity of the intervention to be performed. Figure 25.3 provides a simple algorithm for planning elective interventions in patients with reduced left ventricular function. When the EF is mildly reduced (35–50%), our practice is to perform a right heart catheterization to evaluate the hemodynamics. If the pulmonary wedge pressure is elevated, intravenous Lasix or afterload-reducing agents are used. The intervention is performed with an IABP unit in the catheterization suite. If the EF is from 20 to 34%, similar measures are adopted with the addition of a size 4 Fr sheath inserted in the contralateral femoral artery for rapid institution of support. If the intervention is for a simple lesion and entails only stenting, IABP standby is the only strategy used. If a complex intervention such as the use of a Rotablator® rotational atherectomy system, complex bifurcation, or unprotected left main stenting is planned, an IABP or an Impella are used. Patients with an EF<20% or with a planned intervention on the only patent conduit, undergo the procedure on Impella support. CPB is not commonly used in such patients, but it is an option.

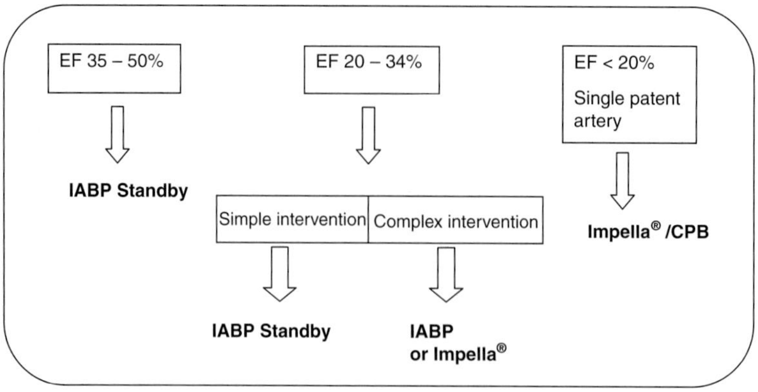

Fig. 25.3 Algorithm for elective supported coronary interventions at the University of Minnesota. *EF* ejection fraction; *IABP* intraaortic balloon pump; *CPB* percutaneous cardiopulmonary bypass

Vascular Remodeling

Vascular remodeling encompasses a complex sequence of morphologic changes in the blood vessel wall in response to various stimuli. Several clinically relevant precipitants of vascular remodeling include inflammation, mechanical disruption of the endothelium, hemodynamic stress and shear force, and hypoxia [44]. In addition, there are several iatrogenic causes of vascular remodeling such as percutaneous intervention, coronary artery bypass grafting, and cardiac transplantation. Gross pathologic specimens have demonstrated that all three layers of the arterial wall are involved in vascular remodeling, including intimal hyperplasia, medial thickening, and adventitial hyperplasia [45, 46].

Laws of physics govern the complex interactions between the arterial wall and blood such as Laplace's law and Poiseuille's law. Poiseuille's law determines shear stress (τ) on the arterial wall and is dependent on blood viscosity, volume of blood flow, and luminal radius ($\tau = 4\eta Q/\pi r^3$), where η is blood viscosity, Q is the volume of blood flow, and r is the radius of the lumen. Based on this physical law, it is evident that even small changes in luminal radius will have significant impact on the shear stress of the vessel wall. The importance of this becomes self-evident when examining the phenomenon first described by Glagov as positive remodeling of the arterial wall. The Glagov phenomenon of vascular remodeling described the changes associated with arterial luminal narrowing in response to atherosclerosis, but is now well recognized in other clinical situations such as angioplasty and hypertension [47]. Prior to Glagov's description, it was generally accepted that atherosclerosis caused stenosis by progressive growth of plaque into the vessel lumen. Alternatively, Glagov described the concept of positive remodeling in which the luminal area remained constant at the cost of increased internal elastic lamina. When the stenosis reached 40%, only then did the vessel luminal area demonstrate a stenosis which was hemodynamically significant [48]. This phenomenon has been described several times subsequently in both human postmortem examinations as well as multiple animal models [49–51].

Vascular remodeling plays a very important role in vivo atherosclerosis, but also has been demonstrated in patients with vascular injury secondary to systemic inflammation, hypertension, and following percutaneous intervention. For example, failure of a vessel lumen to enlarge following balloon dilation was traditionally believed to be secondary to intimal hyperplasia, however, studies have demonstrated that remodeling of the vessel positively was due to an increase in intima–media thickening, thus conserving the vessel lumen. Failure of the vessel to remodel positively resulted in compromised vessel lumen due solely to failure of this mechanism [52–55].

The biology of vascular remodeling has enjoyed tremendous investigation in recent years, and morphologic changes have been influenced by leukocyte recruitment, vascular smooth muscle cell proliferation, and endothelial recovery [45]. Smooth muscle apoptosis, which occurs about 30 min following balloon dilation of an artery, leads to apoptosis and an increased demand for vascular repair which is mediated through local progenitor stem cell recruitment [56–58]. In addition, there is an intense inflammatory cell recruitment composed primarily of monocytes and T-Cells, modulated by several chemokines, which augment disease progression in vascular remodeling [59].

Vascular remodeling remains a very intense area of both basic science and clinical investigation. The ability of an artery to maintain blood flow essential for perfusion requires a complex interplay of several biologic mechanisms. The failure of this system results in progression of atherosclerosis, restenosis following percutaneous transluminal coronary angioplasty, and vascular injury due to hypertension. Clinical solutions to promote ideal vascular remodeling will play an integral role in the treatment of cardiovascular disease.

Impella[R] is a registered trademark of Abiomed: www.abiomed.com/about_abiomed/Terms_of_Use.cfm

TandemHeart™ is a trademark of Cardiac Assist, Inc.: www.cardiacassist.com

Rotablator® is a registered trademark of Boston Scientific: www.bostonscientific.com/Device.bsci?page=HCP_Overview&navRelId=1000.1003&method=DevDetailHCP&id=10081831&pageDisclaimer=Disclaimer.ProductPage

Copyright info: www.bostonscientific.com/SectionData.bsci/,,/navRelId/1008.1027/seo.serve

References

1. Hurst JW. The first coronary angioplasty as described by Andreas Gruentzig. Am J Cardiol. 1986;57:185–6.
2. Gruntzig A. Transluminal dilatation of coronary-artery stenosis. Lancet. 1978;1:263.
3. Gruntzig AR, Senning A, Siegenthlaer WE. Nonoperative dilatation of coronary-artery stenosis. Percutaneous transluminal coronary angioplasty. N Engl J Med. 1979;301:61–8.
4. Kantrowitz A, Tjonneland S, Freed PS, et al. Initial clinical experience with intraaortic balloon pumping in cardiogenic shock. JAMA. 1968; 203:135–40.
5. Talpins NL, Kripke DC, Goetz RH. Counterpulsation and intraaortic balloon pumping in cardiogenic shock. Circ Dynam Arch Surg. 1968; 97:991–9.
6. Scheidt S, Wilner G, Mueller H, et al. Intraortic balloon pumping in cardiogenic shock. Report of a cooperative clinical trial. N Engl J Med. 1973;288:979–84.
7. Willerson JT, Curry GC, Watson JT, et al. Intra-aortic balloon counterpulsation in patients with cardiogenic shock, medically refractory heart failure, and/or recurrent ventricular tachycardia. Am J Med. 1975;58:183–91.
8. DeWood MA, Notske RN, Hensley GR, et al. Intra-aortic balloon counterpulsation with and without reperfusion for myocardial infarction shock. Circulation. 1980;61:1105–12.
9. Nanas JN, Moulopoulos SD. Counterpulsation: historical background, technical improvements, hemodynamic and metabolic effects. Cardiology. 1994;84:156–67.
10. Kern MJ. Cardiac support devices: intra-aortic balloon pump. In: The cardiac catheterization handbook. 4th ed. St. Louis: Mosby; 2003. p. 479–94.
11. Shawl FA, Domanski MJ, Hernandez TJ, et al. Emergency percutaneous cardiopulmonary bypass with cardiogenic shock from acute myocardial infarction. Am J Cardiol. 1989;64:967–70.
12. Vogel RA, Shawl FA, Tommaso CL, et al. Initial report of the national registry of elective cardiopulmonary bypass SUPPORTED coronary angioplasty. J Am Coll Cardiol. 1990;15:23–9.
13. Shawl FA, Domanski MJ, Punja S. Percutaneous cardiopulmonary bypass support in high risk patients undergoing percutaneous transluminal coronary angioplasty. Am J Cardiol. 1989;64:1258–63.
14. Lincoff AM, Popma JJ, Ellis SG, et al. Abrupt vessel closure complicating coronary angioplasty. Clinical, angiographic, and therapeutic profile. J Am Coll Cardiol. 1992;19:926–35.
15. Bauters C, Van Belle E, Lablanche JM et al. Predictive factors of primary success after coronary angioplasty. Arch Mal Coeur Vaiss. 1994 Feb; 87(2); 193–9
16. Meier B. Percutaneous coronary intervention. In: Topel EJ, editor. Textbook of cardiovascular medicine. 2nd ed. Philadelphia: Lippincott Williams & Wilkins; 2002. p. 1665–76.
17. Brigouri C, Sardis C, Pagnotta P, et al. Elective versus provisional intra-aortic balloon pumping in high-risk percutaneous transluminal coronary angioplasty. Am Heart J. 2003;145:700–7.
18. Mishra S, Chu WC, Torguson R, et al. Role of prophylactic intra-aortic balloon pump in high-risk patients undergoing percutaneous coronary intervention. Am J Cardiol. 2006;98:608–12.
19. Stone GW, Marsalese D, Brodie BR, et al. A prospective, randomized evaluation of prophylactic intraaortic balloon counterpulsation in high risk patients with acute myocardial infarction treated with primary angioplasty. J Am Coll Cardiol. 1997;29:1459–67.
20. Mackensie DJ, Wagner WH, Kulber DA, et al. Vascular complications of the intra-aortic balloon pump. Am J Surg. 1992;164:517–21.
21. Cook L, Pillar B, McCord G, et al. Intra-aortic balloon pump complications: a five-year retrospective study of 283 patients. Heart Lung. 1999;28:195–202.
22. Cohen M, Dawson MS, Kopistansky C, et al. Sex and other predictors of intra-aortic balloon conterpulsation-related complications: prospective study of 1119 consecutive patients. Am Heart J. 2000;139:282–7.
23. Meisel S, Shocat M, Sheikha SA, et al. Utilization of low profile intraaortic balloon catheters inserted by the sheathless technique in acute cardiac patients: clinical efficacy with a very low complication rate. Clin Cardiol. 2004;27:600–4.
24. Vogel RA, Tommaso CL, Gundry SR. Initial experience with coronary angioplasty and aortic valvuloplasty using elective semi-percutaneous cardiopulmonary support. Am J Cardiol. 1988;62:811–3.
25. Phillips SJ, Zeff RH, Kongtahworn C, et al. Percutaneous cardiopulmonary bypass: application and indication for use. Ann Thorac Surg. 1989;47:121–3.
26. Vogel RA, Shawl FA, Tommasso CL, et al. Initial report of the national registry of elective cardiopulmonary bypass supported coronary angioplasty. J Am Coll Cardiol. 1990;15:23–9.
27. Schreiber TL, Kodali UR, O'Neill WW, et al. Comparison of acute results of prophylactic intraaortic balloon pumping with cardiopulmonary support for percutaneous transluminal coronary angioplasty (PTCA). Cathet Cardiovasc Diagn. 1998;45:115–9.
28. Cyrus T, Mathews SJ, Lasala JM, et al. Use of mechanical assist during high- risk PCI and STEMI with cardiogenic shock. Catheter Cardiovasc Interv. 2010;75:S1–6.

29. de Souza CF, de Souza BF, De Lima VC, et al. Percutaneous mechanical assistance for the failing heart. J Interv Cardiol. 2010;23:195–202.
30. Sjauw KD, Remmelink M, Baan JR, et al. Left ventricular unloading in acute ST-segment elevation myocardial infarction patients is safe and feasible and provides acute and sustained left ventricular recovery. J Am Coll Cardiol. 2008;51:1044–6.
31. Henriques JP, Remmelink M, Baan Jr J, et al. Safety and feasibility of elective high-risk percutaneous coronary intervention procedures with left ventricular support of the Impella® Recover 2.5. Am J Cardiol. 2006;97:990–2.
32. Dixon SR, Henriques JP, Mauri L, et al. A prospective feasibility trial investigating the use of the Impella® 2.5 System in patients undergoing high-risk percutaneous coronary intervention (the PROTECT I trial): initial U.S. experience. JACC Cardiovasc Interv. 2009;2:91–6.
33. Seyfarth M, Sibbing D, Bauer I, et al. A randomized clinical trial to evaluate the safety and efficacy of a percutaneous left ventricular assist device versus intra-aortic balloon pumping for treatment of cardiogenic shock caused by myocardial infarction. J Am Coll Cardiol. 2008;52:1584–8.
34. Cheng JM, den Uil CA, Hoeks SE, et al. Percutaneous left ventricular assist device vs. intra-aortic balloon pump counterpulsation for treatment of cardiogenic shock: a meta-analysis of controlled trials. Eur Heart J. 2009;30:2102–8.
35. Pulido JN, Park SJ, Charenjit S, et al. Percutaneous left ventricular assist devices: clinical uses, future applications and anesthetic considerations. J Cardiothorac Vasc Anesth. 2010;24:478–86.
36. Aragon J, Lee MS, Kar S, et al. Percutaneous left ventricular assist device: "TandemHeart™" for high-risk coronary intervention. Catheter Cardiovasc Interv. 2005;65:346–52.
37. Vranckx P, Meliga E, De Jaegere PP, et al. The TandemHeart™ percutaneous transseptal left ventricular assist device: a safeguard in high-risk percutaneous coronary interventions. The six-year Rotterdam experience. EuroIntervention. 2008;4:331–7.
38. Atiemo AD, Conte JV, Heldman AW. Resuscitation and recovery from acute right ventricular failure using a percutaneous right ventricular assist device. Catheter Cardiovasc Interv. 2006;68:78–82.
39. Prutkin JM, Strote JA, Stout KK. Percutaneous right ventricular assist device as support for cardiogenic shock due to right ventricular infarction. J Invasive Cardiol. 2008;20:E215–6.
40. Thiele H, Sick P, Boudriot E, et al. Randomized comparison of intra-aortic balloon support with a percutaneous left ventricular assist device in patients with revascularized acute myocardial infarction complicated by cardiogenic shock. Eur Heart J. 2005;26:1276–83.
41. Burkhoff D, Cohen H, Brunckhorst C, et al. A randomized multicenter clinical study to evaluate the safety and efficacy of the TandemHeart™ percutaneous ventricular assist device versus conventional therapy with intraaortic balloon pumping for treatment of cardiogenic shock. Am Heart J. 2006;152:469e1–4698.
42. Rajdev S, Krishnan P, Irani A, et al. Clinical application of prophylactic percutaneous left ventricular assist device (TandemHeart™) in high-risk percutaneous coronary intervention using an arterial preclosure technique: single-center experience. J Invasive Cardiol. 2008;20:67–72.
43. Al-Husami W, Yturralde F, Mohanty G, et al. Single-center experience with the TandemHeart™ percutaneous ventricular assist device to support patients undergoing high-risk percutaneous coronary intervention. J Invasive Cardiol. 2008;20:319–22.
44. Gibbons GH, Dzau VJ. The emerging concept of vascular remodeling. N Engl J Med. 1994;330:1431–8.
45. Schober A, Zercecke A. Chemokines in vascular remodeling. Thromb Haemost. 2007;97:730–7.
46. Mitchell RN, Libby P. Vascular remodeling in transplant vasculopathy. Circ Res. 2007;100:967–78.
47. Korshunov VA, Schwartz SM, Berk BC. Vascular remodeling: hemodynamic and biochemical mechanisms underlying Glagov's phenomenon. Arterioscler Thromb Vasc Biol. 2007;27:1722–8.
48. Glagov S, Weisenberg E, Zarins CK, et al. Compensatory enlargement of human atherosclerotic coronary arteries. N Engl J Med. 1987;316: 1371–5.
49. Bond MG, Adams MR, Bullock BC. Complicating factors in evaluating coronary artery atherosclerosis. Artery. 1981;9:21–9.
50. Bonthu S, Heistad DD, Chappel DA, et al. Atherosclerosis, vascular remodeling, and impairment of endothelium-dependent relaxation in genetically altered hyperlipidemic mice. Arterioscler Thromb Vasc Biol. 1997;17:2333–40.
51. Armstrong ML, Heistad DD, Marcus ML, et al. Structural and hemodynamic response of peripheral arteries of macque monkeys to atherogenic diet. Arteriosclerosis. 1985;5:336–46.
52. Courtman DW, Schwartz SM, Hart CE. Sequential injury of the rabbit abdominal aorta induces intramural coagulation and luminal narrowing independent of intimal mass: extrinsic pathway inhibition eliminates luminal narrowing. Circ Res. 1998;82:996–1006.
53. Cote G, Tardif JC, Lesperance J, et al. Effects of probucol on vascular remodeling after coronary angioplasty. Multivitamins and Probucol Study Group. Circulation. 1999;99:30–5.
54. Nobuyoshi M, Kimura T, Nosaka H, et al. Restenosis after successful transluminal coronary angioplasty: serial angiographic follow-up of 229 consecutive patients. J Am Coll Cardiol. 1988;12:616–23.
55. Tardif JC, Cote G, Lesperance J, et al. Probucol and multivitamins in the prevention of restenosis after coronary angioplasty: multivitamins and Probucol Study Group. N Engl J Med. 1997;337:365–72.
56. Korbling M, Estrov Z. Adult stem cells for tissue repair: a new therapeutic concept? N Engl J Med. 2003;349:570–82.
57. Ross JJ, Hong Z, Willenbring Z, et al. Cytokine-induced differentiation of multipotent adult progenitor cells Into functional smooth muscle cells. J Clin Invest. 2006;116:3139–49.
58. Shober A. Chemokines in vascular dysfunction and remodeling. Arterioscler Thromb Vasc Biol. 2008;28:1950–9.
59. Schmauss D, Weis M. Cardiac allograft vasculopathy: recent developments. Circulation. 2008;17:2131–41.
60. Hasdai D, Berger PB, Battler A, Holmes Jr DR, editors. Cardiogenic shock: diagnosis and treatment. Totowa: Humana Press; 2002.

Chapter 26
Surgical Mechanical Circulatory Support

Forum Kamdar and Ranjit John

Approximately 5.7 million Americans have heart failure, and every year about 300,000 of them die from it. The prevalence of heart failure continues to rise and increases with age [1]. During the last 20 years, hospital admissions for this disease have increased almost threefold, and heart failure now is the most frequent cause of hospital admissions in patients greater than 65 years-old (Fig. 26.1). The management of heart failure is one of the largest single expenses for Medicare, and in 2008, it exceeded $34 billion in direct and indirect costs [1].

Advances in medical therapy, implantable cardioverter defibrillators, and cardiac resynchronization therapy have changed the management of heart failure and brought about decreased progression of disease. Despite these advances, and even with optimal medical management, the prognosis is poor for patients with New York Heart Association class III and class IV heart failure [2–6].

In end-stage heart failure, given the limited medical options and high mortality, orthotopic cardiac transplantation is the definitive therapy. However, a discrepancy exists between the limited availability of donor organs and the ever-increasing number of patients with heart failure. Based on data from the United Network for Organ Sharing (UNOS), 2,163 transplants were performed in the USA in 2008. Yet thousands more patients would benefit from this therapy. Similarly, for those patients with advanced age and comorbid conditions, cardiac transplantation is often not an option to address advanced heart failure.

Historical Perspective

The advent of mechanical circulatory support (MCS) occurred in 1953 when cardiopulmonary bypass (CPB) was used for short-term support to allow for cardiac surgery. The modern era of MCS started in the 1960s with the development of the artificial heart program at the National Institutes of Health [7]. While multiple devices have been developed, including total artificial hearts, ventricular-assist devices were developed to "unload" a failing heart, maintain forward cardiac output, and vital organ perfusion. Refinement of technology, allowing for implantable pumps, led to the HeartMate® being the first FDA-approved device for bridge-to-transplantation in 1994 and, subsequently, the updated HeartMate XVE in 1998. The landmark REMATCH trial in 2002 clearly demonstrated and established the survival and quality of life advantages of implanted ventricular-assist devices in end-stage heart failure (Fig. 26.2) [3].

The clear benefit of left ventricular-assist devices (LVADs) over optimal medical therapy alone for those patients with advanced heart failure has led to the increasing use of LVADs [8, 9]. Further, the excellent medium-term results with LVADs have led to the use of permanent LVAD implantation for patients with end-stage heart failure [3]. Since their inception, mechanical technology has evolved substantially, which has allowed for LVADs to become an accepted treatment modality for patients with end-stage heart failure. Improvement in device design and a better understanding of indications for device insertion has enabled increased applicability and excellent results with LVADs, which has revolutionized the treatment options available for patients with end-stage heart failure (Fig. 26.3).

R. John MD (✉)
Division of Cardiothoracic Surgery, University of Minnesota Medical Center-Fairview, Minneapolis, MN, USA
e-mail: johnx008@umn.edu

Z. Vlodaver et al. (eds.), *Coronary Heart Disease: Clinical, Pathological, Imaging, and Molecular Profiles*,
DOI 10.1007/978-1-4614-1475-9_26, © Springer Science+Business Media, LLC 2012

Fig. 26.1 Hospital discharges for heart failure by sex (USA: 1979–2005). Note: hospital discharges include people discharged alive, dead, and "status unknown." [1] Adapted from Rosamond et al. [1]. Copyright 2008 by American Heart Association

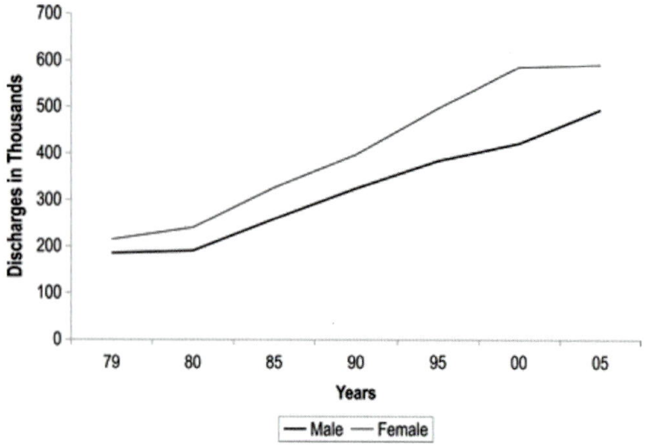

Fig. 26.2 Kaplan–Meier survival estimates from the REMATCH trial demonstrating significant survival benefit of LVADs over optimal medical therapy. Adapted from Rose et al. [3]. Copyright 2001 by Massachusetts Medical Society

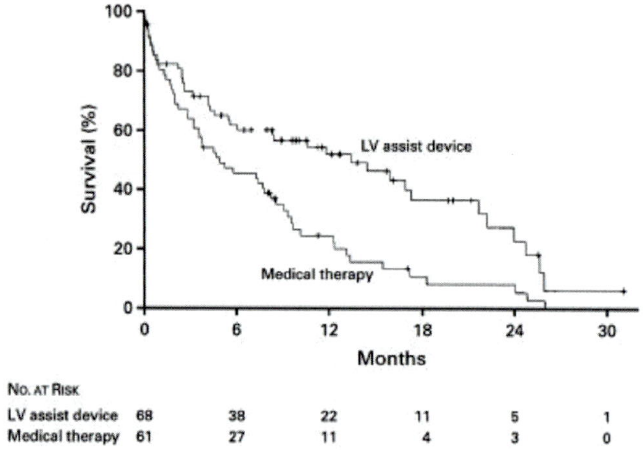

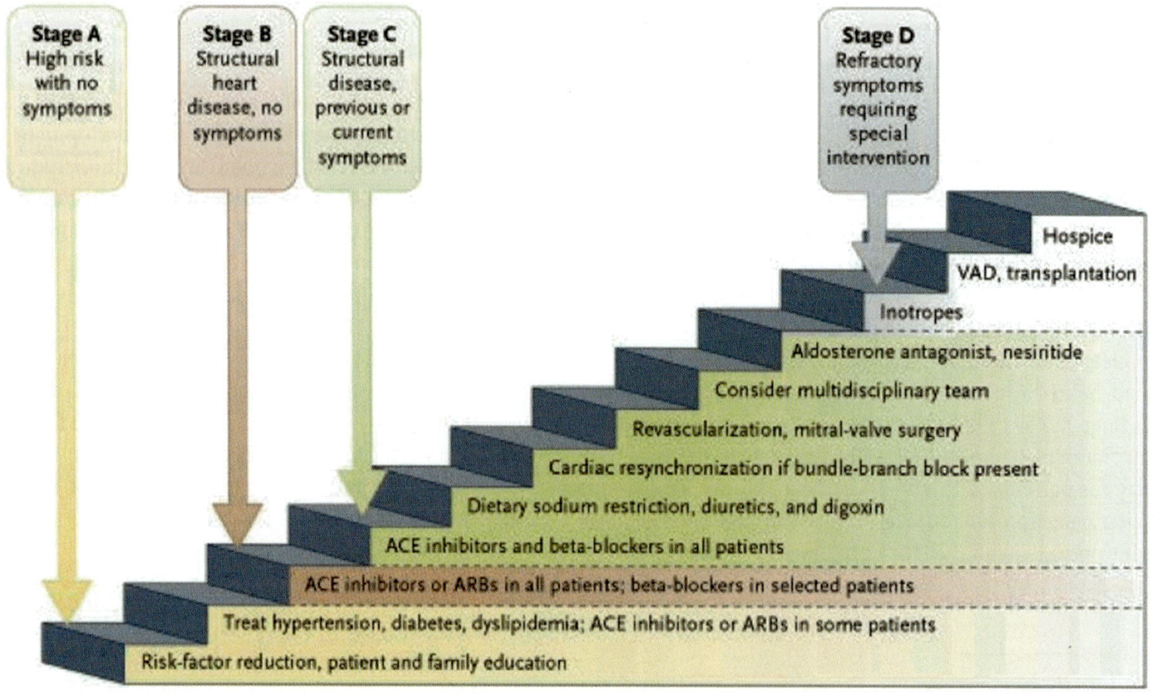

Fig. 26.3 Heart failure treatment modalities based on stage of heart failure. Adapted from Jessup et al. [45]. Copyright by Massachusetts Medical Society

Classification of Ventricular Assist Devices (VADs)

The purpose of VADs are to reduce myocardial work by completely unloading the ventricle while maintaining its output. The classifications are many and can be based on site of support (either left ventricular, right ventricular, or biventricular support), duration of support (temporary vs. permanent), or type of device (continuous vs. pulsatile flow). Clinically, VAD use can be categorized into groups for indication of VAD support including bridge-to-decision, bridge-to-bridge, bridge-to-transplant (BTT), and destination therapy (DT).

Bridge-to-Decision

In patients with acute cardiogenic shock and multisystem organ failure, their condition does not allow evaluation of transplant eligibility due to unclear neurologic status and reversibility of myocardial and end-organ function. The outcomes of permanent LVAD implantation in this group are exceptionally poor [10]. Placement of a temporary or short-term VAD as a bridge-to-decision enables establishment of hemodynamic stability and end-organ recovery to plan further definitive treatment such as a bridge-to-bridge for long-term device placement or, more rarely, bridge-to-recovery (Fig. 26.4). Devices designed for this group of patients are easily and quickly implantable and cost-efficient.

Bridge-to-Transplant (BTT)

Bridge-to-transplant therapy is the most traditional of LVAD clinical uses. Patients have irreversible ventricular failure and meet standard criteria for heart transplantation. Positive outcomes with this clinical application have been important for expanding the field of MCS.

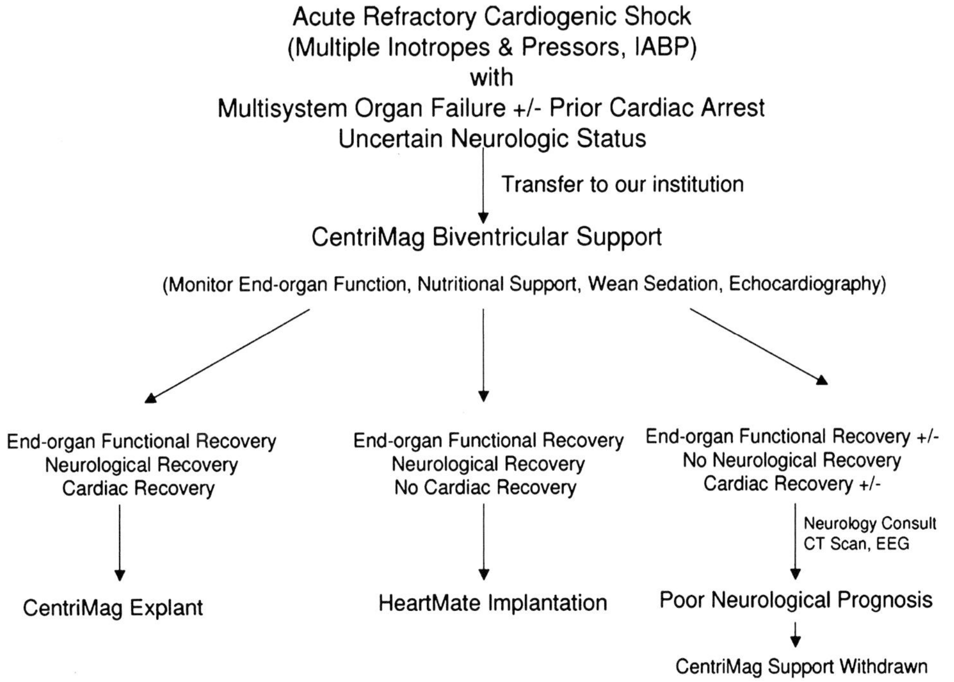

Fig. 26.4 University of Minnesota algorithm for bridge-to-decision. Adapted from John et al. [10]. Copyright by Elsvier publishers

Destination Therapy (DT)

Finally, DT exists for patients with chronic heart failure who are transplant-ineligible. DT evolved from encouraging results with VADs as bridge-to-transplant therapy. Currently, two devices – the HeartMate XVE and HeartMate II – are FDA approved for DT. Device-related adverse events including infection, gastrointestinal bleeding, and thromboembolism have limited the application of current devices as DT. As devices improve, the indications for DT and the demand are expected to grow to help meet the growing number of patients with end-stage heart failure.

Short-Term Support Devices

Indications for short-term MCS are essentially contraindications for permanent support, including: unknown neurological status, significant coagulopathy, multisystem organ dysfunction, severe hemodynamic instability, respiratory failurc, and high probability of early recovery. Both percutaneous and surgically implanted devices exist and the use of device type depends on multiple factors including device availability, patient's status, and the center's experience. Two common surgically implanted devices are the CentriMag® System (Levitronix, Wiltham, MA, USA) and Abiomed® BVS 5000 (ABIOMED, Inc, Danvers, MA, USA).

CentriMag

The CentriMag system is composed of a single-use, extracorporeal, centrifugal blood pump, a motor, console, and flow probe (Fig. 26.5) [11, 12]. Its unique design enables operation without bearings or seals. The impeller is magnetically levitated, allowing unidirectional rotation with minimal friction and thermal generation in the blood flow path. The rotor surface is uniformly washed, which minimizes the area of blood stagnation and turbulence in the pump, thereby reducing thrombus formation and hemolysis [10, 13]. It can be operated from 500 to 5,000 revolutions per minute and generates flow of up to 10 L/min under normal physiologic conditions.

The CentriMag is implanted via a standard median sternotomy with or without the assistance of CPB (Fig. 26.6). For LVAD support, the inflow cannula is placed into the left atria via the interatrial septal groove, adjacent to the right superior pulmonary vein. The outflow cannula is placed in the ascending aorta. For RVAD support, the inflow cannula is positioned in the right atrial appendage, with the outflow cannula in the pulmonary artery. It can be used for either single ventricle- or biventricular support. After insertion, the patient should be anticoagulated with heparin to keep activated clotting time (ACT) of 160–180 s. Patients who have CentriMag support can be weaned to recovery, bridged to permanent VAD, or bridged to transplant [14, 15, 46]. In the University of Minnesota experience, 75% of the 24 patients were successfully explanted or bridged to a permanent device [10].

Abiomed BVS 5000

The Abiomed BVS 5000 is an extracorporeal, pneumatic pulsatile-assist device for temporary support that is composed of single-use blood pumps [15]. It was the first heart-assist device approved by the FDA for the support of postcardiotomy patients. The pump has two polyurethane chambers: an atrial chamber that fills via gravity and a ventricular chamber that pneumatically pumps the blood to the systemic circulation. Two trileaflet valves separate the atrial and ventricular chambers. This device can produce blood flow of up to 5 L/min.

This device can also be used for unilateral or biventricular support, and is inserted via sternotomy. For LVAD support, the inflow cannula is placed into the left atrium and outflow graft in the ascending aorta. For RVAD support, the cannula is placed in the right atrium and outflow graft in the pulmonary artery (Fig. 26.7).

Heparinization to maintain an ACT of 180–200 s is essential after implantation as thrombi can form along the valve surface or outflow cannula. The pump requires exchange weekly or sooner if evidence of fibrin or clot formation appears.

Fig. 26.5 CentriMag pump

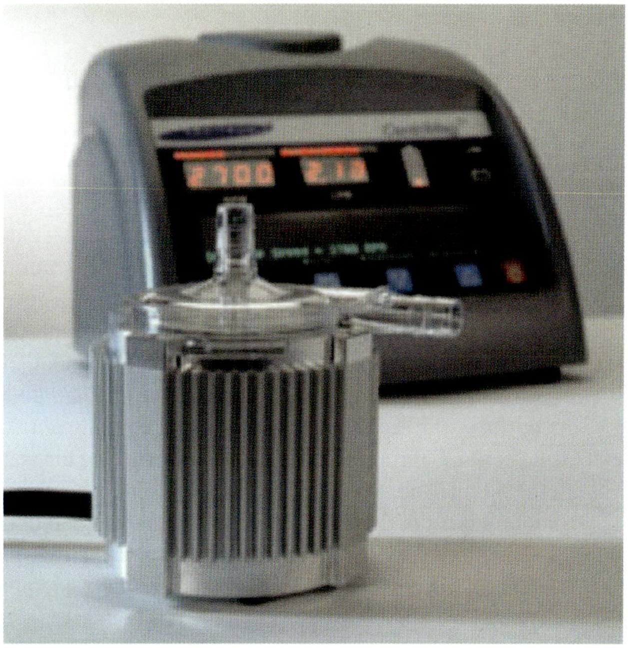

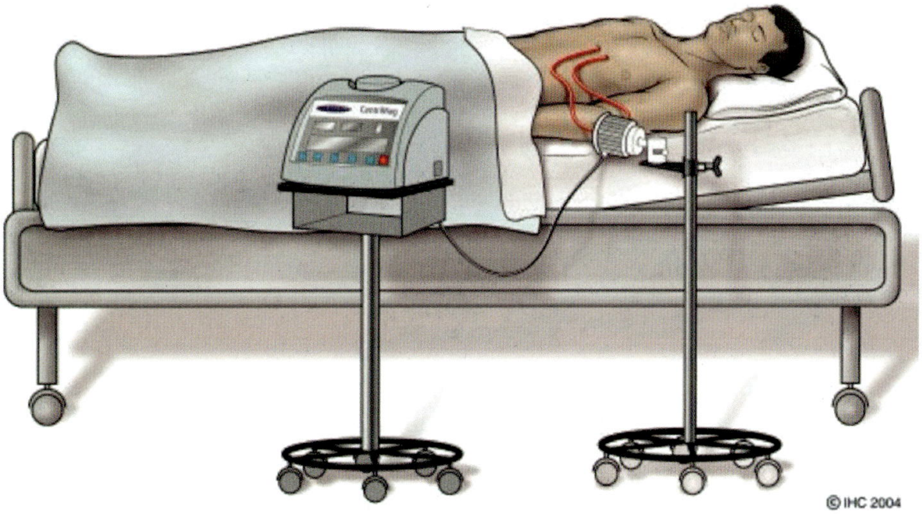

Fig. 26.6 CentriMag LVAD: patient and primary console

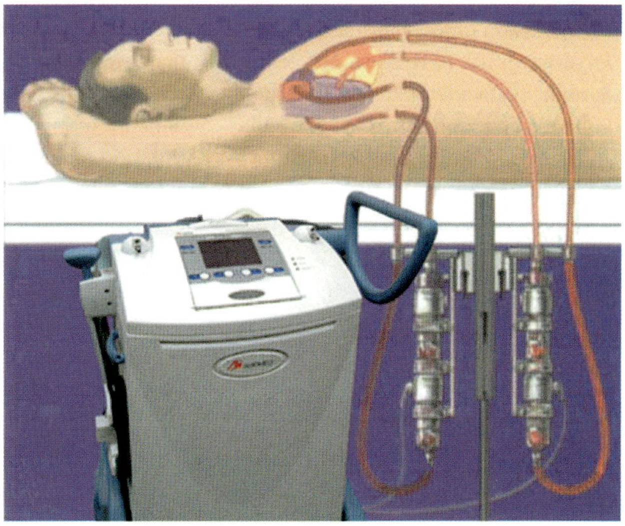

Fig. 26.7 Abiomed BVS 5000 pump and console

Long-Term, Implanted Devices

Pulsatile

Pulsatile devices mimic the physiologic volume displacement mechanism of the human heart. A first-generation pulsatile device, the HeartMate XVE LVAD (Thoratec Corporation, Pleasanton, CA) has been one of the most commonly used LVADs worldwide. It is FDA-approved for both bridge-to-transplant and as DT. The device is a positive-displacement pulsatile pump made of titanium with a polyurethane diaphragm and a pusher-plate actuator. It is driven by an electric motor but can be also driven pneumatically. The HeartMate XVE is an implantable device that can be placed either within a preperitoneal pocket or within the peritoneal cavity (Figs. 26.8 and 26.9). The inflow cannula is inserted into the apex of the LV; the outflow graft is anastomosed to the ascending aorta. The pumping chamber is connected to the battery packs and to electronic controls through a driveline that carries the air vent and electric cable. The HeartMate XVE has a maximum stroke volume of 83 mL and can be operated at up to 120 beats/min, resulting in flow rates of up to 10 L/min [16].

A unique aspect of this device is that it has a textured titanium interior surface. The titanium microspheres, which contact the blood, promote the formation of a pseudointima that resists the formation of thrombi. The rates of thromboembolism are 2–4% with this device, even with anticoagulation therapy with aspirin alone [3, 17], which is an important consideration for patients who cannot tolerate warfarin. While the REMATCH trial demonstrated a clear survival benefit with this device over optimal medical management, several limitations exist. Applicability is limited to those patients with a body surface area (BSA) of 1.5 m^2 or greater. The durability of this device is also a critical limitation, with valve and motor failure occurring after 12 months of support. Even with revisions to the design, durability at 2 years is only 5% [18].

Continuous Flow Devices

Until recently, most patients have been supported with pulsatile, first-generation devices. Continuous-flow devices are second-generation devices that were developed to be smaller, more reliable devices for long-term MCS. Continuous-flow devices incorporate either axial or centrifugal pump technology that generates high-speed rotation of the blood. The hemocompatibility of these devices was questioned due to the high-speed impeller rotation and subsequent hemolysis. The Hemopump® was the first to demonstrate the clinical feasibility of implantable continuous-flow LVADs without significant hemolysis [19].

Two examples of continuous flow devices are the HeartMate II LVAD (Thoratec, Pleasanton, CA), an axial flow pump, and the VentrAssist™ (Ventracor, NSW, Australia), a centrifugal pump.

HeartMate II Axial Flow Pump

The HeartMate II is connected in a similar way as the HeartMate XVE; parallel with the native heart. The inflow cannula is connected to the LV apex; the outflow graft is connected to the ascending aorta. The impeller, the pump's only moving part, spins on blood-lubricated bearings powered by an electromagnetic motor. The inlet and outlet cannulae include woven polyester grafts (CR Bard, Haverhill, PA) that require preclotting. The pump motor and associated blood tube have smooth titanium surfaces; in an effort to duplicate the excellent biocompatibility of the original pulsatile HeartMate XVE, the inlet, outlet elbows, and the intraventricular cannula are textured with titanium microsphere coatings.

The pump has an implant volume of 63 mL and generates up to 10 L/min of flow at a mean pressure of 100 mmHg. The HeartMate II is one seventh the size and one fourth the weight of its predecessor, the HeartMate XVE (Fig. 26.10). The axial flow design and absence of blood sac eliminate the need for venting, currently required for the first generation of implantable pumps, thus reducing the size of the percutaneous driveline and also eliminating the need for internal one-way valves [20]. Several single-center and multicenter studies have shown improved outcomes with the HeartMate II (Figs. 26.11, 26.12, and 26.13) [21–24].The HeartMate II BTT trial included 281 patients enrolled at 33 centers from March 2005 to April 2008. The median duration of device support was 155 days, and the cumulative patient support in the trial was 181 years. Survival to cardiac transplantation, recovery, or ongoing on HeartMate II was 79% at 18 months. Significant improvements were observed across all measures of functional status and quality of life as compared to baseline status. The incidence of

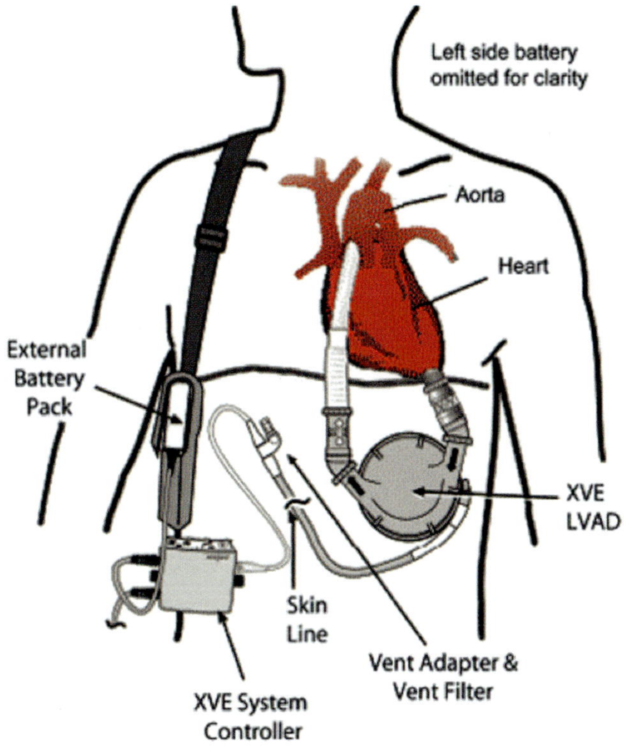

Fig. 26.8 HeartMate XVE

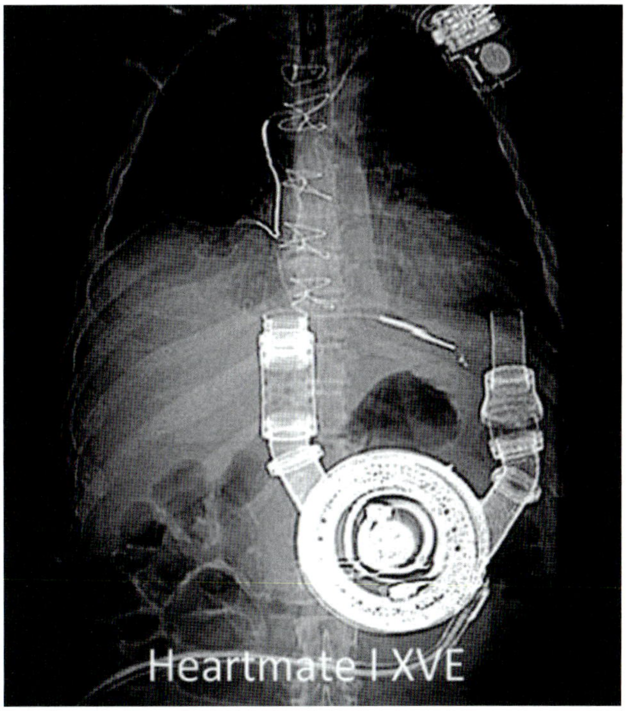

Fig. 26.9 Radiograph of implanted HeartMate XVE

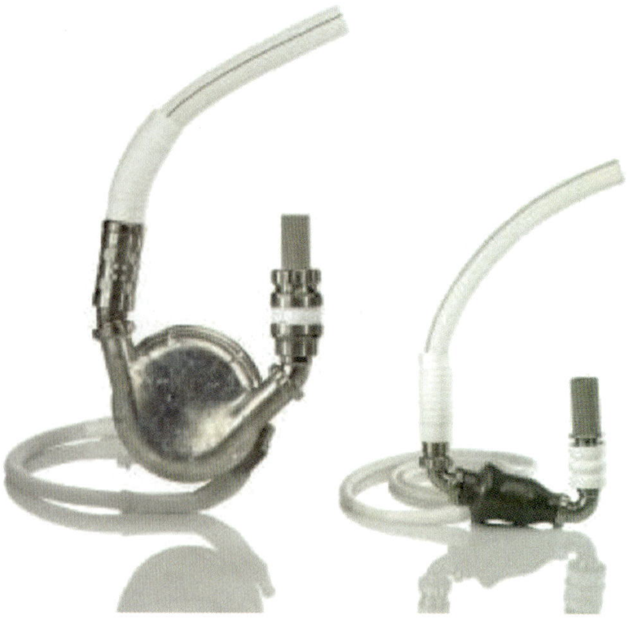

Fig. 26.10 Comparison of HeartMate XVE (*left*) and HeartMate II (*right*)

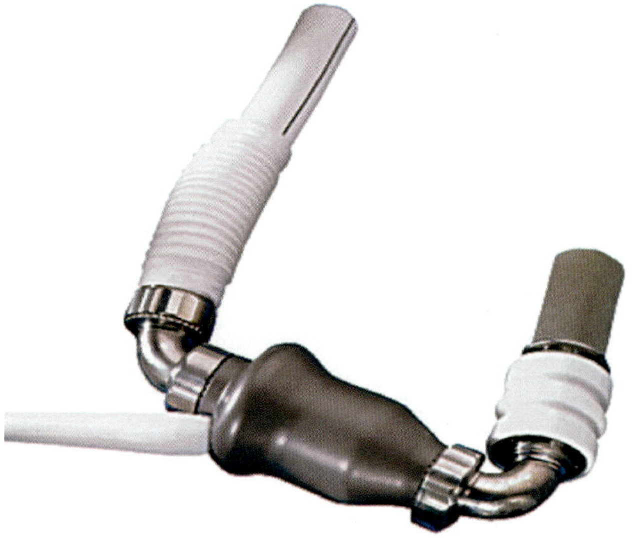

Fig. 26.11 HeartMate II LVAD

major adverse events with comparable definitions – including infections, strokes, and bleeding requiring surgery – was significantly lower than what was clinically observed in the previous bridge-to-transplantation study of the HeartMate I [24]. The HeartMate II DT pivotal clinical trial was a prospective, randomized evaluation of the HeartMate II LVAD. Patients were randomized to HeartMate XVE (control) or Heart Mate II on a 2-1 basis. A total of 192 patients were enrolled at 40 sites. Survival with the HeartMate II was 68% at 1 year (Fig. 26.14). The level of adverse events, including infection, sepsis, and right heart failure in DT patients implanted with the HeartMate II was lower in major categories vs. patients in the control group who were implanted with the XVE. No failures of the pumping mechanism were reported among the HeartMate II DT trial patients (Fig. 26.15) [21].

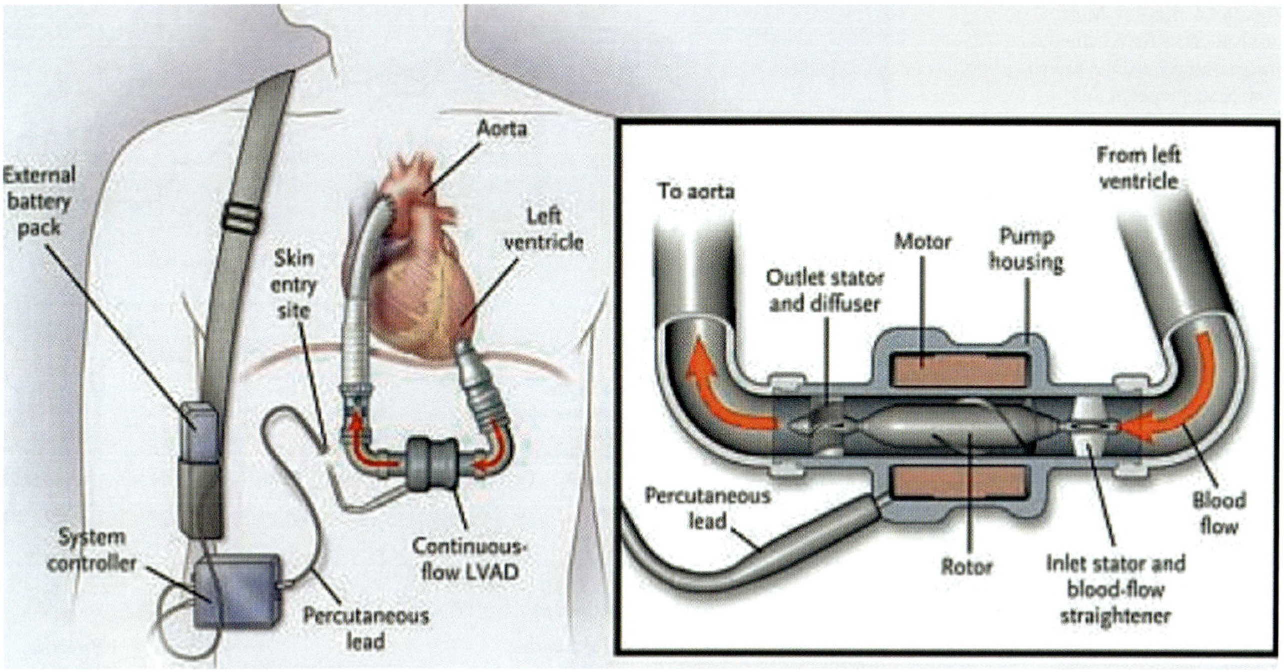

Fig. 26.12 HeartMate II schematic

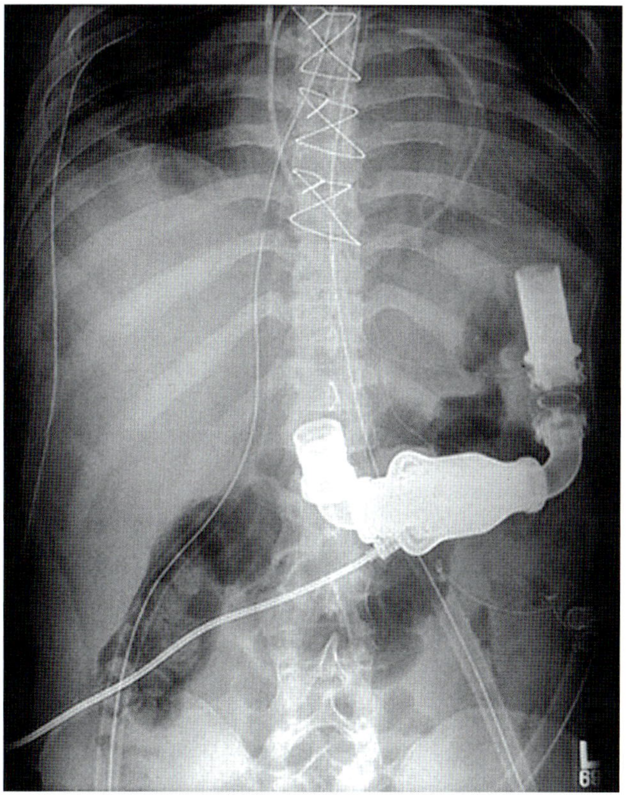

Fig. 26.13 Radiograph of implanted HeartMate II

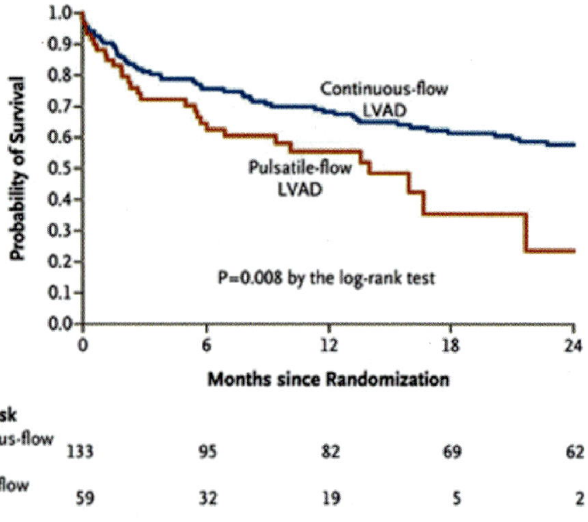

Fig. 26.14 Kaplan–Meier survival curve for continuous and pulsatile LVAD. Adapted from Slaughter et al. [21]. Copright 2009 by Massachusetts Medical Society

	Continuous-Flow LVAD (N=133) (211 patient-yr)		Pulsatile-Flow LVAD (N=59) (41 patient-yr)			
Subgroup	*no. (%)*	*no. of Events/ Patient-Yr*	*no. (%)*	*no. of Events/ Patient-Yr*	**Relative Risk (95% CI)**	**P Value for Interaction**
Pump replacement	12 (9)	0.06	20 (34)	0.51		<0.001
Stroke	24 (18)	0.13	8 (14)	0.22		0.21
Ischemic	11 (8)	0.06	4 (7)	0.10		0.38
Hemorrhagic	15 (11)	0.07	5 (8)	0.12		0.33
LVAD-related infection	47 (35)	0.48	21 (36)	0.90		0.01
Local non-LVAD infection	65 (49)	0.76	27 (46)	1.33		0.02
Sepsis	48 (36)	0.39	26 (44)	1.11		<0.001
Bleeding						
Bleeding requiring PRBC	108 (81)	1.66	45 (76)	2.45		0.06
Bleeding requiring surgery	40 (30)	0.23	9 (15)	0.29		0.57
Other neurologic event	29 (22)	0.17	10 (17)	0.29		0.14
Right heart failure						
Managed with extended use of inotropes	27 (20)	0.14	16 (27)	0.46		<0.001
Managed with RVAD	5 (4)	0.02	3 (5)	0.07		0.12
Cardiac arrhythmia	75 (56)	0.69	35 (59)	1.31		0.006
Respiratory failure	50 (38)	0.31	24 (41)	0.80		<0.001
Renal failure	21 (16)	0.10	14 (24)	0.34		<0.001
Hepatic dysfunction	3 (2)	0.01	0	0.00		
LVAD thrombosis	5 (4)	0.02	0	0.00		
Rehospitalization	107 (94)	2.64	42 (96)	4.25		0.02

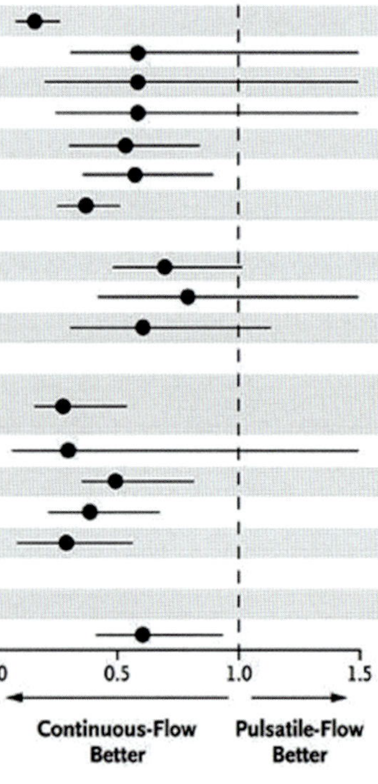

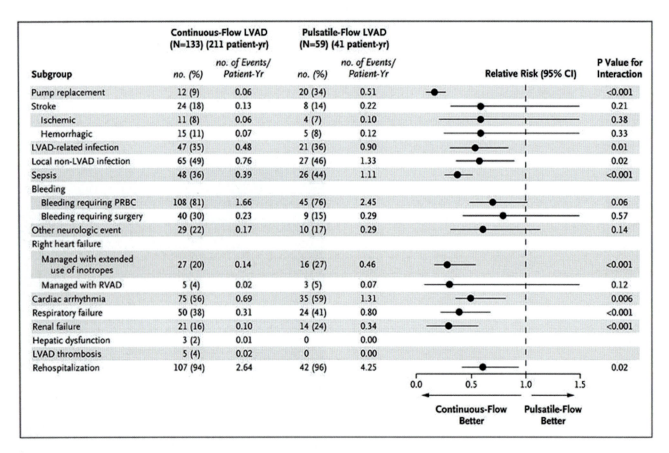

Fig. 26.15 Adverse events in the HeartMate II Destination Therapy trial. Adapted from Slaughter et al. [21]. Copyright 2009 by Massachusetts Medical Society

VentrAssist Centrifugal Pump

Implantable centrifugal pumps are considered the third generation of LVADs. The VentrAssist is a centrifugal pump with hydrodynamic bearings and an electromagnetically driven impeller (Fig. 26.16). It has only one moving part, the impeller, which has four small blades embedded within permanent magnets. The impeller blades spin when an electric current is sequentially switched between three pairs of coils contained within the pump's titanium housing. The impeller is suspended by a thin cushion of blood within the gap of eight hydrodynamic bearings.

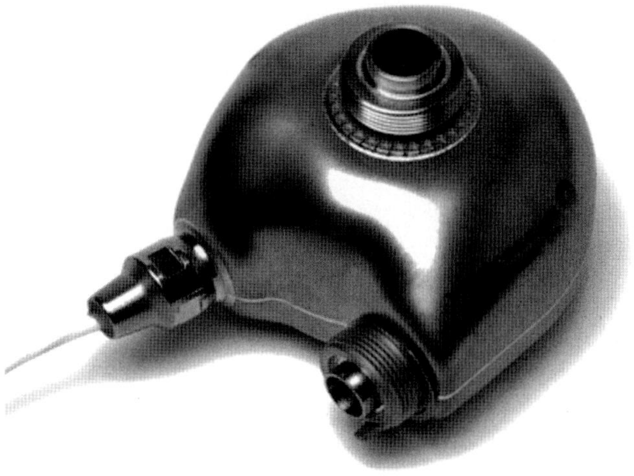

Fig. 26.16 VentrAssist LVAD pump

The pump is treated with a diamond-like carbon coating on blood-contacting surfaces. The pump is small, measuring 67 mm in diameter and weighing 298 g. It can provide flows from 2 to 10 L/min, with average pressure from 50 to 160 mmHg.

Recently, published trials have supported the safety and efficacy of the VentrAssist LVAD as a bridge-to-transplant therapy [21, 25, 47]. Among 33 bridge-to-transplant patients at 1 year, greater than 80% received transplants or became transplant eligible. Additionally, the incidence of adverse events was comparable to other LVADs currently used.

Complications

Recent studies of patients who have been supported by continuous-flow LVADs indicated a decreasing incidence of complications and improved outcomes [21, 23, 24]. However, complications during LVAD support, such as thromboembolism, bleeding, infections, and right ventricular failure remain an issue for long-term LVAD use.

Thromboembolism

The development of novel materials used for implant operations and the increasing use of implanted devices have made it clear that no material is biologically inert. Commonly used biomaterials, including so-called inert compounds such as titanium, polytetrafluoroethylene, and acrylics can trigger an array of iatrogenic effects, including inflammation, fibrosis, coagulation, and infection. In the case of LVADs, in which the biomaterial is in direct contact with the blood circulation, significant changes in systemic immunologic and thrombostatic functions have been well documented. Like most other implanted devices, LVADs activate the coagulation system, resulting in device-related thrombus [26–28].

The older pulsatile device, the HeartMate XVE, had a textured blood contacting surface which allowed for formation of a neointimal layer. This neoitimal layer decreased the risk of thromboembolism, which obviated the need for systemic anticoagulation.

The initial concern about continuous flow devices was the risk of blood trauma and resultant thromboembolism, however a number of studies have demonstrated a low incidence of thromboembolism in these devices (21, 24, 48). Devices such as the HeartMate II have textured inlet and outlet surfaces to duplicate the biocompatibility of the older devices. In the HeartMate II clinical trial, the incidence of "pump thrombosis" was 4% in DT patients and 1.4% in bridge-to-transplant (BTT) patients [21, 24]. Figure 26.17 demonstrates an explanted HeartMate II device that shows no evidence of thrombus. Figure 26.18 shows an example of a pump-related thrombus when using the HeartMate II that required device exchange.

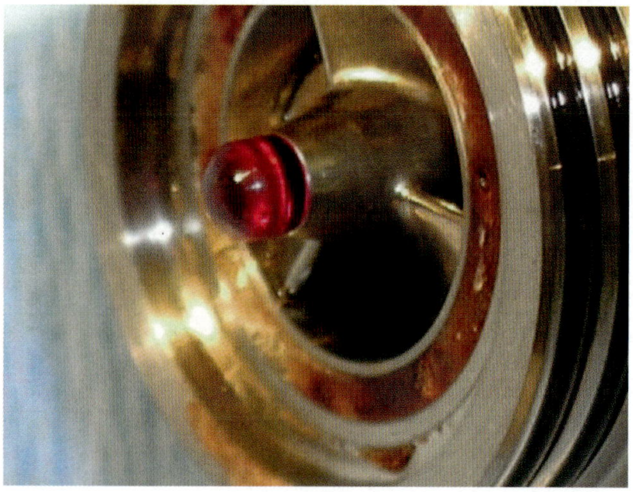

Fig. 26.17 Photograph of an explanted HeartMate II LVAD with no evidence of thrombus deposition at the forward ruby bearing from a patient supported successfully for 164 days

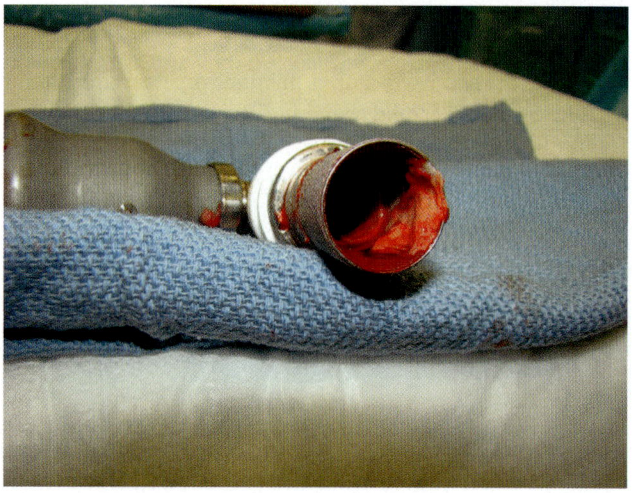

Fig. 26.18 Pump thrombus of HeartMate II requiring device exchange

Bleeding

The standard strategy to reduce the risk of thromboembolism has been systemic anticoagulation. Yet anticoagulation therapy exacerbates the risk of bleeding after LVAD implantation. Anticoagulation for continuous-flow devices, such as the HeartMate II, were initially aggressive and included heparin, antiplatelet medications, and warfarin with a goal INR of 2.5–3.5 [29, 30]. However, recent studies have shown that thrombotic events are lower than the risk of bleeding, which remains a common adverse event. Other studies have confirmed this observation, which has resulted in reduced anticoagulation therapy at the most experienced centers [31, 32].Gastrointestinal (GI) bleeding is a complication of continuous-flow pump support that may be severe and require reducing or discontinuing anticoagulation therapy [32–35]. Two hypotheses of the cause of GI bleeding during LVAD support that are being studied are acquired von Willebrand disease caused by increased shear stress, and reduced pulsatility of the continuous-flow device [36–39].

Infection

In the REMATCH trial, 28% of patients receiving LVADs had an LVAD-related infectious complication by 3 months. While moving to smaller continuous-flow devices that require much less surgical dissection and have smaller drivelines has reduced infections, it remains a major morbidity related to LVADs. The range of LVAD-related infections, which includes driveline infections, LVAD-related blood stream infection, and pump pocket infection, in more recent clinical trials of the

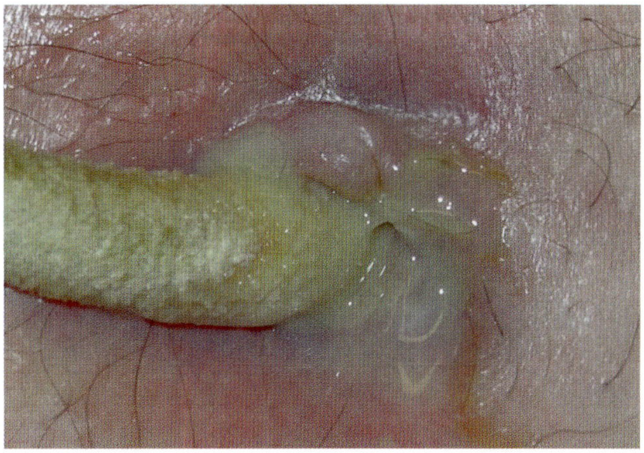

Fig. 26.19 Patient with a driveline exit site infection demonstrating erythema and purulent drainage from the exit site

HeartMate II, has shown a range from 15% (DT) to 35% (BTT) [21, 25]. Preoperative factors such as obesity and malnutrition have been identified as risk factors for LVAD-related infections.The most common presentation of LVAD-related infection is driveline exit site infection (Fig. 26.19). Local inflammatory changes and purulent drainage are frequently seen. Device pocket infection is another localized form of LVAD-related infection. Skin and soft tissues overlying a device pocket may exhibit frank inflammatory changes. Infection of the valves or other blood-contacting surfaces of the LVAD occurs less often. *Staphyloccus aureus* and coagulase-negative staphylococci account for more than 50% of cases of LVAD-related infections. Enterococci, *Enterobacter* spp., and *Pseudomonas aeruginosa* are other commonly isolated bacterial pathogens in LVAD-related infections [40, 41]. Strategies to treat LVAD-related infections include long-term suppressive antibiotics, localized debridement, and device exchange or removal. Preventive measures such as perioperative antibiotics, vancomycin beads, and meticulous driveline care are important in reducing the risk of infection.

In our evaluation of 89 patients with LVAD's, at the University of Minnesota, 24 (27%) were identified with having an infection, of which 11 had bacteremia (12.4%) and 13 had driveline infections (14.6%). The average onset of bacteremia was 121 days from implant, with a range of 5–497 days. Consistent with prior studies, the predominant organism was coagulase negative staphylococcus (8 of 11, 72%). In patients with driveline infections, the average onset was 305 days from LVAD placement, with a range of 15–893 days. Thirty-one percent of driveline exit site cultures demonstrated methicillin-sensitive *Staphylococcus aureus* (MSSA, 4 of 13) and 15.4% were *Enterobacter* species. Two patients had persistent driveline infections requiring continuous IV antibiotics and surgical intervention. (Organisms included *Stenotrophomonas* and MSSA).

In the BTT group, the patients with infection had a significantly longer duration of support 410 ± 342 days vs. those without infection, who had a mean duration of 250 ± 213 days ($p = 0.014$). The 1-year survival was 75% in those with infection vs. 82% in those without infection.

Infectious complications including driveline infections and bacteremia are a major morbidity of LVAD therapy and increase the duration of support in patients awaiting transplantation. To allow these devices to be a long-term alternative to heart transplantation, further investigation into identifying infectious risk factors and focused strategies on treatment of driveline infections is critical.

Right Ventricular Failure

Right ventricular (RV) failure is a leading cause of morbidity and death after LVAD implant due to the inability of the RV to pump sufficient blood through the pulmonary circuit to adequately fill the left side of the heart. It is a major contributing factor to other serious adverse events such as bleeding, renal failure, and prolonged hospitalization. RV function is a major consideration for both volume displacement and continuous-flow devices.

Studies have reported a large range of RV failure requiring RVAD. In the HeartMate XVE study, 11% received RVADs [42]. In the HeartMate II BTT trial, the incidence of postoperative RV failure, defined as need for RVAD support or inonotropic support for 14 days, was 20% [21].

Kormos et al. demonstrated that among 484 patients in the HeartMate II trial, 6% required RVAD and that RV failure was associated with worse outcomes [43]. In our experience at the University of Minnesota Medical School, RV failure after HMII implantation occurred in 2 of 40 patients (5%). Significant improvements occurred in cardiac index, with reductions in right atrial pressure, RV stroke work index, tricuspid annular motion, mean pulmonary artery pressure, and pulmonary vascular resistance after HMII support. A trend toward reduction in tricuspid regurgitation after LVAD support was shown ($p=0.075$) [44].These observations indicate the need for better patient selection for those at high risk for right ventricular failure or potentially providing preoperative RVAD support.

Future Directions

MCS has evolved significantly over the last 2 decades from an experimental strategy for the moribund to an accepted therapy for patients with advanced heart failure. Many devices are available worldwide for a variety of uses and durations of support. The long-term use of LVADs is of interest as a replacement for heart transplantation and remains an area of intense research. Complications associated with LVADs including thrombogenicity, bleeding, infection, and RV failure remain limitations of the devices. Advances in device design, miniaturization of pumps, and patient selection will continue to play a pivotal role in the wider application of LVADs.

References

1. Rosamond W, Flegal K, Furie K, et al. Heart disease and stroke statistics 2008 update: a report from the American Heart Association Statistics Committee and Stroke Statistics Subcommittee. Circulation. 2008;117(4):e125–46.
2. O'Connor C, Gattis W, Zannad F, et al. Beta-blocker therapy in advanced heart failure: clinical characteristics and long-term outcomes. Eur J Heart Fail. 1999;1:81–8.
3. Rose EA, Gelijns AC, Moskowitz AJ, et al. Long-term use of a left ventricular assist device for end-stage heart failure. N Engl J Med. 2001;345:1435–43.
4. Califf RM, Adams KF, McKenna WJ, et al. A randomized controlled trial of epoprostenol therapy for severe congestive heart failure: the Flolan International Randomized Survival Trial (FIRST). Am Heart J. 1997;134:44–54.
5. The SOLVD Investigators. Effect of enalapril on survival in patients with reduced left ventricular ejection fractions and congestive heart failure. N Engl J Med. 1991;325:293–302.
6. Packer M, Coats AJS, Fowler MB, et al. Effect of carvedilol on survival in severe chronic heart failure. N Engl J Med. 2001;344:1651–8.
7. Sandeep J. The artificial heart. N Engl J Med. 2004;350:522–44.
8. Aaronson KD, Eppinger MJ, Dyke DB, Wright S, Pagani FD. Left ventricular assist device therapy improves utilization of donor hearts. Ann Thorac Surg. 2004;39:1247–54.
9. Morgan JA, John R, Rao V, et al. Bridging to transplant with the HeartMate left ventricular assist device: the Columbia Presbyterian 12-year experience. J Thorac Cardiovasc Surg. 2004;127:1309–16.
10. John R, Liao K, Lietz K, et al. Experience with the Levitronix CentriMag circulatory support system as a bridge to decision in patients with refractory acute cardiogenic shock and multisystem organ failure. J Thorac Cardiovasc Surg. 2007;134(2):351–8.
11. De Robertis F, Birks EJ, Rogers P, Dreyfus G, Pepper JR, Khagani A. Clinical performance with the Levitronix CentriMag short-term ventricular assist device. J Heart Lung Transplant. 2006;25:181–6.
12. Mueller JP, Kuenzli A, Reuthebuch O, et al. The CentriMag: a new optimized centrifugal blood pump with levitating impeller. Heart Surg Forum. 2004;7:E477–80.
13. Shuhaiber JH, Jenkins D, Berman M, et al. The Papworth Experience with the Levitronix CentriMag ventricular assist device. J Heart Lung Transplant. 2008;27(2):158–64.
14. De Robertis F, Rogers P, Amrani M, et al. Bridge to decision using the Levitronix CentriMag short-term ventricular assist device. J Heart Lung Transplant. 2008;27:474–8.
15. Samuels LE, Holmes EC, Thomas MP, et al. Management of acute cardiac failure with mechanical assist: experience with the ABIOMED BVS 5000. Ann Thorac Surg. 2001;71:S67–72.
16. Westaby S, Banning AP, Saito S, et al. Circulatory support for long-term treatment of heart failure: experience with an intraventricular continuous flow pump. Circulation. 2002;105:2588–91.
17. Slater JP, Rose EA, Levin HR, et al. Low thromboembolic risk without anticoagulation using advanced design left ventricular assist devices. Ann Thorac Surg. 1996;62:1321–8.
18. Pagani FD, Long JW, Dembitsky WP, et al. Improved mechanical reliability of the HeartMate XVE left ventricular assist system. Ann Thorac Surg. 2006;82:1413–9.
19. Wampler RK, Moise JC, Frazier OH, et al. In vivo evaluation of a peripheral vascular access axial flow blood pump. Trans Am Soc Artif Intern Organs. 1988;34:450–4.
20. Goldstein DJ, Zucker MJ, Pagani FD, et al. Rotary ventricular assist devices: ISHLT Monograph series. In: Frazier OK, Kirklin JK, editors. Mechanical circulatory support. Oxford: Elsevier; 2006. p. 77–104.
21. Slaughter MS, Rogers JG, Milano CA, et al. Advanced heart failure treated with continuous-flow left ventricular assist device. N Engl J Med. 2009;361:2241–51.

22. John R, Kamdar F, Liao K, et al. Improved survival and decreasing incidence of adverse events using the HeartMate II left ventricular assist device as a bridge-to-transplant. Ann Thorac Surg. 2008;86:1227–34.
23. Miller LW, Pagani FD, Russell SD, et al. Use of a continuous-flow device in patients awaiting heart transplantation. N Engl J Med. 2007;357:885–96.
24. Pagani FD, Miller LW, Russell SD. Extended mechanical circulatory support with a continuous flow rotary left ventricular assist device. J Am Coll Cardiol. 2009;54:312–20.
25. Esmore D, Kaye R, Salamonsen M, et al. First clinical implant of the VentrAssist left ventricular assist system as destination therapy for end-stage heart failure. J Heart Lung Transplant. 2005;24:1150–4.
26. Spanier TB, Oz MC, Levin HR, et al. Activation of coagulation and fibrinolytic pathways in patients with left ventricular assist devices. J Thorac Cardiovasc Surg. 1996;112:1090–7.
27. Menconi MJ, Prockwinse S, Owen TA, Dasse KA, Stein GS, Lian GB. Properties of blood contacting surfaces of clinically implanted cardiac assist devices: gene expression, matrix composition, and ultrastructural characterization of cellular linings. J Cell Biochem. 1995;57:557.
28. John R, Panch S, Hrabe J, et al. Activation of endothelial and coagulation system in left ventricular assist device recipients. Ann Thorac Surg. 2009;88(4):1171–9.
29. Amir AW, Bracey FW, Smart RM, Delgado 3rd RM, Shah N, Kar B. A successful anticoagulation protocol for the first HeartMate II implantation in the United States. Tex Heart Inst J. 2005;32:399–401.
30. Frazier OH, Delgado RM, Kar B, Patel V, Gregoric ID, Meyers TJ. First clinical use of the redesigned HeartMate II left ventricular assist system in the United States: a case report. Tex Heart Inst J. 2004;31:157–9.
31. Boyle AJ, Russell SD, Teuteberg JJ, et al. Low thromboembolism and pump thrombosis with the HeartMate II left ventricular assist device: analysis of outpatient anti-coagulation. J Heart Lung Transplant. 2009;28(9):881–7.
32. Tulchinsky M. Lower gastrointestinal bleeding diagnosed by red blood cell scintigraphy in a patient with a left ventricular assist device. Clin Nucl Med. 2008;33:856–8.
33. Daas AY, Small MB, Pinkas H, Brady PG. Safety of conventional and wireless capsule endoscopy in patients supported with nonpulsatile axial flow Heart-Mate II left ventricular assist device. Gastrointest Endosc. 2008;68:379–82.
34. Garatti A, Bruschi G, Girelli C, Vitali E. Small intestine capsule endoscopy in magnetic suspended axial left ventricular assist device patient. Interact Cardiovasc Thorac Surg. 2006;5:1–4.
35. Letsou GV, Shah N, Gregoric ID, Meyers TJ, Delgado R, Frazier OH. Gastrointestinal bleeding from arteriovenous malformations in patients supported by the Jarvik 2000 axial-flow left ventricular assist device. J Heart Lung Transplant. 2005;24:105–9.
36. Malehsa D, Meyer AL, Bara C, Struber M. Acquired von Willebrand syndrome after exchange of the HeartMate XVE to the HeartMate II ventricular assist device. Eur J Cardiothorac Surg. 2009;35:1091–3.
37. Klovaite J, Gustafsson F, Mortensen SA, Sander K, Nielsen LB. Severely impaired von Willebrand factor-dependent platelet aggregation in patients with a continuous-flow left ventricular assist device (HeartMate II). J Am Coll Cardiol. 2009;53:2162–7.
38. Geisen U, Heilmann C, Beyersdorf F, et al. Non-surgical bleeding in patients with ventricular assist devices could be explained by acquired von Willebrand disease. Eur J Cardiothorac Surg. 2008;33:679–84.
39. Crow S, Milano C, Joyce L, et al. Comparative analysis of von Willebrand Factor profiles in pulsatile and continuous left ventricular assist device recipients. ASAIO J. 2010;56:441–5.
40. Gordon SM, Schmitt SK, Jacobs M, et al. Nosocomial bloodstream infections in patients with implantable left ventricular assist devices. Ann Thorac Surg. 2001;72:725–30.
41. Simon D, Fischer S, Grossman A, et al. Left ventricular assist device-related infection: treatment and outcome. Clin Infect Dis. 2005;40:1108–15.
42. Frazier OH, Rose EA, Oz MC, et al. Multicenter clinical evaluation of the HeartMate vented electric left ventricular assist system in patients awaiting heart transplantation. J Thorac Cardiovasc Surg. 2001;122:1186–95.
43. Kormos RL, Teuteberg JJ, Pagani FD, et al. HeartMate II Clinical Investigators. Right ventricular failure in patients with the HeartMate II continuous-flow left ventricular assist device: incidence, risk factors, and effect on outcomes. J Thorac Cardiovasc Surg. 2010;139(5):1316–24.
44. Lee S, Kamdar F, Madlon-Kay R, et al. Effects of the HeartMate II continuous-flow left ventricular assist device on right ventricular function. J Heart Lung Transplant. 2010;29(2):209–15.
45. Jessup M, Brozena S. Heart failure. N Engl J Med. 2003;348:2007–18.
46. Haj-Yahia S, Birks EJ, Amrani M, et al. Bridging patients after salvage from bridge to decision directly to transplant by means of prolonged support with the CentriMag short-term centrifugal pump. J Thorac Cardiovasc Surg. 2009;138:227–30.
47. Esmore D, Kaye D, Spratt P, et al. A prospective, multicenter trial of the VentrAssist left ventricular assist device for bridge to transplant: safety and efficacy. J Heart Lung Transplant. 2008;27(6):579–88. Epub 2008 Apr 23.
48. John R, Kamdar F, Liao K, et al. Low thromboembolic risk for patients with the HeartMate II left ventricular assist device. J Thorac Cardiovasc Surg. 2008;136:1318–23.

Websites

CentriMag is a registered trademark of Levitronix LLC – http://www.levitronix.com/Brochures.html.
Abiomed is a registered trademark of Abiomed – http://www.abiomed.com/about_abiomed/index.cfm.
HeartMate is a registered trademark of Thoratec Corporation – http://www.thoratec.com/medical-professionals/vad-product-information/heartmate-xve-lvad.aspx.
Hemopump is a registered trademark of [not sure – see references to Medtronic and Johnson and Johnson.
VentrAssist is a trademark of Ventracor – http://biotechnology-innovation.com.au/innovations/devices_or_implants/ventrassist.html.

Chapter 27
Diabetes and Coronary Heart Disease

Graham T. McMahon

Introduction

The epidemic of type 2 diabetes continues unabated, with some 25 million patients living with this disease in the United States. Diabetes confers a substantially increased risk for cardiovascular morbidity and mortality [1–5]. Even with the best medical therapies to control blood glucose, diabetic patients have poorer cardiovascular outcomes than nondiabetic individuals. Type 2 diabetes exacerbates traditional, modifiable risk factors for vascular disease; each additional risk factor caused a greater, incremental rise in risk among individuals with diabetes than those without [6].

Adults with diabetes but without known cardiac disease have a similar risk of a cardiovascular event as nondiabetic adults with a history of a prior myocardial infarct [7]. Although these risks can be substantially reduced with careful attention to risk factor modification, less than 10% of patients with diabetes reach their glucose, blood pressure, and cholesterol targets [8, 9].

Hyperglycemia contributes to cardiovascular risk in patients with diabetes, but the relationship between hyperglycemia and cardiovascular disease is more complex than its more easily evident association with microvascular complication. For example, data from the United Kingdom Prospective Diabetes Study (UKPDS) demonstrated that cardiovascular risk rises with increasing hemoglobin A1c (HbA1c), but at a slower incremental rate than that for microvascular disease [10]. Even people with mild impairment of fasting plasma glucose level have excess risk [11]. The Honolulu Heart Program showed during 23 years of follow-up that impaired glucose tolerance doubled the risk of subsequent cardiovascular disease and suggested that much of the cardiovascular risk accrues before the onset of clinical diabetes [12].

Several additional components contribute to the cardiovascular risk profile of patients with diabetes. For example, a longer duration of diabetes during adulthood (the years of exposure to diabetes before age 20 add little to the risk of macrovascular disease), and the greater degree of hyperglycemia correlate with greater risk of macrovascular disease. Microalbuminuria is an indicator of the degree of endothelial dysfunction: Patients with diabetes and microalbuminuria have a 2–3-fold higher risk of cardiovascular events and death than those without this finding, but a similar duration of diabetes [13–15]. Cardiovascular risk for a particular patient can be estimated from online tools such as the Archimedes model or the UKPDS Risk Engine [16].

Atherosclerosis and Diabetes

The etiology of cardiovascular disease in patients with diabetes is multifactorial. Although the principal cause of diabetes' microvascular complications appears to be hyperglycemia, the exact cellular or molecular basis of the macrovascular diabetes complications, including accelerated atherosclerosis, has not yet been elucidated.

Increased glucose concentrations can activate nuclear factor-κB, a key mediator that regulates multiple proinflammatory and proatherosclerotic target genes in vascular smooth muscle cells, endothelial cells, and macrophages [17]. Through this

G.T. McMahon, MD, MMSc (✉)
Division of Endocrinology, Harvard Medical School, Diabetes and Hypertension,
Brigham and Women's Hospital, 221 Longwood Avenue, Boston, MA 02115, USA
e-mail: gmcmahon@partners.org

Z. Vlodaver et al. (eds.), *Coronary Heart Disease: Clinical, Pathological, Imaging, and Molecular Profiles*,
DOI 10.1007/978-1-4614-1475-9_27, © Springer Science+Business Media, LLC 2012

Table 27.1 Treatment goals for adults with type 2 diabetes

Risk factor	Target
Glycemic control	
Glycosylated hemoglobin	<7.0%
Preprandial plasma glucose	90–130 mg/dL
Peak postprandial plasma glucose	<180 mg/dL
Blood pressure	<130/80 mmHg
Lipids	<100 mg/dL
Low-density lipoproteins	<150 mg/dL
Triglycerides	>40 mg/dL
High-density lipoproteins	
Cigarette smoking	Cessation
Overweight or obese	10% weight loss

Adapted from American Diabetes Association [22]. Copyright 2011 by American Diabetes Association

activation of nuclear factor-κB, hyperglycemia enhances monocyte adhesion to the endothelium to promote atherosclerosis [18]. Furthermore, glucose may also activate matrix-degrading metalloproteinases, enzymes implicated in plaque rupture and arterial remodeling [17, 19].

Hyperglycemia is closely associated with inflammation [20]. High levels of tumor necrosis factor-alpha appear to lead to insulin resistance, and insulin resistance in turn is inflammatory. Increased levels of markers and mediators of inflammation and acute-phase reactants such as fibrinogen, C-reactive protein, IL-6, plasminogen activator inhibitor-1 (PAI-1), and others correlate with the onset of diabetes [19, 20].

The effects of glucose on tissue are attributable in part to the formation of sugar-derived substances called advanced glycation end products (AGEs). AGEs form at a constant but slow rate, and accumulate with time, but their formation is accelerated in diabetes because of the increased availability of glucose [21]. AGEs are created from a nonenzymatic reaction between sugars and the free amino groups of proteins, lipids, and nucleic acids, and result in disturbed function of these molecules. These initial reactions are reversible, depending on the concentration of the reactants [21].

A large body of evidence suggests that AGEs are important pathogenetic mediators of almost all diabetes complications, including vascular disease. Increased AGE accumulation in the diabetic vascular tissues has been associated with changes in endothelial cell, macrophage, and smooth muscle cell function. In addition, AGEs can modify low-density lipoprotein (LDL) cholesterol in such a way that it tends to become easily oxidized and deposited within vessel walls, causing streak formation and, in time, atheroma. AGE-crosslink formation results in arterial stiffening with loss of elasticity of large vessels [17, 19].

Reducing Cardiovascular Risk in Diabetes

Increasing evidence shows that cardiovascular disease risk can be reduced in patients with diabetes. Although glycemic control remains the key component of diabetes care, identifying and managing other cardiovascular disease risk factors such as hypertension and dyslipidemia are also vital. The American Diabetes Association (ADA) recommends at least annual screening for cardiovascular disease risk factors (dyslipidemia, hypertension, family history of premature coronary disease, presence of microalbuminuria) as well as tight treatment goals for glycemia, blood pressure, and serum lipid levels (Table 27.1) [22]. The American Heart Association [23] and National Cholesterol Education Program (NCEP) [24, 25] have released similar guidelines recommending that patients with diabetes be treated as high risk and advocating more rigorous lipid and blood pressure targets for both primary and secondary prevention of cardiovascular events if these screening tests reveal abnormalities.

Lifestyle Management

Weight Reduction

Medical nutrition therapy can result in substantial improvements in glycemia, blood pressure, and lipid levels in individuals with diabetes. However, success with lifestyle intervention requires a coordinated team effort that empowers the patient.

Weight loss of as little as 5% of body weight can substantially reduce insulin resistance and blood pressure, and improve glycemic control [26]. Several trials have demonstrated the efficacy of intensive lifestyle modification in patients with diabetes, namely, weight loss; substantial improvements in HbA1c, lipid profile, and urine albumin to creatinine ratio; and reduced dependency on mediations [27–29]. These interventions need not be expensive, typically costing about $350 per participant [27]. Weight loss and reduced use of saturated fats appeared to be the main determinants of successful treatment results [28].

Pharmacologic approaches to weight loss are not routinely recommended. Rimonabant is a selective cannabinoid receptor (CB1) blocker that has been shown to reduce body weight and improve cardiometabolic risk factors in overweight and obese patients. Although effective in patients with diabetes, the drug caused an increased risk of adverse psychiatric effects and never reached the American market [30–32]. Sibutramine and orlistat have been investigated in patients with diabetes and each has been associated with modest reductions in body weight; however, sibutramine is associated with increases in systolic blood pressure [33], and orlistat (now available over the counter) is generally not well tolerated [34]. Sibutramine has recently been associated with an increase in cardiovascular events and has been withdrawn from the American and European markets.

Since medical approaches to weight management have had such limited success, patients and their clinicians are more frequently turning to bariatric surgery as an option. Obese individuals are candidates for weight-loss surgery if medical therapy has failed and if they have a body mass index ≥40 kg/m^2 or a body mass index ≥35 kg/m^2 with comorbid conditions [35]. The laparoscopic silicone gastric banding procedure and gastric restriction combined with diversion such as the Roux-en-Y gastric bypass are now frequently performed, and the perioperative mortality rate has dropped to less than 1% [36]. Sustained weight loss through bariatric surgical intervention is associated both with prevention of progression of impaired glucose tolerance, the clinical remission of type 2 diabetes (in some 60% of patients with diabetes who have the procedure), but also with an estimated reduction in mortality of approximately 20% [37, 38]. Nevertheless, patients considering bariatric surgery should be carefully evaluated by an experienced team, understand the lifetime commitment to dietary measures, and be willing to accept the permanence of the intervention.

Exercise

Physical inactivity is a significant risk factor for cardiovascular events in both men and women. In diabetic women, physical inactivity (activity <1 h/week) is associated with a doubling of cardiovascular event rates when compared with exercise for 7 h/week [39]. Men with diabetes share similar risks: Low cardiorespiratory fitness increased overall mortality by a factor of 2.9 when compared with moderately or highly fit counterparts [40].

Physical activity is a fundamental element of cardiovascular risk reduction in high-risk patients. Exercise influences several aspects of diabetes, including blood glucose concentrations, insulin action, blood pressure, and lipid concentrations, and contributes to successful weight loss. While exercise produces many benefits, patients should be thoughtful when engaging in a new exercise program. Rarely, exercise can precipitate a cardiac symptom or event, and autonomic neuropathy may predispose patients to exercise-induced arrhythmias. Clinicians may prefer to refer patients planning an exercise program of moderate intensity or greater for evaluation with exercise treadmill testing.

During exercise, hyperglycemia can result from excess hepatic glucose output, and ketogenesis can ensue. By contrast, hypoglycemia can result from excess glucose uptake due to either increased insulin concentrations, enhanced insulin action, or impaired carbohydrate absorption during exercise; consequently, insulin doses should generally be reduced prior to exercise, although some insulin is typically still needed. Blood glucose monitoring before and after exercise is particularly important for those with hypoglycemia unawareness. Appropriate foot care and shoe selection can protect diabetics from developing podiatric complications as a result of their activity.

For patients with diabetes, the overall benefits of exercise are significant. A study examining multiple healthy lifestyle habits which include smoking cessation, adequate leisure-time physical activity, and consumption of ≥5 portions of fruits and vegetables per day associated those habits with significantly better quality of life among diabetics [41]. Identifying and preventing potential problems can mitigate complications and promote this valuable approach to healthy living.

Smoking Cessation

Smoking is likely to have at least as detrimental an effect on cardiovascular health in patients with diabetes as it does in those without diabetes. Smoking predicts incident diabetes, and is an independent risk factor for myocardial infarction, stroke, and all-cause mortality in patients with type 2 diabetes [42, 43]. Diabetic smokers are also at higher risk for accelerated microvascular disease. Data show that cigarette smoking and increased urine albumin excretion are interrelated predictors of nephropathy progression in patients with type 1 and type 2 diabetes, and that smoking increases urine albumin excretion in these patients despite improved blood pressure control and pharmacologic inhibition of the angiotensin-converting enzyme (ACE) [44, 45].

Smoking cessation programs reduce tobacco use and are cost-effective [46]. Furthermore, the risks of macrovascular disease can be reduced by quitting smoking, with significant societal cost savings [47, 48]. The most effective smoking cessation programs unite physician and the patient with scheduled follow-ups to review progress and provide support [49]. Discussing reasons for smoking triggers and preferred quit strategy can be useful in negotiating a quit date.

Glycemic Control

Chronic hyperglycemia is associated with a higher cardiovascular event rate, and evidence supports the assertion that reducing glucose levels reduces the risk of developing diabetes-specific complications. However, it has been much more difficult to demonstrate that improved glycemia reduces cardiovascular risk.

Although type 1 and type 2 diabetes differ in many respects, evaluating the role of hyperglycemia control in patients with type 1 diabetes can be mechanistically informative. In the Diabetes Control and Complications Trial, 1,441 patients with type 1 diabetes who were free of documented cardiovascular disease, obesity, hypertension, and hypercholesterolemia were randomized to conventional or intensive diabetes management and followed for a mean of 6.5 years. Intensive management targeted HbA1c of 6%. Those years of lower glucose levels were ultimately shown to be associated with significant cardiovascular risk reduction, as illustrated by the study's follow-up trial, the Epidemiology of Diabetes Interventions and Complications. Intensive treatment during the trial was ultimately associated with a 57% lower long-term cardiovascular risk [50]. The beneficial effect of lower glucose levels was reinforced by the finding that coronary artery calcification, an index of atherosclerosis measured by computed tomography, was found to be significantly lower in the intensive therapy group [51].

The beneficial effect of lowering glucose is more complicated in patients with type 2 diabetes who typically have multiple comorbidities that contribute to elevated cardiovascular risk. The UKPDS recruited 3,867 subjects with type 2 diabetes who were suboptimally controlled on diet alone, and randomized them to conventional treatment (diet unless fasting glucose >270 mg/dL), or intensive treatment with either a sulfonylurea or insulin [52]. Another group of 1,704 overweight patients (>120% ideal) were randomized to diet, metformin, sulfonylurea, or insulin [53]. The intensively treated patients had lower HbA1c levels and fewer microvascular endpoints, but the lower rates of cardiovascular events did not quite reach statistical significance.

The ACCORD and ADVANCE studies were two large trials that sought to determine the effect on cardiovascular risk of lowering glucose to near-normal levels [54, 55]. Both trials compared intensive and standard glucose-lowering targets in type 2 diabetes. Many in the diabetes community were surprised by the major findings that near-normal glycemic control for a median of 3.5–5 years did not reduce cardiovascular events within that time frame. A troubling finding from the ACCORD trial was that near-normal glucose control (achieved with the use of combination therapy incorporating heavy use of thiazolidinediones, sulfonylureas, metformin, and insulin) was associated with a significantly increased risk of death from any cause and death from cardiovascular causes – the very outcomes the trial was designed to prevent [55].

While the results were disappointing, they do not undermine the importance of meeting current guidelines for care, and they should not be interpreted as diminishing the importance of glycemic control in patients with diabetes [56]. The lower-than-anticipated rate of cardiovascular events seen in these trials is an affirmation of the success of modern therapeutics, even when incompletely implemented.

Diabetes Medications and Cardiovascular Disease Risk

Metformin

Metformin reduces blood glucose levels by reducing hepatic glucose production and improving insulin sensitivity in patients with diabetes. Independent of its glycemic effect, metformin lowers total cholesterol, LDL, and particularly triglycerides, but has no effect on high-density lipoprotein (HDL) [57]. Metformin has proven clinical benefit for cardiovascular risk reduction in patients with diabetes and has emerged as a first-line drug for the treatment of type 2 diabetes [58]. In the

UKPDS, overweight patients given metformin had fewer atherosclerotic complications, with a particular decrement in myocardial infarction rates. Results were better for metformin than for sulfonylurea or insulin. With intensive therapy (target glucose of 108 mg/dL), metformin reduced the myocardial infarction rate by 39% ($p=0.01$) while sulfonylurea or insulin use was associated with a nonsignificant risk reduction of 21% [53]. Although increasing evidence exists regarding the safety of metformin and the extremely low risk of lactic acidosis (less than 8 cases per 100,000 patient-years), metformin should nevertheless be avoided in patients with renal, hepatic, pulmonary, or heart failure [59, 60].

Sulfonylureas

There is a theoretical reason why sulfonylureas may have an adverse effect on diabetic patients with epicardial coronary disease. Sulfonylureas act by inhibiting potassium channels, which are present not only in the beta cells but also in the heart and vascular smooth muscle [61]. This class of medications has been shown to prevent cardiac preconditioning, the ability of the heart to recover more quickly after repeated ischemic insults [62]. The UKPDS is often cited in defense of the safety of these agents, as glibenclamide was associated with a reduction in myocardial infarction rates, which was almost statistically significant ($p=0.056$). Although sulfonylureas, like insulin, increase the risk of weight gain and hypoglycemia, the onset of their effect is relatively quick [63]. These drugs remain second-line agents for treatment of type 2 diabetes.

Thiazolidinediones

Thiazolidinediones (TZDs) improve insulin sensitivity and glycemic control, and might preserve insulin secretion and beta cell health in patients with type 2 diabetes [64]. These drugs activate the PPAR-γ receptor, which is involved in the process of atherosclerosis, and its modulation for cardioprotection is an active area of investigation. Some beneficial effects attributed to TZDs include a decrease in blood pressure, improvement of fibrinolysis, correction of diabetic dyslipidemia, a decrease in free fatty acid levels, a reduction in inflammatory markers, and a decrease in carotid artery intimal thickness [65, 66]. TZDs increase LDL cholesterol levels, although this effect may be offset by favorable changes in LDL particle size and susceptibility to oxidation [67].

Despite these pathobiologic effects that would be expected to be associated with substantial reductions in cardiovascular events among treated patients, these drugs have been unable to demonstrate that their use results in any cardiovascular protection; in fact, there have been some indications that the medications from this class can increase the risk of subsequent cardiovascular events [68].

In the PROactive study, addition of 45 mg of pioglitazone to other glucose-lowering drugs in patients with type 2 diabetes reduced some subgroups (all-cause mortality, myocardial infarction, and stroke) but there was no difference in the study's primary endpoint [66, 69]. Additional data from studies of TZDs have indicated that these medications increase the risk of heart failure and fractures, and appear to be associated with an increased risk of myocardial infarction [70]. Consequently prescription of rosiglitazone is restricted by the Food and Drug administration [71].

Incretin Mimetics and DPP-4 Inhibitors

Glucagon-like peptide 1 (GLP-1) stimulates postprandial insulin release; however, it is rapidly degraded by the activity of dipeptidyl peptidase IV (DPP 4). Exenatide and liraglutide are synthetic GLP-1 agonists and have demonstrated glycemic efficacy (HbA1c reductions of between 0.7 and 2%) associated with mild weight loss; nausea is frequent and can be problematic [72, 73]. Longer acting (such as once-weekly) formulations saxagliptin, linagliptin, and sitagliptin of this class have been shown to more effectively control glucose and reduce weight, while being substantially more tolerable [74].

Orally administered DPP-4 inhibitors saxagliptin and sitagliptin (given once daily) have also shown consistent, although moderate improvements in the glycemic profile of type 2 diabetic patients [75–78]. These medications are especially useful in patients with compromised renal function. These drugs are weight-neutral. It remains unclear whether they will be associated with improved cardiovascular outcomes.

Insulin

Insulin remains the most efficacious method of improving glycemic control. However, insulin exposes the user to a risk of hypoglycemia and induces weight gain. Individuals receiving intensive insulin management as part of the UKPDS gained an average of 8.8 lb; 2.3% of the patients had a severe hypoglycemic event in each year of the study [52]. Nevertheless, intensive insulin therapy has a positive effect on lipoproteins, and on lowering triglycerides, LDL, and total cholesterol levels [79]. The independent cardiovascular benefits of insulin have not been convincingly demonstrated [52]. In the UKPDS study, the risk of myocardial infarction in the conventional and intensively treated arms was 17.4 and 14.7 events per 1,000 patient-years, respectively ($p=0.052$).

Among patients who have had a myocardial infarction, aggressive insulin management has been associated with a reduction in mortality of up to 30% [80]. It is unclear whether the effect was due to the immediate insulin-glucose infusion or the long-term improvements in glycemic control resulting from ongoing insulin administration.

Newer, long-acting insulin analogs such as insulin glargine and insulin detemir can be safely introduced to patients on oral hypoglycemic agents. A forced titration schedule starting at 10 units daily and increasing weekly to a target of a fasting glucose of no more than 100 mg/dL is highly effective in reducing the hemoglobin A1c to 7% with minimal risk of hypoglycemia [81, 82]. Results from the ACCORD study suggest caution in aiming for excessively low glucose values.

Blood Pressure Control

Hypertension affects up to 60% of patients with diabetes and rises in prevalence with age and increasing levels of obesity. Hypertension is a major risk factor in the development of both macro- and microvascular complications of diabetes. In type 1 diabetes, hypertension is often secondary to underlying nephropathy, while hypertension in type 2 diabetes often forms part of the metabolic syndrome. As soon as blood pressure rises above 120/80 mmHg, cardiovascular risk in diabetic patients appreciates, and treatment is recommended when blood pressure exceeds 130/80 mmHg [18, 83]. Before starting antihypertensive therapy, patients should be reexamined within 1 month for confirmation, unless the initial diastolic value is greater than 110 mmHg. Many of these patients require multidrug therapy for control. Many classes of antihypertensives have had demonstrated efficacy in diabetics.

ACE Inhibitors and ARBs

ACE inhibitors and angiotensin receptor blockers (ARBs) have been shown to reduce blood pressure, reduce cardiovascular events, and slow the progression of nephropathy [40, 53, 84–89].

The Heart Outcomes Protection Evaluation (HOPE) trial reported on 3,577 people with diabetes out of 9,541 people age 55 or older who also had another vascular risk factor such as smoking, hypertension, or microalbuminuria. The trial found that 10 mg of ramipril vs. placebo over 4.5 years reduced cardiovascular mortality by 37%, myocardial infarction by 22%, and stroke by 33% among individuals with diabetes [40]. A subgroup from the HOPE study underwent carotid ultrasound to evaluate carotid intimal medial thickness. Those being treated with ramipril had a 37% reduction in the rate of thickening, reflecting healthier endothelial function [90]. The relative benefit of ramipril was present in all subgroups regardless of hypertensive status, microalbuminuria, type of diabetes, and nature of diabetes treatment (diet, oral agents, or insulin). The mean reduction in blood pressure with treatment (3/2 mmHg) appeared to be too small to independently account for the risk reductions achieved. Patients with creatinine concentrations >1.4 mg/dL had an even greater benefit than those with more normal renal function.

Diuretics

Diuretics have proven efficacy in blood pressure control. Their benefits outweigh the mild increases in serum glucose associated with their use, and drugs from this class are generally endorsed to reach target blood pressure goals [91, 92]. The Antihypertensive and Lipid Lowering Treatment to Prevent Heart Attack Trial was stopped early after interim analysis revealed a substantial benefit of thiazide diuretics over α-blocking agents [93]. Furthermore, chlorthalidone provided twice as much benefit in reducing cardiovascular events to diabetic patients as nondiabetics with hypertension [94].

Calcium Channel Blockers

Calcium channel blockers are increasingly used ahead of beta-blockers, given evidence of efficacy in patients with diabetes [95]. While calcium channel blockers appear to be inferior to ACE inhibitors in cardiovascular protection, they are often good choices as additional therapy given their ability to lower systolic blood pressure, particularly in African American patients [96].

As a result of these and other studies, major professional organizations recommend ACEIs or ARBs with or without thiazide diuretics as first-line therapy for patients with type 2 diabetes. Calcium channel blockers tend to be used as third-line drugs, with additional therapy individualized.

Lipid Management

The typical lipid profile associated with type 2 diabetes comprises an abnormally low level of HDL cholesterol, an elevated triglyceride level, and a relatively normal LDL cholesterol level. Though the LDL level is often within the normal range or only slightly elevated, the LDL itself is abnormally dense and atherogenic. This combination of abnormal lipids contributes to the cardiovascular risk of patients with type 2 diabetes [97–100]. Generally speaking, LDL levels are neither higher nor more often elevated in diabetic patients than in nondiabetic individuals, but the presence of abnormally high LDL levels should be regarded as an additional risk factor to address in diabetic patients.

The NCEP Adult Treatment Panel III (ATP III) designation of diabetes as a "coronary heart disease risk equivalent" justifies aggressive lipid lowering in patients with diabetes, as if they already have cardiovascular disease [101]. The ATP III recommended that pharmacologic therapy be initiated in diabetic patients whose LDL levels are 130 mg/dL or greater, and that patients be treated to target LDL levels less than 100 mg/dL. A goal of 70 mg/dL or lower is an appropriate target for patients at especially high risk. The ADA recommends the additional goals of raising HDL levels above 40 mg/dL in men and 45 mg/dL in women, and lowering triglycerides below 150 mg/dL.

Statins

Despite the characteristic lipid profile, current guidelines for managing diabetic dyslipidemia typically target LDL cholesterol, as the strongest evidence in support of lipid-lowering therapy for diabetic patients comes from studies showing the benefit of HMG-CoA reductase inhibitors (statins). Statin therapy has proven to be particularly useful in treating dyslipidemia and has resulted in significant reductions in coronary events according to several large primary and secondary trials. A few of these early statin trials included a relatively small number of patients with diabetes.

The most important trial to date examining the relationship between cardiovascular disease, diabetes, and statins is the Collaborative Diabetes Study [102]. Atorvastatin calcium (10 mg/day) was given as primary prevention to 2,838 patients with type 2 diabetes and one other risk factor (hypertension, albuminuria, retinopathy, or current smoking). The LDL at recruitment was required to be <160 mg/dL. After a mean follow-up of 3.9 years, death rates among those on atorvastatin were 27% lower; in addition, acute coronary event rates were reduced by 36%, revascularizations by 31%, and stroke rates by 48%. Patients with an LDL <100 mg/dL had the same magnitude of benefit as those with a higher LDL. This result has challenged the recommendation that statins be introduced to patients with diabetes only when the LDL is above a threshold.

The Heart Protection Study recruited 20,536 individuals on the basis of having established coronary artery disease (65%), diabetes (19%), peripheral vascular disease (13%), or a history of cerebrovascular disease (9%), and randomly assigned them to simvastatin (40 mg/day) or placebo [103]. A relative risk reduction of 25% was observed for coronary and cerebrovascular events, whether the diabetic subjects already had coronary disease or not, confirming the role of statins for primary prevention of cardiac events [103].

Two negative studies are worthy of note. In the Anglo-Scandinavian Cardiac Outcomes Trial–Lipid Lowering Arm (ASCOT–LLA) trial [104], investigators randomized 2,532 subjects with diabetes and hypertension, but without known cardiac disease, to atorvastatin (10 mg/day) or placebo. Atorvastatin did not reduce the risk of nonfatal myocardial infarction and coronary heart disease death in patients with diabetes and hypertension, despite a reduction of 40–50 mg/dL in LDL cholesterol. The lack of demonstrable effect may have been confounded by a noted increase in statin utilization in the placebo group. The Antihypertensive and Lipid-Lowering Treatment to Prevent Heart Attack Trial (ALLHAT–LLT) was non-blinded and pravastatin (40 mg/day) also did not reduce incidence of nonfatal myocardial infarction and coronary heart disease death among 3,638 patients with diabetes; however, only a modest 15–23 mg/dL reduction in LDL cholesterol concentrations was achieved in the treated vs. the usual-care group [105].

The role of statins for secondary prevention of cardiovascular disease is more clearly established. Although large trials of patients with cardiovascular disease were recruited for these landmark studies, they contained relatively small numbers of subjects with diabetes; nevertheless, the large effect size noted is worthy of notice. The landmark Scandinavian Simvastatin Survival Study (4S) included 202 patients with diabetes and a previous myocardial infarction or angina, and a mean LDL cholesterol level of 187 mg/dL [106]. The study followed subjects for a median of 5.4 years and tracked mortality, coronary death, acute coronary syndromes, and coronary revascularization. In the 4S, individuals with diabetes benefited from the medication as much as those without diabetes. Over the course of the trial, in the simvastatin-treated diabetic patients, the mean changes from baseline in total LDL and HDL cholesterol, and triglycerides were −27, −36, +7, and −11%, respectively. As a result, mortality was reduced by 43%, major coronary events by 55%, and any atherosclerotic event by 37%.

The Cholesterol and Recurrent Events (CARE) trial evaluated the effect of pravastatin on 586 diabetic patients with a history of myocardial infarction and a mean LDL cholesterol level of 136 mg/dL [107]. In diabetic patients randomized to treatment, LDL cholesterol was reduced to a mean of 98 mg/dL and the recurrent coronary event rate (coronary death, myocardial infarction, bypass grafting, or angioplasty) was reduced 25% over 5 years; however, the event rates in treated diabetic patients remained higher than event rates in nondiabetic patients, whether randomized to treatment or not.

Fibrates

Epidemiologic evidence links the combined abnormality of elevated triglyceride levels and low HDL levels with adverse cardiovascular outcomes, independent of LDL cholesterol concentrations [108]. While earlier studies such as the Veterans Affairs HDL Intervention Trial (VA-HIT) demonstrated a 32% reduction in cardiovascular events using gemfibrozil therapy, more recent data has been more circumspect about the use of fibrate therapy to reduce cardiovascular disease event rates [109–112]. In the Fenofibrate Intervention and Endpoint Lowering in Diabetes (FIELD) study, fenofibrate did not significantly reduce the risk of the primary outcome of coronary events [111]. Similarly, in the lipid trial of the ACCORD study, combined treatment with fenofibrate and a statin provided no additional protection beyond treatment with a statin alone [112].

Among patients with elevated triglycerides and low HDL levels, fibrates can be useful in combination with statins [112, 113]. When using combination therapy, many practitioners choose fluvastatin or pravastatin, as these agents are not metabolized by cytochrome P450 3A4, are hydrophilic, and are only 50% protein bound – all factors that reduce adverse drug interactive effects such as rhabdomyolysis, a known risk of combining statins with fibrates [114]. Furthermore, fenofibrate appears to be safer in combination with statins than gemfibrozil [115].

Niacin

Niacin is distinct from other lipid-lowering agents in that it has a broad spectrum of beneficial effects on lipids and atherogenic lipoprotein subfraction levels [116]. Extended-release niacin is associated with a reduction in the more common, adverse effects of flushing and diarrhea seen with crystalline niacin, and the beneficial effects on the lipid profile are maintained [117]. Niacin treatment most substantially increases HDL cholesterol and reduces triglyceride levels – common problems in patients with diabetes. However, niacin also induces increased insulin resistance and causes hyperglycemia. In the Arterial Disease Multiple Intervention Trial, which evaluated immediate-release niacin in the treatment of dyslipidemia associated with diabetes and peripheral vascular disease, 125 subjects with diabetes were randomized to receive crystalline niacin 3 g/day (or the maximally tolerated dose) or placebo [118]. Niacin use significantly increased HDL (by 29%) and decreased triglycerides (by 23%), but increased insulin use [118]. Since there is little evidence of efficacy for cardiovascular risk reduction, niacin use remains limited among patients with diabetes.

Colesevelam

Bile acid sequestrants lower cholesterol, but have also been observed to lower glucose levels modestly in patients with type 2 diabetes. Two trials noted improvements in HbA1c of approximately 0.5% in treated patients after 6 months, with concomitant changes in LDL, high-sensitivity c-reactive protein, and apolipoprotein B [119, 120]. There is no evidence of cardiovascular risk reduction with this drug.

Ezetimibe

Ezetimibe selectively inhibits intestinal absorption of dietary cholesterol. The agent is typically used in patients on a high-dose statin as additive therapy, and in that context is indeed more effective at lowering LDL than the statin alone (mean reduction in LDL level of 27%) [121]. Ezetimibe appears to be safe for use in diabetic patients, but large-scale trials have not been reported, and it remains unclear whether its use is associated with the cardiovascular benefit that would be expected from this degree of lipid improvement [121, 122]. Indeed, the results from a study that examined the effect on carotid intimal media thickness suggest that ezetimibe treatment is not associated with the regression of atherosclerosis as might have been expected [123].

Polyunsaturated Fatty Acids

A highly purified formulation of omega-3 polyunsaturated fatty acids (eicosapentaenoic acid, 465 mg, and docosahexaenoic acid, 375 mg) in a 1 g capsule along with 4 mg of vitamin E has been formulated [124]. In combination with statins, this formulation (Lovaza) has been shown to effectively reduce plasma triglycerides and also increase the potentially less atherogenic form of LDL cholesterol while decreasing the small, dense, and atherogenic LDL particles. In patients with a history of myocardial infarction, this formulation in combination with a statin has been associated with a 14% lower risk of death, nonfatal myocardial infarction, and stroke. Four capsules of the formulation must be administered daily for clinical effect [125].

Antiplatelet Therapy

Evidence from controlled clinical trials generally supports the routine use of low-dose, enteric-coated aspirin, such as 81 mg/day, as a primary and a secondary prevention strategy in adults over the age of 30 who have diabetes.

The recommendation to use aspirin for primary prevention is based on several large trials that included patients with diabetes as a subgroup. The Physician's Health Study, which randomized 22,701 physicians to aspirin or placebo, contained a subgroup of 533 diabetic doctors. After 5 years, 325 mg of aspirin daily reduced the risk of acute myocardial infarction from 10 to 4% [126]. The Hypertension Optimal Treatment (HOT) trial also demonstrated benefit to postinfarction aspirin administration, a benefit that was also seen in its subgroup of 1,501 diabetics [83]. Similarly, in the Early Treatment of Diabetic Retinopathy study, aspirin produced a 28% reduction in myocardial infarctions over 5 years [127]. The Primary Prevention Project evaluated the effect of low-dose aspirin (100 mg/day) on subsequent cardiovascular events in 4,495 individuals with at least one of the following risk factors: hypertension, hypercholesterolemia, diabetes, obesity, a family history of premature myocardial infarction, or being elderly. After a mean follow-up of 3.6 years, aspirin was found to significantly lower the frequency of cardiovascular death (from 1.4 to 0.8%) and total cardiovascular events (from 8.2 to 6.3%) [128].

More recent interventions to reduce cardiovascular risk in diabetes have generated substantial protection. Consequently, a benefit to aspirin treatment has been more difficult to detect. For example, in an open-label trial of 2,539 patients with diabetes in Japan, there was no reduction in risk when aspirin was provided in primary prevention [129]. Several meta-analyses have supported the absence of proven benefit, noting small reductions in overall events, but proportionate increases in bleeding events overall [130, 131].

Retrospective analysis of the diabetic subgroup in the Clopidogrel vs. Aspirin in Patients at Risk of Ischemic Events (CAPRIE) study showed that of the 3,866 diabetic patients randomized, 15.6% of those in the clopidogrel arm and 17.7% of those in the aspirin arm had the composite vascular primary endpoint [132]. Clopidogrel appears to be an effective antiplatelet agent for secondary prevention in patients with diabetes, although aspirin is more cost-effective.

Conclusions

As the leading cause of death among patients with diabetes, cardiovascular disease should be a primary concern for patients with type 2 diabetes and the physicians who care for them. Clinicians need to be sensitive to the challenges these patients face in making therapeutic lifestyle changes and be adept at navigating the polypharmacy that follows from targeting multiple cardiovascular disease risk factors.

Most patients with diabetes will require at least one oral hypoglycemic drug and many will ultimately require insulin. Until further data emerge, the most appropriate initial choices remain metformin and a sulfonylurea, moving to metformin and long-acting insulin when glycemic control is suboptimal on maximal dose therapy.

Achieving a systolic blood pressure less than 130 mmHg in patients with diabetes remains challenging. Almost all should be treated with an ACE inhibitor or ARB. Rational additive treatment includes a thiazide diuretic and calcium channel blockers as needed. Most patients will require at least three drugs for control. In the absence of contraindications, 81 mg of aspirin should be given to patients with diabetes who are age 40 or older who have at least one additional risk factor.

For patients with diabetes whose lipids are not at target range, nonpharmacologic interventions (diet and exercise) remain first-line therapies. Lowering LDL cholesterol is the first priority in treating diabetic dyslipidemia. Statins are the agents of first choice. Fibrates may be useful for patients with low HDL levels and elevated triglycerides, but the benefit appears to be modest.

As confirmed by the STENO-2 study, an integrated approach to diabetes management can halve the rate of cardiovascular events [133]. Online tools, case management, and close follow-up can help clinicians avoid the inertia that often accompanies the management of complex patients, such as those with diabetes [134, 135]. Reducing cardiovascular disease in these high-risk patients is challenging, but thoughtful management can meaningfully improve the quality of life and longevity of patients with diabetes.

References

1. Goldstein LB, Adams R, Becker K, et al. Primary prevention of ischemic stroke: a statement for healthcare professionals from the Stroke Council of the American Heart Association. Stroke. 2001;32(1):280–99.
2. Berry JD, Dyer A, Carnethon M, Tian L, Greenland P, Lloyd-Jones DM. Association of traditional risk factors with cardiovascular death across 0 to 10, 10 to 20, and >20 years follow-up in men and women. Am J Cardiol. 2008;101(1):89–94.
3. The Bypass Angioplasty Revascularization Investigation (BARI) Investigators. Comparison of coronary bypass surgery with angioplasty in patients with multivessel disease. N Engl J Med. 1996;335(4):217–25.
4. Miettinen H, Lehto S, Salomaa V, et al. Impact of diabetes on mortality after the first myocardial infarction. The FINMONICA Myocardial Infarction Register Study Group. Diabetes Care. 1998;21(1):69–75.
5. Capes SE, Hunt D, Malmberg K, Pathak P, Gerstein HC. Stress hyperglycemia and prognosis of stroke in nondiabetic and diabetic patients: a systematic overview. Stroke. 2001;32(10):2426–32.
6. Stamler J, Vaccaro O, Neaton JD, Wentworth D. Diabetes, other risk factors, and 12-yr cardiovascular mortality for men screened in the Multiple Risk Factor Intervention Trial. Diabetes Care. 1993;16(2):434–44.
7. Haffner SM, Lehto S, Ronnemaa T, Pyorala K, Laakso M. Mortality from coronary heart disease in subjects with type 2 diabetes and in nondiabetic subjects with and without prior myocardial infarction. N Engl J Med. 1998;339(4):229–34.
8. Cheung BM, Ong KL, Cherny SS, Sham PC, Tso AW, Lam KS. Diabetes prevalence and therapeutic target achievement in the United States, 1999 to 2006. Am J Med. 2009;122(5):443–53.
9. Saydah SH, Fradkin J, Cowie CC. Poor control of risk factors for vascular disease among adults with previously diagnosed diabetes. JAMA. 2004;291(3):335–42.
10. Opara JU, Levine JH. The deadly quartet – the insulin resistance syndrome. South Med J. 1997;90(12):1162–8.
11. Coutinho M, Gerstein HC, Wang Y, Yusuf S. The relationship between glucose and incident cardiovascular events. A metaregression analysis of published data from 20 studies of 95,783 individuals followed for 12.4 years. Diabetes Care. 1999;22(2):233–40.
12. Rodriguez BL, Lau N, Burchfiel CM, et al. Glucose intolerance and 23-year risk of coronary heart disease and total mortality: the Honolulu Heart Program. Diabetes Care. 1999;22(8):1262–5.
13. Messent JW, Elliott TG, Hill RD, Jarrett RJ, Keen H, Viberti GC. Prognostic significance of microalbuminuria in insulin-dependent diabetes mellitus: a twenty-three year follow-up study. Kidney Int. 1992;41(4):836–9.
14. Geluk CA, Tio RA, Tijssen JG, et al. Clinical characteristics, cardiac events and coronary angiographic findings in the prospective PREVEND cohort: an observational study. Neth Heart J. 2007;15(4):133–41.
15. Gerstein HC, Mann JF, Yi Q, et al. Albuminuria and risk of cardiovascular events, death, and heart failure in diabetic and nondiabetic individuals. JAMA. 2001;286(4):421–6.
16. Eddy DM, Schlessinger L. Validation of the Archimedes diabetes model. Diabetes Care. 2003;26(11):3102–10.
17. Orasanu G, Plutzky J. The pathologic continuum of diabetic vascular disease. J Am Coll Cardiol. 2009;53 Suppl 5:S35–42.
18. Piga R, Naito Y, Kokura S, Handa O, Yoshikawa T. Short-term high glucose exposure induces monocyte-endothelial cells adhesion and transmigration by increasing VCAM-1 and MCP-1 expression in human aortic endothelial cells. Atherosclerosis. 2007;193(2):328–34.
19. Mazzone T, Chait A, Plutzky J. Cardiovascular disease risk in type 2 diabetes mellitus: insights from mechanistic studies. Lancet. 2008; 371(9626):1800–9.
20. Shoelson SE, Lee J, Goldfine AB. Inflammation and insulin resistance. J Clin Invest. 2006;116(7):1793–801.
21. Peppa M, Uribarri J, Vlassara H. The role of advanced glycation end products in the development of atherosclerosis. Curr Diab Rep. 2004; 4(1):31–6.
22. American Diabetes Association. Standards of medical care in diabetes – 2010. Diabetes Care. 2010;33 Suppl 1:S11–61.
23. Gibbons RJ, Balady GJ, Bricker JT, et al. ACC/AHA 2002 guideline update for exercise testing: summary article: a report of the American College of Cardiology/American Heart Association Task Force on Practice Guidelines (committee to update the 1997 exercise testing guidelines). Circulation. 2002;106(14):1883–92.

24. National Cholesterol Education Program. Executive Summary of The Third Report of The National Cholesterol Education Program (NCEP) Expert panel on detection, evaluation, and treatment of high blood cholesterol in adults (Adult Treatment Panel III). JAMA. 2001;285(19): 2486–97.
25. Grundy SM, Cleeman JI, Merz CN, et al. Implications of recent clinical trials for the National Cholesterol Education Program Adult Treatment Panel III guidelines. Circulation. 2004;110(2):227–39.
26. Appel LJ, Moore TJ, Obarzanek E, et al. A clinical trial of the effects of dietary patterns on blood pressure. DASH Collaborative Research Group. N Engl J Med. 1997;336(16):1117–24.
27. Wolf AM, Conaway MR, Crowther JQ, et al. Translating lifestyle intervention to practice in obese patients with type 2 diabetes: Improving Control with Activity and Nutrition (ICAN) study. Diabetes Care. 2004;27(7):1570–6.
28. Uusitupa MI. Early lifestyle intervention in patients with non-insulin-dependent diabetes mellitus and impaired glucose tolerance. Ann Med. 1996;28(5):445–9.
29. Pi-Sunyer X, Blackburn G, Brancati FL, et al. Reduction in weight and cardiovascular disease risk factors in individuals with type 2 diabetes: one-year results of the look AHEAD trial. Diabetes Care. 2007;30(6):1374–83.
30. Despres JP, Golay A, Sjostrom L. Effects of rimonabant on metabolic risk factors in overweight patients with dyslipidemia. N Engl J Med. 2005;353(20):2121–34.
31. Pi-Sunyer FX, Aronne LJ, Heshmati HM, Devin J, Rosenstock J. Effect of rimonabant, a cannabinoid-1 receptor blocker, on weight and cardiometabolic risk factors in overweight or obese patients: RIO-North America: a randomized controlled trial. JAMA. 2006;295(7):761–75.
32. Hollander P. Endocannabinoid blockade for improving glycemic control and lipids in patients with type 2 diabetes mellitus. Am J Med. 2007;120(2 Suppl 1):S18–28; discussion S29–32.
33. Fujioka K, Seaton TB, Rowe E, et al. Weight loss with sibutramine improves glycaemic control and other metabolic parameters in obese patients with type 2 diabetes mellitus. Diabetes Obes Metab. 2000;2(3):175–87.
34. Berne C. A randomized study of orlistat in combination with a weight management programme in obese patients with Type 2 diabetes treated with metformin. Diabet Med. 2005;22(5):612–8.
35. Burguera B, Agusti A, Arner P, et al. Critical assessment of the current guidelines for the management and treatment of morbidly obese patients. J Endocrinol Invest. 2007;30(10):844–52.
36. Choban PS, Jackson B, Poplawski S, Bistolarides P. Bariatric surgery for morbid obesity: why, who, when, how, where, and then what? Cleve Clin J Med. 2002;69(11):897–903.
37. Sjostrom L, Narbro K, Sjostrom CD, et al. Effects of bariatric surgery on mortality in Swedish obese subjects. N Engl J Med. 2007; 357(8):741–52.
38. Sjostrom L, Lindroos AK, Peltonen M, et al. Lifestyle, diabetes, and cardiovascular risk factors 10 years after bariatric surgery. N Engl J Med. 2004;351(26):2683–93.
39. Hu FB, Stampfer MJ, Solomon C, et al. Physical activity and risk for cardiovascular events in diabetic women. Ann Intern Med. 2001;134(2): 96–105.
40. Wei M, Gibbons LW, Kampert JB, Nichaman MZ, Blair SN. Low cardiorespiratory fitness and physical inactivity as predictors of mortality in men with type 2 diabetes. Ann Intern Med. 2000;132(8):605–11.
41. Li C, Ford ES, Mokdad AH, Jiles R, Giles WH. Clustering of multiple healthy lifestyle habits and health-related quality of life among US adults with diabetes. Diabetes Care. 2007;30(7):1770–6.
42. Yeh HC, Duncan BB, Schmidt MI, Wang NY, Brancati FL. Smoking, smoking cessation, and risk for type 2 diabetes mellitus: a cohort study. Ann Intern Med. 2010;152(1):10–7.
43. Mikhailidis DP, Papadakis JA, Ganotakis ES. Smoking, diabetes and hyperlipidaemia. J R Soc Health. 1998;118(2):91–3.
44. Sawicki PT, Didjurgeit U, Muhlhauser I, Bender R, Heinemann L, Berger M. Smoking is associated with progression of diabetic nephropathy. Diabetes Care. 1994;17(2):126–31.
45. Chuahirun T, Khanna A, Kimball K, Wesson DE. Cigarette smoking and increased urine albumin excretion are interrelated predictors of nephropathy progression in type 2 diabetes. Am J Kidney Dis. 2003;41(1):13–21.
46. Fiore M, Bailey W, Cohen S. Smoking cessation: clinical practice guideline number 18. Rockville: US Department of Health and Human services, Public Health Service, Agency for Health Care Policy and Research; 1996.
47. Gerber Y, Rosen LJ, Goldbourt U, Benyamini Y, Drory Y. Smoking status and long-term survival after first acute myocardial infarction a population-based cohort study. J Am Coll Cardiol. 2009;54(25):2382–7.
48. Lightwood JM, Glantz SA. Short-term economic and health benefits of smoking cessation: myocardial infarction and stroke. Circulation. 1997;96(4):1089–96.
49. Haire-Joshu D, Glasgow RE, Tibbs TL. Smoking and diabetes. Diabetes Care. 1999;22(11):1887–98.
50. Nathan DM, Cleary PA, Backlund JY, et al. Intensive diabetes treatment and cardiovascular disease in patients with type 1 diabetes. N Engl J Med. 2005;353(25):2643–53.
51. Cleary PA, Orchard TJ, Genuth S, et al. The effect of intensive glycemic treatment on coronary artery calcification in type 1 diabetic participants of the Diabetes Control and Complications Trial/Epidemiology of Diabetes Interventions and Complications (DCCT/EDIC) Study. Diabetes. 2006;55(12):3556–65.
52. UK Prospective Diabetes Study (UKPDS) Group. Intensive blood-glucose control with sulphonylureas or insulin compared with conventional treatment and risk of complications in patients with type 2 diabetes (UKPDS 33). Lancet. 1998;352(9131):837–53.
53. UK Prospective Diabetes Study (UKPDS) Group. Effect of intensive blood-glucose control with metformin on complications in overweight patients with type 2 diabetes (UKPDS 34). Lancet. 1998;352(9131):854–65.
54. Patel A, MacMahon S, Chalmers J, et al. Intensive blood glucose control and vascular outcomes in patients with type 2 diabetes. N Engl J Med. 2008;358(24):2560–72.
55. Gerstein HC, Miller ME, Byington RP, et al. Effects of intensive glucose lowering in type 2 diabetes. N Engl J Med. 2008;358(24): 2545–59.
56. Dluhy RG, McMahon GT. Intensive glycemic control in the ACCORD and ADVANCE trials. N Engl J Med. 2008;358(24):2630–3.
57. DeFronzo RA, Goodman AM. Efficacy of metformin in patients with non-insulin-dependent diabetes mellitus. The Multicenter Metformin Study Group. N Engl J Med. 1995;333(9):541–9.

58. Nathan DM. Thiazolidinediones for initial treatment of type 2 diabetes? N Engl J Med. 2006;355(23):2477–80.
59. Hamnvik OP, McMahon GT. Balancing risk and benefit with oral hypoglycemic drugs. Mt Sinai J Med. 2009;76(3):234–43.
60. Salpeter SR, Greyber E, Pasternak GA, Salpeter EE. Risk of fatal and nonfatal lactic acidosis with metformin use in type 2 diabetes mellitus: systematic review and meta-analysis. Arch Intern Med. 2003;163(21):2594–602.
61. Engler RL, Yellon DM. Sulfonylurea KATP blockade in type II diabetes and preconditioning in cardiovascular disease. Time for reconsideration. Circulation. 1996;94(9):2297–301.
62. Cleveland Jr JC, Meldrum DR, Cain BS, Banerjee A, Harken AH. Oral sulfonylurea hypoglycemic agents prevent ischemic preconditioning in human myocardium. Two paradoxes revisited. Circulation. 1997;96(1):29–32.
63. Kahn SE, Haffner SM, Heise MA, et al. Glycemic durability of rosiglitazone, metformin, or glyburide monotherapy. N Engl J Med. 2006; 355(23):2427–43.
64. Martens FM, Visseren FL, Lemay J, de Koning EJ, Rabelink TJ. Metabolic and additional vascular effects of thiazolidinediones. Drugs. 2002;62(10):1463–80.
65. Mazzone T, Meyer PM, Feinstein SB, et al. Effect of pioglitazone compared with glimepiride on carotid intima-media thickness in type 2 diabetes: a randomized trial. JAMA. 2006;296(21):2572–81.
66. Dormandy JA, Charbonnel B, Eckland DJ, et al. Secondary prevention of macrovascular events in patients with type 2 diabetes in the PROactive Study (PROspective pioglitAzone Clinical Trial In macroVascular Events): a randomised controlled trial. Lancet. 2005; 366(9493):1279–89.
67. Parulkar AA, Pendergrass ML, Granda-Ayala R, Lee TR, Fonseca VA. Nonhypoglycemic effects of thiazolidinediones. Ann Intern Med. 2001;134(1):61–71.
68. Nissen SE, Wolski K. Effect of rosiglitazone on the risk of myocardial infarction and death from cardiovascular causes. N Engl J Med. 2007;356(24):2457–71.
69. Fonseca V, Jawa A, Asnani S. The PROactive study – the glass is half full [commentary]. J Clin Endocrinol Metab. 2006;91(1):25–7.
70. Home PD, Pocock SJ, Beck-Nielsen H, et al. Rosiglitazone evaluated for cardiovascular outcomes in oral agent combination therapy for type 2 diabetes (RECORD): a multicentre, randomised, open-label trial. Lancet. 2009;373(9681):2125–35.
71. Home PD, Pocock SJ, Beck-Nielsen H, et al. Rosiglitazone evaluated for cardiovascular outcomes – an interim analysis. N Engl J Med. 2007;357(1):28–38.
72. Pratley RE, Nauck M, Bailey T, et al. Liraglutide versus sitagliptin for patients with type 2 diabetes who did not have adequate glycaemic control with metformin: a 26-week, randomised, parallel-group, open-label trial. Lancet. 2010;375(9724):1447–56.
73. Drucker DJ, Nauck MA. The incretin system: glucagon-like peptide-1 receptor agonists and dipeptidyl peptidase-4 inhibitors in type 2 diabetes. Lancet. 2006;368(9548):1696–705.
74. Diamant M, Van Gaal L, Stranks S, et al. Once weekly exenatide compared with insulin glargine titrated to target in patients with type 2 diabetes (DURATION-3): an open-label randomised trial. Lancet. 2010;375(9733):2234–43.
75. DeFronzo RA, Hissa MN, Garber AJ, et al. The efficacy and safety of saxagliptin when added to metformin therapy in patients with inadequately controlled type 2 diabetes with metformin alone. Diabetes Care. 2009;32(9):1649–55.
76. Kleppinger EL, Helms K. The role of vildagliptin in the management of type 2 diabetes mellitus. Ann Pharmacother. 2007;41(5):824–32.
77. Ristic S, Byiers S, Foley J, Holmes D. Improved glycaemic control with dipeptidyl peptidase-4 inhibition in patients with type 2 diabetes: vildagliptin (LAF237) dose response. Diabetes Obes Metab. 2005;7(6):692–8.
78. Herman GA, Stein PP, Thornberry NA, Wagner JA. Dipeptidyl peptidase-4 inhibitors for the treatment of type 2 diabetes: focus on sitagliptin. Clin Pharmacol Ther. 2007;81(5):761–7.
79. Taskinen MR, Kuusi T, Helve E, Nikkila EA, Yki-Jarvinen H. Insulin therapy induces antiatherogenic changes of serum lipoproteins in noninsulin-dependent diabetes. Arteriosclerosis. 1988;8(2):168–77.
80. Davies MJ, Lawrence IG. DIGAMI (Diabetes Mellitus, Insulin Glucose Infusion in Acute Myocardial Infarction): theory and practice. Diabetes Obes Metab. 2002;4(5):289–95.
81. Riddle MC, Rosenstock J, Gerich J. The treat-to-target trial: randomized addition of glargine or human NPH insulin to oral therapy of type 2 diabetic patients. Diabetes Care. 2003;26(11):3080–6.
82. Janka HU, Plewe G, Riddle MC, Kliebe-Frisch C, Schweitzer MA, Yki-Järvinen H. Comparison of basal insulin added to oral agents versus twice-daily premixed insulin as initial insulin therapy for type 2 diabetes. Diabetes Care. 2005;28(2):254–9.
83. Hansson L, Zanchetti A, Carruthers SG, et al. Effects of intensive blood-pressure lowering and low-dose aspirin in patients with hypertension: principal results of the Hypertension Optimal Treatment (HOT) randomised trial. HOT Study Group. Lancet. 1998;351(9118):1755–62.
84. Laffel LM, McGill JB, Gans DJ. The beneficial effect of angiotensin-converting enzyme inhibition with captopril on diabetic nephropathy in normotensive IDDM patients with microalbuminuria. North American Microalbuminuria Study Group. Am J Med. 1995;99(5):497–504.
85. The Microalbuminuria Captopril Study Group. Captopril reduces the risk of nephropathy in IDDM patients with microalbuminuria. Diabetologia. 1996;39(5):587–93.
86. Mathiesen ER, Hommel E, Hansen HP, Smidt UM, Parving HH. Randomised controlled trial of long term efficacy of captopril on preservation of kidney function in normotensive patients with insulin dependent diabetes and microalbuminuria. BMJ. 1999;319(7201):24–5.
87. The EUCLID Study Group. Randomised placebo-controlled trial of lisinopril in normotensive patients with insulin-dependent diabetes and normoalbuminuria or microalbuminuria. Lancet. 1997;349(9068):1787–92.
88. Ravid M, Brosh D, Levi Z, Bar-Dayan Y, Ravid D, Rachmani R. Use of enalapril to attenuate decline in renal function in normotensive, normoalbuminuric patients with type 2 diabetes mellitus. A randomized, controlled trial. Ann Intern Med. 1998;128(12):982–8.
89. Chaturvedi N, Sjolie AK, Stephenson JM, et al. Effect of lisinopril on progression of retinopathy in normotensive people with type 1 diabetes. The EUCLID Study Group. EURODIAB controlled trial of lisinopril in insulin-dependent diabetes mellitus. Lancet. 1998;351(9095):28–31.
90. Hansson L, Lindholm LH, Niskanen L, et al. Effect of angiotensin-converting-enzyme inhibition compared with conventional therapy on cardiovascular morbidity and mortality in hypertension: the Captopril Prevention Project (CAPPP) randomised trial. Lancet. 1999;353(9153): 611–6.
91. Asfaha S, Padwal R. Antihypertensive drugs and incidence of type 2 diabetes: evidence and implications for clinical practice. Curr Hypertens Rep. 2005;7(5):314–22.

92. Gress TW, Nieto FJ, Shahar E, Wofford MR, Brancati FL. Hypertension and antihypertensive therapy as risk factors for type 2 diabetes mellitus. Atherosclerosis Risk in Communities Study. N Engl J Med. 2000;342(13):905–12.
93. Messerli FH. Implications of discontinuation of doxazosin arm of ALLHAT. Antihypertensive and Lipid-Lowering Treatment to Prevent Heart Attack Trial. Lancet. 2000;355(9207):863–4.
94. Curb JD, Pressel SL, Cutler JA, et al. Effect of diuretic-based antihypertensive treatment on cardiovascular disease risk in older diabetic patients with isolated systolic hypertension. Systolic Hypertension in the Elderly Program Cooperative Research Group. JAMA. 1996; 276(23):1886–92.
95. Dahlof B, Sever PS, Poulter NR, et al. Prevention of cardiovascular events with an antihypertensive regimen of amlodipine adding perindopril as required versus atenolol adding bendroflumethiazide as required, in the Anglo-Scandinavian Cardiac Outcomes Trial-Blood Pressure Lowering Arm (ASCOT-BPLA): a multicentre randomised controlled trial. Lancet. 2005;366(9489):895–906.
96. Estacio RO, Jeffers BW, Hiatt WR, Biggerstaff SL, Gifford N, Schrier RW. The effect of nisoldipine as compared with enalapril on cardiovascular outcomes in patients with non-insulin-dependent diabetes and hypertension. N Engl J Med. 1998;338(10):645–52.
97. Reaven GM. Pathophysiology of insulin resistance in human disease. Physiol Rev. 1995;75(3):473–86.
98. Austin MA, Edwards KL. Small, dense low density lipoproteins, the insulin resistance syndrome and noninsulin-dependent diabetes. Curr Opin Lipidol. 1996;7(3):167–71.
99. Gordon T, Castelli WP, Hjortland MC, Kannel WB, Dawber TR. High density lipoprotein as a protective factor against coronary heart disease. The Framingham Study. Am J Med. 1977;62(5):707–14.
100. Fontbonne A, Eschwege E, Cambien F, et al. Hypertriglyceridaemia as a risk factor of coronary heart disease mortality in subjects with impaired glucose tolerance or diabetes. Results from the 11-year follow-up of the Paris Prospective Study. Diabetologia. 1989;32(5):300–4.
101. National Cholesterol Education Program. Third report of the National Cholesterol Education Program (NCEP) expert panel on detection, evaluation, and treatment of high blood cholesterol in adults (Adult Treatment Panel III) final report. Circulation. 2002;106(25):3143–421.
102. Colhoun HM, Betteridge DJ, Durrington PN, et al. Primary prevention of cardiovascular disease with atorvastatin in type 2 diabetes in the Collaborative Atorvastatin Diabetes Study (CARDS): multicentre randomised placebo-controlled trial. Lancet. 2004;364(9435):685–96.
103. Heart Protection Study Collaborative Group. MRC/BHF Heart Protection Study of cholesterol lowering with simvastatin in 20,536 high-risk individuals: a randomised placebo-controlled trial. Lancet. 2002;360(9326):7–22.
104. Sever PS, Dahlof B, Poulter NR, et al. Prevention of coronary and stroke events with atorvastatin in hypertensive patients who have average or lower-than-average cholesterol concentrations, in the Anglo-Scandinavian Cardiac Outcomes Trial – Lipid Lowering Arm (ASCOT-LLA): a multicentre randomised controlled trial. Lancet. 2003;361(9364):1149 58.
105. ALLHAT Collaborative Research Group. Major outcomes in moderately hypercholesterolemic, hypertensive patients randomized to pravastatin vs usual care: the Antihypertensive and Lipid-Lowering Treatment to Prevent Heart Attack Trial (ALLHAT-LLT). JAMA. 2002;288(23): 2998–3007.
106. Pyorala K, Pedersen TR, Kjekshus J, Faergeman O, Olsson AG, Thorgeirsson G. Cholesterol lowering with simvastatin improves prognosis of diabetic patients with coronary heart disease. A subgroup analysis of the Scandinavian Simvastatin Survival Study (4S). Diabetes Care. 1997;20(4):614–20.
107. Goldberg RB, Mellies MJ, Sacks FM, et al. Cardiovascular events and their reduction with pravastatin in diabetic and glucose-intolerant myocardial infarction survivors with average cholesterol levels: subgroup analyses in the cholesterol and recurrent events (CARE) trial. The Care Investigators. Circulation. 1998;98(23):2513–9.
108. Assmann G, Schulte H. Relation of high-density lipoprotein cholesterol and triglycerides to incidence of atherosclerotic coronary artery disease (the PROCAM experience). Prospective Cardiovascular Munster study. Am J Cardiol. 1992;70(7):733–7.
109. Rubins HB, Robins SJ, Collins D, et al. Gemfibrozil for the secondary prevention of coronary heart disease in men with low levels of high-density lipoprotein cholesterol. Veterans Affairs High-Density Lipoprotein Cholesterol Intervention Trial Study Group. N Engl J Med. 1999; 341(6):410–8.
110. Rubins HB, Robins SJ, Collins D, et al. Diabetes, plasma insulin, and cardiovascular disease: subgroup analysis from the Department of Veterans Affairs high-density lipoprotein intervention trial (VA-HIT). Arch Intern Med. 2002;162(22):2597–604.
111. Keech A, Simes RJ, Barter P, et al. Effects of long-term fenofibrate therapy on cardiovascular events in 9795 people with type 2 diabetes mellitus (the FIELD study): randomised controlled trial. Lancet. 2005;366(9500):1849–61.
112. Ginsberg HN, Elam MB, Lovato LC, et al. Effects of combination lipid therapy in type 2 diabetes mellitus. N Engl J Med. 2010;362(17): 1563–74.
113. Athyros VG, Papageorgiou AA, Athyrou VV, Demitriadis DS, Kontopoulos AG. Atorvastatin and micronized fenofibrate alone and in combination in type 2 diabetes with combined hyperlipidemia. Diabetes Care. 2002;25(7):1198–202.
114. Corsini A. The safety of HMG-CoA reductase inhibitors in special populations at high cardiovascular risk. Cardiovasc Drugs Ther. 2003; 17(3):265–85.
115. Davidson MH, Armani A, McKenney JM, Jacobson TA. Safety considerations with fibrate therapy. Am J Cardiol. 2007;99(6A):3C–18.
116. Meyers CD, Kamanna VS, Kashyap ML. Niacin therapy in atherosclerosis. Curr Opin Lipidol. 2004;15(6):659–65.
117. Carlson LA. Niaspan, the prolonged release preparation of nicotinic acid (niacin), the broad-spectrum lipid drug. Int J Clin Pract. 2004; 58(7):706–13.
118. Elam MB, Hunninghake DB, Davis KB, et al. Effect of niacin on lipid and lipoprotein levels and glycemic control in patients with diabetes and peripheral arterial disease: the ADMIT study: a randomized trial. Arterial Disease Multiple Intervention Trial. JAMA. 2000;284(10):1263–70.
119. Bays HE, Goldberg RB, Truitt KE, Jones MR. Colesevelam hydrochloride therapy in patients with type 2 diabetes mellitus treated with metformin: glucose and lipid effects. Arch Intern Med. 2008;168(18):1975–83.
120. Goldberg RB, Fonseca VA, Truitt KE, Jones MR. Efficacy and safety of colesevelam in patients with type 2 diabetes mellitus and inadequate glycemic control receiving insulin-based therapy. Arch Intern Med. 2008;168(14):1531–40.
121. Simons L, Tonkon M, Masana L, et al. Effects of ezetimibe added to on-going statin therapy on the lipid profile of hypercholesterolemic patients with diabetes mellitus or metabolic syndrome. Curr Med Res Opin. 2004;20(9):1437–45.
122. Stroup JS, Kane MP, Busch RS. The antilipidemic effects of ezetimibe in patients with diabetes. Diabetes Care. 2003;26(10):2958–9.
123. ENHANCE Study. In brief: Zetia and Vytorin: the ENHANCE study. Med Lett Drugs Ther. 2008;50(1278):5.
124. Bays H. Clinical overview of Omacor: a concentrated formulation of omega-3 polyunsaturated fatty acids. Am J Cardiol. 2006;98(4A):71i–6.

125. GISSI-Prevenzione Trial. Dietary supplementation with n-3 polyunsaturated fatty acids and vitamin E after myocardial infarction: results of the GISSI-Prevenzione trial. Gruppo Italiano per lo Studio della Sopravvivenza nell'Infarto miocardico. Lancet. 1999;354(9177):447–55.
126. Steering Committee of the Physicians' Health Study Research Group. Final report on the aspirin component of the ongoing Physicians' Health Study. N Engl J Med. 1989;321(3):129–35.
127. ETDRS Investigators. Aspirin effects on mortality and morbidity in patients with diabetes mellitus, Early Treatment Diabetic Retinopathy Study report 14. JAMA. 1992;268(10):1292–300.
128. de Gaetano G. Low-dose aspirin and vitamin E in people at cardiovascular risk: a randomised trial in general practice. Collaborative Group of the Primary Prevention Project. Lancet. 2001;357(9250):89–95.
129. Ogawa H, Nakayama M, Morimoto T, et al. Low-dose aspirin for primary prevention of atherosclerotic events in patients with type 2 diabetes: a randomized controlled trial. JAMA. 2008;300(18):2134–41.
130. De Berardis G, Sacco M, Strippoli GF, et al. Aspirin for primary prevention of cardiovascular events in people with diabetes: meta-analysis of randomised controlled trials. BMJ. 2009;339:b4531.
131. Baigent C, Blackwell L, Collins R, et al. Aspirin in the primary and secondary prevention of vascular disease: collaborative meta-analysis of individual participant data from randomised trials. Lancet. 2009;373(9678):1849–60.
132. Bhatt DL, Marso SP, Hirsch AT, Ringleb PA, Hacke W, Topol EJ. Amplified benefit of clopidogrel versus aspirin in patients with diabetes mellitus. Am J Cardiol. 2002;90(6):625–8.
133. Gaede P, Vedel P, Larsen N, Jensen GV, Parving HH, Pedersen O. Multifactorial intervention and cardiovascular disease in patients with type 2 diabetes. N Engl J Med. 2003;348(5):383–93.
134. McMahon GT, Gomes HE, Hickson Hohne S, Hu TM, Levine BA, Conlin PR. Web-based care management in patients with poorly controlled diabetes. Diabetes Care. 2005;28(7):1624–9.
135. Perlin JB, Pogach LM. Improving the outcomes of metabolic conditions: managing momentum to overcome clinical inertia. Ann Intern Med. 2006;144(7):525–7.

Chapter 28
Cardiovascular Disease in Women

Margo Tolins-Mejia

For many years, women were considered more resistant to developing cardiovascular disease (CVD). Yet researchers are discovering that CVD is, in many ways, an equal opportunity disease. In fact, statistics report a greater number of CVD deaths each year for women compared to men [1]. Despite the high mortality rate in both sexes, many features of CVD do show a gender difference.

Women and men differ not only in the prevalence of CVD but also in presenting symptoms and pathophysiology of their disease. To fully understand CVD in women, we must take into account the unique ways in which it manifests in the female body. Only then can we target our diagnostic techniques and treatments to better serve female patients.

Gender Bias

Historically, CVD was thought to be a man's disease. This myth existed in both the public sector and the medical community, which meant that women were not targeted for CVD diagnosis. Several studies have shown that women themselves believe the greatest threat to their health is breast cancer. Over a lifetime, a woman is much more likely to develop CVD than breast cancer (Fig. 28.1).

Female gender has been shown to be associated with delayed presentation and delayed treatment of acute myocardial infarction [2]. Essentially, female patients are not conscious of their CVD risk, and physicians have not considered women as potential cardiac patients. Through increased awareness and early symptom recognition, proven therapies can be provided early in the disease process. The timing of these therapies is crucial for maximum benefit.

Gender Differences

Bias aside, real biological gender differences exist in the progression of CVD. Since 1984, the total number of CVD deaths for women has exceeded those for men. Medical and technological advances have resulted in a reduced total number of CVD deaths per year; however, the reduction for women has lagged behind that seen for men (Fig. 28.2).

Early observational studies from both coronary artery bypass surgery and percutaneous coronary interventional procedures reported higher morbidity and mortality in women. In one study, the 6-month survival rate after a first myocardial infarction was considerably lower in women than in men. This is also true in diabetic patients, where 30-year trends show a marked decrease in CVD mortality in diabetic men, but not for diabetic women [3]. Several explanations for this phenomenon are possible.

M. Tolins-Mejia, MD, FACC (✉)
Department of Cardiology, Mercy/Unity Medical Centers, Minneapolis, MN, USA
e-mail: margo.mejia@metrocardiology.com

Z. Vlodaver et al. (eds.), *Coronary Heart Disease: Clinical, Pathological, Imaging, and Molecular Profiles*,
DOI 10.1007/978-1-4614-1475-9_28, © Springer Science+Business Media, LLC 2012

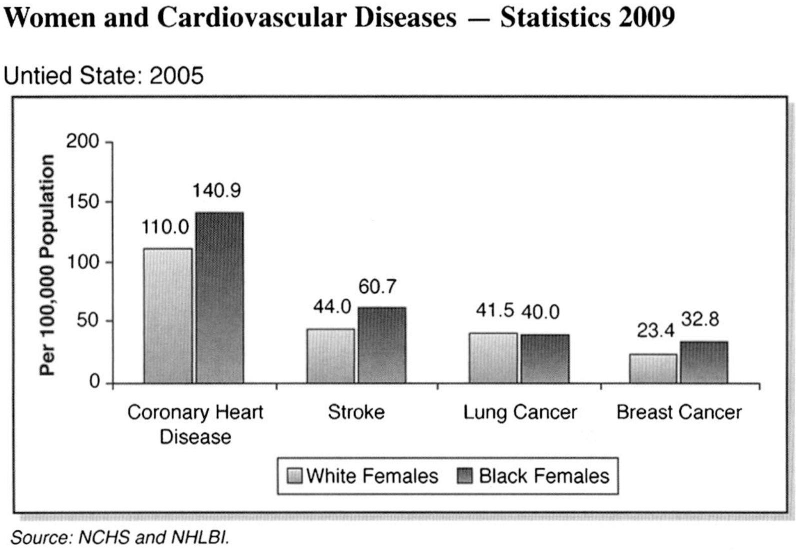

Fig. 28.1 Age-adjusted death rates for coronary heart diease, stroke, and lung and breast cancer. American Heart Association Web site [32]

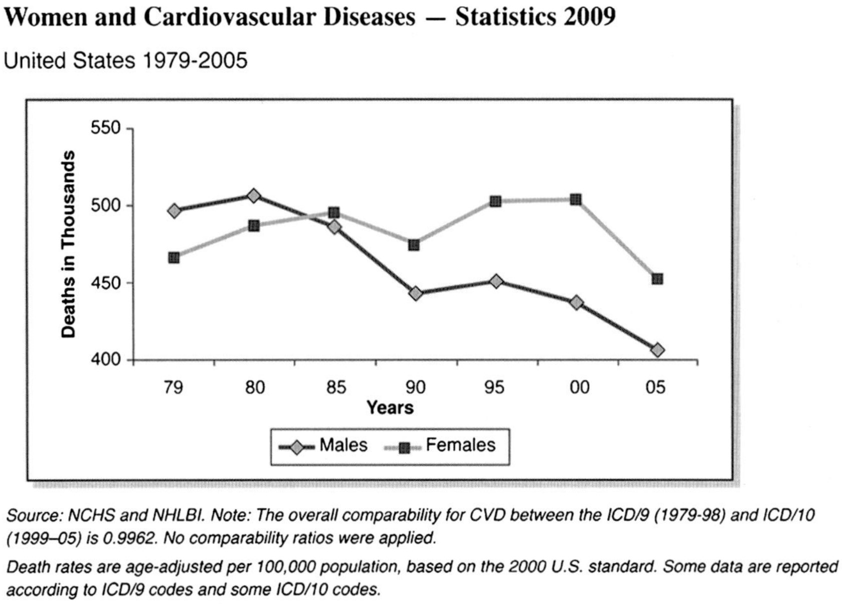

Fig. 28.2 Cardiovascular disease mortality trends for males and females. American Heart Association Web site [32]

Research Participation

The development of new cardiac therapies and devices depends on clinical research trials. Unfortunately, study enrollment, until the 1990s, was almost exclusively male. This changed in 1991 when Bernadine Healy became the first woman to head the National Institutes of Health. Healy believed that heart disease was also a woman's disease, "not a man's disease in disguise." While director, she established a policy whereby the NIH would fund only those clinical trials that included both men and women when the condition being studied affected both genders. This mandate ensured the enrollment of female subjects in cardiac trials. Since that time, much more information has been available on sex-specific diagnosis, management, and treatment of heart disease.

However, although now included in cardiac studies, women remain in the minority. While the reasons for continued, limited enrollment of women in research trials remain unclear, to this day, women have a much lower rate of participation

Variable	Women's health study	Physicians' health study
Sex of participants	Female	Male
Study period	1993–2004	1982–1988[a]
No. of participants	39,876	22,071
Age of participants (year)		
Mean	54.6	53.2
Range	45–89	40–84
Alternate-day dose of aspirin (mg)	100	325
Follow-up (year)		
Mean	10.1	5.0
Range	8.2–10.9	3.8–6.4[a]
Rate of myocardial infarction in the placebo group (no./100,000 person – year)	97.3	439.7
Rate of stroke in the placebo group (no./100,000 person – year)	134.3	179.4

Adapted from Levin [34]. Copyright 2005 by the Massachusetts Medical Society
[a] Randomization began in August 1981 for 124 participants in the pilot study

Fig. 28.3 Comparison of selected features of the aspirin components of the women's health study and the physicians' health study

in cardiac research studies. New cardiac medications and devices are therefore developed from research based primarily on men, and may not be directly applicable to women. This is significant because men differ biologically on many levels. Compared to women, men on average have larger hearts, increased coronary arterial diameters, and a completely different hormonal milieu. These gender differences may require sex-specific therapies for effective treatment of CVD in women.

It was not until 1999, when the realization that cardiac data from men would not always generalize to women prompted publication of the first female-specific recommendations for preventive cardiology [4]. The first evidence-based guidelines for CVD prevention in women was not published until 2004 [5].

An example that exemplifies gender differences involves the beneficial effects of a well-known medication, aspirin. Aspirin prevents thrombotic vascular events primarily through its mechanism as a permanent inhibitor of cyclooxygenase. As described in two landmark studies, investigators of the Physicians' Health Study [6] and the Women's Health Study [7] show results that segregate according to sex.

In the Physicians' Health Study, all enrollees were men. In these men, aspirin significantly reduced the risk of myocardial infarction: The reduction was 44% in men 50 years or older who did not have clinical evidence of coronary disease. There was no significant reduction in the risk of stroke in these male subjects.

The Women's Health Study showed opposite results. In these female subjects, 65 years or older and without a history of CVD, aspirin had no effect on the risk of myocardial infarction. Surprisingly, aspirin therapy in these women was associated with an overall 17% reduction in the risk of stroke (Fig. 28.3). This conundrum of markedly disparate effects of aspirin that separate on the basis of gender remains a mystery. It also clearly demonstrates the danger of applying male-derived data to women.

Comorbid States

Another distinguishing factor that determines prognosis in CVD patients is age at time of presentation. Among patients diagnosed with CVD, women are generally 10–15 years older than men [8]. Advanced age is associated with a higher incidence of diabetes, obesity, hypertension, hyperlipidemia, and heart failure. The classic Framingham cardiac risk factors, which predict the probability of future cardiac events, increase with age. More than 80% of postmenopausal women have one or more of these risk factors [9]. The burden of these comorbidities portends a poorer prognosis.

Vascular Risk Factors

The mechanism of ischemic heart disease may be different in women compared to men. The clinical course of women is characterized by a higher number of office visits and hospitalizations [10]. Paradoxically, despite a higher usage of medical facilities, women with CVD have a more malignant clinical course compared to men. Women have higher rates of sudden cardiac death and increased mortality after myocardial infarction than do men [1].

Even in patients being evaluated for chest pain, women are less likely than men to present with typical angina [11]. Atypical symptoms often delay the diagnosis and treatment of the female patient. And yet, even when women present with typical symptoms, their diagnosis and treatment often differ from those of men. In a recent Minnesota-based study, women presenting with typical evidence of acute myocardial infarction were 46% less likely than men to undergo investigative coronary angiography [12].

When coronary angiography is performed, angiographic results show gender disparity. Women have less obstructive coronary artery disease compared to men. When angina is the preprocedure diagnosis, women statistically have less obstructive coronary artery disease than men presenting with similar symptoms [13]. This is also true for patients presenting with acute coronary syndrome or ST-elevation myocardial infarction. Coronary angiography in patients with an acute coronary event often demonstrates a higher number of normal test results in women compared to men [14].

A recent study on sudden cardiac arrest (SCA) indicated important sex-based differences in presentation and clinical course. Women, compared to men, were significantly less likely to have a history of structural heart disease, either left ventricular (LV) dysfunction or obstructive coronary artery disease, before SCA. In the absence of LV dysfunction, fewer women may be eligible for prophylactic, implantable cardioverter-defibrillators (ICDs) based on current guidelines and therefore may not have equal opportunity for prevention of sudden cardiac death [15].

Obviously, obstructive coronary artery disease alone does not explain the higher CVD mortality found in women. Unique to women are their lifelong changing hormonal states. Since the incidence of CVD increases significantly in postmenopausal women, hormonally mediated factors may play a significant causative role. Basic research has shown vascular integrity to be affected directly by estrogen. Furthermore, clinical studies of premenopausal women with menstrual irregularities, presumably due to fluctuations in their estrogen levels, have shown an increase in CVD risk [16].

One possible mechanism observed in animal studies is the inductive effect of estrogen on prostacyclin production [17], a vascular factor that is protective against CVD. Thus, declining estrogen levels in postmenopausal women could translate into increased risk of CVD. Despite the beneficial effects of endogenous estrogen, hormone replacement therapy does not reduce the risk of CVD events in women.

Menopause is also associated with weight gain, development of metabolic syndrome, and a deleterious change in a woman's cholesterol status [18]. All of these are cardiac risk factors for CVD.

The relationship between menopause, aging, and CVD risk is complex. Recently, Matthews et al. [19] studied the higher cardiovascular risk of perimenopausal women in an effort to determine if these negative changes were due to aging or menopause itself, with its associated loss of endogenous estrogen. Regardless of causation (aging or menopause), this time in a woman's life is characterized by a significant rise in CVD risk. Could unique features of the female gender impact not only the known cardiac risk factors but also a woman's vascular function?

As stated above, women have a lower incidence of obstructive coronary artery disease at time of CVD presentation compared to men. In one study of patients with chest pain, a diagnosis of normal coronary arteries was 5 times more common in women than men [20]. The "typical" angina patient presents with obstructive coronary artery disease, and yet a large proportion of women have chest pain or evidence of ischemia without fixed coronary artery disease. Possible explanations for this phenomenon include coronary artery spasm, coronary artery thrombosis, microvascular disease, and endothelial dysfunction; evidence supports the increased incidence of these physiologies in women.

The human arterial wall contains a smooth muscle layer. Vasospasm is the result of contraction of this smooth muscle layer. Vascular smooth muscle contraction can cause a narrowing in the arterial lumen, which limits blood flow. Migraines and Raynaud phenomenon are believed to be caused by vasospasm and occur more frequently in women than men. These vascular disorders may be associated with coronary reactivity that is modulated by the woman's female hormonal status. Coronary artery vasospasm resulting in angina has been termed variant angina, also called Prinzmetal angina. This type of angina is produced by a narrowing of the coronary arteries caused by vasospasm, rather than by fixed obstructive coronary artery disease. Known risk factors associated with variant angina include female gender.

Chronic autoimmune diseases also affect the vasculature and, in general, have a higher incidence in women. Rheumatoid arthritis, an example of a systemic inflammatory disorder, occurs most often in middle-aged women. Women with rheumatoid arthritis have a significantly higher incidence of myocardial infarction as compared to female controls. This increase in CVD has been explained by the detrimental effects of chronic inflammation on the vascular endothelium, and in turn, the vessel wall. The endothelium is the local regulator of vascular function. Inflammation alters endothelial function and, in turn, negatively impacts many functions of the vessel wall, causing release of mediators and tissue factors that promote thrombosis and vasoconstriction. These effects on vascular biology can eventually lead to myocardial ischemia and adverse structural changes in the coronary arteries.

Case Studies

Supporting the importance of vascular biology are three cardiac conditions that occur predominantly or exclusively in women, and cause myocardial ischemia or injury in the absence of obstructive coronary disease. These include cardiac syndrome X, apical ballooning syndrome, and peripartum cardiomyopathy. Examination of these disorders may provide answers to the mechanisms involved in CVD in women.

Cardiac Syndrome X

CP is a 48-year-old firefighter. She was admitted after developing chest pain while at a house fire. During chest pain, her electrocardiogram (ECG) showed ST abnormalities in the inferior leads V5 and V6 (Fig. 28.4a). Sublingual nitroglycerin relieved her symptoms. Her repeat ECG, in the absence of symptoms, normalized (Fig. 28.4b). Serial troponin levels were upper-normal to minimally elevated.

The patient initially declined invasive cardiac evaluation. A nuclear stress test reproduced her chest pain symptoms and ECG abnormalities. Her perfusion study was normal. She had a recurrent episode of vague chest discomfort in-hospital. Stat ECG during symptoms again showed ST abnormalities. She was then taken to the heart catheterization laboratory. Her coronary angiograms were normal (Figs. 28.5a, b). Her left ventriculogram showed normal LV function and normal wall motion (Fig. 28.6a shows heart function in diastole, and Fig. 28.6b, in systole).

The patient was treated with aspirin, long-acting nitroglycerin, and calcium-channel blocker therapy. Her hyperlipidemia was treated with statin therapy. Despite these modalities, she continues to have frequent episodes of chest pain.

This patient fits the criteria for cardiac syndrome X, which is reported much more frequently in women than in men. Cardiac syndrome X was initially described in 1973 [21] to explain the puzzle of patients with classic chest pain symptoms and evidence of ischemia, yet angiographically normal coronary arteries. ST abnormalities with reproduction of chest pain symptoms on treadmill testing have been reported. Potential mechanisms to explain chest pain and ST-segment depression during exercise in cardiac syndrome X patients include functional abnormalities of the coronary microvasculature during stress.

Abnormal coronary dilator responses and increased reactivity to vasoconstrictors have been reported in these patients. Some studies show limited changes in coronary blood flow in response to rapid pacing and to dilators such as dipyridamole and adenosine [22]. These studies demonstrate the importance of vascular biology in the pathogenesis of angina in women with cardiac syndrome X. Alternative explanations for these observations are possible and the etiology of cardiac syndrome X remains controversial.

Apical Ballooning Syndrome

JP is a 67-year-old anxious woman who was under intense financial stress; she had spent a particular day signing for a new line of credit and anguished about possibly defaulting on the loan. Dull, anterior chest discomfort started that evening. Due to continued symptoms, she sought medical attention the next morning. In the ER, her ECG was markedly abnormal and changed from an earlier tracing (Fig. 28.7). Her chest X-ray (CXR) was consistent with mild, interstitial, pulmonary edema. Brain natriuretic peptide (BNP) and troponin levels were elevated. Creatine kinase-MB was also increased. Stat echocardiography showed a large wall motion abnormality with severe anterior and apical hypokinesia.

An emergency heart catheterization was performed. Coronary angiography showed only minimal luminal irregularities and no evidence of plaque rupture or thrombus (Fig. 28.8a, b). Left ventriculography showed a large anterior-apical wall motion abnormality (Fig. 28.9a, in diastole, and Fig. 28.9b, in systole). Systolic LV function was depressed, and calculated ejection fraction was only 30%.

The patient was started on appropriate medications and discharged on her third hospital day. Follow-up echocardiogram 3 months after admission showed normal LV function and wall motion.

This patient highlights the features of apical ballooning syndrome, also called Takotsubo cardiomyopathy or stress-induced cardiomyopathy, another difficult-to-explain syndrome that affects women disproportionately. The disorder occurs after an intense life stress or acute medical illness, and results in myocardial injury. Stress cardiomyopathy is 9 times as frequent in women as it is in men [23].

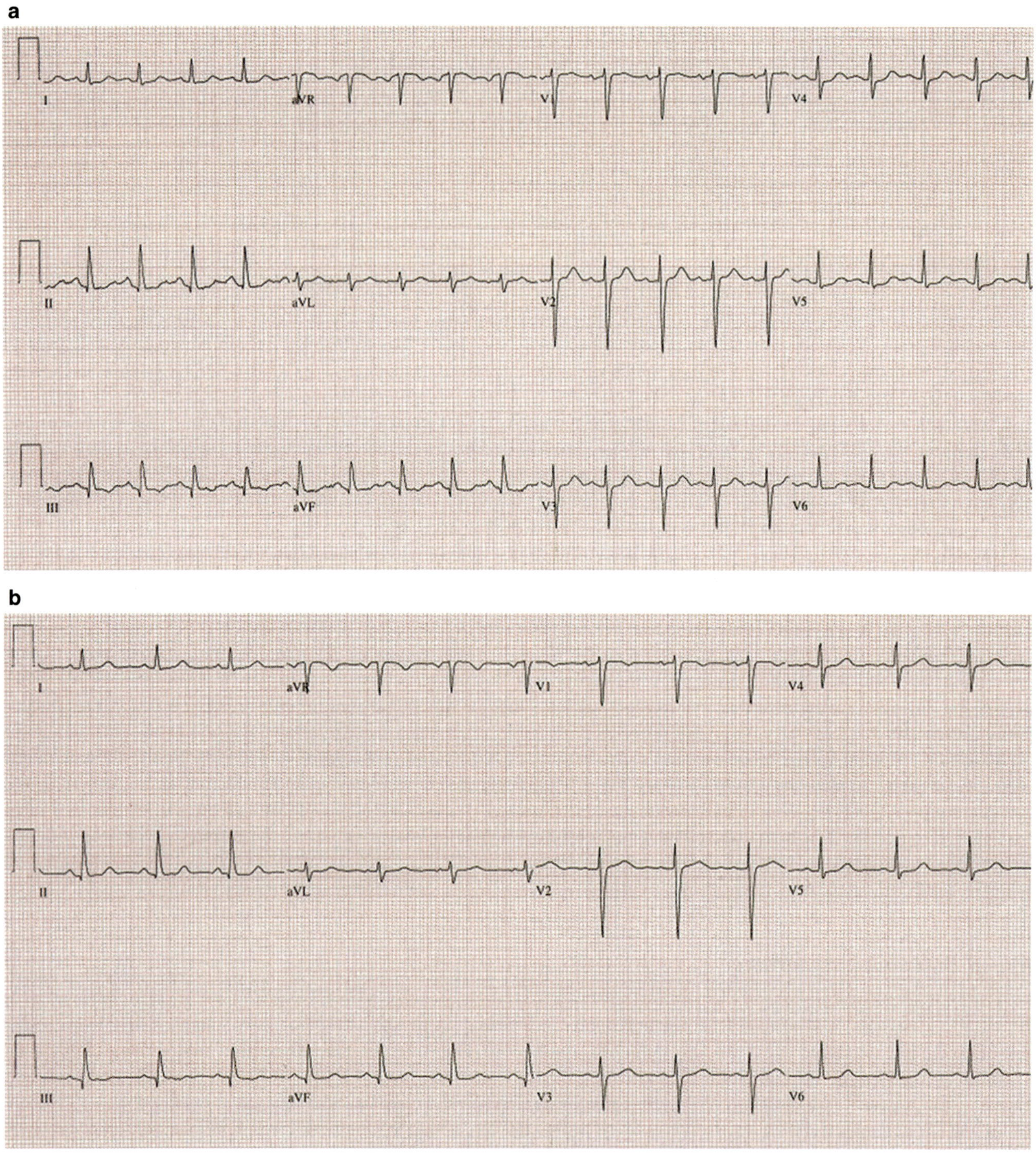

Fig. 28.4 (**a**) Electrocardiogram for patient reporting chest pain. ST-T changes observed in the anterior lateral leads. (**b**) Electrocardiogram without chest pain: results within normal

Patients present with chest pain, ECG abnormalities, and congestive heart failure symptoms. Left ventriculography and echocardiographic studies show a large wall motion abnormality, usually with a significant reduction in overall LV function. Coronary angiograms in these women are usually within normal limits. Patients generally have an excellent prognosis with full recovery of LV function expected. Possible mechanisms for myocardial injury in apical ballooning syndrome include catecholamine excess effects, coronary spasm, and microvascular dysfunction induced by extreme stress. Severe stress appears to affect the vasculature of women more potently than men, leading to this unusual syndrome.

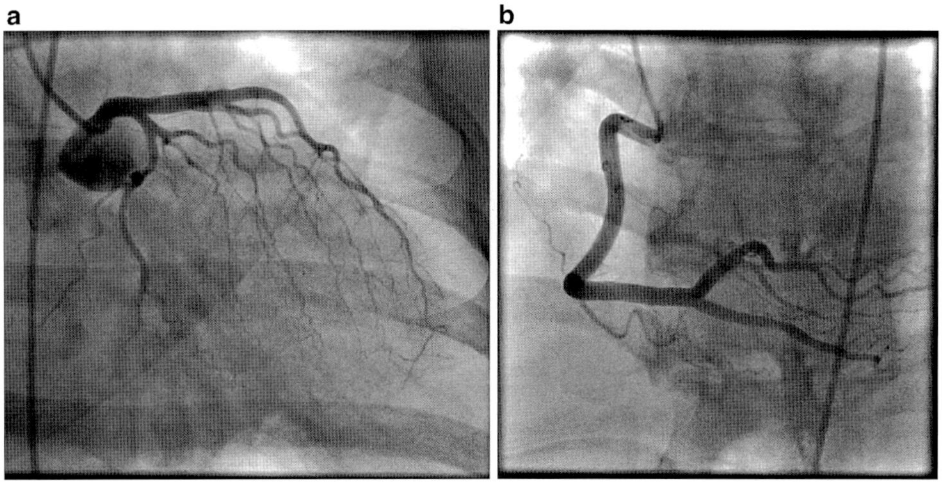

Fig. 28.5 (**a**) Left coronary angiogram: right anterior oblique (RAO) 30, caudal (CAU) 30: within normal. (**b**) Right coronary angiogram: left anterior oblique (LAO) 20, cranial 20: within normal

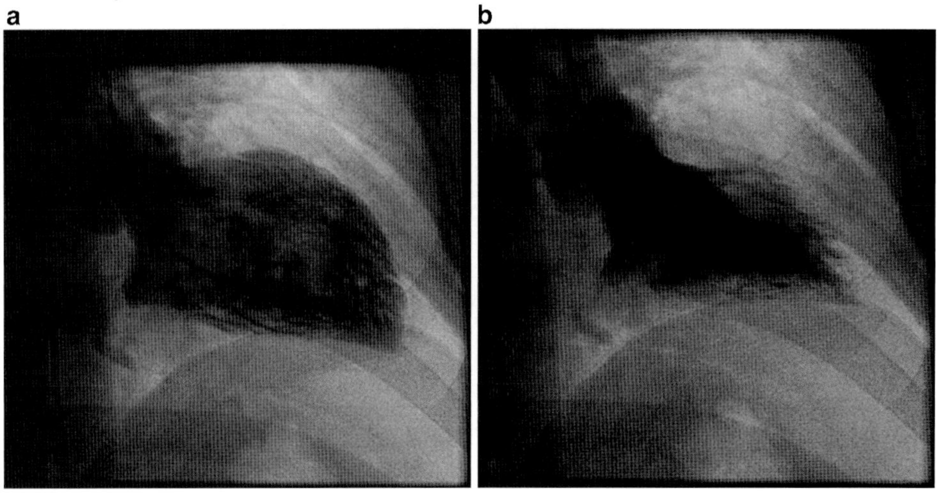

Fig. 28.6 Left ventriculogram: RAO 30. (**a**) In diastole and (**b**). In systole. Normal function, no wall motion abnormalities

Peripartum Cardiomyopathy

TK, a 35-year-old woman, was admitted to the hospital because of extreme dyspnea in her 35th week of pregnancy. Her symptoms consisted of chest tightness, orthopnea, and increased peripheral edema. BNP was elevated. ECG showed sinus tachycardia without acute changes. Figure 28.10a shows her ECG 5 weeks prior to admission. Figure 28.10b shows her ECG at admission. A CXR revealed increased interstitial markings and perihilar haziness – findings consistent with pulmonary edema. Stat echocardiography showed LV enlargement and global hypokinesia with an ejection fraction of 30% (Fig. 28.11a, in diastole, and Fig. 28.11b, in systole).

The patient's respiratory distress worsened rapidly and she was intubated. An emergency C-section was then performed with delivery of a healthy 7 lb. 11 oz. infant. IV diuretics were administered. The patient was extubated 8 h after delivery. She responded to an aggressive medical regimen and was discharged on the eighth postoperative day. Breastfeeding was discouraged, given her need for continued therapy with cardiac medications. She was also counseled about the high risk of having maternal and/or fetal problems with any subsequent pregnancies, and was strongly advised against future pregnancies.

Patient was last seen in clinic 1 year after her delivery. Her most recent echocardiogram shows normal LV size with an ejection fraction of 45–50%. She continues to be asymptomatic.

Peripartum cardiomyopathy is a form of dilated cardiomyopathy that occurs during late pregnancy or in the first 5 months postpartum. The woman experiences congestive heart failure symptoms and her echocardiographic findings include increased LV size with a significant decrease in LV systolic function. The exact pathophysiology of this disorder is unclear. The development of peripartum cardiomyopathy appears to begin with an unknown trigger that initiates an inflammatory process. This inflammation ultimately results in myocardial injury and the development of a cardiomyopathy. Peripartum cardiomyopathy represents another example of a systemic inflammatory state that results in myocardial injury in the absence of obstructive coronary artery disease and is, by nature, unique to women.

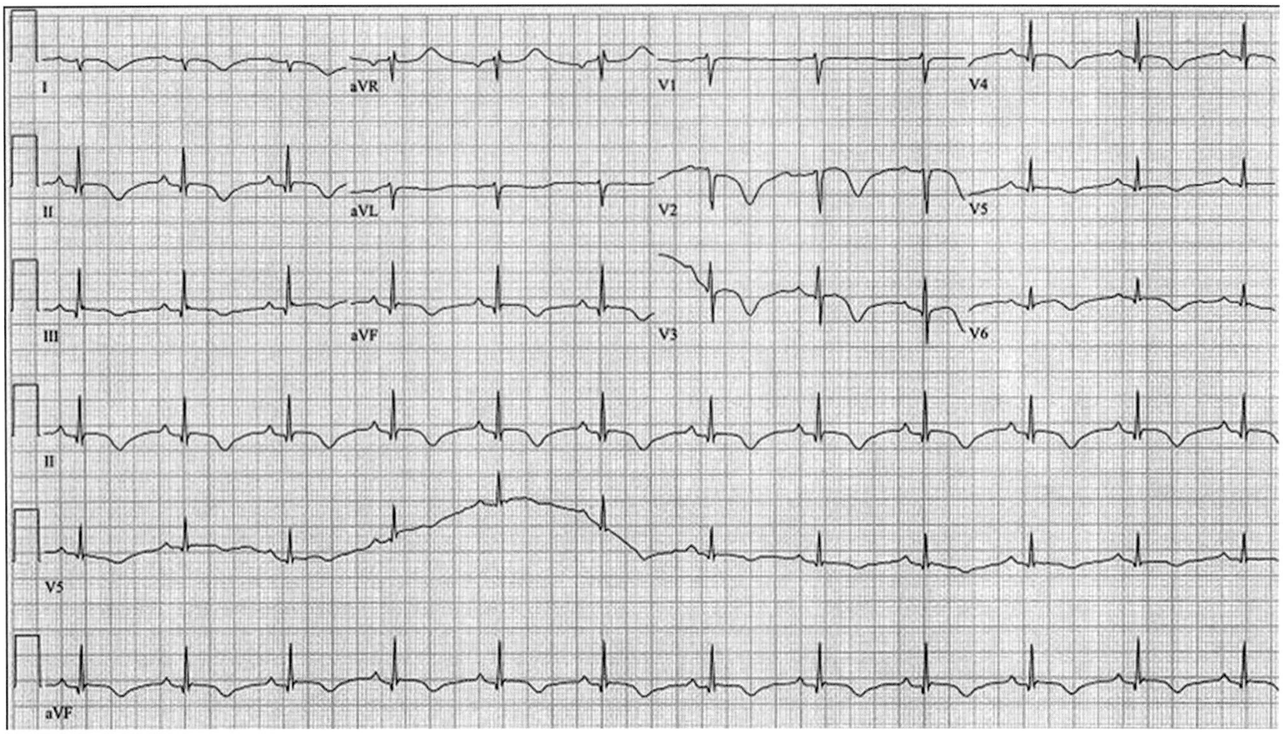

Fig. 28.7 Electrocardiogram on admission markedly abnormal, with ST-T inferior and anterior lateral changes

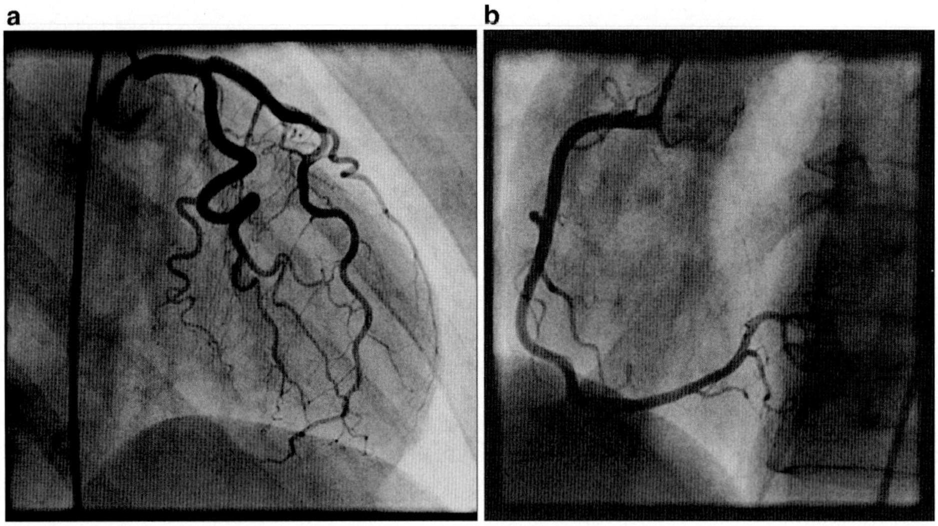

Fig. 28.8 (**a**) Left coronary arteriogram RAO 30, CAU 30. (**b**) Right coronary arteriogram: LAO 35. Minimal luminal irregularities. No evidence of plaque rupture or thrombus

Tests of Vascular Biology

Because vasospasm, endothelial dysfunction, and microvascular disease may play a more prominent role in the pathophysiology of CVD in women, certain tests of vascular biology may be more diagnostic for women than for men. Medical tests for inflammatory states include erythrocyte sedimentation rate (ESR) and C-reactive protein (CRP). Interestingly, basal ESR and CRP levels are slightly higher in women than men [24]. Elevations in CRP have been associated with an increased risk

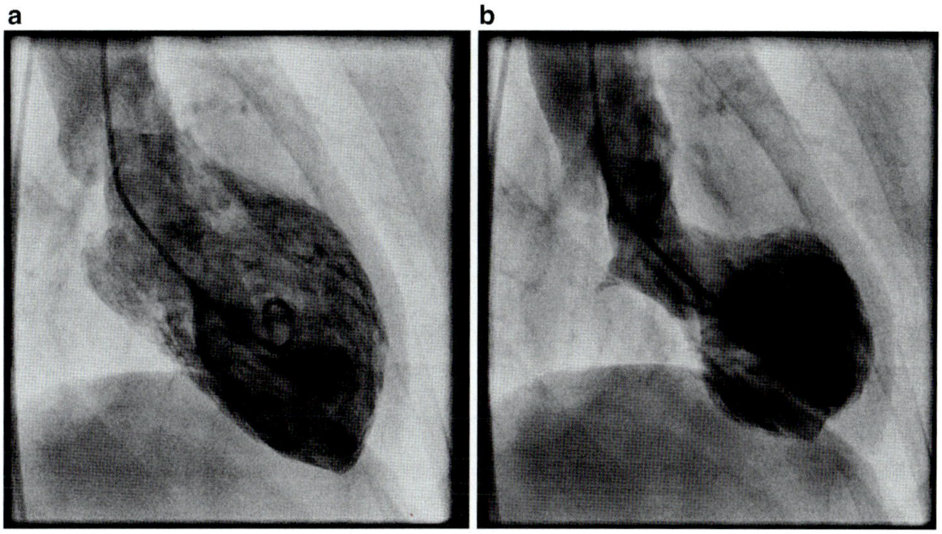

Fig. 28.9 Left ventriculogram: RAO 30. (**a**) Diastole. (**b**) Systole. Large anterior apical wall motion abnormality

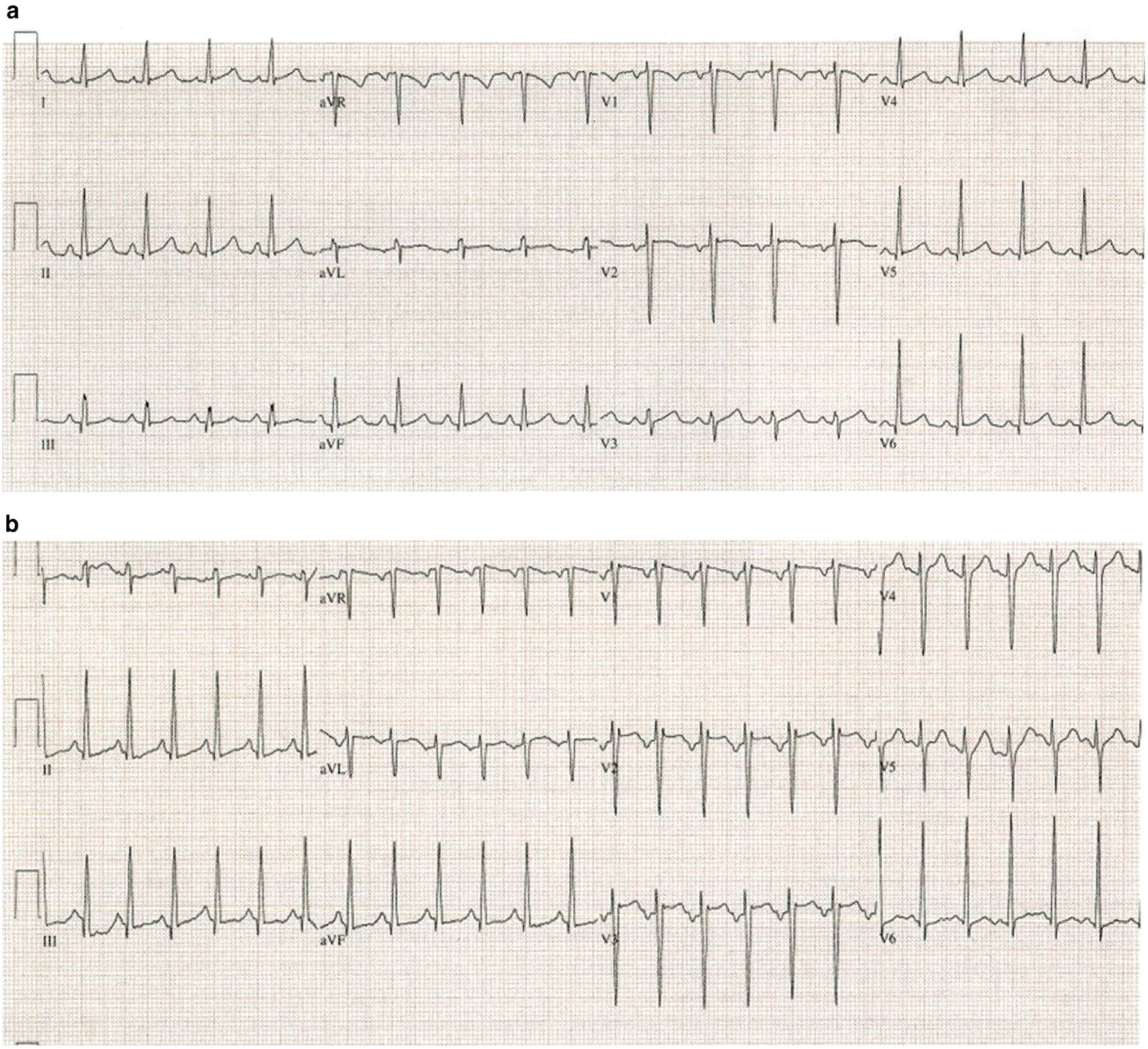

Fig. 28.10 (**a**) Electrocardiogram prior to development of cardiomyopathy: normal. (**b**) Electrocardiogram at admission. Sinus tachycardia without acute changes

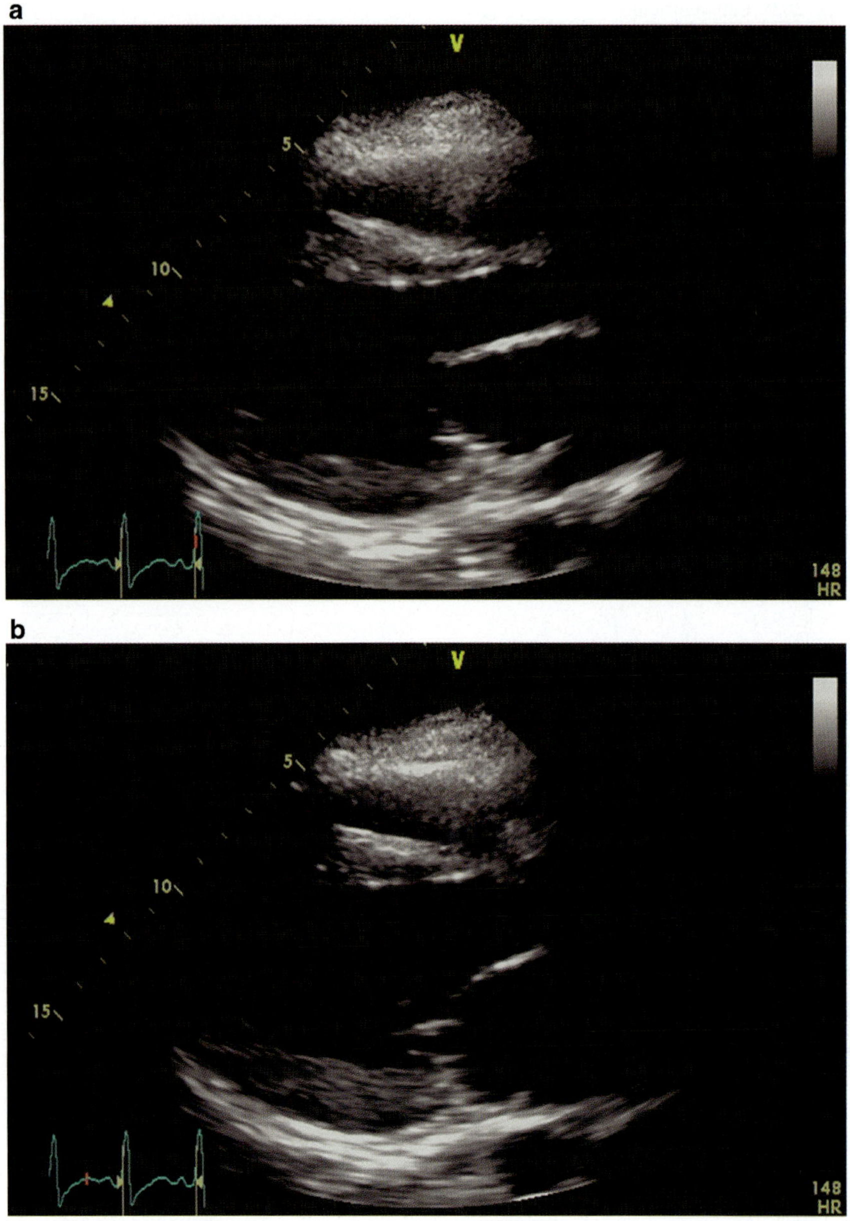

Fig. 28.11 Two-dimensional echocardiogram, parasternal axis view. (**a**) Diastole. (**b**) Systole. LV enlarged, global hypokinesis. Ejection fraction, 30%

of CVD. CRP also correlates with coronary microvascular dysfunction [25] and may therefore be a more important marker of CVD in women than in men.

Endothelial dysfunction is characterized by the inability of arteries to dilate fully in response to an appropriate stimulus. Several methods for measuring this response have been described. If the blood vessel is stressed, the endothelium responds by releasing vasodilators, such as nitric oxide. These vasoactive chemicals cause the vascular smooth muscle to relax, producing vasodilatation. One popular technique for testing endothelial function is brachial artery flow-mediated dilation, a noninvasive technique for measuring endothelial function. In this technique, a blood pressure arm cuff is inflated to high pressures and then released. The subsequent hyperemic response is then measured by ultrasound.

One study found endothelial dysfunction present in approximately 50% of the women who presented with chest pain, in the absence of overt blockages in large coronary arteries [26]. In another study, impaired brachial artery flow-mediated dilation in postmenopausal women was associated with a marked increase in CVD risk [27]. These tests of vascular function could represent important prognostic markers for CVD in women.

Cost Issues

Unfortunately, many symptomatic women without obstructive coronary artery disease continue to have frequent clinic visits and hospitalizations for evaluation and treatment of their chest pain. Some women, despite normal coronary angiograms, continue to have findings of ischemia or myocardial injury [28]. These women also report a higher level of functional disability as compared to men.

The burden of care for women with signs and symptoms of ischemia in the absence of obstructive coronary artery disease is high and can be extremely frustrating to their health care providers. A significant proportion of health care dollars is spent due to the uncertainty surrounding the correct diagnosis and therapy for these patients [29].

Poor Prognosis

The Women's Health Initiative data show that women with nonspecific chest pain have a significantly greater risk for nonfatal myocardial infarction than asymptomatic women [30]. The Women's Ischemia Syndrome Evaluation shows increased mortality in women with chest pain and normal coronary angiograms as compared to those without chest pain [31]. Both of these studies demonstrate that chest pain symptoms, even in the absence of obstructive coronary artery disease, can indicate an increased risk of CVD morbidity and mortality in women. Chest pain symptoms in women, even without definitive coronary artery disease, should not be dismissed; these symptoms could portend a poor prognosis.

Conclusion

While some women do present with typical symptoms of CVD and obstructive coronary artery disease, many others present with atypical symptoms and normal coronary anatomy. To correctly diagnose these atypical patients, the gender-specific pathophysiology of CVD in women must be understood.

Sex differences in the endothelial response to injury can lead to differences in arterial remodeling and repair. Ultimately, this leads to varying degrees of microvascular disease, myocardial ischemia, and myocardial injury. Detrimental disease processes in women may be compounded by their smaller-caliber coronary arteries. Diminutive vessel size may also have played a significant role in the results of women treated with "standard equipment" during coronary revascularization procedures. Currently, women follow the same recommended pathways for percutaneous coronary intervention or coronary artery bypass graft surgery as do their male counterparts.

Despite the similarities of treatment options for obstructive coronary artery disease, women have a higher morbidity and mortality than men. Ongoing basic research and clinical trials will help define the pathophysiology involved in a woman's development of chest pain and her more malignant clinical course. Increased knowledge of these sex-specific differences could lead to better and earlier CVD diagnosis in women, which would translate into a better prognosis and higher quality of care.

References

1. Centers for Disease Control and Prevention. State-specific mortality from sudden cardiac death – United States. Centers for Disease Control and Prevention Web site. 1999. http://www.cdc.gov/mmwr/preview/mmwrhtml/mm5106a3.html. Published Feb. 15, 2002. Accessed 19 July 2010.
2. Jenkins JS, Flaker GC, Nolte B, et al. Causes of higher in-hospital mortality in women than in men after acute myocardial infarction. Am J Cardiol. 1994;73(5):319–22.
3. Gregg EW, Gu Q, Cheng YJ, Narayan KM, Cowie CC. Mortality trends in men and women with diabetes. Ann Intern Med. 2007;147:149–55.
4. Mosca L, Grundy SM, Judelson D, et al. Guide to preventative cardiology for women. AHA/ACC scientific statement. Circulation. 1999;99:2480–4.
5. Mosca L, Appel L, Benjamin E, et al. Evidence-based guidelines for cardiovascular disease prevention in women. Circulation. 2004;109: 672–93.
6. Steering Committee of the Physicians' Health Study Research Group. Final report on the aspirin component of the ongoing Physicians' Health Study. N Engl J Med. 1989;321:129–35.
7. Ridker PM, Cook NR, LeeI M, et al. A randomized trial of low-dose aspirin in the primary prevention of cardiovascular disease in women. N Engl J Med. 2005;352:1293–304.

8. Kannel WB, Vokonas PS. Demographics of the prevalence, incidence and management of coronary heart disease in the elderly and in women. Ann Epidemiol. 1992;2(1):5–14.
9. Mokdad AH, Ford ES, Bowman BA, et al. Prevalence of obesity, diabetes, and obesity-related health risk factors, 2001. JAMA. 2003; 289:76–9.
10. Shaw LJ, Sharaf BL, Johnson BD, et al. The economic burden of angina in women with suspected ischemic heart disease: results from the National Institutes of Health–National Heart, Lung, and Blood Institue-Sponsored Women's Ischemia Syndrome Evaluation (WISE). Circulation. 2006;114:894–904.
11. Alexander KP, Shaw LJ, Delong ER, et al. Value of exercise treadmill testing in women. J Am Coll Cardiol. 1998;32:1657.
12. Nguyen JT, Berger AB, Duval S, Luepker RV. Gender disparity in cardiac procedures and medication use for acute myocardial infarction. Am Heart J. 2008;155(5):862–8.
13. Shaw LJ, Shaw RE, Bairey Merz CN, et al. Impact of ethnicity and gender differences on angiographic coronary artery disease prevalence and in-hospital mortality in the American College of Cardiology – National Cardiovascular Data Registry. Circulation. 2008;117:1787–801.
14. Hochman JS, Tamis JE, Thompson TD, et al. For the global use of strategies to open occluded coronary arteries in acute coronary syndromes IIb investigators. Sex, clinical presentation, and outcome in patients with acute coronary syndromes. N Engl J Med. 1999;341:226–32.
15. Chugh SS, Uy-Evanado A, Teodorescu C, et al. Women have a lower prevalence of structural heart disease as a precursor to sudden cardiac arrest. J Am Coll Cardiol. 2009;54(22):2006–11.
16. BaireyMerz CN, Johnson BD, Sharaf BL, et al. Hypoestrogenemia of hypothalamic origin and coronary artery disease in women evaluated for suspected ischemia: a report from the NHLBI-sponsored WISE study. J Am Coll Cardiol. 2003;41:413–9.
17. Egan KM, Lawson JA, Fries S, et al. COX-2-derived prostacyclin confers atheroprotection on female mice. Science. 2004;306:1954–7.
18. Tannebaum C, Barrett-Connor E, Laughlin GA, Platt RW. A longitudinal study of dehydroepiandrosterone sulphate (DHEAS) change in older men and women: the Rancho Bernardo Study. Eur J Endocrinol. 2004;151:717–25.
19. Matthews KA, Crawford SL, Chae CU, et al. Are changes in cardiovascular disease risk factors in midlife women due to chronological aging or to the menopausal transition? J Am Coll Cardiol. 2009;54:2366–73.
20. Lerner DJ, Kannel WB. Patterns of coronary heart disease morbidity and mortality in the sexes: a 26-year follow-up of the Framingham population. Am Heart J. 1986;111:383–90.
21. Kemp Jr HG. Left ventricular function in patients with the anginal syndrome and normal coronary angiograms. Am J Cardiol. 1973;32:375–6.
22. Panting JR, Gatehouse PD, Grothues F, et al. Abnormal subendocardial perfusion in cardiac syndrome X detected by cardiovascular magnetic resonance imaging. N Engl J Med. 2002;346:1948–53.
23. Wittstein IS, Thiemann DR, Lima JAC, et al. Neurohumoral features of myocardial stunning due to sudden emotional stress. N Engl J Med. 2005;352:539–48.
24. Wong ND, Pio J, Valencia R, et al. Distribution of C-reactive protein and its relation to risk factors and coronary heart disease risk estimation in the National Health and Nutrition Examination Survey (NHANES) III. Prev Cardiol. 2001;4:109–14.
25. Teragawa H, Fukuda Y, Matsuda K, et al. Relation between C-reactive protein and coronary microvascular endothelial function. Heart. 2004; 90(7):750–4.
26. Reis SE, Holubkov R, Smith AJC, et al. Coronary microvascular dysfunction is highly prevalent in women with chest pain in the absence of coronary artery disease: results from the NHLBI WISE Study. Am Heart J. 2001;141(5):735–41.
27. Rossi R, Nuzzo A, Origliani G, Modena MG. Prognostic role of flow-mediated dilation and cardiac risk factors in post-menopausal women. J Am Coll Cardiol. 2008;51:997–1002.
28. Olson MB, Kelsey SF, Matthews K, et al. Symptoms, myocardial ischaemia, and quality of life in women: results from the NHLBI-sponsored WISE study. Eur Heart J. 2003;24:1506–14.
29. Johnson BD, Bairey Merz CN, Kelsey SF, et al. Persistent chest pain predicts cardiovascular events in women with and without obstructive coronary artery disease: results from the NHLBI-sponsored WISE study. Eur Heart J. 2006;27:1408–15.
30. Robinson JG, Wallace R, Limacher M, et al. Cardiovascular risk in women with non-specific chest pain (from the Women's Health Initiative Hormone Trials). Am J Cardiol. 2008;102:693–9.
31. Gulati M, Cooper-DeHoff RM, McClure C, et al. Adverse cardiovascular outcomes in women with nonobstructive coronary artery disease: a report from the National Institutes of Health – National Heart, Lung, and Blood Institute-Sponsored Women's Ischemia Syndrome Evaluation (WISE) study and the St. James Women Take Heart (WTH) project. Arch Intern Med. 2009;169:843–50.
32. American Heart Association Web site. 2010. http://www.americanheart.org/downloadable/heart/1236184538758WOMEN.pdf. Accessed 16 July 2010.
33. Marrugat J, Sala J, Masia R, et al. Mortality differences between men and women following first myocardial infarction. JAMA. 1998;280: 1405–9.
34. Levin RI. The puzzle of aspirin and sex [editorial]. N Engl J Med. 2005;352:1366–8.

Chapter 29
Prevention of Coronary Artery Disease

Daniel Duprez

Abbreviation

ACCORD	Action to control cardiovascular risk in diabetes
ACE-inhibitor	Angiotensin-converting enzyme inhibitor
ACS	Acute coronary syndrome
AHA	American heart association
ARB	Angiotensin receptor blocker
ATP	Adult treatment panel
CABG	Coronary artery bypass graft
CAD	Coronary artery disease
CAMELOT Study	Comparison of amlodipine vs. enalapril to limit occurrences of thrombosis study
CETP	Cholesteryl ester transfer protein
CHARISMA	Clopidogrel for high atherothrombotic risk and ischemic stabilization management and avoidance
CHD	Coronary heart disease
CLAS	Cholesterol lowering atherosclerosis study
CURE	Clopidogrel in unstable angina to prevent recurrent events
CVD	Cardiovascular disease
DBP	Diastolic blood pressure
DHA	Docosahexaenoic acid
EPA	Eicosapentaenoic acid
EUROPA trial	EURopean trial on reduction of cardiac events with perindopril in stable coronary artery disease trial
FATS	Familial atherosclerosis treatment study
GI	Gastrointestinal tract
HATS	HDL-atherosclerosis treatment study
HDL-cholesterol	High-density lipoprotein cholesterol
HOPE trial	Heart outcomes prevention evaluation trial
HOT trial	Hypertension optimal treatment trial
HRT	Hormone replacement therapy
IMPROVE-IT	Examining outcomes in subjects with acute coronary syndrome: Vytorin (ezetimibe–simvastatin) vs. Simvastatin
INVEST	International verapamil–trandolapril study
LDL-cholesterol	Low-density lipoprotein cholesterol
Lp a	Lipoprotein a
MI	Myocardial infarction
PCI	Percutaneous intervention
PPI	Proton pump inhibitor

D. Duprez, MD, PhD (✉)
Cardiovascular Division, University of Minnesota, Minneapolis, MN, USA
e-mail: dupre007@umn.edu

Z. Vlodaver et al. (eds.), *Coronary Heart Disease: Clinical, Pathological, Imaging, and Molecular Profiles*,
DOI 10.1007/978-1-4614-1475-9_29, © Springer Science+Business Media, LLC 2012

SBP	Systolic blood pressure
SHARP	Study of heart and renal protection
THRIVE	Treatment of HDL to reduce the incidence of vascular events
US Public Health Service	United States public health service
VAHIT	Veterans administration HDL intervention trial
VLDL	Very low-density lipoprotein

Introduction

Cardiovascular risk factors are very well established in the pathogenesis of coronary artery disease (CAD): family history of premature cardiovascular disease (CVD), sedentary lifestyle, smoking, obesity, hypercholesterolemia, hypertension, diabetes, renal insufficiency, and early menopause. The American Heart Association (AHA), American College of Cardiology (ACC), European Society of Cardiology (ESC), and several other cardiovascular societies have developed guidelines for the treatment of patients with CAD [1, 2].

Dyslipidemia, hypertension, and diabetes mellitus are established predictors of CVD. Lifestyle risk factors for these conditions including dietary habits, physical inactivity, smoking, and adiposity strongly influence the established cardiovascular risk factors and also affect novel pathways of risk such as inflammation/oxidative stress, endothelial function, and thrombosis/coagulation [3].

Despite the classic risk factors for CAD being well known, evidence-based therapies for CAD are applied less frequently in women compared to men [4]. Similarly, treatment guideline adherence is significantly decreased in elderly patients compared to younger CAD patients.

Risk Factors for CAD

Cardiovascular risk factors can be divided into three categories: (1) lifestyle risk factors such as unhealthy diet, sedentary lifestyle, obesity, and smoking, (2) established risk factors such as hypercholesterolemia, hypertension, and diabetes, and (3) novel risk factors such as inflammation, metabolic syndrome, and thrombotic risk factors (Fig. 29.1). With aging and increasing incidence of diabetes, renal impairment will also accelerate the process of CAD. A family history of premature coronary heart disease should also urge a closer follow-up of these patients.

Lifestyle Risk Factors

Modest alterations of lifestyle risk factors are achievable and can have substantial effects on cardiovascular risk. Thus, basic lifestyle habits should be considered fundamental risk factors for CVD. The clinical evaluation and treatment of dietary,

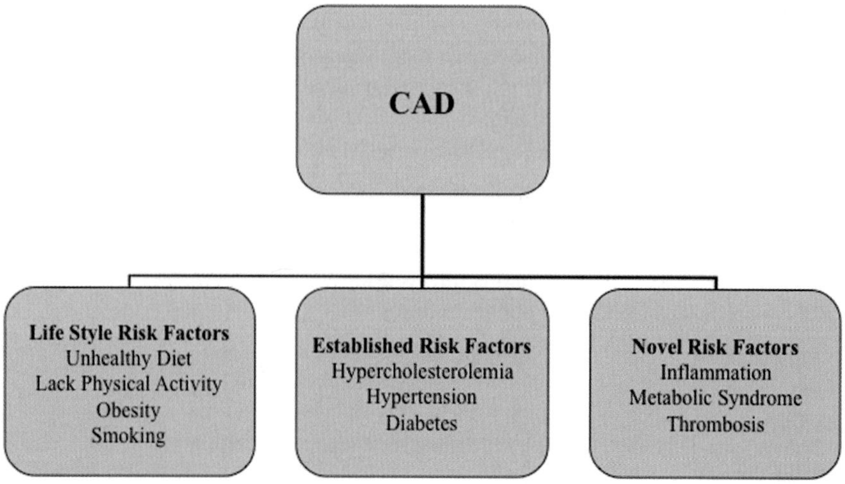

Fig. 29.1 Lifestyle, established, and novel risk factors for coronary artery disease (CAD)

Table 29.1 Diet and lifestyle goals for CAD risk reduction

Consume an overall healthy diet
Be physically active
Avoid use of and exposure to tobacco products
Aim for a healthy body weight
Aim for a normal blood pressure
Aim for recommended levels of low-density lipoprotein (LDL) cholesterol, high-density lipoprotein (HDL) cholesterol, and triglycerides
Aim for a normal blood glucose

physical activity, and smoking habits must become as routine and familiar as assessment of blood pressure (BP), cholesterol, and glucose levels.

Clinicians need to make time to discuss home "self-care" with CAD patients. We need to emphasize that the most important and powerful way to reduce the risk of CAD is under the patient's control. The phenomenal drop in CHD death rate over the past 30 years has been more due to reducing risk factors than due to advances in treatment [5]. It is important that the cardiologist or other health care provider (internist, primary care provider) emphasizes the information to the CAD patient.

Heart-Healthy Diet (Table 29.1)

The AHA recommends a heart-healthy diet for people at risk of developing CAD [6, 7]. The recommendations are to balance caloric intake and physical activity to achieve and maintain a healthy body weight; to consume a diet rich in vegetables and fruits; choose whole-grain, high-fiber foods; to consume fish, especially oily fish, at least twice a week; to limit intake of saturated fat to <7% of energy, trans fat to <1% of energy, and cholesterol to <300 mg/day by choosing lean meats and vegetable alternatives, fat-free (skim) or low-fat (1% fat) dairy products, and by minimizing intake of partially hydrogenated fats; to minimize intake of beverages and foods with added sugars; and to choose and prepare foods with little or no salt. Alcohol may be taken in moderation. To raise high-density lipoprotein (HDL) cholesterol, no more than two alcoholic drinks per day for men and no more than one drink per day for women are recommended. However, some people should not drink alcohol. People who have liver or kidney problems, certain other medical problems, or who are taking certain medications should not use alcohol.

Smoking Cessation

Smoking cessation has proven to be a very effective and cost-effective intervention. The US Public Health Service recommends that clinicians counsel all patients who use tobacco to permanently quit Encompassed in this evaluation are current and past smoking status, with particular emphasis on smoking cessation within the prior 12 months [8]. Exposure to secondhand smoke also should be ascertained. The readiness for smoking cessation should be determined, with intervention by education, counseling, and social support as needed, and pharmacologic support (including nicotine replacement, bupropion, varenicline) as warranted. Relapse-prevention skills should be taught and practiced. Smoking cessation can reduce cardiovascular risk by about one third in patients with CVD [9].

Exercise

The main components of cardiac rehabilitation are described in a scientific statement from the AHA and the American Association of Cardiovascular and Pulmonary Rehabilitation [10–12]. The objectives of cardiac rehabilitation include improvement in exercise habits and exercise tolerance. Attention should also be devoted to the emotional responses to living with heart disease, specifically, amelioration of stress and anxiety, and lessening of depression. In elderly patients, attention should be focused on functional independence. The return to an appropriate and satisfactory occupation is considered to be beneficial to both individual patients and society.

It is very important to counsel CAD patients about physical activity levels and exercise capacity. Attention needs to focus on potential barriers to increasing physical activity and to making behavioral changes. Moreover, referral to an exercise program should be implemented. Recommendations are for a minimum of 30 min and up to 60 min of moderate physical activity on most if not all days of the week, with strategies to incorporate increased physical activity into usual daily activities. Activities should initially be low impact, with gradual increases in activity duration and intensity.

Table 29.2 Antihypertensive drugs and coronary artery disease

ACE-inhibitor (ARB as alternative)
Beta-blocker (angina pectoris, post-MI, post-PCI, post-CABG)
Calcium antagonist
Diuretic (thiazide)
Vasodilator (long-acting nitrates)

ACE angiotensin-converting enzyme; *ARB* angiotensin receptor blocker; *MI* myocardial infarction; *PCI* percutaneous intervention; *CABG* coronary artery bypass graft

A 20–30% reduction in all-cause mortality has been documented in patients with CVD who adhere to a regular physical activity regimen [13].

The risk of cardiovascular complications from exercise should be assessed before initiation of exercise training, using a standardized assessment to identify patients who may have unstable symptoms or other factors that characterize them as at increased risk for adverse cardiovascular events. Symptom-limited exercise testing may be warranted before enrollment in an exercise-based cardiac rehabilitation program, with exercise test performance guiding the level of supervision required for exercise training. Energy expenditure is related to the intensity and duration of exercise. An individualized exercise prescription should incorporate aerobic and resistance training, and address specific patient comorbidities.

Weight Reduction

Obesity is an independent risk factor for CAD and adversely impacts cardiovascular risk factors. Measurement of weight, height, waist circumference, and calculation of body mass index provides the basis for establishing both short- and long-term weight goals. Baseline data regarding daily caloric intake and dietary content of saturated fat, trans fat, cholesterol, sodium, and alcohol consumption are needed to establish the education and counseling needed regarding dietary goals and individualized dietary changes.

The body mass index goal for most adults is 18.5–24.9 kg/m^2, with a waist circumference of <40 in. for men and <35 in. for women [14, 15]. Effective weight loss involves a combination of diet, physical activity/exercise, and a behavioral program. While a 30-min daily exercise regimen is suitable as a global recommendation, exercise designed for weight reduction or maintenance of such weight reduction requires 60–90 min of daily exercise.

Established Risk Factors

Blood Pressure Management (Table 29.2)

Lowering arterial blood pressure reduces the risk for CAD. But several key questions related to blood pressure have caused a lot of debate: (1) What is the optimal blood pressure in patients with CAD? (2) Is there a J-shaped curve, which means that blood pressure that's too low could harm the hypertensive patient with CAD? (3) Is it the blood pressure-lowering effect or the choice of antihypertensive drug that leads to the most cardiovascular protection?

Overwhelming data show that CAD can be prevented or its progression can be delayed when aggressive targets are achieved for major CVD risk factors. As in primary and secondary prevention, the effectiveness of the blood pressure-lowering therapy is evaluated by the degree of blood pressure lowering and the ability of the chosen regimen to reduce clinical end points: myocardial infarction, unstable angina, and ischemic heart disease in general [16–18].

The current consensus target for BP is <140/90 mmHg in general and <130/80 mmHg in individuals with diabetes mellitus or chronic kidney disease [16]. At present, no clinical trials are designed to answer the question about the most appropriate BP target(s) for individuals with latent or overt CAD.

The results of the ACCORD (Action to Control Cardiovascular Risk in Diabetes) trial have intensified the debate about an optimal blood pressure goal [19]. This trial studied patients with type 2 diabetes at high risk for cardiovascular events, targeting a systolic blood pressure (SBP) of less than 120 mmHg, compared with less than 140 mmHg. The trial demonstrated that there was no difference between these two blood pressure levels in reducing the rate of a composite outcome of fatal and nonfatal major cardiovascular events.

The CAMELOT (Comparison of Amlodipine vs. Enalapril to Limit Occurrences of Thrombosis) substudy analyzed results from 274 patients with CAD who completed the coronary intravascular ultrasound substudy [20]. Results showed that subjects with a normal blood pressure according to the definition given in the Seventh Report of the Joint National Committee (JNC) on Prevention, Detection, Evaluation, and Treatment of High Blood Pressure (<120/80 mmHg) had a mean decrease in atheroma volume of 4.6 mm [3], those considered prehypertensive (120–139/80–89 mmHg) had no significant change in atheroma volume, and those considered hypertensive (≥140/90 mmHg) had a mean increase in atheroma volume of 12.0 mm [3]. This study showed the importance of achieving blood pressure goals, especially in those patients with CAD. However, the controversy remains about specific blood pressure treatment goals for individuals with nascent or overt CAD. From a pathophysiological perspective, it can be argued that very low SBP values (<120 mmHg) may be appropriate to reduce myocardial workload. This contrasts with the concern that excessive lowering of diastolic blood pressure (DBP) may impair coronary perfusion.

Whether lowering DBP improves cardiovascular outcome only when coronary perfusion is maintained above the lower limit of coronary autoregulation remains the subject of debate. Data from controlled trials have not shown a J curve. The Hypertension Optimal Treatment (HOT) trial randomized 18,790 patients with an average pretreatment blood pressure of 170/105 mmHg to three treatment groups with different DBP targets: ≤90, ≤85, or ≤80 mmHg [21]. At the study's end, little separation existed in the achieved DBP (mean values 85.2, 83.2, and 81.1 mmHg, respectively), which impaired the ability to detect any meaningful difference among treatment groups. Lower blood pressure did not further decrease or increase the incidence of adverse cardiovascular events, except for a small increase in mortality in those whose diastolic pressures were reduced to <70 mmHg.

The International Verapamil–Trandolapril Study (INVEST) included 22,576 patients with known CAD and hypertension [22]. Subjects with DBP values lower than 70 mmHg were associated with increased risk for myocardial infarction; however, subjects with DBP <70 mmHg were older than those with higher diastolic blood and were more likely to have a history of myocardial infarction, bypass surgery and angioplasty, diabetes mellitus, heart failure, and cancer.

Although lower SBP values are associated with better ischemic heart disease outcomes, the evidence that excessive lowering of DBP may compromise cardiac outcomes (J-shape curve) is inconsistent. So, for patients with an elevated DBP and occlusive CAD with evidence of myocardial ischemia, it seems prudent that their blood pressure should be lowered slowly, and caution is advised in inducing falls of DBP below 60 mmHg if the patient has diabetes mellitus or is over age 60.

The effect of blood pressure-lowering drugs in reducing the risk of disease is entirely or largely due to blood pressure reduction, with one main exception – a special, extra effect of beta-blockers in people who have had a recent myocardial infarction [18].

In patients with CAD, the heart outcomes prevention evaluation trial (HOPE trial) (ramipril-based regimen) and the EUROPA (EURopean trial on reduction of cardiac events with perindopril in stable coronary artery disease trial) (perindopril-based regimen) study provided evidence-based medicine data that angiotensin converting enzyme inhibitor (ACE-inhibitors) for patients with CAD further reduced significantly the risk for a cardiovascular event [23, 24].

The AHA scientific statement regarding "treatment of hypertension in the prevention and management of ischemic heart disease" recommends aggressive blood pressure-lowering for the primary prevention of CAD in hypertensive patients. The recommended target blood pressure is <130/80 mmHg in individuals with any of the following: diabetes mellitus, chronic renal disease, CAD risk equivalents, carotid artery disease (carotid bruit, or abnormal carotid ultrasound or angiography), peripheral arterial disease, or abdominal aortic aneurysm [17]. The choice of drugs remains controversial. There is a general consensus that the amount of blood pressure reduction, rather than the choice of antihypertensive drug, is the major determinant of reduction in cardiovascular risk; however, sufficient evidence from comparative clinical trials supports the use of an ACE inhibitor (or angiotensin receptor blocker), calcium channel blocker, or thiazide diuretic as first-line therapy, supplemented by a second drug if blood pressure control is not achieved by monotherapy. Most patients will require two or more drugs to reach the goal, and when their blood pressure is >20/10 mmHg above goal, two drugs usually should be used from the outset. In an asymptomatic postmyocardial infarction patient, a beta-blocker is a more appropriate choice for secondary prevention for at least 6 months after the infarction and is the drug of first choice if the patient has angina pectoris.

Lipid Management (Table 29.3)

LDL Cholesterol and Statin Therapy

Statins should be considered as first-line drugs when LDL-lowering drugs are indicated to achieve LDL treatment goals.

LDL cholesterol plays a key role in the process of coronary atherosclerotic disease. Since the publication of the adult treatment panel (ATP) III guidelines in 2002 regarding the treatment of high blood cholesterol [14], results from several landmark trials with statin therapy have led to additional recommendations [5, 25].

Findings from additional lipid reduction trials involving more than 50,000 patients resulted in new, optional therapeutic targets, which were outlined in the 2004 update of the National Heart, Lung, and Blood Institute's ATP III report.

Table 29.3 Lipid-lowering drugs

Statins
Low potency; simvastatin, pravastatin, lovastatin, fluvastatin, pitavastatin
High potency: atorvastatin, rosuvastatin
Bile acid sequestrants
Cholestyramine
Colesevalam
Colestipol
Nicotinic acid/niacin
Fibrates
Gemfibrozil
Fenofibrate
Bezafibrate, Ciprofibrate, Clofibrate
Ezetimibe
n-3 (omega) fatty acids

These changes defined optional, lower target cholesterol levels for very high-risk coronary heart disease patients, especially those with acute coronary syndromes (ACSs), and they expanded indications for drug treatment. These trials called for alterations in treatment guidelines, such that LDL-C should be <100 mg/dL for all patients with coronary heart disease and other clinical forms of atherosclerotic disease, but in addition, that it is reasonable to treat to LDL-C <70 mg/dL in such patients. When the <70-mg/dL target is chosen, it may be prudent to increase statin therapy in a graded fashion to determine a patient's response and tolerance. Furthermore, if it is not possible to attain LDL-C <70 mg/dL because of a high baseline LDL-C, it generally is possible to achieve LDL-C reductions of >50% with either statins or LDL-C-lowering drug combinations.

A meta-analysis of 26 trials with 170,000 subjects clearly showed that the size of the proportional reduction in major vascular events is directly proportional to the absolute low-density lipoprotein cholesterol (LDL-cholesterol) reduction that is achieved, with further benefit from more intensive statin therapy, even if LDL cholesterol is already lower than 70 mg/dL [26]. These findings suggest that the primary goal for patients at high risk of occlusive vascular events should be to achieve the largest LDL-cholesterol reduction possible without materially increasing myopathy risk. Current therapeutic guidelines tend to emphasize the need to reach a particular LDL cholesterol target – for example, US National Cholesterol Education Program guidelines suggest that the objective in high-risk patients generally should be to reduce LDL cholesterol to below 100 mg/dL or, optionally, for very high-risk patients, to below 70 mg/dL. By contrast, the results of this meta-analysis suggest that lowering LDL cholesterol further in high-risk patients who achieve such targets would produce additional benefits without an increased risk of cancer or nonvascular mortality.

Guidelines have proposed that high doses of generic statins (e.g., 80 mg simvastatin daily) be used to achieve these benefits, but such regimens may be associated with higher risk of myopathy. Instead, these benefits may be achieved more safely with newer, more potent statins (e.g., 80 mg atorvastatin or 40 mg rosuvastatin daily) and, potentially, by combination of standard doses of generic statins (e.g., 40 mg simvastatin or pravastatin daily) with other LDL-cholesterol-lowering therapies. Serial measurement of lipid levels and of creatine kinase and liver function test levels are based on recommendations of the National Cholesterol Education Program Adult Treatment Panel.

If transaminase levels persist at more than 3 times the upper limit of normal, the FDA recommends discontinuation of therapy. If a patient does not tolerate statin therapy and develops myopathy, one needs to consider other therapies for CAD patients: fibrates, nicotinic acid. In case of statin drug interaction, (e.g., warfarin, cyclosporine, macrolide antibiotics and certain antifungal drugs) pravastatin is the safest statin to use because it does not interfere with the cytochrome P-450 3A (CYP3A)-dependent metabolism.

Bile Acid Sequestrants

One of the oldest cholesterol-lowering medications is the bile acid sequestrant.

Bile acid sequestrants moderately reduce LDL cholesterol and reduce CHD risk [27, 28]. They are additive in LDL cholesterol-lowering in combination with other cholesterol-lowering drugs.

Bile acid sequestrants should be considered as LDL-lowering therapy for persons who cannot tolerate either statin therapy or other lipid-lowering medication, and for combination therapy with statins in persons with very high LDL-cholesterol levels.

A moderate dose of a sequestrant to a statin can further lower LDL cholesterol by 12–16%. Cholestyramine and colestipol are bile acid sequestrants available in the USA. They remain unabsorbed in their passage through the gastrointestinal tract and lack systemic toxicity. They also cause various gastrointestinal symptoms, notably constipation. They can decrease the absorption of a number of drugs that are administered concomitantly. The general recommendation is that other drugs should be taken either an hour before or 4 h after administration of the sequestrant. Bile sequestrants have a tendency to raise triglycerides.

Nicotinic Acid/Niacin

Nicotinic acid (niacin) favorably affects all lipids and lipoproteins. These compounds may not be confused with nicotinamide, which has only a vitamin function and does not affect lipid and lipoprotein levels. Niacin lowers total cholesterol, LDLcholesterol and triglyceride levels, and also raises HDL-cholesterol levels. Niacin typically reduces LDL cholesterol by 10–25%.

The Coronary Drug Project demonstrated that niacin reduced the risk of recurrent myocardial infarction and total mortality during 15 years of follow-up [29]. This trial was performed before the development of statin therapy. The THRIVE study, also known as HPS-THRIVE, is an international study which investigates whether combining niacin with a new drug (MK-0524A) that minimises the facial flushing of niacin, will reduce CVD events in patients with a history of MI, stroke, peripheral arterial disease already treated with a statin-based therapy. Decreased rates of atherosclerotic progression were also observed in three quantitative angiographic trials. In all of these trials (familial atherosclerosis treatment study [FATS] [30], HDL-atherosclerosis treatment study [HATS] [31], and cholesterol lowering atherosclerosis study [CLAS] [32]), nicotinic acid was combined with other LDL-lowering drugs and the effects were compared to placebo.

Niacin is the only lipid-lowering compound shown to reduce lipoprotein a (Lp a) up to 30% with high doses [33]. Whether Lp(a) lowering by nicotinic acid therapy reduces risk for CHD is not known and is under investigation in the THRIVE study.

Niacin-like compounds also raise HDL cholesterol by 15–30% and reduce triglycerides by 20–50%.

The major side effect of niacin is flushing, which is less with the slow- or extended-release drug. Less-severe flushing generally occurs when the drug is taken during or after meals, or if aspirin is administered prior to drug ingestion. Other major side effects are hyperuricemia, gout, and hyperglycemia. Niacin can also increase liver function test results, with a minimal risk for hepatotoxicity.

Nicotinic acid or niacin can be used in CAD patients in combination with statins if LDL cholesterol is not at goal and in case of dyslipidemia (low HDL cholesterol and high triglycerides). It can be an alternative therapy when CAD patients do not tolerate statin therapy.

Fibrates

Fibrates reduce triglycerides by 25–50%, with the most reduction in patients with severe hypertriglyceridemia. Fibrate therapy will raise HDL cholesterol by 10–15%, but greater increases can occur in persons with very high triglyceride levels and very low HDL-cholesterol levels. Fibrates are generally well tolerated in most persons. Gastrointestinal complaints are the most common. Fibrates do increase the likelihood of cholesterol gallstones. Fibrates bind strongly to albumin and, consequently, can cause a rise in plasma concentrations of concomitant drugs such as warfarin, leading to an increased anticoagulant effect. Serum creatinine can rise in patients treated with fenofibrate. In cases of CHD patients with renal impairment, fibrate dosage needs to be reduced. Gemfibrozil in combination with statin therapy has a higher risk for myopathy than the combination of fenofibrate with statin therapy.

Clinical trials with fibrates have been less robust than trials with statin therapy in primary and secondary CHD prevention therapy. In the Veterans Administration HDL Intervention Trial (VAHIT), a secondary prevention trial, gemfibrozil therapy reduced risk for CHD death and nonfatal myocardial infarction by 22%; stroke rates also were reduced by gemfibrozil therapy [34]. The Helsinki Heart Study, a primary prevention trial comparing gemfibrozil vs. placebo, showed a 37% reduction in fatal and nonfatal myocardial infarctions and no change in total mortality during the course of the study [35]. After 8.5–10 years of follow-up, noncardiac death and all-cause mortality were numerically higher, but not statistically significant in the group that received gemfibrozil during the study. More recently, the ACCORD study demonstrated that the combination of fenofibrate and simvastatin did not reduce the rate of fatal cardiovascular events, nonfatal myocardial infarction, or nonfatal stroke, as compared with simvastatin alone in the majority of high-risk patients and those with type 2 diabetes [36].

N-3 (Omega) Fatty Acids

N-3 fatty acids (linolenic acid, docosahexaenoic acid [DHA], and eicosapentaenoic acid [EPA]) lower serum triglycerides by reducing hepatic secretion of triglyceride-rich lipoproteins. They can be used as an alternative therapy for fibrates or nicotinic acid for treatment of hypertriglyceridemia, particularly chylomicronemia. However, a recent meta-analysis regarding a large number of studies about the effect of omega-3 fatty acids on CHD mortality and restenosis showed a modest reduction in mortality and restenosis [37]. Caution must be exercised in interpreting these benefits, as results were attenuated in higher-quality studies, suggesting that bias may be at least partially responsible. Additional high-quality studies are required to clarify the role of omega-3 fatty acid supplementation for the secondary prevention of CVD.

Ezetimibe

Ezetimibe represents a new class of hypolipidemic drugs that inhibit cholesterol absorption in the small intestine [38]. The combination of ezetimibe with statins has been more effective than monotherapy alone in many randomized trials. Ezetimibe has been used in addition to statin therapy or in case patients who are intolerant of statins. Ezetimibe further lowers LDL cholesterol and is generally well tolerated.

The results of the IMPROVE-IT trial are expected in 2012. The IMPROVE-IT trial is a randomized, active-control, double-blind study of subjects with stabilized, high-risk ACS. Its primary objective is to evaluate the clinical benefit of a 10:40-mg ezetimibe-simvastatin combination, compared with simvastatin 40 mg. If the LDL-C response is inadequate, the dose of simvastatin in the ezetimibe–simvastatin combination or simvastatin arm, as appropriate, may be increased to 80 mg. Clinical benefit will be defined as the reduction in the risk of the occurrence of the composite endpoint of CV death, major coronary events, and stroke. Recently, the final results of the Study of Heart and Renal Protection (SHARP) were announced. SHARP showed that cholesterol lowering with a combination of simvastatin and ezetimibe in patients with kidney disease significantly reduced the risk of major atherosclerotic events by 17% and the primary end point for the study, major vascular events, by almost the same amount.

Interval Follow-Up

Maximum lowering of LDL and triglycerides, and rising of HDL cholesterol is achieved within 6 weeks of initiating drug therapy. Thus, the first follow-up visit should occur 6–8 weeks after initiating drug therapy. If the dose is increased, monitoring should be continued at 6–8 weeks until the final dose is determined.

If the initial dose of the drug must be increased or another drug added in an effort to reach the treatment goal(s), the patient should be seen in another 6–8 weeks for follow-up evaluation of the new drug regimen. Once the patient has achieved the treatment goal(s), follow-up intervals may be reduced to every 4–6 months. The primary focus of these visits is encouragement of long-term adherence with therapy. Once the therapy is established, the patient is at goal, and there is a good therapeutic adherence, then follow-up checks of lipid levels and liver function are necessary once a year. If the patient has symptoms of myalgia, CK should be checked.

Antiplatelet Therapy

Aspirin

Aspirin is the milestone therapeutic step in the primary and secondary prevention of coronary heart disease [39, 40]. Aspirin should be administered in a dose of 325 mg in an ACS. In primary and secondary prevention, the mean dose of aspirin is about 81 mg/day. Regarding healthy women, the more recent Women's Health Study randomized controlled trial found no significant benefit from aspirin in reducing cardiac events. However, stroke was significantly reduced [41]. Subgroup analysis showed that all benefit was confined to women over age 65. AHA guidelines recommend to "consider" aspirin in "healthy women" <65 years of age "when benefit for ischemic stroke prevention is likely to outweigh adverse effects of therapy" [42].

Despite proven benefits of aspirin, recurrent vascular events still occur. This has led to the concept of "aspirin resistance." [43] Measurement of platelet response to aspirin is made possible using a number of in vitro laboratory assays of platelet function. The phenomenon of aspirin resistance is important as it raises the possibility of developing strategies to identify those who respond best to a particular antiplatelet regimen.

Thienopyridines

Thienopyridine therapy has been evaluated as an alternative to or in addition to aspirin treatment (dual antiplatelet therapy) to reduce CV events [44]. The absolute risk reduction from thienopyridines is greater in patients at higher CV risk, particularly those with ACSs or patients who have had a coronary stent implanted. The potential benefits of antiplatelet therapy for CAD have been amply demonstrated over the past 2 decades, especially regarding the role of thienopyridine drugs, such as ticlopidine, clopidogrel, and prasugrel. Ticlopidine has been replaced by clopidogrel because of the risk of leucopenia induced by ticlopidine.

Adding clopidogrel to aspirin may produce additional benefit for those at high risk and those with established CVD. A meta-analysis was performed where all randomized controlled trials compared long-term use of aspirin plus clopidogrel, with aspirin plus placebo or aspirin alone in patients with coronary disease, ischemic cerebrovascular disease, peripheral arterial disease, or who were at high risk of atherothrombotic disease [45].

The CHARISMA and clopidogrel in unstable angina to prevent recurrent events (CURE) studies were the most important. The CURE study only enrolled patients with a recent non-ST segment elevation ACS [46]. The use of clopidogrel plus aspirin, compared with placebo plus aspirin, was associated with a lower risk of cardiovascular events (*OR*: 0.87, 95% CI [0.81, 0.94]; $p<0.01$) and a higher risk of major bleeding (*OR* 1.34, 95% CI [1.14, 1.57]; $p<0.01$). Overall, we would expect 13 cardiovascular events to be prevented for every 1,000 patients treated with the combination, but six major bleeds would be caused. In the CURE trial, for every 1,000 people treated, 23 events would be avoided and 10 major bleeds would be caused. In the CHARISMA trial, for every 1,000 people treated, five cardiovascular events would be avoided and three major bleeds would be caused [47].

This analysis demonstrated that the use of clopidogrel plus aspirin is associated with a reduction in the risk of cardiovascular events and an increased risk of bleeding compared with aspirin alone. Benefits outweigh harms only in patients with acute non-ST coronary syndrome.

Dual antiplatelet therapy with aspirin and clopidogrel reduces stent thrombosis following percutaneous coronary intervention (PCI). Patients who are implanted with a bare metal stent are recommended to receive at least 1 month of clopidogrel, and patients receiving a drug-eluting stent are recommended to receive dual therapy for at least 12 months.

Antiplatelet agents increase the risk of bleeding associated with mucosal breaks in the upper and lower gastrointestinal (GI) tracts. It is well known that CAD patients taking aspirin with or without a thienopyridine often take a proton pump inhibitor (PPI). The magnitude of reducing the antiplatelet effect of clopidogrel in case patient takes a PPI is still controversial [47]. Large, well-controlled randomized trials are necessary.

A number of nonthienopyridine oral antiplatelet drugs are under development, including ticagrelor, which is a novel, reversible, direct-acting P2Y12 receptor blocker. Several studies are underway to compare these agents with a thienopyridine.

Frequently Asked Questions

Should We Pay More Attention to Non-HDL Cholesterol?

In CAD patients with high triglycerides, the combination of LDL cholesterol and very-low-density lipoprotein (VLDL) cholesterol – "non-HDL cholesterol" – represents atherogenic cholesterol. It is calculated routinely as total cholesterol minus HDL cholesterol. Non-HDL cholesterol is a secondary target for CAD patients with elevated triglycerides. Changes in lifestyle habits are primary therapy for elevated triglycerides. Special treatment will be considered for different triglyceride categories.

Are Vitamin Supplements Beneficial to CAD Patients?

Despite a large number of CAD patients who take vitamin supplements, no scientific clinical trial with vitamin B6 and folic acid has shown any beneficial effect on CAD progression or in reducing cardiovascular morbidity and mortality.

Recently, vitamin D deficiency has been linked to coronary heart disease. Anderson et al. [48] prospectively analyzed a large electronic medical records database that included 41,504 patients with at least one measured vitamin D level. The prevalence of vitamin D deficiency (≤30 ng/mL) was 63.6%, with only minor differences by gender or age. Vitamin D deficiency was associated with highly significant increases in the prevalence of diabetes, hypertension, hyperlipidemia, and peripheral vascular disease. Also, those without risk factors but with severe vitamin D deficiency had an increased likelihood of developing diabetes, hypertension, and hyperlipidemia. Vitamin D levels were also highly associated with CAD, myocardial infarction, heart failure, and stroke (all $p<0.0001$), as well as with incidence of death, heart failure, CAD/myocardial infarction (all $p<0.0001$), stroke ($p=0.003$), and their composite ($p<0.0001$). These observations lend strong support to the hypothesis that vitamin D might play a primary role in CV risk. No studies indicate that vitamin D supplementation reduces CHD risk.

Vitamin D has been used to prevent and treat statin myopathy; however, clinical trial evidence demonstrating its efficacy is limited.

What About Hormone Replacement Therapy (HRT)?

HRT was used for many years to prevent coronary heart disease and heart attack in women who had gone through menopause. Replacing certain hormones was thought to provide a heart-protective effect enjoyed by women before menopause. A research study that ended in 2002 found, however, that women who took HRT actually had higher rates of heart disease and stroke than women who did not take HRT. HRT is no longer recommended for prevention of heart disease [49].

Therapeutic Adherence

Although the different cardiovascular risks are well known, and the benefits of treatment are well established, many persons are not adequately controlled. Efforts to bring arterial blood pressure and lipids to goal must address barriers to effective adherence. These include doctor–patient communication, cost of therapy, and side effects of medications.

Physicians and CAD patients must be mutually committed to the goals of therapy and achieving control of risk factors. Physicians must communicate instructions clearly and recommend therapies that are effective, affordable and have minimal or no adverse effects on the patient's quality of life or overall cardiac risk profile.

Future

Large clinical trials have demonstrated repeatedly that a large residual risk exists in primary and secondary CHD prevention. The following questions still need to be addressed for CAD patients:

1. What is the optimal blood pressure level?
2. What is the optimal RAAS blocker: ACE-inhibitor, angiotensin II receptor blocker, or a direct renin inhibitor or even an aldosterone antagonist?
3. Will there ever be a statin therapy that will not be associated with myalgia?
4. What is the optimal antiplatelet therapy in monotherapy or in combination with a minimal bleeding risk in the CAD patient in primary and secondary prevention, postangioplasty with stent, or postcoronary bypass graft?
5. Where will the position of the cholesteryl ester transferase protein (CETP) inhibitors?

Several novel HDL-C therapies are in the research pipeline; however, only one class of medication is relatively close to clinical use – CETP inhibitors. Although the first clinically studied CETP inhibitor, torcetrapib, has received much negative attention from a large randomized trial showing increased mortality associated with its use, the overall class of therapeutic agents may still hold some benefit [50]. Currently, two new CETP inhibitors without the off-target effects of torcetrapib are undergoing clinical research.

In addition to specific therapies in development, guidelines such as JNC VII and ATP III urgently need to be updated.

Last but not the least, we need a more personalized and global preventive approach for patients with CAD, leading to continued reduction in CVD morbidity and mortality, a better quality of life, and cost savings.

References

1. Smith Jr SC, Allen J, Blair SN, et al. AHA/ACC; National Heart, Lung, and Blood Institute. AHA/ACC guidelines for secondary prevention for patients with coronary and other atherosclerotic vascular disease: 2006 update: endorsed by the National Heart, Lung, and Blood Institute. Circulation. 2006;113:2363–72.
2. Graham I, Atar D, Borch-Johnsen K, et al. European guidelines on cardiovascular disease prevention in clinical practice: executive summary: Fourth Joint Task Force of the European Society of Cardiology and Other Societies on Cardiovascular Disease Prevention in Clinical Practice (constituted by representatives of nine societies and by invited experts). Eur Heart J. 2007;28:2375–414.
3. Mozaffarian D, Wilson PWF, Kannel WB. Beyond established and novel risk factors. Lifestyle risk factors for cardiovascular disease. Circulation. 2008;117:3031–8.
4. Mosca L, Banka CL, Benjamin EJ, For the Expert Panel/Writing Group, et al. Evidence-based guidelines for cardiovascular disease prevention in women: 2007 update. Circulation. 2007;115:1481–501.
5. Smith Jr SC, Allen J, Blair SN, et al. AHA/ACC guidelines for secondary prevention for patients with coronary and other atherosclerotic vascular disease: 2006 update. Circulation. 2006;113:2363–72.
6. Johnson RK, Appel LJ, Brands M, et al. Dietary sugars intake and cardiovascular health: a scientific statement from the American Heart Association. Circulation. 2009;120:1011–20.
7. Lichtenstein AH, Appel LJ, Brands M, et al. Diet and lifestyle recommendations revision 2006: a scientific statement from the American Heart Association Nutrition Committee. Circulation. 2006;114:82–96.
8. Tonstad S. Smoking cessation: how to advise the patient. Heart. 2009;95:1635–40.
9. Critchley JA, Capewell S. Mortality risk reduction associated with smoking cessation in patients with coronary heart disease: a systematic review. JAMA. 2003;290:86–97.
10. Balady GJ, Williams MA, Ades PA, et al. Core components of cardiac rehabilitation/secondary prevention programs: 2007 update. A scientific statement from the American Heart Association Exercise, Cardiac Rehabilitation, and Prevention Committee; the Council on Clinical Cardiology; the Councils on Cardiovascular Nursing, Epidemiology and Prevention, and Nutrition, Physical Activity, and Metabolism; and the American Association of Cardiovascular and Pulmonary Rehabilitation. Circulation. 2007;115:2675–82.
11. Thompson PD, Franklin BA, Balady GJ, et al. Exercise and acute cardiovascular events: placing the risks into perspective. A scientific statement from the American Heart Association Council on Nutrition, Physical Activity, and Metabolism and the Council on Clinical Cardiology. Circulation. 2007;115:2358–68.
12. Leon AS, Franklin BA, Costa F, et al. Cardiac rehabilitation and secondary prevention of coronary heart disease. An American Heart Association scientific statement from the Council on Clinical Cardiology (Subcommittee on Exercise, Cardiac Rehabilitation, and Prevention) and the Council on Nutrition, Physical Activity, and Metabolism (Subcommittee on Physical Activity), in Collaboration with the American Association of Cardiovascular and Pulmonary Rehabilitation. Circulation. 2005;111:369–76.
13. Linke A, Erbs S, Hambrecht R. Exercise and the coronary circulation – alterations and adaptations in coronary artery disease. Prog Cardiovasc Dis. 2006;48:270–84.
14. National Cholesterol Education Program (NCEP) Expert Panel on Detection, Evaluation, and Treatment of High Blood Cholesterol in Adults (Adult Treatment Panel III). Third Report of the National Cholesterol Education Program (NCEP) Expert Panel on Detection, Evaluation, and Treatment of High Blood Cholesterol in Adults (Adult Treatment Panel III) final report. Circulation. 2002;106:3143–421.
15. Alberti KG, Eckel RH, Grundy SM, et al. Harmonizing the metabolic syndrome: a joint interim statement of the International Diabetes Federation Task Force on Epidemiology and Prevention; National Heart, Lung, and Blood Institute; American Heart Association; World Heart Federation; International Atherosclerosis Society; and International Association for the Study of Obesity. Circulation. 2009;120:1640–5.
16. Chobanian AV, Bakris GL, Black HR, et al. National High Blood Pressure Education Program Coordinating Committee. The seventh report of the Joint National Committee on Prevention, Detection, Evaluation, and Treatment of High Blood Pressure: the JNC 7 Report. JAMA. 2003;289:2560–72.
17. Rosendorff C, Black HR, Cannon CP, et al. Treatment of hypertension in the prevention and management of ischemic heart disease: a scientific statement from the American Heart Association Council for High Blood Pressure Research and the Councils on Clinical Cardiology and Epidemiology and Prevention. Circulation. 2007;115:2761–88.
18. Law MR, Morris JK, Wald NJ. Use of blood pressure-lowering drugs in the prevention of cardiovascular disease: a meta-analysis of 147 randomized trials in the context of expectations from prospective epidemiological studies. BMJ. 2009;338:b1665.
19. ACCORD Study Group, Cushman WC, Evans GW, Byington RP, et al. Effects of intensive blood-pressure control in type 2 diabetes mellitus. N Engl J Med. 2010;362:1575–85.
20. Nissen SE, Tuzcu EM, Libby P, et al. Effect of antihypertensive agents on cardiovascular events in patients with coronary disease and normal blood pressure: the CAMELOT study: a randomized controlled trial. JAMA. 2004;292:2217–25.
21. Hansson L, Zanchetti A, Carruthers SG, et al. Effects of intensive blood-pressure lowering and low-dose aspirin in patients with hypertension: principal results of the Hypertension Optimal Treatment (HOT) randomized trial. HOT Study Group. Lancet. 1998;351:1755–62.
22. Pepine CJ, Handberg EM, Cooper-DeHoff RM, et al. A calcium antagonist vs a non-calcium antagonist hypertension treatment strategy for patients with coronary artery disease. The International Verapamil-Trandolapril Study (INVEST): a randomized controlled trial. JAMA. 2003; 290:2805–16.
23. Yusuf S, Sleight P, Pogue J, Bosch J, Davies R, Dagenais G. Effects of an angiotensin-converting-enzyme inhibitor, ramipril, on cardiovascular events in high-risk patients. The Heart Outcomes Prevention Evaluation Study Investigators. N Engl J Med. 2000;342:145–53.
24. Fox KM. European trial on reduction of cardiac events with Perindopril in stable coronary Artery disease Investigators. Efficacy of perindopril in reduction of cardiovascular events among patients with stable coronary artery disease: randomized, double-blind, placebo-controlled, multicentre trial (the EUROPA study). Lancet. 2003;362:782–8.
25. Grundy SM, Cleeman JI, Merz CN, et al. National Heart, Lung, and Blood Institute; American College of Cardiology Foundation; American Heart Association. Implications of recent clinical trials for the National Cholesterol Education Program Adult Treatment Panel III guidelines. Circulation. 2004;110(2):227–39.

26. Cholesterol Treatment Trialists' (CTT) Collaboration. Efficacy and safety of more intensive lowering of LDL cholesterol: a meta-analysis of data from 170,000 participants in 26 randomized trials. Lancet. 2010;376:1670–81.
27. Lipid Research Clinics Program. The lipid research clinics coronary primary prevention trial results. I. Reduction in the incidence of coronary heart disease. JAMA. 1984;251:351–64.
28. Lipid Research Clinics Program. The lipid research clinics coronary primary prevention trial results. II. The relationship of reduction in incidence of coronary heart disease to cholesterol lowering. JAMA. 1984;251:365–74.
29. Coronary Drug Project Research Group. Clofibrate and niacin in coronary heart disease. JAMA. 1975;231:360–81.
30. Brown G, Albers JJ, Fisher LD, et al. Regression of coronary artery disease as a result of intensive lipid-lowering therapy in men with high levels of apolipoprotein B. N Engl J Med. 1990;323:1289–98.
31. Brown BG, Zhao XQ, Chait A, et al. Simvastatin and niacin, antioxidant vitamins, or the combination for the prevention of coronary disease. N Engl J Med. 2001;345:1583–92.
32. Blankenhorn DH, Nessim SA, Johnson RL, Sanmarco ME, Azen SP, Cashin-Hemphill L. Beneficial effects of combined colestipol-niacin therapy on coronary atherosclerosis and coronary venous bypass grafts. JAMA. 1987;257:3233–40.
33. Carlson LA, Hamsten A, Asplund A. Pronounced lowering of serum levels of lipoprotein Lp(a) in hyperlipidaemic subjects treated with nicotinic acid. J Intern Med. 1989;226:271–6.
34. Rubins HB, Robins SJ, Collins D, For the Veterans Affairs High-Density Lipoprotein Cholesterol Intervention Trial Study Group, et al. Gemfibrozil for the secondary prevention of coronary heart disease in men with low levels of high-density lipoprotein cholesterol. N Engl J Med. 1999;341:410–8.
35. Frick MH, Elo MO, Haapa K, et al. Helsinki Heart Study: primary prevention trial with gemfibrozil in middle-aged men with dyslipidemia: safety of treatment, changes in risk factors, and incidence of coronary heart disease. N Engl J Med. 1987;317:1237–45.
36. ACCORD Study Group (Members of the ACCORD Study Group writing committee are Henry N. Ginsberg, Marshall B. Elam, Laura C. Lovato, John R. Crouse III, Lawrence A. Leiter, Peter Linz, William T. Friedewald, John B. Buse, Hertzel C. Gerstein, Jeffrey Probstfield, Richard H. Grimm, Faramarz Ismail-Beigi, J. Thomas Bigger, David C. Goff, Jr., William C. Cushman, Denise G. Simons-Morton, and Robert P. Byington, Ph.D). Effects of combination lipid therapy in type 2 diabetes mellitus. N Engl J Med. 2010;362:1563–74.
37. Filion KB, El Khoury F, Bielinski M, Schiller I, Dendukuri N, Brophy JM. Omega-3 fatty acids in high-risk cardiovascular patients: a meta-analysis of randomized controlled trials. BMC Cardiovasc Disord. 2010;10:24.
38. Bays HE, Neff D, Tomassini JE, Tershakovec AM. Ezetimibe: cholesterol lowering and beyond. Expert Rev Cardiovasc Ther. 2008;6:447–70.
39. Berger J, Roncaglioni M, Avanzini F, Pangrazzi I, Tognoni G, Brown D. Aspirin for the primary prevention of cardiovascular events in women and men: a sex-specific meta-analysis of randomized controlled trials. JAMA. 2006;295:306–13.
40. Campbell CL, Smyth S, Montalescot G, Steinhubl SR. Aspirin dose for the prevention of cardiovascular disease: a systematic review. JAMA. 2007;297:2018–24.
41. Ridker P, Cook N, Lee I, et al. A randomized trial of low-dose aspirin in the primary prevention of cardiovascular disease in women. N Engl J Med. 2005;352:1293–304.
42. Mosca L, Banka CL, Benjamin EJ. Evidence-based guidelines for cardiovascular disease prevention in women: 2007 update. Circulation. 2007;115:1481–501.
43. Rafferty M, Walters MR, Dawson J. Anti-platelet therapy and aspirin resistance – clinically and chemically relevant? Curr Med Chem. 2010; 17:4578–86.
44. Agewall S, Badimon L, Drouet L, et al. Oral antiplatelet agents in ACS: from pharmacology to clinical differences. Fundam Clin Pharmacol. 2011;25:564–71.
45. Squizzato A, Keller T, Romualdi E, Middeldorp S. Clopidogrel plus aspirin versus aspirin alone for preventing cardiovascular disease. Cochrane Database Syst Rev. 2011;(1):CD005158.
46. Bhatt DL, Fox KA, Hacke W, For the CHARISMA Investigators, et al. Clopidogrel and aspirin versus aspirin alone for the prevention of atherothrombotic events. N Engl J Med. 2006;354:1706–17.
47. Abraham NS, Hlatky MA, Antman EM, et al. ACCF/ACG/AHA. ACCF/ACG/AHA 2010 expert consensus document on the concomitant use of proton pump inhibitors and thienopyridines: a focused update of the ACCF/ACG/AHA 2008 expert consensus document on reducing the gastrointestinal risks of antiplatelet therapy and NSAID use: a report of the American College of Cardiology Foundation Task Force on Expert Consensus Documents. Circulation. 2010;122:2619–33.
48. Anderson JL, May HT, Horne BD, et al. Relation of Vitamin D deficiency to cardiovascular risk factors, disease status, and incident events in a general healthcare population. Am J Cardiol. 2010;106:963–8.
49. Executive Writing Committee (Members of the American Heart Association Executive Writing Committee are Lori Mosca, Emelia J. Benjamin, Kathy Berra, Judy L. Bezanson, Rowena J. Dolor, Donald M. Lloyd-Jones, L. Kristin Newby, Ileana L. Piña, Véronique L. Roger, Leslee J. Shaw, Dong Zhao, Theresa M. Beckie, Cheryl Bushnell, Jeanine D'Armiento, Penny M. Kris-Etherton, Jing Fang, Theodore G. Ganiats, Antoinette S. Gomes, Clarisa R. Gracia, Constance K. Haan, Elizabeth A. Jackson, Debra R. Judelson, Ellie Kelepouris, Carl J. Lavie, Anne Moore, Nancy A. Nussmeier, Elizabeth Ofili, Suzanne Oparil, Pamela Ouyang, Vivian W. Pinn, Katherine Sherif, Sidney C. Smith Jr, George Sopko, Nisha Chandra-Strobos, Elaine M. Urbina, Viola Vaccarino and Nanette K. Wenger). Effectiveness-based guidelines for the prevention of cardiovascular disease in women – 2011 update: a guideline from the American Heart Association. Circulation. 2011;123:1243–62.
50. Kappelle PJ, van Tol A, Wolffenbuttel BH, Dullaart RP. Cholesteryl ester transfer protein inhibition in cardiovascular risk management: ongoing trials will end the confusion. Cardiovasc Ther. 2010 Jul 14; [Epub ahead of print].

Chapter 30
Innovations in Twenty-First Century Cardiovascular Medicine

Mary G. Garry, Joseph M. Metzger, Xiaozhong Shi, and Daniel J. Garry

Promoting Innovation

Our history is replete with examples of innovation and discovery that emerge out of need or necessity, and ultimately reshape our lives and our world (Fig. 30.1). The discovery of fire, the printing press, the steam engine, the concept of gravity, electric lights, telephones, the concept of relativity, the automobile, the airplane, the computer, the cell phone, and countless other innovations cumulatively has changed our lives and our view of life and the world in which we live. These innovations arose from an idea, a need, or a call to action. One example that resulted in innovation was delivered by President John F. Kennedy in his September 12, 1962, speech at Rice University (Houston, TX). In this speech, he called the country to action [3]:

> If … our progress teaches us anything, it is that man, in his quest for knowledge and progress, is determined and cannot be deterred. The exploration of space will go ahead, whether we join in it or not, and it is one of the great adventures of all time, and no nation which expects to be the leader of other nations can expect to stay behind in this race for space. …We choose to go to the moon. We choose to go to the moon in this decade and do the other things, not because they are easy, but because they are hard, because that goal will serve to organize and measure the best of our energies and skills, because that challenge is one that we are willing to accept, one we are unwilling to postpone, and one which we intend to win, and the others, too.

A call to action – whether natural or in times of crisis – fuels innovation, invention, and discoveries. Innovations typically require a supportive environment that values discovery and embraces change (Fig. 30.1). Leaders need to speak regularly about the need for a program to focus on big questions and make an impact in the world. The "top 10" lessons associated with success and innovation include programs:

1. That have a visible and clearly stated need for change and innovation
2. That have shared values
3. That promote communication and a clearly articulated mission
4. That celebrate their success and their innovations
5. That emphasize simplicity – a simple change or innovation is valued over the complex
6. That value quality over quantity
7. That encourage creative solutions to common problems – seeing the world filled with opportunities and not obstacles
8. That recognize and know the customer
9. That have a sense of history and historical excellence
10. That recognize that failures lead to discoveries

The combination of leaders who embrace change, a supportive infrastructure, a collection of resources, and a clear need or crisis – such as cardiovascular disease – collectively fuel discoveries and paradigm shifts that have a profound impact on our patients' lives and our world (Fig. 30.1).

M.G. Garry, PhD (✉) • X. Shi, PhD
Lillehei Heart Institute, University of Minnesota, Minneapolis, MN, USA
e-mail: garry002@umn.edu

J.M. Metzger, PhD
Department of Integrative Biology and Physiology, University of Minnesota, Minneapolis, MN, USA

D.J. Garry, MD, PhD
Division of Cardiovascular Medicine, University of Minnesota, Minneapolis, MN, USA

Z. Vlodaver et al. (eds.), *Coronary Heart Disease: Clinical, Pathological, Imaging, and Molecular Profiles*,
DOI 10.1007/978-1-4614-1475-9_30, © Springer Science+Business Media, LLC 2012

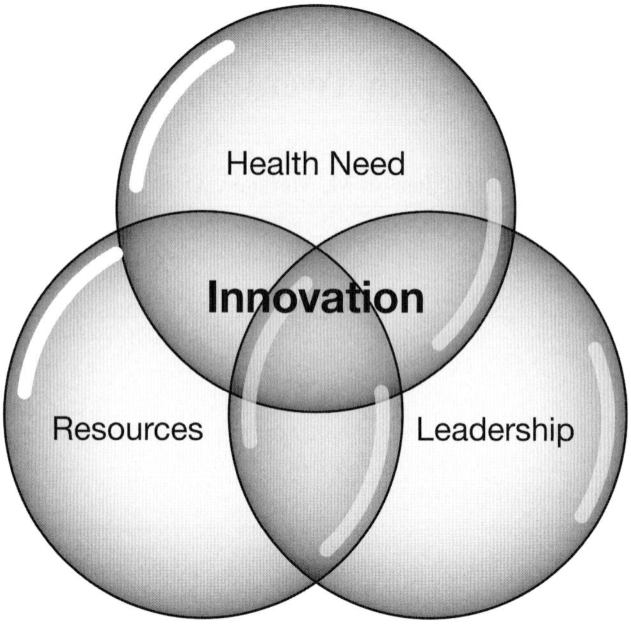

Fig. 30.1 Strategic investments fuel innovation. Strategic investments directed toward a clearly stated healthcare need (i.e., cardiovascular disease) with supportive, forward-looking leadership fuel innovation and paradigm shifts related to treatment of cardiovascular disease

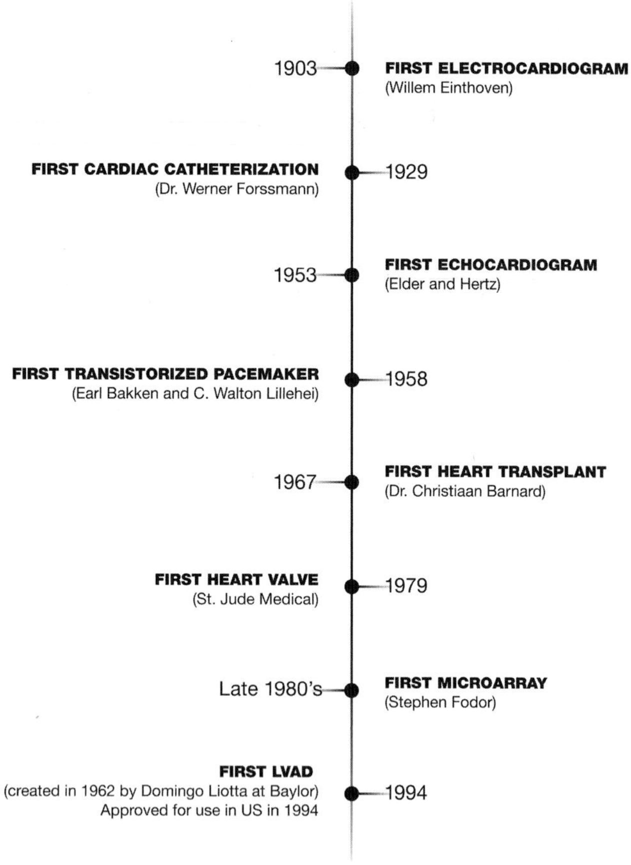

Fig. 30.2 Innovations promote new treatments for cardiovascular disease. This timeline highlights cardiovascular innovations, their pioneering investigators, and dates of the discoveries

Innovative Firsts

Cardiovascular medicine has a rich history of innovation (Fig. 30.2) and the University of Minnesota has had a palpable impact on the healthcare field through its cardiovascular discoveries. As the world's first "heart hospital" [4], the Variety Club Heart Hospital at the University of Minnesota was home to a number of young, pioneering cardiovascular surgeons (Fig. 30.3). Together, these surgeons, led by F. John Lewis, MD, successfully performed the world's first open heart surgical

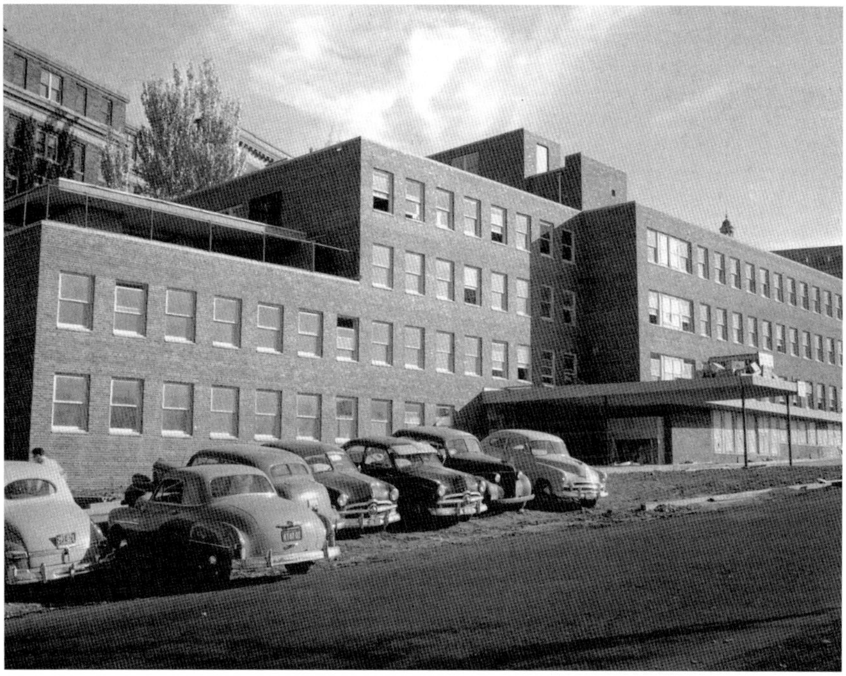

Fig. 30.3 The University of Minnesota was the site of the country's first heart hospital. The Variety Club Heart Hospital at the University of Minnesota served both pediatric and adult patients, and opened on March 18, 1951 (courtesy of University of Minnesota Archives)

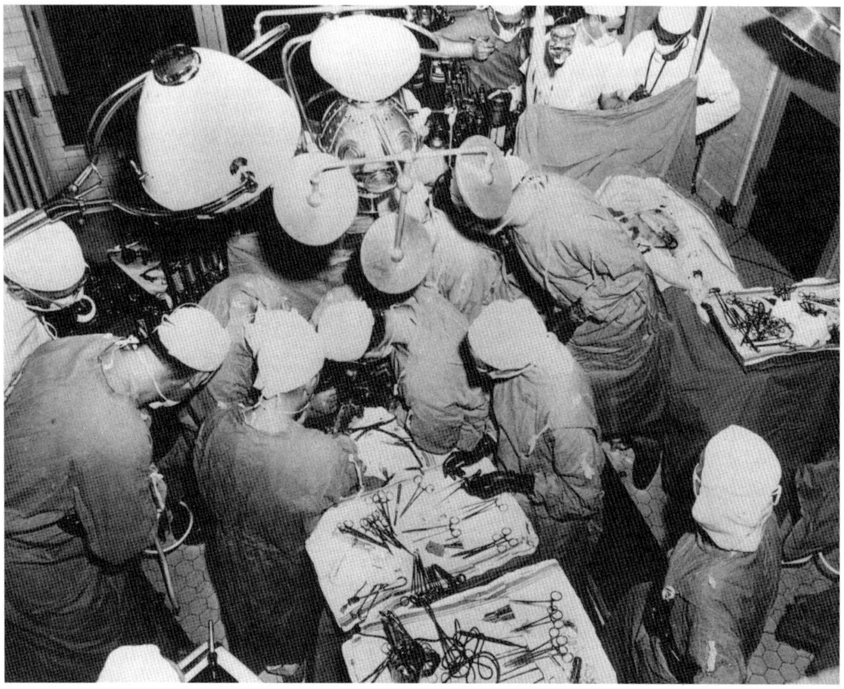

Fig. 30.4 The world's first open heart surgical procedure was performed at the University of Minnesota. Using hypothermia, the world's first open heart surgery (surgical closure of an ASD) was performed by F. John Lewis, MD, at the Variety Club Heart Hospital at the University of Minnesota on September 2, 1952 (courtesy of University of Minnesota Archives)

procedure on September 2, 1952 with the repair of an atrial septal defect (ASD) in a 4-year-old child [5] (Fig. 30.4). Using hypothermia to limit bleeding, University of Minnesota surgeons – Lewis, Varco, Lillehei, and others – proceeded to perform more than 50 additional ASD closures during the next several years [5].

In order to perform more complex surgical repairs in patients with congenital heart disease, University of Minnesota surgeon C. Walton Lillehei, MD, assisted by physicians Richard Varco, Herbert Warden, and Morley Cohen, used cross-circulation. This enabled the adult, ABO-compatible parent to serve as the biological oxygenator for the child undergoing surgical repair of the congenital heart defect (March 26, 1954) (Fig. 30.5). Some believed this cross-circulation procedure to be high risk, stating that a procedure with a possible 100% mortality now became a procedure with a possible 200% mortality [5–8]. Despite these risks, Lillehei treated more than 45 patients using this technology and successfully performed the world's first atrial ventricular canal repair, the world's first tetralogy of Fallot repair, and the world's first mitral valve repair [7].

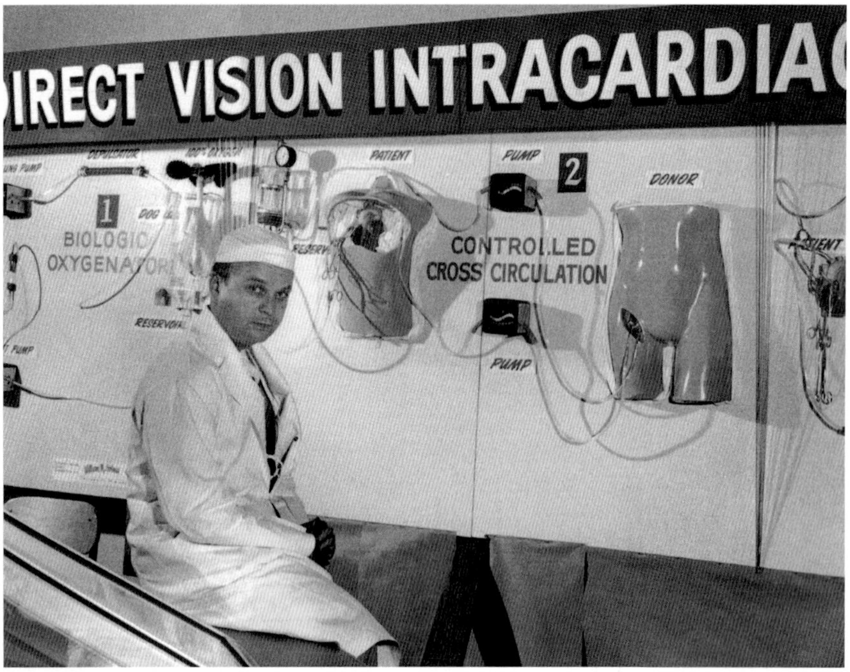

Fig. 30.5 Cross-circulation surgical procedures allowed for more significant cardiovascular surgical procedures to be performed. C. Walton Lillehei, MD, pioneered cross-circulation where the ABO-compatible parent served as the biological oxygenator for the child (the patient). This procedure enabled the world's first successful repair of a ventricular septal defect, tetralogy of Fallot, mitral valve repair, and more, at the University of Minnesota (courtesy of University of Minnesota Archives)

Moreover, even in the absence of an ABO-compatible parent, the innovative surgeons successfully utilized dog lungs to oxygenate the patient's blood [4].

While these were bold initiatives, cross-circulation was not broadly used – rather, it served as a platform for the successful use of the first heart–lung machine, the DeWall–Lillehei Bubble Oxygenator (May 13, 1955) [6]. This bubble oxygenator was a simple machine assembled with parts from the local hardware store and cost $15. Today, this discovery is used in more than 1,000,000 open heart surgical procedures.

These innovations allowed for new, unimaginable surgical interventions. Further innovations arose from the need to have portable, transistorized pacemaker support, as an electrical blackout resulted in the death of a postoperative, pacemaker-dependent patient. One month later, an electrical engineer named Earl Bakken emerged with a transistorized pacemaker that was implanted in a University of Minnesota patient [4, 9]. This technology ultimately fueled the growth of Medtronic which, in its own right, has revolutionized the cardiovascular field.

In addition, the close collaborative interactions between University of Minnesota physicians and biomedical industry leaders resulted in the implantation of the first St. Jude Medical prosthetic valve at the University of Minnesota, which further impacted the field of prosthetic valves [4, 8]. Dr. Lillehei further contributed to the field with the discovery of prosthetic heart valves (Lillehei–Nakib toroidal disk valve, Lillehei–Kaster tilting valve, and Kalke–Lillehei rigid bileaflet valve) and contributed to the culture focused on discovery and invention.

Following the arrival of Jay Cohn, MD, to the University of Minnesota in 1974, new initiatives spurred development of clinical trials to guide therapies for heart failure (V-HeFT studies) [10]. These emerging pharmacotherapies had a major impact on survival for patients with heart failure, and a new subspecialty heart failure field was founded. Today, these therapies, coupled with mechanical circulatory support devices, are associated with increased quality of life in patients with advanced heart failure. These University of Minnesota faculty members are accompanied by legions of discoverers that continue to impact our cardiovascular field and the lives of our patients. One additional measure of innovative products is the number of patents awarded for new devices and pharmacotherapies for patients with heart disease (Fig. 30.6).

Today, we have a growing cardiovascular epidemic that provides a mandate for knowledge and innovation. The goal of this chapter is to highlight emerging technologies that will impact the field and help guide us in improving therapies and, ultimately, finding a cure for this common and devastating disease.

Data Management and Coordination

Data accumulation has the potential to lead to new information and, ultimately, impact our knowledge about cardiovascular health and disease. The value of data accumulation has been recognized for thousands of years. Examples of data collection include various census recordings (population census, birth census, marriage census, death census, etc.) and, more recently,

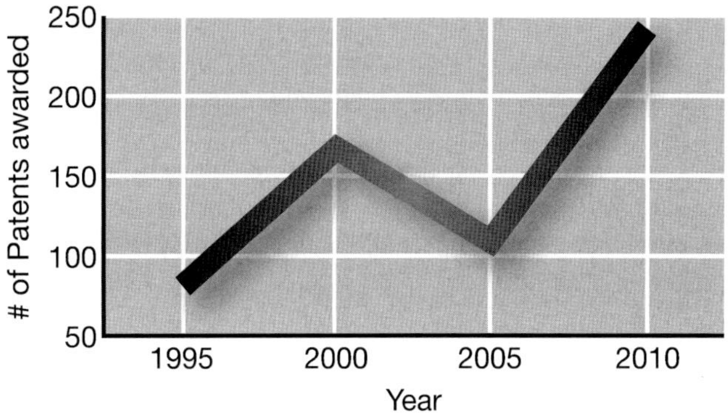

Fig. 30.6 Increased discoveries for cardiovascular disease. Graphic depiction of the number of US patents for the treatment of cardiovascular disease

US personal databases, US criminal databases, World Political Database (information on current leaders from 185 countries), World Intellectual Property Organization (legal databases and information on patent systems), Art Guide (data on artists and museums), Thesaurus of Geographic Names (database of structured vocabulary of one million place names and 900,000 places around the world), and countless others.

The seismic growth in data collection and management has been fueled by the discovery of the computer. Many inventors contributed to the genesis and evolution of the computer including Konrad Zuse (1936: first freely programmable computer), John Atanasoff (1942), John Bardeen, William Schockley, and Walter Brattain (1947: discovery of the transistor), John Backus and International Business Machines (1953/1954: first computer language – FORTRAN computer programming), Jack Kilby and Robert Noyce (1958: discovered the chip known as the integrated circuit), Douglas Engelbart (1964: discovered the computer mouse and "windows"), Intel (1970: discovered the first RAM chip), Alan Shugart and IBM (1971: discovered the floppy disk), Robert Metcalfe and Xerox (1973: established Ethernet computer networking), IBM (1981: the personal computer), Microsoft (1981: discovered MS-DOS computer operating system), Apple (1984: Apple Macintosh computer), and others [11]. The evolution of the computer further led to the development of the Internet by DARPA (the Defense Advanced Research Projects Agency) in order to share information on defense research between academic university laboratories and defense research facilities. This network capability (originally termed ARPANET, for Advanced Research Projects Agency NETwork) has proven to be a platform for information storage and impacts virtually every aspect of our lives today.

Electronic medical records: While our healthcare system relies on databases (i.e., PubMed, which includes more than nine million citations in MEDLINE; Pharmaceutical Information Network; AMA files on American Doctors, etc.), the implementation of this technology for patient care has not been fully realized [12]. Most US physicians and hospitals continue to rely on paper-based records. This is in part due to the challenges associated with changing the practice and behavior of busy professionals, and the associated costs to hospitals and practices to implement a comprehensive electronic medical record (EMR) – estimated between $20 M and $200 M per institution [13].

Paper records have certain challenges; most states require that medical records be stored for a minimum of 7 years. Collation of paper-based health records for review by a provider can be time-consuming and complicated, and paper records can be associated with decreased quality of care for patients, sometimes resulting from medical errors due to poor legibility of handwritten orders. With the increasing mobility of our society, comprehensive implementation of an EMR will be essential to improve quality of care and to improve the efficiency and cost of care.

As of 2009, fewer than 10% of US hospitals have a fully integrated EMR [12]. Common barriers to achieving comprehensive implementation of a hospital EMR include inadequate financial resources for purchase of an EMR, resistance of healthcare workers (i.e., physicians), lack of information technology expertise, and unclear return on investment. Moreover, hospitals that adopt a comprehensive EMR will experience challenges during the transition from a paper-based system to an electronic system (as healthcare workers may expend too much time on the details of this transition, as opposed to the delivery of patient care, and the transition requires training the users – physicians, nurses, lab personnel, pharmacists, and everyone else with a patient-related role – on documentation [12]). For example, the ability to "cut and paste" electronically may result in a 500-page electronic chart as opposed to a 50-page paper chart. In an attempt to encourage the adoption of an EMR in US hospitals, the Bush administration ($30B) and the Obama administration ($19B in a stimulus bill) have provided subsidies to hospital for implementing an EMR [14].

Adopting a synchronized, comprehensive EMR that links every hospital in the United States is expected to result in more efficient (i.e., decreased healthcare costs), safer (decreased medical errors), and higher quality of patient care. This will represent a major innovation and technological advancement for our field. In addition to these improvements, electronic healthcare records will enable databases that can be mined for methods aimed at quality improvement, outcome measures (epidemiological studies), resource management, and surveillance (i.e., public health monitoring of communicable diseases).

Moreover, the ability to build and link biorepositories to these EMRs such that every patient encounter is associated with a tissue specimen will be an unprecedented resource to examine a patient's cellular and molecular profiles to predict, triage, and treat patients more effectively and to increase our knowledge about cardiovascular disease. This will truly lead to "personalized medicine."

These strategies are already being adopted by CTSA (Clinical and Translational Science Awards, launched in 2006) institutions in order to form a network to promote clinical research and improve informatics communication. More than 55 member institutions in 28 states and the District of Columbia use an electronic network aimed at promoting research toward preventing, treating, and curing disease. The CTSA Federation garners more than 3% of the National Institutes of Health (NIH) budget ($467 M allocated for the CTSA program in FY2010, from a $31B NIH budget), and is aimed at transforming clinical and translation research in our country [12].

Surveillance Medicine

US healthcare costs continue to surge, with an estimated $1.3 trillion directed at caring for chronic diseases such as heart failure [15]. In response to these meteoric healthcare expenditures, home monitoring systems that help improve quality of life and decrease hospitalization are becoming more commonplace. Coordinated systems already exist to monitor pacemaker life span, arrhythmias, pacemaker mode, and body weights, and allow for in-home analysis, diagnosis, and initiation of treatment plans for patients with heart disease prior to the arrival at a medical facility. Surveillance will expand to include blood pressure monitoring, hemodynamics monitoring, total body fluid status, and other cardiovascular metrics.

For example, percutaneous delivery of in vivo sensors to measure blood pressure, cardiovascular hemodynamics, or volume status would allow continuous monitoring, with the transmission of information using a standard telephone system to a secure website for review by the patient's physician. Examples of such systems already being used for monitoring patients include the Reveal Loop Recorder to assess heart rate and rhythm disturbances, the Medtronic CareLink Network which allows patients with ICDs to transmit information using a portable monitor connected to their telephone line [16], the OptiVol Fluid Status Monitoring System that evaluates thoracic fluid fluctuations [17], and CardioMEMS for blood pressure monitoring [18]. Further advances are evident in real-time, wireless cardiovascular monitoring of patients using mobile devices, which will enable immediate lifesaving diagnoses and treatments with the use of a cellular telephone (Mednet Healthcare Technologies and AT & T Collaborations). These new initiatives may provide cross talk between the patient's EMR and the in-home monitoring system. This is an embryonic field but has a significant capacity for growth and the potential to limit hospitalizations.

The greatest impact may be felt by patients with heart failure, a diagnosis that accounts for more than one million annual hospitalizations. Increased control and regulation of the patient's heart rhythm and fluid status could have a significant impact on quality of life and healthcare expenditures.

Telemedicine: Telemedicine includes both remote surveillance and interactive services. Closely related to in-home surveillance monitoring systems is the use of telemedicine strategies which will allow for increased collaborative, real-time interactions between physicians in remote rural clinics and cardiovascular subspecialists. Such technologies allow patients to remain in their communities as opposed to traveling to quaternary medical centers in urban settings.

Telemedicine also facilitates the transfer of medical information through interactive, audiovisual media for the purpose of examinations, collaborations, or consultative initiatives. Telemedicine provides further support for primary care physicians located in rural communities, allowing more rapid interventions and initiation of medical therapies [19]. Collectively, these technologies increase efficiencies, decrease expenditures, and improve patient satisfaction.

Examples of telemedicine include efforts directed toward telecardiovascular systems that transmit an ECG or use electronic stethoscopes in delivering cardiovascular care. Teleradiological systems enable transmission of digital radiological images between locations, and connect with telepharmacy systems that facilitate interaction between providers and those providing pharmaceutical care to patients in a remote location.

These innovations will have a significant impact on the delivery of health care to patients in their homes. In a sense, telemedicine represents the return of the house call by healthcare providers, whether physician or physician extender.

Personalized Medicine

Genomics is the study of the entire human genome and how it relates to function and disease. Following the sequence analysis of the human genome in 2001, additional tools have been developed to further define the role of molecular medicine and

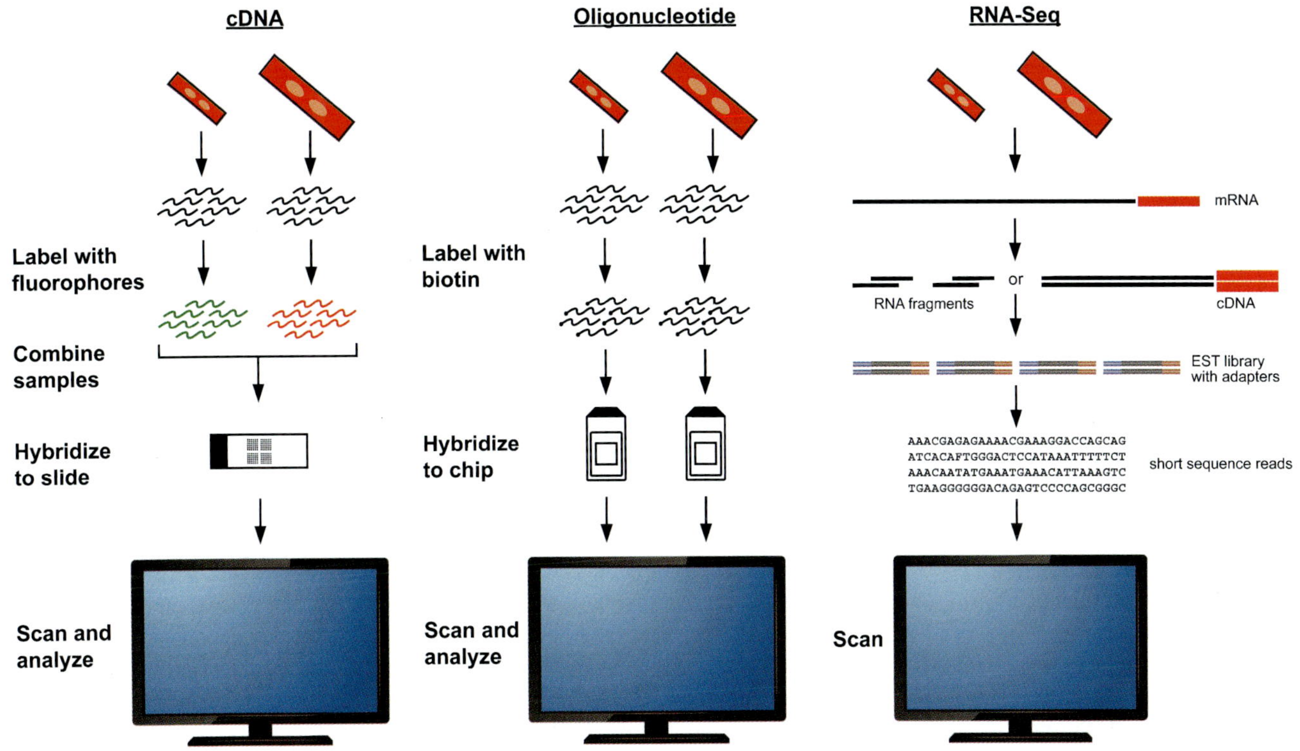

Fig. 30.7 Transcriptome analysis promotes new knowledge for cardiovascular disease. Schematic comparison of cDNA, oligonucleotide, and RNA-Seq array analysis

emerging therapies. The Human Genome Project identified three billion nucleotide bases that were assembled to produce 20,000–25,000 genes [20, 21]. New tools were developed to rapidly examine the mammalian transcriptome. Initially, microarray technologies emerged to evaluate gene expression. These technologies were sensitive, specific, and highly reproducible.

The first generation of microarray technologies used complementary DNA (cDNA) chips or microarrays [22]. This platform uses polymerase chain reaction techniques to amplify cDNA libraries and the individual amplicons spotted onto microscope slides. These cDNA libraries were generated from genetically modified cells, transgenic mouse models, or diseased tissues including congenital or acquired heart specimens. Usually, two total RNA samples are compared (normal vs. diseased) and each one is labeled with a unique fluorescent dye (Cy5 or Cy3), and equal amounts of RNA are hybridized for competitive binding to the chip. The chip is then washed, scanned, and analyzed for the signal intensity of the two RNA samples for each spotted amplicon (Fig. 30.7). The primary advantage of the cDNA microarray analysis is the ability for gene discovery and the relatively low cost. The major limitations for this technique include the relatively large amount of RNA that is required and the inability to compare more than two samples (Table 30.1).

Oligonucleotide microarrays: An alternative transcriptome analysis uses high-density oligonucleotide arrays where synthesized oligomers (25–50 oligonucleotides in length) are spotted or printed on a slide. Both Affymetrix GeneChip and Luminex commercially produce oligonucleotide arrays for mouse and humans that allow for whole genome analysis.

Expression of each transcript is represented by pairs of overlapping oligonucleotide probes that is integrated and normalized to the housekeeping genes (preselected) [23]. Typically, total RNA undergoes first- and second-strand synthesis to generate cDNA, which is biotin-labeled. The biotin-labeled cRNA is then fragmented, hybridized to the chip, washed, scanned, and analyzed. The advantage of the oligonucleotide arrays is the ability to compare many samples, as only one RNA sample is hybridized to one chip (Fig. 30.7). The limitation of the oligonucleotide array is cost, limited use for gene discovery, and the amount of RNA required for analysis (Table 30.1).

RNA-Seq: A recent, new, revolutionary tool for transcriptome analysis includes RNA-Seq which uses deep-sequencing technologies (30–400 bp) [24, 25] (Fig. 30.7). This technology provides a more quantitative level of transcripts and their isoforms compared to other conventional microarray analyses (Table 30.1). Moreover, this technique has increased sensitivity compared to DNA microarrays, and is highly reproducible but limited by cost, transcript complexity, and the requirement of bioinformatics support. Overall, RNA-Seq is expected to replace microarrays for transcriptome analyses [25].

Table 30.1 Technologies for gene expression analysis

	Differential display	SAGE	cDNA microarray	Oligonucleotide microarray	RNA-Seq
Sample comparisons	Any	Any	Two	Any	Any
Amount of starting RNA	~5 μg total	~5 μg poly-A	~1 μg Ply-A	~1–8 μg	~10 μg total RNA
Cost	Low	Medium	High	Medium to high	Low
Complexity of technique	Low	High	High	Medium	High
Reproducibility	Medium	Medium	Medium	High	High
Detection of novel genes	Yes	Yes	Possible	No	Yes
Global genetic profiling	No	Yes	Yes	Yes	Yes
Detection of differential splicing	Yes	No	Possible	Possible	Yes
Customization	Yes	Yes	Yes	No	Yes

Using these new technologies, global gene expression analysis has been performed in mouse and human hearts. These technologies have unveiled molecular signatures of stem cells that "daughter" cardiomyocytes, and they have been instrumental in deciphering transcriptional networks that govern fate decisions and perturbations that result in congenital heart defects and acquired cardiomyopathy [26–28].

These transcriptome analyses have further defined molecular mechanisms that are associated with cardiac hypertrophy and failure of the adult heart. For example, these whole genome analyses were used to examine the molecular response of the adult failing human heart prior to and following hemodynamic unloading using mechanical circulatory support (i.e., left ventricular assist device [LVAD]) [29–32]. These studies revealed that the LVAD-supported heart had decreased scar formation and increased vasculoneogenesis. Future studies will continue to gather voluminous amounts of data that will ultimately be used to direct hypotheses and new therapies for patients with advanced heart failure.

Further uses of transcriptome analysis will be to predict disease, triage patients to specific therapies (personalized medicine), and serve as a prognostic indicator [33, 34]. For example, previous studies used transcriptome analysis to triage patients with node-positive breast cancer to either aggressive chemotherapeutic regimens or conventional chemotherapy [35]. These studies identified a signature of gene expression that was associated with a good or poor outcome. Using these new technologies, patients with a good molecular signature would not be exposed to the side effects of aggressive chemotherapeutic regimens.

Similar protocols are being evaluated to tailor therapies for patients with cardiovascular diseases. For example, whole genome analysis is being used for patients with early-onset heart failure to discern which patients may rapidly progress to advanced heart failure and need more aggressive therapies. In addition, studies are in progress to examine whether cardiac transplant patients (based on their signature of gene expression) are likely to progress toward graft failure (i.e., chronic allograft vasculopathy) and warrant more aggressive immunosuppression agents, or if they are at low risk for vasculopathy (with a favorable signature of gene expression) and would receive decreased immunosuppression agents, limiting future malignancies associated with long-term immunosuppression use. Overall, transcriptome analysis will continue to revolutionize care and triage patients to conventional or aggressive therapies in the near future.

Regenerative Cardiovascular Therapies

In response to a severe injury, many mammalian tissues have the capacity for complete regeneration and restoration of cellular architecture [36–38]. Skeletal muscle, skin, liver, bone marrow, gastrointestinal tract, and other tissues have this regenerative capacity [39–51]. For example, an injury to skeletal muscle that destroys up to 90% of the tissue is associated with complete cellular regeneration within a 2–4-week period – with the cellular architecture indistinguishable from uninjured (normal) tissue [52]. (This regenerative capacity is due to a rare stem cell population, the myogenic stem cells that are resident in adult skeletal muscle).

In contrast to skeletal muscle, the heart has a more limited regenerative capacity. Recent studies using genetic mouse models, bromodeoxy uridine pulsing techniques, or ^{14}C-radiolabeling techniques suggest that the mouse and human heart are capable of cardiomyocyte renewal. A recent study by Bergmann et al. relied on the integration of carbon 14 into DNA as a measure of cellular (cardiac or vascular lineages) turnover [53]. This pulse of carbon 14 was due to above-ground nuclear tests that were ultimately discontinued in 1963 (Limited Nuclear Test Ban Treaty) and served to label cardiomyocytes such that the turnover of heart cells could be estimated by comparing the estimated age of the DNA of the cardiomyocytes with the chronological age of the patient. Using the carbon 14 labeling strategy, an estimated 1% of the cardiomyocytes turned over each year, resulting in the renewal of about half of the cardiomyocytes in a 50-year-old heart (since birth) [53].

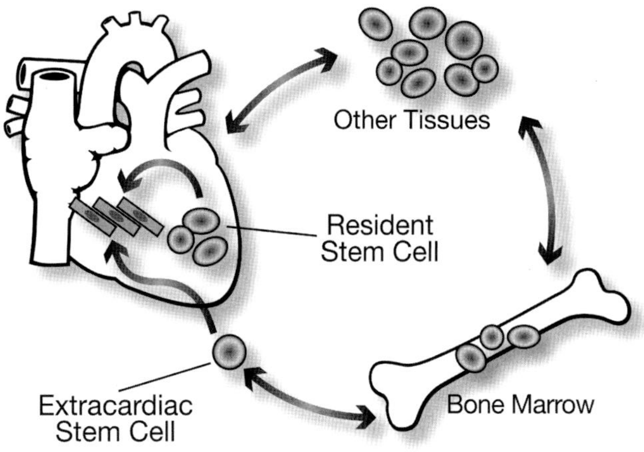

Fig. 30.8 Endogenous and exogenous progenitor/stem cells promote cardiac repair and regeneration. Resident stem cells and noncardiac stem cells may participate in cardiac repair (i.e., promote reverse remodeling) and regeneration

These genetic and radiolabeling studies suggest that limited cardiomyocyte renewal or cardiomyocyte regeneration is possible in the adult human heart.

Cardiac stem/progenitor cell populations: Previous studies have identified stem or progenitor cells that reside in the adult heart [54] (Fig. 30.8). More than six distinct cell populations have been isolated and characterized based on gene expression or cellular characteristics. These stem/progenitor cells include cardiospheres, c-kit$^+$ cells, Sca-1$^+$ cells, SP cells, Isl1$^+$ cells, and SSEA-1$^+$ cells that have all been isolated from the adult heart and shown to have multipotency and increased proliferative capacity, and are capable of differentiating into cardiomyocytes [55–66].

The c-kit positive cells have been isolated from the adult heart and clonal studies support the notion that these stem/progenitor cells have the capacity to daughter all lineages of the adult heart. A second stem/progenitor cell population that resides in the adult mouse and human heart is the side population or SP cells [57, 59, 65]. These cells are isolated using flow cytometry, are rare, and have a multidrug resistance protein (Abcg2) responsible for effluxing dye and allows for their identification and isolation. These cardiac SP cells have a tremendous proliferative capacity and are capable of forming cardiomyocytes [57, 59, 65].

The characterization of these two stem/progenitor cell populations and others provides further support for cardiac regeneration by an endogenous cell population. Future studies will focus on defining signaling pathways and small molecules that can be delivered during the postinjury period (i.e., following a myocardial infarction) that will serve to enhance this regenerative process.

Cell therapy for heart disease: In contrast to the endogenous repair strategy, which is dependent on resident somatic (adult) stem cells in the adult heart, new strategies have focused on cell therapy initiatives to promote cardiac repair (Fig. 30.8). Cell therapy strategies in the form of bone marrow transplantation are proven therapies. Ever since the world's first and second successful bone marrow transplants, which were performed at the University of Minnesota in 1967, this therapy has been used to treat more than 50,000 patients worldwide each year [67].

Cell therapy trials using autologous bone marrow mononuclear cells have been used in a number of European trails (TOP CARE-AMI, BOOST, REPAIR-AMI, ASTAMI, etc.) following ischemic insult (AMI or STEMI) [68–72]. More recently, the National Heart, Lung, and Blood Institute funded the Cardiovascular Cell Therapy Research Network which has undertaken clinical trials using autologous bone marrow mononuclear cells at five participating institutions across the United States [73]. Collectively, these European and US trials support the notion that cell therapy in response to an ischemic cardiovascular insult is safe and may be important in preventing cardiac remodeling. Future studies will examine whether cell therapy promotes cardiac regeneration, limits programmed cell death, and/or promotes neovascularization via a paracrine-mediated effect. Studies will also be needed to determine whether small molecules can be substituted for cells and their effectiveness in promoting cardiac repair.

Human iPSCs: An alternative cell source for cardiovascular cell therapeutic initiatives includes the induced pluripotent stem cell population. Previous studies have demonstrated that mouse and human skin fibroblasts can be reprogrammed to a pluripotent stem cell population [74–77]. Using forced gene expression (SOX2, NANOG, OCT4, and LIN28), Jamie Thomson's laboratory demonstrated the capacity to reprogram human fibroblasts to a pluripotent stem cell population [76, 77]. Further studies have demonstrated the capacity of these iPSCs to differentiate to a cardiomyocyte fate. These technologies offer significant insights as a model for human diseases, as a cell population to assess the efficacy of personalized therapies, and as a potential donor source for regenerative therapies.

Molecular band-aid for the failing heart: The prospect of translating to the clinic mechanistic insights derived from molecular cardiology studies has reached new heights in recent years. Cell-, gene-, and chemical-based technological advances have led to a wave of human clinical trials seeking new approaches to remediate acquired and inherited forms of cardiovascular disease. Highlighted below are two molecular cardiology advances that may one day serve as unique tools to effect positive outcomes in the course of human heart disease.

The roads to heart failure are complex and incompletely understood. There is growing evidence that one facet of failing heart muscle is the progressive loss of cardiac muscle membrane integrity owing to, at least in part, the loss of the key cytoskeletal protein dystrophin [78–82]. The complete loss of dystrophin is well known to cause Duchenne muscular dystrophy (DMD), a progressive and fatal disease of weakened skeletal and cardiac muscle [83–85]. In DMD, membrane instability in muscle underlies the molecular basis of disease pathogenesis in this uniformly fatal condition [86–88]. Membrane damage is especially evident when muscles are subjected to conditions of increased mechanical stress. Animal models of DMD have shown strong evidence of stress-induced membrane micro-tears/damage in the dystrophic cardiac myocytes [86]. Dystrophin deficiency has also been reported in acquired forms of cardiac muscle dysfunction and disease, including aging and ischemia [81, 89, 90]. The confluence of altered cytoskeleton integrity and membrane instability in acquired heart disease leads to a new hypothesis that preservation of normal membrane function is central to preserving overall cardiac muscle performance.

At present, there are no effective treatments for cardiac muscle dysfunction resulting from acquired or inherited forms of muscle membrane instability. This underscores the significance in designing and testing new strategies to prevent membrane instability in cardiac muscles with reduced membrane integrity owing to loss of dystrophin. Recently, the synthetic copolymer, poloxamer 188 (P188), an off-the-shelf Pluronic developed over a half-century ago for industrial applications, has been shown to have unique chemical properties in conferring striated muscle membrane sealant functionality [86, 87, 91]. The unique chemical properties of copolymer P188, in which a hydrophobic central core of polypropylene oxide residues are flanked on either end by hydrophilic polyethylene oxide moieties, enable this structure to engage with damaged muscle membrane, effectively preventing deleterious entities to enter (e.g., Ca^{2+}) or key cell constituents to leave (e.g., cTnI). The unique properties of P188 form a chemical-based molecular band-aid to preserve fragile membrane function and heart performance under stress. The P188 molecular band-aid was recently shown in chronic, large, animal preclinical trials to block heart failure markers and the development of dilated cardiomyopathy in vivo [91]. Future studies seeking rational design of chemical-based molecular band-aid structures are ongoing and will serve to establish a new pipeline chemical with membrane reparative functionalities.

Cardiac guardian angel: Single histidine-modified troponin I: Myocardial infarction causes marked decrement in heart performance owing in part to the deleterious effects of myoplasmic acidification on the cellular contractile apparatus [92]. Here the thin myofilaments, the very agents that govern the regulation of sarcomeric contraction in response to intracellular Ca^{2+} transients, markedly downregulate their responsiveness to activating Ca^{2+} in ischemia [93, 94]. This Ca^{2+} desensitization of the sarcomere is related in part to the troponin I molecular switch mechanism of the thin filament [93, 95]. Hence, troponin I forms a central element in cardiac muscle dysfunction in ischemia, hypoxia, and acidosis [93, 94].

During human heart development, two isoforms of troponin I are expressed. In fetal and early neonatal life, the slow skeletal troponin I isoform is expressed. Shortly after birth, expression of this embryonic isoform is extinguished and at the same time, with exquisite stoichiometric control, expression of the adult cardiac troponin I gene is activated. This developmental switch has profound physiologic consequences, including rendering the adult heart much more sensitive to acidosis-mediated sarcomeric Ca^{2+} desensitization compared to neonatal/fetal myocardial [93–95].

Recent molecular deconstruction of the primary structures of the embryonic and adult troponin I isoforms has revealed a pH-sensitive "histidine button" that dictates in large measure the pH-dependent desensitization of the cardiac sarcomere [94, 96–99]. The histidine button is naturally present in all embryonic cardiac troponin isoform, and lost in the adult version in vertebrate evolution [99]. Genetic addition of this histidine button in the mammalian adult troponin I isoform produces a marked gain of function in the face of numerous pathophysiological challenges to the heart [96]. Unique features of this gain-in-function mechanism are that, under baseline conditions, heart performance is not altered by the engineered histidine button; it is only under stress conditions that new troponin-based functionality is revealed. In essence, this single histidine serves as a molecular guardian angel in the sarcomere, sustaining systolic and diastolic function under dire conditions of ischemia/hypoxia.

Future studies elucidating the molecular mechanism of sarcomeric regulation with this troponin modification will enable potential gene- or chemical-based approaches to redesign the underpinnings of sarcomeric structure and function in heart health and disease [100].

Cardiovascular Devices

Numerous cardiovascular devices have been used to promote rhythm control and hemodynamic stability. Ever since the first implantation of the transistorized pacemaker at the University of Minnesota in 1958, new technologies have improved the quality of life and improved survival in patients with heart disease [4]. For example, the development of the dual-chambered pacemaker, the biventricular pacemaker, the implantable cardioverter defibrillator, and others have been implanted in millions of patients worldwide [101]. These devices emphasize the role of minimally invasive strategies to deploy and maintain (i.e., generator changes) these technologies. Future studies may include the development of extended-life batteries, miniaturization of generators, development of the bioartificial pacemaker, or use of other cardiovascular devices that can be deployed percutaneously.

Percutaneous heart valves: Intense interest has focused on the percutaneous deployment of cardiac valves. Increasing patient age, decreased functional status, medical comorbidities, and decreased cardiac function have fueled the development of nonsurgical, catheter-based delivery and placement of prosthetic heart valves. Examples of percutaneous heart valves include the Sapien (Edwards Lifesciences), the CoreValve (Medtronic), and the Melody Pulmonic Valve (Medtronic) [102]. A recent review of this emerging technology recorded a 30-day survival of 89%. Associated adverse events included life-threatening arrhythmias, ventricular perforation, and vascular access complications. Overall, this new technology is a promising therapeutic alternative in patients who have severe valvular disease and are poor surgical candidates.

Septal occlude devices: While the world's first open heart surgical procedure was undertaken to repair an ASD in a patient at the University of Minnesota (1952), today such procedures are routinely performed nonsurgically [4, 5]. In addition to percutaneous valve replacements, septal occluder devices have been developed to nonsurgically repair (close) atrial and ventricular septal defects. These devices are now placed in a cardiac catheterization laboratory. The treatment of structural heart disease will increasingly rely on nonsurgical, percutaneous strategies.

Mechanical circulatory support: Other cardiovascular devices provide mechanical circulatory support for acute and chronic advanced heart failure [103]. The limited success of the total artificial heart has resulted in development of ventricular assist devices that allow for retention of the failed heart and rerouting of the blood from the left ventricle (apex) to the ascending aorta. The pumps support the right (RVAD), left (LVAD), or both (BiVAD) ventricles. These continuous-flow pumps offer lifesaving technology and improved quality of life as a destination or bridge to transplant support. A limitation of this technology is the exteriorization of the driveline resulting in increased incidence of infections. Future product developments will focus on a smaller pump; internalization of the driveline; production of extended-life, battery-powered devices; and percutaneous placement of high-output VADs.

Bioartificial heart: Recent bioengineering studies support the notion that a bioartificial heart or sections (slices) of heart may be used for regenerative therapeutic applications. Using detergents, the entire adult rat, porcine, and human heart have been decellularized and repopulated with stem cell populations that differentiate to form all lineages of the heart (i.e., cardiomyocytes, smooth muscle cells, endothelial cells, etc.) [104]. Such a strategy emphasizes the role of the extracellular matrix and its supportive role as a scaffold in rebuilding the heart. Using such a strategy, investigators at the University of Minnesota have proposed the use of human cadaveric hearts to rebuild patches or the generation of a total bioartificial heart from the recipient's stem cell population [104]. While such an initiative could provide an alternative tissue source for orthotopic heart transplantation (i.e., solid organ transplantation), these technologies may also provide new insights regarding tissues for repairing structural heart disease, as opposed to replacing the entire organ. Overall, the biomedical engineering field has revolutionized the cardiovascular field and will continue to impact the field of structural heart disease and advanced heart failure.

Minimally Invasive Surgical Procedures

Conventional cardiac surgical procedures require median sternotomy in order to fully expose the heart and great vessels. Recent efforts have used minimally invasive strategies without cardiac standstill or use of the heart–lung machine. Minimally invasive surgical procedures are used for valvular repair/replacement or coronary artery surgical revascularization (MIDCAB), and require smaller incisions (2–4-in. incisions) [105]. Robot-assisted cardiac surgery is a minimally invasive surgical procedure that uses a computer console and the surgeon controlling the robot's arms with small levers [106]. The advantage of this procedure is an even smaller incision (<2 cm), thus liming the risks of infection, bleeding, stroke, or prolonged hospital stay. These technologies will expand the procedures provided to elderly patients and those who have more significant comorbidities.

Preventive Cardiovascular Medicine

Increasing efforts are focusing on prevention as opposed to the costly treatment of end-stage, advanced heart failure. Focusing on smoking cessation, diet control, physical activity, blood pressure control, and cholesterol control has had a significant impact on cardiovascular disease prevention.

The Framingham Heart Study was launched in 1948 to identify common factors that contribute to cardiovascular disease [107]. The initial cohort included 5,209 men and women living in the town of Framingham, MA, and now includes study participants spanning multiple generations [107]. Results from these studies helped formulate the Framingham Risk Score as a predictor (low vs. intermediate vs. high risk) for myocardial infarction. While issues suggest that such a score may not be broadly applied – as the study group was largely Caucasian and did not completely address issues surrounding gender and metabolic syndrome – this study population has provided a foundation for further studies. The Rasmussen Risk Score (University of Minnesota) and the Dallas Heart Study (University of Texas Southwestern Medical Center) are complementary study populations that use a series of noninvasive clinical tests and have increased diversity of study participants [108, 109]. The use of genotyping strategies in conjunction with these risk scores may further advance the predictive scores and tailor medical therapies to treat patients at risk for an adverse cardiovascular event, namely stroke or myocardial infarction.

Disclosure: J.M. Metzger is on the scientific advisory board of and holds shares in Phrixus Pharmaceuticals Inc., a company developing novel therapeutics for heart failure.

References

1. Lloyd-Jones D, Adams RJ, Brown TM, et al. Heart disease and stroke statistics – 2010 update: a report from the American Heart Association. Circulation. 2010;121:e46–215.
2. Lloyd-Jones D, Adams R, Carnethon M, et al. Heart disease and stroke statistics – 2009 update: a report from the American Heart Association Statistics Committee and Stroke Statistics Subcommittee. Circulation. 2009;119:480–6.
3. Kennedy JF. Presidential speech at Rice University [transcript]. Armed Forces Radio and Television Service, AFRTS Collection (Library of Congress), 12 Sept 1962. Los Angeles: Armed Forces Radio and Television Service.
4. Garry DJ. The Lillehei Heart Institute: building on the shoulders of giants. J Cardiovasc Transl Res. 2008;1:273–7.
5. Gott VL. Lillehei, Lewis, and Wangensteen: the right mix for giant achievements in cardiac surgery. Ann Thorac Surg. 2005;79:S2210–3.
6. Dewall RA, Warden HE, Melby JC, Minot H, Varco RL, Lillehei CW. Physiological responses during total body perfusion with a pump-oxygenator; studies in one hundred twenty patients undergoing open cardiac surgery. J Am Med Assoc. 1957;165:1788–92.
7. Lillehei CW, Varco RL, Cohen M, Warden HE, Patton C, Moller JH. The first open-heart repairs of ventricular septal defect, atrioventricular communis, and tetralogy of Fallot using extracorporeal circulation by cross-circulation: a 30-year follow-up. Ann Thorac Surg. 1986;41:4–21.
8. Cooley DA. A tribute to C. Walton Lillehei, the "father of open heart surgery". Tex Heart Inst J. 1999;26:165–6.
9. Gott VL. C. Walton Lillehei and his trainees: one man's legacy to cardiothoracic surgery. J Thorac Cardiovasc Surg. 1989;98:846–51.
10. Katz AM. The "modern" view of heart failure: how did we get here? Circ Heart Fail. 2008;1:63–71.
11. Spencer DD. The timetable of computers: a chronology of the most important people and events in the history of computers. Ormond Beach: Camelot Publishing Company; 1999.
12. Jha AK, DesRoches CM, Campbell EG, et al. Use of electronic health records in U.S. hospitals. N Engl J Med. 2009;360:1628–38.
13. Boonstra A, Broekhuis M. Barriers to the acceptance of electronic medical records by physicians from systematic review to taxonomy and interventions. BMC Health Serv Res. 2010;10:231.
14. Steinbrook R. Health care and the American Recovery and Reinvestment Act. N Engl J Med. 2009;360:1057–60.
15. Orszag PR, Emanuel EJ. Health care reform and cost control. N Engl J Med. 2010;363:601–3.
16. Schoenfeld MH, Compton SJ, Mead RH, et al. Remote monitoring of implantable cardioverter defibrillators: a prospective analysis. Pacing Clin Electrophysiol. 2004;27:757–63.
17. Yamokoski LM, Haas GJ, Gans B, Abraham WT. OptiVol fluid status monitoring with an implantable cardiac device: a heart failure management system. Expert Rev Med Devices. 2007;4:775–80.
18. Abraham WT, Adamson PB, Bourge RC, et al. Wireless pulmonary artery haemodynamic monitoring in chronic heart failure: a randomised controlled trial. Lancet. 2011;377:658–66.
19. Singh SN, Wachter RM. Perspectives on medical outsourcing and telemedicine – rough edges in a flat world? N Engl J Med. 2008;358:1622–7.
20. Venter JC, Adams MD, Myers EW, et al. The sequence of the human genome. Science. 2001;291:1304–51.
21. International Human Genome Sequencing Consortium. Finishing the euchromatic sequence of the human genome. Nature. 2004;431:931–45.
22. Schena M, Shalon D, Davis RW, Brown PO. Quantitative monitoring of gene expression patterns with a complementary DNA microarray. Science. 1995;270:467–70.
23. Gallardo TD, Hammer RE, Garry DJ. RNA amplification and transcriptional profiling for analysis of stem cell populations. Genesis. 2003;37:57–63.
24. Wang Z, Gerstein M, Snyder M. RNA-Seq: a revolutionary tool for transcriptomics. Nat Rev Genet. 2009;10:57–63.
25. Ozsolak F, Milos PM. RNA sequencing: advances, challenges and opportunities. Nat Rev Genet. 2011;12:87–98.
26. Onda H, Poulin ML, Tassava RA, Chiu IM. Characterization of a newt tenascin cDNA and localization of tenascin mRNA during newt limb regeneration by in situ hybridization. Dev Biol. 1991;148:219–32.

27. Masino AM, Gallardo TD, Wilcox CA, Olson EN, Williams RS, Garry DJ. Transcriptional regulation of cardiac progenitor cell populations. Circ Res. 2004;95:389–97.
28. Naseem RH, Meeson AP, Michael Dimaio J, et al. Reparative myocardial mechanisms in adult C57BL/6 and MRL mice following injury. Physiol Genomics. 2007;30:44–52.
29. Blaxall BC, Tschannen-Moran BM, Milano CA, Koch WJ. Differential gene expression and genomic patient stratification following left ventricular assist device support. J Am Coll Cardiol. 2003;41:1096–106.
30. Chen Y, Park S, Li Y, et al. Alterations of gene expression in failing myocardium following left ventricular assist device support. Physiol Genomics. 2003;14:251–60.
31. Hall JL, Grindle S, Han X, et al. Genomic profiling of the human heart before and after mechanical support with a ventricular assist device reveals alterations in vascular signaling networks. Physiol Genomics. 2004;17:283–91.
32. Kittleson MM, Hare JM. Molecular signature analysis: using the myocardial transcriptome as a biomarker in cardiovascular disease. Trends Cardiovasc Med. 2005;15:130–8.
33. Bullinger L, Dohner K, Bair E, et al. Use of gene-expression profiling to identify prognostic subclasses in adult acute myeloid leukemia. N Engl J Med. 2004;350:1605–16.
34. Dave SS, Wright G, Tan B, et al. Prediction of survival in follicular lymphoma based on molecular features of tumor-infiltrating immune cells. N Engl J Med. 2004;351:2159–69.
35. Rosenwald A, Wright G, Chan WC, et al. The use of molecular profiling to predict survival after chemotherapy for diffuse large-B-cell lymphoma. N Engl J Med. 2002;346:1937–47.
36. Menthena A, Deb N, Oertel M, et al. Bone marrow progenitors are not the source of expanding oval cells in injured liver. Stem Cells. 2004; 22:1049–61.
37. Vig P, Russo FP, Edwards RJ, et al. The sources of parenchymal regeneration after chronic hepatocellular liver injury in mice. Hepatology. 2006;43:316–24.
38. Gennero L, Roos MA, Sperber K, et al. Pluripotent plasticity of stem cells and liver repopulation. Cell Biochem Funct. 2010;28:178–89.
39. Mauro A. Satellite cell of skeletal muscle fibers. J Biophys Biochem Cytol. 1961;9:493–5.
40. McCulloch EA, Till JE. Regulatory mechanisms acting on hemopoietic stem cells. Some clinical implications. Am J Pathol. 1971;65:601–19.
41. Cheng H, Leblond CP. Origin, differentiation and renewal of the four main epithelial cell types in the mouse small intestine. V. Unitarian theory of the origin of the four epithelial cell types. Am J Anat. 1974;141:537–61.
42. Wilson C, Cotsarelis G, Wei ZG, et al. Cells within the bulge region of mouse hair follicle transiently proliferate during early anagen: heterogeneity and functional differences of various hair cycles. Differentiation. 1994;55:127–36.
43. Osawa M, Hanada K, Hamada H, Nakauchi H. Long-term lymphohematopoietic reconstitution by a single CD34-low/negative hematopoietic stem cell. Science. 1996;273:242–5.
44. Garry DJ, Yang Q, Bassel-Duby R, Williams RS. Persistent expression of MNF identifies myogenic stem cells in postnatal muscles. Dev Biol. 1997;188:280–94.
45. Johansson CB, Svensson M, Wallstedt L, Janson AM, Frisen J. Neural stem cells in the adult human brain. Exp Cell Res. 1999;253:733–6.
46. Kim CF, Jackson EL, Woolfenden AE, et al. Identification of bronchioalveolar stem cells in normal lung and lung cancer. Cell. 2005;121: 823–35.
47. Weaver CV, Garry DJ. Regenerative biology: a historical perspective and modern applications. Regen Med. 2008;3:63–82.
48. Gracz AD, Ramalingam S, Magness ST. Sox9 expression marks a subset of CD24-expressing small intestine epithelial stem cells that form organoids in vitro. Am J Physiol Gastrointest Liver Physiol. 2010;298:G590–600.
49. Hoffman AM, Shifren A, Mazan MR, et al. Matrix modulation of compensatory lung regrowth and progenitor cell proliferation in mice. Am J Physiol Lung Cell Mol Physiol. 2010;298:L158–68.
50. Krampert M, Chirasani SR, Wachs FP, et al. Smad7 regulates the adult neural stem/progenitor cell pool in a transforming growth factor beta- and bone morphogenetic protein-independent manner. Mol Cell Biol. 2010;30:3685–94.
51. Sotiropoulou PA, Candi A, Mascre G, et al. Bcl-2 and accelerated DNA repair mediates resistance of hair follicle bulge stem cells to DNA-damage-induced cell death. Nat Cell Biol. 2010;12:572–82.
52. Shi X, Garry DJ. Muscle stem cells in development, regeneration, and disease. Genes Dev. 2006;20:1692–708.
53. Bergmann O, Bhardwaj RD, Bernard S, et al. Evidence for cardiomyocyte renewal in humans. Science. 2009;324:98–102.
54. Garry DJ, Olson EN. A common progenitor at the heart of development. Cell. 2006;127:1101–4.
55. Beltrami AP, Barlucchi L, Torella D, et al. Adult cardiac stem cells are multipotent and support myocardial regeneration. Cell. 2003;114: 763–76.
56. Oh H, Bradfute SB, Gallardo TD, et al. Cardiac progenitor cells from adult myocardium: homing, differentiation, and fusion after infarction. Proc Natl Acad Sci USA. 2003;100:12313–8.
57. Martin CM, Meeson AP, Robertson SM, et al. Persistent expression of the ATP-binding cassette transporter, Abcg2, identifies cardiac SP cells in the developing and adult heart. Dev Biol. 2004;265:262–75.
58. Messina E, De Angelis L, Frati G, et al. Isolation and expansion of adult cardiac stem cells from human and murine heart. Circ Res. 2004;95: 911–21.
59. Pfister O, Mouquet F, Jain M, et al. CD31- but Not CD31+ cardiac side population cells exhibit functional cardiomyogenic differentiation. Circ Res. 2005;97:52–61.
60. Moretti A, Caron L, Nakano A, et al. Multipotent embryonic isl1+ progenitor cells lead to cardiac, smooth muscle, and endothelial cell diversification. Cell. 2006;127:1151–65.
61. Wang X, Hu Q, Nakamura Y, et al. The role of the sca-1+/CD31- cardiac progenitor cell population in postinfarction left ventricular remodeling. Stem Cells. 2006;24:1779–88.
62. Bearzi C, Rota M, Hosoda T, et al. Human cardiac stem cells. Proc Natl Acad Sci USA. 2007;104:14068–73.
63. Ott HC, Matthiesen TS, Brechtken J, et al. The adult human heart as a source for stem cells: repair strategies with embryonic-like progenitor cells. Nat Clin Pract Cardiovasc Med. 2007;4 Suppl 1:S27–39.
64. Smith RR, Barile L, Cho HC, et al. Regenerative potential of cardiosphere-derived cells expanded from percutaneous endomyocardial biopsy specimens. Circulation. 2007;115:896–908.

65. Martin CM, Ferdous A, Gallardo T, et al. Hypoxia-inducible factor-2alpha transactivates Abcg2 and promotes cytoprotection in cardiac side population cells. Circ Res. 2008;102:1075–81.
66. Johnston PV, Sasano T, Mills K, et al. Engraftment, differentiation, and functional benefits of autologous cardiosphere-derived cells in porcine ischemic cardiomyopathy. Circulation. 2009;120:1075–83.
67. Goldman JM, Horowitz MM. The international bone marrow transplant registry. Int J Hematol. 2002;76 Suppl 1:393–7.
68. Schachinger V, Assmus B, Britten MB, et al. Transplantation of progenitor cells and regeneration enhancement in acute myocardial infarction: final one-year results of the TOPCARE-AMI Trial. J Am Coll Cardiol. 2004;44:1690–9.
69. Meyer GP, Wollert KC, Lotz J, et al. Intracoronary bone marrow cell transfer after myocardial infarction: eighteen months' follow-up data from the randomized, controlled BOOST (BOne marrOw transfer to enhance ST-elevation infarct regeneration) trial. Circulation. 2006;113:1287–94.
70. Menasche P, Alfieri O, Janssens S, et al. The Myoblast Autologous Grafting in Ischemic Cardiomyopathy (MAGIC) trial: first randomized placebo-controlled study of myoblast transplantation. Circulation. 2008;117:1189–200.
71. Beitnes JO, Hopp E, Lunde K, et al. Long-term results after intracoronary injection of autologous mononuclear bone marrow cells in acute myocardial infarction: the ASTAMI randomised, controlled study. Heart. 2009;95:1983–9.
72. Schachinger V, Assmus B, Erbs S, et al. Intracoronary infusion of bone marrow-derived mononuclear cells abrogates adverse left ventricular remodelling post-acute myocardial infarction: insights from the reinfusion of enriched progenitor cells and infarct remodelling in acute myocardial infarction (REPAIR-AMI) trial. Eur J Heart Fail. 2009;11:973–9.
73. Traverse JH, Henry TD, Vaughan DE, et al. Rationale and design for TIME: a phase II, randomized, double-blind, placebo-controlled pilot trial evaluating the safety and effect of timing of administration of bone marrow mononuclear cells after acute myocardial infarction. Am Heart J. 2009;158:356–63.
74. Takahashi K, Yamanaka S. Induction of pluripotent stem cells from mouse embryonic and adult fibroblast cultures by defined factors. Cell. 2006;126:663–76.
75. Meissner A, Wernig M, Jaenisch R. Direct reprogramming of genetically unmodified fibroblasts into pluripotent stem cells. Nat Biotechnol. 2007;25:1177–81.
76. Park IH, Zhao R, West JA, et al. Reprogramming of human somatic cells to pluripotency with defined factors. Nature. 2008;451:141–6.
77. Zhang J, Wilson GF, Soerens AG, et al. Functional cardiomyocytes derived from human induced pluripotent stem cells. Circ Res. 2009;104:e30–41.
78. Toyo-oka T, Kawada T, Xi H, et al. Gene therapy prevents disruption of dystrophin-related proteins in a model of hereditary dilated cardiomyopathy in hamsters. Heart Lung Circ. 2002;11:174–81.
79. Vatta M, Stetson SJ, Perez-Verdia A, et al. Molecular remodelling of dystrophin in patients with end-stage cardiomyopathies and reversal in patients on assistance-device therapy. Lancet. 2002;359:936–41.
80. McMahon CJ, Vatta M, Fraser Jr CD, Towbin JA, Chang AC. Altered dystrophin expression in the right atrium of a patient after Fontan procedure with atrial flutter. Heart. 2004;90(12):e65.
81. Toyo-oka T, Kawada T, Nakata J, et al. Translocation and cleavage of myocardial dystrophin as a common pathway to advanced heart failure: a scheme for the progression of cardiac dysfunction. Proc Natl Acad Sci USA. 2004;101:7381–5.
82. Vatta M, Chang AC, McMahon CJ. Altered expression of dystrophin within the thoracic aorta in coarctation. Cardiol Young. 2005;15:73–4.
83. Hoffman EP, Brown Jr RH, Kunkel LM. Dystrophin: the protein product of the Duchenne muscular dystrophy locus. Cell. 1987;51:919–28.
84. Emery AE. Clinical and molecular studies in Duchenne muscular dystrophy. Prog Clin Biol Res. 1989;306:15–28.
85. Hoffman EP. Muscular dystrophy: identification and use of genes for diagnostics and therapeutics. Arch Pathol Lab Med. 1999;123:1050–2.
86. Yasuda S, Townsend D, Michele DE, Favre EG, Day SM, Metzger JM. Dystrophic heart failure blocked by membrane sealant poloxamer. Nature. 2005;436:1025–9.
87. Townsend D, Blankinship MJ, Allen JM, Gregorevic P, Chamberlain JS, Metzger JM. Systemic administration of micro-dystrophin restores cardiac geometry and prevents dobutamine-induced cardiac pump failure. Mol Ther. 2007;15:1086–92.
88. Townsend D, Yasuda S, Metzger J. Cardiomyopathy of Duchenne muscular dystrophy: pathogenesis and prospect of membrane sealants as a new therapeutic approach. Expert Rev Cardiovasc Ther. 2007;5:99–109.
89. Armstrong SC, Latham CA, Shivell CL, Ganote CE. Ischemic loss of sarcolemmal dystrophin and spectrin: correlation with myocardial injury. J Mol Cell Cardiol. 2001;33:1165–79.
90. Vatta M, Stetson SJ, Jimenez S, et al. Molecular normalization of dystrophin in the failing left and right ventricle of patients treated with either pulsatile or continuous flow-type ventricular assist devices. J Am Coll Cardiol. 2004;43:811–7.
91. Townsend D, Turner I, Yasuda S, et al. Chronic administration of membrane sealant prevents severe cardiac injury and ventricular dilatation in dystrophic dogs. J Clin Invest. 2010;120:1140–50.
92. Lee JA, Allen DG. Mechanisms of acute ischemic contractile failure of the heart. Role of intracellular calcium. J Clin Invest. 1991;88:361–7.
93. Metzger JM, Westfall MV. Covalent and noncovalent modification of thin filament action: the essential role of troponin in cardiac muscle regulation. Circ Res. 2004;94:146–58.
94. Davis J, Westfall MV, Townsend D, et al. Designing heart performance by gene transfer. Physiol Rev. 2008;88:1567–651.
95. Metzger JM, Michele DE, Rust EM, Borton AR, Westfall MV. Sarcomere thin filament regulatory isoforms. Evidence of a dominant effect of slow skeletal troponin I on cardiac contraction. J Biol Chem. 2003;278(15):13118–23.
96. Day SM, Westfall MV, Fomicheva EV, et al. Histidine button engineered into cardiac troponin I protects the ischemic and failing heart. Nat Med. 2006;12(2):181–9.
97. Palpant NJ, Day SM, Herron TJ, Converso KL, Metzger JM. Single histidine-substituted cardiac troponin I confers protection from age-related systolic and diastolic dysfunction. Cardiovasc Res. 2008;80:209–18.
98. Palpant NJ, D'Alecy LG, Metzger JM. Single histidine button in cardiac troponin I sustains heart performance in response to severe hypercapnic respiratory acidosis in vivo. FASEB J. 2009;23:1529–40.
99. Palpant NJ, Houang EM, Delport W, et al. Pathogenic peptide deviations support a model of adaptive evolution of chordate cardiac performance by troponin mutations. Physiol Genomics. 2010;42:287–99.

100. Turner I, Belema-Bedada F, Martindale J, et al. Molecular cardiology in translation: gene, cell and chemical-based experimental therapeutics for the failing heart. J Cardiovasc Transl Res. 2008;1:317–27.
101. Lamas GA, Lee KL, Sweeney MO, et al. Ventricular pacing or dual-chamber pacing for sinus-node dysfunction. N Engl J Med. 2002;346: 1854–62.
102. Feldman T, Leon MB. Prospects for percutaneous valve therapies. Circulation. 2007;116:2866–77.
103. Rose EA, Gelijns AC, Moskowitz AJ, et al. Long-term use of a left ventricular assist device for end-stage heart failure. N Engl J Med. 2001; 345:1435–43.
104. Ott HC, Matthiesen TS, Goh SK, et al. Perfusion-decellularized matrix: using nature's platform to engineer a bioartificial heart. Nat Med. 2008;14:213–21.
105. Diegeler A, Thiele H, Falk V, et al. Comparison of stenting with minimally invasive bypass surgery for stenosis of the left anterior descending coronary artery. N Engl J Med. 2002;347:561–6.
106. Barbash GI, Glied SA. New technology and health care costs – the case of robot-assisted surgery. N Engl J Med. 2010;363:701–4.
107. Levy D, Garrison RJ, Savage DD, Kannel WB, Castelli WP. Prognostic implications of echocardiographically determined left ventricular mass in the Framingham Heart Study. N Engl J Med. 1990;322:1561–6.
108. Victor RG, Haley RW, Willett DL, et al. The Dallas Heart Study: a population-based probability sample for the multidisciplinary study of ethnic differences in cardiovascular health. Am J Cardiol. 2004;93:1473–80.
109. Cohn JN, Duprez DA. Time to foster a rational approach to preventing cardiovascular morbid events. J Am Coll Cardiol. 2008;52:327–9.

Index

Z. Vlodaver et al. (eds.), *Coronary Heart Disease: Clinical, Pathological, Imaging, and Molecular Profiles*,
DOI 10.1007/978-1-4614-1475-9, © Springer Science+Business Media, LLC 2012

D

E

F

Q

R

V

Y